RESPIRATORY INFECTIONS IN ALLERGY AND ASTHMA

LUNG BIOLOGY IN HEALTH AND DISEASE

Executive Editor

Claude Lenfant
Director, National Heart, Lung, and Blood Institute
National Institutes of Health
Bethesda, Maryland

56. Physiological Adaptations in Vertebrates: Respiration, Circulation, and Metabolism, *edited by S. C. Wood, R. E. Weber, A. R. Hargens, and R. W. Millard*
57. The Bronchial Circulation, *edited by J. Butler*
58. Lung Cancer Differentiation: Implications for Diagnosis and Treatment, *edited by S. D. Bernal and P. J. Hesketh*
59. Pulmonary Complications of Systemic Disease, *edited by J. F. Murray*
60. Lung Vascular Injury: Molecular and Cellular Response, *edited by A. Johnson and T. J. Ferro*
61. Cytokines of the Lung, *edited by J. Kelley*
62. The Mast Cell in Health and Disease, *edited by M. A. Kaliner and D. D. Metcalfe*
63. Pulmonary Disease in the Elderly Patient, *edited by D. A. Mahler*
64. Cystic Fibrosis, *edited by P. B. Davis*
65. Signal Transduction in Lung Cells, *edited by J. S. Brody, D. M. Center, and V. A. Tkachuk*
66. Tuberculosis: A Comprehensive International Approach, *edited by L. B. Reichman and E. S. Hershfield*
67. Pharmacology of the Respiratory Tract: Experimental and Clinical Research, *edited by K. F. Chung and P. J. Barnes*
68. Prevention of Respiratory Diseases, *edited by A. Hirsch, M. Goldberg, J.-P. Martin, and R. Masse*
69. *Pneumocystis carinii* Pneumonia: Second Edition, *edited by P. D. Walzer*
70. Fluid and Solute Transport in the Airspaces of the Lungs, *edited by R. M. Effros and H. K. Chang*
71. Sleep and Breathing: Second Edition, *edited by N. A. Saunders and C. E. Sullivan*
72. Airway Secretion: Physiological Bases for the Control of Mucous Hypersecretion, *edited by T. Takishima and S. Shimura*
73. Sarcoidosis and Other Granulomatous Disorders, *edited by D. G. James*
74. Epidemiology of Lung Cancer, *edited by J. M. Samet*
75. Pulmonary Embolism, *edited by M. Morpurgo*
76. Sports and Exercise Medicine, *edited by S. C. Wood and R. C. Roach*
77. Endotoxin and the Lungs, *edited by K. L. Brigham*
78. The Mesothelial Cell and Mesothelioma, *edited by M.-C. Jaurand and J. Bignon*
79. Regulation of Breathing: Second Edition, *edited by J. A. Dempsey and A. I. Pack*
80. Pulmonary Fibrosis, *edited by S. Hin. Phan and R. S. Thrall*
81. Long-Term Oxygen Therapy: Scientific Basis and Clinical Application, *edited by W. J. O'Donohue, Jr.*
82. Ventral Brainstem Mechanisms and Control of Respiration and Blood Pressure, *edited by C. O. Trouth, R. M. Millis, H. F. Kiwull-Schöne, and M. E. Schläfke*
83. A History of Breathing Physiology, *edited by D. F. Proctor*
84. Surfactant Therapy for Lung Disease, *edited by B. Robertson and H. W. Taeusch*
85. The Thorax: Second Edition, Revised and Expanded (in three parts), *edited by C. Roussos*

ADDITIONAL VOLUMES IN PREPARATION

The opinions expressed in these volumes do not necessarily represent the views of the National Institutes of Health.

RESPIRATORY INFECTIONS IN ALLERGY AND ASTHMA

Edited by
Sebastian L. Johnston
Imperial College London
London, England

Nikolaos G. Papadopoulos
University of Athens
Athens, Greece

MARCEL DEKKER, INC.   NEW YORK · BASEL

Library of Congress Cataloging-in-Publication Data
A catalog record for this book is available from the Library of Congress.

ISBN: 0-8247-4126-9

This book is printed on acid-free paper.

Headquarters
Marcel Dekker, Inc.
270 Madison Avenue, New York, NY 10016
tel: 212-696-9000; fax: 212-685-4540

Eastern Hemisphere Distribution
Marcel Dekker AG
Hutgasse 4, Postfach 812, CH-4001 Basel, Switzerland
tel: 41-61-260-6300; fax: 41-61-260-6333

World Wide Web
http://www.dekker.com

The publisher offers discounts on this book when ordered in bulk quantities. For more information, write to Special Sales/Professional Marketing at the headquarters address above.

INTRODUCTION

The Preface to this monograph begins with the words ". . . asthma is as old as the history of medicine." The same can be said about infections, especially those of the respiratory system. Thus, it should not be surprising that the association between asthma (and allergy) and respiratory infections became a matter of considerable interest in the research community. The complexity of this association is almost limitless: the infection can be viral, garden-variety bacterial, or more atypical, such as mycobacteria. Each appears to elicit different questions. For example, whether viral infections are protective or causative of asthma depends on the age when the infection occurs and what the virus is!

Although these are indeed very old questions and problems, it was only in the second half of the last century that we started to see major research efforts in this area. Inflammatory processes and mediating molecules were actively studied and new observations led to further questions.

The first volume in the Lung Biology in Health and Disease series of monographs appeared 26 years ago, in 1977. Its title was *Immunologic and Infectious Reaction in the Lung.* In a way, that volume is analogous to the first steps of a toddler, and since its publication, many studies have been completed and reported. This new volume, *Respiratory Infections in Allergy and Asthma,* edited by Drs. Sebastian L. Johnston and Nikolaos G. Papadopoulos, presents a field that has matured and is truly vibrant, as the editors rightly acknowledge. Many well-known experts have contributed to this volume and among them many will be recognized by the readership of the series.

The purpose of this series of monographs is to help advance the field of respiratory medicine: this volume illustrates this goal and how it can be reached. Workers in the field of asthma and respiratory infections will find inspiration, clinicians will acquire a broader view of the diseases that concern them, and all of this will, in turn, lead to better care.

As the Executive Editor of the series, I thank the editors and the contributors for the opportunity to present this volume to our readership.

Claude Lenfant, M.D.
Bethesda, Maryland

FOREWORD

Twenty years ago it might have seemed odd to write a book with this title, so it is instructive to look back and see why this was so. Asthma was, of course, widely recognized, but it was seen as a small part of the subject of chronic chest diseases. Since then, asthma has increased in prevalence in many parts of the world and is often underdiagnosed and inadequately managed.

Allergy was another neglected specialty—almost unrepresented in Britain. Diseases of the skin and intestinal tract were thought to be due to sensitization to external substances, ranging from metals to food ingredients, and produced by immunological mechanisms. Allergic illnesses, such as eczema and hay fever, were known to be associated with asthma (either in the same patient or in the family), and this was ascribed to genetic factors. But sensitization to allergens was also involved and the question arose as to how the immune system damaged the skin in one person or at one time and the respiratory tract at another—and in such apparently different ways.

Thirty years ago our understanding of respiratory viruses had just begun to blossom. Influenza and adenovirus infections had become easy to recognize in the laboratory, while respiratory syncytial (RSV) or parainfluenza virus infections could be diagnosed almost at presentation. Tests for rhinoviruses and coronaviruses could perhaps reveal the cause of one cold in three, but what caused the other two?

Some viruses, such as RSV, commonly caused wheezy illnesses like bronchiolitis in infants. But almost any virus could be found in a wide range of syndromes, and some infections that had been ascribed to viruses turned out to be the result of fastidious bacteria, such as mycoplasmas, which were not easy to detect. It was all distinctly confusing.

However, these discoveries did not answer all the questions. They did not explain to the clinician (1) whether a wheezy child had a virus infection or asthma; (2) why a dose of an antihistamine could stop the running nose and sneezing of hay fever but not the same symptoms of a cold; and (3) why the immune system clearly produced antibodies that protected from and seemed to terminate virus infections but the same system was apparently capable of producing harm as well.

Since then, molecular techniques have been applied to viruses, allergy, and asthma and have opened our eyes to the intricacies of the cellular biology that underlies these types of diseases. This can all be very confusing, but we have been able to use molecular techniques to probe different aspects of the mechanisms of these diseases and, in the process, we have have discovered that the bodily responses to the external environment use certain basic cellular processes that can interact with each other.

For instance, in Southampton, molecular methods of detecting virus nucleic acid were used to study children suffering from recurrent episodes of wheezing; it was shown that these episodes were almost always accompanied by infection with a cold virus of some sort. Similar techniques enable us to look for the genes that are activated in the cells of the respiratory mucosa or in a tissue culture infected with a rhinovirus, and the products can be identified by immunoassays. This can further lead to looking for the cytokines that might emerge from virus-infected cells in the nasal mucosa, or an activated immunocyte nearby, and to discovering whether it explains the inflammation and the mucus secretion that occurs. As a final example, molecular techniques have revealed that there are two populations of lymphocytes, type 1 and type 2, which can orient the immune system: type 1 toward an antiviral response to an infection or type 2 to an allergic sensitization. Patients infected early in life seem to be less vulnerable to sensitization and allergy in general.

Combining the insights from all these fields of study can give a clinician a more comprehensive understanding of the nature and pattern of his or her patients' illness. It can also widen the scope of someone specializing in a narrow segment of research. There is more to be discovered about how genetics, allergen exposure, airborne pollution, and infections interact. Such a combination might also reveal a topic that is ripe for research but is as yet unrecognized. For example, we know that psychological stress increases vulnerability to cold viruses. Even though no study has yet uncovered an immunological or physiological mechanism for this, it might explain the old clinical impression that psychological issues seem to lead to attacks of asthma. Likewise, we know that certain molecules such as IL-6 and IL-8 are released during colds and are powerful mediators of inflammatory responses, but no one has yet shown that specifically blocking their effect improves the symptoms of colds or affects the nature or scale of the immune response.

Starting from a molecular understanding of the interaction between influenza virus neuraminidase and the carbohydrates of the cell surface, new specific anti-influenza drugs have been developed. Let us hope that similar therapeutic benefits will follow as we unravel the biology of allergy, asthma, and the respiratory viruses.

These are all complex issues and we should not be carried away by attractive and oversimplified generalizations. We need expert guidance to reach a balanced overview and summary. We need to know what reliable evidence there is and what conclusions we can safely draw. Then we can integrate this information with what we already know from our own reading and experience. I believe this book will be invaluable for this purpose. It will also encourage us to take a more in-depth view, to formulate new questions, and to use new techniques to discover the answers.

David Tyrrell

PREFACE

Although asthma is as old as the history of medicine, its dramatic increase during the last few decades has made it an important public health concern. Each year, more money is spent on treating asthma than tuberculosis and AIDS combined! Although clearly a complex subject, there is increasing evidence that the increase in asthma in westernized countries may be related to responses to changing environmental stimuli regulating immune responses. Important questions relating to this phenomenon are which factors mediate the increase and, more importantly, which are amenable to treatment? To answer these questions, we clearly need to improve our understanding of the pathogenesis of asthma.

In addition to the importance of increasing our understanding of asthma itself, the importance of understanding the association between respiratory viral infections, common colds, and asthma exacerbations has also recently become clear; however, the mechanisms involved are far from resolved. Most respiratory viruses were isolated less than half a century ago, and, over the last 10 years, improved detection technologies have greatly contributed to our increased understanding of the diseases they cause. In addition, human and animal models of respiratory infections and asthma have proved invaluable in developing an understanding of the underlying mechanisms of these diseases and their interconnectedness.

This volume comprehensively reviews the complex role of respiratory infections both in the development of asthma as a disease and in the exacerbation of the disease once established. We hope to stimulate interest in this exciting field by bringing together a group of contributors whose knowledge and expertise provide a growing body of evidence that supports a major, but complex role for respiratory infections in asthma and clearly delineate future research trends.

The years ahead will certainly be exciting and, hopefully, beneficial to asthma patients. We hope that the research reviewed in this book and developing from it in the future will enhance our ability to (1) halt the increase in prevalence of asthma that is currently so worrisome and (2) treat exacerbations of the disease when it does occur.

We would like to take this opportunity to express our gratitude to all those who have contributed to this comprehensive reference text. This field is reaching a stage of maturity and their contributions will be helpful to both scientists and clinicians who deal with the asthma epidemic on a daily basis.

Sebastian L. Johnston
Nikolaos G. Papadopoulos

CONTRIBUTORS

Ian Adcock, Ph.D.   Department of Thoracic Medicine, National Heart and Lung Institute, Imperial College London, London, England

Luigi Allegra, M.D.   Institute of Respiratory Diseases, Policlinico Hospital, University of Milan, Milan, Italy

Philip G. Bardin, Ph.D., F.R.A.C.P.   Department of Respiratory and Sleep Medicine, Monash Medical Centre and University, Melbourne, Australia

Susanne Becker, Ph.D.   National Health and Environmental Effects Laboratory, U.S. Environmental Protection Agency, Research Triangle Park, North Carolina, U.S.A.

Cinzia M. Bellettato, Ph.D.   Department of Clinical and Experimental Medicine, University of Ferrara, Ferrara, Italy

Peter N. Black, M.B., Ch.B., F.R.A.C.P.   Department of Medicine, University of Auckland, Auckland, New Zealand

Francesco Blasi, M.D., Ph.D.   Institute of Respiratory Diseases, Policlinico Hospital, University of Milan, Milan, Italy

Rosemary J. Boyton   Imperial College London, London, England

G. Daniel Brooks, M.D.   Department of Medicine, University of Wisconsin, Madison, Wisconsin, U.S.A.

William W. Busse, M.D. Department of Medicine, University of Wisconsin, Madison, Wisconsin, U.S.A.

Gaetano Caramori, M.D., Ph.D. Asthma Research Center, University of Ferrara, Ferrara, Italy

Roberto Cosentini Policlinico Hospital, University of Milan, Milan, Italy

Richard W. Costello, M.D., F.R.C.P. Department of Medicine, Royal College of Surgeons in Ireland, Dublin, Ireland

Dean D. Creer, M.B.Ch.B. Department of Respiratory Medicine, Royal London Hospital, London, England

Iolo J. M. Doull, D. M., F.R.C.P.H. Cystic Fibrosis Respiratory Unit, University Hospital of Wales, Cardiff, Wales

Gert Folkerts, Ph.D. Department of Pharmacology and Pathophysiology, University of Utrecht, Utrecht, The Netherlands

Colin M. Gelder, M.B. Department of Infection and Immunity, University of Wales College of Medicine, Cardiff, Wales

Erwin W. Gelfand, M.D. Department of Pediatrics, National Jewish Medical and Research Center, Denver, Colorado, U.S.A.

James E. Gern, M.D. Department of Pediatrics, University of Wisconsin, Madison, Wisconsin, U.S.A.

Jonathan Grigg, M.D. Department of Child Health, University of Leicester, Leicester, England

Jack M. Gwaltney, Jr. Division of Epidemiology and Virology, University of Virginia, Charlottesville, Virginia, U.S.A.

David L. Hahn, M.D., M.S. Department of Family Medicine, University of Wisconsin Medical School, Madison, Wisconsin, U.S.A.

Frederick Henderson U.S. Environmental Protection Agency, Research Triangle Park, North Carolina, U.S.A.

J. Owen Hendley Division of Epidemiology and Virology, University of Virginia, Charlottesville, Virginia, U.S.A.

Stephen T. Holgate, B.Sc., M.D., D.Sc., Infection, Inflammation, and Repair Division, Department of Respiratory Cell and Molecular Biology, University of Southampton, Southampton, England

Ian Humphreys, B.Sc.   Department of Biological Sciences, Imperial College London, London, England

Tracy Hussell, Ph.D.   Department of Biological Sciences, Imperial College London, London, England

Sebastian L. Johnston, M.D., F.R. C. P.   Department of Respiratory Medicine, National Heart and Lung Institute, Imperial College London, London, England

Robert F. Lemanske, Jr., M.D.   Departments of Pediatrics and Medicine, University of Wisconsin, Madison, Wisconsin, U.S.A.

Patrick Mallia, M.D., M.R.C.P. (UK)   Department of Respiratory Medicine, National Heart and Lung Institute, Imperial College London, London, England

Richard J. Martin, M.D.   Department of Medicine, National Jewish Medical and Research Center, Denver, Colorado, U.S.A.

Fernando D. Martinez, M.D.   Arizona Respiratory Center, University of Arizona, Tucson, Arizona, U.S.A.

Mike McKean, M.D.   Department of Child Health, University of Leicester, Leicester, England

Richard B. R. Muijsers   University of Utrecht, Utrecht, The Netherlands

Niels Mygind, M.D., Ph.D.   Department of Medicine, Vejle Hospital, Vejle, Denmark

Steven Myint, M.D., Ph.D.   GlaxoSmithKline, Harlow, Essex, England

Karl G. Nicholson, M.D., F.R.C.P., F.R.C.Path.   Infectious Diseases Unit, Leicester Royal Infirmary, Leicester, England

Frans P. Nijkamp   University of Utrecht, Utrecht, The Netherlands

Terry L. Noah, M.D.   Division of Pulmonology, Department of Pediatrics, University of North Carolina, Chapel Hill, North Carolina, U.S.A.

Peter J. M. Openshaw   National Heart and Lung Institute, Imperial College London, London, England

Nikolaos G. Papadopoulos, M.D., Ph.D.   Allergy Unit, Second Pediatric Clinic, University of Athens, Athens, Greece

Alberto Papi, M.D.   Department of Clinical and Experimental Medicine, University of Ferrara, Ferrara, Italy

Philip K. Pattemore, M.D., F.R.A.C.P.   Department of Paediatrics, Christchurch School of Medicine and Health Sciences, University of Otago, Christchurch, New Zealand

Stelios Psarras, Ph.D.   Allergy Unit, Second Pediatric Clinic, University of Athens, Athens, Greece

Louis A. Rosenthal, Ph.D.   Department of Medicine, University of Wisconsin, Madison, Wisconsin, U.S.A.

Pekka Saikku, M.D., Ph.D.   Department of Medical Microbiology, University of Oulu, Oulu, Finland

Gwendolyn Sanderson, B.Sc.   Department of Respiratory Medicine, Imperial College London, London, England

Jürgen Schwarze, M.D.   Department of Respiratory Medicine, National Heart and Lung Institute, Imperial College London, London, England

Michael Silverman, M.D., F.R.C. P.   Department of Child Health, University of Leicester, Leicester, England

Ronald L. Sorkness, Ph.D.   Departments of Medicine and Pediatrics and School of Pharmacy, University of Wisconsin, Madison, Wisconsin, U.S.A.

Iain Stephenson, M.A., M.R.C.P.   Infectious Diseases Unit, Leicester Royal Infirmary, Leicester, England

E. Rand Sutherland, M.D., M.P.H.   Department of Medicine, National Jewish Medical and Research Center, Denver, Colorado, U.S.A.

Paolo Tarsia   Policlinico Hospital, University of Milan, Milan, Italy

Erika von Mutius   University Children's Hospital, Munich, Germany

Gerhard Walzl, M.D.   Department of Biological Sciences, Imperial College London, London, England

Robert C. Welliver, M.D.   Children's Hospital and State University of New York at Buffalo, Buffalo, New York, U.S.A.

Birgit Winther   Division of Epidemiology and Virology, University of Virginia, Charlottesville, Virginia, U.S.A.

CONTENTS

1

Overview on Asthma and the Role of the Airway Epithelium

STEPHEN T. HOLGATE

University of Southampton
Southampton, England

I. Geographical Variation in Asthma Prevalence: Gene–Environmental Interactions

The last two decades have witnessed a consistent and worrying increase in the occurrence of allergic diseases of all types. A series of cohort studies in which similar survey methods have been used, reveal increases not only in the developed world but also in those countries where adoption of aspects of the western lifestyle is prominent. There have been numerous attempts to link these trends to particular aspects of the western lifestyle, but no single one satisfactorily explains the changes and differences in disease demography. In some countries, such as Papua, New Guinea and Australia, increased exposure to indoor allergens, such as house dust mite, has been strongly incriminated while, in others, it is stated that reduced exposure to gastrointestinal or respiratory infections in early childhood is responsible. Alterations in diet, overuse of antibiotics in infancy, exposure to air pollutants inside and outside the home, and differences in exposure to microbial products such as CpG oligonucleotides and lipopolysaccharide all have their advocates. While all of these environmental factors are capable of influencing the emergence of atopic disease, it seems most likely that a combination of factors interfacing with a susceptible genotype is where the answers are most likely to lie. Major advances will occur when a clearer understanding is obtained about the multiple susceptibility genes that underlie atopic sensitization and its expression in specific organs.

Until this time we must be satisfied with further carefully conducted epidemiological studies in which appropriate biomarkers are followed. In this regard, the second and third phases of the International Study of Asthma and Allergy in Children (ISAAC) will be especially informative. From longitudinal epidemiological knowledge gained to date, it seems clear that the increasing trends in allergic disease exhibit a cohort effect. This strongly indicates that, whatever environmental factors are operating, they are doing so at a time when the immune response is "plastic" and can be deviated from its normal course of development to produce enhanced susceptibility to sensitizing stimuli. The fact that up to 50% of a western population are now atopic points to common factors operating early in life or even prenatally. Understanding the factors that regulate the way food and inhalant allergens are recognized and processed into an allergen response is paramount if we are able to translate epidemiological findings into disease pathogenesis. Certainly, the nature of allergens (e.g., the biological activities) and the concomitant environmental insults that accompany their access to the immune response, like exposure to pollutants such as diesel particulates or passive tobacco smoke are likely to be important in determining whether an individual mounts an allergic response, ignores the stimulus, or evolves a protective tolerizing reaction. Thus, it may be that atopic disease develops as a result of lack of tolerance acquisition rather than as a purely active process.

Key among the events that may subvert the immune response at mucosal surfaces is exposure to microorganisms or products derived from them. In the late 1980s, David Strachan put forward the idea that repeated infections in early life may prevent the development of hay fever. He subsequently extended this idea to suggest that the most significant cause of the increase in atopic disease in western countries is the decreased exposure to cross-infection among younger siblings created by a reduced family size. This "hygiene hypothesis" has gained much popularity as an explanation for the rising trends in atopic disease. Several studies have provided supportive evidence that certain "invasive" infections, such as tuberculosis, hepatitis A, toxoplasmosis, and measles in early childhood, provide some protection against the acquisition of atopy and atopic disease later in life. More recently, it has been suggested that infection per se may not be critical, but what is important is how the developing mucosal immune response responds to bacterial products presented to the gastrointestinal or respiratory tracts. For example, it has been argued that one factor accounting for the large difference in the prevalence of atopy between Sweden and Estonia is a difference in the repertoire of gastrointestinal bacteria in infancy which influences the shape and magnitude of systemic immunity via the gut-associated lymphoid tissue and that, in turn, family structure and size and infant diets in part determine this. An important role played by microorganism exposure is further supported by the low prevalence of atopy found in children raised on livestock farms resulting from their early contact with fecal microbes and their products.

While these ideas have fueled an active debate about the role of lifestyle in the pathogenesis of chronic inflammatory disease, this has sometimes drawn on the most tenuous of data. For example, it has been argued that respiratory virus infections in early infancy exert a protective influence over atopy and asthma and that the increased transfer of respiratory viruses in children's day-care centers might account for the East–West difference in the incidence of asthma and allergy. However, a relatively cursory review of the literature in this field reveals considerable controversy, some studies revealing protection while others show enhanced risk of asthma and atopy. The existence of multiple confounding factors that influence the emergence of atopy in these environments are difficult to control for could easily explain divergent results observed in these studies. Examples include differences in diet, early exposure to pets and livestock, less use of antibiotics and more sedentary lifestyle. While not yet providing clear answers, what studies of this type show is that there is no substitute for capturing as much information as possible about the environment to which children are exposed during their early development and to supplement this with important maternal factors that may operate in pregnancy (fetal programming) and in the intimate fetomaternal relationship.

II. The Immunology of Asthma

While the concept that allergic diseases and asthma have an inflammatory basis has been advocated for many years, a clear appreciation of what this means in terms of disease pathogenesis and evolution has had to await discovery of immune mechanisms that direct the type of inflammatory response characteristic of these diseases. Although immunoglobulin (Ig) E, mast cells, basophils, and eosinophils all contribute to the inflammatory milieu, a clear understanding of how this is orchestrated in response to allergen and other types of environmental exposure has not become clear until the role of the T-lymphocyte was understood and, more specifically, the Th2-like subtype defined. A major breakthrough in understanding occurred when it was shown that at sites of chronic allergic inflammation, $CD4^+$ T cells polarized to secrete an array of cytokines encoded on a cluster on chromosome 5q 31-33. Together, these cytokines (IL-3, -4, -5, -9, -13 and GM-CSF) have the capacity to drive the allergic response. Conversely, the Th1 like T-cell, with its capacity to produce IL-2, IFN-γ, and TNF-β, has an opposing effect in suppressing the Th-2 response in part through the actions of IFN-γ. The environmental, genetic, and pathophysiological factors that direct immunity along one route or another have become a major focus for modern research. The dendritic cell has emerged at the forefront as the principal initiator of these responses, the polarity of which is under the influence of the nature of the allergen, the secretion (or not) of IL-12 and IL-18, and engagement of the various forms of intercellular costimulation that accompanies antigen presentation for the subsequent propagation of an effective T-cell-proliferative, survival, and cytokine response. In the presence of IL-12 or IL-18 the immune response is directed toward a Th1 response. Conversely, in the presence of low levels of IL-12, high levels of prostaglandin E_2 (which suppresses IL-12 production) or when selective costimulatory molecules become engaged (T-1/ST-2 or ICOS) then there is expansion of T- cells expressing a Th2 phenotype. A further level of complexity has recently been introduced by the discovery of subpopulations of regulatory T cells that are sensitive to environmental exposure and capable of shutting down or deviating components of the immune response. There is also considerable debate over those factors that influence the maturation of dendritic cells in favor (or not) of being able to elicit Th1- or Th2-dominant responses and, under certain circumstances, their role in superimposing Th1 and Th2 responses.

Having a clearer immunological basis upon which to hang some of the epidemiological and therapeutic studies has greatly enhanced understanding of the way that environmental risk factors may influence the development and expression of atopy. There are many studies showing that children who progress to develop atopy have impaired production of the Th1 cytokine IFN-γ by cord blood mononuclear cells at birth, which may have a genetic basis. Over the first 18 months of life, this impaired Th1 response is modified by environmental factors that shape immune competency; however, available information from cohort studies would suggest that reduced responsiveness of Th1 pathways most likely account for the persistence of the Th2 profile. At this time, it is not clear whether the same immunological abnormalities predict the development of asthma, although several short studies strongly point to early (i.e., during the first year of life) sensitization to foods (e.g., egg and milk) and aeroallergens as a major risk factor for persistent asthma in childhood. Early sensitization is clearly an important factor in the inception of asthma but whether alone this is sufficient for chronic asthma to emerge is uncertain. The recent German MAS study (1) has clearly shown that, in a large cohort of newborn children followed until age 7 years, sensitization to indoor allergens was associated with asthma, wheeze, and increased bronchial responsiveness, but there was no relationship between the level of early indoor allergen exposure and the prevalence of asthma and its partial phenotypes other than atopy. The authors conclude that the induction of specific IgE responses and the development of childhood asthma are determined by independent genetic and environmental factors influencing structural abnormalities regarding growth and elasticity of airways and lung parenchyma.

Pearce and colleagues have approached the question of atopy and asthma from a different perspective by reviewing the literature carefully and deriving from these the population attributable risk of atopy contributing to asthma (2). They have concluded that the proportion of asthma cases in both children and adults that are attributable to atopy is less than 50%. The same authors have recently applied a similar approach to investigate the contribution of early-life allergen exposure to the development of asthma and found it was as low as 4 to11% (3).

If allergen exposure and atopy are not linearly linked to the development of asthma, then there must be other important mechanisms underlying the onset, consolidation, and possible progression of this airways disorder. The bronchial epithelium and the way that it communicates with cells in the airway wall would seem to be a good place to start because it is this structure that provides the initial airway mucosal interface with the external environment and becomes host to the Th2-linked inflammatory response. It is becoming evident that inflammation alone is unable to explain many of the features of asthma such as the incomplete resolution of disease with inhaled corticosteroids, the slow reversal and persistence of bronchial hyperresponsiveness in the presence of inhaled corticosteroids, the superior efficacy of adding a long-acting inhaled β_2-adrenoceptor agonist to a topical corticosteroid in preference to increasing the dose of corticosteroid in controlling moderate-to-severe disease, the tracking of asthma severity from childhood throughout life, and the progressive decline in pulmonary function over time that occurs when asthma is studied at a population level.

Among inflammatory cells, eosinophils have been assumed to play a central role in disease pathogenesis; however, studies with an anti-IL-5-blocking monoclonal antibody (4) and rhIL-12 (5) have failed to reveal efficacy despite markedly reducing circulating and airway eosinophil numbers. Thus, while being associated with asthma and atopy, airway eosinophilia would not seem to be critical requirements for disease expression. Genetic studies have also demonstrated that atopy and bronchial hyperresponsiveness (BHR) have different patterns of inheritance. These findings imply that *locally* operating factors play an important role in predisposing individuals to asthma and provide an explanation for the epidemiological evidence that identifies environmental factors such as pollutant exposure, diet, and respiratory virus infection, which all increase oxidant stress in the airways, as important disease risk factors. Thus, rather than IgE-mediated inflammation being the initiation of asthma, the epithelium itself may be abnormal and in this way predispose this airway toward local allergen sensitization, and at the same time create the necessary microenvironment to encourage restructuring of the airways with goblet-cell hyperplasia, smooth muscle hypertrophy, increased deposition of matrix and proliferation of microvessels and nerves–events that reflect remodeling of the airways.

III. Asthma: An Epithelial Disease

Morphometry has revealed that mucosal and adventitial thickening of asthmatic airways is able to account for a large component of BHR and excessive airway narrowing observed in established disease. At best, these structural changes are poorly responsive to corticosteroids and, although with prolonged treatment some improvement in BHR is evident, it frequently remains abnormal. This failure of corticosteroids is reflected in the findings of our recent European Network For Understanding the Mechanisms Of Severe Asthma (ENFUMOSA) study, which has revealed that these patients exhibit a greatly impaired quality of life (6), a component of fixed airflow obstruction, and have clear evidence of airway wall remodeling (7). In such patients, there was evidence of persistent matrix turnover with higher levels of cleaved tenascin C, matrix metalloproteinase-2 (MMP-2), and collagen VI indicating active matrix turnover. Airway remodeling also provides an explanation for corticosteroid-resistant BHR and the accelerated decline in lung function observed over time in adult asthma. In 5- to 11-year-old children, the recent CAMP study (8) has shown that the initial beneficial effect of an inhaled corticosteroid on the post-bronchodilator improvement in airway function observed during the first year of treatment was lost over the following 3 years. This is best explained by an alteration occurring in tissue structure and function that is insensitive to corticosteroids. The importance of tissue remodeling as an early and consistent component of childhood asthma has been emphasized in a recent biopsy study that describes collagen deposition in the *lamina reticularis* and underlying fibroblast proliferation, rather than eosinophil infiltration, as diagnostic features of this disease (9). Although remodeling has been considered to be secondary to long-standing inflammation, airway biopsy studies in young children have shown tissue restructuring up to 4 years before the onset of symptoms (10), indicating that these processes may occur early in the development of asthma and may even be a primary requirement for the establishment of persistent inflammation.

Epithelial disruption is characteristically increased in the asthmatic bronchial epithelium. It has been proposed that this damage is artefactual; however, our findings of enhanced expression of the epidermal growth factor receptor (EGFR) (11) and the epithelial isoform of CD44 indicate that injury has occurred in vivo (12). We have also revealed increased epithelial expression of Fas and Fas ligand in patients who have died with asthma (13) while, in bronchial biopsies in ongoing asthma, there is markedly increased immunostaining of asthmatic columnar (but notably not basal) epithelial cells for p85, the caspase-3 cleavage product of poly(ADP-ribose) polymerase (PARP) (14), indicating that epithelial apoptosis is increased in this disease. While such observational studies are able to identify differences between asthmatic and normal subjects, they are unable to differentiate whether the changes are a cause or consequence of inflammation. To address this, we have established primary cultures using bronchial epithelial cells brushed from the airways of normal and asthmatic subjects in order to compare responses under identical conditions in vitro. Although no difference in the rate of proliferation of these cultures under optimal growth conditions have been found, when rendered quiescent by growth factor depletion, those cells from asthmatic airways exhibit a significantly greater sensitivity to oxidant-induced apoptosis in the face of a normal apoptotic response to the DNA and RNA synthesis inhibitor, actinomycin D (14). In being preserved through several generations *in vitro*, this susceptibility to oxidants is unlikely to be a secondary effect of airway inflammation. Since epidemiological studies have identified multiple interacting risk factors for asthma, including diets low in antioxidants and inhalant pollutants (15), it seems plausible that the effect of environmental oxidants on a susceptible epithelium provides a plausible triggering mechanism for the induction of epithelial activation and damage in asthma. Once initiated, the resulting inflammatory cell influx causes secondary damage through production of endogenous reactive oxygen species resulting in chronic tissue injury and persistent inflammation.

The extent of epithelial shedding in asthma is not observed in other inflammatory diseases such as COPD, where the epithelium becomes multilayered due to squamous metaplasia while the underlying lamina reticularis remains normal. While these differences may reflect the quality of inflammation, airway eosinophilia is observed in the absence of asthma and, as in COPD, neutrophils may dominate inflammation in severe asthma. EGFR expression in asthma increases with disease severity and is evident throughout the epithelium, suggesting that damage is widespread (11). Significantly, EGFR overexpression is insensitive to the action of corticosteroids and is positively correlated with the thickness of the lamina reticularis thereby linking epithelial injury to underlying remodeling changes.

In vitro studies point to a central role for activation of EGFR signaling in the restoration of the bronchial epithelium following injury, since mechanical damage induces rapid phosphorylation of the EGFR regardless of the presence of exogenous ligand and wound closure is enhanced by EGF or heparin binding EGF-like growth factors (HB-EGF) but not by the unrelated ligand keratinocyte growth factor [FGF7]. Recognizing that EGF is a potent mitogen, the increase in epithelial EGFR in asthma is paradoxical because it is *not* matched by increased proliferation to replace columnar cells that have been shed (16) and, in this way, contrasts with the hyperproliferative state of the epithelium seen in COPD. Using bronchial biopsies from patients with severe asthma, the cyclin-dependent kinase inhibitor p21^{waf} has been shown to be overexpressed in basal as well as in columnar epithelial cells, pointing to a potential mechanism for reduced EGFR-mediated proliferation (17).

IV. Asthma: A Disorder of Airway Wall Remodeling

High-resolution computed tomography (HRCT), postmortem and biopsy studies in chronic asthma have all revealed airway wall thickening in relation to disease severity and chronicity (18). This involves deposition of interstitial collagens in the *lamina reticularis*, matrix deposition in the submucosa, smooth muscle hyperplasia, and microvascular and neuronal proliferation. Thickening of the *lamina reticularis* is a highly characteristic feature of this disease (19, 20) and, on the basis of measurements made in human airways (21) and, in a guinea pig model of chronic antigen exposure, it appears to reflect events linked to thickening of the entire airway wall (22). A layer of subepithelial mesenchymal cells with features of myofibroblasts have been described in asthma whose number was increased in asthma in proportion to the thickness of the reticular collagen layer (23). These cells correspond to the attenuated fibroblast sheath described by Evans and coworkers (24) lying adjacent to the lamina reticularis and forming a network similar to hepatic stellate cells which, when activated by liver damage, are the key effector cells responsible for fibrosis (25). As the bronchial epithelium is in intimate contact with the attenuated fibroblast sheath, these two cellular layers are in a key position to coordinate responses to challenges from the inhaled environment into the deeper layers of the submucosa (26). Injury to epithelial monolayers in vitro results in increased release of fibroproliferative and fibrogenic growth factors that are increased in asthma (27,28). To further establish the relationship between EGFR signaling in the repair and remodeling processes, we have used an EGFR-selective tyrosine kinase inhibitor to inhibit epithelial repair in vitro with a resultant increase in release of profibrogenic cytokines such as TGF-β_2 by the damaged epithelial cells (11). This points to parallel pathways operating in repairing epithelial cells, some of which direct efficient restitution and are regulated by the EGFR, while others control profibrogenic growth factor production and are independent of the EGFR. In asthma, impaired epithelial proliferation causes the bronchial epithelium to spend longer in a repair phenotype resulting in increased secretion of profibrogenic growth factors (11). Using a coculture model, there is direct evidence that epithelial injury causes myofibroblast activation (29). Thus, polyarginine (a surrogate for eosinophil basic proteins) or mechanical damage to confluent monolayers of bronchial epithelial cells grown on a collagen gel seeded with human myofibroblasts leads to enhanced proliferation and increased collagen gene expression due to the combined effects of a number of profibrogenic growth factors.

Communication between the epithelium and the subepithelial fibroblast sheath is reminiscent of the processes that drive physiological remodeling of the airways during embryogenesis, where the epithelium and mesenchyme act as a trophic unit to regulate airway growth and branching (30). The epithelial-mesenchymal trophic unit (EMTU) has the appearance of being reactivated in asthma to drive pathological remodeling and to create a microenvironment to support airways inflammation. In subjects with asymptomatic BHR, longitudinal studies have shown that those who progress to asthma show parallel changes in inflammation and remodeling (31). Thickening of the *lamina reticularis* in bronchial biopsies from young children is also present several years before asthma becomes clinically manifest (10). During lung development, epithelial and mesenchymal growth is in part regulated by the balance of EGF and TGF-β signaling pathways as appears also to occur in chronic asthma. It follows that in early life, in susceptible individuals, environmental factors interact with the EMTU to initiate structural changes in the airways that could account for the decrease in lung function observed in young children who are susceptible to early wheezing (32) and for the loss of corticosteroid responsiveness on baseline lung function observed in the CAMP study (8). On this basis, it is probable that bronchial epithelial susceptibility either precedes or occurs in parallel with factors that predispose to Th2 mediated inflammation and is an absolute requirement for the persistence of inflammation and for remodeling to occur.

If a susceptible epithelium is accepted as a plausible start for asthma, then it becomes easier to understand how and why exposure to environmental factors other than allergens might be linked to disease induction and exacerbation. The complex cellular events that are linked to altered stress responses in the epithelium on exposure to pollutants or respiratory viruses is only just being appreciated (15,33). Many, if not all, of these activate oxidant pathways that could lead to accelerated epithelial damage through increased apoptosis. There are numerous studies linking asthma with a reduced antioxidant status and, as such, asthmatic individuals may be especially susceptible to dietary deficiencies in such antioxidants as vitamins A, E, and C. Functional polymorphisms of the antioxidant enzymes or their expression could also provide an essential genetic component to this aspect of asthma.

V. Virus Interactions with Asthmatic Airways

Among the potential environmental factors that are strongly linked to asthma is infection by respiratory viruses. Rhinoviruses are responsible for the majority of common colds which are usually self-limiting and not accompanied by lower airways disease (34). Of importance, however, is the fact that in adults and children with asthma respiratory viruses, rhinoviruses, especially, can cause profound exacerbations of asthma and are responsible for the majority of hospital admissions for childhood asthma and a rather lower proportion in adults. The recent demonstration that rhinoviruses can directly infect the epithelium of the lower airways (35) provides the direct concrete evidence as to why this normally relatively innocuous virus type can lead to severe asthma attacks. Once inside the epithelial cell, and especially if replicating, this results in a wide range of cellular events linked to the propagation of an inflammatory response. These include the secretion of a range of chemokines and cytokines, the increased expression of MHC and costimulatory molecules and the augmented cell surface expression of ICAM-1, the adhesion molecule that enables rhinovirus entry to the cell. The ability of rhinoviruses to also infect inflammatory cells (e.g., monocytes and structural cells, like fibroblasts) directly provides added mechanisms for driving an asthmatic response. The important question that requires answering is why the asthmatic epithelium is more susceptible than the normal epithelium to virus infection? The answer to this may probably be through a combination of factors including the constitutionally increased expression of viral receptors such as ICAM-1, the "damage" already present in the stressed and repairing epithelium in asthma and the intrinsic susceptibility of the epithelium to injury, which is probably accelerated by virus infection.

Whether or not virus infection in early life is a key event in the inception of asthma is a key question that requires vigorous perusal. The powerful effects that respiratory viruses have to initiate inflammatory and tissue damaging responses place them high up the league of potential environmental factors that could drive the asthmatic process. If, as has been suggested, normal individuals can tolerate lower airway infection with respiratory viruses but those predisposed to asthma cannot, then a search for differences that may exist in the regulatory pathways operating in the epithelium and the EMTU in normal and asthmatic subjects and the subsequent ability of these to resist virus infection or generate an inflammatory response is required. Whether such mechanisms or different ones are also involved in the powerful effects that respiratory viruses have in initiating or worsening some forms of asthma is likely to be a field of intense future research, especially if linked to the identification of novel therapeutic targets.

References

1. Lau S, Illi S, Sommerfield C, Niggemann B, Bergmann R, von Mutius E, Wahn U. Early exposure to house dust mite and cat allergens and development of childhood asthma: a cohort study. Multi Centre Allergy Study Group. Lancet 2000; 356:1392–1397.
2. Pearce N, Pekkanen J, Beasley R. How much asthma is really attributable to atopy? Thorax 1999; 54:268–272.
3. Pearce N, Douwes J, Beasley R. Is allergen exposure the major primary cause of asthma? Thorax 2000; 55:424–431.

4. Leckie MJ, Brinke AT, Khan J, Diamant Z, O'Connor B, Walls CM, et al. Effects of an interleukin-5 blocking monoclonal antibody on eosinophils, airways hyper-responsiveness, and the late asthmatci response. Lancet 2000; 356:2144–48.

5. Bryan SA, Kanabar V, Matti S, Leckie MJ, Khan J, Rolfe L, et al. Effect of recombinant human interleukin-12 on eosinophils, airway hyper-responsiveness and the late asthmatic response. Lancet 2000; 356:2149–2153.

6. ENFUMOSA Study Group. Quality of life in severe asthma. Am J Respir Crit Care Med 2000; 161(3):A923.

7. ENFUMOSA Study Group. Clinical, Physiological and Pathological Features of Chronic Severe Asthma: A Multicentre European Study–ENFUMOSA. Eur Respir J (submitted).

8. The Childhood Asthma Management Program Research Group. Long-term effects of budesonide or nedocromil in children with asthma. N Engl J Med 2000; 343:1054–1063.

9. Cokugras H, Akcakaya N, Seckin, Camcioglu Y, Sarimurat N, Aksoy F. Ultrastructural examination of bronchial biopsy specimens from children with moderate asthma. Thorax 2001; 56:25–29.

10. Pohunek P, Roche WR, Tarzikova J, Kurdman J, Warner JO. Eosinophilic inflammation in the bronchial mucosa of children with bronchial asthma. Eur Resp J 1997; 10 (Suppl 25):160s (abstr).

11. Puddicombe SM, Polosa R, Richter A, Krishna MT, Howarth PH, Holgate ST et al. The involvement of the epidermal growth factor receptor in epithelial repair in asthma. FASEB J 2000; 14:1362–1374.

12. Lackie PM, Baker JE, Gunthert U, Holgate ST. Expression of CD44 isoforms is increased in the airway epithelium of asthmatic subjects. Am J Respir Cell Mol Biol 1997; 16(1):14–22.

13. Dorscheid DR, Wilson SJ, Hamann KJ, Rabe KF, Beasley R, Holgate ST et al. Expression of Fas (CD95) and Fas Ligand (CD95L) in airway epithelium of subjects with fatal asthma. J Allergy Clin Immunol (submitted).

14. Bucchieri F, Lordan JL, Richter A, Buchanan D, Wilson SJ, Howarth PH et al. Asthmatic bronchial epithelium is more susceptible to oxidant-induced apoptosis. Am J Respir Cell Mol Biol 2002; 17:179–185.

15. Nel AE, Diaz-Sanchez D, Li N. The role of particulate pollutants in pulmonary inflammation and asthma: evidence for the involvment of organic chemicals and oxidative stress. Curr Opin Pulm Med 2001; 7:20–26.

16. Demoly P, Simony-Lafontaine J, Chanez P, Pujol JL, Lequeux N, Michel FB et al. Cell proliferation in the bronchial mucosa of asthmatics and chronic bronchitics. Am J Respir Crit Care Med 1994; 150:214–217.

17. Torres-Lozano C, Puddicombe SM, Richter A, Bucchieri F, Howarth PH, Vrugt R et al. Impaired epithelial proliferation and expression of the cyclin dependent kinase inhibitor, p21^{waf}, in asthmatic bronchial epithelium. Am J Respir Cell Mol Biol (submitted).

18. Busse WW, Banks-Schlegel S, Wenzel SE. Pathophysiology of severe asthma. J Allergy Clin Immunol 2000; 106:1033–1042.

19. Roche WR, Beasley R, Williams JH, Holgate ST. Subepithelial fibrosis in the bronchi of asthmatics. Lancet 1989; 1(8637):520–524.

20. Boulet LP, Laviolette M, Turcotte H, Cartier A, Dugas M, Malo JL et al. Bronchial subepithelial fibrosis correlates with airway responsiveness to methacholine. Chest 1997; 112(1):45–52.

21. Chetta A, Foresi A, Del Donno M, Bertorelli G, Pesci A, Olivieri D. Airways remodeling is a distinctive feature of asthma and is related to severity of disease. Chest 1997; 111:852–857.

22. Toda M, Yoshida M, Nakano Y, Cheng G, Motojima S, Fukada T. An animal model for airway wall thickening. J Allergy Clin Immunol 1997; 99:S409 (abstr).

23. Brewster CE, Howarth PH, Djukanovic R, Wilson J, Holgate ST, Roche WR. Myofibroblasts and subepithelial fibrosis in bronchial asthma. Am J Respir Cell Mol Biol 1990; 3:507–511.

24. Evans MJ, van Winkle LS, Fanucchi MV, Plopper CG. The attenuated fibroblast sheath of the respiratory tract epithelial-mesenchymal trophic unit. Am J Respir Cell Mol Biol 2000; 21:655–657.

25. Arthur MJ, Mann DA, Iredale JP. Tissue inhibitors of metalloproteinases, hepatic stellate cells and liver fibrosis. J Gastroenterol Hepatol 1998; 13 (Suppl):S33-S38

26. Holgate ST, Davies DE, Lackie PM, Wilson SJ, Puddicombe SM, Lordan JL. Epithelial-mesenchymal interactions in the pathogenesis of asthma. J Allergy Clin Immunol 2000; 105:193–204.

27. Redington AE, Roche WR, Holgate ST, Howarth PH. Co-localization of immunoreactive transforming growth factor-beta 1 and decorin in bronchial biopsies from asthmatic and normal subjects. J Pathol 1998; 186:410–415.

28. Shute J, Redington AE, McConnell W, Howarth P. Binding and release of FGF-2 from heparan sulphate proteoglycans in bronchial tissue. Am J Pathol 2000 (submitted).

29. Zhang S, Smartt H, Holgate ST, Roche WR. Growth factors secreted by bronchial epithelial cells control myofibroblast proliferation: an in vitro co-culture model of airway remodeling in asthma. Lab Invest 1999; 79:395–405.

30. Warburton D, Schwarz M, Tefft D, Flores-Delgado G, Anderson KD, Cardoso WV. The molecular basis of lung morphogenesis. Mech Dev 2000; 92:55–81.

31. Laprise C, Laviolette M, Boutet M, Boulet LP. Asymptomatic airway hyperresponsiveness: relationships with airway inflammation and remodelling. Eur Respir J 1999; 14: 63–73.

32. Stick S. The contribution of airway development to paediatric and adult lung disease. Thorax 2000; 55:587–594.

33. Papi A, Stanciu LA, Papadopoulos NG, Teran LM, Holgate ST, Johnston SL. Rhinovirus infection induces major histocompatibility complex class I and costimulatory molecule upregulation on respiratory epithelial cells. J Infect Dis 2000; 181:1780–4

34. Johnston S, Holgate S. Epidemiology of viral respiratory tract infections. In: Myint S, Taylor-Robinson D, eds. Viral and Other Infections of the Human Respiratory Tract. London: Chapman & Hall, 1996: 1–38.

35. Papadopoulos NG, Bates PJ, Bardin PG, Papi A, Leir SH, Fraenkel DJ, Meyer J, Lackie PM, Sanderson G, Holgate ST, Johnston SL. Rhinoviruses infect the lower airways. J Infect Dis 2000; 181:1875–1884.

2

Microbiology and Epidemiology of Upper Respiratory Tract Infections

STEVEN MYINT

GlaxoSmithKline
Harlow, Essex, England

I. Introduction

Respiratory tract infections are the most common cause of acute physical illness in the developed world. Upper respiratory tract infections (URTI) constitute the bulk of the morbidity (Fig. 1). In the United States the rate of outpatient visits for URTI has been estimated as 200:100,000 of the population per year (3).

In developing countries acute respiratory infections are an even greater health burden. It is estimated that approximately 15 million children and adolescents under the age of 15 years die from acute respiratory tract infections, mainly starting as upper respiratory tract illnesses that progress to pneumonia (39). There are huge variations from country to country, with death rates six times higher in Paraguay than in Costa Rica, which in turn has a five times higher death rate than that of the United States (76). Data suggest that incidence of infection is not significantly greater in developing countries but that severity of illness is responsible for the increased mortality.

Despite advances in medicine and environmental improvement, this pre-eminence of respiratory tract infection has not changed over the last century. Recent decades have defined the specific causes as new pathogens and technologies are introduced. No doubt, this will continue to evolve and be redefined with the advent of respiratory antiviral therapy and new vaccines.

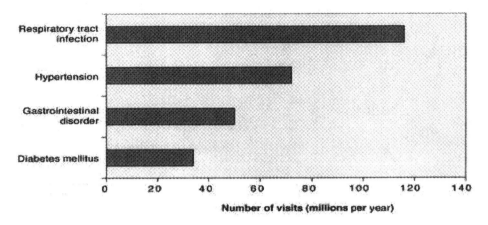

Figure 1   Relative frequency of common illnesses in the United States.

II. Basic Concepts

The upper respiratory tract (URT) is generally defined as that part of the airways above the cricoid cartilage. This includes the nose, pharynx, larynx, paranasal sinuses, Eustachian tube, and middle ear. The respiratory tract should, however, be considered a continuum with infectious agents that initially colonize the upper parts of the airway but may spread to other parts: in general, host factors are responsible for the eventual localization of infection. At all ages, however, fewer than 10% of infections also affect the lower respiratory tract (53). In addition, it is well recognized that viral invaders predispose to certain bacterial secondary infections.

Much of the upper airways have a normal microbiological flora. These include most classes of infectious agents (Table 1).

The most common pathogens of the upper respiratory tract are viruses, with most clinical syndromes being viral in cause (Fig. 2). Bacteria are significant pathogens for sore throat, sinusitis, and otitis media, although even in these infections there is often a viral component. Although there is some evidence that bacteria play a role in the genesis and precipitation of asthma, with the exception of mycoplasma and chlamydia, this is far less robust than that for viruses. This chapter will focus on viruses since the other contributions in this volume have remained focussed on this area. It is not intended to be a comprehensive review (see Refs. 19,71), but will provide sufficient detail to allow an understanding of subsequent chapters.

III. Common Clinical Syndromes and Their Epidemiology

The common clinical syndromes are what are termed common colds, influenza, sinusitis, pharyngitis, otitis media, laryngitis, and laryngotracheitis. The frequent pathogens responsible for these syndromes are shown in Figure 2. Conditions such

Table 1 Normal Flora of the Upper Respiratory Tract

Common (>50%)	*Streptococcus mutans* and other α-hemolytic streptococci
	Neisseria spp.
	Corynebacterium spp.
	Bacteroides spp.
	Veillonella spp.
	Other anaerobic cocci
	Fusiform bacteria
	Candida albicans
	Haemophilus influenzae
	Entamoeba gingivalis
Less common (<50%)	*Streptococcus pyogenes*
	Streptococcus pneumoniae
	Neisseria meningitidis
	Staphylococcus aureus
	Others

Source: Ref. 72.

as epiglottitis, tonsillitis, and adenoiditis are usually related to pharyngitis, with a common viral cause and group A β-hemolytic streptococci being the characteristic bacterial pathogens.

A. Common Colds

Common colds are viral infections of the nasal and paranasal airways: acute rhinosinusitis. The clinical presentation is of rhinorrhea, nasal congestion, and sneezing, with fever, general malaise, and sore throat being less frequent. Most are trivial infections in developed countries, although there are rare case reports of complications such as fatal cardiac arrhythmias. In developing countries they are more often harbingers of lower respiratory tract illness, secondary bacterial infection, and mortality. The main issues in developed countries now derive from such infections' economic importance and sequelae such as exacerbations of underlying chronic lung disease. In the United States, it is estimated that 26 million days of absence from school and 23 million days of absence from work are attributable to common colds and sore throats per year. There are also estimated to be 27 million consultations of physicians and $2 billion of over-the-counter remedies bought. This puts the total cost to the economy in the United States at over $15 billion per annum (18). There is currently not a specific treatment.

The causes of common colds are viral, with rhinoviruses and coronaviruses being the most frequent (Table 2); indeed these two viruses are often termed "the common cold viruses." Although in experimental infections there is variation in the likelihood of symptoms produced by the different viral causes (Table 3), in an individual it is not possible to determine the specific causes based on symptoms or their severity. In epidemiological terms, the differences in incubation period are, however,

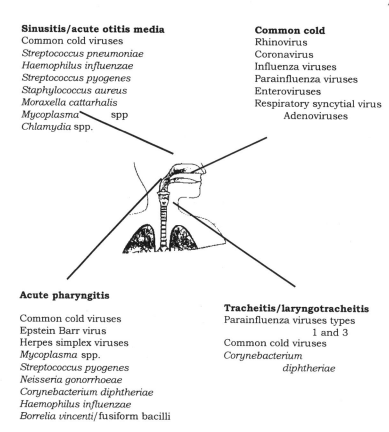

Sinusitis/acute otitis media
Common cold viruses
Streptococcus pneumoniae
Haemophilus influenzae
Streptococcus pyogenes
Staphylococcus aureus
Moraxella cattarhalis
Mycoplasma spp
Chlamydia spp.

Common cold
Rhinovirus
Coronavirus
Influenza viruses
Parainfluenza viruses
Enteroviruses
Respiratory syncytial virus
    Adenoviruses

Acute pharyngitis

Common cold viruses
Epstein Barr virus
Herpes simplex viruses
Mycoplasma spp.
Streptococcus pyogenes
Neisseria gonorrhoeae
Corynebacterium diphtheriae
Haemophilus influenzae
Borrelia vincenti/fusiform bacilli

Tracheitis/laryngotracheitis
Parainfluenza viruses types
    1 and 3
Common cold viruses
Corynebacterium
    diphtheriae

Figure 2   Common causes of infections of the upper respiratory tract.

Table 2   Relative Frequency of Pathogens
in Common Colds in Adults

Pathogen	%
Rhinoviruses	40–50
Coronaviruses	20–30
Influenza virus	10–15
Adenoviruses	5
Parainfluenza viruses	5
Respiratory syncytial virus	1
Enteroviruses and other viruses	1–10

Table 3 Relative Frequency (%) of Symptoms by Virus Challenge in Adult Volunteers

Clinical feature	Coronavirus 229E	Rhinovirus 2	Influenza A
Fever	9–23	7–16	98
Rhinorrhea and/or obstruction	94–100	64–100	20–30
Headache	32–85	28–50	85
General malaise	46–47	28–43	80
Sneezing	85	50	30
Sore throat	54–68	87–93	50–60
Cough	21–31	64–68	90
Hoarseness	12	57	10
Myalgia	9	21	60–75
Watery/sore eyes	29	43	60–70
Chills	18	21	90

Source: Ref. 90.

useful markers with, for example, coronavirus colds having a longer mean incubation period than rhinoviruses. In addition there is variation in the profile of possible causes depending on age and setting. In the elderly, respiratory syncytial virus influenza A, and coronavirus are the most common agents in daycare centers (25). The other group with respiratory syncytial virus commonly found are children under the age of 2 years.

The incubation period varies from 12 to 72 h, depending on causative virus, although this may be shorter in experimental inoculation directly into the nose. Transmission may be by either fomites or airborne spread. Young children and mothers have high secondary attack rates, with spread in communities occurring most frequently in schools, daycare centers, and in the home. The median duration of illness is a week, but 25–30% of cases persist, with any symptom, for 2 weeks or more. Although methods do exist to make a specific diagnosis the clinical features are usually used to do this in the absence of specific therapy (except for influenza, see below). Differential diagnosis is mainly from acute bacterial rhinosinusitis in longer-duration cases, since this is a complication that may require antibiotic therapy.

On average, adults suffer two to four acute upper respiratory tract infections per year, and children experience them more often, with up to 6–12 attacks per year in the preschool-age group (53,64–66). This frequency in early life means that the preschool child is symptomatic 20% of the time (i.e., 2.5 months of the year). There is no evidence that breastfeeding is protective. Although this varies by population studied, it appears that males are more susceptible under the age of 3 years (65), but a slight preponderance in females occurs in older children and adults (36). It is suggested that the increased female susceptibility in adults may be due to mothers having greater exposure to children (27). In the elderly, there are no gender differences in incidence but men are more likely to develop subsequent pneumonia (35). Cigarette smokers have the same or greater frequency of colds and are more likely to have symptoms of greater severity (14,36). Parental smoking does not appear to increase the susceptibility to common colds in children (31). Moderate alcohol consumption appears to have no influence on incidence rates in smokers, but is associated with both decreased incidence and risk of illness in nonsmokers (14). Tonsillectomy does not seem to affect the prevalence of colds, although children seem to be more likely to have one around the time of a tonsillectomy and adenoidectomy (17). The effect of air pollution on common colds and other upper respiratory tract illness is unclear. During episodes of high external air pollution, upper respiratory tract illness symptoms are common but probably represent toxic effects, although episodes of infectious bronchitis and pneumonia do seem to be more common. This increased morbidity has been correlated with particulates and sulfur dioxide (92). Exposure to a cold or wet environment does not influence the incidence of colds (21), although high indoor humidity appears to be a major risk factor (81).

Studies have also shown that psychosocial factors are important in the susceptibility to common colds and influenza. In experimental virus challenge studies, patients with cognitive dissonance and stress had increased virus shedding and higher symptom scores (87).

Lower birthweight, smaller head circumference, higher socioeconomic class, and a positive family history also seem to correlate with increased risk of colds (12). There are also genetic factors: acute respiratory infections are more common among Malays than other ethnic groups in Malaysia, African-Americans and Native Americans than white Americans (5,54). They are also more frequent among children with allergy and bronchial hyperreactivity (13,47).

Common colds and the other acute upper respiratory tract infections occur throughout the year but are relatively less frequent in summer than in the other seasons (65). Common colds peak in the United States in September and October, predominantly due to the seasonality of rhinovirus infections. This shows a correlation with low temperature and higher humidity but is most commonly attributed to crowding indoors, which is postulated to facilitate transmission. This notion is supported by the finding that the peak in tropical countries is during the rainy season. There is a second peak in countries such as the United States in early spring. This is usually attributed to the reopening of schools as a major factor (27). Low body temperature has not been shown to increase susceptibility (21).

B. Influenza

Influenza illness is caused predominantly by influenza A and B viruses. Even if confined to the upper respiratory tract, characteristics of the illness allow it to be differentiated from other causes of common colds: abrupt onset, marked malaise, and more severe myalgia. In addition, there is almost always a fever, a feature that occurs in only a minority of common colds due to other viruses. Influenza, like respiratory syncytial virus and adenoviruses, are also more likely to result in lower respiratory tract illness.

Influenza has a winter predominance in temperate climates in nonpandemic years. During the season, there is usually excess morbidity and mortality, which, in addition to that due to pneumonia, is associated with cardiovascular events such as myocardial and cerebral infarction. Attack rates are highest in the young, but more severe morbidity and mortality are highest in those over 65, especially those with chronic underlying conditions such as chronic lung disease, renal disease, diabetes mellitus, hemoglobinopathies, and immunodeficiency. About one-third of all hospitalized patients in the developed world have an underlying chronic condition and one-quarter of them are over 65 years of age. In addition to the medical burden, there is an economic burden: each case is estimated to be associated with, on average, 3 days absence from work or school, 3–4 days of restriction to bed, and 5–6 days of restricted general activity (82). Infection, however, occurs in all age groups except for infants, and in all parts of the world. The timing of the influenza season appears to be different in tropical climates, with multiple outbreaks not being unusual.

It is generally accepted that aerosol and direct transmission are both important in the spread of infection. The former may be responsible for more rapid dissemination, as outbreaks have shown. An example is the dissemination within a 4.5 h detainment of a commercial aircraft without auxiliary ventilation from an index case to 72% of susceptible individuals. Since most passengers did not have direct contact, transmission is likely to have been via aerosol dispersion (68).

Schoolchildren have the highest attack rates and most likely are the primary source of spread in most communities. In most epidemics, 35–50% of affected persons are initially of school age. As the days pass, this percentage declines and preschool-age children and the elderly become infected. Race and gender differences do not seem to be important for susceptibility, but children in lower socioeconomic groups appear to be at greater risk of infection than those in higher socioeconomic classes (33).

Epidemics and pandemics occur because of the changing nature of the virus (see below). The old adage that pandemics occurred in 10–14 year cycles appears to have been broken since there has not been one since the 1977–1978 season, but the world gears up each year for the anticipated next one. Four influenza pandemics have occurred in the 20th century. The 1918 Spanish influenza was the most devastating: it killed 550,000 persons in the United States and 20 million persons worldwide. The 1977 Russian influenza had a relatively minor effect and did not increase mortality. The 1957 Asian influenza and the 1968 Hong Kong influenza had effects in between those of the Spanish and Russian episodes.

In pandemic years, the season tends to be extended beyond the winter and spreads from a focus, over a period of weeks and months, globally. The last threat of a pandemic was in 1997 when human cases of a new strain, an H5N1 virus subtype, were detected in Hong Kong. However, there was not efficient person-to-person transmission of the virus and the human infections were controlled when mass destruction of chickens from markets and their breeding farms was instituted. In March 1999, H9N2 viruses were isolated from two hospitalized children in Hong Kong. Molecular analyses indicated that the HA and NA genes of these isolates are avian in origin and prevalent in poultry in Hong Kong. This virus was a human-adapted virus, giving it the potential for rapid spread in a human population. The next pandemic is expected to originate from southeast Asia because new strains regularly appear from this region. Many theories purport to explain this part of the world as the epicenter, with perhaps the most plausible being the close proximity of human to avian species. This encourages the development of avian–human reassortants.

C. Sinusitis, Pharyngitis, Acute Otitis Media, Laryngitis

These conditions have a mixed viral and bacterial cause, with viruses probably being the original invader but subsequent bacterial infection, in a minority, resulting in enhanced symptoms. They are most commonly preceded by the common cold, as evidenced by radiography, but if the cause is viral it is usually clinically inapparent (38). The epidemiology therefore reflects that of common colds as described above.

All these infections are common, with 2–35% of cases of common colds being complicated with one or more of these clinical complications. Cases tend to be most prevalent during the winter months, with children under the age of 15 years more commonly affected than older age groups. Indeed the peak incidence is in the first 3 years of life, with another peak at the age of school entry. Like most infectious diseases, males are more often affected than females and there may be some genetic susceptibility in cases of recurrent infection. Patients with atopic disease also seem to be more prone to recurrent sinusitis and there is a belief that this is akin to asthma of the upper airways. This genetic component is also reflected in specific racial groups: Australian aborigines and Canadian Inuits have a high frequency of both infection and recurrence.

Breastfeeding in the first few months of life seems to be associated with a reduced risk of infection (85). As with common colds, psychosocial factors appear to play a role in susceptibility to these infections. In a longitudinal study of 16 families, stressful life events were four times more likely to precede an episode of streptococcal pharyngitis than to follow it (60). Passive smoking and exposure to environmental air pollutants such as sulfur dioxide also predispose to these infections, although some symptoms may be due to direct irritant effects (24,48).

Patients with white cell defects, hypogammaglobulinemia, and acquired immunodeficiency syndromes are more prone to infection. The importance of ciliary function is illustrated by the fact that patients with ciliary defects, such as those with cystic fibrosis, also have a higher prevalence.

IV. The Major Viral Pathogens

A. Rhinoviruses

Structure and Replication

Human rhinoviruses (HRV) are members of the virus family Picornaviridae, which also includes polioviruses, enteroviruses, and hepatitis A. These are all small (30 nm diameter) nonenveloped viruses with single-stranded positive-sense RNA genomes.

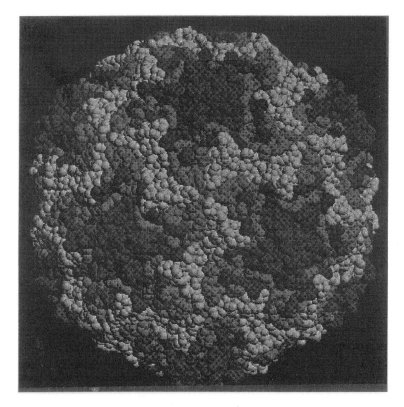

Figure 3 Computerized image of rhinovirus structure. In the original, different protein units are shown in different colors with the pentameric vertices in blue. A fourth protein unit is not visible: it is on the inner surface of the capsid.

There are over 100 immunotypes recognized with the first of these, rhinovirus 1A, being described in 1956.

The 7.2 kb uncapped genome is translated into a single 250 kDa polyprotein with two proteinases (2A and 3C) that almost immediately post-translation cleave this precursor into immediate and structural proteins. Structural proteins (VP1, VP0, and VP3) are assembled as 60 protomer subunits into 12 pentamers to form a capsid with icosahedral symmetry (Fig. 3). As the virion matures, VP0 is itself cleaved into VP2 and VP4 to form the infectious particles. The viral genome is also replicated and covalently bound to another product of the polyprotein, VPg. This entire replication cycle takes place in the cytoplasm in 5–10 h (80).

X-ray crystallography has shown that the capsid has a depression, so-called canyon, in the apex region of viral pentamers. This region is involved in receptor binding to host cells prior to infection. There appear to be two receptors utilized by different rhinovirus subgroups. The major group rhinoviruses, typified by the HRV-

14, bind to intracellular adhesion molecule type 1 (ICAM-1) whereas the minor group rhinoviruses, typified by HRV-1a, bind to a low-density lipoprotein (43,83). The major group appears, at least in vitro, to be able to upregulate the expression of ICAM-1, which may aid cell-to-cell spread (6,86).

Rhinoviruses can be differentiated from other members of the Picornaviridae by their resistance to solubilization in ether and lability to acid conditions at pH 3–5. They also have an optimal temperature of replication of 33–35°C, a feature they share with coronaviruses. Although there is replication at 37°C, the viral yield in cell culture is only 10–50% of that at the lower temperature (84). This feature is an important facet in examining the pathogenesis of these viruses in acute asthma.

Epidemiology

Rhinoviruses are the most common cause of common colds, and possibly the most common cause of infection. Estimates, from predominantly U.S.-based studies, put rhinovirus infection rates in adults at 0.5–0.8 per person per year (15,36,41). Infants have a higher rate of 1.21 per person per year.

Because immunity to a single serotype is long-lasting (see below), the most naive individuals (i.e., children) are the major reservoir of infection. There are not animal, not even primate, reservoirs. It has been debated for decades whether aerosol or fomite transmission of rhinovirus infections is the predominant mode. Aerosol transmission has been documented in the experimental situation using insufflators and in rebreathing experiments. This appears, however, to be less efficient than might be predicted. Nasal washings from experimentally infected individuals contain on the order of 10^2–10^3 tissue culture infection dose (TCID$_{50}$)/ml, with a log or more reduction pharyngeal washings (20). Since sneeze aerosols are a mixture of these, the likely mean titer is estimated to be on the order of 1–10 TCID$_{50}$/ml. Only a fraction of the sneeze aerosol is of the 3–16 μm size that deposits in the anterior and middle turbinates. Experimental infection with aerosols of this size suggests that 10–20 TCID$_{50}$/ml concentration is required to cause infection (22). On the other hand, only 0.032–0.75 TCID$_{50}$/ml appears to be required for direct inoculation. In addition, 60–90% of infected individuals has infectious virus recoverable from their hands for several hours (2,37), and infectious virus can be found on environmental objects (78). The use of virucidal hand treatment in an experimental transmission model reduced secondary contacts by 60%, which suggests that both routes of transmission may occur naturally (42). The direct route is possibly more important since manual air ventilation and disinfection appear to have little influence on prevalence rates in an office setting (49). Direct inoculation into the mouth and kissing are inefficient methods of transmission (50). Secondary attack rates in family and school settings are on the order of 30–50% with continuous exposure over a week or more (63). The duration of exposure is important in raising secondary attack rates (59).

Pathogenesis and Immunology

The incubation period in experimental infection is typically 16–24 h, but may be 2–3 days. The usual initial site of infection is likely to be the nasal epithelium of the anterior nares, although infection can also be induced by inoculation of the conjunctiva. There is little detectable damage to the nasal epithelium, although cilial function is reduced (45). Ultrastructural studies show that foci of infection are isolated and scattered (4,88). There is some inflammation with a predominant neutrophil influx that occurs within 24 h of infection (29,73).This subsides by day 4 after experimental infection. Infection tends to be localized to the nasal cavity, pharynx, paranasal sinuses, and middle ear. Viremia has been reported, but this was an unusual case of sudden infant death syndrome (91). It is thought that symptoms arise because of the host response, a topic that is discussed in detail in subsequent chapters. Over 60% of infections are symptomatic (51,52). A proinflammatory cytokine cascade and local IgG and IgA are induced early (8). A detectable serum neutralizing antibody response occurs later at 2–3 weeks. Virus shedding peaks on days 2 and 3, and may persist for 14 days or more.

Little detail is known about the immune response to rhinovirus infections. Serum N antibody titers appear to have an inverse correlation with subsequent infection and rise in 75–80% of cases postinfection (10). N antibody is detectable two weeks postinfection in naive volunteers, peaking at 3–4 weeks, and falling over subsequent months. IgA is the predominant component of neutralizing activity in the nose. The humoral response appears to be disease-modifying but interferon is thought to be the principal mechanism for recovery (11). Even less is known about the cell-mediated immune response.

B. Coronaviruses

Structure and Replication

Coronaviruses are roughly spherical, enveloped particles, approximately 100 nm in diameter with a characteristic fringe of 20 nm long surface projections that are round or petal-shaped. This crown gives the viruses their name. The nucleocapsid structure is extended and helical.

The HCV 229E genomic RNA is a single molecule of positive strand RNA composed of about 27,300 nucleotides and a 3′ poly-A tract of not less than 50 residues with 8 major open reading frames. The total number of HCV 229E gene products is, however, unknown. The hallmark of the coronavirus gene expression is the production of a 3′ coterminal set of subgenomic mRNAs in the infected cell. With the exception of the smallest mRNA, all mRNAs are structurally polycistronic but only the information encoded in the 5′ unique region of the RNA (i.e., the region absent from the next smallest RNA) is translated to protein. In the majority of cases, a single polypeptide is translated from each mRNA. The mechanism by which coronavirus subgenomic mRNAs are generated is complex and the details are beyond the scope of this chapter. This involves a process of discontinuous transcription and each mRNA has a leader RNA derived from the 5′ end of the genomic RNA.

Epidemiology

Studies of coronaviruses as causes of clinical illness have shown that coronaviruses are second only to rhinoviruses as causes of the common cold. In the U.S. and

England 229E and OC43 are responsible for 15–30% of all clinical cases (70), with an approximately equal number of subclinical infections. Typically either a 229E or OC43 serotype dominates in one year, with alternation from year to year in dominance. Peak incidence is in the winter months, although summer outbreaks have also been described.

Pathogenesis and Immunology

Little is known of the detail of pathogenic mechanisms in human coronavirus infection, principally because humans are the only model of infection. Infection can be induced experimentally by direct inoculation of virus into the nose but this is unlikely to be the natural route. By analogy with rhinoviruses, transmission is likely to be either by aerosols or fomites, with the former a more likely explanation for the frequent simultaneous transmission to those exposed. In support of this is the finding that 229E survives well in an atmosphere of high humidity and low temperature (46).

Once in the nose the virus is thought to enter by a specific receptor: aminopeptidase N (CD13) in the case of 229E and a sialic-acid containing receptor in the case of OC43. Ultrastructural studies suggest that it is ciliated cells, not goblet cells, that are infected (1). Replication then takes place over the next 8–24 h. In MRC-c and WI-38 cells, 229E virus can be found in rough endoplasmic reticulum 12 h after infection, and in cytoplasmic vesicles and extracellularly 24–36 h after infection. Replication is optimal at 32–33°C: the temperature in the superficial layers of the nasal mucosa. Virus budding then takes place from Golgi apparatus with little loss of cells. Cilia appear to be withdrawn into the cell and this may be associated with rhinorrhea, although increased plasma exudation of proteins such as fibrinogen, which may be histamine-responsive, must also play a role. Serum antibody levels rise after about a week but it is not clear whether it is this response or cell-mediated mechanisms that clear infection (9). Certainly there is some inverse correlation of the severity and likelihood of disease with preexisting serum antibody, but the mere presence of such antibody is not protective. Serum antibody levels peak about 2 weeks after infection and decline to low or undetectable levels at 12–18 months. The serum antibody response is mainly directed against the surface protein but there is also an, albeit lesser, antibody response directed to the nucleoprotein and membrane proteins.

Interferon, specific nasal secretory IgA, and total nasal secretory protein appear to play a role in protection from infection (89). Other nonspecific factors, such as the rise in local temperature that occurs during nasal blockage, may be important not in resistance but in aborting an infection because they may induce the production of heat shock proteins, activate lymphocytes, and inhibit viral replication.

The cell-mediated immune response has not been investigated in natural infections but sera from volunteers have been shown to possess antibody that can elicit antibody-dependent cellular toxicity (ADCC) in vitro.

Whatever the relative importance of different arms of the immune response in clearing coronavirus infection, reinfections are common and can occur within a year to the same serotype or within 2 months to a heterologous serotype.

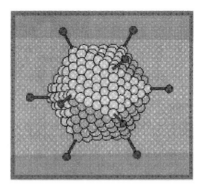

Figure 4 Model of adenovirus.

C. Adenoviruses

Structure and Replication

Adenoviruses are so called because they were first isolated from adenoid tissue. They, however, cause a wide spectrum of disease affecting most bodily systems. They are medium-sized nonenveloped DNA-containing viruses. They have a capsid with icosahedral symmetry composed of 240 nonvertex hexon capsomeres and 12 vertex capsomeres (Fig. 4). Protruding from the vertex penton is a stalklike structure: the fiber. This capsid encloses a genome of linear single-stranded DNA of 30–38 kb pairs encoding 30–40 genes.

There are 10 structural proteins whose putative properties are shown in Table 4.

On the basis of antigenic (and functional) differences in the hexon, penton,

Table 4 Adenovirus Proteins

Name	Location	Known functions
II	Hexon monomer	Structural
III	Penton base	Penetration
IIIa	Associated with penton base	Penetration
IV	Fiber	Receptor binding; hemagglutination
V	Core associated with DNA and penton base	Histonelike; packaging
VI	Hexon minor polypeptide	Stabilization/assembly of particle
VII	Core	Histonelike
VIII	Hexon minor polypeptide	Stabilization/assembly of particle
IX	Hexon minor polypeptide	Stabilization/assembly of particle
TP	Genome—terminal protein	Genome replication

Table 5 Human Adenovirus Classification

Subgroup	Type	Oncogenic potential	Hemagglutination Rhesus	Rat
A	12, 18, 31	High	−	+/−
B	3, 7, 11, 14, 21, 34, 35	Weak	+	−
C	1, 2, 5, 6	None	−	+/−
D	8–10, 13, 15, 17, 19, 20, 22–30, 32, 33, 36–39	None	+/−	+
E	4	None	−	+/−
F–G	40, 41	?	−	+/−

and fiber proteins, the 49 human serotypes are classified into 6 subgenera, A–F, with one or more serotypes in each (Table 5).

Replication, which takes place in the nucleus of the host cell, is classified into an early and a late phase, the latter defined as beginning with the onset of DNA replication. Initial infection is a two-stage process involving, first, interaction of the fiber protein with a range of cellular receptors, which include the major histocompatibility class (MHC) class I molecule and the coxsackievirus–adenovirus receptor. The penton base protein then binds to the integrin family of cell surface heterodimers, allowing internalization via receptor-mediated endocytosis. Most cells express primary receptors for the adenovirus fiber coat protein; however, internalization is more selective. After uncoating steps, and transport of genome to the nucleus immediate early and early mRNAs are transcribed from the viral DNA. This is regulated by virus-encoded *trans*-acting regulatory factors. Products of the immediate early genes regulate expression of the early genes. Multiple protein products are made from each gene by alternative splicing of mRNA transcripts. The first mRNA protein to be made is termed E1A. This protein is a *trans*-acting transcriptional regulatory factor whose precise mode of action is not known (not a DNA-binding transcription factor) but is necessary for transcriptional activation of early genes. The second protein made is E1B. E1A + E1B together (and independently of other virus proteins) are capable of transforming primary cells in vitro.

At the onset of DNA replication, the pattern of transcription changes from that of early to the late genes. There is *cis*-acting control of this switch (i.e., only newly replicated DNA is used for late gene transcription). The late genes are transcribed from the major late promoter; at least 13 species of mRNA are produced by alternative splicing. Assembly of protein units occurs in the nucleus, but begins in the cytoplasm when individual monomers form into hexon and penton capsomers. Empty immature capsids are assembled from these protomers in the nucleus, where the core is formed from genomic DNA + associated core proteins. Although host cell macromolecular synthesis ceases earlier in the infection, infection does not result in lysis of the cell. Virus particles tend to accumulate in the nucleus and are visible in the microscope as inclusion bodies; these are thought to be the basis of latent infections: reactivation is caused by accidental lysis of infected cells, releasing virus particles from the nuclei; effectively forming a reinfection.

Epidemiology

Adenovirus infections are very common, and most people have been infected with at least one type by adolescence. Virus can also be isolated from the majority of surgically removed tonsils/adenoids.

The prevalence of adenovirus infections in a community setting have been investigated in the Virus Watch programs undertaken in several sites including New York and Seattle (28). Data from the Seattle and New York studies indicate that the infection rate in infants is 179: 100 person years for all adenovirus serotypes (57: 100 person years for types 1 and 2), with the rate of infection declining in the older child up to the age of 9 years, but increasing again thereafter. The so-called epidemic serotype 7 was an exception to this pattern and infection rates increased progressively with age. Thirty-six percent of infections resulted in persistence of virus shedding for longer than a month, 14% lasted longer than 1 year, and occasional patients excreted the same virus serotype for over 2 years. However, it was also noted that although virus excretion could be prolonged, it appeared to be finite (the maximum documented time was 906 days). Thus, life-long persistence of the virus does not occur, and the virus is probably not transmitted vertically. There were no clear differences between the common serotypes (types 1, 2, 3, 5) in their ability to establish this persistent excretion.

Data from the Virus Watch studies also suggested that 51–56% of new infections are asymptomatic without clear differences in relation to age or virus type. Isolation of virus from the respiratory tract correlated better with clinical disease: 65% of such patients were symptomatic in contrast to 31% of patients whose virus excretion was confined to the feces. There was indirect evidence to suggest that less virus was present in the respiratory tract compared with feces, in which the virus concentration may have been boosted by multiplication in the gut cells. Thus it was possible that virus isolation from the respiratory tract was successful only from patients with a higher virus load. In those individuals who became ill, respiratory symptoms predominated, the majority being confined to the upper respiratory tract. Of 184 episodes of illness documented, only 10 involved the lower respiratory tract.

In a large hospital-based study of 18,096 children in Washington, adenoviruses were isolated from 1792 (9.9%) (7). When compared to the isolation rate in a control population, the authors estimated that approximately 7% of respiratory diseases in hospitals are causatively linked to adenoviruses. In over 54% of patients with respiratory disease from whom adenovirus was isolated from the throat, the virus appeared to be causally related to concurrent illness. However, isolation of virus types 1, 3, 6, or 7 appeared to be more clinically significant, and virus isolation from the throat was more relevant than virus isolation from the feces. They also observed that when throat swabs were cultured, adenovirus cytopathic effect appeared earlier (mean of 9 days vs. 12 days) in patients with disease compared to controls, suggesting a larger virus load in the former.

Adenovirus infections are found throughout the world, but underdeveloped countries appear to have a higher prevalence; in developed countries, higher prevalence is also seen in lower socioeconomic groups. Most children have been exposed to respiratory virus serotypes by school entry and this age group remains the focus for spread of infections. Spread of respiratory illness may be by both the respiratory and fecal–oral routes. Epidemics also occur, with febrile acute respiratory disease in military recruits and adenovirus 3–associated swimming outbreaks being well recognized. Both epidemics and endemic disease have a higher incidence in the late winter, spring, and early summer. People with deficient cell-mediated immunity are also at higher risk of severe adenoviral infection.

Pathogenesis and Immunity

The majority of infections are asymptomatic but result in so-called latent, or, more accurately, occult infection. This property has suggested that the virus has a role in the genesis of asthma. It is not known how long the virus can persist in the body, or whether it is capable of reactivation after long periods of time.

In symptomatic illness, the incubation period is 6–9 days, although this is more commonly only 2 days in viral challenge studies. The initial site of infection may be either the respiratory or gastrointestinal mucosa. In bronchial, bronchiolar, and alveolar epithelium, acidophilic intranuclear inclusions are seen that most likely represent aggregates of viral material. Characteristically there is also loss of definition of the nuclear membrane on histological examination, this composite picture being referred to as a smudge cell. In respiratory infection, virus has also been isolated from lymphocytes and kidney, thus suggesting that there may be several sites of possible latency.

The host response varies depending on the primary site of viral localization. There is an inverse correlation between nasal IgA and disease severity (55). Humoral immunity plays at least a partial response in the normal immune response, and patients with poor cell-mediated immunity, such as those with malnutrition, have more severe disease.

Adenovirus persistence and latency are of particular interest in chronic respiratory disease. Virus has been recovered from bronchoalveolar washings of children with asthma 12 months or more after acute infection (56). Adenovirus E1A, a viral factor involved in persistence, has also been found more often in patients with chronic obstructive pulmonary disease (COPD) than in controls (57). It has been hypothesized that this persistence has had a role in the continuing inflammation seen in these patients.

D. Influenza Viruses

Structure and Replication

Influenza viruses are members of the Orthomyxoviridae family. They are enveloped viruses with a segmented RNA genome. They are highly pleiomorphic (variable),

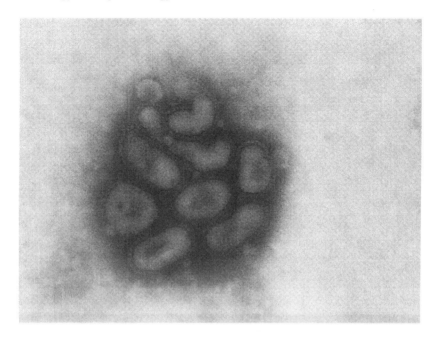

Figure 5   Electron micrograph of influenza virus.

mostly spherical/ovoid, 80–120 nm diameter, but many forms occur, including long filamentous particles (up to 200 nm long × 80–120 nm diameter) (Fig. 5).

The outer surface of the particle consists of a lipid envelope from which project prominent glycoprotein spikes of two types: a hemagglutinin (HA), and a neuraminidase (NA); apart from influenza C (see below), which has a single hemagglutinin–esterase fusion (HEF) glycoprotein. The envelope is composed of matrix (M) protein. These encapsidate a genome of RNA and nucleoprotein (N) in a helical form with three polymerase proteins associated with each segment.

There are three species of influenza virus, termed A, B, and C. Influenza A viruses infect a wide variety of mammals, including humans, horses, pigs, ferrets, and birds. They are the main virus found in epidemic and pandemic episodes. There are 15 known hemagglutinin (H) serotypes and nine known neuraminidase (N) serotypes Pigs and birds are believed to be particularly important reservoirs, generating pools of genetically/antigenically diverse viruses that are transferred back to the human population via reassortment. Influenza B viruses infect humans only and cause less severe disease as influenza A. There is a single serotype. Influenza C viruses also infect humans only, but are an uncommon cause of symptomatic illness.

The genomes of influenza A and B viruses consist of 8 segments of single-strand RNA of negative polarity. The entire genome contains approximately 13,500 nucleotides and 8 segments of influenza A and B encode 10 polypeptides (Table 6).

Table 6   Major Polypeptides of Influenzas A and B

Segment	Size(nt)	Polypeptide(s)	Function
1	2341	PB2	Transcriptase: cap binding
2	2341	PB1	Transcriptase: elongation
3	2233	PA	Transcriptase: protease activity
4	1778	HA	Hemagglutinin
5	1565	NP	Nucleoprotein: RNA binding; part of transcriptase complex; nuclear/cytoplasmic transport of vRNA
6	1413	NA	Neuraminidase: release of virus
7	1027	M1	Matrix protein: major component of virion
		M2	Integral membrane protein–ion channel
8	890	NS1	Nonstructural: nucleus; effects on cellular RNA transport, splicing, translation. Anti-interferon protein
		NS2	Nonstructural: nucleus+cytoplasm, function unknown

The multisegmented nature of the virus is responsible for continuing epidemics and pandemics. There have been several worldwide major pandemics in which the vast majority of the world's population has been susceptible to a new strain of influenza. The immunological naivete is due to a major change in the antigenicity of the H and N proteins, so-called antigenic shift. More subtle changes in the antigenic nature of influenza viruses have occurred during interpandemic periods, often resulting in epidemics, and these changes have been termed antigenic drift.

Antigenic shift is due to the segmented nature of the rival genome, as genotypic reassortment of the segments readily occurs during a mixed infection. This has readily been observed in vitro, and evidence also exists that it has occurred in vivo between swine and human strains and between swine and avian strains. One or more of the genome segments, including those coding for the surface glycoproteins of the prevalent strain, is replaced by the corresponding segment(s) from the avian (or other source) reservoir of influenza viruses. In 1957, the H2N2 viruses obtained their HA, NA, and PB1 genome segments from an avian virus, with the other five segments deriving from the preexisting H1N1 viruses. In 1968, the H2N2 viruses obtained novel HA and PB1 segments, again from the avian pool, generating the H3N2 strains. This is not, however, the only way of generating new viruses. Sequencing studies have revealed a nonreassortment mechanism for the appearance of new human strains: direct adaptation of an avian virus to humans (30). Phylogenetic analyses of gene products, with the exception of those replaced by reassortment during 1957 and 1968, provide convincing evidence that all current human influenza viruses, and also the classic H1N1 swine viruses, were derived directly from an avian virus 80–100 years ago. Indeed, the infamous Spanish flu pandemic of 1918 may have been the result of this adaptation of a nonhuman strain to humans, with a concurrent increase in virulence and subsequent devastating effects.

Antigenic drift results from the substitution of a small number of critical amino acid residues within antigenic sites of the HA. In common with all RNA viruses, influenza virus populations are described as quasispecies in that they consist of a complex mixture of microvariants due to the inherent, relatively high, error rate of the viral RNA polymerase. Any variant virus can readily become dominant if an appropriate selection pressure is applied. It is assumed that variant viruses cause epidemics when the antigenicity of the HA has altered sufficiently for the virus to escape neutralization by a sufficient proportion of the population. Sequencing studies indicate that, in general, epidemic strains have amino acid changes in at least two antigenic sites of the HA molecule.

Epidemiology

This has been discussed previously.

Pathogenesis and Immunity

The virus is highly infectious, with fewer than five infectious particles required to infect the lower respiratory tract in volunteers; however, 100 times this amount seems to be required to infect the nasopharynx experimentally (16). It is possible that the lower, not the upper, respiratory tract is the initial site of infection. After an incubation period of 1–5 days, there is an abrupt onset of illness although viral shedding is typically 24 h before the onset of illness. Duration of viral shedding is 3–5 days in volunteers but appears to be longer and of greater virus yield in natural infections, especially if pneumonia is a clinical feature. Viremia is hard to detect, but does appear to occur in fatal cases.

The virus infects columnar epithelial cells in the respiratory tract and peripheral blood mononuclear cells that are attracted as part of the host response. Entry into the cell is facilitated by binding of the HA spikes to mucoproteins containing terminal N-acetyl neuraminic acid. Virus is then internalized by receptor-mediated endocytosis. In the mature endosome the HA undergoes a low pH-induced conformational change that induces fusion of the virion and endosome membranes permitting the ribonucleoprotein (RNP)/transcriptase complex of the virus to enter the cytoplasm. The M2 protein appears to play a role in this process. After entry into the cytoplasm and uncoating from matrix, the RNP cores are transported to the nucleus where the negative sense genome is transcribed and replicated by the three virion RNA-dependent RNA polymerases. During transcription of mRNA, the viral polymerases cannibalize host cell 5′-methylated cap structures for priming viral mRNA synthesis, while polyadenylation occurs at a stretch of uridine residues approximately 20 residues from the 5′ end of genomic RNA. Thus mRNA is not a complete copy of vRNA. For vRNA replication a full-length complementary RNA is synthesized as an intermediate from which molecules of vRNA are transcribed. The two surface glycoproteins, HA and NA, are synthesized in the endoplasmic reticulum and transported to the cell surface through the Golgi network where processing takes place. Nascent RNP associated with matrix protein exit from the nucleus and interact at the internal plasma membrane at regions where HA and NA have accumulated. Mature virions are formed when nucleocapsids bud through the plasma membrane at these sites. Polarized budding occurs from the apices in the epithelial cells in vivo, which may contribute to restricting the infection to the respiratory epithelium.

The immune response to the influenza involves strong T- and B-cell responses. The serum antibody response to HA is influenza-subtype-specific and includes antibodies directed to cross-reactive as well as strain-specific determinants of the HA molecule. The nature of the humoral responses in humans depends upon age and previous experience of influenza infection or immunization. In 1977, when influenza A(H1N1) subtype re-emerged after 25 years, the antibody response to A/USSR/77 (H1N1) vaccine in young people was much weaker than the corresponding response in adults over the age of 25 years (75). This was due to anamnestic responses in the older people. Children naturally infected with influenza virus respond by producing serum antibodies that are predominantly strain-specific. In adults the predominant antibodies to infection or vaccination are cross-reactive or strain-specific to earlier virus strains. This is known as the phenomenon of original antigenic sin, whereby the humoral response is directed to conserved regions of the HA molecule shared by early and more modern virus strains. Although this cross-reacting antibody is inefficient at virus neutralization, it still appears to play a role in immunity by enhancing uptake of virus by Fc receptor–bearing cells such as antigen-presenting cells. Neutralization of infection is by immunoglobulin G (IgG), IgA, secretory IgA and IgM, and each class of antibody probably contributes to protection. It is likely that the antibody response to NA, and other proteins, does play a part in immunity to influenza but its importance is probably less than that of antibody to HA.

Infection with influenza virus causes a significant T-cell response involving both helper T (Th) cells and cytotoxic T (Tc) cells. Th cells, with a Th1 cytokine profile, have a pivotal role in the development of the protective antibody response both postinfection and postvaccination with inactivated vaccine, and also appear to function in aiding the Tc response. A Th2 response is associated with a failure to clear virus in mice (34). Tc cells are stimulated by and function in the destruction of virus infected cells, so they are not induced by inactivated vaccine but have been shown to aid recovery from virus infection. The human Th response is directed mainly at the major structural components of the virus (HA, NA, NP, and M) and is fairly evenly divided between them. Th clones against the surface glycoproteins tend to be strain-specific while clones that recognize the internal components are generally cross-reactive. The regions of the HA recognized by Th clones appear to be sequential epitopes, although there is evidence that conformational epitopes also exist. Several specific HA peptides that stimulate Th cells have been defined and are located on both surface and internal regions of the HA1. Regions within HA2 also stimulate Th cells, although these are less well defined. The Tc response is cross-reactive among influenza A viruses, but not influenza B, and is directed primarily toward the NP.

E. Respiratory Syncytial Virus

Structure and Replication

Respiratory syncytial virus was first isolated from a chimpanzee with a common cold-like illness (67). It is a medium-sized, 80–350 nm diameter, pleomorphic enveloped virus in a genus *Pneumovirus* within the Paramyxoviridae family. The nonsegmented negative-sense RNA genome has 10 genes coding for 10 separate proteins. The coding sequence is 3′ NS1-NS2-N-P-M-SH-G-F-M2-L 5′.

There are two major and one minor transmembrane proteins, all involved in pathogenesis. The heavily glycosylated G protein is important for viral infectivity and virulence. Antibody to G is neutralizing. The second major transmembrane protein, F (for fusion protein), is involved in virus–cell and cell–cell fusion. The third transmembrane protein, SH, also contributes to fusion.

Two membrane-associated matrix proteins, M and M2, are thought to be important for virus assembly and membrane stabilization.

The genome also codes for its own replicative machinery: an N protein, a phosphorylated P protein, and a large (L) polymerase. NS1 and NS2 are nonstructural proteins of uncertain function. In vitro, virus binds slowly to cell membranes, taking up to 2 h for maximal attachment, with replication occurring entirely in the cytoplasm. Virus release starts at 24 h postinfection.

The virus is thermolabile, with 99% of infectivity lost at 37°C in 48 h.

Two subgroups of RSV are recognized based on characteristic reaction patterns with monoclonal antibody pools. These two subgroups, designated A and B, have different antigenic properties in G, F, N, M, and P proteins. The major differences occur in the G protein where only one epitope is shared between the serogroups.

Epidemiology

Humans are the only natural host of human RSV, although other RS viruses infect cattle and sheep; sheep, rodents, and primates can also be experimentally infected. Annual winter epidemics in the children and elderly begin in late autumn and continue to early spring in temperate zones. Infections rates are highest in the first 2 years of life, with 50–70% being infected in the first year and the remainder by the end of the second (69). Peak incidence is at 2 months of age for both RS virus bronchiolitis and pneumonia. Few children have bronchiolitis after the first year of life. This pattern appears to be worldwide, except that the epidemics tend to occur in the rainy season in the tropics (82a). In developed countries, incidence of infection is also higher in urban areas than rural areas, which might represent either proximity or people, and possibly the negative impact of air pollution. It is known that the risk factors for infection with RSV in early infancy include the number of older siblings and the level of overcrowding in the household.

Children with bronchopulmonary dysplasia or congenital heart disease with pulmonary hypertension show enhanced susceptibility to life-threatening RSV infection. Twenty years ago mortality rates of 30–70% were reported in such children.

Despite intensive virological research the morbidity of RSV infection in these children remains unchanged. Indeed advances in intensive care management and surgical correction procedures are responsible for the markedly decreased mortality rate of RSV infection in these compromised children (62).

Pathogenesis and Immunity

Studies on outbreaks of RSV infection in closed communities and experimentally challenged adult volunteers indicate an incubation period of 4–6 days. Initially RSV replication is confined to the nasopharynx, reaching titers of 10^4–10^6 $TCID_{50}$/ml in secretions. In severe disease viral shedding persists for many days. Spread of virus may be cell-to-cell as in vitro RSV-infected cells fuse to form syncytia. About 40% of infants infected with RSV develop symptoms of lower airways disease. Clinical evidence of lung infection usually appears 1–3 days after the onset of nasopharyngeal infection.

Such a time scale suggests that inhalation of virus and/or infected cells with embolization to the terminal airways is the likely route of spread.

The initial docking of RSV to the mucosal surface of respiratory tract epithelial cells is mediated by the G protein. Fusion of the RSV with the host-cell membrane occurs at the cell surface and is mediated by F protein dimers. Filamentous viral processes bud from the cytoplasmic membrane of infected cells, protruding to a final length of 10 µm. The rapid and synchronized budding from localized regions of the membrane indicates a directed process of recruitment of viral components to areas selected for virus maturation overlying regions where the cytoplasm is undergoing hectic motion. Filaments extend at a rate of 110–250 nm/s and shedding of a complete virus takes less than 1 min. An interesting feature of RSV replication is that host-cell protein synthesis is not downregulated.

Several features in the natural history of RSV infections suggest that severe disease has an immunopathological basis. Thus bronchiolitis occurs while maternal IgG to RSV persists and enhanced disease was seen in children vaccinated with formalin-inactivated virus when subsequently exposed to natural infection. Furthermore, replication in vitro does not induce dramatic cell pathology and syncytial formation is reputedly rare in the lungs of infants dying of RSV infection. Taken together, these facts suggest that tissue destruction as a direct consequence of virus replication is not the major determinant of disease causation in RSV infection. However, we do not yet have a full understanding of the immunopathology of terminal airways disease.

Perhaps the most important determinant of the age-related severity of RSV bronchiolitis is the incomplete development of the terminal airways in infancy. At age 3 months the terminal two generations of bronchioles are still developing and the numbers of alveoli are only one-quarter the adult value. The implication is that partial bronchiolar obstruction due to filament production by RSV-infected cells, the sloughing of dead cells into the lumen, plus syncytial formation cause a marked increase in terminal airways resistance given the highly cellular, immature lungs of infants. A postmortem study of infants dying of RSV infection has confirmed the shedding of viral-infected epithelial cells into the bronchial lumen and the presence of giant syncytial cells in the alveoli (74). mRNA for proinflammatory cytokines (interleukin [IL]-1β, IL-6, tumor necrosis factor [TNF-α]) together with adhesion molecules (ICAM-1, ELAM-1, and VCAM-1) are present in the middle ear exudates of children infected with RSV, but these mediators may have been induced by the direct interaction of virus with epithelial cells and/or mucosal lymphocytes and macrophages. Alveolar macrophages in bronchoalveolar lavage (BAL) from RSV-infected children were shown to be infected with RS virus and to coexpress class II human leukocyte antigen (HLA) DR, IL-1β, and TNF-α proteins (61). Thus the key features of RS virus-mediated damage to the terminal airways may be explained as both due to viral induced pathology and immunopathology.

The role of antibody in immunity to RSV infection has been extensively studied and the overwhelming weight of evidence clearly indicates a beneficial role for antibody in both prophylaxis and therapy. In contrast, relatively little attention has been paid to cell-mediated immunity in RSV infection and disease. Furthermore, the studies that have attempted to assign a protective or pathogenic role to immune cells have yielded equivocal results. Since much of this is directed to understanding lower respiratory tract disease, it will not be further discussed here.

In older children and healthy adults RSV infection typically presents as what is termed a heavy cold. The recurrence of upper respiratory tract infections throughout life suggests that protective immunity in the nasopharynx is short-lived, but that useful immunity in lower airways is more lasting. However, this protection is not lifelong since RSV pneumonia is a significant problem in the elderly.

F. Parainfluenza Viruses

Structure and Replication

Parainfluenza viruses (PIV) belong to the family Paramyxoviridae. There are 5 subtypes: parainfluenza viruses 1, 2, 3, 4a, and 4b. Parainfluenza viruses 1 and 3 belong to the paramyxovirus genus, whereas parainfluenza viruses 2, 4a, and 4b belong to the rubella virus genus along with mumps. They possess a single-stranded negative-sense RNA genome and are enveloped viruses with helical symmetry. The virions are 150–200 nm in diameter with hetical nucleocapsids (Fig. 6). A virion transcriptase initiates transcription into five to eight mRNAs.

No common group antigen exists, but some degree of cross-reactivity can be demonstrated with the different serotypes and with mumps virus. They possess both a hemagglutinin and neuraminidase that differentiates them from respiratory syncytial virus.

Epidemiology

These viruses appear to be ubiquitous in all populations irrespective of their size, degree of isolation, or socioeconomic status. Recurrent reinfections are a characteristic feature of the biology of these viruses. Subtype 3 has a propensity to be endemic.

Although understudied compared to other respiratory viral pathogens, they

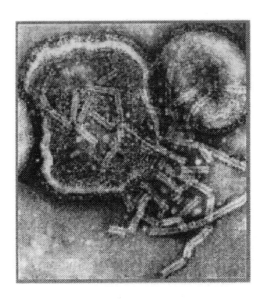

Figure 6   Electron micrograph of parainfluenza virus.

are not uncommon. In a longitudinal study of 1500 American children with febrile respiratory disease, 17% of children under the age of 2 years had a parainfluenza virus isolated (77) with PIV 3 being found in more than half of these cases. All the cases of PIV1 were associated with croup. Infection is uncommon before the age of 4 months, suggesting a role for maternal antibody, and rises until school age. Infections are less common, and more likely to be asymptomatic, in adults and adolescents, although the parents of school-age children seem more prone to infection than the general adult population. Croup is more common in males but this is thought to be due more to the host than any difference in virus prevalence between the genders (32).

Transmission is by the respiratory route. Unlike rhinoviruses, infectious parainfluenzavirus does not seem to survive on hands longer than 1 h, so this route of transmission is less likely (2). There is tittle evidence of animal reservoirs, although related viruses are found in sheep and cattle.

Pathogenesis and Immunity

PIV utilizes sialic acid receptors which are widespread but replication is confined to respiratory epithelial cells, macrophages, and dendritic cells. The immune response to infection is not well characterized but IgA appears to be important for the termination of infection (58). Nasal antibody is, possibly, more important than serum antibody.

A feature of this group of viruses, which it shares with the closely related measles virus, is the ability to persist. This is seen in vitro with PIV3 and in immunocompromised patients.

V. Concluding Remarks

The majority of respiratory virus pathogens have probably been identified but new ones such as respiratory Hantaan ("sin nombre") virus are periodically found. It is unlikely that there will be a clear cause-and-effect role determined for any known or novel viruses, but it is likely that some or all play an important role in both the precipitation of the acute attack and the pathogenesis of chronic lung disease.

References

1. Afzelius BA. Ultrastructure of human nasal epithelium during an episode of coronavirus infection. Virchows Arch 1994; 424:295–300.
2. Ansari SA, Springthorpe VS, Sattar SA, Rivard S, Rahman M. Potential role of hands in the spread of respiratory viral infections: studies with human parainfluenza virus 3 and rhinovirus 14. J Clin Microbiol 1991; 29:2115–2119.
3. Armstrong GL, Pinner RW. Outpatient visits for infectious diseases in the United States 1980–1996. Arch Intern Med 1999; 159:2531–2536.
4. Arrunda E, Boyle TR, Winther B. Localisation of human rhinovirus replication in the upper respiratory tract by in-situ hybridisation. J Infect Dis 1995; 171:1329–1333.
5. Azizi BH, Zulkifi HI, Kasim MS. Protective and risk factors for infections in hospital-ised urban Malaysian children: a case control study. Southeast Asian J Trop Med Public Health 1995; 26:280–285.
6. Bianco A, Sethi SK, Allen JT, Knight RA. Th2 cytokines exert a dominant influence on epithelial cell expression of the major group human rhinovirus receptor, ICAM-1. Eur Respir J 1998; 12:619–626.
7. Brandt CD, Kim HW, Vargosko AJ, et al. Infections in 18000 infants and children in a controlled study of respiratory tract disease. I. Adenovirus pathogenicity in relation to serologic type and illness syndrome. Am J Epidemiol 1969; 90:484–500.
8. Butler WT, Waldmann TA, Rossen RD. Changes in IgA and IgG concentrations in nasal secretions prior to the appearance of antibody during viral respiratory infections in man. J Immunol 1970; 105:584–591.
9. Callow KA. Effect of specific humoral immunity and some non-specific factors on resis-tance of volunteers to respiratory coronavirus infections. J Hyg 1985; 95:173–189.
10. Cate TR, Couch RB, Johnson KM. Studies with rhinoviruses in volunteers. Production of illness, effect of naturally acquired antibody and demonstration of a protective effect not associated with serum antibody. J Clin Invest 1964; 43:56–65.
11. Cate TR, Douglas RG, Couch RB. Interferon and resistance to upper respiratory tract virus illness. Proc Soc Exp Biol Med 1969; 131:631–636.
12. Cauwenberge P. Epidemiology of common cold. Rhinology 1985; 23:273–282.
13. Cerquerio MC, Murtagh P, Halac A, Aila M, Weissenbacher M. Epidemiologic risk factors for children with acute lower respiratory tract infection in Buenos Aires, Argen-tina: a matched case control study. Rev Infect Dis 1990; 12:1021–1028.
14. Cohen S, Tyrrell DAJ, Russell MAH, Jarvis MJ, Smith AP. Smoking, alcohol consump-tion, and susceptibility to the common cold. Am J Public Health 1993; 83:1277–1283.
15. Cooney MK, Hall CE, Fox JP. The Seattle Virus Watch. III. Evaluation of isolation methods and summary of infections detected by virus isolations. Am J Epidemiol 1972; 96:286–305.

16. Couch RB, Cate TR, Douglas RG, Gerone PJ, Knight V. Effect of route of inoculation on experimental respiratory viral disease in volunteers and evidence of airborne transmission. Bacteriol Rev 1966; 30:517–529.

17. Dingle JH, Badger GF, Jordan WS Jr. Illness in the Home: Study of 25000 Illnesses in a Group of Cleveland Families. Cleveland: The Press of Case Western University, 1964:1–12.

18. Dixon RE. Econimic costs of respiratory tract infections in the United States. Am J Med 1985; 78 (suppl. 6B):45–51.

19. Dolin R, Wright PF, eds. Viral infections of the respiratory tract. In: Lenfant C, ed. Lung Biology in Health and Disease. New York: Marcel Dekker, 1999.

20. Douglas RG Jr, Cate TR, Gerone PJ, Couch RB. Quantitative rhinovirus shedding patterns in volunteers. Am Rev Respir Dis 1966; 94:159–167.

21. Douglas RG Jr, Lingram KM, Couch RB. Exposure to cold environment and rhinovirus cold. Failure to demonstrate an effect. N Engl J Med 1968; 279:742–747.

22. Douglas RG. Pathogenesis of rhinovirus common colds in human volunteers. Ann Otol Rhinol Laryngol 1970; 79:563–571.

23. Enarson DA, Chretien J. Epidemiology of respiratory infectious diseases. Curr Opin Pulmon Dis 1999; 5:128–135.

24. Etzel RA, Pattishall EN, Haley NJ. Passive smoking and middle ear effusion among children in day care. Pediatrics 1992; 90:228–232.

25. Falsey AR, McCann RM, Hall WJ, Tanner MA, Criddle MM, Formica MA, Irvine CS, Kolassa JE, Barker WH, Treanor JJ. Acute respiratory tract infection in daycare centers for older persons. J Am Geriatric Soc 1995; 43:30–36.

26. Fox JP, Hall CE, Cooney MK, Luce RE, Kronmal RA. The Seattle Virus Watch. II. Objectives, study population and its observation, data processing and summary of illnesses. Am J Epidemiol 1972; 96:270–285.

27. Fox JP, Cooney MK, Hall EE. The Seattle Virus Watch. V. Epidemiologic observations of rhinovirus infections, 1965–1969, in families with young children. Am J Epidemiol 1975; 101:122–143.

28. Fox JP, Hall CE, Cooney MK. The Seattle Virus Watch. VIII. Observations of adenovirus infections. Am J Epidemiol 1977; 105:362–386.

29. Fraenkel DJ, Bardin PG, Sanderson G, Lampe F, Johnston SL, Holgate ST. Immunohistochemical analysis of nasal biopsies during rhinovirus experimental colds. Am J Respir Crit Care Med 1994; 150:1130–1136.

30. Gammelin M, Altmuller A, Reinhardt U, et al. Phylogenetic analysis of nucleoproteins suggests that human influenza A viruses emerged from a 19th-century avian ancestor. Mol Biol Evol 1990; 7:194–200.

31. Gardner G, Frank AL, Taber LH. Effects of social and family factors on viral respiratory infection and illness in the first year of life. J Epidemiol Commun Health 1984; 38:42–48.

32. Glezen WP, Loda FA, Clyde WA Jr, Senior RJ, Sheaffer CI, Conley WG, Denny FW. Epidemiologic patterns of acute lower respiratory tract disease of children in pediatric group practice. J Pediatr 1971; 78:397–406.

33. Glezen WP, Frank AL, Taber LH, Tristan MP, Valbona C, Paredes A, Allison JE. Influenza in childhood. Pediatr Res 1983; 17:1029–1032.

34. Graham MB, Braciale VL, Braciale TJ. Influenza virus-specific CD4+ helper type 2 T lymphocyctes do not promote recovery from experimental virus infection. J Exp Med 1994; 180:1273–1282.

35. Graham N. Epidemiology of acute respiratory infections. Epidemiol Rev 1990; 12:149–178.
36. Gwaltney JM Jr, Hendley JO, Simon G, Jordan WS Jr. Rhinovirus infections in an industrial population. I. The occurrence of illness. N Engl J Med 1966; 275:1261–1268.
37. Gwaltney JM Jr, Moskalski PB, Hendley JO. Hand-to-hand transmission of rhinovirus colds. Ann Intern Med 1978; 88:463–467.
38. Gwaltney JM Jr, Phillips CD, Miller RD, Riker DK. Computed tomographic study of the common cold. N Engl J Med 1994; 330:25–30.
39. Gwatkin DR. How many will die? A set of demographic estimates of the annual number of infant and child deaths in the world. Am J Public Health 1980; 70:1286–1289.
40. Hamre D, Procknow JJ. Viruses isolated from natural common colds among young medical students. Am Rev Respir Dis 1963; 88:277–282.
41. Hamre D, Connelly AP Jr, Procknow JJ. Virologic studies of acute respiratory disease in young adults. IV. Virus isolations during four years of surveillance. Am J Epidemiol 1966; 83:238–249.
42. Hendley JO, Gwaltney JM Jr. Mechanisms of transmission of rhinovirus infections. Epidemiol Rev 1988; 10:243–258.
43. Hofer F, Gruenberger M, Kowalski H, Machat H, Huettinger M, Kuechler E, Blass D. Members of the low density lipoprotein receptor family medicate cell entry of a minor-group common cold virus. Proc Natl Acad Sci USA 1994; 91:1839–1842.
44. Holmes MJ, Callow KA, Childs RA, Tyrrell DAJ. Antibody dependent cellular cytotoxicity against coronavirus 229E-infected cells. Br J Exp Pathol 1986; 67:581–586.
45. Hoorn M, Tyrrell DA. Effects of some viruses on ciliated cells. Am Rev Respir Dis 1966; 93:156–161.
46. Ijaz MK, Brunner AH, Sattar SA, Nair RC, Johnson-Lussenberg CM. Survival characteristics of airborne human coronavirus 229E. J Gen Virol 1985; 66:2743–2748.
47. Jedrychowski W, Flak E. Atopy and low birth weight as deteminants of susceptibility to acute respiratory tract infections. Przegl Epidemiol 1996; 50:315–322.
48. Kim PE, Musher DM, Glezen WP. Association of invasive pneumococcal disease with season, atmospheric condition, air pollution, and the isolation of respiratory viruses. Clin Infect Dis 1996; 22:100–106.
49. Kingston D, Lidwell OM, Williams REO. The epidemiology of the common cold. III. The effect of ventilation, air disinfection and room size. J Hyg Camb 1962; 60:341–352.
50. Jennings L. Catching the common cold. Microbiol Aust 1996; 32–36.
51. Johnson KM, Bloom HH, Forsyth BR, Chanock RM. Relationship of rhinovirus infection to mild upper respiratory disease. II. Epidemiologic observations in male military trainees. Am J Epidemiol 1965; 81:131–138.
52. Ketler A, Hall CE, Fox JP, Elveback L, Cooney MK. The Virus Watch program: a continuing surveillance of viral infections in metropolitan New York families, VII. Rhinovirus infections: observations of virus excretion, intrafamilial spread and clinical response. Am J Epidemiol 1969; 90:244–254.
53. Loda FA, Glezen WP, Lyde WA Jr. Respiratory disease in group day care. Paediatrics 1972; 49:428–437.
54. Losonsky GA, Santosham M, Sehgal VM, Zwahlen A, Moxon ER. Haemophilus influenzae disease in White Mountain Apaches: molecular epidemiology of a high risk population. Pediatr Infect Dis 1984; 3:539–547.

55. McCormick DP, Wenzel RP, Davies JA, Beam WE. Nasal secretion protein responses in patients with wild-type adenovirus infections. Infect Immun 1972; 6:282–288.

56. Macek V, Sorli J, Kopriva S, Marin J. Persistent adenoviral infection and chronic airway obstruction in children. Am Rev Respir Dis 1994; 150:7–10.

57. Matsuse T, Hayashi S, Kuwano K, Kuenecke H, Jeffries WA, Hogg JC. Latent adenoviral infection in the pathogenesis of chronic airway obstruction. Am Rev Respir Dis 1992; 146:177–184.

58. Mazanec MB, Huang YT, Pimplikar SW, Lamm ME. Mechanisms of inactivation of repiratory viruses by IgA, including intraepithelial neutralization. Semin Virol 1996; 7:285–292.

59. Meschievitz CK, Schultz SB, Dick EC. A model for obtaining predictable natural transmission of rhinoviruses in human volunteers. J Infect Dis 1984; 150:195–201.

60. Meyer RJ, Haggerty RJ. Streptococcal infections in families: factors altering susceptibility. Pediatrics 1962; 29:539–549.

61. Midulla F, Villani A, Panuska JR, et al. Respiratory syncytial virus lung infection in infants: immunoregulatory role of infected alveolar macrophages. J Infect Dis 1993; 168:1515–1519.

62. Moler FW, Khan AS, Meliones JN. Respiratory syncytial virus morbidity and mortality estimates in congenital heart disease patients: a recent experience. Crit Care Med 1992; 20:1406–1413.

63. Monto AS. A community study of respiratory infections in the tropics. 3. Introduction and transmission of infections within families. Am J Epidemiol 1968; 88:69–79.

64. Monto AS, Napier JA, Metzner HL. The Tecumseh study of Respiratory Illness. I. Plan of study and observations on syndromes of acute respiratory disease. Am J Epidemiol 1971; 94:269–279.

65. Monto AS, Ullman BM. Acute respiratory illness. in an American community: the Tecumseh study. JAMA 1974; 227:164–169.

66. Monto AS, Ross H. Acute respiratory illness in the community: frequency of illness and the agents involved. Epidemiol Infect 1993; 110:145–160.

67. Morris JA, Blount RE Jr, Savage RE. Recovery of cytopathogenic agent from chimpanzees with coryza. Proc Soc Exp Biol Med 1956; 92:544–562.

68. Moser MR, Bender TR, Marelolis NS, Noble GR, Kendal AP, Ritter DG. An outbreak of influenza aboard a commercial airliner. Am J Epidemiol 1979; 110:406–416.

69. Mufson MA, Levine HD, Wasil RE, Mocega-Gonzalez HE, Krause HE. Epidemiology of respiratory syncytial virus infection among infants and children in Chicago. Am J Epidemiol 1973; 98:88–95.

70. Myint S. Human coronavirus infections. In: Siddell S, ed. The Coronaviridae. New York: Plenum Press, 1995:389–401.

71. Myint S, Taylor-Robinson D, eds. Viral and Other Infections of the Human Respiratory Tract. London: Chapman & Hall, 1996.

72. Myint S, Kilvington S, Maggs A, Swann RA. Medical Microbiology Made Memorable. Edinburgh: Churchill Livingstone, 2000.

73. Naclerio RM, Proud D. Kinins are generated during experimental rhinovirus colds. J Infect Dis 1988; 157:133–142.

74. Neilson KA, Yunis EJ. Demonstration of respiratory synctial virus in an autopsy series. Paediatr Pathol 1990; 10:491–502.

75. Nicholson KG, Tyrrell DAJ, Harrison P. Clinical studies of monovalent inactivated whole virus and subunit A/USSR/77 (H1N1) vaccine; serological responses and clinical reactions. J Biol Stand 1979; 7:123–136.

76. Pio A, Leowski J, Ten Dam HG. The magnitude of the problem of acute respiratory infections. In: Douglas RM, Kerby-Beaton E, eds. Acute Respiratory Infections: Proceedings of an International Workshop. Australia: University of Adelaide, 1985:3–16.

77. Reed G, Jewett PH, Thompson J, Tollefson S, Wright PF. Epidemiology and clinical impact of parainfluenxzavirus infections in otherwise healthy infants and young children less than 5 years old. J Infect Dis 1996; 175:807–813.

78. Reed SE. An investigation of the possible transmission of colds through indirect contact. J Hyg (Camb) 1975; 75:249–258.

79. Reed SE. The etiology and epidemiology of common colds and the possibility of prevention. Clin Otolaryngol 1981; 6:379–387.

80. Rueckert RR. In: Field BN, Knipe DM, Howley PM, Chanock RM, Monath TP, Melnick JL, Roizman B, eds. Fields Virology. Philadelphia: Lippincott, 1996:609–654.

81. Rylander R, Megevand Y. Enviromental risk factors for respiratory infections. Arch Environ Health 2000; 55:300–303.

82. Schoenbaum SC. Impact of influenza in persons and populations. In: Brown LE, Hampson AW, Webster RG, eds. Options for the Control of Influenza III. New York: Elsevier, 1996:17–25.

82a. Spence L, Barratt N. Respiratory syncytial virus associated with acute respiratory infections in Trinidadian patients. Am J Epidemiol 1968; 88:257–266.

83. Staunton DE, Merluzzi VJ, Rothlein R, Barton R, Marlin SD, Springer TA. A cell adhesion molecule, ICAM-1, is the major cell surface receptor molecule for rhinoviruses. Cell 1989; 56:849–853.

84. Stott EJ, Killington RA. Rhinoviruses. Annu Rev Microbiol 1972; 26:503–524.

85. Teale DW, Klein JO, Rosner B. Epidemiology of otitis media in the first seven years of life in children in Greater Boston: a prospective cohort study. J Infect Dis 1989; 160: 83–94.

86. Terajima M, Yamaya M, Sekizawa K. Rhinovirus infection of primary cultures of human tracheal epithelium: role of ICAM-1 and IL-1. Am J Physiol 1997; 273:L749–759.

87. Totman R, Reed SE, Craig JW. Cognitive dissonance, stress and virus-induced common colds. J Psychosom Res 1977; 21:51–61.

88. Turner RB, Winther B, Henley JO. Sites of virus recovery and antigen detection in epithelial cells during experimental rhinovirus infection. Acta Otolaryngol 1984; 413: 9–14.

89. Tyrrell DAJ. Rhinoviruses and coronaviruses—virological aspects of their role in causing colds in man. Eur J Respir Dis 1983; 64:332–335.

90. Tyrrell DA, Cohen S, Schlarb JE. Signs and symptoms in common colds. Epidemiol Infect 1993; 111:143–156.

91. Urquhart GE, Grist NR. Virological studies of sudden, unexplained infant deaths in Glasgow 1967–1970. J Clin Pathol 1972; 25:443–446.

92. Ware JM, Ferris BJ, Dockery DW, Spengler JD, Strum DO. Effects of ambient sulfur oxides and suspended particles in respiratory health of preadolescent children. Am Rev Respir Dis 1983; 133:834–839.

3

Epidemiology and Diagnosis of Virus-Induced Asthma Exacerbations

PHILIP K. PATTEMORE

Christchurch School of Medicine and Health Sciences
University of Otago
Christchurch, New Zealand

I. Introduction

Attacks of asthma are a major cause of respiratory morbidity and mortality worldwide. Most asthma attacks do not fit the characteristic features of inhaled allergen response: rapid onset within 30 min of exposure to an allergen, and a biphasic response, recovering within 24 h. Upper respiratory signs, particularly nasal symptoms, precede many attacks with a latency of 24–48 h, and many asthma attacks involve symptoms lasting several days to a week, and deterioration in lung function that may last 2 weeks (1–3). Whereas day-to-day asthma symptoms precipitated by allergens, exercise, or cold air are brought readily under control with inhaled steroids, asthma attacks are often not as easily prevented (4). These observations of common clinical experience indicate that there are reasons for asthma attacks other than allergen exposure or dehydration of the airway epithelium secondary to exercise or dry air inhalation.

If mechanisms other than classic allergic pathways cause many or most asthma attacks, this has implications for the design of treatment and preventive strategies. Since asthma attacks constitute a major part of the morbidity and cost of asthma, specific means of reducing the risk of attacks may be important alongside research efforts into primary prevention of allergy, atopy, and asthma.

43

In the 1950s doctors talked of bacterial infections as precipitants of asthma attacks, and believed that this phenomenon was a manifestation of bacterial allergy. From the mid-1970s until now there have been an increasing number of investigations of viruses as triggers of these attacks. Investigations conducted in the 1970s and 1980s, using techniques of viral culture, serology, and immunofluorescent antigen detection, demonstrated that viruses could be isolated or identified during many asthma attacks (5). These studies were performed in many different ways, some of which lessened the chances of viral recovery. Some studies studied spontaneous presentations of asthma attacks in patients admitted to a hospital or emergency department in an extended cross-sectional design. Hospital admission for acute asthma often occurs some days after the onset of respiratory symptoms. Thus specimens collected in the hospital may be taken when virus excretion has fallen, making virus isolation more difficult. Cohort studies following children prospectively with early reporting of symptoms have generally found higher identification rates.

The studies in the 1970s and 1980s used a great variety of identification methods, sensitive to varying degrees to different viruses. Often these were based on what was available in a nearby clinical diagnostic laboratory. Conventional diagnostic laboratories use sensitive identification methods for respiratory viruses that are serious or epidemic strains such as respiratory syncytial virus (RSV) and influenza; these methods are not usually sensitive to the common cold viruses: rhinoviruses and coronaviruses. Sensitive culture methods for rhinoviruses have been available since the early 1970s but were not always used in the studies of patients with wheezing episodes. Precise techniques and expertise are also important in rhinovirus culture. Antigen and antibody detection tests are too difficult for rhinovirus because of the large number of serotypes. There has been limited availability of sensitive coronavirus culture media and antibody immunoassays for the two human coronaviruses 229E and OC43 and these have rarely been used in the studies mentioned.

The advent of molecular identification of viral nucleotides using methods of nucleotide binding, amplification and reverse transcription (polymerase chain reaction [PCR] and reverse transcriptase RT-PCR) have now greatly enhanced this research. The methods are much more sensitive to small numbers of viruses. The full range of respiratory viruses including rhinoviruses and coronaviruses, as well as *Chlamydia pneumoniae, Mycoplasma pneumoniae*, and *Legionella* sp. can now be identified by PCR.

This chapter focuses on the epidemiological evidence for a link between virus infections and asthma attacks and summarizes the findings of the contributory studies.

II. What Is the Evidence That Virus Infections Trigger Asthma Attacks?

In 1992 we (5) reviewed the available evidence that respiratory virus infection was a primary trigger of asthma attacks. No studies of asthma using viral PCR had been published at that time. That evidence can be summarized as follows:

1. Respiratory viruses have been identified in similar proportions in both asthma attacks and respiratory infections in control subjects at the same period. This applies both to the overall viral identification rates and to the identification rates of individual viruses.
2. On the other hand, viruses are identified in only small proportions of asthmatic subjects when they are asymptomatic. Bacteria, however, are found in the upper respiratory tract of asthmatic subjects in similar proportions during symptomatic and asymptomatic periods.
3. If a person with asthma develops an infection in which a rhinovirus, coronavirus, or RSV is cultured, the likelihood of an associated asthma attack is remarkably predictable at around 50–70% in the prospective studies in which this could be estimated.
4. Studies that have compared the seasonal variation of asthma admissions and of multiple variables including levels of pollution, allergens, and infections have generally only found relationships with seasonal patterns of infection.
5. There is a close relationship between timing of respiratory virus identifications and asthma attacks in individuals followed prospectively.
6. The associations between viruses and asthma are stronger in patients with more severe infections and with more severe asthma.

These categories of evidence, and others, will be examined in the light of further published studies, including those using viral PCR. In many cases, data for relevant categories has been extracted from the figures given in studies where this was not explicitly given.

A. Respiratory Virus Isolation Rates in Extended Cross-Sectional Studies

These are studies (Table 1) in which an event such as a hospital admission or a doctor visit for an asthma attack was the sampling unit. In some of the studies control subjects admitted or seen for other reasons were also tested.

The quality of the studies can be compared by examining the following:

Number of subjects included
Number of episodes studied
Relevance of the source of cases
Description of the episodes studied
Period over which samples were collected
Range and sensitivity of the virus identification methods used
For PCR studies, demonstration of lack of cross-contamination

The study of control subjects or asymptomatic samples is also important and will be discussed later.

In Table 1 the studies have been divided into those involving infants, children, and adults. Weighted average identification rates in each age-group are shown separately for studies using conventional methods and those using PCR.

Table 1 Identification Rates of Viruses and Atypical Bacteria in wheezy Episodes Extended Cross-Sectional Studies Sampling Unsolicited Presentations with RTI/Asthma

First author (Ref.)	Subjects			Source of cases	Presenting condition (no.)	Study period	Wheezy episodes studied			Methods[a]			
	Year	No.	age (y)				Description given	No.	Spec	Culture	Serum	ag-D	RT-PCR
Infants													
Duff (6)	1993	20	0–2	ED	Wheezing illness	24 m	Wheezing	20	4	d'eg'		x	
Rylander (7)	1996	103	0–18 m	Admission	Wheezing bronchitis	15 m	Breathing diff. & wheezing	103	1	bd'gg'il			
Rakes (8)	1999	22	0–2	ED	Wheezing illness		Auscultatory wheeze	22	4	d'eg'		x	PCR
Children													
Tyrrell (13)	1965	1888	0–17+	Home/admissions	RTI (1888)	36 m	Bronchitis/iolitis c̄ wheeze	225	12	abd'eg			
Disney (14)	1971	51	?0–14	Admissions	Asthma	12 m	Asthma attacks	51	12	d'h	lm		
Glezen (15)	1971	2000	0–15+	Ped. practice	LRTI (3000)	66 m	"Bronchiolitis" c̄ wheeze	855	12	d'egk			
Horn (16)	1975	919	0–13	General practice	RTI (1934)	60 m	Wheezy bronchitis/iolitis	561	12	d'ehk			
Mitchell (17)	1976	192	1–12	Admissions	Asthma/wheezy br.	36 m	Asthma/wheezy bronchitis	267	125	d'eh	?lm		
Henderson (18)	1979	3–6000	0–15	Ped. practice	LRTI (6165)	132 m	Wheeze-associated RTI	1851	2	d'eghk			
Horn (19)	1979	163	0–12	General practice	Wheezy bronchitis	62 m	Wheezy bronchitis	554	12	d'ehk			
Horn (20)	1979	22	5–15	General practice	Wheezy bronchitis	16 m	Wheezy bronchitis	72	123	d'fg'hk			
Carlsen (21)	1984	169	2–15	Ped. clinic/adm's	Asthma	24 m	Asthma attacks	256	5	d'gg'	mo	x	
Jennings (22)	1987	204	0–12	Admissions	Asthma	12 m	Asthma attacks	204	125	d'd''ehi	mn	x	
Duff (6)	1993	70	2–16	ED	Wheezing illness		Wheezing	70	4	d'eg'			
Rylander (7)	1996	78	18–48 m	Admission	Wheezing bronchitis	24 m	Breathing diff. and wheezing	78	1	bd'gg'il			PCR
Rakes (8)	1999	48	2–16	ED	Wheezing illness	15 m	Auscultatory wheeze	48	4	d'eg'		x	PCR
Freymuth (23)	1999	75	0–14	Admissions	Asthma	60 m	Severe asthma attacks	132	5	fil		x	PCR
Infants and children: weighted averages: pre-PCR studies[c]							12 studies	5167	1257+ve				
Infants and children: weighted averages: PCR studies							2 studies	202	166+ve				
Adults													
Allegra (27)	1994	74	Adults	Outpatients	Asthma	18 m	Asthma exacerbation	74	2	d''hil	o	x	
Ross (28)	1994	112	Adults	Admissions	Asthma	12 m	Asthma exacerbation	142	5	d'eg	m	xy	
Abramson (29)	1994	38	>10	ED	Asthma	6 m	Asthma attack	38	5	d'eg		x	
Sokhandan (30)	1995	33	>17	ED	Asthma exacerbation	6 m	Asthma exacerbation	35	1	d'f	m	x	
Teichtahl (31)	1997	79	>16	Admissions	Asthma exacerbation	12 m	Asthma exacerbation	79	5	(?eg)	m	x	
Atmar (32)	1998	122	>16	ED	Asthma exacerbation	18 m	Asthma exacerbation	148	4	d''ehi	lno	x	PCR
Wark (33)	2002	49	>15	ED	Asthma exacerbation	11 m	Asthma exacerbation	49	3	fil	o	x	PCR
Adults: weighted averages: pre-PCR studies[c]							5 studies	368	87+ve				
Adults: weighted averages: PCR studies[d]							2 studies	197	119+ve				

ED = emergency department; RTI = respiratory tract infection; LRTI = lower RTI; O/P = outpatient; Rhin = rhinovirus; Cor = coronavirus; RSV = respiratory syncytial virus; Par = parainfluenza virus; Inf = influenza virus; Ad = adenovirus; Ent = enterovirus; H.S. = Herpes simplex.; M.P. = *Mycoplasma pneumoniae*; C.P. = *Chlamydia pneumoniae*.

[a] Methods:

Spec (specimen): 1 = nose swab; 2 = throat swab; 3 = sputum; 4 = nasal washings; 5 = nasal aspirate; 6 = rectal swab.

Culture (cell line): a = embryonated egg; b = human embryonic kidney; c = human amniotic cells; d^1/d^2 = 1°/2° monkey kidney; d'' = LLC-MK2; e = human embryonic lung (incl WI38); f = MRC-5; g = Hela; g' = Ohio Hela; h = Hep-2; i = Clone16; j = MDCK; k = Mycoplasma culture 1 = other.

Serum: 1 = hemagglutination inhibition; m = complement fixation; n = neutralization; o = antibody-enzyme immunoassay.

Ag-D (antigen detection): x = immunofluorescence microscopy; y = antigen-enzyme immunoassay; z = electron microscopy.

RT-PCR (reverse transcriptase polymerase chain reaction). PCR = PCR used specific for those viruses whose results are shown boxed.

Total and specific viral identification rates (%) in wheezy episodes

First author (Ref.)	Year	Any virus	Rhin	Cor	RSV	Par	Inf	Ad	Ent	H.S.	M.P.	C.P.	Other	Dual[b]
Infants														
Duff (6)	1993	70.0	15.0		50.0		5.0		5.0					?
Rylander (7)	1996	33.0	1.9	0.0	19.4	7.8		2.9	1.0					(27.2)
Rakes (8)	1999	81.8	45.5		68.2				4.5					
Children														
Tyrrell (13)	1965	28.4	3.1		8.0	3.6		4.0	5.3	0.9			0.9	
Disney (14)	1971	9.8			2.0	5.9					2.8		2.0	
Glezen (15)	1971	25.1	1.8		8.8	8.3		1.8	0.7				0.4	
Horn (16)	1975	27.4	12.1		2.7	3.2	1.1	0.9	3.0	1.1	1.6			1.1
Mitchell (17)	1976	17.2	6.0		3.7	1.1	2.0	3.0	2.2	1.5			0.7	1.1
Henderson (18)	1979	21.4	1.3		7.3	5.7	1.1	2.3			2.5			
Horn (19)	1979	26.4	12.6		2.2	4.0	2.0	0.9	4.0		1.8			1.1
Horn (20)	1979	48.6	31.9		1.4	4.2	11.1	1.4			1.4			
Carlsen (21)	1984	28.5	12.9	1.6	5.5	3.9	1.6	3.1						
Jennings (22)	1987	18.6	1.5		6.4	0.5	2.9	2.0	5.4					
Duff (6)	1993	31.4	22.9		4.3		1.4		2.9					
Rylander (7)	1996	19.2	11.5		1.3	5.1			1.3					?
Rakes (8)	1999	83.3	72.9	6.3	6.3		2.1		2.1					(4.2)
Freymuth (23)	1999	81.8	46.9	4.5	21.2	3.7	5.1	4.5	9.8		2.3	4.5		(20.4)
Infants and children: weighted averages: pre-PCR studies[c]		24.3	5.6	1.6	6.6	5.0	2.0	2.0	3.2	1.1	2.2	0.0	0.6	(0.3)
Infants and children: weighted averages: PCR studies		82.2	53.0	4.5	21.2			4.5	9.8		2.3	4.5		(17.3)

Table 1 Continued

First author (Ref.)	Year	Any virus	Rhin	Cor	RSV	Par	Inf	Ad	Ent	H.S.	M.P.	C.P.	Other	Dual[b]
Adults														
Allegra (27)	1994	20.3		2.7	5.4	1.4				1.4	9.5			
Rossi (28)	1994	28.9		6.3	9.2	4.2	9.9			2.1			(3.5)	
Abrahamson (29)	1994	21.1		•	•	•			0.7					
Sokhandan (30)	1995	0.0							•					
Teichtahl (31)	1997	29.1	11.4	[14.2]	1.3		19.0	2.5		1.3				(6.3)
Atmar (32)	1998	55.4	[35.8]		2.7		8.1	0.7					2.0	(8.1)
Wark (33)	2002	75.5	[8.2]	[4.1]	38.8	[0.0]	[24.5]	[0.0]			0.0			
Adults: weighted averages: pre-PCR studies[c]		23.6	11.4	0.0	3.6	7.9	7.5	4.6	0.0	0.9	1.8	9.5	2.0	(2.7)
Adults: weighted averages: PCR studies[d]		60.4	28.9	11.7	38.8	0.0	12.2	0.0						(5.8)

[b] Numbers in parentheses for dual infections indicate that the viruses concerned are also included under the individual virus rates.

[c] For the pre-PCR studies, the weighted averages identification rates for each virus were calculated using only those studies that identified that virus. The averages include data from studies that are labeled as PCR studies but did not use PCR specific for that virus.

[d] For the PCR studies, the weighted average rates for each virus were calculated using only those studies that used PCR specific for that virus.

• Abramson's study did not allow calculation of individual virus rates during asthma episodes. Viruses that were found are shown as a dot (•).

A. Infant Studies

There have been many studies of RSV in infancy, but the studies of infants in the table are included (6–8) because they were part of a wider study of all respiratory viruses in children with wheeze episodes in which the results in infants were reported separately.

Two studies were recruited from the emergency department and one from hospital admissions. The first and third studies listed used nasal washings for viral culture and immunofluorescence, and a similar range of cell lines for viral culture including Ohio Hela cells (which are usually sensitive for rhinoviruses). The second study (7) used only cell culture of nasal swabs with a wide variety of cell lines including Ohio Hela cells. The third study (8) in addition used PCR for picornaviruses and coronaviruses. Control infants with nonrespiratory problems were also sampled in the third study. Aside from this and comparison of PCR with viral culture for rhinovirus, there is no documentation of within-study specificity and lack of contamination in this study.

Overall these studies identified viruses in 39.0% of wheezy episodes in the two studies using conventional virology and 81.8% in the study using PCR. The likelihood of any virus identified was significantly higher in the PCR study (odds ratio = 7.03, 95% confidence interval [CI]: 2.24, 22.04). All three studies not surprisingly found RSV to be the predominant virus, but the third study using PCR identified rhinoviruses much more commonly than the other two studies (odds ratio 19.67, 95% CI: 5.77, 67.07). Using PCR, other studies have found that rhinoviruses are more important as pathogens in infancy than was previously thought. They have been identified in up to 24% of cases of otitis media (9,10) and in serious illnesses of infants (11,12).

B. Studies in Children Older Than 2 Years

This is the age-group most frequently studied and includes studies reported over a time span of 35 years (6–8,13–23), during which technology has evolved and changes in the epidemiology of asthma have taken place. This included, in particular, a significant increase in the prevalence of asthma (24), and a very large increase in the use of preventive inhaled therapy.

In spite of this time span and the diversity of the studies, there are important similarities in the results achieved, and the differences can be largely explained by the methods used. In particular, the studies that used conventional virology share certain features with each other, as do the two studies that used PCR. All studies covered a period of at least 12 months, which allows for sampling during all seasons.

In the studies that used conventional virology, the overall viral identification rates range from 9.8% to 48.6%. Only three studies, those of Disney (14), Mitchell (17), and Jennings (22), identified viruses in less than 20% of cases. These three studies sampled hospital admissions, in which, as mentioned in the Introduction, there may be a delay between the onset of symptoms and taking of virus samples, and a significant fall off in virus excretion. Horn and colleagues (16) found viruses in 33% of specimens obtained in the first 3 days of illness, but in only 18% of specimens obtained after 5 days. Mitchell and colleagues in a later prospective study (25) likewise isolated viruses in 17% of samples taken within 48 h of onset and in 10% of samples taken after 48 h.

Earlier studies used nose and throat swabs, whereas more recent studies have tended to use nasal aspirates and washings. The latter methods potentially include more virus, although this is not in itself reflected in the identification rates. The gradual replacement of serology in earlier studies with antigen immunofluorescence in later studies also did not appreciably affect relevant virus (such as RSV and parainfluenza) recovery rates, but immunofluorescence has the advantage of rapid identification.

The biggest factor in the overall rates of identification before the advent of PCR seems to have been the choice of cell lines used for viral culture. Most early studies cultured with primary monkey kidney cells, human embryonic lung fibroblasts, and Hep-2 cells; some also used Hela cells. Overall viral identification rates in these studies range from 9.8% to 28.4%. The addition of MRC-5 or Ohio Hela cells (coded f and g' under Culture in Table 1) in four later studies (6,7,20,21) increased the overall viral identification rates to between 19.2 and 48.6%. This increase was due to increased recovery of rhinoviruses (Table 2) from approximately 4.5% to 14.4% (including infant and child studies), a significant increase with an odds ratio of 3.60 (95% CI:2.76, 4.71). Rhinovirus was the most common virus identified overall in these studies.

No studies used coronavirus-sensitive cells such as clone 16 cells; not surprisingly coronavirus was only identified in four cases in a single study (21). Most studies identified relatively small proportions of cases with RSV, parainfluenza, influenza, adenovirus, and enteroviruses. Positive tests for *Mycoplasma pneumoniae* were found in some cases, but *Chlamydia pneumoniae* was not sought.

The weighted average rates of viral identification for the 11 pre-PCR studies are shown in Table 1. Because of the differences in sensitivity of studies for different viruses, the weighted average for each particular virus is calculated using figures from only those studies that found any cases of that virus. It does include figures from studies that used PCR for other viruses but not for that virus. This gives the most optimistic average identification figures for pre-PCR studies. The overall identification rate for any virus was 24.3% and for rhinovirus 5.6%.

One other study in Japan (26) that studied RSV (using antigen immunoassay) found RSV in 3 of 33 (9.1%) asthma attacks leading to hospitalisation in children aged 0–13. This was lower than the rate in bronchiolitis (64.1%) in the same study but similar to the overall RSV identification rate in the other conventional virology studies shown in Table 1 (6.6%).

Two studies published in 1999 have used nucleic acid detection methods for viruses (8,23). These studies used RT-PCR; one of these included picornavirus and coronavirus primers and the other used PCRs for rhinovirus, coronavirus, RSV, adenovirus, enterovirus, *M. pneumoniae* and *C. pneumoniae*. Quality assurance issues in the work by Rakes and colleagues (8) have been discussed above. In the study of Freymuth and colleagues (23) it is stated that known negative and positive samples were included in-line for the PCR analysis, although the results in these

Table 2 Extended Cross-Sectional Studies: Comparison of Methods of Recovery of Rhinovirus in Infants and Children with Episodes of Wheeze

Method	No. of studies	No. of samples	Samples +ve for rhinovirus	% +ve for rhinovirus	Comparison of rhinovirus identification rates	Odds ratio	95% CI
Culture without Ohio HeLa cells	8	4568	203	4.44			
Culture with Ohio HeLa cells	4	599	86	14.36	Culture with vs. without Ohio HeLa cells	3.60	2.76, 4.71
RT-PCR for picornavirus[a]	3	202	107	52.97	RT-PCR vs. culture with Ohio HeLa cells	6.72	4.69, 9.62

[a] >90% found to be rhinovirus in some studies.

samples are not confirmed. Both studies also used viral antigen immunofluorescence and viral culture. The two studies have a weighted average identification rate of 82.2%, which is a highly significant increase compared to the weighted average for pre-PCR studies (Table 3) with an odds ratio of 14.67 (95% CI: 9.96, 21.62). Most of this increase comes from increased identification of rhinoviruses, which was by far the most common virus detected in these studies. When figures for infants and children are combined, RT-PCR offered a nearly sevenfold increase in rhinovirus detection (odds ratio 6.72, 95% CI 4.69, 9.62) over studies using culture in Ohio Hela cells (Table 2), and a 19-fold increase over all non-PCR studies combined (odds ratio 18.81, 95% CI:13.93, 25.41).

There were smaller changes in rates of identification of other viruses in the study of Freymuth and colleagues (23), which used PCR for viruses other than rhinovirus and coronavirus. This was the only study to find representatives from every group of respiratory viruses including coronaviruses. Weighted averages for each particular virus in PCR studies were calculated using figures from only those studies that used PCR for that virus. Odds ratios (OR) for virus identification in PCR vs. the most optimistic average of non-PCR studies (Table 4) were statistically significant for RSV (OR = 3.81), enteroviruses (OR = 3.95), and *C. pneumoniae* (no conventional studies looked for this organism). Odds ratios were greater than 2.0 but not significant for coronaviruses and adenoviruses, and close to unity for *M. pneumoniae*.

C. Studies in Adults

Extended cross-sectional studies of viruses and asthma in adults have only been reported since 1994 (27–33). All except three of the listed studies extended for at least 12 months. Figures for total but not specific virus identification in asthma attacks were extractable from the study of Abramson and colleagues (29). The types of virus found in this study are shown by dots in Table 1. Sokhandan and colleagues (30) did not identify any viruses in 35 exacerbations of asthma, whereas they stated that using the same methods they were identifying cases of RSV, parainfluenza virus, influenza virus, and adenovirus in other hospitalized patients. The study extended for 6 months. The authors used only two cell culture lines, and although one of these was MRC-5 (which is sensitive to rhinovirus) the techniques used were probably inadequate to detect rhinovirus because this organism was not reported in any of their hospital patients. It does not appear that they included any known positive samples in-line in the viral identification methods to check on its sensitivity at the time.

Apart from the study of Sokhandan and colleagues, studies without PCR in adults show very similar identification rates: between 20.3 and 29.1%. The weighted average rate of identification (23.6%) is not significantly different from the pre-PCR weighted average rate in childhood studies (24.3%; 95% CI on difference in proportions: −3.81%, 5.18%). However, there was much less consistency in the viruses identified. No studies used Ohio Hela cells or coronavirus-sensitive cell cultures. The predominant organism was different in each study, and included *Chla-*

Table 3 Extended Cross-Sectional Studies: Overall Rates of Virus Identification with and Without PCR in Infants, Children, and Adults

	No. of studies	No. of samples	No. of virus +ve samples	Percent of samples +ve for virus	Odds ratio studies with vs. without PCR	95% CI
Infants						
Studies without PCR	2	123	48	39.0		
Studies with PCR	1	22	18	81.8	7.03	2.24, 22.04
Children						
Studies without PCR	12	5044	1209	24.0		
Studies with PCR	2	180	148	82.2	14.67	9.96, 21.62
Adults						
Studies without PCR	5	368	87	23.6		
Studies with PCR	2	197	119	60.4	4.93	3.39, 7.16

Table 4 Extended Cross-Sectional and Prospective Studies: Likelihood of Specific Virus Identification in Studies Using PCR Versus Conventional Virology

	Children cross-sectional		Children prospective		Adult cross-sectional		Adult prospective	
	Odds ratio	95% CI	Odds ratio	95% CI	Odds ratio	95% CI	Odds ratio	95% CI
Rhinovirus	**18.81**	**13.93, 25.41**	**9.15**	**5.26, 15.90**	**3.17**	**1.48, 6.77**	**11.01**	**5.44, 22.28**
Coronavirus	2.94	0.89, 9.68	0.82	0.34, 2.00	↑↑		N/A	
RSV	**3.81**	**2.47, 5.86**	N/A		**16.90**	**7.90, 36.18**	N/A	
Parainfluenza	N/A		N/A		↓↓		N/A	
Influenza	N/A		N/A		1.72	0.94, 3.17	N/A	
Adenovirus	2.29	0.98, 5.31	N/A		↓↓		N/A	
Enterovirus	**3.34**	**1.82, 6.14**	N/A		N/A		N/A	
M. pneumoniae	1.05	0.33, 3.38	N/A		N/A		N/A	
C. pneumoniae	↑↑		N/A		N/A		N/A	

↑↑ Odds ratio too high to be calculated (denominator = 0).

↓↓ Odds ratio too low to be calculated (numerator = 0).

Odds ratio for each virus is based on data from: (a) conventional virology studies that identified any of that virus and (b) PCR studies that used PCR primers for that virus.

Boldface type indicates odds ratios that are statistically significant (i.e., the 95% confidence interval does not include unity).

mydia pneumoniae in one study, enterovirus and parainfluenza virus in another, and influenza and rhinovirus in another.

Two recent adult studies (32,33) used PCR, one of them for picornaviruses, coronaviruses, and influenza viruses, the other used multiple PCRs including rhinoviruses, coronaviruses, RSV, parainfluenza viruses, influenza viruses, and adenoviruses. Wark et al. (33) documented the lack of contamination using in-line control samples.

The weighted average viral identification rate (Table 3) was significantly higher in the adult studies using PCR than those without PCR (60.4% vs. 23.6% respectively; odds ratio 4.93; 95% CI 3.39, 7.16).

Weighted averages and odds ratios for particular virus identifications have been calculated in studies using and not using PCR for that virus as described in the section on Studies in Children Older than 2 Years above. The odds ratio for the identification rate in individual viruses in PCR versus non-PCR studies (Table 4) were significantly increased for rhinoviruses (OR = 3.17), coronavirus (no pre-PCR studies identified coronavirus), RSV (OR = 16.90), and influenza virus (OR = 1.72). The study of Wark and colleagues (33) did not identify any parainfluenza viruses or adenoviruses, despite using PCR for these viruses.

B. Respiratory Virus Isolation Rates in Prospective Studies

Table 5 shows methods and results in studies in which children or adults with asthma were followed prospectively and asked to report wheezy illnesses or infections for virological study. Once again, a variety of virological methods have been used and cases have been followed for periods of 3–24 months. Only three studies in total used Ohio Hela cell cultures, and two of these studies also used PCR. The intensity of follow-up also varied greatly. One study (2), which used only serology and consequently did not identify any rhinovirus or coronavirus, nonetheless achieved a high overall identification rate of 48.9%. This was undoubtedly because these children, managed in a Swiss mountain resort for difficult asthmatics, were examined every day by a physician and had serology and spirometry done with every identified infection. The fact that such a high rate of identification could be achieved by intense surveillance even without finding rhinovirus or coronavirus is itself suggestive that the other studies, using less intense follow-up, may be missing some virus infections.

Prospective Studies in Children

The weighted average viral identification rate in prospective pre-PCR studies in children (1–3,25,34–39) was higher than the corresponding figure in the cross-sectional studies (31.9% vs. 24.3%) (Table 6). This higher overall rate was the result of higher identification rates of rhinovirus, coronavirus, and influenza virus, which, in that order, were the most common viruses found. The increase in identification rate probably reflects the potential for virus sampling earlier in the illness in the prospective studies, since the virology methods used in these studies were no more

Table 5 Identification Rates of Viruses and Atypical Bacteria in Wheezy Episodes: Prospective Studies of Subjects with Asthma

First author	Subjects			Source of cases	Entry condition	Study period	Episodes studied			Methods[a]			
	Year	No.	Age (y)				Description given	No.	Spec	Culture	Serum	Ag-D	RT-PCR
Children													
Berkovich (34)	1970	84	0.5–16	Ped clinic	Asthma	6m	Wheezing episodes	108	16	bcd'e	?lm		
Lambert (35)	1970	2	7–25	?General practice	Asthma	24m	Exacerbations	11	123	bd'e	m		
McIntosh (36)	1973	32	1–7	Hospital	Asthma	15m	RTI with wheezing	139	12	d'ehk	lm		
Minor (37)	1974	16	3–11	Allergy clinic	Asthma	7m	Exacerbations	61	12	d'ehk	?lm		
Minor (38)	1976	49	3–60	General practice	Asthma (41 children)	8m	Asthma episodes	71	12	d'eh	l		
Mitchell (25)	1978	16	2–6	Ped resp clinic	Asthma	12m	Wheezing episodes	91	12	d²eh	?lm		
Roldaan (2)	1982	32	9–16	Asthma resort	Asthma	3–30m	Exacerbations	45			lm		
Mertsola (1)	1991	54	1–6	Hospital	Wh. bronchitis	3m	Wheezing episodes	76	5	eg'	o	y	
Johnston (39)	1995	108	9–11	General practice	Wheeze/cough	13m	Wheezing episodes	82	5	d'' g'hij	o	x	PCR
Children: weighted averages: pre-PCR studies[c]							8 studies	602	192+ve				
Children: weighted averages: PCR studies							1 study	82	66+ve				
Adults													
Huhti (4)	1974	63	15–77	Admission	Asthma	12m	Asthma admission	142			m		
Hudgel (41)	1979	19	24–67	O/P/private pract.	Asthma	8–19m	Exacerbations	76	4	d'eh	lm		
Clarke (42)	1979	51	adult	O/P Clinic	Asthma	18m	Exacerbations	27	1	?d'eh			
Clarke (42)	1979	51	adult	O/P Clinic	Asthma	18m	Exacerbations	102			m		
Beasley (43)	1988	31	15–156	O/P Clinic	Asthma	11m	Exacerbations	178	5	d'ee'	lm	xz	
Nicholson (44)	1993	138	19–46	Multiple	Asthma	rolling	Asthma exacerbation	61	12	fg'ij	mo		PCR
Atmar (32)	1998	29	19–50	Pulm. clinic.	Asthma	mean 19.5m	Asthma exacerbation	87	4	d''ehi	lno		PCR
Elderly													
Nicholson (45)	1997	291	>60	Country	All	24m	URTI with wheeze	291	12		lmo		PCR
Adults including elderly: weighted averages: pre-PCR studies[c]							5 studies	525	61+ve				
Adults including elderly: weighted averages: PCR studies[d]							3 studies	439	217+ve				

ED = emergency department; RTI = respiratory tract infection; LRTI = lower RTI; O/P = outpatient; Rhin = rhinovirus; Cor = Coronavirus; RSV = respiratory syncytial virus; Par = parainfluenza virus; Inf = influenza virus; Ad = adenovirus; Ent = Enterovirus; H.S. = Herpes simplex.; M.P. = *Mycoplasma pneumoniae*; C.P. = *Chlamydia pneumoniae*.
[a] Methods:
Spec (Specimen): 1 = nose swab; 2 = throat swab; 3 = sputum; 4 = nasal washings; 5 = nasal aspirate; 6 = rectal swab.
Culture (cell line): a = embryonated egg; b = human embryonic kidney; c = human amniotic cells; d'/d² = 1/2° monkey kidney; d'' = LLC-MK2; e = human embryonic lung (incl WI38);
f = MRC-5; g = Hela; g' = Ohio Hela; h = Hep-2; i = MDCK; j = Clone16; k = Mycoplasma culture.
Serum: 1 = haemagglutination inhibition; m = complement fixation; n = neutralisation; o = antibody-enzyme immunoassay.
Ag-D (Antigen detection): x = immunofluorescent microscopy; y = antigen-enzyme immunoassay; z = electron microscopy.
RT-PCR (Reverse transcriptase polymerase chain reaction). PCR = PCR used specific for those viruses whose results are shown boxed.

Total and specific viral identification rates (%) in wheezy episodes

First author	Year	Any virus	Rhin	Cor	RSV	Par	Inf	Ad	Ent	H.S.	M.P.	C.P.	Other	Dual[b]
Children														
Berkovich (34)	1970	22.2		2.8	6.5	10.2	0.9	9.0		4.6				
Lambert (35)	1970	45.5	27.0			18.0								
McIntosh (36)	1973	41.7		9.4	17.3	14.4	0.7	4.3		3.3	0.7			(7.2)
Minor (37)	1974	37.7	24.6				9.8							
Minor (38)	1976	23.9	9.9		2.8	1.4	5.6	1.4					2.8	
Mitchell (25)	1978	14.3	5.5		1.1	1.1		2.2	4.4					
Roldaan (2)	1982	48.9			2.2	4.4	37.8	2.2			2.2			6.6
Mertsola (1)	1991	39.5	10.5	11.8		6.6	1.3	1.3			1.3			6.6
Johnston (39)	1995	80.5	56.1	8.5	4.9	7.3	9.8							(6.1)
Children: weighted averages: pre-PCR studies[c]		31.9	12.3	10.2	6.5	7.1	8.2	2.4	4.4	3.3	2.2	0.0	2.8	(2.5)
Children: weighted averages: PCR studies		80.5	56.1	8.5										(6.1)
Adults														
Huhti (40)	1974	19.0		4.2	4.2	7.7	0.7		0.7	3.5		0.7	(2.8)	
Hudgel (41)	1979	10.5	2.6		1.3	2.6	3.9							
Clarke (42)	1979	14.8	11.1			2.9	1.0							
Clarke (42)	1979	3.9				1.7	1.1		3.7					
Beasley (43)	1988	10.0	2.2		4.5					0.6				
Nicholson (44)	1993	44.3	27.8	8.2	1.6	6.6	3.3							(1.6)
Altmar (32)	1998	43.7	•	•		•	•	•						
Elderly														
Nicholson (45)	1997	52.1	26.6	9.6	7.4	0.0	8.5							
Adults including elderly: weighted averages: pre-PCR studies[c]		11.6	3.2	9.4	5.1	3.3	5.4	0.8	3.7	0.8	3.5	0.0	0.7	0.8
Adults including elderly: weighted averages: PCR studies		49.4	26.7											(0.3)

b Numbers in parentheses for dual infections indicate that the viruses concerned are also included under the individual virus rates.

c For the pre-PCR studies, the weighted averages identification rates for each virus were calculated using only those studies that identified that virus. The averages include data from studies that are labeled as PCR studies but did not use PCR specific for that virus.

d For the PCR studies, the weighted average rates for each virus were calculated using only those studies that used PCR specific for that virus.

• The study of Atmar did not allow calculation of individual virus rates during asthma episodes. Viruses found are shown as a dot (•).

Table 6 Virus Identification Rates in Prospective Versus Cross-Sectional Studies

	No. of studies	No. of samples	No. of virus +ve samples	Percent of samples +ve for virus	Odds ratio prospective vs. cross-sectional studies	95% CI
Children: studies without PCR						
Cross-sectional	12	5167	1257	24.3		
Prospective	8	602	192	31.9	1.46	1.21, 1.75
Children: studies with PCR						
Cross-sectional	2	202	166	82.2		
Prospective	1	82	66	80.5	0.89	0.46, 1.72
Adults: studies without PCR						
Cross-sectional	4	368	87	23.6		
Prospective	5	525	61	11.6	0.42	0.30, 0.61
Adults: studies with PCR						
Cross-sectional	2	197	119	60.4		
Prospective	3	439	217	49.4	0.64	0.46, 0.90

extensive or sensitive than those used in the cross-sectional studies. Two studies identified coronavirus.

Only one study used PCR (3). Extensive testing and controls to demonstrate lack of contamination were used. The overall rate of identification was 80.5%, more than double the weighted average rate for pre-PCR studies (Table 7) with a highly significant odds ratio of 8.81 (95% CI: 4.97, 15.61). A very large increase in identification of rhinoviruses (56.1% vs. 12.3%, odds ratio 9.15) was the only significant increase that led to the higher overall identification rate (Table 4). Coronaviruses were detected in a similar proportion in the PCR study (8.5%) and the two pre-PCR studies that used appropriate serology for coronavirus (9.4% and 11.8%). The virus detection rates for any viruses, rhinoviruses, and coronaviruses in Johnston and colleagues (3,39) were very similar to the corresponding rates in the cross-sectional studies that used PCR (Table 6).

Prospective Studies in Adults

The methods and intensity of follow-up in these studies (32,40–45) were very variable. In one study (42), the results for serology were presented in the paper separately and with a different denominator from the results for viral culture, and thus these two results are presented on different lines in Table 5. Atmar and colleagues (32) presented overall figures for viral detection in asthma attacks but specific virus identification was shown for all respiratory illnesses in the cohort, whether these were asthma attacks or not. For this study the viruses detected in the study are indicated by dots in Table 5.

In the studies using only conventional virology, viral detection rates are low, ranging from 3.9 to 19.0%. The studies with the highest and the lowest rates both used only serology for identification. Few rhinoviruses and no coronaviruses were cultured, again owing to lack of use of sensitive cell culture lines for these viruses.

The three PCR studies shown, two in adults up to middle age and one in elderly people, all show much higher viral detection rates of 43.7–52.1%. The two studies by Nicholson and colleagues (44,45) documented quality control measures using known positive and negative samples in-line, whereas this is not clear in the study of Atmar et al. (32). The increased weighted average identification rate of 49.4% in these three studies is highly significant compared to the rate of 11.6% in pre-PCR studies (odds ratio 7.44; 95% CI 5.37, 10.30) (Table 7). Once again (Table 4), this increase is made up of increases in identification of rhinoviruses (OR 9.98). As is the case in infants, rhinoviruses are increasingly identified as significant pathogens in the elderly (46).

Atmar and colleagues (32) reported finding coronavirus by PCR in 7% of all respiratory illnesses in their asthma cohort. This is similar to the weighted average identification rate of coronavirus in asthma episodes in the two studies of Nicholson and others (44,45), which identified coronavirus only by conventional virology (8.2% and 9.6% respectively). Thus in both children and adults it appears that coronavirus can be found as readily (although perhaps not so conveniently) by sensitive conventional studies as by PCR.

Table 7 Prospective Studies: Overall Rates of Virus Identification with and Without PCR in Children and Adults

	No. of studies	No. of samples	No. of virus +ve samples	Percent of samples +ve for virus	Odds ratio studies with vs. without PCR	95% CI
Children						
Studies without PCR	8	602	192	31.9		
Studies with PCR	1	82	66	80.5	8.81	4.97, 15.61
Adults						
Studies without PCR	5	525	61	11.6		
Studies with PCR	3	439	217	49.4	7.44	5.37, 10.30

C. Summary of Findings from Review of Cross-Sectional and Prospective Studies

The major points arising from the above studies can be summarized as follows:

1. Cross-sectional and prospective studies have shown that a considerable proportion of asthma attacks or wheezing episodes is associated with virus or atypical bacterial infections. Studies that included PCR primers for rhinovirus and coronavirus have found that 80–82% of childhood exacerbations of wheezing and 50–60% of adult exacerbations are associated with identifiable viruses or atypical bacteria.

2. The organisms associated include all the known respiratory viruses, as well as *Mycoplasma pneumoniae* and *Chlamydia pneumoniae*, although the frequency of particular organisms vary from study to study.

3. Rhinoviruses are the most common viruses associated with episodes of wheeze in children and adults, in studies that employed adequate identification methods for these viruses. In infants, RSV is the most common associated virus, but the contribution of rhinovirus is still substantial.

4. The virology methods that are most often associated with increased viral detection rates are those most sensitive to rhinovirus infections (Table 2). Ohio Hela cells appear to be much more sensitive than any other cell lines for rhinovirus culture. RT-PCR for rhinovirus is several-fold more sensitive again than Ohio Hela cell culture. RT-PCR for coronavirus, RSV, influenza viruses, and enteroviruses is also more sensitive than other identification methods for these viruses.

5. There is lack of documentation in some conventional studies of the sensitivity of their virology methods. Conversely, there is lack of documentation in some PCR studies of specificity and lack of contamination. However it is true that the latter studies have identified viruses at very similar rates regardless of whether or not they documented specificity and use of internal control samples (e.g., 83.3% overall in Rakes et al. (8) vs. 81.8% overall in Freymuth et al. (23). Findings of case–control studies are discussed below.

6. More intensive and early sampling during infections such as occurs in prospective studies appears to confer an advantage at least in studies of children using conventional virology (Table 6). This advantage is not seen in adult or child studies using PCR, which suggests that the sensitivity of PCR compensates for the fall-off in virus excretion in samples obtained some days after the onset of symptoms. For adults conventional prospective studies achieved lower identification rates than cross-sectional ones. The reason for this is not apparent except that these studies were very variable in the virological methods they used.

7. We do not know what triggers may be associated with the 20–50% of exacerbations of wheezing in which viruses are not identified by PCR. Allergen or other environmental exposures, and nonspecific asthma triggers (dry air or exercise), are possibilities. Some studies (7,8,20) have suggested that virus-negative children with wheeze are more likely to show various atopic features (allergic history, skin test positivity, high serum IgE, or high levels of sputum eosinophils) than virus-

positive children. Others (6,17,21,28) suggest that there is little difference. This will be further considered below.

It is also possible that unidentified organisms are involved. Bacteria have been looked for in a number of studies (2,14,20,25,31,34,36–38,41,42,47) with no convincing evidence of association with acute wheezing. It is notable that in many of the prospective studies the episodes with a virus or atypical bacteria identified were described as very similar to episodes with no identification in regard to either the symptom pattern (1,2,25,28,32,34,36,37,40,44) or the seasonal pattern (18,21,36). Thus it is entirely plausible that more of these episodes are associated with viruses than were identified.

D. Case–Control Studies of Viral Identification Rates in Asthma Attacks

A number of cross-sectional and prospective studies have compared viral identification rates in acute wheezing episodes and in either a separate control group (external controls) or in the cases at times when they had respiratory infections without wheeze or were asymptomatic (internal controls). Odds ratios are used here to describe the likelihood of viral isolation in episodes of wheeze.

Studies of Cases and External Controls

These studies were all extended cross-sectional studies (6,8,13,14,16,22,29,31). The studies are organized into three groups in Table 8 according to the type of controls, which included children with nonrespiratory illnesses (e.g., admission for surgical procedures), children with respiratory infections who did not wheeze (usually admitted and investigated at the same time as the cases), and children with asthma who were asymptomatic (in an asthma outpatient clinic).

All but one of the studies using nonrespiratory controls found significantly higher rates of virus isolation in asthmatic subjects with wheeze than in nonrespiratory cases. The exceptional instance was the subset of Rakes et al. (8) that studied children under 2 years. It found a high odds ratio, but with only 22 cases and 17 controls it lacked statistical power. If these results are combined with those of the older children in the same study, the result is highly significant (odds ratio 6.57; 96% CI: 2.93, 14.75). The overall odds ratios for both conventional and PCR studies are very similar and both highly significant (respectively 6.85; 95% CI 3.64, 12.90 and 6.57; 95% CI 3.14, 7.23).

The second group of studies using control cases with nonwheezing respiratory infections all used conventional virology. None of these studies showed a significant difference in virus identification rates between cases and controls. The overall rates were similar (25.0% and 26.8%, respectively) and the overall odds ratio was close to 1.0. The study of Horn and colleagues (19) (not listed in Table 8), showed that the age distribution of various respiratory viruses was similar whether these were identified during wheezy episodes or nonwheezy respiratory episodes in control children.

Table 8 Overall Virus Identification Rates in Case-Control Studies: Cross-Sectional Studies with Separate (External) Control Group

Study (Ref.)	Year	Virology[a]	Age group	ID rate in cases (exacerbations of wheeze or asthma)	ID rate in controls (for description see group headings)	Odds ratio of +ve virus in wheeze vs. control	95% CI
Controls = subjects with nonrespiratory illness							
Duff (6)	1993	Conventional	Infants <2	14/20 = 70%	2/10 = 20%	9.33	1.51, 57.66
Duff (6)	1993	Conventional	Children >2	22/70 = 31%	5/45 = 11%	3.67	1.27, 10.56
Abramson (29)	1994	Conventional	Adults	8/38 = 21%	2/90 = 2%	11.73	2.36, 58.35
Teichtahl (31)	1997	Conventional	Adults	23/79 = 29%	4/54 = 7%	5.13	1.66, 15.86
Rakes (8)	1999	With PCR	Infants <2	18/22 = 82%	9/17 = 53%	4.00	0.95, 16.93
Rakes (8)	1999	With PCR	Children >2	40/48 = 83%	16/42 = 38%	8.13	3.04, 21.69
Overall		Conventional		67/207 = 32%	13/199 = 7%	6.85	3.64, 12.90
Overall		With PCR		58/70 = 83%	25/59 = 42%	6.57	2.93, 14.75
Controls = subjects with nonwheezy respiratory infections							
Tyrrell (13)	1965	Conventional	Children	64/225 = 28%	94/437 = 21%	1.45	1.00, 2.10
Disney (14)	1971	Conventional	Children	5/51 = 10%	15/47 = 32%	0.23	0.08, 0.70
Horn (16)	1975	Conventional	Children	152/554 = 27%	71/244 = 29%	0.92	0.66, 1.29
Jennings (22)	1987	Conventional	Children	38/204 = 19%	110/356 = 31%	0.51	0.34, 0.78
Overall*		Conventional		259/1034 = 25.0%	290/1084 = 26.8%	0.91	0.75, 1.11
Controls = subjects with asthma sampled during asymptomatic periods							
Jennings (22)	1987	Conventional	Children	38/204 = 19%	4/123 = 3.3%	6.81	2.37, 19.59

[a] "Conventional" refers to studies that did not use PCR for virus identification.

Only one study used a separate group of asymptomatic asthmatic subjects as controls (22). In this study viruses were identified in approximately 19% of cases and 3% of asymptomatic asthmatic controls, with an odds ratio for association of 6.81 (95% CI: 2.31, 19.59). This odds ratio is comparable to those found in the first group of studies.

Studies of Cases with Internal Control Samples

All (3,19,25,32,35,38,41,43,44,48) but one (19) of these studies are prospective studies (Table 9). Control samples were taken from cases either during nonwheezy respiratory infections or during asymptomatic periods.

All studies that took control samples during nonwheezy respiratory infections found similar rates of virus identification in control and wheezy samples. The overall odds ratios were 0.82 (95% CI: 0.57, 1.18) for studies using only conventional virology methods and 1.13 (95% CI: 0.63, 1.15) for studies using PCR. These figures match closely the results previously described for the corresponding studies with external controls.

Virus identification during asymptomatic periods varied from 0.8 to 7% for conventional studies and from 0 to 21% for PCR studies. The odds ratios indicate a significantly increased likelihood of virus detection during wheeze episodes than during asymptomatic periods in every one of these studies. The lowest odds ratio was 2.87 (95% CI:1.27, 6.50) and the highest was unmeasurable because of a zero isolation rate in controls. Two studies (3,48) that tested only for rhinovirus (by PCR) during asymptomatic periods shared very similar odds ratios of 9–10 with similar confidence intervals. These were included in the overall figures for PCR studies since rhinovirus was the most common virus identified in any of these studies. The overall odds ratio for conventional studies was 6.77 (95% CI: 4.59, 9.99) and that for PCR studies was 10.17 (95% CI: 6.17, 16.73).

E. Summary of Case-Control Study Findings

Thus in every one of the reported studies, using either external control subjects or internal control samples, viruses can be found during wheezing episodes at the same rate as is prevalent during symptomatic respiratory infections in children of the same age at the same time. However, viruses are 6–10 times more likely to be associated with wheezing episodes than with nonrespiratory illness or with asymptomatic periods in asthmatic children. These comparisons, involving large numbers of children and including studies with highly sensitive methods, argue very strongly that the viruses causing prevalent respiratory infections also trigger attacks of wheezing in susceptible individuals, and that this is not an artifact of the methods (e.g., contamination) nor does it indicate chronic carriage of these viruses in asthmatic subjects.

Two recent studies (49,50) that did not sample episodes of wheezing appear to contradict these conclusions. West and colleagues (49) used a sensitive seven-virus PCR panel with careful controls to ensure sensitivity and lack of contamination of specimens. They sampled 21 children with diagnosed asthma, 16 children with exercise-induced bronchoconstriction, and 33 of their classmates who did not have

Table 9 Overall Virus Identification Rates in Case-Control Studies: Studies (Mostly Prospective) Using Asthmatic Cases as Their Own (Internal) Controls

Study (Ref.)	Year	Virology[a]	Age group	ID rate in case episodes (exacerbations of wheeze or asthma)	ID rate in control samples (for description see group headings)	Odds ratio of +ve virus in wheeze vs. control	95% CI
Control samples = samples taken during nonwheezy respiratory infections							
Lambert (35)	1972	Conventional	Child and adult	5/11 = 45%	9/22 = 41%	1.20	0.28, 5.18
Minor (38)	1976	Conventional	Children	17/71 = 24%	16/57 = 28%	0.81	0.36, 1.79
Horn (19)	1979	Conventional	Children	146/554 = 26%	31/105 = 30%	0.85	0.54, 1.35
Atmar (32)	1998	With PCR	Adults	38/87 = 44%	19/50 = 38%	1.27	0.62, 2.58
Kuga (48)	2000	With PCR (picornavirus only)	Adults	16/52 = 31%	8/25 = 32%	0.94	0.34, 2.64
Overall		Conventional		168/636 = 26%	56/184 = 30%	0.82	0.57, 1.18
Overall		With PCR		54/139 = 39%	27/75 = 36%	1.13	0.63, 2.02
Control samples = samples taken during asymptomatic periods							
Lambert (35)	1972	Conventional ("infectious agent")	Child and adult	6/11 = 55%	7/98 = 7%	15.60	3.79, 64.16
Mitchell (25)	1978	Conventional	Children	13/91 = 14%	1/120 = 0.8%	19.83	2.54, 154.67
Horn (19)	1979	Conventional	Children	146/554 = 26%	1/31 = 3%	10.74	1.45, 79.43
Huhti (40)	1974	Conventional	Adults	27/142 = 19%	10/189 = 5%	4.20	1.96, 9.01
Hudgel (41)	1979	Conventional	Adults	8/84 = 10%	8/243 = 3%	3.09	1.12, 8.52
Beasley (43)	1988	Conventional	Adults	18/178 = 10%	4/161 = 2%	4.42	1.46, 13.34
Nicholson (44)	1993	With PCR	Adults	27/44 = 61%	0/61 = 0%	↑↑↑	
Atmar (32)	1998	With PCR	Adults	38/87 = 44%	10/47 = 21%	2.87	1.27, 6.50
Johnston (39)	1993	With PCR	Children	46/82 = 56%	8/65 = 12%	9.10	3.86, 21.49
Kuga (48)	2000	With PCR (picornavirus only)	Adults	16/52 = 31%	4/92 = 4%	9.78	3.06, 31.26
Overall		Conventional		218/1060 = 21%	31/842 = 4%	6.77	4.59, 9.99
Overall		With PCR (picornavirus only)		127/265 = 49%	22/265 = 8%	10.17	6.17, 16.73

↑↑↑ = too high to estimate (denominator = 0).
[a] "Conventional" refers to studies that did not use PCR for virus identification.

asthma. None of the children had identifiable symptoms of respiratory infection at the time of sampling by nasal swab. The respiratory virus identification rates were 62% in asthmatic children, 62% in those with exercise-induced bronchoconstriction, and 60% in controls. They have suggested that respiratory viruses are commonly carried in asymptomatic children.

Macek and others (50) using PCR found respiratory viruses in 19 of 20 post-mortem airway samples in 10 adults dying of asthma, 4 adults with asthma dying of other causes, and 6 adults without asthma. Seven of the 10 who died of nonasthma causes died from vascular (coronary or cerebral) events. Again careful quality assurance of PCR technique was performed with in-line testing of known positive and negative controls. This group has previously published studies suggesting that latent adenovirus infection may contribute to persistent refractory asthma (51–53).

What is not clear from the recent studies of Macek and West and their colleagues is whether any of these subjects had had symptoms of virus infection in the recent past, or (in West et al.) were followed up to see if they subsequently developed such symptoms and may have been sampled during an incubation phase. Small numbers of residual or incubating viruses may have been picked up by PCR in such cases.

It is also possible that studying postmortem cases gives rise to selection bias. Influenza infections are well known to be associated with cardiovascular and pulmonary mortality (54–56) and rhinovirus and other virus infections may also be involved. Visseren and colleagues (57) have found that a number of respiratory viruses cause endothelial tissues to shift from anticoagulant to procoagulant activity. Thus patients dying from cardiopulmonary disease may be more likely to have had respiratory virus infection at the time of death than asymptomatic living subjects.

Aside from the studies of West and colleagues, and Hogg et al., chronic carriage of respiratory viruses has not been convincingly demonstrated. The balance of evidence from 265 asthmatic subjects studied in a prospective fashion and using RT-PCR is that only a small proportion of tests are positive during asymptomatic periods.

F. Temporal Variation of Infections and of Asthma Attacks

Seasonal Variation

The variation of frequency of asthma attacks over a year has been the subject of study by a number of authors. One of the most enlightening studies was that of Storr and Lenney (58), which examined the childhood asthma admission rates in Brighton, England. For each week of the calendar year, the average of admission rates in that week over 10 consecutive years was calculated. The resulting graphs (Fig. 1) showed that there was a major drop in asthma admissions during school holiday periods, and a sharp rise to a peak of asthma admissions after the beginning of each school term. It is difficult to explain this trend in terms of environmental exposure to allergens or irritants such as tobacco smoke since these exposures tend to be lower at school than at home. The child population of Brighton, a holiday

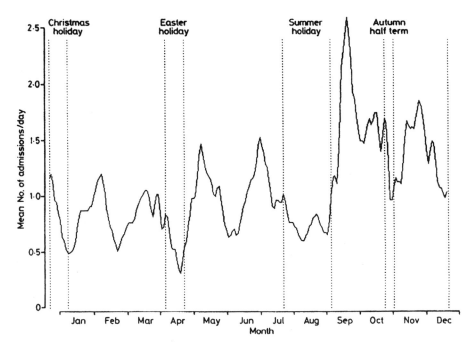

Figure 1 Variation in hospital admissions for childhood asthma by week of the year in Brighton, England. Figures for each week of the year have been averaged over the 10 years 1975–1985. The periods of school holidays are shown. (From Ref. 58.)

resort, would not be expected to decrease during vacations. Mass exposure to new viruses introduced at the beginning of school terms by children who have acquired viruses during the vacation would explain these data very well.

This explanation was supported by our study (59) in children in Southampton, England. We found a very similar pattern to that described by Storr and Lenney in the numbers of virus identifications in the cohort of children we were following (Fig. 2). Furthermore, pediatric hospital admissions in children in Southampton and in the wider Wessex region (also shown in Fig. 2) followed a remarkably similar pattern. The numbers each half-month of virus identifications in the cohort were significantly correlated with pediatric hospital admission numbers for asthma in the same half-month periods (correlation coefficient 0.67, $p < 0.001$ for correlation with Wessex region). There was also a significant but weaker correlation with adult hospital admissions for asthma (correlation coefficient 0.5, $p = 0.013$).

Thus there are two associations: an association between the school calendar and the number of viruses found in our cohort, and a correlation between the half-monthly number of viruses in the cohort and the number of hospital admissions for asthma in the region. The implication is that hospital admissions for asthma are triggered by the respiratory viruses prevalent in the community, and peak at the

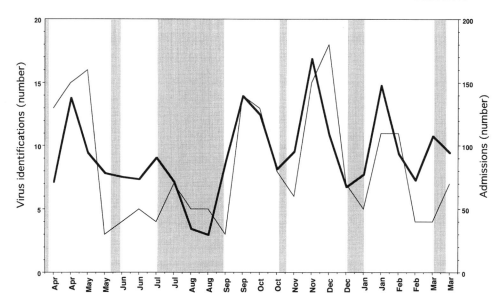

Figure 2 Variation over 1 year of hospital admissions for childhood asthma in the Wessex region, England (heavy line), and numbers of viruses isolated from a cohort of 108 children with respiratory illness in Southampton, Wessex, England (light line). Figures are shown for each half-month of the year from April, 1989, to March, 1990. The periods of school holidays are shown by shaded bars. (Adapted and redrawn from Ref. 59.)

same times, which tends to be just after the beginning of school terms. It follows that viruses trigger severe attacks of asthma as well as the milder episodes of wheezing seen in our cohort (of which 80.5% were associated with viruses (Table 5).

Disney and colleagues (14) found no correlation between the peak of viral infections in winter and the autumn peak in asthma attacks in 51 children in 1971. However, no rhinoviruses were identified, since they did not use sensitive cell lines, and only five viruses in total were found. McIntosh and co-workers (36), who identified viruses (none of them rhinovirus) in 41.7% of 139 episodes of wheezing, found a clear seasonal relationship between wheezing illnesses and virus infections. In the first year of study of the cohort of 32 children, peaks of wheezing illness coincided with peaks of RSV and parainfluenza 2 infections, and the same viruses as well as coronaviruses were associated with wheezing illness in the second year. Mitchell and co-workers (25) also showed a relationship between the seasonal pattern of asthma exacerbations and that of viral isolations, in that the proportion of episodes associated with viruses was similar throughout the year. Henderson and colleagues (18) found strong coincidence of peaks of RSV infections with so-called "wheezing-associated respiratory infections" in children less than 2 years of age. In older children, peaks of wheezing illness coincided with peaks of parainfluenza 3 and *M. pneumoniae* isolations.

Carlsen and Ørstavik (60) did not find a relationship between the seasonal distribution of acute asthma episodes and the occurrence of rhinovirus in 33 of these episodes; rhinovirus infections occurred throughout the year. The study may have been underpowered for this analysis, since on average fewer than three rhinovirus infections were found each month, and there were slightly more infections in the last half of the year when asthma episodes were also more common. Rylander and co-workers in 1996 reported that peaks of admission for wheezing bronchitis coincided with peaks of RSV infection in March–April in children less than 18 months old, and with peaks of rhinovirus in September for older children.

Three studies have examined the seasonal pattern of asthma attacks in relationship to allergens, other environmental triggers, and virus infections. Carlsen and colleagues (21) found strong relationships between the seasonal incidence of asthma attacks over a 2 year period and virus infections, particularly rhinovirus infections (May–June and August–September) and RSV infections (November–December). There was no correlation between asthma attacks and spore counts for *C. herbarum*, or pollen counts for birch or grasses in subjects allergic to these various allergens. They concluded that the "single precipitating factor most frequently associated with acute asthma was respiratory virus infection."

Potter and colleagues (61) performed a careful study of 40 asthmatic children aged 2–14 years consecutively admitted to hospital, and 40 known asthmatics who did not have an attack, selected from the outpatient department on the same day as the cases. Meteorological and pollen data were obtained for the entire 4 months of the study, and compared to time of onset of symptoms. Cases and controls had a questionnaire administered for recent behavioral, socioeconomic, and domestic factors (including recent emotional events and home use of environmental chemicals). Recent allergen exposure was enquired for, and allergies were documented by history and by either skin prick test or radioallergosorbent test (RAST). Medication compliance was assessed and cases and controls were examined for signs of infection. None of the meteorological, pollen count, socioeconomic, home exposure, or compliance factors were associated with attacks. Seven cases and seven controls had recently been exposed to a known allergen. Thirty-two cases and 33 controls had evidence on examination of nasal allergy. On the other hand, 23 cases and 5 controls had coryza on examination ($p < 0.001$), 18 cases and 1 control had x-ray evidence of pneumonia or bronchitis ($p < 0.001$), 3 cases and no control had acute otitis media, and 18 cases, and 1 control had a red, inflamed throat ($p < 0.001$). More of the cases than controls had shared a bed with a relative. The authors concluded: "the majority of severe asthma attacks were associated with infection of the respiratory tract."

Dales and coworkers (62) investigated the autumn increase in hospital admissions for asthma in preschool children in Canada between 1981 and 1989. They analyzed meteorological, air pollution, and aerobiological data over the period, as well as admissions for croup, bronchitis/bronchiolitis, and pneumonia. They collected data on a nonrespiratory group of admissions for comparison (diseases of cerebral vasculature, esophagus, appendix, intestine, gallbladder, biliary tree, pancreas, kidney, and urinary tract). There was a large autumn peak of asthma admissions but not of nonrespiratory admissions every year of the study in October or

November. Data for each week from August to December were averaged over the 9 years of the study for admissions and for environmental data.

Admissions for asthma rose from a low at weeks 29–34 of the year to peak at weeks 38–48. By contrast, ozone, sulfates, and particulates peaked at weeks 28–32 and had dropped to a low by week 44 when admissions were at their peak. Ragweed pollen peaked in week 32 and was low by week 39. Basidiospores peaked at week 36 and were low by week 39. Neither temperature nor humidity was correlated with the autumn peak in admissions, although monthly average temperature fell steadily and relative humidity increased steadily during the latter half of the year. However, averaged weekly admissions for croup bore a strong association with admissions for asthma, and admissions for pneumonia and bronchitis increased steadily through the autumn. Admissions for respiratory infection unadjusted explained 20% of the variance in asthma admissions; after adjustment for climate, air pollution, and aeroallergen levels, respiratory infection explained 14% of the variance. Week-to-week changes in infection also correlated with week-to-week changes in asthma admissions. The conclusion of the authors was: "Based on seasonal patterns, respiratory infection is the major identifiable risk factor for the large autumnal increase in asthma admissions."

Temporal Associations in Individuals

At least three prospective studies (3,36,37) have documented over prolonged periods the temporal association of virus identifications in individuals with daily records of symptoms of asthma, asthma medication use, or deteriorations in lung function. In the study of Minor and colleagues (37), virology samples were taken every 2 weeks, in that of McIntosh and colleagues (36) virology was performed monthly as well as with each acute episode (results from McIntosh et al. shown in Fig. 3). In these two studies, the majority of virus isolations occurred at times of asthma symptoms or use of asthma relief medication.

Roldaan and Masural (2) showed that the temporal profile of forced expiratory volume in 1 s (FEV1) followed a very similar pattern in three children with influenza after aligning the first day of symptoms (Fig. 4). In all three children, on the first day of symptoms FEV1 had already dropped slightly but it fell dramatically to a trough 1–2 days later, and slowly recovered over approximately 14 days.

The very strong seasonal link between virus respiratory infections and asthma attacks together with the close temporal association of virus infections in individuals with the onset of asthma symptoms and lung function deterioration together provide very strong corroborative (albeit circumstantial) evidence that viruses are the chief triggers of asthma attacks.

Associations with Age

The predominant viruses associated with episodes of wheezing at different ages are the same as those associated with all respiratory infections at those ages (see Tables 1 and 5). Thus RSV infections associated with asthma are most common in the first year of life (6,8) and decrease in incidence thereafter, although they are still found

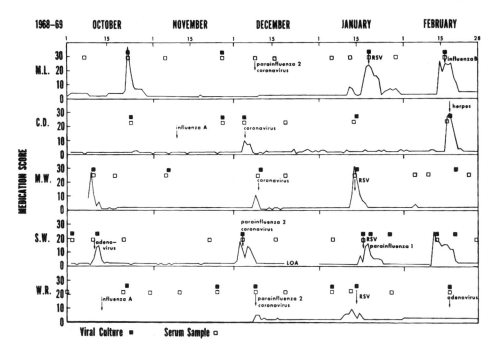

Figure 3 Daily medication scores of five children over 5 months in relation to respiratory viral infection. Samples taken for virology are indicated by open boxes □ for serum samples, and solid boxes ■ for nasopharyngeal and throat swabs for viral cultures. Virus isolations are shown by the arrows and the names of the viruses. (From Ref 36.)

with wheezing episodes in adults and the elderly (45). Influenza and *Mycoplasma pneumoniae* infections become more commonly in wheezing episodes in late childhood. Rhinoviruses are commonly associated with wheezing at all ages and become the predominant organism found in wheezy episodes from 2 years of age onward.

Between childhood and adulthood there is a decrease in the rate of virus detection in wheezing episodes. In cross-sectional studies using PCR the overall rates of virus detection (Table 1) were 82.2% in children and 61.4% in adults (95% CI on difference in proportions: -12.35%, -29.30%). In prospective studies using PCR the overall rates of virus detection (Table 5) were 80.5% in children and 49.4% in adults (95% CI on difference in proportions: -21.29%, -40.83%).

G. The Likelihood That a Virus Infection in an Asthmatic Will Trigger an Episode of Wheeze

Data are shown in Figure 5 from prospective studies of asthmatic subjects that allow estimation of the risk of wheezing if an asthmatic subject gets a virus infection (1,32,36–38,43,45,63). Studied that were not informative were those in which inves-

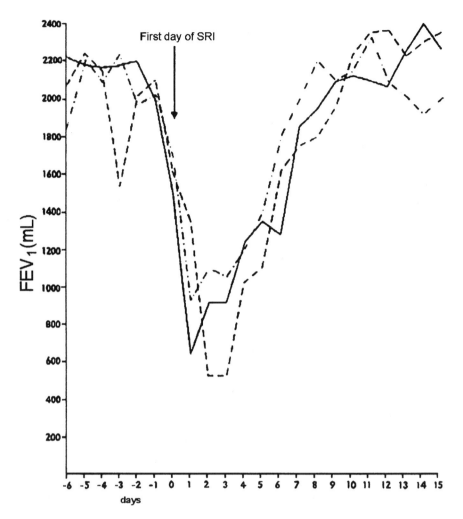

Figure 4 Graphs show FEV₁ of three asthmatic children who had an episode of asthma and demonstrated seroconversion to influenza A virus during the episode. The graphs have been aligned by the first day of symptoms in each of the subjects as indicated by the arrow. (From Ref. 2.)

tigations were only performed during episodes of wheezing and not during non-wheezy infections or asymptomatic periods. The denominator for each data point is the number of specific virus-positive episodes of respiratory infection in asthmatic subjects followed for varying periods. The numerator is the number of episodes of wheezing during these specific virus infections.

The weighted average rate of wheezing if any virus was identified was very similar in child and adult studies when these are matched by the use or nonuse of

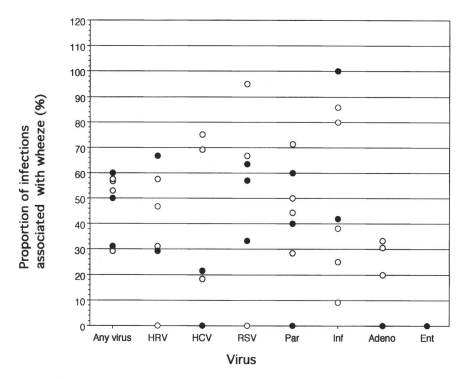

Figure 5 The proportion of asthmatic subjects who wheeze during an infection with any virus and with specific viruses. Open circles ○ = studies of children; solid circles ● = studies of adults. Figures were obtained from studies cited in the text. (Adapted and redrawn with additional data from Ref. 5.)

PCR. For studies using conventional virology, 55.2% of all asthmatic children who had a respiratory virus wheezed, compared to 56.5% of asthmatic adults. During any virus infection identified by PCR, 29.2% of children and 31.2% of adults wheezed. That the rates are lower in PCR studies is to be expected as a greater proportion of infections were identified (denominator), without a proportional increase in recognition of wheezing (numerator). This applies to most of the specific virus rates as well as to the rates for any virus (Fig. 6).

Among the specific viruses, 50–70% of rhinovirus and coronavirus infections identified by conventional means were associated with wheezing, compared to 20–30% of these infections identified in PCR studies. Results for other viruses were not as consistent, but RSV caused relatively high rates of wheezing in both children and adults (50–100% for conventional studies and 30–45% for PCR studies). The rates of wheezing for parainfluenza and influenza ranged between 30 and 100%. Wheezing was universally less common in adenovirus and enterovirus infections, but the numbers here were small, and numbers for other organisms were too small and erratically reported to be included.

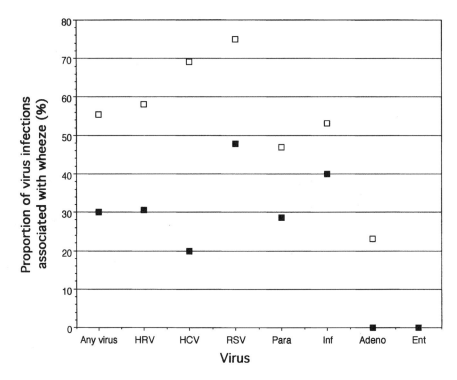

Figure 6 The proportion of asthmatic subjects who wheeze during an infection with any virus and with specific viruses: weighted averages for non-PCR studies (open squares □) and PCR studies (solid squares ■). Figures calculated from the same studies as in Figure 5.

The level of consistency among studies that used conventional virology and among those that used PCR is remarkably good for rhinovirus and coronavirus infections, considering the diversity of the study years, and detailed methods. One could speculate that an individual's own immune and inflammatory response to a particular virus as well as virus subtypes will affect the likelihood of an asthma exacerbation occurring during a given infection. The relationship between severity of the infection and the likelihood and severity of asthma depends to some extent on these factors. This has been examined in a small number of studies, which will be discussed next.

H. Dose–Response Effects of Viruses in Asthma

Three types of partial dose–response relationships between viruses and asthma have been examined, as illustrated in the figurative representations of contingency tables in Figure 7. The first type is demonstrated by the strong association between virus identification and asthma attacks, as demonstrated in those case–control studies with internal controls discussed above. The second type concerns the likelihood that severe virus respiratory infections trigger asthma (of any severity) more commonly

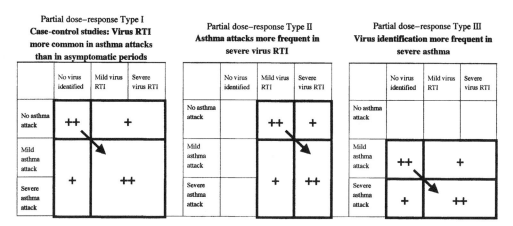

Figure 7 Representations of contingency tables indicating three types of partial dose–response relationships demonstrated in the literature (see text). Heavy lines indicate the cells for the groups studied. For instance, if the comparison group includes all virus respiratory tract infections (RTI) regardless of severity, the cell will be shown to include both the mild and severe categories of RTI. High cell frequencies are indicated by + +, low cell frequencies by +. The arrow shows the direction of increasing dose and increasing response.

than mild infections. The third type concerns the likelihood that acute asthma associated with virus-positive infections (of any severity) is more severe than acute asthma with no infection identified, or its corollary that viruses can be identified more commonly during severe asthma attacks than mild asthma attacks. The evidence for the second and third types of partial dose–response relationship is provisional since the numbers depend on the sensitivity of viral identification and studies examining these ideas have used only conventional virology to date.

With regard to the severity of respiratory infections, Minor and colleagues (37) in 1974 found that 21 of 23 (91%) severe virus infections were accompanied by an asthma attack compared to only 2 of 12 (17%) mild virus infections. This yields a high odds of wheezing in severe vs. mild infections of 52.50 (95% CI: 6.43, 428.59). No asthma attacks occurred in 12 asymptomatic periods when virus or *M. pneumoniae* was identified. In a study closely supervised by physicians on a daily basis and with regular serological testing, Roldaan and Masural documented wheezing in 7 of 19 (37%) symptomatic respiratory infections and 1 of 12 (8%) mild respiratory infections. The odds ratio of 6.42 is not significant (95% CI: 0.68, 60.84). These authors, however, also documented several cases of seroconversion to a virus at the time of an asthma exacerbation with no other signs of respiratory infection, suggesting that even subclinical infections can trigger asthma. Combining the results of Minor et al. and Roldaan et al. yields a risk of asthma in 67% of severe infections and 13% of mild infections (odds ratio: 14.00; 95% CI: 3.56, 55.06).

With regard to the severity of asthma, Mitchell and colleagues (17) isolated 39 viruses in a sample of 267 children hospitalized with wheezy bronchitis. The virus-positive subjects had more blood gas measurements performed and a greater tendency to respiratory acidosis than the virus-negative subjects did. Horn and colleagues (20) found viruses in 14 of 22 (64%) severe attacks and 21 of 50 (42%) mild attacks. Put the other way, asthma was severe in 14 of 35 (40%) of virus-positive episodes and 8 of 37 (21.6%) virus-negative episodes. The odds ratio is not significant for this association of virus positivity with severe attacks (2.42; 95% CI: 0.86, 6.80). In an adult prospective study of 31 patients, Beasley and colleagues (43) found viruses in 10 of 28 (36%) severe exacerbations of asthma and 8 of 150 (5%) milder exacerbations (odds ratio 9.86; 95% CI: 3.45, 28.21). That is, 56% of virus-positive exacerbations were severe, compared to 11% of virus-negative exacerbations. Combining the results of Horn et al. and Beasley et al. shows that 24 of 53 (45%) virus-positive exacerbations were severe, compared to 26 of 197 (13%) virus-negative exacerbations (odds ratio: 5.44; 95% CI: 2.76, 10.75).

All of the studies mentioned have used conventional virology, and data are not readily extractable from any of the papers using PCR to date. The evidence at face value suggests that an asthma attack is 14 times more likely to occur during a severe than a mild virus-positive infection, and that an asthma attack is five times more likely to be severe in a virus-positive exacerbation than a virus-negative exacerbation. These figures, although tentative, do indirectly suggest an association between the severity of virus infections and the severity of the asthma attack.

There is as yet no study showing a true dose–response relationship: that the severity of the virus infection determines the severity of the associated asthma (Fig. 8). There is also no study examining severity of asthma or of respiratory infection in anything other than binary form (mild vs. severe). Quantitative measures of severity, such as lung function or inflammatory markers, would theoretically enable more

Severe asthma attack more common in severe virus RTI			
	No virus identified	Mild virus RTI	Severe Virus RTI
Mild asthma attack		++	+
Severe asthma attack		+	++

Figure 8 Figurative representations of contingency table indicating the type of cell groupings needed to demonstrate a true dose–response effect. Markings are as for Figure 7.

detailed analysis of response, although such measures represent only particular aspects of severity. The dose of infecting virus, or the degree of viral-induced local or systemic inflammatory response, might be considered more valid measures of dose than a score for mild or severe symptoms of infection. However, we lack the tools to measure infecting dose of virus, and inflammatory response to viruses is complex and difficult to differentiate reliably from asthmatic inflammation. Thus it is (and will remain) difficult to be certain whether a true dose-response effect exists or, alternatively, whether there is an all-or-none response of asthmatics to virus infection.

I. Are Asthmatics Particularly Prone to Viral Infections?

Subjects with asthma, particularly in childhood, often appear to develop more frequent respiratory infections than their nonasthmatic siblings or spouses. Furthermore, many children who are referred for specialist review with recurrent infections turn out to have asthma. There are two possible hypotheses (which are not mutually exclusive) to explain these observations:

1. People with asthma are more susceptible to virus infection than people without asthma.
2. People with asthma manifest symptoms of respiratory infection more readily (because they wheeze) than people without asthma and thus have fewer episodes of subclinical infection.

In support of the first hypothesis (greater susceptibility to virus infection), Minor and co-workers (37) found a greater incidence of identifiable viral infections in asthmatic children than in their nonasthmatic siblings, attributable mostly to an excess of rhinovirus infections. Tarlo and colleagues (64) found that asthmatic adults reported more symptomatic respiratory infections than their nonasthmatic spouses, but had a lower viral identification rate.

Isaacs and others (65) compared 30 preschool children who presented with recurrent respiratory infection to a control group of children. The index children had higher incidence of respiratory illnesses (9.3 episodes per year vs. 5.4 episodes per year in controls, $p < 0.001$). Index children had lower respiratory symptoms in 33% of their episodes vs. 10% in control subjects ($p < 0.01$). The virus isolation rate (by conventional means) was similar in index subjects (40%) and in controls (36%); thus a higher annual rate of virus infections was experienced by the index children. Although asthma was not specified in this study, the predominance of wheeze among index subjects suggests that many of these were asthmatic. If so, this would lend support to the first hypothesis.

We obtained very similar findings to Isaacs et al. in a cohort of 108 children, of whom 42 had a diagnosis of asthma (3,63). We found that the median annual rate of respiratory illnesses reported by the children with diagnosed asthma was significantly higher (2.78) than that reported by children without asthma (1.84; 95% CI on median difference 0.18, 1.83). However viruses were identified by PCR or conventional means in a similar proportion of reported illnesses in both groups (asthma: 76.6%, no asthma 80.8%; odds ratio 0.78; 95% CI 0.44, 1.37). By computerized searching of the children's daily symptom records over 13 months, we found a large number of unreported episodes of significant increase in symptom scores (782 episodes of upper respiratory symptoms and 576 episodes of lower respiratory symptoms in the cohort) (3). The annual rates of upper respiratory and lower respiratory episodes were significantly higher in subjects with diagnosed asthma than in those without asthma, but a similar proportion of these were reported by children with and without asthma (63). Combining these results suggests that compared to children without asthma, the children with asthma experience higher annual rates of computer-defined respiratory illnesses, reported infections, and virus-positive infections. On the other hand asthmatic children do not seem more likely to report increases in symptoms than nonasthmatic children.

The second hypothesis (more obvious symptoms of infection) is supported by the fact that in the prospective study of Roldaan and Masural (2) two subjects had an asthma attack with no other respiratory symptoms at the time of seroconversion to influenza A virus. Four subjects had an asthma attack with very mild upper respiratory symptoms, associated with seroconversion to influenza A in one subject and parainfluenza 3 virus in the other three subjects. The implication is that these subjects would have had subclinical infections that would not be noticed, but for the fact that they had an asthma attack at the time.

The second hypothesis is further supported by the study of Horn and Gregg (66), who found a higher overall incidence of symptoms among asthmatic children with rhinovirus infection than in rhinovirus infection in other groups. Rhinovirus infection in asthmatics was most commonly associated with so-called bronchitis with wheeze, whereas rhinovirus infection among other groups was associated predominantly with upper respiratory symptoms. In the case of RSV infection, asthmatics exhibited a higher rate of wheeze than other groups, but the overall incidence of symptoms was lowest in asthmatics, and highest in those children with no history of respiratory illness. With parainfluenza virus infection the results were more variable. Reporting bias may be a contributing factor to these differences, but it is not self-evident that this is the whole explanation.

There is thus some evidence for both hypotheses and both may be true, but the evidence is more robust for the first: that asthmatic subjects are more susceptible to virus infections than nonasthmatic subjects. It has been suggested that this may be due to virus binding, since the epithelial receptor for rhinovirus, ICAM-1 may be more highly expressed in asthmatic subjects although this is not proven (67–69). The second hypothesis is more difficult to establish without comparing asthmatic and nonasthmatic subjects who have an identical wild-type virus. Nonetheless the study of Roldaan and Masural (2) strongly suggests that an asthma attack may be the only symptom of a virus infection in an asthmatic subject.

J. Relationships Between Virus Infections and Markers of Atopy

Table 10 shows the results of studies that have compared viral detection rates in atopic and nonatopic subjects (20,21,28,33,63,70). Atopy has been mostly defined

Table 10 Overall Virus Identification Rates in Atopic and Nonatopic Subjects

Author (Ref.)	Year	Virology method[a]	Atopy criteria	Atopic virus identification rate		Nonatopic virus identification rate		Odds ratio	95% CI
Horn (20)	1979	Conventional	SPT	25/58	43.1%	10/14	71.4%	0.30	0.09, 1.08
Cogswell (70)	1982	Conventional	SPT/eczema	23/43	53.5%	28/49	57.1%	0.86	0.38, 1.97
Carlsen (21)	1984	Conventional	SPT, IgE, RAST	48/179	26.8%	25/76	32.9%	0.75	0.42, 1.34
Duff (6)	1993	Conventional	RAST	14/44	31.8%	8/24	33.3%	0.93	0.32, 2.69
Rossi (28)	1994	Conventional	SPT	17/44	38.6%	24/68	35.3%	1.15	0.53, 2.53
Pattemore (63)		With PCR	SPT	119/154	77.3%	109/136	80.1%	0.84	0.48, 1.48
Rakes (8)	1999	With PCR	RAST	14/24	58.3%	20/24	83.3%	0.28	0.07, 1.08
Wark (33)	2002	With PCR	SPT	21/29	72.4%	16/20	80.0%	0.66	0.17, 2.57
Weighted averages		Conventional		127/368	34.5%	95/231	41.1%	0.75	0.54, 1.06
Weighted averages		With PCR		154/207	74.4%	145/180	80.6%	0.70	0.43, 1.14
Weighted averages		All studies		281/575	48.9%	240/140	58.4%	0.68	0.53, 0.88

[a] "Conventional" refers to studies that did not use PCR for virus identification.

by skin prick testing and in a few studies by various combinations of high IgE, positive RAST tests, and the presence of atopic eczema. Virus identification rates in atopic subjects range from 26.8 to 53.5%, with a weighted average of 34.5% in studies using conventional virology, and a weighted average of 74.4% in three studies using PCR. The rates in nonatopic subjects were slightly higher in all but the study of Rossi and colleagues (28) (weighted averages 41.1% and 81.6% for conventional and PCR studies respectively). Looked at the other way, the proportion of subjects who were atopic was slightly higher among those who were virus negative (63.9% and 60.2% for conventional and PCR studies, respectively) than among those who were virus positive (57.2% and 51.5%, respectively).

None of the individual studies or the weighted averages of conventional or of PCR studies had significant odds ratios, but when all studies were combined the odds ratio was significant at 0.68 (95% CI: 0.53, 0.88). Although it is probably not valid to combine study results with different virology methods in this way, the consistent tendency in all studies does suggest a weak association between viral infection and being nonatopic or between absence of infection and being atopic. None of the individual studies in Table 10 is powered enough to detect the small difference, but the trend is consistent and would be expected to be significant in a study with more than 375 subjects of whom 50% are atopic. It could be hypothesized that in atopic subjects allergen exposure accounts for a proportion of attacks, and thus virus infection triggers a smaller proportion of attacks than in nonatopic subjects. The evidence for this hypothesis is not strong enough to reach firm conclusions at this point.

Other studies have documented similar viral detection rates in atopic and nonatopic subjects (1) or in subjects with so-called "extrinsic" and "intrinsic" asthma (40). Trigg and colleagues (71), however, in a study with PCR of nonasthmatic subjects, found that those with atopy had fewer viruses identified than those without atopy, which is consistent with the conclusions above.

Two studies in different subjects from the same research group, one study using conventional virology and one using PCR, have documented that the risk of wheezing is highest in subjects who both are atopic and virus positive. Duff and colleagues (6) found that in children over age 2, the odds ratio for wheezing was 4.5 (95% CI: 2.0, 10.2) if there was a positive RAST test, 3.7 (95% CI: 1.3, 10.6) if a virus was identified, and 10.8 (95% CI: 1.9, 59.0) if both were present. Rakes and colleagues (8) showed a similar relationship for rhinovirus infection and RAST positivity, nasal eosinophilia, and elevated nasal levels of eosinophil cationic protein (ECP). Rhinovirus infection gave an odds ratio of wheezing in 2–16-year-old children of 4.4 ($p < 0.002$), and positive RAST gave an odds ratio of 3.2 ($p < 0.02$). The combination of rhinovirus infection and any one of RAST positivity, nasal eosinophilia, or elevated nasal ECP gave odds ratios of, respectively, 17, 21, and 25 (all $p < 0.001$).

Thus although the likelihood of infection may be slightly less in atopic than in nonatopic subjects during a wheezing episode, the combination of atopy and virus infection gives an highly increased risk of acute wheezing.

K. Do Viruses Trigger Asthma When Inoculated into Volunteers?

Experimental inoculation of viruses, particularly laboratory-cultured rhinoviruses such as human rhinovirus-16, has been undertaken in asthmatic, atopic, and normal subjects (all of whom have been adult volunteers) to try to determine the precise effects of rhinovirus infection on airway narrowing, bronchial hyperresponsiveness, and airway cytological and cytokine response. Most studies (72–75) have not shown a significant drop in spirometry readings, but bronchial responsiveness increased in asthmatic and sometimes normal subjects in the same studies. Grunberg and colleagues (76) studied mild atopic asthmatics with RV-16 inoculation and documented decreases in FEV_1 on home spirometry. Bardin and co-workers (77) found decreases in peak expiratory flow (PEF) in 2 of 11 normal subjects, 1 of 3 atopic subjects, and 3 of 6 atopic asthmatic subjects, again in association with RV-16 colds.

Airway eosinophils and IL-8 levels have been found to be increased by rhinovirus colds (73,74). One study found no difference between asthmatic and healthy subjects in their response to RV-16 infection (75). Bardin and colleagues, in a study of atopic and normal subjects, showed heightened severity of infection in atopic subjects with rhinovirus colds (78). The study of Trigg et al. of naturally occurring colds in atopic and nonatopic individuals (71) found an increase in activated airway eosinophils only in atopic subjects and those who were virus-negative during a common cold.

The studies available to date do not lead to a clear conclusion about the effect of experimental inoculation of rhinoviruses on asthma. These experimentally induced infections may differ substantially from naturally occurring colds because the prior exposure and immunity to RV-16 may vary considerably between adult subjects and cause differences in their response. Furthermore, the repeated passage of these viruses through laboratory culture media may result in lower virulence than wild-type rhinovirus.

III. Do Virus Infections Trigger Asthma Attacks?

A. Koch's Postulates

The evidence presented in this chapter for the causative role of respiratory viruses in asthma exacerbations can be examined against Koch's postulates. For a single agent-specific disease the postulates are that to be a proven agent of the disease the following conditions must be met:

The agent must be present in every case of the disease.

The agent must be isolated from the host and grown in vitro.

The disease must be reproduced when a pure culture of the agent is inoculated into a healthy susceptible host.

The same agent must be recovered again from the experimentally infected host.

These criteria obviously have limitations when applied to a multifactorial disease, when a heterogeneous group of agents (rather than a single agent) is in question, and when the technology for isolating agents is in evolution. However, if one accepts "agents" rather than "agent" and "most cases" instead of "every case" the case for viruses causing (triggering) attacks of asthma is as follows:

> Respiratory viruses (and atypical bacteria) have been identified by sensitive means in upwards of 80% of episodes of wheezing or asthma exacerbations in infants and school-aged children and in 40–60% of such episodes in adults and the elderly.

> These sensitive tests (PCR) are pure in that they detect specific nucleic acid for a particular virus species. Many studies have also isolated viruses by culture, serology, and immunofluorescence in up to 50% of episodes of wheezing in children and in up to 30% of episodes of wheezing in adults.

> The disease has not been reliably reproduced after experimental inoculations of human rhinovirus-16. However experimental inoculation of this virus may substantially differ from naturally occurring colds with wild-type virus. Inoculation of an asthmatic subject with freshly isolated virus from another asthmatic subject with an acute episode of wheeze has not been performed. These days such a procedure may face barriers of an ethical nature because of concerns about transferring body fluids or infectious agents. In addition, there is no adequate animal model of asthma in which to study this.

> For the same reasons, virus identification in a secondary inoculated case has not been performed as yet. Indirect evidence of this might be acquired from naturally occurring cross-infection among asthmatic subjects (e.g., siblings) with demonstration of the same virus by genetic fingerprinting.

B. Other Criteria of Biological Causality

Other evidence that viruses trigger asthma attacks can be listed as follows:

1. The notion that viruses infecting the respiratory tract could trigger respiratory tract obstruction in susceptible individuals is both biologically plausible and consistent with clinical experience.
2. Very high and significant odds ratios (weighted average 6.77 in conventional virology studies and 10.17 in PCR studies) have been obtained for the association of virus infection with asthma exacerbations in case–control studies performed with asymptomatic or nonrespiratory cases as controls. Every study for which these figures are available has a significant, high odds ratio.
3. The rate of viral identification is similar (odds ratio not significant) in cases with wheeze and in controls with nonwheezy respiratory infection in all studies performed.
4. The age-related changes in predominant virus are the same for viruses associated with wheeze episodes and those prevalent in all respiratory infections.
5. The seasonal variation in asthma attacks very closely follows that of virus infections in populations of adults and children.

6. The seasonal variation in asthma attacks does not follow that of any other environmental influence studied, including aeroallergen levels, air pollution, and climatic changes.

7. The time course of an asthma exacerbation associated with viral sero-conversion is very similar to the time course of respiratory virus infection (2).

8. Asthma attacks are very closely temporally related to virus infections in individuals and symptoms of viral infection almost always precede symptoms of asthma during exacerbations.

9. The risk of wheezing is substantial (30–55%) in asthmatic subjects who have an identified respiratory virus infection, (particularly rhinovirus, coronavirus or RSV). The risk is especially high in atopic subjects.

10. There is a suggestion of a dose–response relationship between severity of infection and severity of asthma, but this is not adequately documented to date.

IV. Conclusions and Suggestions for Further Study

The epidemiological evidence presented leaves very little room for doubt that viruses are causally linked to asthma exacerbations and are the most common triggers of asthma attacks in children and in adults. Further epidemiological studies of this association will add very little to this conclusion, except to document new organisms that may be associated with asthma attacks.

The only weak link in the chain of evidence is the incomplete reproduction of asthma attacks in adult volunteers inoculated with rhinovirus-16. As explained previously, there are very good reasons why this may be so. To get around these obstacles and complete Koch's criteria, a study would have to inoculate asthmatic subjects with a virus to which they are immunologically naive and that has been freshly recovered in pure culture from an asthmatic subject during an asthma attack. This study will be difficult to perform since most adult subjects will have experienced many rhinovirus, coronavirus, and RSV infections, and ethical considerations would bar experimental inoculation in children. An animal model of asthma would be of great assistance here.

Notwithstanding this area of weak data, I would argue that the combined weight of epidemiological evidence for biological causation is such that no other conclusion can be sustained. The importance of this finding is that viruses are recognized as the most common triggers of asthma, and that their contribution to asthma morbidity is acknowledged.

Two studies of United Kingdom doctors' views on and prescribing habits for asthma attacks reported high rates of antibiotic use. Connolly and colleagues (79) found that 91% of general practitioners, 71% of general physicians, 100% of chest physicians, and 100% of pediatricians believed that viruses were the most likely type of infection associated with acute asthma. The risk of bacterial infection was listed as greater than 20% by up to 50% of general practitioners, 83% of general physicians, 43% of chest physicians, and 10% of pediatricians, more so in intrinsic than extrinsic asthma. Antibiotics were prescribed for asthma frequently by 42% and sometimes by 92% of general practitioners. For general physicians the figures were 69% and 60%, for chest physicians 29% and 29%, and for pediatricians 6% and 63%. The authors noted also that "there was a tendency for frequent prescribers of antibiotics to withhold corticosteroids." Jones and Gruffydd-Jones (80) in 1996 surveyed general practitioners regarding their management of constructed histories of asthma attacks in a child and in an adult. Antibiotics would have been prescribed by 66% of the doctors for the adult case and by 58% of the doctors for the child.

These two studies indicate that antibiotics are being inappropriately prescribed for attacks of asthma although bacterial infection (other than atypical bacteria in a small proportion of attacks) has been shown *not* to be associated with asthma attacks in many studies. This practice is of concern as it will unnecessarily increase antibiotic use and bacterial resistance in the community. As the study of Connolly and others (79) suggested, more appropriate treatments may not be used if antibiotics are prescribed.

The large contribution of virus infections to asthma morbidity that is implied by their role in triggering up to 80% of attacks needs also to be understood. This morbidity makes a strong case for investigating measures aimed at preventing virus infections in asthmatic subjects and blocking the ability of viruses to trigger asthma (81). This needs to be undertaken in addition to work to prevent the development of asthma. Simple measures that are easily available (such as regular handwashing with soap, and avoiding or keeping at least 1 m distance from people with colds) can be recommended to asthmatic subjects now, since they are safe and have evidence from cross-infection control studies to commend them.

Work to prevent binding of virus to the airway epithelium, and preventing its activation and reproduction, is in progress, and new ways of pre-empting an attack in asthmatic subjects who already have an infection should be explored. The practice of doubling the dosage of inhaled steroids at the onset of an attack has been shown not to be useful in children who are taking maintenance inhaled steroids (82). However, the use of inhaled steroids episodically for "viral wheeze" in children who are not using them as maintenance lowered the risk of requiring oral corticosteroids (relative risk 0.53, 95% CI: 0.27, 1.04) in two studies reported in the Cochrane review by McKean and Ducharme (4).

To further our understanding of the relationship between asthma and viruses beyond what we can ascertain from the studies so far, an ideal epidemiological study would need to have the following characteristics.

Prospective design

Intensive daily follow-up of symptoms and lung function over a period of at least 12 months

Large number of cases (300 or more) with clearly defined asthma

Control group without asthma drawn from the same sampling population studied in parallel

Reporting of all respiratory episodes

Regular surveillance of induced nasal secretions with PCR for all respiratory viruses, and atypical bacteria

Study of all respiratory episodes with PCR as above, and consideration given to viral culture (to confirm the presence of live virus) and serology (to confirm infection rather than carriage)

Similar handling of control and case specimens

Internal positive and negative controls for each virus included in-line with all PCR specimens and PCR analysis assessed in blinded fashion

Such studies are very expensive and time-consuming and it is often difficult to recruit control subjects for a prospective study. However, a study that was able to meet these criteria would allow more definite conclusions especially in regard to subgroup analysis, for instance, the relationship of atopy to virus infection.

In conclusion, viruses are the most common and important triggers of asthma attacks and episodes of wheezing in infants, children, adults, and the elderly. It is vital to improving the health of asthmatics that we aim to prevent or ameliorate virus-induced asthma.

Acknowledgments

I am grateful to my colleagues Fiona Lampe and Sebastian Johnston for providing further data from the Southampton cohort study for this chapter.

References

1. Mertsola J, Ziegler T, Ruuskanen O, Vanto T, Koivikko A, Halonen P. Recurrent wheezy bronchitis and viral respiratory infections. Arch Dis Child 1991; 66:124–129.
2. Roldaan AC, Masural N. Viral respiratory infections in asthmatic children staying in a mountain resort. Eur J Respir Dis 1982; 63:140–150.
3. Johnston SL, Pattemore PK, Sanderson G, Smith S, Lampe F, Josephs L, Symington P, O'Toole S, Myint SH, Tyrrell DA, Holgate ST. Community study of role of viral infections in exacerbations of asthma in 9–11 year old children. Br Med J 1995; 310: 1225–1229.
4. McKean M, du Charme F. Inhaled steroids for episodic viral wheeze of childhood (Cochrane Review). In: The Cochrane Library, 4, 2000. Oxford: Update Software.
5. Pattemore PK, Johnston SL, Bardin PG. Viruses as precipitants of asthma symptoms. I. Epidemiology. Clin Exp Allergy 1992; 22:325–336.
6. Duff AL, Pomeranz ES, Gelber LE, Price GW, Farris H, Hayden FG, Platts-Mills TA, Heymann PW. Risk factors for acute wheezing in infants and children: viruses, passive smoke, and IgE antibodies to inhalant allergens. Pediatrics 1993; 92:535–540.
7. Rylander E, Eriksson M, Pershagen G, Nordvall L, Ehrnst A, Ziegler T. Wheezing bronchitis in children. Incidence, viral infections, and other risk factors in a defined population. Pediatr Allergy Immunol 1996; 7:6–11.
8. Rakes GP, Arruda E, Ingram JM, Hoover GE, Zambrano JC, Hayden FG, Platts-Mills TA, Heymann PW. Rhinovirus and respiratory syncytial virus in wheezing children

requiring emergency care. IgE and eosinophil analyses. Am J Respir Crit Care Med 1999; 159:785–790.

9. Pitkaranta A, Virolainen A, Jero J, Arruda E, Hayden FG. Detection of rhinovirus, respiratory syncytial virus, and coronavirus infections in acute otitis media by reverse transcriptase polymerase chain reaction. Pediatrics 1998; 102:291–295.

10. Pitkaranta A, Jero J, Arruda E, Virolainen A, Hayden FG. Polymerase chain reaction-based detection of rhinovirus, respiratory syncytial virus, and coronavirus in otitis media with effusion. J Pediatr 1998; 133:390–394.

11. McMillan JA, Weiner LB, Higgins AM, Macknight K. Rhinovirus infection associated with serious illness among pediatric patients. Pediatr Infect Dis J 1993; 12:321–325.

12. Gatchalian SR, Quiambao BP, Morelos AM, Abraham L, Gepanayao CP, Sombrero LT, Paladin JF, Soriano VC, Obach M, Sunico ES. Bacterial and viral etiology of serious infections in very young Filipino infants. Pediatr Infect Dis J 1999; 18:S50–55.

13. Tyrrell DAJ. A collaborative study of the aetiology of acute respiratory infections in Britain 1961–4. Br Med J 1965; 2:319–326.

14. Disney ME, Matthews R, Williams JD. The role of infection in the morbidity of asthmatic children admitted to hospital. Clin Allergy 1971; 1:399–406.

15. Glezen WP, Loda FA, Clyde WA Jr, Senior RJ, Sheaffer CI, Conley WG, Denny FW. Epidemiologic patterns of acute lower respiratory disease of children in a pediatric group practice. J Pediatr 1971; 78:397–406.

16. Horn ME, Brain E, Gregg I, Yealland SJ, Inglis JM. Respiratory viral infection in childhood. A survey in general practice, Roehampton 1967–1972. J Hyg (Lond) 1975; 74: 157–168.

17. Mitchell I, Inglis H, Simpson H. Viral infection in wheezy bronchitis and asthma in children. Arch Dis Child 1976; 51:707–711.

18. Henderson FW, Clyde WA Jr, Collier AM, Denny FW, Senior RJ, Sheaffer CI, Conley WG III, Christian RM. The etiologic and epidemiologic spectrum of bronchiolitis in pediatric practice. J Pediatr 1979; 95:183–190.

19. Horn ME, Brain EA, Gregg I, Inglis JM, Yealland SJ, Taylor P. Respiratory viral infection and wheezy bronchitis in childhood. Thorax 1979; 34:23–28.

20. Horn ME, Reed SE, Taylor P. Role of viruses and bacteria in acute wheezy bronchitis in childhood: a study of sputum. Arch Dis Child 1979; 54:587–592.

21. Carlsen KH, Ørstavik I, Leegaard J, Hoeg H. Respiratory virus infections and aeroallergens in acute bronchial asthma. Arch Dis Child 1984; 59:310–315.

22. Jennings LC, Barns G, Dawson KP. The association of viruses with acute asthma. NZ Med J 1987; 100:488–490.

23. Freymuth F, Vabret A, Brouard J, Toutain F, Verdon R, Petitjean J, Gouarin S, Duhamel JF, Guillois B. Detection of viral, Chlamydia pneumoniae and Mycoplasma pneumoniae infections in exacerbations of asthma in children. J Clin Virol 1999; 13:131–139.

24. Landau LI. Asthma: Prognosis. In: Taussig LM, Landau LI, eds. Pediatric Respiratory Medicine. St Louis: Mosby, 1999:935.

25. Mitchell I, Inglis JM, Simpson H. Viral infection as a precipitant of wheeze in children. Combined home and hospital study. Arch Dis Child 1978; 53:106–111.

26. Saijo M, Ishii T, Kokubo M, Takimoto M, Takahashi Y. Respiratory syncytial virus infection in lower respiratory tract and asthma attack in hospitalized children in North Hokkaido, Japan. Acta Paediatr Jpn 1993; 35:233–237.

27. Allegra L, Blasi F, Centanni S, Cosentini R, Denti F, Raccanelli R, Tarsia P, Valenti V. Acute exacerbations of asthma in adults: role of Chlamydia pneumoniae infection. Eur Respir J 1994; 7:2165–2168.

28. Rossi OV, Kinnula VL, Tuokko H, Huhti E. Respiratory viral and Mycoplasma infections in patients hospitalized for acute asthma. Monaldi Arch Chest Dis 1994; 49:107–111.

29. Abramson M, Pearson L, Kutin J, Czarny D, Dziukas L, Bowes G. Allergies, upper respiratory tract infections, and asthma. J Asthma 1994; 31:367–374.

30. Sokhandan M, McFadden ER Jr, Huang YT, Mazanec MB. The contribution of respiratory viruses to severe exacerbations of asthma in adults. Chest 1995; 107:1570–1574.

31. Teichtahl H, Buckmaster N, Pertnikovs E. The incidence of respiratory tract infection in adults requiring hospitalization for asthma. Chest 1997; 112:591–596.

32. Atmar RL, Guy E, Guntupalli KK, Zimmerman JL, Bandi VD, Baxter BD, Greenberg SB. Respiratory tract viral infections in inner-city asthmatic adults. Arch Intern Med 1998; 158:2453–2459.

33. Wark AB, Johnston SL, Moric I, Simpson JL, Hensley MJ, Gibson PG. Neutrophil degranulation and cell lysis is associated with clinical severity in virus-induced asthma. Eur Respir J 2002; 19:68–75.

34. Berkovich S, Millian SJ, Snyder RD. The association of viral and mycoplasma infections with recurrence of wheezing in the asthmatic child. Ann Allergy 1970; 28:43–49.

35. Lambert HP, Stern H. Infective factors in exacerbations of bronchitis and asthma. Br Med J 1972; 3:323–327.

36. McIntosh K, Ellis EF, Hoffman LS, Lybass TG, Eller JJ, Fulginiti VA. The association of viral and bacterial respiratory infections with exacerbations of wheezing in young asthmatic children. J Pediatr 1973; 82:578–590.

37. Minor TE, Dick EC, DeMeo AN, Ouellette JJ, Cohen M, Reed CE. Viruses as precipitants of asthmatic attacks in children. JAMA 1974; 227:292–298.

38. Minor TE, Dick EC, Baker JW, Ouellette JJ, Cohen M, Reed CE. Rhinovirus and influenza type A infections as precipitants of asthma. Am Rev Respir Dis 1976; 113 :149–153.

39. Johnston SL, Pattemore PK, Sanderson G, Smith S, Lampe F, Josephs L, Symington P, O'Toole S, Myint SH, Tyrrell DA, Holgate ST. Unpublished data, 1995.

40. Huhti E, Mokka T, Nikoskelainen J, Halonen P. Association of viral and mycoplasma infections with exacerbations of asthma. Ann Allergy 1974; 33:145–149.

41. Hudgel DW, Langston L Jr, Selner JC, McIntosh K. Viral and bacterial infections in adults with chronic asthma. Am Rev Respir Dis 1979; 120:393–397.

42. Clarke CW. Relationship of bacterial and viral infections to exacerbations of asthma. Thorax 1979; 34:344–347.

43. Beasley R, Coleman ED, Hermon Y, Holst PE, O'Donnell TV, Tobias M. Viral respiratory tract infection and exacerbations of asthma in adult patients. Thorax 1988; 43:679–683.

44. Nicholson KG, Kent J, Ireland DC. Respiratory viruses and exacerbations of asthma in adults. Br Med J 1993; 307:982–986.

45. Nicholson KG, Kent J, Hammersley V, Cancio E. Acute viral infections of upper respiratory tract in elderly people living in the community: comparative, prospective, population based study of disease burden. Br Med J 1997; 315:1060–1064.

46. Pitkaranta A, Hayden FG. Rhinoviruses: important respiratory pathogens. Ann Med 1998; 30:529–537.

47. Berman SZ, Mathison DA, Stevenson DD, Tan EM, Vaughan JH. Transtracheal aspiration studies in asthmatic patients in relapse with "infective" asthma and in subjects without respiratory disease. J Allergy Clin Immunol 1975; 56:206–214.

48. Kuga H, Hoshiyama Y, Kokubu F, Imai T, Tokunaga H, Matsukura S, Kawaguchi M, Adachi M, Kawaguchi T. [The correlation between the exacerbation of bronchial asthma and Picornavirus (human rhino virus) infection in throat gargles by RT-PCR]. Arerugi 2000; 49:358–364.

49. West JA, Dakhama A, Khan MA, Vedal S, Hegele RG. Community study using a polymerase chain reaction panel to determine the prevalence of common respiratory viruses in asthmatic and nonasthmatic children. J Asthma 1999; 36:605–612.

50. Macek V, Dakhama A, Hogg JC, Green FH, Rubin BK, Hegele RG. PCR detection of viral nucleic acid in fatal asthma: is the lower respiratory tract a reservoir for common viruses? Can Respir J 1999; 6:37–43.

51. Hogg JC. Persistent and latent viral infections in the pathology of asthma. (Review). Am Rev Respir Dis 1992; 145:S7–9.

52. Hogg JC. Adenoviral infection and childhood asthma [editorial; comment]. Am J Respir Crit Care Med 1994; 150:2–3.

53. Macek V, Sorli J, Kopriva S, Marin J. Persistent adenoviral infection and chronic airway obstruction in children. Am J Respir Crit Care Med 1994; 150:7–10.

54. Engblom E, Ekfors TO, Meurman OH, Toivanen A, Nikoskelainen J. Fatal influenza A myocarditis with isolation of virus from the myocardium. Acta Med Scand 1983; 213:75–78.

55. Kron J, Lucas L, Lee TD, McAnulty J. Myocardial infarction following an acute viral illness. Arch Intern Med 1983; 143:1466–1467.

56. Tillett HE, Smith JW, Gooch CD. Excess deaths attributable to influenza in England and Wales: age at death and certified cause. Int J Epidemiol 1983; 12:344–352.

57. Visseren FL, Bouwman JJ, Bouter KP, Diepersloot RJ, de Groot PH, Erkelens DW. Procoagulant activity of endothelial cells after infection with respiratory viruses. Thromb Haemost 2000; 84:319–324.

58. Storr J, Lenney W. School holidays and admissions with asthma. Arch Dis Child 1989; 64:103–107.

59. Johnston SL, Pattemore PK, Sanderson G, Smith S, Campbell MJ, Josephs LK, Cunningham A, Robinson BS, Myint SH, Ward ME, Tyrrell DA, Holgate ST. The relationship between upper respiratory infections and hospital admissions for asthma: a time-trend analysis. Am J Resp Crit Care Med 1996; 154:654–660.

60. Carlsen KH, Ørstavik I. Bronchopulmonary obstruction in children with respiratory virus infections. Eur J Respir Dis 1984; 65:92–98.

61. Potter PC, Weinberg E, Shore SC. Acute severe asthma. A prospective study of the precipitating factors in 40 children. S Afr Med J 1984; 66:397–402.

62. Dales RE, Schweitzer I, Toogood JH, Drouin M, Yang W, Dolovich J, Boulet J. Respiratory infections and the autumn increase in asthma morbidity. Eur Respir J 1996; 9:72–77.

63. Pattemore PK, Lampe FC, Smith S, Clough JB, Holgate ST, Johnston SL. Unpublished data, 2000.

64. Tarlo S, Broder I, Spence L. A prospective study of respiratory infection in adult asthmatics and their normal spouses. Clin Allergy 1979; 9:293–301.

65. Isaacs D, Clarke JR, Tyrrell DA, Valman HB. Selective infection of lower respiratory tract by respiratory viruses in children with recurrent respiratory tract infections. Br Med J (Clin Res Ed) 1982; 284:1746–1748.

66. Horn ME, Gregg I. Role of viral infection and host factors in acute episodes of asthma and chronic bronchitis. Chest 1973; 63(suppl):44S–48S.

67. Vignola AM, Campbell AM, Chanez P, Bousquet J, Paul-Lacoste P, Michel FB, Godard P. HLA-DR and ICAM-1 expression on bronchial epithelial cells in asthma and chronic bronchitis. Am Rev Respir Dis 1993; 148:689–694.
68. Johnston SL. Viruses and asthma. Allergy 1998; 53:922–932.
69. Gern JE, Busse WW. Association of rhinovirus infections with asthma. Clin Microbiol Rev 1999; 12:9–18.
70. Cogswell JJ, Halliday DF, Alexander JR. Respiratory infections in the first year of life in children at risk of developing atopy. Br Med J (Clin Res Ed) 1982; 284:1011–1013.
71. Trigg CJ, Nicholson KG, Wang JH, Ireland DC, Jordan S, Duddle JM, Hamilton S, Davies RJ. Bronchial inflammation and the common cold: a comparison of atopic and non-atopic individuals. Clin Exp Allergy 1996; 26:665–676.
72. Cheung D, Dick EC, Timmers MC, de Klerk EP, Spaan WJ, Sterk PJ. Rhinovirus inhalation causes long-lasting excessive airway narrowing in response to methacholine in asthmatic subjects in vivo. Am J Respir Crit Care Med 1995; 152:1490–1496.
73. Fraenkel DJ, Bardin PG, Sanderson G, Lampe F, Johnston SL, Holgate ST. Lower airways inflammation during rhinovirus colds in normal and in asthmatic subjects. Am J Respir Crit Care Med 1995; 151:879–886.
74. Grunberg K, Kuijpers EA, de Klerk EP, de Gouw HW, Kroes AC, Dick EC, Sterk PJ. Effects of experimental rhinovirus 16 infection on airway hyperresponsiveness to bradykinin in asthmatic subjects in vivo. Am J Respir Crit Care Med 1997; 155:833–838.
75. Fleming HE, Little FF, Schnurr D, Avila PC, Wong H, Liu J, Yagi S, Boushey HA. Rhinovirus-16 colds in healthy and in asthmatic subjects: similar changes in upper and lower airways. Am J Respir Critical Care Med 1999; 160:100–108.
76. Grunberg K, Timmers MC, de Klerk EP, Dick EC, Sterk PJ. Experimental rhinovirus 16 infection causes variable airway obstruction in subjects with atopic asthma. Am J Respir Crit Care Med 1999; 160:1375–1380.
77. Bardin PG, Fraenkel DJ, Sanderson G, van Schalkwyk EM, Holgate ST, Johnston SL. Peak expiratory flow changes during experimental rhinovirus infection. Eur Respir J 2000; 16:980–985.
78. Bardin PG, Fraenkel DJ, Sanderson G, Dorward M, Lau LC, Johnston SL, Holgate ST. Amplified rhinovirus colds in atopic subjects. Clin Exp Allergy 1994; 24:457–464.
79. Connolly CK, Murthy NK, Prescott RJ, Alcock RM. Infection in exacerbations of asthma: views of different groups of practitioners. Postgrad Med J 1991; 67:892–896.
80. Jones K, Gruffydd-Jones K. Management of acute asthma attacks associated with respiratory tract infection: a postal survey of general practitioners in the U.K. Respir Med 1996; 90:419–425.
81. Openshaw PJ, Lemanske RF. Respiratory viruses and asthma: can the effects be prevented? Eur Respir J Suppl 1998; 27:35s–39s.
82. Garrett J, Williams S, Wong C, Holdaway D. Treatment of acute asthmatic exacerbations with an increased dose of inhaled steroid. Arch Dis Child 1998; 79:12–17.

4

Role of Viral Infection in the Inception of Asthma

FERNANDO D. MARTINEZ

University of Arizona
Tucson, Arizona, U.S.A.

The role of viral infection in the inception of asthma is not well understood. The empirical observation of a temporal association between an acute lower respiratory illness (LRI) attributed to viruses and the subsequent development of persistent or recurrent episodes of airway obstruction has suggested to many clinicians and patients a causal relationship. There is what is termed proof of concept for this potential deleterious effect of viruses in the confirmed role of adenoviral infection as a cause of *bronchiolitis obliterans* in early life (1). This has suggested the possibility that this same role may be played by other viruses and, by analogy with *bronchiolitis obliterans*, by those that are more frequently observed during the first years of life.

The most plausible example of this potential association between viral respiratory illness in early life and the subsequent development of asthma is that of the respiratory syncytial virus (RSV). The knowledge that children who have confirmed episodes of RSV–LRI are at increased risk of subsequent wheezing illnesses is solidly supported by both epidemiological evidence and clinical practice. Post-RSV wheezing is a label that many pediatricians use to describe symptoms in infants who have had severe episodes of RSV and, during the subsequent months, seem to develop acute airway obstruction with most viral infections. The label implies some form of causal relation. The nature of this potential causation pathway has been the matter of considerable debate and extensive research, both in humans and in animal models.

This chapter will examine the evidence for a causal association between infection with RSV (and potentially with other respiratory viruses) and the subsequent development of asthma in children. This issue is of great relevance for public health, because of the high morbidity and health care costs attributable to asthma in childhood (2). If the connection were to be confirmed, prevention of viral respiratory infection in early life could become a major strategy for the prevention of asthma.

I. RSV, LRI, and Subsequent Wheezing: Two Possible Scenarios

Before the purpose of this chapter can be pursued any further, it is important to clarify some methodological issues. There is now quite convincing evidence that, by the age of 2 years, the great majority of children show immunological evidence of having encountered and weathered RSV (3). Thorough, prospective studies with stringent surveillance have shown that in two-thirds of all these cases no clinical manifestation or overt episode of LRI became evident (4). Therefore, being universal, it is obviously not RSV infection itself that can be considered the risk factor for subsequent asthma. In this context, the factors that determine acute illness during an RSV infection become, by definition, one of the determinants of the association between RSV infection and asthma. These factors may be of two types: sufficient and interactive. Sufficient factors are defined here as those that would have determined asthma regardless of the incidence of RSV infection. For example, if RSV infection were to prompt the first clinical manifestation of atopic asthma, RSV would be a mere trigger of mechanisms that are essentially independent of it. This could be one explanation for the association between RSV and asthma: it is subjects with subjacent asthma who develop RSV-related *illness*. On the other hand, RSV could interact with other factors: a predisposing genetic background; concomitant exposure to certain environmental factors that increase the risk of LRI; or occurrence of the infection at a critical period in the development of the immune system, lung, or airways. This may trigger a peculiar response to RSV that is associated with acute LRI and subsequent recurrent wheezing. What differentiates this scenario from the first is that, in this case, without RSV illness there would be no subsequent wheezing. However, it is important to stress here that only a small proportion of infants who develop acute RSV-LRI go on to develop recurrent wheezing. Thus, in this second scenario, RSV illness cannot be by itself a sufficient factor for the development of subsequent asthma; factors other than those determining risk for acute LRI must be at work.

II. "Transient" Wheezers and "Persistent" Wheezers

Our group has been particularly interested in determining if there was evidence supporting the existence of these two possible scenarios. For this purpose, we used the data from the Tucson Children's Respiratory Study, a longitudinal assessment of the risk factors for and the long-term consequences of acute LRI in infants (5). In almost 900 children enrolled at birth in 1980–1984, LRIs were ascertained directly by the children's pediatricians, and clinical, immunological, and virological studies were performed at the time of the acute LRI. Follow-up of these children is continuing, and extensive surveys have been performed at 2–4 year intervals for the past 18–22 years. One of our first reported findings was that children who had confirmed LRIs during the first 3 years of life could be classified into two groups: those who were still having reported wheezing illnesses at the age of 6 years (persistent wheezers) and those who were not (transient wheezers) (6). The former group is particularly relevant for this discussion. We will thus concentrate on the risk factors for a persistent wheezer after viral infection in early life.

Several characteristics were found to be different between these two groups: persistent wheezers were more likely to have parental history of asthma, a personal history of eczema and so-called allergic rhinitis, higher levels of total serum IgE at 9 months and at 6 years of age, and a history of wheezing apart from colds during the first 2 years of life. Moreover, over 60% of persistent wheezers were skin test positive (atopic) at age 6 compared with less than 25% of transient wheezers. This proportion was not different from that observed among children who had no reports of wheezing during the first 6 years of life. It is interesting to note that, in our data, persistent wheezers were not more likely to be atopic than children who were also wheezing at age 6 but had not had LRIs (late wheezers). Late wheezers were also as likely to have a family history of asthma as persistent wheezers. These results suggested to us that indeed factors predisposing to asthma could predispose certain children to LRI *and* to subsequent wheezing. An interesting finding was that this association was independent of the cause of the LRI: both infants who had RSV-LRI and those in whom RSV was not isolated at the time of the acute LRI were at increased risk for wheezing at the age of 6 if they had the risk factors associated with persistent wheezing. There was thus no evidence in our data that RSV played a specific role in the association between LRI and subsequent asthma-like symptoms among children at risk for asthma.

III. Heterogeneity of Persistent Wheezing

However, it was also clear in our data that persistent wheezers were not a homogeneous group: up to 40% were not skin test positive at age 6 and most had no personal or family history of allergy or asthma. In order to study further the risk factors that could determine the persistence of symptoms in these children, we performed a longitudinal analysis of the data from the Tucson Children's Respiratory Study (7). We classified children who had LRIs during the first 3 years of life into 4 hierarchical and mutually exclusive groups based on the causes of the first reported LRI: RSV, parainfluenza, other microbial agents, and no isolation of a causative agent. We then studied the outcome of these children as assessed by the reported occurrence of wheezing episodes at ages 6, 8, 11, and 13. The goal of the study was to determine if, after adjusting for other known risk factors (including parental history of asthma, atopic dermatitis, allergic sensitization, and breastfeeding, among others), RSV could still be a risk factor for wheezing during the school years. Our results showed that children who had RSV-LRI in early life were three to four times more likely to have both frequent (more than three episodes in the previous year) and infrequent wheezing at age 6, but this risk decreased markedly with age and was only of borderline significance at age 13. LRIs in which viruses other than RSV were isolated showed similar trends, albeit less consistent due to small numbers of affected children. Skin test reactivity to allergens was unrelated to the occurrence of RSV illness in early life. These results thus suggested that persistent wheezers are part of a heterogeneous group of subjects and that an atopic background is not the only mechanism that underlies the connection between RSV-LRI and wheezing by age 6. Other mechanisms must be at play, because the increased risk of asthma-like symptoms in subjects with a history of RSV-LRI was independent of a family history of asthma and allergies.

IV. Role of Bronchial Hyperresponsiveness

Some indication as to the nonatopic mechanisms that predispose to post-RSV wheezing was provided by the data from the Tucson Children's Respiratory Study. Confirming observations from other studies, it was observed that children with a history of RSV-LRI had significantly lower levels of several parameters derived from spirometric curves, and specifically, low ratios of forced expiratory volume to functional vital capacity (FEV_1/FVC ratios), when compared with children with no such history. These diminished levels of lung function were almost completely reversed by a single dose of albuterol, administered with a metered-dose inhaler (7). These results thus suggested that one possible mechanism by which a history of RSV-LRI may increase the likelihood of subsequent wheezing is a preexisting or acquired alteration in the regulation of airway tone.

Reports from a longitudinal study in western Australia (8–11) have recently provided support for the contention that airway hyperresponsiveness present shortly after birth and before any LRI is a risk factor for post-RSV wheezing. In this study, responses to histamine were assessed during the first months of life and again at age 6. These measures were correlated with the risk of wheezing and with baseline lung function in infancy, with these same phenotypes at age 6, and with the likelihood of being atopic at age 6. There was no association between histamine hyperresponsiveness measured shortly after birth and wheezing in infancy (8), nor was there any relation between baseline lung function in infancy and bronchial hyperresponsiveness (BHR) to histamine measured concomitantly (10). Since level of lung function measured shortly after birth was strongly associated with wheezing during infancy in this same cohort (9), it was clear from these data that BHR and level of lung function were measuring different characteristics of the lung at this very early stage of life. When children were seen again at the age of 6 years, BHR measured at that age was unrelated to BHR at birth (10). However, BHR measured shortly after birth was strongly associated both with lung function and with the likelihood of wheezing at the age of 6 years. Moreover, BHR measured at the age of 6 years was also strongly associated with the likelihood of wheezing at the same age, but independently of BHR measured shortly after birth. BHR at birth was unrelated to allergic sensitization at age 6, whereas BHR at age 6 has been shown to be associated with allergic sensitization at that same age (12). These results thus suggest that at least two separate alterations in the regulation of airway tone could be present in children who wheeze at age 6: one appears to be congenital and unrelated to allergic sensitization, and the other is most likely acquired and strongly associated to skin test reactivity to allergens. Although rates of RSV infection were not measured in the Australian cohort, it is tempting to speculate that both these mechanisms may contribute to the connection between RSV-LRI and subsequent wheezing: children with congenital (and perhaps inherited) BHR may be more prone to wheeze during viral episodes both during the first years of life and at age 6. Children who have abnormal responses to RSV infection may also be left with alterations in the regulation of airway tone that predispose them to subsequent wheezing.

V. Altered Responses to RSV and Subsequent Wheezing

Although many studies have addressed the nature of the response to RSV and its association with the severity of acute RSV-LRI, the immune factors that may explain the increased risk of subsequent wheezing in children with a history of RSV-LRI have not been as extensively explored. In the early 1980s, Welliver et al. (13) reported increased prevalence of RSV-specific IgE in nasal secretions of infants who wheezed during RSV infection and subsequently developed recurrent wheezing episodes. Although these findings are controversial (14), it is plausible to surmise that subjects who are predisposed to have a response to infection that is characterized by a predominance of the T-helper-(Th-)2 cytokines may be more likely to wheeze during RSV infection and to develop the atopic form of the disease later in life.

Our own studies have provided support for this hypothesis. As part of the Tucson Children's Respiratory Study, we measured total serum IgE levels and eosinophil counts at the time of acute LRI and during the convalescent period (approximately 30 days later) for the same LRI ascertained before age 3 (15). We observed that children whom we later classified as persistent wheezers (as defined above) had significantly higher total serum IgE levels and higher eosinophil counts at the time of the acute illness than children who were later classified as transient wheezers. Total serum IgE levels were also significantly higher during the acute phase than those observed during the convalescent phase in persistent wheezers but not in transient wheezers. These associations were observed both for LRI due to RSV and in those due to other viruses or for which no agent was isolated. Similar results to those of our study have been reported by researchers who measured markers of eosinophil activation in serum of patients with acute RSV-LRI: children with high levels of circulating eosinophilic cationic protein are more likely to have subsequent wheezing than those who show low levels of this protein (16,17). These studies have not definitely established if infants who have alterations in these markers of a Th-2 response do so as a consequence of RSV-LRIs, or if these alterations are only markers of an early predisposition to asthma, which would have been detected even in the absence of a LRI. There is, however, little doubt that the presence of immune responses to viral infection skewed towards a Th-2 phenotype during infancy clearly predict the subsequent development of persistent wheezing and could partially explain the association between the latter and RSV-LRI.

Nevertheless, as explained earlier, this cannot be the only mechanism involved in this association. Recent observations also suggest that, in some children, persistence of wheezing after RSV may be the consequence of alterations in immune responses to the virus that do not involve the Th-1/Th-2 paradigm. Bont and co-workers (18) studied cytokine responses of peripheral blood mononuclear cells to nonspecific stimuli (lipopolysaccharide, interferon-γ [IFN-γ] and phytohemagglutinin) during the acute and convalescent phase of RSV requiring hospitalization. They compared these responses in children who did or did not have episodes of wheezing during the subsequent year. The risk of subsequent wheezing was unrelated to interleukin-12 (IL-12) or IFN-γ/IL-4 responses during the acute or convalescent phase of the RSV-LRI. The IFN-γ/IL-4 responses were negatively associated with a family history of allergy, suggesting that at least in this group of children, a predisposition to atopic asthma did not explain the association between RSV-LRI and subsequent wheezing. However, children who had episodes of wheezing after RSV had significantly higher IL-10 responses during the convalescent phase of the LRI than those observed in children who did not have subsequent wheezing episodes. Moreover, there was a strong positive correlation between the number of wheezing episodes during the subsequent year and the intensity of the IL-10 response. These results thus suggested that factors that predispose to high IL-10 responses during the convalescent period of RSV-LRI may predispose to the development of post-RSV wheezing.

The mechanisms by which IL-10 responses during acute infection could predispose to persistent wheezing after RSV remain unresolved. Bont et al. (18) did not specifically determine the cells responsible for the production of IL-10 in their studies, but speculated that most likely these were antigen-presenting cells, since the results were obtained after stimulation with lipopolysaccharide and IFN-γ. A paradoxical finding is that more recent studies of IL-10 responses by peripheral blood mononuclear cells to mitogens measured before the development of any LRI show an inverse association with the likelihood of having wheezing LRIs during the first year of life (19). No studies have assessed if there is an association between pre-LRI IL-10 responses and IL-10 responses during the convalescent phase of a LRI, but it is plausible to surmise that different cells and different mechanisms may be involved in one and the other. IL-10 is a potent downregulator of both Th-1 and Th-2 responses in humans (20). It is thus possible that individuals with strong preexisting IL-10 responses may have attenuated inflammatory reactions to RSV and may thus be less likely to develop acute LRI. On the other hand, strong IL-10 responses during the LRI may foster the activity of an invasive virus such as RSV by excessive downregulation of the immune response to the infectious agent.

Recent studies in animal models suggest that an alternative explanation is also possible: IL-10 may have a direct effect in airway smooth muscle and in the regulation of airway tone (21,22). Wild-type mice infected with RSV showed significant subsequent increases in BHR compared with sham-infected animals. This increase in BHR was not observed when the same experiments were performed in animals in which the IL-10 gene had been rendered dysfunctional and, therefore, these animals were unable to produce IL-10. These results suggested that IL-10 may not only have direct activity on immune cells but may also have a direct role in the regulation of airway tone (22). The mechanisms involved are not well understood, but open a new field in our understanding of the potential role of cytokines that, until recently, were not known to be able to exert their function in cells other than those of the immune system.

The finding of a potential role of interleukins such as IL-10 on airway function/responsiveness independent of the Th-1/Th-2 paradigm may offer a new basis for our understanding of those forms of recurrent wheezing during childhood that are not associated with increased risk of allergic sensitization.

VI. Conclusions

The mechanisms that determine the association between RSV-LRI and the subsequent development of persistent episodes of wheezing are complex and heterogeneous. In certain children, a predisposition to atopic asthma may explain both the development of acute RSV-LRI and the subsequent development of IgE-associated asthma. Children with congenital BHR unrelated to the atopic phenotype may also be more prone to present with acute airway obstruction during viral LRI and to develop recurrent episodes of wheezing thereafter. Finally, abnormal responses to RSV and other viruses may prime the airways for the development of alterations in the regulation of airway tone. Although each of these three mechanisms may separately explain post-RSV wheezing in different children, they may also overlap in the same child, thus determining the wide spectrum of severity and chronicity of this condition in the general population.

References

1. Murtagh P, Kajon A. Chronic pulmonary sequelae of adenovirus infection. Pediatr Pulmon 1997; 16:150–151.
2. Sears MR. Consequences of long-term inflammation. The natural history of asthma. Clin Chest Med 2000; 21(2):315–329.
3. Glezen WP, Taber LH, Frank AL, Kasel JA. Risk of primary infection and reinfection with respiratory syncytial virus. Am J Dis Child 1986; 140(6):543–546.
4. Wright AL, Taussig LM, Ray CG, Harrison HR, Holberg CJ. The Tucson Children's

Respiratory Study. II. Lower respiratory tract illness in the first year of life. Am J Epidemiol 1989; 129(6):1232–1246.

5. Taussig LM, Wright AL, Morgan WJ, Harrison HR, Ray CG. The Tucson Children's Respiratory Study. I. Design and implementation of a prospective study of acute and chronic respiratory illness in children. Am J Epidemiol 1989; 129(6):1219–1231.

6. Martinez FD, Wright AL, Taussig LM, Holberg CJ, Halonen M, Morgan WJ, The Group Health Medical Associates. Asthma and wheezing in the first six years of life. N Engl J Med 1995; 332(3):133–138.

7. Stein RT, Sherrill D, Morgan WJ, Holberg CJ, Halonen M, Taussig LM, Wright AL, Martinez FD. Respiratory syncytial virus in early life and risk of wheeze and allergy by age 13 years. Lancet 1999; 353:541–545.

8. Stick SM, Arnott J, Turner DJ, Young S, Landau LI, Le Souef PN. Bronchial responsiveness and lung function in recurrently wheezy infants. Am Rev Respir Dis 1991; 144(5):1012–1015.

9. Young S, Arnott J, O'Keeffe PT, Le Souef PN, Landau LI. The association between early life lung function and wheezing during the first 2 yrs of life. Eur Respir J 2000; 15(1):151–157.

10. Palmer LJ, Rye PJ, Gibson NA, Burton PR, Landau LI, Le Souef PN. Airway responsiveness in early infancy predicts asthma, lung function, and respiratory symptoms by school age. Am J Respir Crit Care Med 2001; 163(1):37–42.

11. Turner SW, Palmer LJ, Rye PJ, Gibson NA, Judge PK, Young S, Landau LI, Le Souef PN. Infants with flow limitation at 4 weeks: outcome at 6 and 11 years. Am J Respir Crit Care Med 2002; 165(9):1294–1298.

12. Lombardi E, Morgan WJ, Wright AL, Stein RT, Holberg CJ, Martinez FD. Cold air challenge at age 6 and subsequent incidence of asthma. A longitudinal study. Am J Respir Crit Care Med 1997; 156(6):1863–1869.

13. Welliver RC, Wong DT, Sun M, Middleton E Jr, Vaughan RS, Ogra PL. The development of respiratory syncytial virus-specific IgE and the release of histamine in nasopharyngeal secretions after infection. N Engl J Med 1981; 305(15):841–846.

14. de Alarcon A, Walsh EE, Carper HT, La Russa JB, Evans BA, Rakes GP, Platts-Mills TA, Heymann PW. Detection IgA and IgG but not IgE antibody to respiratory syncytial virus in nasal washes and sera from infants with wheezing. J Pediatr 2001; 138(3):311–317.

15. Martinez FD, Stern DA, Wright AL, Taussig LM, Halonen M. Differential immune responses to acute lower respiratory illness in early life by subsequent development of persistent wheezing and asthma. J Allergy Clin Immunol 1998; 102:915–920.

16. Reijonen TM, Korppi M, Kuikka L, Savolainen K, Kleemola M, Mononen I, Renes K. Serum eosinophil cationic protein as a predictor of wheezing after bronchiolitis. Pediatr Pulmonol 1997; 23(6):397–403.

17. Pifferi M, Ragazzo V, Caramella D, Baldini G. Eosinophil cationic protein in infants with respiratory syncytial virus bronchiolitis: predictive value for subsequent development of persistent wheezing. Pediatr Pulmonol 2001; 31(6):419–424.

18. Bont L, Heijnen CJ, Kavelaars A, van Aalderen WM, Brus F, Draaisma JT, Geelen SM, Kimpen J. Monocyte IL-10 production during respiratory syncytial virus bronchiolitis is associated with recurrent wheezing in a one-year follow-up study. Am J Respir Crit Care Med 2000; 161(5):1518–1523.

19. Tesse R, Wright AL, Martinez FD, Halonen M. IL-10 responses associated with risk of recurrent wheeze in infancy and IL-10 gene single nucleotide polymorphisms (SNPs). Am J Respir Crit Care Med 2002; 165(8):A796.

20. Rennick D, Berg D, Holland G. Interleukin 10: an overview. Prog Growth Factor Res 1992; 4(3):207–227.

21. Makela MJ, Kanehiro A, Dakhama A, Borish L, Joetham A, Tripp R, Anderson L, Gelfand EW. The failure of interleukin-10-deficient mice to develop airway hyper-responsiveness is overcome by respiratory syncytial virus infection in allergen-sensitized/challenged mice. Am J Respir Crit Care Med 2002; 165(6):824–831.

22. Makela MJ, Kanehiro A, Borish L, Dakhama A, Loader J, Joetham A, Xing Z, Jordana M, Larsen GL, Gelfand EW. IL-10 is necessary for the expression of airway hyper-responsiveness but not pulmonary inflammation after allergic sensitization. Proc Natl Acad Sci USA 2000; 97(11):6007–6012.

5

Respiratory Viruses
Do They Protect From or Induce Asthma?

PATRICK MALLIA and SEBASTIAN L. JOHNSTON

National Heart and Lung Institute
Imperial College London
London, England

Asthma is a chronic, inflammatory disease of the airways in which both genetic and environmental factors contribute to disease development and expression. Sensitization to aeroallergens with the subsequent formation of allergen-specific IgE antibodies in individuals with a genetic predisposition to atopy is believed to be central to the pathogenesis of the disease. This abnormal immune response to inhaled allergens leads to chronic airway inflammation with a characteristic eosinophilic infiltrate. There is also increasing evidence that T lymphocytes expressing a predominantly type 2 pattern of cytokine production orchestrate this inflammatory response. Despite the central role of allergic mechanisms in asthma pathogenesis, it is recognized that other nonallergic factors influence the asthmatic phenotype, including exercise, airborne pollutants, psychological factors, and respiratory tract infections.

The role of virus respiratory tract infections as the main cause of asthma exacerbations is well established, although the mechanisms of the effect of viruses in this context remain under investigation. However, the effect of early-life infections on the development of asthma continues to be a source of controversy and debate. This arises from the fact that two completely opposing mechanisms of action have been proposed: that infections can both protect against and induce the development of asthma. In this chapter we will review the evidence regarding the interactions between respiratory virus infections and asthma and how these conflicting points of view can be reconciled.

I.   Studies Showing an Association with Increased Risk of Asthma

A temporal association between respiratory virus infection and the development of allergic sensitization in children was first reported in a small study in 1979 (1). Subsequent to this initial report data from further animal studies led to the prevailing view that virus infections promoted the development of asthma and allergic sensitization (2). Human studies evaluating the relationship between respiratory tract infections in early life and the development of asthma appeared to confirm a positive association between the two.

A study of a cohort of Norwegian children aged 6–16 years used parental questionnaires to record episodes of respiratory tract infection before the age of 3 years. The authors noted that increased reporting of early respiratory tract infections was associated with an increased risk of asthma after the age of 3 years (3). Similar results were seen in a Finnish study, which found that parental reports that their children "had more respiratory infections on average than other children of the same age" was associated with a greater risk of asthma (4). However, both these studies were retrospective and the accuracy of such recall data can be questioned. To overcome this disadvantage a number of groups have recruited cohorts of children from birth and used prospective questionnaires and diaries to record episodes of respiratory infections. Studies from Australia (5,6) and Norway (7), using a prospective study design, also found a positive association between reported episodes of respiratory tract infection in early life and the risk of developing asthma. In a further study from the United States, parents reported any symptoms suggestive of respiratory tract infection in the first 3 years of life and symptomatic children were assessed by a pediatrician to obtain an objective diagnosis of lower respiratory tract infection (8). The prevalence of asthma at ages 6 and 11 in this cohort was higher in those children with a doctor's diagnosis of pneumonia or lower respiratory tract infection in the first 3 years of life compared to those with no infectious episodes.

These studies suggest that increased numbers of respiratory tract infections in early life are associated with a higher risk of developing asthma and therefore they may play a causative role in the pathogenesis of the disease.

II.   Studies Reporting a Protective Effect on Asthma

A possible inverse relationship between infection and allergy was first proposed in 1976 from studies on white families and Native Americans in northern Canada (9). The authors reported that elevated serum IgE levels and the prevalence of asthma and eczema were higher in the white population, whereas helminthic, viral, and bacterial infections were more common in the Native Americans. They suggested that atopic disease was the price paid for lower levels of infectious diseases. These observations remained relatively unnoticed until this hypothesis was resurrected in 1989 by Strachan, who observed an inverse relationship between the prevalence of hay fever and family size (10). Because the presence of siblings results in more frequent childhood infections, he suggested that increased infections in early childhood confer a protective effect against the later development of allergy, a premise that came to be known as the "hygiene hypothesis." Since this study there have been numerous publications reporting a protective effect of early life infections on the development of allergic diseases in later life. The reunification of Germany provided investigators with the opportunity to study populations that had been exposed to different environmental exposures but had a similar genetic background. Due to the widespread use of childcare at an early age, larger families, and overcrowded housing conditions, children from the former East Germany had more respiratory tract infections than those in the West (11). When the prevalence of current asthma in the two populations was measured it showed a significant inverse relationship, with a prevalence of 5.9% in the West compared to 3.9% in the East.

III. Daycare and Family Size

Other studies have utilized factors within the same population that affect the exposure of children to respiratory viruses to study their effect on asthma. Daycare and larger family size, both of which have been shown to increase the incidence of respiratory infections in children (12–14), have been used in such studies. These two factors can be used to define cohorts of children with varying levels of exposure to respiratory viruses in early life.

A protective effect of attendance at daycare on the development of asthma was first reported in a retrospective study of schoolchildren in Australia (15). Subsequently there have been two large studies confirming this finding in populations in the United States and Germany. In a study of 1035 children in the Tucson Children's Respiratory Study, an inverse relationship between the age of entering daycare and a diagnosis of asthma at ages 6–13 years was seen (16). By age 13, 12% of children who had attended daycare or had two or more older siblings had developed asthma, compared to 21% in those with one or no siblings or who had not attended daycare. Kramer et al. reported similar results in a study of children in whom the prevalence of asthma at ages 5–14 was related to the age of entry to daycare (17). They found an increased prevalence of doctor-diagnosed asthma among children who entered daycare over the age of 2 years compared to those who entered in the first year of life. The protective effect of early entry into daycare was stronger in small families with fewer than four people living together.

The protective effect of siblings seen in the Tucson cohort has been replicated in a number of other studies. A study of children aged 5–11 in the United Kingdom found that the prevalence of asthma was negatively associated with the number of children in the family (18). Children in families having more than three children were 50% less likely to have asthma than those with no siblings. An Australian study also showed a significant protective trend with increasing numbers of siblings but no further protective effect for three or more siblings (19). The protective effect was greater for the presence of older siblings than for younger siblings. This protective effect of multiple siblings has also been reported for adult asthmatics (20).

In these studies, therefore, when exposure to respiratory viruses is measured using surrogate markers such as daycare and large families, a protective effect on the subsequent development of asthma is found.

IV. Respiratory Syncytial Virus and Asthma

One of the most common viruses to infect the human respiratory tract in infancy is respiratory syncytial virus (RSV). It usually causes a self-limiting upper respiratory tract infection and there is evidence of almost universal infection in children by age 2. In a small percentage of infants RSV can cause a more severe lower respiratory tract infection, bronchiolitis, which is a significant cause of hospitalization in infants. RSV bronchiolitis has been linked with an increased risk of wheezing and asthma in later life for many years; however, its role in inducing asthma remains an area of controversy and debate.

Links between RSV bronchiolitis and recurrent wheezing were first reported in 1959 (21). Numerous studies have been published since then and the majority found that children with RSV bronchiolitis in the first year of life have an increased prevalence of wheezing in later childhood. A systematic review of studies of RSV and asthma found a prevalence of wheezing in the first 5 years after the initial episode of 40% in the bronchiolitis group vs. 11% in the control group ($p < 0.001$) (22). The prevalence of wheeze in the bronchiolitis group was double that of the control group (21% vs. 10%) between 5 and 10 years of follow-up, although this difference was not statistically significant. No association between RSV bronchiolitis and allergic sensitization was found.

Because childhood asthma is strongly associated with atopy, this suggests that other mechanisms may be responsible for postbronchiolitis wheezing. However, further follow-up data from one of the studies included in this review did report a strong association between RSV bronchiolitis and both atopic sensitization and asthma (23). Children who have been hospitalized for RSV bronchiolitis were followed prospectively with an age-matched control group recruited simultaneously. When assessed at age 7 the cumulative prevalence of asthma in the RSV group was 30% compared to 3% in the control group ($p < 0.0001$). The figures for any positive allergy test were 41% and 22%, respectively ($p = 0.039$). This study was notable for the low prevalence of asthma reported in the control group of children, especially in those with a positive family history of asthma (prevalence 0%), suggesting that the method of selection of the control group may have involved negative selection for the risk of asthma. This may have occurred as the controls were age-matched and recruited contemporaneously from the same city as the index cases. Thus the control children were very likely exposed to RSV since they were well during the annual RSV epidemic, yet they did not develop bronchiolitis. This suggests that children negatively selected for bronchiolitis are also negatively selected for asthma.

Supporting this conclusion is a report that infants with a family history of atopy are more likely to develop bronchiolitis and have a higher rate of hospitalization (24). From these data it appears that selecting RSV-infected infants who develop bronchiolitis selects those already at highest risk of developing asthma and allergic sensitization.

A further important question is whether RSV is unique in this relationship with asthma or whether this relationship also exists with other viruses that infect the respiratory tract. Some of the studies that have found a positive association between bronchiolitis and subsequent wheezing did not obtain a virological diagnosis, but used a clinical diagnosis based on lower respiratory tract symptoms and signs. Recent reports have found that in a substantial proportion of cases of infants with a clinical diagnosis of acute bronchiolitis the causative agent was rhinovirus (25,26), highlighting the fact that although RSV is detected in 70–80% of cases of bronchiolitis cases, bronchiolitis is not equivalent to infection with RSV. Rhinovirus as a single agent was detected in 19% (25) and 29% (26) of cases of bronchiolitis and in one of the studies detection of rhinovirus was significantly associated with increased disease severity (26).

Other studies have also suggested that the relationship of RSV with asthma may not differ from that of other respiratory viruses. A study of wheezing in children hospitalized during concurrent epidemics of RSV and influenza A lower respiratory tract infections (27) found that 60% of the children had two or more episodes of subsequent wheezing, but there was no difference in the risk associated with the two viruses. A report from the Tucson group, in which virological sampling was performed during all reported lower respiratory tract infections in the first 3 years of life, found an increased prevalence of wheeze between 3 and 11 years of age in those with RSV detected during acute lower respiratory tract infection before 3 years of age (28). However, similar relationships were also seen for lower respiratory tract illnesses caused by other respiratory viruses.

It may therefore be that the relationship of RSV with the subsequent development of asthma is no different from that of other respiratory viruses and the number of publications highlighting the role of RSV may simply reflect the following:

1. Diagnostic testing for other respiratory viruses was simply not carried out.
2. At the time these studies were carried out, diagnostic methods for other respiratory viruses were insensitive or unavailable (especially so for rhinoviruses).
3. RSV is the most common viral respiratory tract infection in children of this age group.

V. Viral Infections and Asthma Exacerbations

In contrast to the controversy regarding the effect of virus infection on the development of asthma, it is now widely accepted that in established asthma respiratory viruses clearly exert a detrimental effect by causing acute exacerbations. The association between colds and asthma exacerbations has been recognized for many years, but low virus detection rates in clinical samples suggested that viruses were responsible for a minority of exacerbations only (29,30). However, this belief was challenged with the advent of techniques allowing for improved virus detection rates, especially for rhinoviruses and coronaviruses, the two most prevalent causative agents of the common cold. Isolation of these two agents is very poor using standard methods of virus culture, and serology is unavailable, so studies using these methods alone are likely to have seriously underestimated the real contribution of viruses to exacerbations. Polymerase chain reaction (PCR)-based methods result in a much higher detection rate and have revealed the contribution of viruses to asthma exacerbations to be much greater than was previously thought. Community-based studies using PCR detected a respiratory virus in 80–85% of asthma exacerbations in children (31) and 44% in adults (32). The most common virus detected was the rhinovirus, accounting for 66% of viral exacerbations in children and 60% in adults. The impact of using PCR was shown by the fact that in one of these studies 82% of rhinovirus infections were detected with PCR only.

A time trend analysis comparing seasonal patterns of respiratory infections and hospital admissions for acute exacerbations of asthma showed a strong correlation between the two, providing indirect evidence that virus infections also contribute to more severe exacerbations (33). This was confirmed in studies of respiratory virus infections in patients presenting to hospital with asthma exacerbations. In a study from the United States, 55% of 148 asthma exacerbations seen in the Emergency Department and 50% of patients requiring hospitalization were associated with the presence of a virus (34). An Australian study of 49 adults presenting with an asthma exacerbation detected a virus in 76% of cases (35), and found that exacerbations in which a virus was detected were associated with a lower forced expiratory volume in 1 s (FEV_1), higher hospital admission rate, and longer hospital stay compared to noninfective exacerbations. Analysis of deaths due to asthma showed a winter peak in children under 5 years and adults over 45 years, suggesting that respiratory virus infections may contribute to asthma mortality in these two age groups (36).

There is evidence that respiratory viruses and allergic sensitization can act together to exacerbate asthma. A study of exacerbations in children showed that the concomitant presence of virus infection and allergy increased the risk of wheezing (37). A study of adult asthmatics hospitalized with acute exacerbations found that admission to hospital with acute asthma was strongly associated with the combination of allergic sensitization, exposure to high levels of an allergen the subject was sensitized to, and concurrent viral infection (38).

VI. Mechanisms of Interaction Between Virus Infections and Asthma

In parallel with the epidemiological studies indicating a protective effect of early life infections on allergic diseases, there is a growing body of evidence exploring the immunological mechanisms that could account for a protective effect of infections on allergy.

Allergic inflammation is characterized by a distinctive subset of CD4+ T lymphocytes, which have been termed T_H2 cells. They are defined by the production of a cytokine profile comprising interleukin 4 (IL-4), IL-5, and IL-13. This pattern of cytokine production favors the development of an allergic inflammatory profile characterized by the recruitment of eosinophils and mast cells and production of IgE. T_H1 lymphocytes, on the other hand, produce the cytokines interferon gamma (IFN-γ) and IL-2 and result in the production of immunoglobulin G (IgG) and IgM and the development of cytotoxic T-cell responses (39). The exact role that T_H2 lymphocytes play in asthma is still debated (40), but there is substantial evidence that they orchestrate the chronic airway inflammation that characterizes asthma (41). This T_H1/T_H2 paradigm has also been extended to CD8+ T cells (42) and therefore, in relation to the overall balance between the two phenotypes, the terms type 1 and type 2 responses are more accurate.

Human adaptive immune responses at birth are significantly different from those of adults and the immune system undergoes marked changes in the first few years of life. Development of the immune system begins in utero where type 1 immunity is downregulated and type 2 responses predominate. This is believed to be essential for a successful pregnancy because IFN-γ is toxic to the placenta (43). At birth the immune response remains skewed toward a type 2 profile, with cord mononuclear cells showing impaired production of IFN-γ. In infants with a family history of atopic diseases this impairment in type 1 immunity is even more pronounced (44,45). Subsequently the capacity to produce IFN-γ increases over the first years of life until it reaches adult levels around 5 years of age (46), but this maturation of the immune system toward type 1 immune responses is delayed in children at high risk of atopy. Therefore, it can be postulated that the chance of this normal maturation failing is greater in high-risk children and they may remain with relatively excessive type 2 patterns of immune response.

It has been shown in animal models that the principal stimulus driving this maturation of the immune system is the presence of microbial stimuli. Animals kept in an environment devoid of microbes fail to downregulate type 2 responses (47). The innate immune system acts as the link between microbial stimulation and development of adaptive immune responses, and the cytokine IL-12 plays a central role in driving the maturation of the system toward an adult phenotype. IL-12 is produced by antigen-presenting cells (APCs) including dendritic cells and monocyte–macrophages and is an obligatory signal for the differentiation of naïve T_H0 cells to T_H1 cells (48). It stimulates T cells and natural killer (NK) cells to produce IFN-γ, which has a positive feedback on IL-12 production. IL-12 and IFN-γ together create a microenvironment in which CD4+ cells are preferentially stimulated to differentiate into T_H1 cells. In the presence of low levels of IL-12, T cells polarize into T_H2 cells that produce IL-4, which further inhibits T_H1 cell development.

Microbial products such as lipopolysaccharide and viral nucleic acid dsRNA induce a rapid maturation of dendritic cells with upregulation of major histocompatibility complex (MHO), adhesion, and costimulatory molecules, production of IL-12, and a strong T_H1 response (49). Therefore the stimulatory effect of infectious agents and bacterial products on IL-12 provides a mechanism by which individuals at high risk of atopy who do not receive adequate microbial stimulation during this crucial time of immune development may maintain persistently elevated type 2 immune responses. The reductions in exposure to infectious agents due to smaller family sizes, improved hygiene, and vaccination that have occurred in industrialized nations over the past 40 years could thereby lead to an increase in the prevalence of allergic diseases such as asthma.

The genetic basis that determines susceptibility to atopy and allergic disease is incompletely understood, but already involves a large number of different genes. However, a genetic polymorphism that influences the response of the innate immune system to lipopolysaccharide (LPS) has shed some light on the interaction between the immune system and viruses. The effect of the LPS mimics that of viruses: increased exposure to LPS in early life has a protective effect on the development of asthma, but exposure to LPS in patients with established asthma exacerbates the disease (50).

A receptor for LPS is the protein CD14 that belongs to the class of pattern-recognition receptors; binding of LPS to CD14 induces the formation of IL-12 by APCs. CD14 and other pattern-recognition receptors provide a link between the innate and adaptive immune responses. Variations in these signaling pathways could contribute to the risk of developing allergic diseases.

There is evidence for this hypothesis in humans with the discovery that a polymorphism in the promoter region for the CD14 gene is associated with varying levels of soluble CD14 and is inversely related to IgE levels. Children homozygous for an allele that resulted in lower levels of CD14 had higher serum IgE levels, higher IL-4 responses, and lower IFN-γ responses in peripheral blood mononuclear cells (PBMC) (51). CD14 has also been shown to act as a receptor for the fusion protein (F protein) of RSV in a murine model (52) and mice deficient for another pattern recognition receptor TLR4 showed impaired clearance of RSV from the lungs. Therefore variations in expression of CD14 and other pattern-recognition receptors may be a common pathway influencing both the severity of viral infection and the development of allergy.

The skewing of the immune response to a type 2 profile not only favors the development of allergic disease such as asthma but also alters the host response to viral infection. The host response to viral infection is regulated by type 1 cytokines such as IFN-γ. If this response is deficient the mechanisms that are essential for viral clearance are impaired. This impairment in antiviral mechanisms may explain the increased symptoms with virus infection seen in atopic subjects. Deficient production of type 1 cytokines in atopic subjects has been documented in vitro and correlated with disease severity and viral clearance in vivo. Papadopoulos et al. showed that PBMCs from atopic asthmatics exposed ex vivo to live rhinovirus produce lower levels of the type 1 cytokines IL-12 and IFN-γ than those of normal controls (53). Another study measured the ex vivo secretion of IFN-γ by PBMCs taken from subjects with allergic rhinitis or asthma. Rhinovirus inoculation was then performed and the quantity of precold rhinovirus-induced IFN-γ produced showed an inverse correlation with peak rhinovirus shedding during the infection (54). Gem et al. assessed mRNA levels of the type 1 and type 2 cytokines IFN-γ and IL-5 in sputum during the acute phase of experimental infection with rhinovirus 16. A low IFN-γ/IL-5 ratio (i.e., a weak type 1 response) correlated with higher peak cold symptoms and a longer duration of viral shedding (55), providing in vivo evidence that impaired type 1 responses can result in impaired viral clearance and increased symptoms.

Impaired type 1 immune responses may also play an important role in the variations in the severity of RSV infection in infants. In a study of 11 infants with RSV bronchiolitis, cytokine levels were measured in stored cord blood taken at birth. Decreased levels of IL-12 were found in the children who subsequently developed bronchiolitis compared to a control group who did not (56). Decreased levels of IFN-γ, IL-12, and IL-18 and impaired viral clearance have also been demonstrated in children with RSV bronchiolitis compared to children who were infected with RSV but developed upper respiratory tract infection only (57).

VII. Can We Explain the Paradox?

What, then, is the true effect of respiratory tract in early life infections on asthma? The evidence is confusing: studies seem to give conflicting results depending on the way exposure to viruses is measured. Although it would seem that assessing use of daycare, family size or reports of respiratory tract infections measure the same denominator (i.e., exposure to respiratory viruses), they result in the opposite conclusions regarding the effect of respiratory virus infections on asthma. This para-doxical effect is seen even within the same study. Studies that assessed the effect of both reported infections and family size found a positive association for the former and a negative association with the latter within the same study cohort (3–5).

Studies measuring overall exposure to viruses at a population level, such as those utilizing family size or daycare as surrogates for frequency of infection, are not confounded by the host response to infection, but measure total exposure levels irrespective of the host response. Host response is a major determinant of the severity of symptoms manifested during a viral infection. The studies that utilize reports of individual infections are confounded by the severity of symptoms that develop in response to infection: more symptomatic infections are more likely to be reported than minimal symptomatic or asymptomatic infections.

Therefore, an alternative explanation for the positive association between re-ported infections and asthma is that children at higher risk of developing asthma are also at a higher risk of developing and reporting symptoms during respiratory tract infections. Thus, rather than being a causative factor, reported infections and asthma are associated through common risk factors. Studies that measure exposure to infections independently of symptoms and therefore host response are unaffected by this interaction and therefore will reflect the true relationship between early life infection and asthma.

There is now evidence emerging that this hypothesis is the correct explanation for the positive relationship between reported infections and asthma. Studies assess-ing the expression of respiratory tract infections in children at high and low risk of atopic disease have found that those with a family history of atopy are in fact at higher risk of developing symptomatic lower respiratory tract infections. A prospective birth cohort study of 4146 children in the Netherlands has explored the interactions between a parental history of allergic disease and childhood infections (58). Infants with a parental history of allergy had a higher incidence of symptomatic lower respiratory tract infections, but not upper respiratory tract infections, than children with no atopic family history. The risk of symptomatic lower respiratory tract infections increased with exposure to greater numbers of children and if both parents were atopic. The risk of doctor-diagnosed lower respiratory tract infections therefore was highest for those children with two allergic parents and who attended large daycare centers, with an adjusted odds ratio of 6.1 compared to the reference group of no childcare and nonallergic parents. By comparison, the adjusted odds ratio for lower respiratory tract infection for children in large daycare centers with nonallergic parents was 3.8. There was no association between parental allergy and upper respiratory tract infections. This differential effect of upper and lower respiratory tract infections was also seen in a study from the German Multicentre Allergy Study (59). The authors reported a strong negative correlation between an increased frequency of upper respiratory viral infections in early life and asthma diagnosis, current wheeze, and bronchial hyperreactivity at age 7. However the number of lower respiratory tract infections in the first 3 years of life was positively associated with the same outcome measures. There was a strong positive association among wheezing, lower respiratory tract infection, and asthma but a nonsignificant association for nonwheezing episodes. The study also assessed the frequency of lower respiratory tract infections in children with a family history of atopy and found a higher rate of frequent lower respiratory tract infections (≥ 2 infections before age 3) than in those with no history of allergy. When lower respiratory tract infections were excluded, there was an inverse relationship between the total burden of infectious diseases and asthma.

This association between lower respiratory tract infection and atopy may be due either to an increased risk of infection or to more respiratory tract symptoms during viral infection. Studies in adults suggest that the latter is the correct explanation. A study of experimental rhinovirus infection in atopic subjects and normal controls found that whereas normal subjects with neutralizing antibodies developed mild symptoms only, atopic subjects with antibodies developed severe colds despite receiving the same dose of virus (60). Studies of airway hyperresponsiveness after experimental rhinovirus infection have also shown that atopics develop significantly greater increases in responsiveness than normal controls (61). A study of cohabiting couples who were discordant for the presence of atopy and asthma measured the frequency and severity of natural rhinovirus infections (62). Regular sampling of the upper respiratory tract for virus detection was performed regardless of whether the subjects had symptoms or not to eliminate the possibility of reporting bias. The frequency of infections in the two groups was the same, but the partners with atopic asthma developed more severe lower respiratory tract symptoms and falls in PEF. Whether these findings in adults with established allergy are applicable to children at high risk of developing allergic disease is not known. However, they do indicate that virus infection in atopic individuals results in more symptoms and changes in airway physiology than in nonatopic controls.

Therefore, if children at high risk of atopy are also at high risk of developing symptomatic lower respiratory tract infection, studies that rely on symptoms will give different results to those that measure exposure independently of the host response. The studies using family size and daycare measure overall infectious burden in the first years of life regardless of the host symptoms and show a protective effect on asthma consistent with the hygiene hypothesis. However, studies using symptomatic lower respiratory tract infections as a measure of infectious burden probably select children at high risk of developing asthma, resulting in a positive association being found between the two. Therefore, symptomatic early-life lower respiratory tract infections should be considered as a predictor for, and not as a causative factor in, the development of asthma.

VIII. Conclusions

The associations between virus respiratory tract infections and asthma are undoubtedly complex. The evidence indicates that an increased overall load of virus infections in early life protects against the later development of asthma, but virus infections exacerbate established asthma. The protective effect of multiple infections is likely mediated through their effect on ensuring normal maturation of the immune system toward a predominantly type 1 pattern of immune responses, especially in infants at high risk of atopy. In addition, impaired antiviral responses seen in high-risk children lead to increased pathology and reporting of lower respiratory tract symptoms with viral infections. Therefore, when reported individual respiratory tract infections are used to measure the burden of infectious disease, a positive association between the two is found but we believe that this reflects common predisposing factors and is not a causative association.

References

1. Frick OL, German DF, Mills J. Development of allergy in children. I. Association with virus infections. J Allergy Clin Immunol 1979; 63(4):228–241.
2. Busse WW. The relationship between viral infections and onset of allergic diseases and asthma. Clin Exp Allergy 1989; 19(1):1–9.
3. Nystad W, Skrondal A, Magnus P. Day care attendance, recurrent respiratory tract infections and asthma. Int J Epidemiol 1999; 28(5):882–887.
4. Pekkanen J, Remes S, Kajosaari M, Husman T, Soininen L. Infections in early childhood and risk of atopic disease. Acta Paediatr 1999; 88(7):710–714.
5. Ponsonby AL, Couper D, Dwyer T, Carmichael A, Kemp A. Relationship between early life respiratory illness, family size over time, and the development of asthma and hay fever: a seven year follow up study. Thorax 1999; 54(8):664–669.
6. Oddy WH, de Klerk NH, Sly PD, Holt PG. The effects of respiratory infections, atopy and breastfeeding on childhood asthma. Eur Resp J 2002; 19(5):899–905.

7. Nafstad P, Magnus P, Jaakkola JJ. Early respiratory infections and childhood asthma. Pediatrics 2000; 106(3):E38.

8. Castro-Rodriguez JA, Holberg CJ, Wright AL, Halonen M, Taussig LM, Morgan WJ, et al. Association of radiologically ascertained pneumonia before age 3 yr with asthma like symptoms and pulmonary function during childhood: a prospective study. Am J Respir Crit Care Med 1999; 159(6):1891–1897.

9. Gerrard JW, Geddes CA, Reggin PL, Gerrard CD, Horne S. Serum IgE levels in white and metis communities in Saskatchewan. Ann Allergy 1976; 37(2):91–100.

10. Strachan DP. Hay fever, hygiene, and household size. Br Med J 1989; 299(6710):1259–1260.

11. von Mutius E, Martinez FD, Fritzsch C, Nicolai T, Roell G, Thiemann HH. Prevalence of asthma and atopy in two areas of West and East Germany. Am J Respir Crit Care Med 1994; 149(2 Pt 1):358–364.

12. Hjern A, Haglund B, Bremberg S. Lower respiratory tract infections in an ethnic and social context. Paediatr Perinat Epidemiol 2002; 14:53–60.

13. Nafstad P, Hagen JA, Oie L, Magnus P, Jaakkola JJ. Day care centers and respiratory health. Pediatrics 1999; 103(4 Pt 1):753–758.

14. Louhiala PJ, Jaakkola N, Ruotsalainen R, Jaakkola JJ. Form of day care and respiratory infections among Finnish children. Am J Public Health 1995; 85(8 Pt 1):1109–1112.

15. McCutcheon H, Woodward A. Acute respiratory illness in the first year of primary school related to previous attendance at child care. Aust NZ J Public Health 1996; 20(1):49–53.

16. Ball TM, Castro-Rodriguez JA, Griffith KA, Holberg CJ, Martinez FD, Wright AL. Siblings, day-care attendance, and the risk of asthma and wheezing during childhood. N Eng J Med 2000; 343(8):538–543.

17. Kramer U, Heinrich J, Wjst M, Wichmann HE. Age of entry to day nursery and allergy in later childhood. Lancet 1999; 353(9151):450–454.

18. Rona RJ, Duran-Tauleria E, Chinn S. Family size, atopic disorders in parents, asthma in children, and ethnicity. J Allergy Clin Immunol 1997; 99(4):454–460.

19. Ponsonby AL, Couper D, Dwyer T, Carmichael A. Cross sectional study of the relation between sibling number and asthma, hay fever, and eczema. Arch Dis Child 1998; 79(4):328–333.

20. Jarvis D, Chinn S, Luczynska C, Burney P. The association of family size with atopy and atopic disease. Clin Exp Allergy 1997; 27(3):240–245.

21. Wittig HJ, Glaser J. The relationship between acute bronchiolitis and childhood asthma. J Allergy 2002; 30:19–23.

22. Kneyber MCJ, Steyerberg EW, de Groot R, Moll HA. Long-term effects of respiratory syncytial virus (RSV) bronchiolitis in infants and young children: a quantitative review. Acta Paediatr 2000; 89(6):654–660.

23. Sigurs N, Bjarnason R, Sigurbergsson F, Kjellman B. Respiratory syncytial virus bronchiolitis in infancy is an important risk factor for asthma and allergy at age 7. Am J Respir Crit Care Med 2000; 161(5):1501–1507.

24. Trefny P, Stricker T, Baerlocher C, Sennhauser FH. Family history of atopy and clinical course of RSV infection in ambulatory and hospitalized infants. Pediatr Pulmonol 2000; 30(4):302–306.

25. Andreoletti L, Lesay M, Deschildre A, Lambert V, Dewilde A, Wattre P. Differential detection of rhinoviruses and enteroviruses RNA sequences associated with classical

immunofluorescence assay detection of respiratory virus antigens in nasopharyngeal swabs from infants with bronchiolitis. J Med Virol 2000; 61(3):341–346.

26. Papadopoulus NG, Moustaki M, Tsolia M, Bossios A, Astra E, Prezerakou A, et al. Association of rhinovirus infection with increased disease severity in acute bronchiolitis. Am J Respir Crit Care Med 2002; 165:1285–1289.

27. Eriksson M, Bennet R, Nilsson A. Wheezing following lower respiratory tract infections with respiratory syncytial virus and influenza A in infancy. Pediatr Allergy Immunol 2000; 11(3):193–197.

28. Stein RT, Sherrill D, Morgan WJ, Holberg CJ, Halonen M, Taussig LM, et al. Respiratory syncytial virus in early life and risk of wheeze and allergy by age 13 years. Lancet 1999; 354(9178):541–545.

29. Tarlo S, Broder I, Spence L. A prospective study of respiratory infection in adult asthmatics and their normal spouses. Clin Allergy 1979; (9(3)):293–301.

30. Minor TE, Dick EC, Baker JW, Ouellette JJ, Cohen M, Reed CE. Rhinovirus and influenza type A infections as precipitants of asthma. Am Rev Respir Dis 1976; 113(2): 149–153.

31. Johnston SL, Pattemore PK, Sanderson G, Smith S, Lampe F, Josephs L, et al. Community study of role of viral infections in exacerbations of asthma in 9–11 year old children. Br Med J 1995; 310(6989):1225–1229.

32. Nicholson KG, Kent J, Ireland DC. Respiratory viruses and exacerbations of asthma in adults [see comments.]. Br Med J 1993; 307(6910):982–986.

33. Johnston SL, Pattemore PK, Sanderson G, Smith S, Campbell MJ, Josephs LK, et al. The relationship between upper respiratory infections and hospital admissions for asthma: a time-trend analysis. Am J Respir Crit Care Med 1996; 154(3 Pt 1):654–660.

34. Atmar RL, Guy E, Guntupalli KK, Zimmerman JL, Bandi VD, Baxter BD, et al. Respiratory tract viral infections in inner-city asthmatic adults. Arch Intern Med 1998; 158(22):2453–2459.

35. Wark PAB, Johnston SL, Moric I, Simpson JL, Hensley MJ, Gibson PG. Neutrophil degranulation and cell lysis is associated with clinical severity in virus-induced asthma. Eur Respir J 2002; 19:68–75.

36. Campbell MJ, Cogman GR, Holgate ST, Johnston SL. Age specific trends in asthma mortality in England and Wales, 1983–95: results of an observational study. Br Med J 1997; 314(7092):1439–1441.

37. Rakes GP, Arruda E, Igram JM, Hoover GE, Zambrano JC, Hayden FG, et al. Rhinovirus and respiratory syncytial virus in wheezing children requiring emergency care. IgE and eosinophil analyses. Am J Respir Crit Care Med 1999; 159(3):785–790.

38. Green RM, Custovic A, Sanderson G, Hunter J, Johnston SL, Woodcock AA. Synergism between allergens and viruses and risk of hospital admission with asthma: case–control study. Br Med J 2002; 324:763.

39. Mosmann TR, Cherwinski H, Bond MW, Giedlin MA, Coffman RL. Two types of murine helper T cell clone. I. Definition according to profiles of lymphokine activities and secreted proteins. J Immunol 1986; 136(7):2348–2357.

40. Salvi SS, Babu KS, Holgate ST. Is asthma really due to a polarized T cell response toward a helper T cell type 2 phenotype? Am J Respir Crit Care Med 2001; 164(8 Pt 1):1343–1346.

41. Hamid Q, Azzawi M, Ying S, Moqbel R, Wardlaw AJ, Corrigan CJ, et al. Interleukin-5 mRNA in mucosal bronchial biopsies from asthmatic subjects. Int Arch Allergy Appl Immunol 1991; 94(1–4):169–170.

42. Cho S-H, Stanciu LA, Begishivili T, Bates PJ, Holgate ST, Johnston SL. Peripheral blood CD4+ and CD8+ T cell type 1 and type 2 cytokine production in atopic asthma and normal subjects. Clin Exp Allergy 2002; 32:427–433.

43. Wegmann TG, Lin H, Guilbert L, Mosmann TR. Bidirectional cytokine interactions in the maternal-fetal relationship: is successful pregnancy a TH2 phenomenon? Immunol Today 1993; 14(7):353–356.

44. Holt PG, Clough JB, Holt BJ, Baron-Hay MJ, Rose AH, Robinson BW, et al. Genetic risk for atopy is associated with delayed postnatal maturation of T-cell competence. Clin Exp Allergy 1992; 22(12):1093–1099.

45. Prescott SL, Macaubas C, Smallacombe T, Holt BJ, Sly PD, Holt PG. Development of allergen-specific T-cell memory in atopic and normal children. Lancet 1999; 353(9148): 196–200.

46. Holt PG. Postnatal maturation of immune competence during infancy and childhood. Pediatr Allergy Immunol 1995; 6(2):59–70.

47. Sudo N, Sawamura S, Tanaka K, Aiba Y, Kubo C, Koga Y. The requirement of intestinal bacterial flora for the development of an IgE production system fully susceptible to oral tolerance induction. J Immunol 1997; 159(4):1739–1745.

48. Macatonia SE, Hosken NA, Litton M, Vieira P, Hsieh CS, Culpepper JA, et al. Dendritic cells produce IL-12 and direct the development of Th1 cells from naïve CD4+ T cells. J Immunol 1995; 154(10):5071–5079.

49. Cella M, Salio M, Sakakibara Y, Langen H, Julkunen I, Lanzavecchia A. Maturation, activation, and protection of dendritic cells induced by double-stranded RNA. J Exp Med 2002; 189:821–829.

50. Reed CE, Milton DK. Endotoxin-stimulated innate immunity: a contributing factor for asthma. J Allergy Clin Immunol 2001; 108(2):157–166.

51. Baldini M, Lohman IC, Halonen M, Erickson RP, Holt PG, Martinez FD. A Polymorphism* in the 5′ flanking region of the CD14 gene is associated with circulating soluble CD14 levels and with total serum immunoglobulin E. Am J Respir Cell Mol Biol 1999; 20(5):976–983.

52. Kurt-Jones EA, Popova L, Kwinn L, Haynes LM, Jones LP, Tripp RA, et al. Pattern recognition receptors TLR4 and CD14 mediate response to respiratory syncytial virus. Nature Immunol 2000; 1:398–401.

53. Papadopoulos NG, Stanciu LA, Papi A, Holgate ST, Johnston S.L. A defective type 1 response to rhinovirus in atopic asthma. Thorax 2002; 57:328–332.

54. Parry DE, Busse WW, Sukow KA, Dick CR, Swenson C, Gern JE. Rhinovirus-induced PBMC responses and outcome of experimental infection in allergic subjects. J Allergy Clin Immunol 2000; 105(4):692–698.

55. Gern JE, Vrtis R, Grindle KA, Swenson C, Busse WW. Relationship of upper and lower airway cytokines to outcome of experimental rhinovirus infection. Am J Respir Crit Care Med 2000; 162(6):2226–2231.

56. Blanco-Quiros A, Gonzalez H, Arranz E, Lapena S. Decreased interleukin-12 levels in umbilical cord blood in children who developed acute bronchiolitis. Pediatr Pulmonol 1999; 28(3):175–180.

57. Legg JP, Hussain IR, Warner JA, Low JL, Johnston S.L, Warner JO. Type 1 and type 2 cytokine imbalance in acute respiratory syncytial virus brochiolitis. Am J Respir Crit Care Med 2002; in press.

58. Koopman LP, Smit AH, Heijnen MLA, Wijga A, van Strien RT, Kerkhof M. Respiratory infection in infants: interaction of parental allergy, child care, and siblings—the PIAMA study. Pediatrics 2002; 108:943–948.

59. Illi S, von Mutius E, Lau S, Bergmann R, Niggemann B, Sommerfeld C, et al. Early childhood infectious diseases and the development of asthma up to school age: a birth cohort study. Br Med J 2001; 322(7283):390–395.
60. Bardin PG, Fraenkel DJ, Sanderson G, Dorward M, Lau LC, Johnston SL, et al. Amplified rhinovirus colds in atopic subjects. Clin Exp Allergy 1994; 24(5):457–464.
61. Gern JE, Calhoun W, Swenson C, Shen G, Busse WW. Rhinovirus infection preferentially increases lower airway responsiveness in allergic subjects. Am J Respir Crit Care Med 1997; 155(6):1872–1876.
62. Come JM, Marshall C, Smith S, Sanderson G, Holgate ST, Johnston SL. Frequency, severity, and duration of rhinovirus infections in asthmatics and non-asthmatics: a longitudinal cohort study. Lancet 2002; 359:831–834.

6

Respiratory Virus Infection of the Lower Airways and the Induction of Acute Asthma Exacerbations

STELIOS PSARRAS and NIKOLAOS G. PAPADOPOULOS

University of Athens
Athens, Greece

I. Introduction

Respiratory viral infections are among the most common causes of physician consultation, especially among the pediatric population. While in most occasions the upper airway is affected (i.e., a common cold), it is frequently difficult to define clinical and/or pathological limits between upper and lower airway involvement. Hence, in the context of viral infections, it is not overstated that the human airways could be viewed as a continuous system starting from the nostrils and ending at the alveoli (1). Although significant differences between anatomical sites could be pointed out, viral agents with a tropism for the respiratory system infect and/or can produce symptoms in both upper and lower airways. In addition to its importance in purely infectious disease states, this observation is relevant to the sequence of events leading from a common cold to the exacerbation of reactive airway disease, mainly asthma. During the last decades, a remarkable increase in the prevalence of asthma in affluent societies has been documented. Asthma now affects over 150 million people worldwide and costs more than tuberculosis and acquired immunodeficiency syndrome (AIDS) combined (2). Although there is no doubt that a multitude of genetic and environmental factors are involved in the induction and progression of asthma, upper respiratory viral infections (URIs) are the most common trigger of acute exacerbations. This correlation has long been suspected, as it is a daily observation of practicing physicians.

During the 1970s and 1980s, over 20 studies sought to isolate respiratory viruses during asthma exacerbations; however, isolation rates were low (3). This was attributed to retrospective study designs as well as the lack of sensitive detection methodologies. With the advent of the polymerase chain reaction (PCR) and the design of prospective studies, it was demonstrated that asthma exacerbations in the community follow virologically confirmed URIs in at least 85% of cases in children (4) and in more than half the cases in adults (5). Furthermore, it was shown that such infections could be responsible for severe exacerbations leading to hospitalization (6). Parallel studies have shown that experimental or natural URIs can lead to airway hyperresponsiveness over a prolonged period of time (7). The definition of pathogenic events leading from a URI to an acute asthma exacerbation is therefore of considerable importance if novel therapeutic targets are to be defined. Crucial to our understanding of such events is the debate over whether asthma exacerbations are the result of direct infection of the bronchial epithelium by respiratory viruses, or indirect mechanisms consequent upon upper respiratory infection alone. In the former case, local immunological and inflammatory responses could initiate a cascade of events ultimately leading to an acute exacerbation. Furthermore, such a sequence of events would increase the possibility that a window of opportunity for the use of specific antiviral agents could exist. Such a model cannot be disputed in principle for respiratory viruses such as influenza or respiratory syncytial virus that are known to be able to infect the bronchial epithelium productively. Nevertheless, the most common agents isolated in both URIs and asthma exacerbations are human rhinoviruses (RVs), which represent approximately 60% of all isolated viruses. It has been commonly held that these viruses are not cytotoxic to the airway epithelium and, due to optimal growth at the temperature of the nasal cavity (33°C), are not able to replicate in the lower airways (8). However, we have recently shown that RVs are able to replicate at central temperature (37°C), and in fact do so in the bronchi of human volunteers after experimentally induced URIs (9,10). As a result of these studies, the direct lower airway infection hypothesis has become more plausible. Of course, the necessity of lower airway viral infection for the development of an acute asthma exacerbation has yet to be demonstrated. Furthermore, both direct and indirect effects could act simultaneously. In the present chapter, evidence for and characteristics of lower airway infection by respiratory viruses, as well as the possible mechanisms that could lead from such an infection to an acute asthma exacerbation, are described.

II. From Bronchial Infection to Asthma: Mechanistic Hypotheses

Asthma is characterized by bronchoconstriction, inflammation, and remodeling. All these events can be influenced by local viral infection (Fig. 1). Cell death is certainly involved in virus-induced bronchoconstriction. However, there are considerable differences in the extent of cytotoxicity caused by different viruses, although no similar differences in the so-called asthma-inducing capacity of these viruses have been observed. Direct cytotoxicity due to viral replication may result in a considerable amount of cellular debris falling into the lumen. At the same time, loss of ciliated cells and/or ciliary function reduces mucus clearance. Occluded bronchi due to necrotic epithelial cells, inflammatory cells, mucus and plasma exudate are not unusual histopathological findings in patients with acute, severe lower respiratory infections, as well as in severe asthma. In addition, a number of epithelial cell functions could be impaired. It is well documented that epithelial cells are able to modulate airway muscle tone by producing bronchodilating substances such as prostaglandin E_2 (11) or nitric oxide (NO). These cells also produce substances that regulate fibroblast proliferation and extracellular matrix production. Furthermore, epithelial cells are a locus of neuropeptide metabolism; neutral endopeptidase 24-11 (NEP 24-11), the major metabolizing enzyme for substance P (SP) and neurokinin A (NK-A), is found abundantly on their surface. Therefore, any acute decrease in the number of epithelial cells may have profound results on the surrounding tissues (Fig. 1). Furthermore, viral infection may render the airways more susceptible to neurogenic inflammation by altering the expression of neuropeptide receptors (e.g., NK-Rs) (12–15). Virus-induced structural changes of the bronchial mucosa may also lead to exposure of the underlying neural tissue to the environment. An extensive network of afferent nerves is situated immediately below the epithelial tight junctions. Allergens, irritants, or inflammatory products present in the area may stimulate these nerves to release bronchoconstricting neuropeptides. In addition, regulatory neural mechanisms affecting bronchoconstriction are altered due to viral infection. Thus, M_2 muscarinic receptors, which serve as negative feedback regulators of acetylcholine release from vagal parasympathetic nerves, are dysfunctional following viral infection (16). Subsequently, M_3 muscarinic receptors may induce acetylcholine-mediated bronchoconstriction, leading to airway hyperresponsiveness (17).

Of major importance is virus-induced inflammation. Inflammation is a fundamental characteristic of asthma, but also it is able to induce a cascade of self-perpetuating or augmenting events that can in principle lead to an acute asthma exacerbation. Inflammation can be the result of a direct response of the respiratory epithelium to viral infection. Indeed, numerous studies have shown, both in vitro and in vivo, that upon infection the respiratory epithelium produces a number of cytokines and chemokines, which are key elements of the inflammatory response. In particular, interleukin-6 (IL-6), IL-8, IL-11, RANTES, MIP-1α, and granulocyte–macrophage colony-stimulating factor (GM-CSF) produced by epithelial cells upon respiratory virus infection (18–21) (10) participate in a number of regulatory processes that may significantly affect airway homeostasis and function (Fig. 1). RANTES, for instance, is a strong eosinophil chemoattractant (22), whereas GM-CSF is a survival factor and stimulates degranulation of these inflammatory cells (23). Moreover, IL-11 may directly affect bronchial hyperresponsiveness (24) and IL-8 is a potent neutrophil chemoattractant and activator, whereas it may also recruit activated eosinophils (25). Finally, proinflammatory molecules, such as tumor necrosis factor-α (TNF-α) and IL-1β, and antiviral agents, such as interferon-γ (IFN-γ), produced by

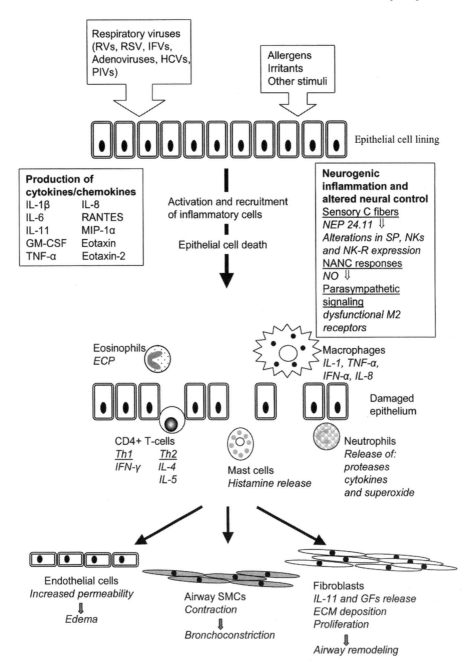

the epithelium or some inflammatory cells upon respiratory viral infection (26), can further mediate airway inflammation and affect cellular distribution in this tissue (e.g., by inducing expression of adhesion molecules in several cell types) (27,28).

In parallel, the local immune surveillance, including macrophages, dendritic cells, as well as locally attracted T cells, can be activated either through direct recognition of the virus or by the local cytokine milieu. Notably, the balance of Th1 and Th2 cytokines (IFN-γ, IL-4, IL-5, and IL-10), which are produced by helper T cells and have been found to be elevated in the lungs upon respiratory viral infection (29,30), may affect antiviral activity and protection, as well as mediate asthmatic inflammation in the airways. Furthermore, acute-phase cytokines secreted by the recruited and activated macrophages can mediate airway infection-associated systemic symptoms. Several respiratory viruses can infect macrophages and this may interfere with their role in antigen presentation (31,32). When peripheral blood mononuclear cells from atopic asthmatic subjects are exposed to RV, they produce IFN-γ and IL-10 at levels significantly lower or higher, respectively, than those produced by normal cells (33). Furthermore, in the same setting, the antigen presentation machinery is activated and once again this is impaired in atopic asthmatic individuals (34). This evidence suggests that differences in RV immunity in atopic individuals may favor a Th2-type inflammation in response to viral infection. Increased numbers of mast cells have been found in the lungs after viral infection characterized by increased release of both basal and stimulated histamine (35). On the other hand, neutrophil proteases released upon degranulation of neutrophils, the predominant cell type detected in nasal secretions during the acute phase of viral infection, are able to increase the mucus production by the airway submucosal glands (36), thus contributing further to airway obstruction. Finally, cytokines and other proteins secreted upon degranulation of recruited granulocytes may trigger further

Figure 1 Summary of major cellular and molecular interactions characterizing viral infection of the airway epithelium. Upon infection of the epithelial tissue by respiratory viruses, a number of cytokines and chemokines are produced by the epithelial cell lining, as well as by resident inflammatory cells, such as macrophages and lymphocytes, which are activated by the viruses. This leads in turn to the recruitment and activation of several types of inflammatory cells, such as eosinophils, neutrophils, mast cells, lymphocytes, and macrophages, which produce additional cytokines, further mediating airway inflammation. In addition, virally mediated cytotoxicity allows the access of other external stimuli such as allergens to the underlying stroma. Such stimuli may then act in conjunction with the viral-mediated responses. Epithelial cell death may also lead to the irritation of the underlying neural tissue and altered neural control. On the other hand, the activated inflammatory cells release a number of molecules, such as the eosinophil cationic protein, histamine, neutrophil proteases, and superoxide, that further mediate airway inflammation and lead to airway hyperresponsiveness and remodeling. Increased permeability of the endothelial cells leads to the development of edema, inflammatory interactions lead to the contraction of airway smooth muscle cells, whereas proliferation and extracellular matrix deposition of stimulated stromal fibroblasts lead to airway remodeling. In the complex network of cellular and molecular interactions prevailing in the virus-infected airway, the balance of Th1 vs. Th2 lymphocytes may also play an important role.

airway inflammatory responses. For example, the increase in eosinophilic cationic protein (ECP) in sputum seems to be correlated with increased airway responsiveness in adults with asthma (37). However, the precise role of eosinophils in airway inflammation, as well as the particular interactions governing the virally triggered recruitment and activation of inflammatory cells in the airways is not yet clear and needs to be determined.

III. Viral Agents Involved in Acute Asthma Exacerbations

Viral agents with a tropism for the respiratory system infect and/or produce symptoms in both upper and lower airways. Notwithstanding the differences between upper and lower airway epithelium, and a relative preference for, and/or different pathology of each virus in either, there is little doubt that the topology of respiratory viral infections supports the so-called united airways hypothesis (38). Although it is frequently mentioned that hundreds of different viruses can produce respiratory symptoms, this is due to the large number of picornavirus (>150) and adenovirus (>50) serotypes. Since there are small differences in clinical presentation between such serotypes, seven or eight types of agents can be separately described. The most prevalent pathogenic micro-organisms throughout the world are probably the human rhinoviruses (RVs). These so-called common cold viruses belong to the picornavirus (small RNA) family, which also includes the enteroviruses, such as polio, echo, and coxsackieviruses, and the cardio- and aphtoviruses (39). Over 100 serotypes of RVs have been identified and numbered. These are classified into major (90% of serotypes) and minor groups; the former use intercellular adhesion molecule-1 (ICAM-1) as their cellular receptor (40), while the latter use the low-density lipoprotein receptor (LDL-R) (41). Comparative titrations of nasal, pharyngeal, and oral titrations have shown that replication is more active in the nose. However, in a study comparing nasal and throat swabs and sputum samples during asthma exacerbations, viral isolation rate was higher in sputum, suggesting that RVs may also replicate in the lower airway (42). The epidemiology of RV colds is closely related to social contact and peaks are usually seen when children return to school after a holiday period (6).

In the first 2 years of life respiratory syncytial virus (RSV) is the most prevalent respiratory virus. RSV belongs to the pneumoviridae and is a medium-size (120–300 nm) RNA virus. There are two major strains, designated A and B, and although it has been reported that A strains are more common and produce more severe disease, this has not been a consistent finding (43). A wide range of species can be experimentally infected with human RSV, but natural infection is species-specific. Similarly to RV, RSV enters the body through the eye or nose and less often through the mouth (44). The virus subsequently spreads along the airway mucosa, mostly by cell-to-cell transfer along intracytoplasmic bridges, but also through aspiration from the upper to the lower airway. RSV follows a well-characterized epidemiological pattern, with yearly outbreaks between October and May in temperate climates (45). At least half of the infant population is infected during their first RSV epidemic, while almost all children have been infected by age 2 (46).

Three types of influenza viruses (IFV) designated A, B, and C, belonging to the orthomyxoviruses, have been identified. They are negative-stranded segmented RNA viruses. Infection with IFV occurs by aspiration of contaminated droplets from infected persons. Infected cells become round and swollen with pyknotic nuclei. Edema and polymorphonuclear infiltration are seen in the surrounding tissues (47). The progressive changes in epithelial cells suggest that infection starts in the trachea and then ascends and/or descends. The epidemiology of IFV is characterized by yearly epidemics, lasting for 6–8 weeks during late winter; each year there is usually only one dominant type or subtype. Illnesses initially appear in children, while later in the epidemic more adults are affected. Viruses are present in the community before and after the epidemic, causing illness at a low frequency (48,49). Pandemics have been occurring every 10–40 years (50).

In contrast to the rest of the respiratory viruses, adenoviruses are DNA viruses. They are a large family of viruses including 6 subgenera and over 50 serotypes. The propensity of adenoviruses to shut off the expression of host mRNA and induce excess synthesis of adenoviral proteins leads to an accumulation of such proteins as intranuclear bodies, which are incompatible with normal cell function. In upper airway epithelial cells, ciliary and microtubular abnormalities lead to a defective mucociliary clearance (51). An important feature of adenovirus is its ability to persist in the host for a long time, through low-grade replication, or even longer with production of adenoviral proteins without replication of a complete virus (52).

The youngest of the respiratory viruses, isolated in the mid-1960s, are human coronaviruses (HCV). Most human coronaviruses studied to date are related to one of two reference strains, designated OC43 and 229E, which differ extensively (53). Human aminopeptidase N, which is present on lung, intestinal, and kidney epithelial cells, has been identified as a receptor for HCV-229E (54). OC43 binds to major histocompatibility class (MHC) class I molecules (55). Viral replication has been demonstrated in the nasal mucosa, inducing inflammation, ciliary damage, and epithelial cell shedding (56). Cytopathic effects are not pronounced, as in the case of RV infections. HCV replication in the lower airway has not been confirmed. Volunteers can be successfully infected by intranasal inoculation (57). HCV causes about 15% of common colds. The disease is generally mild and there is evidence that HCV colds may induce milder symptoms than other viruses (4). However, there have been reports of lower respiratory tract involvement in young children and the elderly (58).

Human parainfluenza viruses (PIV) include four members, numbered 1–4 and belong to the paramyxovirus genus, together with mumps, and were also isolated in the late 1950s. Each PIV has distinct epidemiological characteristics. PIV-1 occurs in biennial epidemics during autumn in both northern and southern hemispheres. Its peak incidence occurs in children between 2 and 3 years of age. PIV-2 epidemics may occur yearly or biennially, affecting mostly children younger than 5 (59). PIV-3 is unique among PIV in its propensity to infect infants younger than 6 months of age in spring epidemics (60). Fewer data are available on PIV-4, which has been isolated from a small number of children and adults. Aerosol spread is considered important (61), although deposition on surfaces and subsequent self-inoculation may also be relevant (62). Virus replication can occur throughout the tracheobronchial tree; however, only mild and rapidly repaired focal tissue destruction is observed in vivo, with the exception of immunocompromised hosts in whom fatal, giant-cell pneumonia may occur.

IV. Viruses in the Lung: Clinical Evidence

Clinical features analyzed in numerous studies clearly indicate that after their initial replication in the nasopharyngeal cavities the majority of the so-called conventional respiratory viruses are spread to the lower respiratory tract. This has been widely accepted for RSV, as well as IFV and PIV (63,64). RSV-caused bronchiolitis, for example, is characterized by necrosis and sloughing of the epithelium of the small airways and induction of mucus secretion, a fact that leads to airway obstruction. Alveolar filling and interstitial infiltration have been observed, especially during fatal cases in adult patients. Restoration of epithelial structures is generally delayed, with ciliated epithelial cells reappearing after 2 weeks, whereas 4–8 weeks are considered as the usual time period for complete recovery in normal cases (65). RSV-mediated respiratory illness is of major importance in infancy, where community-acquired infection rates can be up to 60% in the first year of life (46).

The consequences of the viruses' ability to spread in the lower respiratory tract are being manifested in statistics concerning virus-associated hospitalizations and death rates, varying between different population groups. In a collective study from 10 developing countries, 70% of the children under 5 years of age exhibiting lower respiratory tract illness had been infected by RSV (66). In the elderly, 10% of hospitalizations during winter are due to RSV infections (67). Notably, another 10% of these cases seems to be fatal. Also, in adult patients, up to 2.4% of community-acquired lower respiratory tract-associated illnesses can be attributed to RSV (68). On the other hand, 15% of PIV infections in children lead to lower-tract-associated complications (69). Furthermore, annual influenza epidemics cause significant morbidity and mortality rates worldwide, due to pneumonia, as well as influenza-related symptoms (63).

The implication of RSV infection for the development of pneumonias and lower respiratory tract disease in early life, as well as the late asthma and/or wheezing concerning pneumonias, has been firmly established through prospective studies (70). Another major contributor in the development of acute respiratory tract infections in children up to 3 years old is RV. Although RSV results in hospitalization of pediatric patients clearly more frequently than RV, rhinovirus's effects are similar, when associated with bronchiolitis (71). Kellner et al. (72), using tissue culture virus isolation techniques, were able to show that in pediatric patients with a normal immune status, 14% of acute obstructive bronchitis and 25% of pneumonia manifestations were associated with rhinovirus infection, not substantially differing from RSV percentages (24% and 25%, respectively). In studies in which the age range was restricted to the first 30 days of life, RSV infections associated with pneumonia were more frequent (55%) than the second more abundant source, that of RV (15%)

(73). In a recent study of infants with bronchiolitis, RV was isolated in about one-third of virally confirmed cases and its presence was associated with increased disease severity (74). The contribution of the remaining respiratory viruses (parainfluenza and influenza viruses, adenoviruses, and enteroviruses) appeared less pronounced for this age group, in these studies (72–74). However, there is no doubt that influenza virus infections can cause primary viral pneumonia characterized by bilateral interstitial infiltrates, as well as that they result in asthma and bronchitis exacerbations in patients with asthma and chronic obstructive pulmonary disease (COPD), respectively (63). In contrast, coronaviruses (both OC43 and 229E types) seem to cause mainly upper respiratory tract infections (75), although lower respiratory tract complications are not excluded under specific conditions, as described below.

Lower respiratory tract complications are of course more prominent in individuals with impaired immune status or chronic disorders. In particular, children with chronic conditions are 4–21 times more likely to be hospitalized for acute respiratory illness, during epidemics of influenza (76). In subjects with cardiopulmonary disorders, infection by influenza A, RSV, RV, and coronavirus led to similar symptoms of lower respiratory illness; however, only the former two forced the individual to undergo hospitalization (77). In patients with pulmonary diseases of different causes (including asthma, COPD, bronchiolitis, and pneumonia), IFV, PIV, and RSV infections likewise made up 75% of the total viral infections detected. Nevertheless, picornaviruses and coronaviruses were also present, with the former showing a preference for pediatric patients, whereas the latter appears only in adults (78). Recent evidence suggests that RVs and coronaviruses can also be associated at high percentages (depending on the age group) with cardiopulmonary diseases. The symptoms of the infection vary, ranging from bronchiolitis and pneumonia in young children to exacerbations of asthma in older children, and COPD and congestive heart failure in the elderly (79). The impact of an RSV infection has been recently assessed in this age group and the virus has been found responsible for as much as 2–9% of pneumonias occurring annually in the United States (80).

The impact of RV infection on lower respiratory illness has gained increasing attention during the last years. Early recovery of rhinoviruses from sputum during acute exacerbation of chronic bronchitis suggested a pivotal role of RV infection in causing lower respiratory tract disease (81). Accordingly, development of pneumonia in infants has been associated with infection by RV serotype 13, which, in addition, was immunohistochemically detected in the lungs (81,82). A significant finding is that rhinovirus is readily detected in the sputum of COPD patients after the onset of COPD exacerbation, clearly correlating RV infection with worsening of this chronic condition of the lower respiratory tract (83). In a recent paper the presence of RV genetic material was documented in lung tissue from patients who died from asthma (84). It should be noted, however, that multiple virus detection is common in samples from asthmatic cadavers, with RSV being the predominant respiratory virus, followed by RV (84,85). Flow cytometric analysis of $CD8^+$ T lymphocytes recovered from these samples revealed a $CD8^+$-mediated Th1/Th2 switch in the bronchi of the patients developing fatal asthma (84).

Immunosuppressed subjects form an important study group since they are frequently infected by viral agents, whereas at the same time lower respiratory tract infections are the most common health complication they face. In a recent 5 year study, respiratory viruses including IFV, PIV, adenoviruses, RSV, enteroviruses, and RV were recovered from bronchoalveolar lavage (BAL) fluid of immunocompromised patients, forming 20% of total viral isolates from these subjects (86). Most of the infected individuals developed pneumonia, with the higher percentages attributed to IF virus, eventually leading to death. In particular, IFV-A infection seems to be largely associated with lower respiratory complications in the majority of adult bone marrow transplant patients and other groups of immunocompromised adults (87). High morbidity and mortality rates of immunocompromised subjects due to pneumonia and other lower respiratory tract diseases have also been reported for PIV (86,88). Although the impact of RSV infection in adulthood is generally characterized as rather mild, when the patient's immune status is suppressed mortality rates as high as 32% of those infected have likewise been reported (89). Several manifestations of RSV and PIV infection are being shared by other opportunistic pathogens infecting immunocompromised patients (e.g., cytomegalovirus). Although this may obscure the primary cause of the structural and functional changes occurring in the lower respiratory tract, focal to diffuse alveolar interstitial infiltrates are generally attributed to the conventional respiratory viruses (64). In a recent study, the majority of myelosuppressed blood and marrow transplant recipients who were infected with RV developed fatal pneumonia (90), once again pointing out that this virus could cause a considerable disease burden. This will need to be re-evaluated in comparison to agents previously considered to have higher impact, such as IFV and RSV.

V. In Vitro Studies of Respiratory Virus Infection in Lower Respiratory Cellular Elements

Numerous in vitro studies have attempted to evaluate the effects of virus infections in cells originating from both upper and lower respiratory tracts. Although these assays were conducted under laboratory conditions not necessarily identical with those prevailing in vivo, experimental data reflect similar functional and structural changes reported from clinical observations as described above, while shedding light on the mechanisms underlying postinfectious alterations in lower respiratory epithelium.

One of the important questions addressed in the respective studies is to what extent respiratory virus infection, especially RV, can mediate epithelial cell death. This is of particular importance in the lower epithelium since necrotic epithelial cells can lead to airway narrowing, thus significantly contributing to asthma exacerbations (91).

Several studies have shown that respiratory viruses are in general able to infect and propagate in cells of respiratory origin. However, although RV, coronavirus, IFV-A, and adenovirus could be propagated in human nasal epithelial cells, only

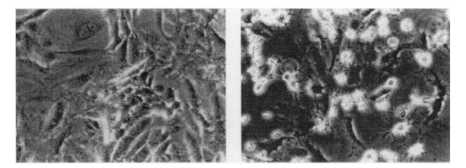

Figure 2 Cytopathic effect produced by rhinovirus on cultured bronchial epithelial cells (right panel). A normal monolayer is shown on the left.

the two last produced cytopathic effect (CPE) (92). On the other hand, RSV readily infects and is propagated in both nasal and bronchial epithelial cells, although the former are able to produce significantly higher viral titers. It is interesting that RSV can also infect bronchoalveolar macrophages, yet this inoculation seems to be less productive than that targeted to the epithelial cells of the respiratory tract (93). RV can also infect human bronchial epithelial cell lines (18), as well as primary human bronchial epithelial cultures (10) (Fig. 2). In the latter case, a CPE could be observed when the cells were cultured at low cell densities (10). Similar results were reported from another recent study; however, in that case RV-mediated CPE was attributed to specific serotypes (94). The evidence suggesting that RVs do attack the lower respiratory epithelium was further supported by our recent finding showing that, in contrast to previous observations (8), RVs replicate readily at 37°C (mean temperature of the lower respiratory tract), and may exceptionally even prefer it to 33°C (mean temperature of the upper tract) (9). Thus, the conditions prevailing in lower respiratory tract do not form an obstacle to RV infection, as previously believed.

Infection by RV is able to stimulate the expression of several cytokines and inflammatory mediators, which can play a significant role in destabilizing the homeostasis of the physiological respiratory epithelium. A number of these mediators can attract eosinophils and other cell types in the inflammatory region, further propagating pathogenetic changes toward the asthmatic phenotype. In characteristic fashion, RV infection induces the production of IL-8, IL-6, and GM-CSF from BEAS-2B epithelial cell line (18). IL-8 promoter activity has been shown to be positively regulated by RV39 through an NF-kB-mediated transcriptional pathway (95). However, a recent report provides evidence that in human bronchial epithelial cells both IL-6- and IL-8 RV-mediated upregulation are NF-kB independent, whereas translocation of this transcription factor seems to be partially responsible for the induction of GM-CSF expression in these cells (96).

The well-established eosinophil chemoattractant RANTES (94), as well as eotaxin and eotaxin-2 (97), are significantly increased following RV infection. Similar increases in RANTES production from human bronchial epithelial cells were also observed during RSV infection, and the effect seems to be mediated through activation and nuclear translocation of the transcription factor NF-κB upon RSV infection (98,99). In this context it was also shown that RSV-infected alveolar epithelial cells (the A549 cell line) are able to trigger eosinophil degranulation, as judged by measurements of released eosinophil cationic protein (ECP) (100). An interesting finding is that RSV-mediated RANTES production by A549 cells, as well as by the normal human bronchial cell line NHBE, decreased when the cells were pretreated with an antibody against ICAM-1. This treatment also protected the epithelial cells from subsequent RSV infection, suggesting that, at least partially, infection by this virus depends on the very same receptor used by the major RV group (101).

ICAM-1 expression is also stimulated by major RVs in primary human bronchial epithelial cells, through an NF-κB-dependent mechanism (102), suggesting a positive auto-regulatory loop during virus infection of the epithelium. Minor RVs are likewise able to upregulate low-density lipoprotein (LDL) receptor in epithelial cells (103). Such loops can be successfully inhibited by corticosteroid treatment (104).

Finally, RV stimulates the antigen-presentation machinery of bronchial and pulmonary epithelial cells by upregulating MHC-I and costimulatory molecule (e.g., B7-1) expression (105). RVs can also infect other cellular units of the respiratory tract and alter important functional characteristics. For example, RV infection of human bronchial smooth muscle cells and rabbit tracheal smooth muscle cells has been shown to increase the smooth muscle constrictor responsiveness and to diminish β-adrenoreceptor-mediated relaxation. This antirelaxative action of RV is probably mediated by upregulation of a component of the signal transduction pathway leading to cAMP accumulation (106). However, it should be noted here that it is doubtful whether RV is able to reach these cellular elements that are more or less hidden underneath the epithelium. Finally, RV, but also RSV and PIV-3, stimulate IL-11 expression from human stromal cells (lung fibroblasts) (24).

The duration of RSV expression may also alter macrophage function, as has been shown in in vitro studies with a macrophage-like cell line in which these inflammatory cells were characterized by increased phagocytosis and production of IL-1β and IL-6 (107).

In conclusion, respiratory viruses are able to infect and activate several lower respiratory cellular elements, most notably bronchial epithelium, suggesting potential steps in the cascade leading from infection to asthma exacerbation and/or perpetuation.

VI. Animal Models of Lower Respiratory Tract Viral Infections

Extensive studies have been conducted with animal models for most respiratory virus infections, with the notable exception of RV, confirming data from in vitro studies and clinical observations in humans. Intranasal inoculation of adenovirus type 5 readily leads to pneumonia in cotton rats and mice, even when the virus fails to replicate (108,109). Primate and murine models of IFV-A infection confirm the ability of this virus to cause pneumonia. The H5N1 subtype, which is of avian origin but results in primary viral pneumonia in humans (and death in some cases) (110), was highly propagated in the lungs of *Cynomolgus* macaques, resulting in extensive loss of alveolar and bronchiolar epithelium, and necrotic lesions in the lungs in some cases (111). Immunohistochemical findings provided evidence that the virus affected both bronchial and bronchiolar epithelial cells, pneumocytes, alveolar macrophages, and neutrophils. However, infection was restricted to the respiratory tract and was not found in the brain or other tissues as seen in rodents, pointing out the importance of the animal model. Similar findings, although of much less severity, were reported for the common H3N2 human subtype (112).

RSV-related studies presented evidence showing that following the initial infection of the upper respiratory tract, RSV is spread in the lower airway (113–115), associated with an increase in airway reactivity (116). Focal severe chronic bronchiolitis was recently induced in a bovine model of aerosol-mediated RSV infection, also associated with alteration of ciliogenesis (117). Lung-localized viral proteins persist for more than 6 weeks in guinea pigs, despite the appearance of anti-RSV antibodies, suggesting that they may be insufficient for clearance of the virus (118). Murine animal models of RSV infection have been also established. In these models RSV inoculation leads to airway damage and airway hyperreactivity 10–12 days postinfection, with IL-13 playing a pivotal role in this response (119).

Asthma-related physiological changes are often described in the airways of virus-infected laboratory animals. Thus, increased airway reactivity to histamine and acetylcholine and airway hyperresponsiveness to metacholine were reported in guinea pigs following PIV-3 infection (115,116,120,121). In dogs, a transient increase of the bronchial reactivity to acetylcholine was observed following IFV-C infection, peaking 1 week later and returning to normal levels 1 month after the inoculation (122).

Viral infection also stimulates chemoattractive functions, leading to recruitment of inflammatory cells to the epithelial tissue. Four days after inoculation, PIV-3 infected guinea pigs showed an influx of inflammatory cells in the airways: mainly alveolar macrophages, a feature associated with the appearance of airway hyperresponsiveness (123). PIV-3- or RSV-infected guinea pigs show increased populations of recruited inflammatory cells, such as macrophages, monocytes, lymphocytes, and eosinophils, in the lower airway (115,116,123). The BAL fluid of PIV-3-infected guinea pigs likewise contains increased numbers of lymphocytes (120,123).

Respiratory virus infections generally lead to activation and redistribution of cell populations that mediate innate immunity. Thus, increased numbers of lung neutrophils and eosinophils, in parallel to airway hyperresponsiveness to metacholine, have been observed in murine models of RSV infection (124), with IL-5 playing a critical role in the development of this inflammatory state (125). Notable is that eosinophilia and infiltration of the lamina propria with lymphoid mononuclear cells, as well as increased airway reactivity to metacholine, are also characteristic features of murine models of asthma (126). On the contrary, the role of neutrophils remains obscure and there is also evidence that the number of neutrophils is not significantly increased in a guinea pig PIV-3 infection model (127).

Mast cell morphology and numbers are altered towards a more activated state following PIV-3 infection of guinea pigs (127). In addition, in a rat model of PIV infection of the lung, mast cells were accumulated in the airways, leading to the development of persistent airway hyperresponsiveness (128,129). Similar findings in calves suggested that increased levels of histamine released by the mast cells play an important role in virus-induced airway hyperresponsiveness (130).

Detailed studies have been conducted to monitor cytokine production following infection of laboratory animals. Thus, mice infected with influenza IL-1 and TNF-α were elevated in BAL fluid (131). Moreover, in a similar model CM-CSF, TNF-α, IL-1α, IL-1β, and IFN-γ concentrations peaked between 36 and 72 h postinfection, whereas IL-6 remained steadily elevated through the infection period. Other cytokines such as G-CSF and M-CSF show more delayed kinetics, reaching maximum values 5 days postinfection (132). Moreover, PIV-3 stimulates IFN-γ production in hamsters and mice (81,132,133).

In all, animal models have been useful in unraveling various links between lower respiratory infection and the development of inflammation and airway responsiveness. Unfortunately, there are no conclusive small-animal model studies concerning human RV infection. A major limitation appears to be the fact that 90% of human rhinoviruses bind to human ICAM-1 to infect target cells (40,134) but are unable to bind to murine ICAM-1 (135). However, minor RVs, using LDL receptor for cell entrance, bind to both the human and the murine version of this protein (41,136). This allows this RV group to infect murine cells of both mesenchymal and epithelial origin (136,137). Moreover, by transfecting mouse fibroblasts with RNA from a major group RV, Lomax and Yin (137) were able to achieve transient viral growth of a major group member in the murine environment. Recent observations showing that major RVs can readily infect murine bronchial epithelial cells, stably transfected with human ICAM-1 (Tuthill TB, Papadopoulos NG et al., manuscript in preparation), suggest that the generation of transgenic animal models of RV infection may be feasible in the near future.

VII. Experimental Human Studies with RV: The Ultimate Evidence

The absence of a reliable animal model for RV infection is counterbalanced by the fact that the mild symptoms caused by these viruses allow the experimental challenge of human volunteers with these pathogens. This renders RV human studies invaluable tools in monitoring and evaluating the impact of respiratory virus infections.

Thus, it has been shown that human rhinoviruses can cause common cold symptoms and induce characteristic damage nasal epithelium (138). Notably, clinical features of tracheobronchitis were apparent after RV inoculation in some of the early studies, suggesting an effect of this virus in the lower epithelium (139). In carefully designed health safety protocols, inoculation (nasal instillation) of 2×10^3–3×10^4 tissue culture-50% infective dose ($TCID_{50}$) of human rhinovirus serotype 16 has been able to cause symptomatic experimental colds in healthy and/or asthmatic individuals, as judged by a number of criteria, including Jackson score (140–142), increased titers of rhinovirus neutralizing antibodies in serum, and others (143). Although a significant increase in metacholine reactivity is reported, Fleming et al. (143) did not observe any significant change in pulmonary function, or any related asthma exacerbation following RV infection under these conditions. Furthermore, these authors did not find any difference regarding bronchial reactivity in asthmatics, nor did rhinovirus inoculation cause asthma exacerbation in their group of asthmatics. These data partially confirmed previous results in which asthmatic subjects inoculated with higher doses of RV16 (3×10^4 $TFID_{50}$), did not show any changes in FEV_1 values compared with the control group (141,142). Infection of healthy individuals with RV39 likewise did not cause any alteration in lower airway function, including bronchial reactivity to metacholine (144). However, the significant increase in response to metacholine observed also in some of the RV16 reports is clearly correlated with a worsening of asthma (141). Furthermore, aerosol- or nasal instillation-mediated inoculation of RV16 causes increased bronchial reactivity to histamine in asthmatics (142,145,146), but not in all cases (147).

Since the conditions of the naturally occurring rhinovirus infection cannot be precisely reproduced, it is possible that differences in inoculation protocols concerning both the quantity of applied virus and application manner might affect the overall viral effects in the lower airway. Moreover, differences among the more than 100 RV serotypes might explain variations in the severity or the type of the effects they cause. Finally, serially passaged RV strains in laboratory cell culture conditions might have accumulated modifications leading to changes in virulence and other growth characteristics compared to the native ancestors.

However, there is no doubt that RV infections cause significant alterations in the lower airways, which can be related to changes in airway responsiveness and asthma exacerbations. In an early study, success in culturing and isolation RV from children with wheezy bronchitis was twice as probable when sputum was used as the initial material, compared to nasal or throat-derived samples (42). In subsequent studies with experimentally infected volunteers, RV cultures were obtained from lower-airway brushings (148). Moreover, with the aid of the RT-PCR technique, the presence of RV genetic material was clearly documented in bronchial lavage cells, and this happened only after experimental inoculation (149). However, lower airway secretions obtained through sputum induction or bronchoscopy may be contaminated with material from the upper airway (150). Recently, the presence of RV genetic material was demonstrated in bronchial biopsies from RV-inoculated volunteers using in situ hybridization (10) (Fig. 3). The implementation of this technique not only excluded the possibility of sample contamination from RV originating from the upper airway but also allowed the detection of the replicative strand of RV in the bronchi, indicating that RV productively infects the lower airways. Furthermore, the identification rates of RV in bronchial biopsies after experimental

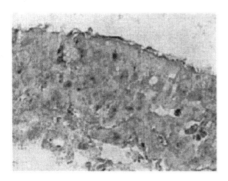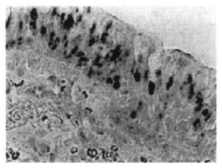

Figure 3 Detection of rhinovirus RNA with in situ hybridization, in a bronchial biopsy of a volunteer experimentally infected with the virus, at baseline (left) and upon an experimentally induced cold (right). No signal is observed at the baseline biopsy. In contrast, an intense signal (black spots) located on the bronchial epithelium can be observed 3 days after nasal inoculation.

inoculation were similar to those reported for nasal samples (151) obtained after experimental or natural infection (50%), consistent with a unique, patchworklike manner of distribution of RV infection, which is similar in both the upper and the lower airways.

Furthermore, bronchial mucosa is infiltrated with lymphocytes and the epithelium is enriched with eosinophils following RV16 infection of asthmatic and healthy individuals (146). However, eosinophilia was apparent in allergic but not in healthy individuals in another RV16 inoculation protocol (147), similar to what is seen in endobronchial allergen challenge (152). In addition, it seems that the effects of RV infection are greatly enhanced in some cases when combined with allergic stimuli. Thus, RV infection increases airway hyperresponsiveness to allergen inhalation and the probability of a subsequent late-phase allergic response (153). Moreover, RV administration leads to increased levels of histamine, released into the lower airways following allergen challenge, as well as to increased numbers of recruited eosinophils and total leukocytes, which can be observed in this tissue 2 days later (147). The fact that these effects are preferentially observed in allergic individuals rather than healthy subjects, suggests a specific induction of allergen-induced airway responsiveness by RV. RV16-inoculated asthmatic subjects are likewise characterized by persistently increased numbers of both eosinophils and T cells recruited in the lower airways (146). In contrast to the healthy control group, the differences observed in the asthmatics in this study were still obvious more than 1 month after the viral infection, indicating that RV can magnify both short- and long-term preexisting allergic responses. Concomitantly, RV39 inoculation was shown to increase total IgE in experimentally infected atopic volunteers, although allergen-specific IgE levels are not affected by this serotype (144,154). Moreover, the well-established RV-mediated increase of histamine release in the lower respiratory tract, observed in the allergic state, seems to be more pronounced in airways characterized by higher baseline FEV_1 values (155). The above findings clearly indicate that RV infections specifically enhance allergen-induced responses in the lower airway. Furthermore, these and other studies suggest that RVs and allergens may not act independently but rather in tandem in the lower respiratory tract, their overall effect depending on, among other factors, the type of immune response (e.g., Th1/Th2 balance) elicited by the host against the viral pathogen (33,156).

VIII. Conclusion

Respiratory viruses, in their great majority, can reach and infect the bronchial epithelium. This is probably a frequent event after upper respiratory infections and has a number of important consequences, including initiation and amplification of inflammatory responses, which can lead to an acute asthma exacerbation. Discerning relative importance of this pathway, as well as its interaction with inflammatory pathways mediated through other stimuli, such as allergens or pollutants, is next step, in understanding the pathogenesis of asthma exacerbations.

References

1. Papadopoulos N, Johnston S. Viral infections of the nose and lung. Eur Respir Mono 2002; in press.
2. Bronchial Asthma. WHO Fact Sheet 2000; 206: http://www.who.int/inf-fs/en/fact206.html.
3. Pattemore PK, Johnston SL, Bardin PG. Viruses as precipitants of asthma symptoms. I. Epidemiology. Clin Exp Allergy 1992; 22:325–336.
4. Johnston SL, Pattemore PK, Sanderson G, Smith S, Lampe F, Josephs L, Symington P, O'Toole S, Myint SH, Tyrrell DAJ, Holgate ST. Community study of role of viral infections in exacerbations of asthma in 9–11-year-old children. Br Med J 1995; 310: 1225–1228.
5. Nicholson KG, Kent J, Ireland DC. Respiratory viruses and exacerbations of asthma in adults. Br Med J 1993; 307:982–986.
6. Johnston SL, Pattemore PK, Sanderson G, Smith S, Campbell MJ, Josephs LK, Cunningham A, Robinson BS, Myint SH, Ward ME, Tyrrell DA, Holgate ST. The relationship between upper respiratory infections and hospital admissions for asthma: a time-trend analysis. Am J Respir Crit Care Med 1996; 154:654–660.
7. Gem JE, Busse WW. The effects of rhinovirus infections on allergic airway responses. Am J Respir Crit Care Med 1995; 152:S40–45.
8. Killington RA, Stott EJ, Lee D. The effect of temperature on the synthesis of rhinovirus type 2 RNA. J Gen Virol 1977; 36:403–411.
9. Papadopoulos NG, Sanderson G, Hunter J, Johnston SL. Rhinoviruses replicate effectively at lower airway temperatures. J Med Virol 1999; 58:100–104.
10. Papadopoulos NG, Bates PJ, Bardin PG, Papi A, Leir SH, Fraenkel DJ, Meyer J, Lackie PM, Sanderson G, Holgate ST, Johnston SL. Rhinoviruses infect the lower airways. J Infect Dis 2000; 181:1875–1884.
11. Butler GB, Adler KB, Evans JN, Morgan DW, Szarek JL. Modulation of rabbit airway

smooth muscle responsiveness by respiratory epithelium. Involvement of an inhibitory metabolite of arachidonic acid. Am Rev Respir Dis 1987; 135:1099–1104.

12. Piedimonte G, Rodriguez MM, King KA, McLean S, Jiang X. Respiratory syncytial virus upregulates expression of the substance P receptor in rat lungs. Am J Physiol 1999; 277:L831–840.

13. Piedimonte G, King KA, Holmgren NL, Bertrand PJ, Rodriguez MM, Hirsch RL. A humanized monoclonal antibody against respiratory syncytial virus (palivizumab) inhibits RSV-induced neurogenic-mediated inflammation in rat airways. Pediatr Res 2000; 47:351–356.

14. Borson DB, Brokaw JJ, Sekizawa K, McDonald DM, Nadel JA. Neutral endopeptidase and neurogenic inflammation in rats with respiratory infections. J Appl Physiol 1989; 66:2653–2658.

15. Dusser DJ, Jacoby DB, Djokic TD, Rubinstein I, Borson DB, Nadel JA. Virus induces airway hyperresponsiveness to tachykinins: role of neutral endopeptidase. J Appl Physiol 1989; 67:1504–1511.

16. Jacoby DB, Fryer AD. Interaction of viral infections with muscarinic receptors. Clin Exp Allergy 1999; 29 Suppl 2:59–64.

17. Empey DW, Laitinen LA, Jacobs L, Gold WM, Nadel JA. Mechanisms of bronchial hyperreactivity in normal subjects after upper respiratory tract infection. Am Rev Respir Dis 1976; 113:131–139.

18. Subauste MC, Jacoby DB, Richards SM, Proud D. Infection of a human respiratory epithelial cell line with rhinovirus. Induction of cytokine release and modulation of susceptibility to infection by cytokine exposure. J Clin Invest 1995; 96:549–557.

19. Arnold R, Humbert B, Werchau H, Gallati H, Konig W. Interleukin-8, interleukin-6, and soluble tumour necrosis factor receptor type I release from a human pulmonary epithelial cell line (A549) exposed to respiratory syncytial virus. Immunology 1994; 82:126–133.

20. Zhu Z, Tang W, Ray A, Wu Y, Einarsson O, Landry M, Gwaltney JJ, Elias J. Rhinovirus stimulation of interleukin-6 in vivo and in vitro. Evidence for nuclear factor kappa B-dependent transcriptional activation. J Clin Invest 1996; 97:421–430.

21. Zhu Z, Tang W, Gwaltney JM, Wu Y, Elias JA. Rhinovirus stimulation of interleukin-8 in vivo and in vitro: role of NF-kappa B. Am J Physiol 1997; 273:L814–824.

22. Kameyoshi Y, Dorschner A, Mallet AI, Christophers E, Schroder JM. Cytokine RANTES released by thrombin-stimulated platelets is a potent attractant for human eosinophils. J Exp Med 1992; 176:587–592.

23. Lopez AF, Williamson DJ, Gamble JR, Begley CG, Harlan JM, Klebanoff SJ, Waltersdorph A, Wong G, Clark SC, Vadas MA. Recombinant human granulocyte-macrophage colony-stimulating factor stimulates in vitro mature human neutrophil and eosinophil function, surface receptor expression, and survival. J Clin Invest 1986; 78:1220–1228.

24. Einarsson O, Geba G, Zhu Z, Landry M, Elias J. Interleukin-11: stimulation in vivo and in vitro by respiratory viruses and induction of airways hyperresponsiveness. J Clin Invest 1996; 97:915–924.

25. Teran LM, Johnston SL, Schroder JM, Church MK, Holgate ST. Role of nasal interleukin-8 in neutrophil recruitment and activation in children with virus-induced asthma. Am J Respir Crit Care Med 1997; 155:1362–1366.

26. Becker S, Quay J, Soukup J. Cytokine (tumor necrosis factor, IL-6, and IL-8) production by respiratory syncytial virus-infected human alveolar macrophages. J Immunol 1991; 147:4307–4312.

27. Tosi MF, Stark JM, Smith CW, Hamedani A, Gruenert DC, Infeld MD. Induction of ICAM-1 expression on human airway epithelial cells by inflammatory cytokines: effects on neutrophil-epithelial cell adhesion. Am J Respir Cell Mol Biol 1992; 7:214–221.

28. Stark JM, Godding V, Sedgwick JB, Busse WW. Respiratory syncytial virus infection enhances neutrophil and eosinophil adhesion to cultured respiratory epithelial cells. Roles of CD18 and intercellular adhesion molecule-1. J Immunol 1996; 156:4774-4782.

29. Baumgarth N, Brown L, Jackson D, Kelso A. Novel features of the respiratory tract T-cell response to influenza virus infection: lung T cells increase expression of gamma interferon mRNA in vivo and maintain high levels of mRNA expression for interleukin-5 (IL-5) and IL-10. J Virol 1994; 68:7575–7581.

30. Sarawar SR, Doherty PC. Concurrent production of interleukin-2, interleukin-10, and gamma interferon in the regional lymph nodes of mice with influenza pneumonia. J Virol 1994; 68:3112–3119.

31. Roberts NJ. Different effects of influenza virus, respiratory syncytial virus, and Sendai virus on human lymphocytes and macrophages. Infect Immun 1982; 35:1142–1146.

32. Gem J, Joseph B, Galagan D, Borcherding W, Dick E. Rhinovirus inhibits antigen-specific T cell proliferation through an intercellular adhesion molecule-1-dependent mechanism. J Infect Dis 1996; 174:1143–1150.

33. Papadopoulos NG, Stanciu LA, Papi A, Holgate ST, Johnston SL. A defective type-1 response to rhinovirus in atopic asthma. Thorax 2002; in press.

34. Papadopoulos NG, Stanciu LA, Papi A, Holgate ST, Johnston SL. Rhinovirus-induced alterations on peripheral blood mononuclear cell phenotype and costimulatory molecule expression in normal and atopic asthmatic subjects. Am J Respir Crit Care Med 2000; 161:A898.

35. Bardin PG, Johnston SL, Pattemore PK. Viruses as precipitants of asthma symptoms II. Physiology and mechanisms. Clin Exp Allergy 1993; 22:809–822.

36. Schuster A, Fahy JV, Ueki I, Nadel JA. Cystic fibrosis sputum induces a secretory response from airway gland serous cells that can be prevented by neutrophil protease inhibitors. Eur Respir J 1995; 8:10–14.

37. Grunberg K, Smits H, Timmers M, de Klerk E, Dolhain R, Dick E, Hiemstra P, Sterk P. Experimental rhinovirus 16 infection. Effects on cell differentials soluble markers in sputum in asthmatic subjects. Am J Respir Crit Care Med 1997; 156:609–616.

38. Passalacqua G, Ciprandi G, Canonica GW. United airways disease: therapeutic aspects. Thorax 2000; 55 Suppl 2:S26–27.

39. Papadopoulos NG, Johnston SL. Rhinoviruses. In: Zuckerman A, Banatvala J, Pattison J, eds. Principles and Practice of Clinical Virology, 4th ed. Chichester: John Wiley & Sons, 1999:329–343.

40. Greve JM, Davis G, Meyer AM, Forte CP, Yost SC, Marlor CW, Kamarck ME, McClelland A. The major human rhinovirus receptor is ICAM-1. Cell 1989; 56:839–847.

41. Hofer F, Gruenberger M, Kowalski H, Machat H, Huettinger M, Kuechler E, Blass D. Members of the low density lipoprotein receptor family mediate cell entry of a minor-group common cold virus. Proc Natl Acad Sci USA 1994; 91:1839–1842.

42. Horn M, Reed S, Taylor P. Role of viruses and bacteria in acute wheezy bronchitis in childhood: a study of sputum. Arch Dis Child 1979; 54:587–592.

43. Peret TCT, Hall CB, Hammond GW, Piedra PA, Storch GA, Sullender WM, Tsou C, Anderson LJ. Circulation patterns of group A and B human respiratory syncytial

virus genotypes in 5 communities in North America. J Infect Dis 2000; 181:1891–1896.

44. Hall CB, Douglas RGJ, Geiman JM. Respiratory syncytial virus infections in infants: quantitation and duration of shedding. J Pediatr 1976; 89:11–15.

45. Hall CB. Respiratory syncytial virus: a continuing culprit and conundrum. J Pediatr 1999; 135:S2–7.

46. Glezen WP, Taber LH, Frank AL, Kasel JA. Risk of primary infection and reinfection with respiratory syncytial virus. Am J Dis Child 1986; 140:543–546.

47. Potter CW. Influenza. In: Zuckerman AJ, Banatvala JE, Pattison JR, eds. Principles and Practice of Clinical Virology. Chichester: John Wiley & Sons, 2000:253–277.

48. Brammer TL, Izurieta HS, Fukuda K, Schmeltz LM, Regnery HL, Hall HE, Cox NJ. Surveillance for influenza—United States, 1994–95, 1995–96, and 1996–97 seasons. MMWR CDC Surveill Summ 2000; 49:13–28.

49. Update: influenza activity—United States and worldwide, 1999–2000 season, and composition of the 2000–01 influenza vaccine. MMWR 2000; 49:375–381.

50. Stamboulian D, Bonvehi PE, Nacinovich FM, Cox N. Influenza. Infect Dis Clin North Am 2000; 14:141–166.

51. Carson JL, Collier AM, Hu SS. Acquired ciliary defects in nasal epithelium of children with acute viral upper respiratory infections. N Engl J Med 1985; 312:463–468.

52. Matsuse T, Hayashi S, Kuwano K, Keunecke H, Jefferies WA, Hogg JC. Latent adenoviral infection in the pathogenesis of chronic airways obstruction. Am Rev Respir Dis 1992; 146:177–184.

53. Myint SH. Human coronaviruses: a brief review. Rev Med Virol 1994; 4:35–46.

54. Yeager CL, Ashmun RA, Williams RK, Cardellichio CB, Shapiro LH, Look AT, Holmes KV. Human aminopeptidase N is a receptor for human coronavirus 229E. Nature 1992; 357:420–422.

55. Collins AR. Human coronavirus OC43 interacts with major histocompatibility complex class I molecules at the cell surface to establish infection. Immunol Invest 1994; 23:313–321.

56. Afzelius BA. Ultrastructure of human nasal epithelium during an episode of coronavirus infection. Virchows Arch 1994; 424:295–300.

57. Callow KA, Parry HF, Sergeant M, Tyrrell DA. The time course of the immune response to experimental coronavirus infection of man. Epidemiol Infect 1990; 105:435–446.

58. Falsey A, McCann R, Hall W, Criddle M, Formica M, Wycoff D, Kolassa J. The "common cold" in frail older persons: impact of rhinovirus and coronavirus in a senior daycare center. J Am Geriatr Soc 1997; 45:706–711.

59. Leogrande G. Studies on the epidemiology of child infections. 3. Parainfluenza viruses (types 1–4) and respiratory syncytial virus infections. Microbios 1992; 72:55–63.

60. Easton AJ, Eglin RP. Epidemiology of parainfluenza virus type 3 in England and Wales over a ten-year period. Epidemiol Infect 1989; 102:531–535.

61. McLean DM, Bannatyne RM, Givan KF. Myxovirus dissemination by air. Can Med Assoc J 1967; 96:1449–1453.

62. Ansari SA, Springthorpe VS, Sattar SA, Rivard S, Rahman M. Potential role of hands in the spread of respiratory viral infections: studies with human parainfluenza virus 3 and rhinovirus 14. J Clin Microsc 1991; 29:2115–2119.

63. Cox NJ, Subbarao K. Influenza. Lancet 1999; 354:1277–1282.

64. Hall CB. Respiratory syncytial virus and parainfluenza virus. N Engl J Med 2001; 344:1917–1928.

65. Hall WJ, Hall CB, Speers DM. Respiratory syncytial virus infection in adults: clinical, virologic, and serial pulmonary function studies. Ann Intern Med 1978; 88:203–205.

66. Selwyn BJ. The epidemiology of acute respiratory tract infection in young children: comparison of findings from several developing countries. Coordinated Data Group of BOSTID Researchers. Rev Infect Dis 12 Suppl 8:S870–888.

67. Simoes EA. Respiratory syncytial virus infection. Lancet 1999; 354:847–852.

68. Dowell SF, Anderson LJ, Gary HE Jr, Erdman DD, Plouffe JF, File TM Jr, Marston BJ, Breiman RF. Respiratory syncytial virus is an important cause of community-acquired lower respiratory infection among hospitalized adults. J Infect Dis 1996; 174:456–462.

69. Reed G, Jewett PH, Thompson J, Tollefson S, Wright PF. Epidemiology and clinical impact of parainfluenza virus infections in otherwise healthy infants and young children <5 years old. J Infect Dis 1997; 175:807–813.

70. Castro-Rodriguez JA, Holberg CJ, Wright AL, Halonen M, Taussig LM, Morgan WJ, Martinez FD. Association of radiologically ascertained pneumonia before age 3 yr with asthmalike symptoms and pulmonary function during childhood: a prospective study Am J Respir Crit Care Med 1999; 159:1891–1897.

71. McMillan J, Weiner L, Higgins A, Macknight K. Rhinovirus infection associated with serious illness among pediatric patients. Pediatr Infect Dis J 1993; 12:321–325.

72. Kellner G, Popow-Kraupp T, Kundi M, Binder C, Kunz C. Clinical manifestations of respiratory tract infections due to respiratory syncytial virus and rhinoviruses in hospitalized children. Acta Paediatr Scand 1989; 78:390–394.

73. Abzug M, Beam A, Gyorkos E, Levin M. Viral pneumonia in the first month of life. Pediatr Infect Dis J 1990; 9:881–885.

74. Papadopoulos NG, Moustaki M, Tsolia M, Bossios A, Astra E, Prezerakou A, Gourgiotis D, Kafetzis D. Association of rhinovirus infection with increased disease severity in acute bronchiolitis. In press 2002.

75. Bradburne AF, Bynoe ML, Tyrrell DA. Effects of a "new" human respiratory virus in volunteers. Br Med J 1967; 3:767-769.

76. Izurieta HS, Thompson WW, Kramarz P, Shay DK, Davis RL, DeStefano F, Black S, Shinefield H, Fukuda K. Influenza and the rates of hospitalization for respiratory disease among infants and young children. N Engl J Med 2000; 342:232–239.

77. Walsh EE, Falsey AR, Hennessey PA. Respiratory syncytial and other virus infections in persons with chronic cardiopulmonary disease. Am J Respir Crit Care Med 1999; 160:791–795.

78. Glezen WP, Greenberg SB, Atmar RL, Piedra PA, Couch RB. Impact of respiratory virus infections on persons with chronic underlying conditions. JAMA 2000; 283:499–505.

79. El Sahly HM, Atmar RL, Glezen WP, Greenberg SB. Spectrum of clinical illness in hospitalized patients with "common cold" virus infections. Clin Infect Dis 2000; 31:96–100.

80. Han LL, Alexander JP, Anderson LJ. Respiratory syncytial virus pneumonia among the elderly: an assessment of disease burden. J Infect Dis 1999; 179:25–30.

81. Craighead J, Meier M, Cooley M. Pulmonary infection due to rhinovirus type 13. N Engl J Med 1969; 281:1403–1404.

82. Imakita M, Shiraki K, Yutani C, Ishibashi-Ueda H. Pneumonia caused by rhinovirus. Clin Infect Dis 2000; 30:611–612.

83. Seemungal TA, Harpe-Owen R, Bhowmik A, Jeffries DJ, Wedzicha JA. Detection of

rhinovirus in induced sputum at exacerbation of chronic obstructive pulmonary disease. Eur Respir J 2000; 16:677–683.

84. O'Sullivan S, Cormican L, Faul JL, Ichinohe S, Johnston SL, Burke CM, Poulter LW. Activated, cytotoxic CD8(+) T lymphocytes contribute to the pathology of asthma death. Am J Respir Crit Care Med 2001; 164:560–564.

85. Macek V, Dakhama A, Hogg JC, Green FH, Rubin BK, Hegele RG. PCR detection of viral nucleic acid in fatal asthma: is the lower respiratory tract a reservoir for common viruses? Can Respir J 1999; 6:37–43.

86. Rabella N, Rodriguez P, Labeaga R, Otegui M, Mercader M, Gurgui M, Prats G. Conventional respiratory viruses recovered from immunocompromised patients: clinical considerations. Clin Infect Dis 1999; 28:1043–1048.

87. Whimbey E, Bodey GP. Viral pneumonia in the immunocompromised adult with neoplastic disease: the role of common community respiratory viruses. Semin Respir Infect 1992; 7:122–131.

88. Lewis VA, Champlin R, Englund J, Couch R, Goodrich JM, Rolston K, Przepiorka D, Mirza NQ, Yousuf HM, Luna M, Bodey GP, Whimbey E. Respiratory disease due to parainfluenza virus in adult bone marrow transplant recipients. Clin Infect Dis 1996; 23:1033–1037.

89. Englund JA, Sullivan CJ, Jordan MC, Dehner LP, Vercellotti GM, Balfour HH. Respiratory syncytial virus infection in immunocompromised adults. Ann Intern Med 1988; 109:203–208.

90. Ghosh S, Champlin R, Couch R, Englund J, Raad I, Malik S, Luna M, Whimbey E. Rhinovirus infections in myelosuppressed adult blood and marrow transplant recipients. Clin Infect Dis 1999; 29:528–532.

91. Hegele RG, Hayashi S, Hogg JC, Pare PD. Mechanisms of airway narrowing and hyperresponsiveness in viral respiratory tract infections. Am J Respir Crit Care Med 1995; 151:1659.

92. Winther B, Gwaltney JM, Hendley JO. Respiratory virus infection of monolayer cultures of human nasal epithelial cells. Am Rev Respir Dis 1990; 141:839–845.

93. Becker S, Soukup J, Yankaskas JR. Respiratory syncytial virus infection of human primary nasal and bronchial epithelial cell cultures and bronchoalveolar macrophages. Am J Respir Cell Mol Biol 1992; 6:369–374.

94. Schroth MK, Grimm E, Frindt P, Galagan DM, Konno SI, Love R, Gem JE. Rhinovirus replication causes RANTES production in primary bronchial epithelial cells. Am J Respir Cell Mol Biol 1999; 20:1220–1228.

95. Zhu Z, Tang W, Gwaltney JMJ, Wu Y, Elias JA. Rhinovirus stimulation of interleukin-8 in vivo and in vitro: role of NF-kappa B. Am J Physiol 1997; 273:L814–824.

96. Kim J, Sanders SP, Siekierski ES, Casolaro V, Proud D. Role of NF-kappa B in cytokine production induced from human airway epithelial cells by rhinovirus infection. J Immunol 2000; 165:3384–3392.

97. Papadopoulos NG, Papi A, Meyer J, Stanciu LA, Salvi SS, Holgate ST, Johnston SL. Rhinovirus infection upregulates eotaxin and eotaxin-2 expression in bronchial epithelial cells. Clin Exp Allergy 2001; 31:1060–1064.

98. Thomas LH, Friedland JS, Sharland M, Becker S. Respiratory syncytial virus-induced RANTES production from human bronchial epithelial cells is dependent on nuclear factor-kappa B nuclear binding and is inhibited by adenovirus-mediated expression of inhibitor of kappa B alpha. J Immunol 1998; 161:1007–1016.

99. Bitko V, Barik S. Persistent activation of RelA by respiratory syncytial virus involves

protein kinase C, underphosphorylated IkappaBbeta, and sequestration of protein phosphatase 2A by the viral phosphoprotein. J Virol 1998; 72:5610–5618.

100. Olszewska-Pazdrak B, Pazdrak K, Ogra PL, Garofalo RP. Respiratory syncytial virus-infected pulmonary epithelial cells induce eosinophil degranulation by a CD18-mediated mechanism. J Immunol 1998; 160:4889–4895.

101. Behera AK, Matsuse H, Kumar M, Kong X, Lockey RF, Mohapatra SS. Blocking intercellular adhesion molecule-1 on human epithelial cells decreases respiratory syncytial virus infection. Biochem Biophys Res Commun 2001; 280:188–195.

102. Papi A, Johnston SL. Rhinovirus infection induces expression of its own receptor intercellular adhesion molecule 1 (ICAM-1) via increased NF-kappa B-mediated transcription. J Biol Chem 1999; 274:9707–9720.

103. Suzuki T, Yamaya M, Kamanaka M, Jia YX, Nakayama K, Hosoda M, Yamada N, Nishimura H, Sekizawa K, Sasaki H. Type 2 rhinovirus infection of cultured human tracheal epithelial cells: role of LDL receptor. Am J Physiol 2001; 280:L409–420.

104. Papi A, Papadopoulos NG, Degitz K, Holgate ST, Johnston SL. Corticosteroids inhibit rhinovirus-induced intercellular adhesion molecule-1 up-regulation and promoter activation on respiratory epithelial cells. J Allergy Clin Immunol 2000; 105:318–326.

105. Papi A, Stanciu LA, Papadopoulos NG, Holgate ST, Johnston SL. Rhinovirus infection induces HLA class I , but not class II, and costimulatory molecules upregulation on respiratory epithelial cells. J Infect Dis 2000; 181:1780–1784.

106. Hakonarson H, Maskeri N, Carter C, Hodinka RL, Campbell D, Grunstein MM. Mechanism of rhinovirus-induced changes in airway smooth muscle responsiveness. J Clin Invest 1998; 102:1732–1741.

107. Guerrero-Plata A, Ortega E, Gomez B. Persistence of respiratory syncytial virus in macrophages alters phagocytosis and pro-inflammatory cytokine production. Vir Immunol 2001; 14:19–30.

108. Ginsberg HS, Moldawer LL, Sehgal PB, Redington M, Kilian PL, Chanock RM, Prince GA. A mouse model for investigating the molecular pathogenesis of adenovirus pneumonia. Proc Natl Acad Sci USA 1991; 88:1651–1655.

109. Pacini DL, Dubovi EJ, Clyde WA. A new animal model for human respiratory tract disease due to adenovirus. J Infect Dis 1984; 150:92–97.

110. Yuen KY, Chan PK, Peiris M, Tsang DN, Que TL, Shortridge KF, Cheung PT, To WK, Ho ET, Sung R, Cheng AF. Clinical features and rapid viral diagnosis of human disease associated with avian influenza A H5N1 virus. Lancet 1998; 351:467–471.

111. Rimmelzwaan GF, Kuiken T, van Amerongen G, Bestebroer TM, Fouchier RA, Osterhaus AD. Pathogenesis of influenza A (H5N1) virus infection in a primate model. J Virol 2001; 75:6687–6691.

112. Rimmelzwaan GF, Baars M, van Beek R, van Amerongen G, Lovgren-Bengtsson K, Claas EC, Osterhaus AD. Induction of protective immunity against influenza virus in a macaque model: comparison of conventional and iscom vaccines. J Gen Virol 1997; 78 (Pt 4):757–765.

113. Prince GA, Horswood RL, Berndt J, Suffin SC, Chanock RM. Respiratory syncytial virus infection in inbred mice. Infect Immun 1979; 26:764–766.

114. Kakuk TJ, Soike K, Brideau RJ, Zaya RM, Cole SL, Zhang JY, Roberts ED, Wells PA, Wathen MW. A human respiratory syncytial virus (RSV) primate model of enhanced pulmonary pathology induced with a formalin-inactivated RSV vaccine but not a recombinant FG subunit vaccine. J Infect Dis 1993; 167:553–561.

115.   Hegele RG, Robinson PJ, Gonzalez S, Hogg JC. Production of acute bronchiolitis in guinea-pigs by human respiratory syncytial virus. Eur Respir J 1993; 6:1324–1331.

116.   Robinson PJ, Hegele RG, Schellenberg RR. Increased airway reactivity in human RSV bronchiolitis in the guinea pig is not due to increased wall thickness. Pediatr Pulmonol 1996; 22:248–254.

117.   Philippou S, Otto P, Reinhold P, Elschner M, Streckert HJ. Respiratory syncytial virus-induced chronic bronchiolitis in experimentally infected calves. Virchows Arch 2000; 436:617–621.

118.   Streckert HJ, Philippou S, Riedel F. Detection of respiratory syncytial virus (RSV) antigen in the lungs of guinea pigs 6 weeks after experimental infection and despite the production of neutralizing antibodies. Arch Virol 1996; 141:401–410.

119.   Tekkanat KK, Maassab HF, Cho DS, Lai JJ, John A, Berlin A, Kaplan MH, Lukacs NW. IL-13-induced airway hyperreactivity during respiratory syncytial virus infection is STAT6 dependent. J Immunol 2001; 166:3542–3548.

120.   Folkerts G, Verheyen A, Nijkamp FP. Viral infection in guinea pigs induces a sustained non-specific airway hyperresponsiveness and morphological changes of the respiratory tract. Eur J Pharmacol 1992; 228:121–130.

121.   Kudlacz EM, Shatzer SA, Farrell AM, Baugh LE. Parainfluenza virus type 3 induced alterations in tachykinin NK1 receptors, substance P levels and respiratory functions in guinea pig airways. Eur J Pharmacol 1994; 270:291–300.

122.   Inoue H, Horio S, Ichinose M, Ida S, Hida W, Takishima T, Ohwada K, Homma M. Changes in bronchial reactivity to acetylcholine with type C influenza virus infection in dogs. Am Rev Respir Dis 1986; 133:367–371.

123.   Folkerts G, Van Esch B, Janssen M, Nijkamp FP. Virus-induced airway hyperresponsiveness in guinea pigs in vivo: study of broncho-alveolar cell number and activity. Eur J Pharmacol 1992; 228:219–227.

124.   Schwarze J, Hamelmann E, Bradley KL, Takeda K, Gelfand EW. Respiratory syncytial virus infection results in airway hyperresponsiveness and enhanced airway sensitization to allergen. J Clin Invest 1997; 100:226–233.

125.   Schwarze J, Cieslewicz G, Hamelmann E, Joetham A, Shultz LD, Lamers MC, Gelfand EW. IL-5 and eosinophils are essential for the development of airway hyperresponsiveness following acute respiratory syncytial virus infection. J Immunol 1999; 162:2997–3004.

126.   Temelkovski J, Hogan SP, Shepherd DP, Foster PS, Kumar RK. An improved murine model of asthma: selective airway inflammation, epithelial lesions and increased methacholine responsiveness following chronic exposure to aerosolised allergen. Thorax 1998; 53:849–856.

127.   Folkerts G, Nijkamp FP. Virus-induced airway hyperresponsiveness. Role of inflammatory cells and mediators. Am J Respir Crit Care Med 1995; 151:1666.

128.   Sorkness R, Lemanske RF, Castleman WL. Persistent airway hyperresponsiveness after neonatal viral bronchiolitis in rats. J Appl Physiol 1991; 70:375–383.

129.   Castleman WL, Sorkness RL, Lemanske RF, McAllister PK. Viral bronchiolitis during early life induces increased numbers of bronchiolar mast cells and airway hyperresponsiveness. Am J Pathol 1990; 137:821–831.

130.   Ogunbiyi PO, Black WD, Eyre P. Parainfluenza-3 virus-induced enhancement of histamine release from calf lung mast cells—effect of levamisole. J Vet Pharm Ther 1988; 11:338–344.

131.   Vacheron F, Rudent A, Perin S, Labarre C, Quero AM, Guenounou M. Production of

interleukin 1 and tumour necrosis factor activities in bronchoalveolar washings following infection of mice by influenza virus. J Gen Virol 1990; 71(Pt 2):477–479.

132. Hennet T, Ziltener HJ, Frei K, Peterhans E. A kinetic study of immune mediators in the lungs of mice infected with influenza A virus. J Immunol 1992; 149:932–939.

133. Harmon AT, Harmon MW, Glezen WP. Evidence of interferon production in the hamster lung after primary or secondary exposure to parainfluenza virus type 3. Am Rev Respir Dis 1982; 125:706–711.

134. Uncapher C, DeWitt C, Colonno R. The major and minor group receptor families contain all but one human rhinovirus serotype. Virology 1991; 180:814–817.

135. Register R, Uncapher C, Naylor A, Lineberger D, Colonno R. Human-murine chimeras of ICAM-1 identify amino acid residues critical for rhinovirus and antibody binding. J Virol 1991; 65:6589–6596.

136. Yin F, Lomax N. Host range mutants of human rhinovirus in which nonstructural proteins are altered. J Virol 1983; 48:410–418.

137. Lomax N, Yin F. Evidence for the role of the P2 protein of human rhinovirus in its host range change. J Virol 1989; 63:2396–2399.

138. Turner RB, Hendley JO, Gwaltney JMJ. Shedding of infected ciliated epithelial cells in rhinovirus colds. J Infect Dis 1982; 145:849–853.

139. Cate TR, Couch RB, Fleet WF, Griffith WR, Gerone PJ, Knight V. Production of tracheobronchitis in volunteers with rhinovirus in a small-particle aerosol. Am J Epidemiol 1965; 81:95–105.

140. Jackson GG, Dowling HF, Spiesman IG, Board AV. Transmission of the common cold to volunteers under controlled conditions. 1. The common cold as a clinical entity. Arch Intern Med 1958; 101:267–278.

141. Cheung D, Dick E, Timmers M, de Klerk E, Spaan W, Sterk P. Rhinovirus inhalation causes long-lasting excessive airway narrowing in response to methacholine in asthmatic subjects in vivo. Am J Respir Crit Care Med 1995; 152:1490–1496.

142. Grunberg K, Timmers M, Smits H, de Klerk E, Dick E, Spaan W, Hiemstra P, Sterk P. Effect of experimental rhinovirus-16 colds on airway hyperresponsiveness to histamine and interleukin-8 in nasal lavage in asthmatic subjects in vivo. Clin Exp Allergy 1997; 27:36–45.

143. Fleming HE, Little FF, Schnurr D, Avila PC, Wong H, Liu J, Yagi S, Boushey HA. Rhinovirus-16 colds in healthy and in asthmatic subjects: similar changes in upper and lower airways. Am J Respir Crit Care Med 1999; 160:100–108.

144. Skoner D, Doyle W, Seroky J, Van Deusen M, Fireman P. Lower airway responses to rhinovirus 39 in healthy allergic and nonallergic subjects. Eur Respir J 1996; 9: 1402–1406.

145. Grunberg K, Kuijpers E, de Klerk E, de Gouw H, Kroes A, Dick E, Sterk P. Effects of experimental rhinovirus-16 infection on airway hyperresponsiveness to bradykinin in asthmatic subjects in vivo. Am J Respir Crit Care Med 1997; 155:833–838.

146. Fraenkel DJ, Bardin PG, Sanderson G, Lampe F, Johnston SL, Holgate ST. Lower airways inflammation during rhinovirus colds in normal and in asthmatic subjects. Am J Respir Crit Care Med 1995; 151:879–886.

147. Calhoun W, Dick E, Schwartz L, Busse W. A common cold virus, rhinovirus 16, potentiates airway inflammation after segmental antigen bronchoprovocation in allergic subjects. J Clin Invest 1994; 94:2200–2208.

148. Halperin SA, Eggleston PA, Hendley JO, Suratt PM, Groschel DH, Gwaltney JMJ. Pathogenesis of lower respiratory tract symptoms in experimental rhinovirus infection. Am Rev Respir Dis 1983; 128:806–810.

149. Gern JE, Galagan DM, Jarjour NN, Dick EC, Busse WW. Detection of rhinovirus RNA in lower airway cells during experimentally induced infection. Am J Respir Crit Care Med 1997; 155:1159–1161.

150. Halperin S, Suratt P, Gwaltney JMJ, Groschel D, Hendley J, Eggleston P. Bacterial cultures of the lower respiratory tract in normal volunteers with and without experimental rhinovirus infection using a plugged double catheter system. Am Rev Respir Dis 1982; 125:678–680.

151. Bardin PG, Johnston SL, Sanderson G, Robinson BS, Pickett MA, Fraenkel DJ, Holgate ST. Detection of rhinovirus infection of the nasal mucosa by oligonucleotide in situ hybridization. Am J Respir Cell Mol Biol 1994; 10:207–213.

152. Teran LM, Carroll MP, Shute JK, Holgate ST. Interleukin 5 release into asthmatic airways 4 and 24 hours after endobronchial allergen challenge: its relationship with eosinophil recruitment. Cytokine 1999; 11:518–522.

153. Lemanske RF Jr, Dick EC, Swenson CA, Vrtis RF, Busse WW. Rhinovirus upper respiratory infection increases airway hyperreactivity and late asthmatic reactions. J Clin Invest 1989; 83:1–10.

154. Skoner D, Doyle W, Tanner E, Kiss J, Fireman P. Effect of rhinovirus 39 (RV-39) infection on immune and inflammatory parameters in allergic and non-allergic subjects. Clin Exp Allergy 1995; 25:561–567.

155. Gern J, Calhoun W, Swenson C, Shen G, Busse W. Rhinovirus infection preferentially increases lower airway responsiveness in allergic subjects. Am J Respir Crit Care Med 1997; 155:1872–1876.

156. Gern JE, Vrtis R, Grindle KA, Swenson C, Busse WW. Relationship of upper and lower airway cytokines to outcome of experimental rhinovirus infection. Am J Respir Crit Care Med 2000; 162:2226–2231.

7

Consequences of Respiratory Viral Infection in Airway Epithelial Cells

SUSANNE BECKER and FREDERICK HENDERSON

U.S. Environmental Protection Agency
Research Triangle Park, North Carolina, U.S.A.

I. Introduction

The airway epithelial cell–mucociliary barrier protects us from infection by inhaled microbes, environmental irritants, and toxic materials. The constitutive epithelial cell defenses include secretion of antioxidants, antiproteases, and antimicrobial substances as well as the regulation of fluid balance. The nasal cavities are protected by squamous and ciliated epithelium. The proximal airways are lined by pseudostratified tall columnar epithelium composed of basal cells, mucus-producing secretory cells, and ciliated cells. The serous and mucous cells of the glands in the large airways are responsible for production of most of the mucous layer, which is essential for mucociliary clearance. In the bronchioles the epithelial lining turns into simple, cuboidal epithelium composed of ciliated cells and Clara cells. When the epithelium is damaged, Clara cells, basal cells, and secretory cells in the airways undergo

Disclaimer: The literature review described in this article has been supported by the United States Environmental Protection Agency. It has been subjected to Agency review and has been approved for publication. Approval does not necessarily reflect the views of the Agency and no official endorsement should be inferred. Mention of trade names and commercial products does not constitute endorsement or recommendation for use.

rapid proliferation, while the ciliated cells appear terminally differentiated and do not divide.

The seasonally occurring human respiratory viruses escape the extracellular epithelial cell defenses by penetrating into airway epithelial cells, using them as their host for replication. Viral replication is often initiated in the cells before the host has a chance to generate protective measures. These will subsequently include production of interferons, mucus hypersecretion, release of inflammatory mediators, and activation of the immune response. The viruses that most commonly infect airway epithelial cells are members of human rhinovirus (HRV) family and primarily target epithelial cells in the nose and upper airways, causing symptoms generally restricted to the upper respiratory tract. Respiratory syncytial virus (RSV) has a preference for both basal and ciliated cells in the lower airways, but also infects upper respiratory tract epithelia. Influenza (flu) can be found in cells throughout the respiratory tract while adenovirus (Adv) is characteristically found in alveolar epithelial cells, and has a preference for replicating cells. The propensity of RSV, Adv, and parainfluenza to infect bronchiolar epithelial cells preferentially is reflected by the disease these viruses cause in infants, where virus-induced bronchiolitis and pneumonia are the most common cause of hospitalization in this age group.

It has been long recognized by patients and clinicians alike that viral respiratory infection is an important trigger of wheezing in infants and of exacerbations of asthma in older children and adults (1–3). The importance of RSV as the single most important cause of virus-induced wheezing in young infants has been recognized since the virus was first isolated in the late 1950s, and this relationship is reaffirmed worldwide annually (4,5). The parainfluenza viruses are also important triggers of virus-associated wheezing (6). Recent use of polymerase chain reaction (PCR) diagnostic methods has solidified the importance of rhinovirus infection in asthma exacerbations (7,8). The principal mediators of viral infection-associated airway obstruction have not been comprehensively or conclusively defined, but the hypothesis is that hyperreactivity involves products of epithelial cells. The infected respiratory epithelial cell may be a source of chemical mediators of bronchoconstriction, such as leukotrienes, prostaglandins, neuropeptides, endothelins, and mucosal edema. Furthermore, infected epithelial cells may secrete proinflammatory molecules and other factors that promote release of pathophysiologically relevant effector molecules from innate and immune host defense cells participating in the response to infection.

In this chapter recent advances in our knowledge of respiratory viral interactions with airway epithelial cells will be reviewed, beginning with studies of the most common respiratory viruses (HRV, RSV, and flu) and the resulting induction of inflammatory mediators, often common with mediators found in asthmatic airways. The role of interferons in respiratory viral infections will then be discussed, since the known molecular signaling events leading to interferon production are likely to serve as guides of events required for regulation of respiratory virus-induced proinflammatory products.

II. Inflammatory Mediators Induced by Viral Infection of Airway Epithelium

A. Respiratory Syncytial Virus

This virus commonly infects the bronchial airways of infants and approximately 1% of infected babies are hospitalized with acute bronchiolitis. The small airways show submucosal mononuclear cell infiltration, epithelial necrosis, and mucous plugging. Viral antigen expression in infected infants is restricted to bronchial and alveolar epithelial cells. The virus repeatedly infects children as well as adults, seemingly because immunity following primary infection is incomplete, and RSV does not appear as dependent on elimination by neutralizing antibody as other respiratory viruses. In older children and adults the infection is manifested as rhinorrhea, bronchitis, fever, and wheezing. Bronchiolitis in infancy has been shown to be a significant risk factor for development of childhood asthma (9-11). The severity of the primary infection, as indicated by the need for treatment in the intensive care unit, has been shown to be correlated with later wheezing (12).

RSV infection of airway epithelial cells involves two proteins in the viral envelope: the attachment G-protein and the fusion F-protein. The G-protein, a highly glycosylated transmembrane protein with structural features similar to mucinous proteins, mediates viral attachment (13). The F-protein mediates membrane fusion and virus entry (14). To be active the F-protein precursor in the infected cell requires proteolytic cleavage to produce the two disulfide-linked glycosylated membrane protein subunits Fl and F2. A recent study has shown that the proprotein convertase furin, which plays an important role in posttranslational protein processing, may be involved in cleavage (15). The cell surface receptor for RSV on epithelial cells has as yet not been identified although information is available about its nature and binding requirements. Heparin inhibits infectivity, suggesting that glycosaminoglycans on the surface of epithelial cells seem to be very important in infection (16). Furthermore, interference with heparan sulfation in the host cell reduces RSV infection. Studies by Hallack et al. (17) have implicated special sulfate N-linked groups on a minimum 10-saccharide chain to be necessary for infection. Martinez and Melero (18) also found that sulfation was essential for infectivity. Both G- and F- proteins contain heparin/heparan sulfate-binding domains (19,20). Surfactant protein A (SP-A), a collectin that strongly binds to carbohydrates on various pathogens, was found to bind to G-protein and greatly enhance the infection of Hep2 cells in an SP-A dose-dependent manner, subsequently increasing release of IL-8 (21). In contrast, another surfactant protein SP-D inhibited infection of Hep2 cells by RSV (22), thus serving as a primary host defense molecule in RSV infection, constitutively present in the airways.

The notion that the host cell for viral replication is an important effector cell in inflammation as well as a player in adaptive immune responses has been most extensively researched with RSV-infected epithelial cells. Studies have been done with various sources of airway epithelial cells, including the type II cell-like tumor line A549, SV40-large T-transfected bronchial epithelial cell line BEAS-2B, confluent primary tracheobronchial epithelial cells, nasal epithelial cells, and differentiated ciliated primary cell cultures. Furthermore, airway biopsies have been obtained from nasal turbinate tissue during acute RSV infection. The primary interest has been to identify proinflammatory cytokines that could explain the cytopathology of the disease.

RSV at multiplicities of infection (MOI) 0.1–3 have been found to induce production of the granulocyte chemoattractant protein IL-8 in all the above-mentioned airway epithelial cells and lines (23–27). Becker et al. (23) found IL-8 mRNA expression and IL-8 release by infected primary nasal epithelial cells, in tracheal epithelial cells, as well as the BEAS-2B cells, within 4 h of exposure to virus. In A549 cells, IL-8 as well as IL-6 was measured early in infection and did not require infectious virus (24,25). Studies by Patel et al. (28, 29) suggested that more long-term production of these cytokines was mediated by IL-1 released by the A549 cells, since IL-1 antibodies and the IL-1 receptor antagonist inhibited IL-6 and IL-8 production. RSV-infected A549 cell also produced, IL-l, TNF, and IL-6 (25,28) while BEAS-2B cultures, neither IL-6, granulocyte–macrophage colony-stimulating factor (GM-CSF), nor TNF-α could be detected within 24 h of infection (26). GM-CSF, but not IL-6 or TNF, was found to depend on viral replication in BEAS-2B and primary epithelial cell cultures, and appeared concomitantly with release of viral particles. In supernatants of cells actively replicating RSV, elevated levels of IL-8 levels were no longer detected, and it was concluded that IL-8 production was an early event associated with virus uptake, but was not influenced by viral replication (30). Tristram et al. (31) studied the development of RSV infection in primary ciliated epithelial cell cultures. These cells were grown on collagen filters with air liquid interphase that promoted development of cilia. RSV infection resulted in loss of cilia, ciliostasis, and sloughing of cells. In contrast to studies in BEAS-2B and undifferentiated primary airway epithelial cells, a significant increase in the release of IL-6 and IL-8 was found in the differentiated cultures, peaking at 72 h after infection.

Asthma disease severity and presence of eosinophils/or released eosinophil cationic protein (ECP) in airways secretions appear to be strongly correlated (32). Since RSV infection is often associated with wheezing and respiratory distress, several groups have investigated the production of chemotactic factors that may attract eosinophils to the site of infection. Nasal lavage fluid of RSV-infected children contain significantly higher levels of the ECP , which is released upon eosinophil activation, than did fluids from healthy children (33,34). The chemokines RANTES, Eotaxin, macrophage chemoattractant protein (MCP-l), and macrophage inflammatory protein (MIP-lα), which have been shown to attract or activate eosinophils were suspected to be produced by RSV-infected epithelial cells. Several studies have shown that RANTES, but not Eotaxin, is produced in various epithelial cell lines in a virus replication-dependent manner; both mRNA and protein levels increased until destruction of infected cells (31,35–37). MIP-lα was produced to a lesser extent, while MCP-1, although constitutively present in airway epithelia, was found to be induced in the A549 cell but not in primary tracheobronchial epithelial cell cultures. In transformed cell lines, increases in RANTES synthesis may not require viral replication (38).

Concomitant with increased release of RANTES by RSV-infected epithelial cells, chemoattraction of eosinophils and monocytes, but not polymorphonuclear neutrophil leukocytes (PMN), could be demonstrated, and migration of both cell types could be blocked by antibodies to RANTES but not MIP-1α (30,36). Yet to be published studies from this laboratory (30) will show that both inflammatory cell types block spread of virus in the epithelial cell monolayer, and decrease production of cytokines GM-CSF, G-CSF, and RANTES, all of which are regulated directly or indirectly by viral burden. A likely mechanism of viral inactivation by the eosinophils is the release of ECP or other eosinophil granule products (39,40), which have been shown to inactivate virus through their RNAse like activity (40,41). Monocytes, on the other hand, phagocytize and thus restrict viral spread. Furthermore, the monocytes exposed to infected epithelial cells obtain the characteristics of activated antigen-presenting cells, including expression of increased levels of CD40, CD86, and HLA-DR, as well as secretion of chemoattractants for lymphocytes.

There is a good association between recovery of RANTES and MIP-1α in airways secretions/lavage and RS viral infection in both children and adults (42, 43). Significantly higher levels of RANTES were recovered from children with RSV disease than other viral airways infection (26). Noah and Becker recently, published a study involving healthy volunteers experimentally infected with RSV (~1000 PFU/person) (42). Note that the viral dose was 100–1000-fold less infectious virus than given to 1 million cultured epithelial cells. Epithelial biopsies were obtained from all subjects and cytokine message as well as cytokines present in the nasal lavage fluids were assessed. Three individuals out of 10 exposed developed a full-fledged infection and shed virus. There was a transient 2.7-fold increase in IL-8 protein following virus instillation in all subjects, followed by a 5.7-fold increase during viral shedding and increased neutrophilic inflammation. However, the epithelial biopsies did not show increased expression of IL-8 mRNA. Increased levels of RANTES, MCP-1, and MIP-1α protein were found in the lavage fluid during viral shedding, but only RANTES was identified in the nasal biopsies, and was found to be significantly increased. MCP-1 and MIP-1α levels were not sufficiently expressed in the epithelial cells to allow satisfactory quantitation and comparison of message between uninfected and infected subjects.

As inflammatory PMN, monocytes, and eosinophils migrate from blood into the infected airway mucosa, adherence receptors CD18/11a and 11b on the inflammatory cells are involved in interactions with endothelial cells and with airway cells, most likely interacting with their counter receptor ICAM-1 on the tissue cells. RSV infection has been shown to induce ICAM-1expression on airway epithelia (44,45). RSV infection resulted in increased adherence of PMN to the epithelial cells, which could be blocked by antibodies to ICAM-1 and CD18 (46). An interesting finding was that eosinophil degranulation induced by the RSV-infected epithelial cells was CD18-dependent but did not require interaction with ICAM-1 (47). Other receptors involved in inflammatory and immune cell interactions are also induced on infected epithelial cells. Expression of selected adhesion molecules and major histocompatibility complex (MHC) class I and II antigens on infected A549 cells was investigated by means of flow cytometry and immunocytochemistry. The results from this study indicated that RSV infection significantly upregulated the expression of ICAM-1, VCAM-1, and MHC class I and II antigens (48). Garofalo et al. (49) demonstrated that infection increased expression of class I MHC molecules on the cell surface, which depended on interferon-β and IL-1α produced by the infected cells, based on experiments in which neutralizing antibodies to these cytokines inhibited induction by supernatants of infected cells.

Various approaches have been taken to understand how viral replication may be limited in airway cells. Although RSV-infected cells produce interferon, inhibition of RS viral replication in the airway cells by exogenous interferons (IFN) have been unsuccessful. Among multiple respiratory viruses assessed, RSV appeared to be the least susceptible (50,51). However, the combination of TNF and IFN-β were shown to reduce, but not completely inhibit, replication (52). Similar studies performed with primary airway epithelial cells and the BEAS-2B line also found TNF by itself to be ineffective (26). A high dosage of NO_2 (1.5 ppm) reduced viral replication in BEAS-2B to a similar extent as the combination of TNF plus interferon (53). RSV infection was found to induce the nitric oxide synthetase (NOS) gene but the relationship of this enzyme to RSV replication or virally induced inflammatory mediators was not explored (54). NOS activation and NO production may be another feature common of virally infected and asthmatic airway cells (55, 56). Epithelial cells apoptosis upon RSV infection could be a possible means of restricting viral replication. Two studies have shown RSV-induced apoptosis, although death occurs late in infection, too late to have an impact on viral proliferation (57, 58). Other studies have shown that apoptosis is not induced in infected epithelial cells despite induction of the interleukin-1 converting enzyme caspase 3 and extensive cell death (59). Domachowske et al. (60) showed that RSV infection protected against TNF-induced apoptosis of airway epithelial cells.

Various groups have identified the expression and release of mediators from RSV-infected epithelial cells, which may have a bearing on airway hyperreactivity. Endothelin I (ET-1) is a potent spasmogen and mitogen of vascular smooth muscle, initially identified in endothelial cells (61). It was recently shown that ET-1 is also produced by airway epithelial cells and was suggested to be a mediator of asthma exacerbation. Its actions include airway smooth muscle contraction, bronchoconstriction, and proliferation, and it has proinflammatory activities and induces mucus hypersecretion. The induction of ET-1 was investigated in RSV-infected A549 cells. mRNA was maximally expressed at 16 h postinfection, while endothelin levels in the infected A549 supernatants peaked at 72 h (62,63). RSV has also been shown to upregulate expression of β_2-adrenergic and muscarinic receptors (64), which may explain the excessive mucus secretion observed during viral disease.

Taken together, RSV infection induces an airway epithelial cell phenotype in common with the perceived epithelial cell phenotype in asthma. How this contributes to airways hyperreactivity, directly or through involvement of inflammatory cells and the immune response, may best be explored in the appropriate animal models.

B. Human Rhinoviruses

Infection of the nasal and tracheal epithelium by human rhinoviruses (HRV) is the cause of the common cold. This disease is first manifested as a burning itch in the throat and nose, followed by sneezing, rhinorrhea, and malaise. Cough is usually mild. Lower respiratory tract symptoms are likely to suggest a cause other than rhinovirus. However, in persons with asthma, bronchitis, or chronic respiratory disease, HRV infection may result in persistent bronchitis and exacerbated airway symptoms (65–68).

The Rhinovirus family is comprised of more than 100 immunologically distinct serotypes. Upon infection, the virus is found in both ciliated and squamous epithelial cell in the nose and throat (69,70). The large majority of rhinoviruses (approx. 90%) binds to the intercellular adhesion molecule ICAM-1 (71,72), the remaining serotypes bind to the receptors for low-density lipoproteins (LDLR) (73,74). In the normal lung, ICAM-1 is expressed on the alveolar epithelium, and on some basal cells of the bronchial epithelium (75). It is suprising, that nasal epithelium, which is perceived as the main target of rhinoinfection, expresses no or very low levels of ICAM-1, although the receptor is expressed when the nasal passages are inflamed (76). Furthermore, ICAM-1 was rapidly induced following culture of nasal cells. Winter et al. (77) followed HRV infection in cultured epithelium from nasal polyps and turbinate tissue. Peak titer occured 24–48 h postinfection with no apparent cytopathology. In a study by Terajima et al. (78), primary cultures of tracheal epithelial cells were infected with HRV-2 and HRV-14. Both the ICAM-1-dependent HRV-14 strain and the independent LDLR-binding strain HRV-2 upregulated receptor expression. On the other hand, antibodies to ICAM-1 inhibited infection only with the appropriate ICAM-1 binding HRV-14 strain. Upregulation of ICAM-1 expression by HRV infection has been demonstrated in several studies with both transformed lines and primary epithelial cells (79–82), while other investigators have been unable to demonstrate that rhinovirus infection alters ICAM-1 expression on primary airway epithelial cell cultures (83).

Various cytokines have been shown to modulate ICAM-1 expression, which may have implications for susceptibility to HRV infection. Bianco et al. (84,85) found that IL-1, IL-8, and TNF increased expression of ICAM-1 while IFN-γ induced persistent downregulation of expression, even overriding the effect of the former cytokines. Exposure of the epithelial cells to TNF, which increased ICAM-1 expression, resulted in increased infection of the cells with HRV14 but not the minor member HRV2. Furthermore, Th2 type cytokines IL-4, IL-5, IL-10, and IL-13 associated with allergic/asthmatic airways were all found to induce ICAM-1 expression (85). These studies were not followed up by actually infecting the susceptible cells, but the investigators speculated that asthmatic airways modulated by Th2 cytokines would therefore be more susceptible to HRV infection. Experimental or natural HRV infection of asthmatic or atopic individuals increased ICAM-1 in bronchial epithelium (86,87). ICAM-1 was assessed by immunohistochemistry; stained cells were given an intensity score showing that HRV-infected airways had increased expression of this receptor compared to uninfected cells (86). Nasal epithelial cells obtained from normal and asthmatic individuals were compared and the basal level of expression was significantly higher in atopic/asthmatic epithelial cells than in normals (88). Relevant allergen exposure of atopic epithelium increased expression of ICAM-1 in vitro, as did infection with HRV-14 (88). Furthermore, polyp cells from atopic individuals released more HRV upon infection in vitro than normal cells.

As with RSV, a better understanding of potential inflammatory events involved in HRV infection of airway epithelium has been obtained through in vitro studies. Proinflammatory cytokine production, especially the production of IL-8 by airway epithelial cells, has received the bulk of attention since PMN inflammation measured by nasal lavage is prominent feature in this disease. HRV infection of A549 resulted in increased IL-8 expression, which persisted for up to 5 days (89). Both viral titers and IL-8 mRNA expression peaked in cell supernatants within the first 24 h following infection. Cytokine induction was also found to be induced by ultraviolet (UV)-inactivated virus, suggesting that viral replication was not required for expression. HRV infection of immortalized and primary cultures of tracheal epithelial cells, results in the production of various cytokines including IL-1, IL-6, IL-8, GM-CSF, and RANTES (82,83,90–93). In a study by Schroth et al. (83) primary human bronchial epithelial cells (BE) were infected with either HRV16 or HRV49, and viral replication, cell viability, and cell activation were measured. Both viral serotypes replicated in BE cells. Infection resulted in increased secretion of IL-8 , GM-CSF, and RANTES, but infection did not alter expression of ICAM-1.

Experimental HRV infection in volunteers may add validity to in vitro experiments implicating the involvement of cytokines and inflammation in the disease. In a study by Fraenkel et al. (94), nasal biopsies taken 4 days following infection were assessed for inflammatory cells. There was no evidence for inflammatory cells associated with the cold, and no difference in inflammatory indices was seen between atopic and normal individuals. Furthermore, there was no difference in inflammatory indices at peak infection compared to convalescent samples obtained 6–18 weeks following infection. The authors suggested that inflammation was not associated with rhinovirus infection. On the other hand, others have shown increased IL-8 staining of nasal epithelium in conjunction with PMN in the nasal lavage fluid in HRV-infected individuals (95–97). Nasal lavage fluid IL-8 and PMN inflammation were strongly correlated, as were PMN inflammation and the presence of G-CSF. However, inflammation assessed in induced sputum, which is believed to recover cells from the central airways was found to be modest compared to the nasal lavage (96,97). Grunberg et al. (96) stained nasal cells from experimentally infected individuals for IL-8 and found that an increase in IL-8 positive cells 2 days following infection was attributable to IL-8-positive neutrophils. However, it is not clear from these studies if IL-8 in the lavage fluid is actually derived from the infected epithelial cells or from inflammatory cells, or both. A study by Fleming et al. (98) showed that unprovoked asthmatics had higher numbers of neutrophils, eosinophils, and interleukin IL-6 in nasal lavage than normal individuals. After inoculation with HRV, both groups showed significant increases in nasal neutrophils, IL-6, and IL-8, and modest increases in sputum neutrophils and IL-6, but not IL-8.

With the exception of studies involving pharmaceutical drug interventions, little research has been done to understand mechanisms by which replication of HRV can be physiologically modulated in epithelial cells. Nitric oxide may inhibit replication of virus. NO donors were shown by Sanders et al. (99,100) to inhibit HRV replication as well as infection-induced production of IL-6, IL-8, and GM-CSF. The laboratory also recently showed that HRV infection induced iNOS in epithelial cells (101). In an earlier study, Kaul et al. (102) infected BEAS-2B cells but found no effect of NO donors or inhibitors of NOS on viral replication. They also could not demonstrate NO production in the infected cells.

C. Influenza Viruses

Influenza viruses are segmented negative-sense strand-enveloped viruses that infect the respiratory tract and cause respiratory symptoms as well as systemic disease, including debilitating fever, nausea, and muscular fatigue. Influenza can also exacerbate asthma, particularly in children (103). Influenza B and C uses the human airways as the sole site of replication, while influenza A infects aquatic birds, chickens, horses, and pigs, as well as humans. The most severe illnesses are caused by type A virus because of mutations in the envelope hemagglutinin (HA) and neuraminidase (NA) permits escape from neutralizing antibodies induced by previous exposure to the virus. The antigenic drift is believed to develop partly by immunological pressures in the various host species (104,105).

Influenza is transmitted through cough and sneeze of respiratory secretions, after the virus infects cells in the airway epithelium. The first cycle of replication takes approximately 6 h, and very high titers of virus are shed during this initial period. Although influenza viral replication appears to be restricted to the respiratory tract, viral antigens and particles are likely to enter the circulation. Autopsy specimens have found viral antigens in endothelial cells, liver, kidney, brain, and intestines (106). It is believed that in uncomplicated infections virus is restricted to the respiratory tract, while more severe disease may be induced by viral penetration into the circulation and nodes (107). However, once established in the airways the extent of viral replication in cells other than airway epithelial cells is not clear.

The ciliated tracheobronchial epithelial cells are believed to be the primary host of influenza viral replication. The viral hemagglutinin serves as the attachment moiety and interacts with terminal sialic acid residues on host cell glycoproteins (108). H3 strain of influenza A has a specificity for the sialic acid terminal residue NeuAcalpha3,6 gal. In a study by Baum and Paulson (109), a lectin specific to this sialic acid linkage was used to demonstrate its expression on the ciliated epithelial cells but not on the surface of goblet cells. Upon entry of the flu into host cell endosomes, acidification of the virus results in a conformational change and exposure of the HA2 domain necessary for assembly and release of infectious virus. Host cell enzymes are vital for proteolytic cleavage of HA, and infectivity (110–114). Clara cells produce a tryptase that functions extracellularly in the lumen of the respiratory tract (111), which can cleave HA to enable viral infection. In pathogenic flu strains this activation may also occur intracellularly. The nature of this cleaving protease in human airway epithelial cells has not been determined, but it is speculated that the absence of suitably active enzymes in other cell types in body determines the host cell specificity and restricts flu replication to the airways. In birds the differentiation between virulent and avirulent influenza A correlates with the sequence of a few amino acids adjacent to the point where the HA is cleaved. The presence of several basic amino acids at the cleavage sequence is associated with high pathogenicity, since these sequences are susceptible to cellular proteases present in cells throughout the body (113,114). Influenza A viruses with these polybasic sequences are highly pathogenic also in humans.

Influenza virus infection (H1N1) and replication have been studied in fetal and adult tracheal and bronchial epithelial cells and in BEAS-2B cells (115–117). Infection is assessed by hemadsorption, and fluorescent staining for viral antigens. Successful infection is ensured when hemadsorbing material increase with time in culture, and supernatants of the infected cells enable infection of new epithelial cell cultures. There is some controversy over the fate of the infected cells. In a study by Reiss et al. (115) the flu did not affect cell proliferation and no cytopathic effects of the virus were observed. On the other hand, Winther et al. (116) performed an interesting comparative study of rhinovirus, flu, and adenovirus on the cytopathology in primary cultures of nasal epithelial cells, Maximal viral titers were obtained between 24 and 48 h but no detectable damage was found in the epithelial cells infected with HRV while both flu and Adv caused cytopathic effects and destruction of the nasal cell monolayer. Ferret airway epithelium resembles that of the human airways. This model was used by Sweet et al. (117) to assess flu replication in different sites of the airways. They examined four different wild type flu isolates and found poor infectivity in bronchial tissue with three of the isolates, while all four isolates replicated well in nasal turbinate tissue. It was suggested that the mildness of the disease caused in humans by these isolates was due to the lack of replication of these viruses in the lower airways, and not to protection by neutralizing antibodies.

As with HRV and RSV, influenza-induced IL-6 and IL-8 have been demonstrated in epithelial cell lines and primary cultures of nasal and bronchial epithelial cells (118–120). In primary airway epithelial cell cultures, a doubling of IL-8 production was induced by H3N2 flu. Release of GM-CSF and RANTES was investigated by Matsukura et. al. (119) in the NCI-H292 cells. RANTES but not GM-CSF was induced in these cells. Furthermore, Eotaxin and RANTES were detected in primary bronchial epithelial cells infected with H3N2 (121,122). Eosinophil chemotaxis was stimulated by supernatants from the infected cells, and activity was blocked by antibodies to RANTES. In contrast, RANTES could not be detected in flu-infected (A/victoria 3/75) BEAS-2B cells, even at viral titers that ensured exposure of every cell, as assessed by hemadsorption. Parallel infection of the cultures with RSV induced high levels of this chemokine (32). Experimental influenza infection of human volunteers may validate the role of cytokines in flu infection. The role for IL-6 and IL-8 in influenza symptoms was investigated in adults who received intranasal inoculation of a drug-sensitive (rimantadine) strain of influenza A in the presence or absence of rimantadine (123). Symptom scores were documented and viral shedding, and concentrations of IL-6 and IL-8 were assessed in nasal lavage fluids. Successful infection, demonstrated by shedding of virus resulted in increases in IL-6 and IL-8. Rimantadine decreased shedding of virus, and decreased IL-8 levels. Viral shedding and IL-6 levels were significantly associated with symptom scores, suggesting a causal association between IL-6, but not IL-8, and viral disease. In another study (124), nasal lavage fluid was collected for up to 8 days from 17 healthy individuals challenged with influenza A H1N1. IL-6 and and IL-4 were analyzed. IL-6, but not IL-4, was significantly increased in individuals who shed virus and correlated with development of nasal symptoms but not systemic symptoms. In a study by Hayden et al. (125) nasal IL-6 and IFN-α levels correlated with systemic symptoms. Viral cytopathology was done comparing biopsies from flu-infected and normal donors. A very similar thickening of the epithelium, epithelial cell damage, and sloughing was seen in both infected and control biopsies (126).

Accumulation of PMN in the airways during flu infection is likely to cause oxidative damage to the epithelium. Antioxidant enzymes are constitutively active in epithelial cells and are activated in inflammatory situations. Jacoby and Choi (127) showed that flu infection led to increased production of manganese-dependent superoxide dismutase but decreased catalase, suggesting that the epithelial cells may protect themselves from extracellular damage. The role of NO in influenza survival and replication in airway epithelial has been investigated in a recent study. Inducible nitric oxide synthetase (NOS_2) induction was found in human airway epithelial cells following exposure of the cells to influenza or synthetic double-stranded RNA (128). NOS_2 mRNA abundance was increased between 8 and 48 h after influenza or dsRNA stimulation; IFN-γ exposure elicited enhanced NOS_2 mRNA expression for up to 6 days. Although not studied in human airway epithelial cells, it was shown that NO donors in the Marvin Darby kidney cell system impaired viral replication. NO affected viral RNA synthesis early in the replicative cycle (129).

D. Adenovirus and Infection of Airway Cells

Adenovirus (Adv) is a common respiratory pathogen that causes a broad range of clinical symptoms ranging from common cold symptoms to bronchitis, croup, and pneumonia. However, it may also cause various other illnesses, such as gastroenteritis, and conjunctivitis. All adenoviruses are transmitted by direct contact, fecal–oral transmission, and occasionally waterborne transmission.

The virus replicates in the lower airways; histopathology finds the virus in type 2 cells, and basal cells in the broncheoli (130). Much has been learned about the interaction of this virus with airway epithelium since replication-defective recombinant adenoviruses have been used to transfer genes such as the cystic fibrosis transmembrane conductance regulator (CFTR) into airway cells. It was found that Adv could readily infect lung epithelial cell lines such as A549, and proliferating primary airway epithelial cell monolayers (131,132). However, in vivo, in mice and human, very large doses of Adv had to be given in vivo to permit infection and CFTR expression of airway cells. These doses caused a substantial inflammatory response in the airways. Noah et al. (132) hypothesized that the inflammatory response was caused by cytokines such as IL-6 and IL-8 produced by the infected/ transfected cells. They infected human bronchial epithelial cells with wildtype Adv5 and a LacZ-containing recombinant Adv5 vector and assessed for release of IL-8 and IL-6. However, culture medium collected for up to 96 h postinfection showed no release of these cytokines by either wildtype Adv or vector despite infection of all cells. In the same study alveolar macrophages showed no increase in cytokine production following exposure. Kaner et al. (133) demonstrated in the transgene expression system that alveolar macrophages are 100–1000 times less effective in accepting the virus than the A549 cells. Using an in vitro model of regenerating airway epithelium, Dupuit et al. (134) showed that Adv only infected poorly differentiated cells, but infection did not require proliferating cells. Another study showed that loss of epithelial cell integrity by interference with cadherin D in the intercellular junctions predisposed the cells to infection transfection with replication-defective Adv (135).

A better understanding of Adv infectivity has recently been obtained as the cellular receptor for this virus has been identified. Adv has a fiber protein that is involved in infection. In 1996, Goldman et al. (136) suggested that the integrin $\alpha_v\beta_5$ binds a RGD motif on the fiber protein. Analysis of $\alpha_v\beta_5$ in human airways found nasal epithelial cells void of this integrin while the epithelial cells in the distal airways expressed it in abundance. Adv binding to Hela cells was inhibited by a monoclonal antibody raised against recombinant Ad5 fiber knob, which by mimeotope analysis of the monoclonal binding sites showed homology with the α_2 of the heavy chain of HLA class I molecule and the fibronectin type III molecules (137).

Infection of human airway epithelial cell cultures grown under conditions favoring development of cilia revealed that binding sites for Adv were absent on the apical surface of the differentiated cells (138). Walters et al. (139) recently showed that class I MHC and Adv binding was present on the basolateral surface of differentiated epithelium. However, binding to the differentiated cells was apparently not inhibited by a mutation in the fiber pentone base that mediates binding to integrin, implying that attachment did not require this interaction. Another study implying that integrin binding per se was not involved in infectivity used $5 knockout mice to demonstrate that infectivity was not impaired (140).

III. Interferons and Respiratory Viral Signaling

A. Role of Interferon in Respiratory Viral Infection

Interferons were the first cytokines demonstrated to be expressed by virus-infected cells. They were identified, using bioassays, as secreted proteins with the capacity to protect noninfected cells from viral infection, or to suppress virus replication in infected cells. Two main species of human interferon molecules were found to be produced by virus-infected cells: interferon and interferon-α (the type I interferons). Interferon-β (type II interferon) is secreted by T lymphocytes and NK cells and mediates antiviral effects, but its production is not elicited directly by viral infection of these cell types. In humans, IFN-α expression is limited to cells of lymphoid dendritic cell and monocyte lineages, while IFN-β is expressed primarily in epithelial cells and fibroblasts. There are at least 14 interferon-α genes and a single IFN- gene, all located in close proximity on chromosome 9p21–22. Type I interferons secreted in response to viral infection have both autocrine effects on the virus-infected cells and paracrine effects on neighboring epithelial cells, antigen-presenting cells, resident or recruited inflammatory cells (mast cells, eosinophils, neutrophils), or responding cells of the innate (NK) and antigen-specific (T or B lymphocyte) antiviral responses.

Endogenous or exogenous interferons mediate their antiviral action at different points in the viral life cycle, including viral penetration and uncoating, transcription of viral mRNA, translation of viral proteins, replication of virion RNA, and assembly and release of virion progeny. Among the best-defined mechanisms of IFN-mediated anti-viral effects are the Mx family of GTPases responsible for inhibiting replication of many RNA viruses including orthomyxoviruses, paramyxoviruses, and arboviruses; dsRNA-dependent 2'-5' oligoadenylate synthetase-mediated activation of RNAse L, which disrupts 28S ribosomal RNA; and dsRNA-dependent protein kinase (PKR), which phosphorylates eukaryotic translation initiation factor 2 (eIF2a) interfering with viral protein translation. In addition, activation of PKR is also central to virus-induced activation of NF-κB, which is fundamental to expression of many genes elicited by viral infection or interferon stimulation including multiple cytokines, chemokines, adhesion molecules, and inflammatory effector molecules, as is discussed below.

In early studies, McIntosh (141) and Hall (142) compared nasal lavage fluid IFN concentrations in young children with infections due to RSV, influenza viruses, and parainfluenza viruses. Both investigators found absent to very low levels of interferon in nasal secretions of infants with RSV infection. In contrast, interferon bioactivity was regularly detected in nasal lavage fluids of children with influenza or parainfluenza virus infections, with median concentrations of approximately 100 U/mL. Hall (143) made similar observations in adults with naturally acquired RSV and influenza virus infections. Interferon is produced in response to rhinovirus infection and rhinoviruses are consistently sensitive, in vitro, to its antiviral effects (144,145).

For survival, viruses have evolved mechanisms to evade the antiviral effects of the interferon system. The extent to which this is successfully achieved can be a correlate not only of successful viral replication but also of viral pathogenicity. Evading antiviral effects of IFN or interfering with IFN synthesis appears to be prominent in respiratory viral infections. Not only is RSV a weak IFN inducer in respiratory epithelial cells (as reflected in the clinical studies cited above), it is also resistant to the cellular antiviral mechanisms activated by pretreatment with exogenous type 1 interferons. In comparison studies, Atreya demonstrated that replication of human parainfluenza virus type 3 (PIV3) was reduced 1000-fold by exogenous type I IFN while replication of RSV was reduced less than 10-fold (146). Pretreatment of cells with interferon followed by coinfection with RSV and PIV3 did not result in loss of antiviral activity against PIV3, suggesting that RSV did not produce factors with the capacity to abrogate interferon's actions against coinfecting, interferon-sensitive viruses. Schlender recently demonstrated that resistance to IFN in bovine RSV was mediated by two viral nonstructural proteins: NS1 and NS2 (147). Pretreatment of MDBK cells with type I IFN markedly impaired replication of NS1, NS2, or NS1/2 deletion mutants of bovine RSV, while growth of wild type virus was not restricted. Thus, both NS1 and NS2 are required to circumvent the antiviral effects of interferon in bovine RSV; deletion of either protein abrogates interferon resistance. Furthermore, NS deletion mutants were effective inducers of type I interferon secretion in MDBK cells while wild type virus was not. An NS1 deletion mutant of human RSV has recently been studied in chimpanzees (148). The human NS1 deletion mutant was attenuated in vivo as reflected by restricted replication in the chimpanzee respiratory tract, but studies regarding interferon induction were not reported. Thus, RSV is a very weak interferon inducer in respiratory tract in vivo and in cultured respiratory epithelial cells. The steps in the interferon activation pathways that are impeded during RSV infection have not been defined. Furthermore, RSV replication is not restricted by prior treatment of cells with exogenous interferon. However, RSV does not interfere with exogenous type I or type II IFN signaling through their respective receptors while many other viruses do (146,149).

As noted above, wild-type influenza viruses are comparatively effective interferon inducers in vivo. However, recent work has shown that influenza viruses also express mechanisms to evade interferon-induced antiviral effects using the NS1 protein. Two mechanisms of anti-interferon action of the influenza NS1 protein have been demonstrated. Talon (150) used comparative studies with wild-type virus and an NS1 deletion mutant to show that NS1 binds dsRNA and inhibits phosphorylation of IRF-3. IFN-β expression was inhibited during infection with wild-type virus but not during NS1 deletion mutant infection. Work by Hatada (151) suggested that influenza NS1 also inhibited viral activation of double-stranded PKR. Viruses expressing NS1 mutant molecules were unable to abrogate PKR-mediated phosphorylation during virus growth. As a consequence eIF2a was phosphorylated and virus protein synthesis was suppressed in cells infected with mutant viruses.

Paramyxoviridae use distinct virus-specific mechanisms to circumvent the interferon response. STAT1 and STAT2 are cellular transcription factors involved in IFN signaling and are thus critical for the IFN-induced antiviral state. Didcock and colleagues demonstrated that the paramyxovirus simian virus 5 (SV5) blocks IFN signaling by targeting STAT1 for proteasome-mediated degradation (152,153). To determine whether this feature was common to all paramyxoviridae, they examined the abilities of SV5, Sendai virus (SeV), RSV, and human parainfluenza viruses types 2 and 3 (hPIV2 and hPIV3, respectively) to block signaling (149). Results showed that in reporter assays SV5, SeV, and hPIV3 blocked both type I and type II IFN signaling; hPIV2 blocked type I but not type II IFN signaling; and RSV failed to block either type I or type II IFN signaling. In agreement with these findings, SV5 and SeV inhibited the formation of the ISGF3 and GAF transcription complexes (essential for type I and type II signaling, respectively). A surprising result was that although hPIV3 inhibited IFN induction of the ISGF3 complex, GAF complexes were detected in hPIV3-infected cells. hPIV2 also blocked the formation of the ISGF3 complex but not the GAF complex, whereas RSV failed to block the induction of either complex. SV5 was the only virus that caused the degradation of STAT1. Indeed, in SeV- and hPIV3-infected cells STAT1 was phosphorylated on tyrosine 701 (Y701), a characteristic of IFN receptor activation. However, consistent with these viruses blocking IFN signaling downstream of receptor activation, the levels of serine 727 (S727)-phosphorylated forms of STAT1-alpha were reduced in SeV- and hPIV3-infected cells. In contrast, both (Y701)- and (S727)-phosphorylated forms of STAT1 were detected in hPIV2-infected cells but there was a specific loss of STAT2. Both STAT1 (including Y701- and S727-phosphorylated forms) and STAT2 could readily be detected in RSV-infected cells. Despite not being able to block type I or type II IFN signaling, RSV was able to replicate in human cells that produce and respond to IFN, suggesting that RSV must have an alternative method(s) for circumventing the IFN response. These results demonstrate that although interference with IFN signaling is a common strategy among paramyxoviruses, distinct virus-specific mechanisms are used to achieve this end.

B. Activation of Cellular Gene Expression by Exogenous Interferons and by Viral Infection

Extracellular interferons mediate their effects on susceptible cells through 2 component interferon receptors, IFN and, utilize the type I interferon receptor composed of IFNAR1 and IFNAR2C. Engagement and cross-linking of type I interferon receptors triggers phosphorylation of JAK1 and Tyk-2, which phosphorylate the transcription factors STAT1 and STAT2. STAT1 and 2 heterodimers translocate to the nucleus in association with p48-forming ISGF3, which serves as a major promoter of transcription of interferon-responsive genes (154). However, stimulation of many of the same genes can be elicited directly by viral infection without the need for an autocrine type I interferon stimulatory loop.

Viral infection or transfection of cells with double-stranded RNA (dsRNA) has been shown to trigger cellular gene expression by activating transcription factors along the pathways demonstrated schematically in Figure 1 (155–162).

In summary, viral infection elicits phosphorylation of constitutively expressed cytoplasmic IRF-3, which is then translocated to the nucleus where DNA binding is accomplished after association with the histone acetyl-transferases CREB binding protein-1 (CBP) and/or p300 (157); synthesis of IRF-1; synthesis and phosphorylation of IRF-7; and activation of PKR, which phosphorylates IKK, which phosphorylates IκB, which dissociates from NF-κB, resulting in nuclear translocation and DNA binding (157). In addition, viral infection or intracellular dsRNA activates 2′-5′ oligoadenylate synthetase, which leads to production of oligoadenylates, which activate RNAse L, which disrupts 18 and 28S ribosomal RNA species. This pathway of protein synthesis inhibition appears related to creation of permissive conditions for activation of MKK3 and MKK6, which activate p38MAPK and MKK4, which

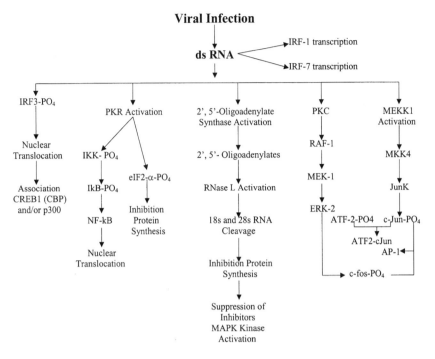

Figure 1   Pathways of transcription factor activation during viral infection.

activates c-Jun NH2 terminal kinase (158). Jun kinase is also activated by dsRNA by a pathway starting with activation of MEK kinase 1 (159). Jun kinase phosphorylates both c-Jun and ATF-2, creating the ATF-2–c-Jun transcription factor complex. Phosphorylated c-Jun is also a component of AP-1. Recent evidence (161) indicates that viral infection can activate isoforms of protein kinase C, initiating a pathway for ERK2 activation that then phosphorylates c-fos, the second component of the AP-1 transcription factor complex. Our understanding of the complexities of these kinase cascades is maturing, but future work will certainly expand on and clarify the outline provided in Figure 1. These components of the viral response system are considered typically stimulatory. There are also inhibitory components of the interferon response system triggered by viral infection including IRF-2 and 4 (155). The balance of contributions from activation and inhibitory pathways to the expression of different interferon-stimulated genes (ISGs) vary substantially and are virus-, infected-cell-, and target-gene-specific. Although these are among the more extensively investigated viral infection-triggered transcription-factor pathways, this list is almost certainly incomplete. The fine detail of cooperation among transcription factors to trigger specific ISGs continues to be elucidated and refined. Involvement of these pathways will be demonstrated in the examples of viral infection-triggered cytokine and chemokine gene expression discussed below.

C. Transcription Factor Utilization in Viral Infection-Induced Expression of Interferons, Chemokines, and Adhesion Molecules

Interferon-β

Infection with specific viruses or transfection of cells with dsRNA has been shown to result in assembly of a functional transcription factor complex (enhanceosome) that is essential for induction of IFN-β transcription. The IFN-β promoter contains a virus inducible enhancer region consisting of four positive regulatory domains (PRD-I to PRD-IV). PRDI and PRDIII are interferon regulatory factor elements (IRF-E), PRDII is an NF-kB binding site, and PRDIV is recognized by ATF2-c-Jun. The IRF-E motifs in the IFN-β regulatory domain are recognized by different members of the IRF family including IRF-1, IRF-3, and IRF-7. Optimum enhancement of IFN-β mRNA synthesis is obtained with a transcription factor complex that includes IRF3, IRF7, ATF2-c-Jun, NF-κB p50–65, and by high-mobility group protein I (HMGI) binding to the transcription factor complex (163).

It would be surprising if the signaling mechanisms and the transcription factor machinery identified in IFN-β, gene activation were not also involved in induction of other proinflammatory genes induced by respiratory viral infection. As an alternative, IFN-β may be an intermediary in several infection-induced host responses, and the interferon-induced activation pathways may guide us in unraveling respiratory virus-induced pathways of cell activation.

Activation of IL-8 Gene Transcription

Transcriptional activation of IL-8 has been investigated in epithelial cells infected with various respiratory viruses. The 5′ untranslated region of the IL-8 gene contains binding sites for IRF-1, AP-1, NF-IL-6, HNF-1, and NF-κB, among others. Mastronarde (162), using CAT reporter constructs, identified AP-1 cooperation with NF-κB for RSV infection-induced IL-8 expression; NF-IL-6 made a smaller contribution to virus-induced activation of IL-8 transcription. The antioxidants n-acetyl cysteine and dimethyl pyrroline oxide inhibited IL-8 synthesis and binding of AP-1 and NF-IL-6 transcription factors to nuclear extracts following RSV infection. The antioxidant compounds had no effect on nuclear binding of NF-κB subunits. Zhu et al. (164, 165) used mutated constructs of the IL-8 NF-κB site in the luciferase reporter assay to demonstrate involvement of NF-κB in gene transcription following HRV infection. They found that HRV infection stimulated both IL-8 and IL-6-promoter-driven luciferase activity, which was blocked by mutations at the cytokine-specific NF-κB site. A mutation in the NF-IL-6 site decreased luciferase production to a lesser extent. Casola and colleagues (166) identified a transcription factor binding domain of the IL-8 promoter region that was termed the RSV response element (RSVRE). This region included a binding site for IRF-1 that was synthesized robustly after RSV infection. Optimum expression of an IL-8-promoter-driven luciferase reporter was obtained when active NF-κB, RSVRE, AP-1, and NF-IL-6-binding domains were present in the promoter. As previously observed by Mastronarde,

(162), intact NF-κB binding was an absolute requirement. Maximal suppression of reporter gene expression was observed with mutations in the AP-1 and RSVRE-binding domains. Activation of MAP-kinases was investigated in A549 cells and it appeared that only ERK-2 was activated by RSV (167). Recently, Monick expanded on this observation by demonstrating activation of multiple protein kinase C isoforms and downstream activation of ERK-2 during RSV infection (160), thus identifying additional steps in the signal transduction cascade initiated and sustained by viral infection.

Other investigators exploring the involvement of NF-κB in HRV-induced IL-8 induction have obtained results that dispute the absolute requirement of this transcription factor. Kim et al. (168) proceeded with performing experiments blocking NF-κB activation by inhibitors such as calpain inhibitor I, and sulfazine, both of which were shown to have no effect on HRV-induced IL-6 and IL-8 mRNA induction. However, although calpain inhibitor had no effect on cytokine protein production, sulfazine inhibited protein production. These results indicated that NF-κB activation was not involved in HRV-induced cytokine production. However, oxidative mechanisms were shown to be necessary for cytokine production. It is interesting that Kaul et al. recently proposed that IL-8 production is independent of virus binding to ICAM-1 (was not blocked by anti ICAM-1), but was dependent on a flavoprotein that may act in concert with p47phox (169).

Respiratory Virus-Induced RANTES Gene Induction

The molecular mechanism for virus-induced RANTES induction has been shown to involve the activation of NF-κB. Thomas observed nuclear translocation of NF-κB following RSV infection; overexpression IκB-alpha mediated using an adenoviral vector inhibited both NF-κB translocation and RANTES production (170). Viral replication was not affected by IκB overexpression. Studies by Koga and colleagues indicated that respiratory syncytial virus-induced RANTES expression may be more dependent on stabilization of RANTES mRNA in primary human tracheobronchial epithelial cells than on newly induced RANTES mRNA transcription (38). Lin (171) studied transcriptional control of RANTES expression following paramyxovirus (Sendai virus) infection of 293 cells. Following Sendai virus challenge, chemokine mRNA expression was surveyed using the ribonuclease protection assay for a panel of human chemokine genes. Strong viral induction was only identified for RANTES mRNA. Viral infection elicited binding of IRF-3 and NF-κB (p65/p50) to the RANTES promoter and these factors were primarily responsible for activation of mRNA transcription. Stimulation of cells with exogenous type I interferon did not elicit RANTES mRNA expression, and culture of cells in interferon-neutralizing antibody did not suppress RANTES expression in virus-infected cells, excluding autocrine interferon effects. Additional experiments by Genin (172) in 293 cells and U937 human myeloid cells provided evidence for participation of IRF-7 in the promoter complex responsible for RANTES transcription. IRF-7 was not constitutively expressed in 293 cells but was expressed after viral infection.

Tripp (173) recently provided evidence that modifications of viral protein expression had an impact on the pattern of pulmonary expression of chemokine mRNAs in mice infected with respiratory syncytial virus. Responses of animals infected with wild-type RSV (antigenic group B) and a mutant virus with deletions of the G and SH proteins were compared. Infection with the G/SH deletion mutant resulted in enhanced expression of multiple chemokine genes in the lung when compared to infection with the wild-type parent virus. Thus, expression of specific viral proteins modulates patterns of cytokine and chemokine expression during viral infection and the consequent recruitment of inflammatory cells to sites of infection.

Activation of ICAM-1 Gene Transcription

Papi et al. (77) demonstrated rhinovirus-induced expression of ICAM-1 in A549 cells and primary human bronchial epithelial cells. Transcription factor utilization was studied in A549 cells. Proteins binding to AP-1 and NF-κB domains in the ICAM promoter were observed following viral infection, but deletion of the AP-1 binding domain suggested that transcription was only dependent on NF-κB activation. Chini studied ICAM-1 expression in A549 cells infected with respiratory syncytial virus (174) and demonstrated participation of NF-κB and C/EBP transcription factors in viral infection-triggered gene expression. The importance of viral infection-activated PKR as the central activator of NF-κB was not addressed in these experiments.

IV. Summary

This chapter has reviewed the state of knowledge about consequences of respiratory virus infection on airway epithelial cells. The current research emphasis is heavily weighted toward responses that result in inflammation and recovery from disease by involvement of the individual's immune defenses. The respiratory viruses vary in their responsiveness to interferons, and most respiratory viruses have evolved mechanisms by which interferon effects aimed at restricting viral replication can be subverted. Thus, the infected cell must mobilize a well-orchestrated inflammatory and immune response to infection to limit and ultimately terminate the spread of viral infection in the respiratory epithelium. A spectrum of proinflammatory genes is activated in infected epithelial cells and their products are directly relevant to recruitment and activation of antigen-presenting cells, mast cells, neutrophils, eosinophils, innate (NK cells), and viral antigen-specific (lymphocyte) cellular responses.

The respiratory epithelial cell is the primary target of the infecting virus, but it remains unclear whether viral infection-elicited epithelial cell gene expression contributes directly to the pathophysiology of acute viral infection triggered asthma. It is unknown, for example, whether bronchoconstricting compounds are secreted directly by virus-infected respiratory epithelial cells. However, inflammatory cells recruited to the site of infection are important potential sources of molecules that could ultimately mediate the pathophysiology of viral infection-induced asthma exacerbations.

References

1. Illi S, von Mutius E, Lau S, Bergmann R, Niggemann B, Sommerfeld C, Wahn U. Early childhood infectious diseases and the development of asthma up to school age: a birth cohort study. Br Med J 2001; 322:390–395.
2. Kimpen JL. Viral infections and childhood asthma. Am J Respir Crit Care Med 2000; 162: S108–112.
3. Sigurs N, Bjarnason R, Sigurbergsson F, Kjellman B. Respiratory syncytial virus bronchiolitis in infancy is an important risk factor for asthma and allergy at age 7. Am J Respir Crit Care Med 2000; 161:1501–1507.
4. Eriksson M, Bennet R, Nilsson A. Wheezing following lower respiratory tract infections with respiratory syncytial virus and influenza A in infancy. Pediatr Allergy Immunol 2000; 11:193-197.
5. Weber MW, Mulholland EK, Greenwood BM. Respiratory syncytial virus infection in tropical and developing countries. Med Int Health 1998; 3:268–280.
6. Tuffaha A, Gern JE, Lemanske RF Jr. The role of respiratory viruses in acute and chronic asthma. Clin Chest Med 2000; 21:289-300.
7. Johnston SL, Pattemore PK, Sanderson G, Smith S, Lampe F, Josephs L, Symington P, O'Toole S, Myint SH, Tyrrell DA, et al. Community study of role of viral infections in exacerbations of asthma in 9–11 year old children. Br Med J 1995 310:1225–1229.
8. Macek V, Dakhama A, Hogg JC, Green FH, Rubin BK, Hegele RG. PCR detection of viral nucleic acid in fatal asthma: is the lower respiratory tract a reservoir for common viruses? Can Respir J 1999, 6:37–43.
9. Stein RT, Sherrill D, Morgan WJ, Holberg CJ, Halonen M, Taussig LM, Wright AL, Martinez FD. Respiratory syncytial virus in early life and risk of wheeze and allergy by age 13 years. Lancet 1999; 354:541–545.
10. Ehlenfield DR, Cameron K, Welliver RC. Eosinophilia at the time of respiratory syncytial virus bronchiolitis predicts childhood reactive airway disease. Pediatrics 2000;105: 79–83.
11. Pullan CR, Hey EN. Wheezing, asthma, and pulmonary dysfunction 10 years after infection with respiratory syncytial virus in infancy. Br Med J Clin Res Ed 1982; 284: 1665–1669.
12. Price JF. Acute and long-term effects of viral bronchiolitis in infancy. Lung 1990; 168(Suppl):414–421.
13. Levine S, Klaiber-Franco R, Paradiso PR. Demonstration that glycoprotein G is the attachment protein of respiratory syncytial virus. J Gen Virol 1987; 68:2521–2524.
14. Walsh EE, Hruska J. Monoclonal antibodies to respiratory syncytial virus proteins: identification of the fusion protein. J Virol 1983; 47:171–177.
15. Bold, G. Pedersen LO, Birdeslund, HH. Cleavage of respiratory syncytial virus fusion protein is required for surface expression: role of furin. Virus Res 2000; 68:25–33.
16. Krusat T, Streckert HJ. Heparin-dependent attachment of respiratory syncytial virus (RSV) to host cells. Arch Virol 1997; 142:1247–1254.

17. Hallak LK, Spillman D, Collins PL, Peebles ME. Glucosaminoglycan sulfation requirements for respiratory syncytial virus infection. J Virol 2000; 74:10508–10513.

18. Martinez I, Melero JA. Binding of human respiratory syncytial virus to cells: implication of sulfated cell surface proteoglycans. J Gen Virol 2000; 81:2715–2722.

19. Feldman SA, Hendry RM, Beeler JA. Identification of a linear heparin binding domain for human respiratory syncytial virus attachment glycoprotein G. Virology 1999; 73: 6610–6617.

20. Feldman SA, Audet S, Beeler JA. The fusion glycoprotein of human respiratory syncytial virus facilitates virus attachment and infectivity via an interaction with cellular heparan sulfate. J Virol 2000; 74:6442–6447.

21. Hickling TP, Malhotra R, Bright H, McDowell W, Blair ED, Sim RB. Lung surfactant protein A provides a route of entry for respiratory syncytial virus into host cells. Viral Immunol. 2000; 13:125–135.

22. Hickling TP, Bright H, Wing K, Gower D, Martin SL, Sim RB, Malhotra R. A recombinant trimeric surfactant protein D carbohydrate recognition domain inhibits respiratory syncytial virus infection in vitro and in vivo. Eur J Immunol 2000; 29:3478–3484.

23. Becker S, Koren HS, Henke DC. Interleukin-8 expression in normal nasal epithelium and its modulation by infection with respiratory syncytial virus and cytokines tumor necrosis factor, interleukin-1, and interleukin-6. Am J Respir Cell Mol Biol 1993; 8: 20–27.

24. Fiedler MA, Wernke-Dollries K, Stark JM. Inhibition of viral replication reverses syncytial virus-induced NF-kappaB activation and interleukin-8 gene expression in A549 cells. J Virol 1996; 70:9079–9082.

25. Mastronarde JG, Monick MM, Gross TJ, Hunninghake GW. Amiloride inhibits cytokine production in epithelium infected with respiratory syncytial virus. Am J Physiol 1996; 271:L201-L207.

26. Noah TL, Becker S. Respiratory syncytial virus-induced cytokine production by a human bronchial epithelial cell line. Am J Physiol 1993; 265:L472-L478.

27. Arnold R, Humbert B, Werchau H, Gallati H, Konig W. Interleukin-8, interleukin-6, and soluble tumour necrosis factor receptor type I from a human pulmonary epithelial cell line (A549) exposed to respiratory syncytial virus. Immunology 1994: 82:126–133.

28. Patel JA, Kunimoto M, Sim TC, Garofalo R, Eliott T, Baron S, Ruuskanen O, Chonmaitree T, Ogra PL, Schmalstieg F. Interleukin-1 alpha mediates the enhanced expression of intercellular adhesion molecule-1 in pulmonary epithelial cells infected with respiratory syncytial virus. Am J Resp Cell Mol Biol 1995; 13:602–609.

29. Patel JA, Jiang Z, Nakajima N, Kunimoto M. Autocrine regulation of interleukin-8 by interleukin-1 alpha in respiratory syncytial virus-infected pulmonary epithelial cells in vitro. Immunology 1998; 95:501–506.

30. Becker S, Soukup JM. Airway epithelial cell-induced activation of monocytes and eosinophils in respiratory syncytial viral infection. Immunobiology 1999; 201:88–106.

31. Tristam DA, Hicks W Jr, Hard R. Respiratory syncytial virus and human bronchial epithelium. Arch Otolaryngol Head Neck Surg 1998; 124:777–783.

32. Fujitaka M, Kawaguchi H, Kato Y, Sakura N, Ueda K, Abe Y. Significance of the eosinophil cationic protein/eosinophil count ratio in asthmatic patients: its relationship to disease severity. Ann Allergy Asthma Immunol 2001; 86:323–329.

33. Garofalo R, Dorris A, Ahlstedt S, Welliver RC. Peripheral blood eosinophil counts and eosinophil cationic protein content of respiratory secretion in bronchiolitis: relationship to severity of disease. Pediatr Allergy Immunol 1994; 5:111–117.

34. Oh JW, Lee HB, Yum MK, Kim CR, Kang JO, Park IK. ECP levels in nasopharyngeal secretions and serum from children with respiratory virus infections and asthmatic children. Allergy Asthma Proc 2000; 21: 97–100.

35. Becker S, Reed W, Henderson FW, Noah TL. RSV infection of human airway epithelial cells causes production of the beta-chemokine RANTES. Am J Physiol 1997; 272: L512-L520.

36. Olszewska-Pazdrak B, Casola A, Saito T, Alam R, Crowe SE, Mei F, Ogra PL, Garofalo RP. Cell-specific expression of RANTES, MCP-1, and MIP-1alpha by lower airway epithelial cells and eosinophils infected with respiratory syncytial virus J Virol 1998; 72:4756–4764.

37. Saito T, Deskin RW, Casola A, Haeberle H, Olszewska B, Ernst PB, Alam R, Ogra PL, Garofalo R. Respiratory syncytial virus induces selective production of the chemokine RANTES by upper airway epithelial cells. J Infect Dis 1997; 175:497–504.

38. Koga T, Sardina E, Tidwell RM, Pelletier M, Look DC, Holtzman MJ. Virus-inducible expression of a host chemokine gene relies on replication-linked mRNA stabilization. Proc Natl Acad Sci USA 1999; 96:5680–5685.

39. Harrison AM, Bonville CA, Rosenberg HF, Domachowske JB. Respiratory syncytial virus-induced chemokine expression in the lower airways; eosinophils recruitment and degranulation. Am J Respir Crit Care Med 1999; 159:1918–1924.

40. Domachowske JB, Dyer KD, Adams AG, Leto TL, Rosenberg HF, Eosinophil cationic protein/RNase 3 is another RNase A-family ribonuclease with direct antiviral activity. Nucleic Acids Res 1998; 26(14):3358–3363.

41. Rosenberg HF, Domachowske JB. Eosinophils, ribonucleases and host defense: solving the puzzle. Immunol Res 1999; 20:261-274.

42. Noah TL, Becker S. Chemokines in nasal secretions of normal adults experimentally infected with respiratory syncytial virus. Clin Immunol 2000; 97:43–49.

43. Bonville CA, Rosenberg HF, Domachowske JB. Macrophage inflammatory protein-1alpha and RANTES are present in nasal secretions during ongoing upper respiratory tract infection. Pediatr Allergy Immunol 1999; 10:39–44.

44. Arnold R, Konig W. ICAM-1 expression and low-molecular-weight G-protein activation of human bronchial epithelial cells (A549) infected with RSV. J Leuk Biol 1996; 60:766–771.

45. Matsuzaki Z, Okamoto Y, Sarashina N, Ito E, Togawa K, Saito I. Induction of intercellular adhesion molecule-1 in human nasal epithelial cells during respiratory syncytial virus infection. Immunology 1996; 88:565–568.

46. Stark JM, Godding V, Sedgwick JB, Busse WW. Respiratory syncytial virus infection enhances neutrophil and eosinophil adhesion to cultured respiratory epithelial cells. Roles of CD18 and intercellular adhesion molecule-1. J Immunol 1996; 156:4774-4782.

47. Olszewska-Pazdrak B, Pazdrak K, Ogra PL, Garofalo RP. Respiratory syncytial virus-infected pulmonary epithelial cells induce eosinophil degranulation by a CD 18-mediated mechanism. J Immunol 1998; 160:4889–4895.

48. Wang SZ, Hallsworth PG, Dowling KD, Alpers JH, Bowden JJ, Forsyth KD. Adhesion molecule expression on epithelial cells infected with respiratory syncytial virus. Eur Respir J 2000; 15:358–366.

49. Garofalo R, Mei F, Espejo R, Ye G, Haeberle H, Baron S, Ogra PL, Reyes VE. Respiratory syncytial virus infection of human respiratory epithelial cells up-regulates class I MHC expression through the induction of IFN-beta and IL-1 alpha. J Immunol 1996, 157:2506–2513.

50. Sperber SJ, Hayden FG. Comparative susceptibility of respiratory viruses to recombinant interferons-α2b and β. J. Interferon Res 1989; 9:285–293.

51. Atreya PL, Kulkarni S. Respiratory syncytial virus strain A2 is resistant to the antiviral effects of type I interferons and human MxA. J Virol 1999; 261:227–241.

52. Merolla R, Rebert NA, Tsiviste PT, Hoffmann SP, Panuska JR. Respiratory syncytial virus replication in human lung epithelial cells: inhibition by tumor necrosis factor alpha and interferon-β. Am J Respir Crit Care Med 1995; 152:1358–1366.

53. Becker S, Soukup JM. Effect of nitrogen dioxide on respiratory viral infection in airway epithelial cells. Environ Res 1999; 81:159–166.

54. Tsutsumi H, Takeuchi R, Ohsaki M, Seki K, Chiba S. Respiratory syncytial virus infection of human respiratory epithelial cells enhances inducible nitric oxide synthase gene expression. J Leuk Biol 1999; 66:99–104.

55. Sanders SP. Asthma, viruses, and nitric oxide. Pro Soc Exp Biol Med 1999; 220:123–132.

56. Redington AE, Meng QH, Springall DR, Evans TJ, Creminon C, Maclouf J, Holgate ST, Howarth PH, Polak JM. Increased expression of inducible nitric oxide synthase and cyclo-oxygenase-2 in the airway epithelium of asthmatic subjects and regulation by corticosteroid treatment. Thorax 2001; 56:351–357.

57. O'Donnell DR, Milligan L, Stark JM. Induction of CD95 (Fas) and apoptosis in respiratory epithelial cell culture following respiratory syncytial virus infection. Virology 1999; 257:198-207.

58. Bitko V, Barik S. An endoplasmic reticulum-specific stress-activated caspase (caspase-12) is implicated in the apoptosis of A549 epithelial cells by respiratory syncytial virus. J Cell Biochem 2001; 80:441–454.

59. Takeuchi R, Tsutsumi H, Osaki M, Haseyama K, Mizue N, Chiba S. Respiratory syncytial virus infection of human alveolar epithelial cells enhances interferon regulatory factor 1 and interleukin-1beta-converting enzyme gene expression but does not cause apoptosis. J Virol 1998; 72:4498–4502.

60. Domachowske JB, Bonville CA, Mortelliti AJ, Colella CB, Kim U, Rosenberg HF. Respiratory syncytial virus infection induces expression of the anti-apoptosis gene IEX-IL in human respiratory syncytial cells. J Infect Dis 2000; 181:824–830.

61. Goldie RG, Fernandes LB. A possible mediator role for endothelin-1 respiratory disease. Monaldi Arch Chest Dis 2000; 55:162–167.

62. Behera AK, Kumar M, Matsuse H, Lockey RF, Mohapatra SS. Respiratory syncytial virus induces the expression of 5-lipoxygenase and endothelin-1 in bronchial epithelial cells. Biochem Biophys Res Commun 1998; 251:704–709.

63. Samransamruajkit R, Gollapudi S, Kim CH, Gupta S, Nussbaum E. Modulation of endothelin-1 expression in pulmonary epithelial cell line (A549) after exposure to RSV. Int J Mol Med 2000; 6:101–105.

64. Tsutsumi H, Ohsaki M, Seki K, Chiba S. Respiratory syncytial virus infection of human respiratory epithelial cells enhances both muscarinic and beta2-adrenergic receptor gene expression. Acta Virol 1999; 43:267–270.

65. Johnston SL. Natural and experimental rhinovirus infections of the lower respiratory tract. Am J Respir Crit Care Med 1995; 152:S46–52.

66. Van Kempen M, Bachert C. Van Cauwenberge P. An update on the pathophysiology of rhinovirus upper tract infection. Rhinology 1999; 37:97–103.

67. Hendley JO. Clinical virology of rhinoviruses. Adv Virus Res 1999; 54:453–66.

68. Gern JE, Busse WW. Association of rhinovirus infections with asthma. Clin Microbiol Rev 1999; 12:9–18.

69. Turner RB, Winther B, Hendley JO, Mygind N, Gwaltney JM Jr. Sites of virus recovery and antigen detection in epithelial cells during experimental rhinovirus infection. Acta Otolaryngol Suppl 1984; 413:9–14.
70. Gwaltney JM Jr. 1995. Rhinovirus infection of the normal human airway. Am J Respir Crit Care Med 1995; 152:536–539.
71. Staunton DE, et al. A cell adhesion molecule ICAM-1 is the major surface receptor for rhinoviruses. Cell 1989; 56, 849-853.
72. Greve JM, et al. The major rhinovirus receptor is ICAM-1. Cell 1989; 56: 839–847.
73. Hofer F. et al. Members of the low density lipoprotein receptor family mediate cell entry of a minor group common cold virus. Proc Natl Acad Sci USA 1984; 91:1839–1842.
74. Suzuki T, Yamaya M, Kamanaka M, Jia YX, Nakayama K, Hosoda M, Yamada N, Nishimura H, Sekizawa K, Sasaki H. Type 2 rhinovirus infection of cultured human tracheal epithelial cells: role of LDL receptor. Am J Physiol Lung Cell Mol Physiol 2001; 280:L409-20.
75. Feuerhake F, Fuchsl G, Bals R, Welsch U. Expression of inducible cell adhesion molecules in the normal lung: immunohistochemical study of their distribution in the pulmonary blood vessels. Histochem Cell Biol 1998, 110:387–394.
76. Demoly P, Sahla M, Campbell AM, Bousquet J, Crampette L. ICAM-1 expression in upper respiratory mucosa is differentially related to eosinophil and neutrophil inflammation according to the allergic status. Clin Exp Allergy 1998; 28:731–738.
77. Winther B, Gwaltney JM, Hendley JO. Respiratory virus infection of monolayer cultures of human nasal epithelial cells. Am Rev Respir Dis 1990; 141:839–845.
78. Terajima M, Yamaya M, Sekizawa K, Okinaga S, Suzuki T, Yamada N, Nakayama K, Ohrui T, Oshima T, Numazaki Y, Sasaki H. Rhinovirus infection of primary cultures of human tracheal epithelium: role of ICAM-1 and IL-1beta. Am J Physiol 1997; 273: L749-L759.
79. Papi A, Johnston SL. Rhinovirus infection induces expression of its own receptor intercellular adhesion molecule 1 (ICAM-1) via increased NF-kappaB-mediated transcription. J Biol Chem 1999; 274:9707–9720.
80. Papi A, Stanciu LA, Papadopoulos NG, Teran LM, Holgate ST, Johnston SL. Rhinovirus infection induces major histocompatibility complex class I and costimulatory molecule upregulation in respiratory epithelial cells. J Infect Dis 2000; 181:1780–1784.
81. Altman LC, Ayars GH, Baker C, Luchtel DL. Cytokines and eosinophil-derived cationic proteins upregulate intercellular adhesion molecule-1 on human nasal epithelial cells. J Allergy Clin Immunol 1993; 92:527–536.
82. Subauste MC, Jacoby DB, Richards SM, Proud D. Infection of a human respiratory epithelial cell line with rhinovirus. Induction of cytokine release and modulation of susceptibility to infection by cytokine exposure. J Clin Invest 1995; 96:549-557.
83. Schroth MK, Grimm E, Frindt P, Galagan DM, Konno SI, Love R, Gern JE. Rhinovirus replication causes RANTES production in primary bronchial epithelial cells. Am J Respir Cell Mol Biol 1999; 20:1220–1228.
84. Bianco A, Spiteri MA. A biological model to explain the association between human rhinovirus respiratory infections and bronchial asthma. Monaldi Arch Chest Dis 1998; 53:83–87.
85. Bianco A, Sethi SK, Allen JT, Knight RA, Spiteri MA. Th2 cytokines exert a dominant influence on epithelial cell expression of the major group human rhinovirus receptor, ICAM-1. Eur Respir J 1998; 12:619–626.

86. Grunberg K, Sharon RF, Hiltermann TJ, Brahim JJ, Dick EC, Sterk PJ, Van Krieken JH. Experimental rhinovirus 16 infection increases intercellular adhesion molecule-1 expression in bronchial epithelium of asthmatics regardless of inhaled steroid treatment. Clin Exp Allergy 2000; 30:1015–1023.

87. Trigg CJ, Nicholson KG, Wang JH, Ireland DC, Jordan S, Duddle JM, Hamilton S, Davies RJ. Bronchial inflammation and the common cold: a comparison of atopic and non-atopic individuals. Clin Exp Allergy 1996; 26:665–676.

88. Bianco A, Whiteman SC, Sethi SK, Allen JT, Knight RA, Spiteri MA. Expression of intercellular adhesion molecule-1 (ICAM-1) in nasal epithelial cells of atopic subjects: a mechanism for increased rhinovirus infection? Clin Exp Immunol 2000; 121:339–345.

89. Johnston SL, Papi A, Bates PJ, Mastronarde JG, Monick MM, Hunninghake GW. Low grade rhinovirus infection induces a prolonged release of IL-8 in pulmonary epithelium. J Immunol 1998; 160:6172–6182.

90. Yamaya M, Sekizawa K, Suzuki T, Yamada N, Furukawa M, Ishizuka S, Nakayama K, Terajima M, Numazaki Y, Sasaki H. Infection of human respiratory submucosal glands with rhinovirus: effects on cytokine and ICAM-1 production. Am J Physiol 1999; 277:L362–371.

91. Zalman LS, Brothers MA, Dragovich PS, Zhou R, Prins TJ, Worland ST, Patick AK. Inhibition of human rhinovirus-induced cytokine production by AG7088, a human rhinovirus 3C protease inhibitor. Antimicrob Agents Chemother 2000; 44:1236–1241.

92. Zhu Z, Tang W, Gwaltney JM, Wu Y, Elias JA. Rhinovirus stimulation of interleukin-8 in vivo and in vitro: role of NF-κB. Am J Physiol 1997; 273:L814–824.

93. Zhu Z, Tang W, Ray A, Wu Y, Einarsson O, Landry ML, Gwaltney J Jr, Elias JA. Rhinovirus stimulation of interleukin-6 in vivo and in vitro. Evidence for nuclear factor kappa B-dependent transcriptional activation. J Clin Invest 1996; 15:421-430.

94. Fraenkel DJ, Bardin PG, Sanderson G, Lampe F, Johnston SL, Holgate ST. Immunohistochemical analysis of nasal biopsies during rhinovirus experimental colds. Am J Respir Crit Care Med 1994; 150:1130–1136.

95. Turner RB, Weingand KW, Yeh CH, Leedy DW. Association between interleukin-8 concentration in nasal secretions and severity of symptoms of experimental rhinovirus colds. Clin Infect Dis 1998; 26:840–846.

96. Grunberg K, Smits HH, Timmers, MC, deKlerk EP, Dolhain RJ, Dick EC, Hiemstra PS, Sterk PJ. Experimental rhinovirus infection. Effect on cell differentials and soluble markers in sputum in asthmatic subjects. Am J Respir Crit Care Med 2000; 156: 609–616.

97. Gern JE, Vrtis R, Grindle KA, Swenson C, Busse WW. Relationship of upper and lower airway cytokines to outcome of experimental rhinovirus infection. Am J Respir Crit Care Med 2000; 162:2226–2231.

98. Fleming HE, Little FF, Schnurr D, Avila PC, Wong H, Liu J, Yagi S, Boushey HA. Rhinovirus-16 colds in healthy and in asthmatic subjects: similar change in upper and lower airways. Am J Respir Crit Care Med 1999; 160:100–108.

99. Sanders SP, Siekierski ES, Porter JD, Richards SM, Proud D. Nitric oxide inhibits rhinovirus-induced cytokine production and viral replication in a human respiratory epithelial cell line. J Virol 1998; 72:934–42.

100. Sanders SP, Kim J, Connolly KR, Porter JD, Siekierski ES, Proud D. Nitric oxide inhibits rhinovirus-induced granulocyte macrophage colony-stimulating factor production in bronchial epithelial cells. Am J Respir Cell Mol Biol 2001; 24:317–325.

101. Sanders SP, Siekierski ES, Richards SM, Porter JD, Imani F, Proud D. Rhinovirus infection induces expression of type 2 nitric oxide synthase in human respiratory epithelial cells in vitro and in vivo. J Allergy Clin Immunol 2001; 107:235–423.

102. Kaul P, Singh I, Turner RB. Effect of nitric oxide on rhinovirus replication and virus-induced interleukin-8 elaboration. Am J Respir Crit Care Med. 1999; 159:1193–1188.

103. Nicholson KG. Clinical features of influenza. Semin Respir Infect 1992; 7:26–37.

104. Zambon MC. Epidemiology and pathogenesis of influenza. J Antimicrob Chemother 1999; 44(Suppl B):3–9.

105. Stamboulian D, Bonvehi PE, Nacinovich FM, Cox N. Influenza. Infect Dis Clin North Am 2000; 14:141–166.

106. Zinserling AV, Aksenov OA, Melnikova VF, Zinserling VA. Extrapulmonary lesions in influenza. Tohoku J Exp Med 1983; 140:259–272.

107. Lyarskaya TY, Ketiladze ES, Zhilina NN, Orlova NN. Detection of viral antigen by autoradiography and immunofluorescence in epithelial cells of the respiratory tract in natural and experimental influenza infection. Acta Virol 1966; 10:521–527.

108. Suzuki Y, Ito T, Suzuki T, Holland RE Jr, Chambers TM, Kiso M, Ishida H, Kawaoka Y. Sialic acid species as a determinant of the host range of influenza A viruses. J Virol 2000; 74:11825-11831.

109. Baum LG, Paulson JC. Sialyloligosaccharide of the respiratory epithelium in the selection of human influenza virus receptor specificity. Acta Histochem Suppl 1990; 40:35–38.

110. Steinhauer DA. Role of hemagglutinin cleavage for the pathogenicity of influenza virus. Virology 1999; 258:1–20.

111. Kido H, Yokogoshi Y, Sakai K, Tashiro M, Kishino Y, Fukutomi A, Katunuma N. Isolation and characterization of a novel trypsin-like protease found in rat bronchiolar epithelial Clara cells. A possible activator of the viral fusion glycoprotein. J Biol Chem 1992; 267:13573–13579.

112. Kido H, Beppu Y, Imamura Y, Chen Y, Murakami M, Oba K, Towatari T. The human mucus protease inhibitor and its mutants are novel defensive compounds against infection with influenza A and Sendai viruses. Biopolymers 1999; 51:79–86.

113. Kido H, Murakami M, Oba K, Chen Y, Towatari T. Cellular proteinases trigger the infectivity of the influenza A and Sendai viruses. Mol Cells 1999; 9:235–244.

114. Goto H, Kawaoka Y. A novel mechanism for the acquisition of virulence by a human influenza A virus. Proc Natl Acad Sci USA 1998; 95:10224–10228.

115. Reiss TF, Gruenert DC, Nadel JA, Jacoby DB. Infection of cultured human airway epithelial cells by influenza A virus. Life Sci 1991; 49:1173–1181.

116. Winther B, Gwaltney JM, Hendley JO. Respiratory virus infection of monolayer cultures of human nasal epithelial cells. Am Rev Respir Dis 1990; 141:839–845.

117. Sweet C, Bird RA, Coates DM, Overton HA, Smith H. Recent H1N1 viruses (A/USSR/90/77, A/Fiji/15899/83, A/Firenze/13/83) replicate poorly in ferret bronchial epithelium. Arch Virol 1985; 85:305–311.

118. Choi AM, Jacoby DB. Influenza virus A infection induces interleukin-8 gene expression in human airway epithelial cells. FEBS Lett 1992; 309:327–329.

119. Matsukura S, Kokubu F, Noda H, Tokunaga H, Adachi M. Expression of IL-6, IL-8, and RANTES on human bronchial epithelial cells, NCI-H292, induced by influenza virus A. J Allergy Clin Immunol 1996; 98:1080–1087.

120. Adachi M, Matsukura S, Tokunaga H, Kokubu F. Expression of cytokines on human bronchial epithelial cells induced by influenza virus A. Int Arch Allergy Immunol 1997; 113:307–311.

121. Kawaguchi M, Kokubu F, Kuga H, Tomita T, Matsukura S, Kadokura M, Adachi M. Expression of eotaxin by normal airway epithelial cells after influenza virus A infection. Int Arch Allergy Immunol 2000; 122:44–49.

122. Matsukura S, Kokubu F, Kubo H, Tomita T, Tokunaga H, Kadokura M,Yamamoto T, Kuroiwa Y, Ohno T, Suzaki H, Adachi M. Expression of RANTES by normal airway epithelial cells after influenza virus A infection. Am J Respir Cell Mol Biol 1998; 18:255–264.

123. Skoner DP, Gentile, DA, Patel, A, Doyle WJ. Evidense for cytokine mediation of disease expression in adults experimentally infected with influenza A virus. J Inf Dis 1999; 180:10–14.

124. Gentile D, Doyle W, Whiteside T, Fireman P, Hayden FG, Skoner D. Increased interleukin-6 levels in nasal lavage samples following experimental influenza A virus infection. Clin Diagn Lab Immunol 1998; 5:604–608.

125. Hayden FG, Fritz R, Lobo MC, Alvord W, Strober W, Straus SE. Local and systemic cytokine responses during experimental human influenza A virus infection. Relation to symptom formation and host defense. J Clin Invest 1998; 101:643–649.

126. Soderberg M, Hellstrom S, Lundgren R, Bergh A. Bronchial epithelium in humans recently recovering from respiratory infections caused by influenza or mycoplasma. Eur Respir J 1990; 3:1023–1028.

127. Jacoby DB, Choi AM. Influenza virus induces expression of antioxidant genes in human epithelial cells. Free Rad Biol Med 1994; 16:821–824

128. Uetani K, Der SD, Zamamian-Daryoush M, de La Motte C, Lieberman BY, Williams BR, Erzurum SC. Central role of double-stranded RNA-activated protein kinase in microbial induction of nitric oxide synthase. J Immunol 2000; 165:988–996.

129. Rimmelzwaan GF, Baars MM, de Lijster P, Fouchier RA, Osterhaus AD. Inhibition of influenza virus replication by nitric oxide. J Virol 1999; 73:8880–8883.

130. Rosman FC, Mistchenko AS, Ladenheim HS, do Nascimento JP, Outani HN, Madi K, Lenzi HL. Acute and chronic human adenovirus pneumonia: cellular and extracellular matrix components. Pediatr Pathol Lab Med 1996; 16:521–541.

131. Rosenfeld MA, Chu CS, Seth P, Danel C, Banks T, Yoneyama K,Yoshimura K, Crystal RG. Gene transfer to freshly isolated human respiratory epithelial cells in vitro using a replication-deficient adenovirus containing the human cystic fibrosis transmembrane conductance regulator cDNA. Hum Gene Ther 1994; 5:331–342.

132. Noah TL, Wortman IA, Hu PC, Leigh MW, Boucher RC. Cytokine production by cultured human bronchial epithelial cells infected with a replication-deficient adenoviral gene transfer vector or wild-type adenovirus type 5. Am J Respir Cell Mol Biol 1996; 14:417–424.

133. Kaner RJ, Worgall S, Leopold PL, Stolze E, Milano E, Hidaka C, Ramalingam R, Hackett NR, Singh R, Bergelson J, Finberg R, Falck-Pedersen E, Crystal RG. Modification of the genetic program of human alveolar macrophages by adenovirus vectors in vitro is feasible but inefficient, limited in part by the low level of expression of the coxsackie/adenovirus receptor. Am J Respir Cell Mol Biol 1999; 20:361–370.

134. Dupuit F, Zahm JM, Pierrot D, Brezillon S, Bonnet N, Imler JL, Pavirani A, Puchelle E. Regenerating cells in human airway surface epithelium represent preferential targets for recombinant adenovirus. Hum Gene Ther 1995; 6:1185–1193.

135. Man Y, Hart VJ, Ring CJ, Sanjar S, West MR. Loss of epithelial integrity resulting from E-caderin dysfunction predisposes airway epithelial cells to adenoviral infection. Am J Respir Cell Mol Biol 2000; 23:610–617.

136. Goldman M, Su Q, Wilson JM. Gradient of RGD-dependent entry of adenoviral vector in nasal and intrapulmonary epithelial: implications for gene therapy of cystic fibrosis. Gene Ther 1996; 3:811–818.

137. Hong SS, Karayan L, Tournier J, Curiel DT, Boulanger PA. Adenovirus type 5 fiber knob binds to MHC class I alpha2 domain at the surface of human epithelial and B lymphoblastoid cells. EMBO J 1997; 16:2294–2306.

138. Zabner J, Freimuth P, Puga A, Fabrega A, Welsh MJ. Lack of high affinity fiber receptor activity explains the resistance of ciliated airway epithelial to adenovirus infection. J Clin Invest 1997; 100:1144–1149.

139. Walters RW, Grunst T, Bergelson JM, Finberg RW, Welsh MJ, Zabner J. Basolateral localization of fiber receptors limits adenovirus infection from the apical surface of airway epithelial. J Biol Chem 1999; 274:10219–10226.

140. Huang X, Griffiths M, Wu J, Farese RV Jr, Sheppard D. Normal development, wound healing, and adenovirus susceptibility in beta5-deficient mice. Mol Cell Biol 2000; 20: 755–759.

141. McIntosh K. Interferon in nasal secretions from infants with viral respiratory tract infections. J Pediatr 1978; 93:33-36.

142. Hall CB, Douglas RG Jr, Simons RL, Geiman JM. Interferon production in children with respiratory syncytial, influenza, and parainfluenza virus infections. J Pediatr 1978; 93:28–32.

143. Hall CB, Douglas RG Jr, Simons RL. Interferon production in adults with respiratory syncytial viral infection. Ann Intern Med 1981; 94:53–55.

144. Henderson FW, Dubovi EJ, Harder S, Seal E Jr, Graham D. Experimental rhinovirus infection in human volunteers exposed to ozone. Am Rev Respir Dis 1988; 137:1124–1128.

145. Sperber SJ, Hayden FG. Comparative susceptibility of respiratory viruses to recombinant interferons-alpha 2b and-beta. J Interferon Res 1989; 9:285–293.

146. Atreya PL, Kulkarni S. Respiratory syncytial virus strain A2 is resistant to the antiviral effects of type I interferons and human MxA. Virology 1999; 261:227–241.

147. Schlender J, Bossert B, Buchholz U, Conzelmann KK. Bovine respiratory syncytial virus nonstructural proteins NS1 and NS2 cooperatively antagonize alpha/beta interferon-induced antiviral response. J Virol 2000; 74:8234–8242.

148. Teng MN, Whitehead SS, Bermingham A, St Claire M, Elkins WR. Murphy BR. Collins PL. Recombinant respiratory syncytial virus that does not express the NS1 or M2–2 protein is highly attenuated and immunogenic in chimpanzees. J Virol 2000; 74: 9317-9321.

149. Young DF, Didcock L, Goodbourn S, Randall RE. Paramyxoviridae use distinct virus-specific mechanisms to circumvent the interferon response. Virology 2000; 269:383-390.

150. Talon J, Horvath CM, Polley R, Basler CF, Muster T, Palese P, Garcia-Sastre A. Activation of interferon regulatory factor 3 is inhibited by the influenza A virus NS1 protein. J Virol 2000; 74:7989–7996.

151. Hatada E, Saito S, Fukuda R. Mutant influenza viruses with a defective NS1 protein cannot block the activation of PKR in infected cells. J Virol 1999; 73:2425–2433.

152. Didcock L, Young DF, Goodbourn S, Randall RE. The V protein of simian virus 5 inhibits interferon signaling by targeting STAT1 for proteasome-mediated degradation. J Virol 1999; 73:9928–9933.

153. Young DF, Chatziandreou N, He B, Goodbourn S, Lamb RA, Randall RE. Single

amino acid substitution in the V protein of simian virus 5 differentiates its ability to block interferon signaling in human and murine cells. J Virol 2001; 75:3363–3370.

154. Stark GR, Kerr IM, Williams BRG, Silverman RH, Schreiber RD. How cells respond to interferons. Annu Rev Biochem 1998; 67:227–264.

155. Mamane Y, Heylbroeck C, Genin P, Algarte M, Servant MJ, LePage C, DeLuca C, Kwon H, Lin R, Hiscott J. Interferon regulatory factors: the next generation. Gene 1999; 237:1–14.

156. Kumar KP, McBride KM, Weaver BK, Dingwall C, Reich NC. Regulated nuclear-cytoplasmic localization of interferon regulatory factor 3, a subunit of double-stranded RNA-activated factor 1. Mol Cell Biol 2000; 20:4159–4168.

157. Zamanian-Daryoush M, Mogensen TH, DiDonato JA, Williams BRG. NF-kB activation by double-stranded-RNA-activated protein kinase (PKR) is mediated through NF-kB-inducing kinase and IkB kinase. Mol Cell Biol 2000; 20:1278–1290.

158. Iordaov MS, Paranjape JM, Ahou A, Wong J, Williams BRG, Meurs EF, Silverman RH, Maung BE. Activation of p38 mitogen-activated protein kinase and c-Jun NH_2-terminal kinase by double-standed RNA and encephalomyocarditis virus: Involvement of Rnase L, protein kinase R, and alternative pathways. Mol Cell Biol 2000; 20:617–627.

159. Xia Y. Makris C. Su B. Li E. Yang J. Nemerow GR. Karin M. MEK kinase 1 is critically required for c-Jun N-terminal kinase activation by proinflammatory stimuli and growth factor-induced cell migration. Proc Natl Acad Sci USA 2000; 97:5243–5248.

160. Monick MM, Staber JM, Thomas KW, and Hunninghake GW. Respiratory syncytial virus infection results in activation of multiple protein kinase C isoforms leading to activation of mitogen-activated protein kinase. J Immunol 2001; 166:2681-2687.

161. Kawasaki H, Schiltz L, Chiu R, Itakura K, Taira K, Nakatani Y, Yokoyama KK. ATF-2 has intrinsic histone acetyltransferase activity which is modulated by phosphorylation. Nature 2000; 405:195–200.

162. Mastronade JG, Monick MM, Mukaida N, Matsushima K, Hunninghake GW. Activator protein-1 is the preferred transcription factor for co-operative interaction with nuclear factor-kB in respiratory syncytial virus-induced interleukin-8 gene expression in airway epithelium. J Infect Dis 1998; 177:1275–1281.

163. Falvo JV, Parekh BS, Lin CH, Fraenkel E, Maniatis T. Assembly of a functional beta-interferon enhanceosome is dependent on ATF-2-c-jun heterodimer orientation. Mol Cell Biol 2000; 20:4814–4825.

164. Zhu Z, Tang W, Gwaltney JM, Wu Y, Elias JA. Rhinovirus stimulation of interleukin-8 in vivo and in vitro: role of NF-kB. Am J Physiol 1997, 273: L814-L824.

165. Zhu Z, Tang W, Ray A, Wu Y, Einarsson O, Landry ML, Gwaltney J Jr, Elias JA. Rhinovirus stimulation of interleukin-6 in vivo and in vitro. Evidence for nuclear factor kappa B-dependent transcriptional activation. J Clin Invest 1996; 15:421-430.

166. Casola A, Garofalo RP, Jamaluddin M, Vlahopoulos S, Brasier AR. Requirement of a novel upstream response element in respiratory syncytial virus-induced IL-8 gene expression. J Immunol 2000; 164:5944–5951.

167. Chen W, Monick MM, Carter AB, Hunninghake GW. Activation of ERK2 by respiratory syncytial virus in A549 cells is linked to the production of interleukin-8. Exp Lung Res 1999; 26:13.

168. Kim J, Sanders SP, Siekierski ES, Casolaro V, Proud D. Role of NF-kappaB in cytokine production induced from human airway epithelia cells by rhinovirus infection. J Immunol 2000; 165:3384–3392.

169. Kaul P, Biaglioli MC, Singh I, Turner RB. Rhinovirus-induced oxidative stress and interleukin-8 elaboration involves p47-phox but is independent of attachment to intercellular adhesion molecule-1 and viral replication. J Infect Dis 2000; 181:1885–1890.

170. Thomas LH, Friedland JS, Sharland M, Becker S. Respiratory syncytial virus induced RANTES production from human bronchial epithelial cells is dependent on nuclear factor-kappa B nuclear binding and is inhibited by adenovirus mediated expression of inhibitor of kappa B alpha. J Immunol 1998; 161:1007–1016.

171. Lin R, Heylbroeck C, Genin P, Pitha PM, Hiscott J. Essential role of interferon regulatory factor 3 in direct activation of RANTES chemokine transcription. Mol Cell Biol 1999; 19:959–966.

172. Genin P, Algarte M, Roof P, Lin R, Hiscott J. Regulation of RANTES chemokine gene expression requires cooperativity between NF- kB and IFN-regulatory factor transcription factors. J Immunol 2000; 164:5352–5361.

173. Tripp RA, Jones L, Anderson LJ. Respiratory syncytial virus G and/or SH glycoproteins modify CC and CXC chemokine mRNA expression in the BALB/c mouse. J Virol 2000; 74:6227–6229.

174. Chini BA, Fiedler MA, Milligan L, Hopkins T, Stark JM. Essential roles of NF-kB and C/EBP in the regulation of intercellular adhesion molecule-1 after respiratory syncytial virus infection of human respiratory epithelial cell cultures. J Virol 1998; 72: 1623–1626.

8

Cytokine Network in Virus Infections and Asthma

TERRY L. NOAH

University of North Carolina
Chapel Hill, North Carolina, U.S.A.

I. Introduction

The respiratory tract is regularly exposed to inhaled micro-organisms. In normal individuals, this rarely results in prolonged lower respiratory illness, but in those with asthma, exacerbations of airway obstruction may result. Epidemiological studies strongly suggest that viral infection is a common cause of significant exacerbations in both children and adults with asthma, as discussed fully elsewhere in this book. Inflammatory and immune responses, which are now believed to be in large part governed by the lung's complex cytokine system, play key roles in producing the clinical features of both asthma and acute viral infection. This chapter will provide an overview of the cytokine network in the lung, how it is altered in asthma, and how viral respiratory infection may further affect cytokine balance to produce exacerbations of airways obstruction.

II. Role of Cytokines in Lung Host Defense

Infectious lung disease is prevented in the normal host through a combination of innate and adaptive immune defense systems. Innate defenses active at the airway surface include physical barriers such as filtering of air at the nose and mucociliary clearance in the conducting airways. Proteins active in innate lung defense include lysozyme, complement, defensins, lactoferrin, transferrin, and the collectins (surfactant proteins A and D)(1). These factors help to prevent infection through direct antimicrobial activity or by enhancing the efficiency of phagocytosis by resident macrophages or neutrophils in the respiratory tract. If microbes are able to overcome the physical, biochemical, and cellular components of innate defense mechanisms, they may trigger activation of the cytokine network, which shapes and further amplifies both inflammatory and adaptive immune responses.

Cytokines are small, soluble peptides that serve as mediators communicating between cells. These peptides transmit messages leading to a variety of target cell responses including differentiation, activation, chemotaxis, or apoptosis (2). A large and ever-growing number of cytokines have been characterized, and an exhaustive description of them is beyond the scope of this chapter. These mediators have varying and overlapping effects determined by the pattern of receptor expression on target cells, as well as other factors including concentration and the influence of other factors in the tissue microenvironment. In the context of lung infection, cytokines are critical for communication between resident cells at the site of infection and effector cells of the inflammatory and immune systems. Under some circumstances tissue damage may allow systemic release of cytokines, but cytokine responses are probably most intense and functionally important at the site of infection. The profile of cytokines produced locally at a site of injury or infection affects both qualitative and quantitative aspects of the inflammatory response.

Cells central to initiation of inflammation in the lung, such as the alveolar macrophage, and effector immune or inflammatory cells themselves, are major sources of cytokines. However, cytokines are also produced by antigen-presenting cells (airway dendritic cells), mast cells, and a variety of resident cell types such as airway epithelium or fibroblasts, after appropriate stimulation. Epithelial cytokines may be especially important in the setting of viral infections, since most respiratory viruses target the epithelial cells lining the respiratory tract. The influence of this interaction on the cytokine network is discussed in detail below.

A. Functional Classification of Cytokines

Cytokines can be classified based on similarities in protein structure (2) or on their general function in inflammation (3). A functional classification is perhaps more helpful in understanding how the cytokine network responds to challenges such as infection. This approach defines cytokines as belonging to a so-called early-response group (tumor necrosis factor alpha [TNF-α] and interleukin 1 beta [IL-1β]) produced by macrophages, monocytes, neutrophils, and lymphocytes, and responsible for the initial amplification of inflammation via proinflammatory effects on many cell types; a so-called recruitment group, which includes the chemokines; an activation group whose members activate the functions of selective subgroups of leukocytes and influence the nature of cell-mediated and humoral immune responses (Table 1); and repair cytokines, which are active in the resolution phase of inflammation. The activities of specific cytokines have been determined using in vitro bioassays, selective

Table 1 Selected "Activation" Cytokines, Their Cellular Sources, and Actions in Inflammatory Responses

Cytokine	Cellular sources	Actions in inflammation
IL-2	T lymphocytes (CD4+)	Th1 differentiation
		Proliferation of T cells
		Proliferation of B cells (with IL-4)
IL-4	T lymphocytes	Th2 differentiation
	NK cells	Proliferation, activation of B lymphocytes
	T lymphocytes	Neutrophil respiratory burst and phagocytosis
	Mast cells/basophils	Mast cell proliferation
IL-5	T lymphocytes	Eosinophil maturation, migration, activation, survival
	Mast cells	Antibody secretion by B cells
	Eosinophils	
IL-6	Alveolar macrophages	B-cell differentiation
	Airway epithelium	T-cell (CD8+) differentiation
	Monocytes	Acute-phase reaction
	Eosinophils	
	T lymphocytes	
	Neutrophils	
	Fibroblasts	
IL-10	Alveolar macrophages	Inhibits Th1 cytokine responses by T cells
	T lymphocytes	Inhibits T cell proliferation
	Monocytes	Chemoattractant for T cells (CD8+)
	Airway epithelium	
IL-11	Fibroblasts	Acute-phase reactant
	Smooth muscle cells	Stimulates B-cell differentiation
	Airway epithelium	Induces cholinergic differentation and tachykinin production
IL-12	B lymphocytes	Stimulation of Th1 cells
	Macrophages	B-cell activation and differentiation
	Dendritic cells	
IL-13	Th2 lymphocytes	Stimulate MHCII expression on macrophages
	Th0 lymphocytes	Increase vascular cell adhesion molecule expression, endothelial cells
	NK cells	
	CD8+ lymphocytes	Stimulates B-cell activation, production of IgE and IgG4
	Mast cells/basophils	Downregulates macrophage cytokine production
	Dendritic cells	
IL-15	Peripheral blood mononuclear cells	Promotes NK maturation
		T-cell proliferation
IL-16	T lymphocytes (CD8+)	T-lymphocyte recruitment and activation
		Migration of eosinophils, monocytes
IL-18	Macrophages	Induces IFN-γ in T cells
		Inhibits IL-10 production in PBMC
		Promotes GM-CSF production in stimulated PBMC
IFNγ	T lymphocytes	Th1 differentiation
	B lymphocytes	Antiviral
	NK cells	Promotes growth of T cells
		Inhibits IL-4-induced B-cell proliferation and antibody production
G-CSF	Alveolar macrophages	Stimulates proliferation of neutrophils
	Monocytes	Enhances phagocytosis, chemotaxis, and bactericidal activity of neutrophils
	Neutrophils	
GM-CSF	Alveolar macrophages	Stimulates growth and differentiation of monocytes, neutrophil, and eosinophil lineages
	T lymphocytes	
	Airway epithelium	Activates mature forms of these cells

Cytokines listed are limited to those discussed in text.
Source: Refs. 1, 3, 105, 106, 134–139.

neutralization in animal models with antibodies or receptor antagonists, localized expression via virus-mediated gene transfer, and, more recently, transgenic (targeted-deletion or overexpression) models. Many in vivo investigations of cytokine function have relied on mouse models, and most murine cytokines have functions analogous to their human counterparts. However, future experiments with so-called humanized mice that have undergone targeted deletion of murine genes with addition (knock-in) of human genes of interest may further refine our understanding of the true in vivo functions of specific cytokines in health and disease (4).

B. Recruitment Cytokines: the Chemokines

A subgroup of cytokines, referred to as the chemokines, appears to be responsible for chemoattractant activity for leukocytes to sites of inflammation. These mediators range in size from 7 to 15 kDa and are biologically active at low concentrations $(10^{-8} - 10^{-10}$ M)(2). The range of target cell types affected by each chemokine is determined by expression of its corresponding receptor(s), many of which have also been cloned and characterized. Four families of chemokines have been defined, based on the position of the first two cysteines in the molecule. Of these families, the best understood currently are the C-X-C chemokines, receptors for which are specifically expressed on neutrophils, and the C-C chemokines, whose receptors are expressed on other leukocytes including eosinophils (see Table 2). The selective activity of certain C-C chemokines toward eosinophils (i.e., regulated on activation, normal T-cell expressed and secreted ([RANTES] and eotaxin) makes them of particular interest in the pathogenesis of asthma and allergy.

C. Cytokine Response to Viral Infection

The initial site of attachment and infection for most of the common human respiratory viruses is with the epithelium lining the airways. It is now known that many

Table 2 Selected C-X-C and C-C Chemokines, Their Receptors, and Leukocyte Target Cells Affected

Chemokine	Family	Receptor	Target cell affected
IL-8	C-X-C	CXC1, CXC2	Neutrophil
GROα,β,γ	C-X-C	CXCR2	Neutrophil
MIP-1α	C-C	CCR1, CCR5	Monocyte, eosinophil, basophil, T lymphocyte
RANTES	C-C	CCR1, CCR3, CCR4, CCR5	Monocyte, eosinophil, basophil, T lymphocyte
MCP-1,2,3,4	C-C	CCR1, CCR2, CCR3, CCR4	Monocyte, eosinophil, basophil, T lymphocyte
Eotaxin	C-C	CCR3	Eosinophil, basophil, T lymphocyte

Chemokines listed are limited to those mentioned in the text.
Source: Ref. 2, p. 133.

of these viruses, including some commonly associated with asthma exacerbation, can directly induce epithelial production of cytokines and chemokines. The mechanisms underlying this induction are discussed fully in Chapter 9. Thus, infected airway epithelial cells probably act as sentinel cells in the cytokine network (5), producing a chemokine increase at the site of viral infection, which helps to regulate initial recruitment of leukocytes from the submucosa and circulation. Chemokine tissue gradients may attract not only nonspecific cellular elements of innate immunity, such as neutrophils and eosinophils, but also cells participating in the adaptive immune response such as lymphocytes and monocytes. Macrophages in the airways and alveoli are also very likely to play important roles in the first responses to viral infection, by virus- or phagocytosis-induced production of the proinflammatory early cytokines TNF-α and IL-1β, and a wide range of other cytokines and chemokines (6).

Dendritic cells are monocyte-derived, antigen-presenting cells that form an important link between innate defense at the mucosal surface and the adaptive immune response. After antigen capture and maturation (promoted by macrophage- or epithelium-derived cytokines such as TNF-α, IL-4, and granulocyte–macrophage colony-stimulating factor [GM-CSF]), dendritic cells can migrate to lymphoid tissues where they stimulate T-cell immune responses. Presentation of viral antigen induces clonal expansion of antigen-specific B and T lymphocytes that confer specific acquired immunity. Virus-infected cells in the airway are thus recognized by memory CD4+ T cells (in association with class II major histocompatibility complex [MHC] or cytotoxic CD8+ T cells (in association with class I MHC). This recognition, as well as recognition of antibody-associated virus antigen by natural killer (NK) cells, leads to killing of the infected cell and release of effector cell activation cytokines (e.g., IFN-γ), which further enhance the antiviral activities of local phagocytes (7).

Together, these cell types thus contribute to a complex network of cytokines that amplifies a rapid, nonspecific response and a subsequent antigen-specific response to viral infection in the airway. A more complete discussion of the cellular immune responses to respiratory viruses is found in Chapter 10 of this book. The precise makeup and duration of the immune/inflammatory response is probably influenced by both the inciting pathogen and by underlying host factors, as discussed below for asthma. It is reasonable to assume that cytokines are also key factors in the resolution of inflammation in the normal host, but this process is at present less well understood.

III. Cytokine Abnormalities in Asthma

Asthma is a chronic inflammatory disorder of the airways in which many cells and cellular elements play a role, including mast cells, macrophages, neutrophils, epithelial cells, and particularly eosinophils and T lymphocytes (8). In susceptible individuals, this inflammation causes recurrent episodes of wheezing, chest tightness, and coughing. These episodes are usually associated with widespread but variable airflow obstruction, due to a combination of smooth muscle contraction, edema, excess mucus, epithelial shedding, and inflammatory cell infiltrates (9). The inflammation is similar to that seen in allergic reactions, and is also associated with bronchial hyperresponsiveness (BHR) to a variety of stimuli (10–13). Over time, remodeling of the airway wall occurs with smooth muscle hypertrophy and basement membrane thickening, further increasing obstruction and BHR (14).

Cytokines produced by inflammatory and structural cells in the asthmatic airway play a central role in prolonging and maintaining the inflammatory process. Since airway eosinophils appear to be closely associated with BHR in both asthma patients and animal models (12,13, 15–17), the components of the cytokine network affecting eosinophil trafficking to the airway have been extensively investigated. As indicated previously, eosinophils express receptors for, and therefore chemoattract to, the C-C chemokines RANTES, eotaxin, macrophage inflammatory protein (MIP-1α), and macrophage chemotactic protein (MCP). Elevated levels of these chemokines have been observed in the asthmatic airway (18). Other cytokines, such as GM-CSF, IL3, and IL-5 appear to prime eosinophils for chemotaxis; in particular, IL-5 and eotaxin appear to be selectively and synergistically involved in promotion of eosinophil chemotaxis (19). Primed (but not unprimed) eosinophils may also chemoattract to the C-X-C chemokine IL-8 (20). Noah et al. (21) found elevated levels of IL-8 and ECP in nasal secretions of asthmatic children at a healthy baseline, and there was significant correlation between levels of these two factors. Interleukin-4 activates endothelium to express VCAM-1, inducing eosinophils to adhere and initiate migration from the bloodstream to the airway surface (22). Local eosinophilia appears to be a better correlate of BHR than systemic eosinophilia (23), and elevated levels of eosinophil products (11) or eosinophil-active cytokines such as RANTES, IL-4, IL-5, and GM-CSF have been noted in bronchoalveolar lavage fluid (BALF) or sputum from asthmatic patients (24). Although this is only circumstantial evidence for a role in asthma, experimental manipulation of these factors in mice appears to confirm their functional importance for the maintenance of allergic inflammation and BHR (25–28). Furthermore, blockage of C-C chemokine receptors has been found to improve airway physiology and reduce inflammation (29).

Murine experiments have given rise to the concept of the Th1 and Th2 subgroups of helper T cells, defined by their unique cytokine production profiles (30). Th1 cells produce IL-2 and IFN-γ but no IL-4 or IL-5, and appear to function in the cell-mediated immune response against intracellular organisms. Th2 cells produce IL-4, IL-5, IL-6, IL-10, and IL-13. The major effects of the Th2 cytokines include attraction and activation of eosinophils, and promotion of B-cell differentiation toward IgE production. Thus, Th2 cells are active against parasitic infection and in allergic reactions. Although it is less certain that a clear differentiation exists in humans between the Th1 and Th2 type responses, in both humans with asthma and in animal models Th2-associated cytokines appear to predominate in the airway and be linked to BHR (25, 31–36). Although allergy is highly associated with asthma, it is apparently not sufficient alone for the development of asthma, because not all allergic individuals develop asthma. Conversely, there are asthmatics who have no demonstrable allergy. Thus, the exact mechanisms and factors required for persistence of the eosinophil-rich, Th2-dominated cytokine milieu in the asthmatic airway are not yet completely clear.

Viral respiratory infection is a common event that may play a role in the initial triggering of asthmatic airway inflammation in susceptible hosts, as well as in exacerbation of existing asthma (37). Virus-induced perturbation of the lung cytokine network, as discussed in the next section, is a likely mechanism for these effects.

IV. Effects of Viral Infection on Cytokines and Airway Inflammation, and Relevance for Asthma

Epidemiological studies strongly implicate viral infection as an important cause of asthma exacerbation. Specific viral pathogens associated with asthma exacerbation include rhinovirus, respiratory syncytial virus, parainfluenza virus, influenza virus, and adenovirus (38–43). Recent investigations have suggested possible mechanisms for the exacerbation of asthma via effects on the cytokine network. General mechanisms by which viral infection at the airway surface influences this network are shown schematically in Figures 1 to 4. Published observations for specific cytokine effects induced by rhinovirus, respiratory syncytial virus, and parainfluenza virus are reviewed in the following sections.

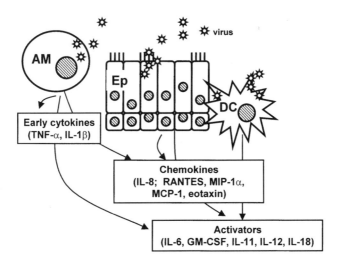

Figure 1 Early events in the cytokine network after virus infection at the airway surface. Virus interacts directly with epithelial cells (Ep), alveolar macrophages (AM), and antigen-presenting dendritic cells (DC) at the mucosal surface. This interaction results in production and release of early cytokines, chemokines, and activators.

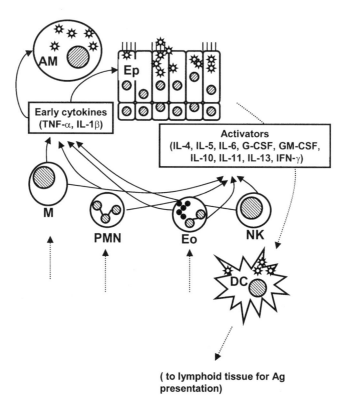

Figure 2 Chemokines elicited by early events (Fig. 1) attract monocytes (M), neutrophils (PMN), eosinophils (Eo), and natural killer cells (NK) to the airway surface. Activation of these cells results in production of more early cytokines, activators, and chemokines, amplifying the inflammatory process. Dendritic cells (DC) migrate to lymphoid tissue where they present antigens to naïve T cells.

A. Rhinovirus

Rhinoviruses (RV) cause the majority of common colds, and are probably the most common cause of virus-induced asthma exacerbations in older children and adults (38). Because of the epidemiological importance of RV, many studies have now addressed its influence on respiratory tract inflammation.

In humans, many studies of RV have used nasal secretions for safety and for ease of repetitive sampling. Several specific cytokines are reported to be increased in nasal secretions of patients with naturally acquired or experimental RV infection. These include IL-8 (44–50), IL-6 (51), eotaxin (47), and, granulocyte colony-stimulating factor (G-CSF) (49). Although IL-8 was elevated in nasal washings from wheezing and nonwheezing infants with RV infection, only the wheezing infants also had elevated RANTES (50). Greiff et al. (48) noted that in allergic rhinitic subjects inoculated with RV-16, increased IL-8 correlated with eosinophilic cationic

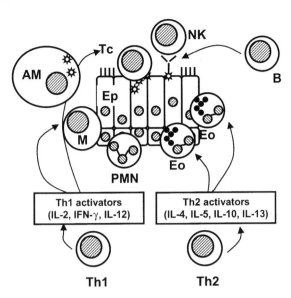

Figure 3 Antigen presentation triggers antigen-specific activation and proliferation of T and B lymphocytes. These include cytotoxic T cells (Tc), which recognize antigen complexed to MHC class I, and helper T cells (Th) that recognize antigen complexed to MHC Class II. Helper T cells may further differentiate into Th1 cells (promoting cell-mediated immunity) or Th2 cells (promoting humoral immunity and allergic type inflammation), depending on host factors and the cytokine milieu. Antibody recognition of viral antigen leads to NK cell-driven lysis of infected cells.

protein (ECP), a marker for eosinophil degranulation. In healthy and asthmatic adults with experimentally induced RV-16 infection, IL-6 and IL-8 were elevated in nasal lavage fluids compared to baseline. However, RANTES, IL-5, and IFN-γ were elevated only in a subgroup of asthmatics having the most severe symptoms (45).

Because the important clinical manifestations of asthma relate to lower airways function, a major question has been whether virus-induced nasal inflammatory changes reflect events in the lower airways. Grunberg et al. (46) found that nasal administration of RV-16 to subjects with mild allergic asthma led to an increase in BHR measured by histamine challenge, and this correlated with nasal IL-8 increases. Jarjour and colleagues (49) found that nasal inoculation of RV-16 in subjects with allergic asthma resulted in an acute increase in IL-8, G-CSF, and neutrophils in nasal secretions; a similar inflammatory response was found in BALF 96 h (but not 48 h) after inoculation. It is possible that a delayed lower airways inflammation after nasal RV infection might be due to immune response factors rather than direct infection. However, recent evidence suggests that RV can infect the lower as well as the upper airways after nasal inoculation of human volunteers (52). Thus, the direct effects of RV infection of nasal mucosa may be reiterated in the tracheobronchial mucosa in normal humans.

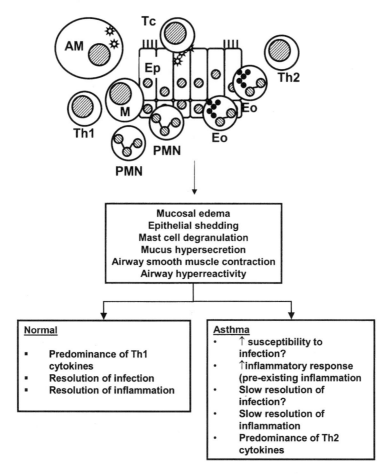

Figure 4 Influx of inflammatory cells to the mucosal surface is associated with release of cytokines and other factors that cause airway edema, epithelial shedding, mast cell degranulation, smooth muscle contraction, mucus hypersecretion, and bronchial hyperreactivity. In asthmatics, resolution of the process may be slow due to the amplifying effect of preexisting inflammation on the cytokine network, as well as inhibitory effects of Th2 inflammation on virus clearance.

RV infects respiratory epithelium via attachment to the intracelluar adhesion molecule (ICAM-1) on the cell surface. A number of recent reports document that RV can induce cytokine production by epithelial cells. Subauste et al. (53) showed enhanced RV-14 infection of a human bronchial epithelial cell line after stimulation with TNF-α, which upregulates ICAM-1 expression. RV infection induced production of IL-8, IL-6, and GM-CSF in this study. Similar experiments by Terajima et al. (54) in primary cultures, and Yamaya et al. (140) using submucosal gland cultures, showed that RV infection may itself upregulate ICAM-1 via autocrine effects of induced IL-1β. It has been noted that in addition to TNF-α and IL-1β, IL-8- and Th2-associated cytokines such as IL-13 upregulate RV-induced epithelial ICAM-1 whereas IFN-γ downregulates ICAM-1 (55). Thus, the Th2-weighted airway cytokine milieu in asthmatics may increase susceptibility to RV infection via effects on ICAM-1. Other in vitro reports have shown epithelial production of RANTES (56) and IL-5-mediated, autocrine IL-1β-stimulated airway smooth muscle cell contraction (57) after RV infection. The precise intracellular signaling pathways responsible for RV-induced cytokine increases remain to be elucidated, but appear to involve activation of NF-κB and the stress-activated protein kinase p38 (58,59).

Inoculation of peripheral blood mononuclear cells (PBMC) with RV caused increased IL-8 expression (60). Incubation of monocytes with RV-14 also has been reported to increase IL-10 production. These in vitro studies suggest that RV may also have direct effects on inflammatory or immune cell cytokine production. Since these cells are chronically present in the asthmatic airway, their activation in the presence of RV may represent another mechanism for amplification of airway inflammation in asthma.

B. Respiratory Syncytial Virus

Respiratory syncytial virus (RSV) is the most common cause of acute lower respiratory infection in young children (61), and is also a common cause of asthma exacerbation at all ages (38). Early RSV infection severe enough to cause hospitalization is associated with an increased risk for recurrent wheezing later in childhood (62). This observation has led to several lines of research investigating how RSV infection might trigger long-term airway hyperresponsiveness. A full discussion of this topic is found elsewhere in this volume. The following paragraphs will review recent work relevant to how RSV affects the cytokine network, immune response patterns, and BHR.

Studies in humans infected with RSV have shown several cytokine changes of potential importance. Most of these studies have been performed in infants and young children, and focus on levels of chemokines in respiratory lavage fluids. Becker et al. (63) noted that, compared to other viral infections, RSV is associated with greater increases in RANTES in nasal secretions. The bronchiolitis syndrome, an acute wheezing illness usually caused by RSV, has been associated with increases IL-8 and neutrophil products in nasal lavage (64,65), and with a polymorphism in the IL-8 gene promoter (IL8–251A) (66). In lower respiratory secretions, IL-8, RANTES, and MIP-1α were elevated, and MIP-1α correlated closely with levels of ECP, suggesting a role for eosinophil degranulation in RSV bronchiolitis (67). RSV-induced chemokine increases in the human respiratory tract have been confirmed in an experimental setting. Experimental nasal inoculation of healthy adults with wild type RSV yielded markedly increased IL-8, MIP-1α, MCP-1, and RANTES in nasal lavage fluids of subjects who developed clinical symptoms and virus shedding, and the increases occurred simultaneously with virus shedding, which started 5–6 days after nasal inoculation (68). In a bovine model, BALF levels of TNF-α were markedly increased starting 6 to 7 days after inoculation (69).

The clinical severity of RSV infection has been noted to correlate with quantity of virus in nasal secretions in hospitalized infants (70). This is of interest because RSV dose-related cytokine effects have been reported in in vitro studies of human alveolar macrophages and respiratory epithelium. Becker and colleagues (71) found that alveolar macrophages produce IL-8, TNF-α, and IL-1β after incubation with RSV in vitro. Noah and Becker (72) reported virus inoculum-dependent increases in mRNA abundance and release of IL-8, IL-6, and GM-CSF by a human bronchial epithelial cell line. Recent reports have focused on RSV-induced epithelial chemokine production. In BALB/c mice, intranasal inoculation of RSV induced a variety of chemokines including MIP-2, IP-10, RANTES, eotaxin, MIP-1α, and MCP-I (73). Chemokine levels paralleled the intensity of inflammation and inoculum dose. MIP-1α was the most abundantly expressed chemokine and primarily localized to airway epithelium. Human epithelial cell lines have produced IL-8, MIP-1α, and RANTES after RSV infection in vitro (67). Compared to other viruses, RSV appears to be an especially potent inducer of RANTES (63, 74). This effect is only partially inhibited by corticosteroids (75) and may result from virus replication-dependent stabilization of RANTES mRNA (76). Coculture of RSV-infected epithelium with leukocytes suggests that epithelial RANTES attracts eosinophils and monocytes, which then produce chemokines MCP-1, MIP-1α, and MIP-1β (77). RSV-infected monocytes may produce factors that stimulate epithelial IL-8 secretion as well (78), and neutrophils incubated with RSV release IL-8, MIP-1α, MIP-1β, and myeloperoxidase (79). Thus, RSV-driven amplification of mucosal inflammation via the cytokine network can be demonstrated in vitro.

RSV may induce immune responses that favor Th2-type inflammation, but data in humans are inconsistent to date. Incubation of PBMC with RSV resulted in a significantly higher IL-10/IFN-γ ratio than when PBMC were incubated with adenovirus (80). Convalescent-phase PBMC from infants hospitalized with RSV infection showed significantly increased IL-10 production in infants with post-RSV recurrent wheezing compared with infants without post-RSV wheezing (81). In another study, stimulated PBMC from RSV-infected infants produced more IL-4 and less IFN-γ than those from controls (82). In contrast, RSV-stimulated T cells from PBMC of infants with RSV showed predominantly IFN-γ production, with only low levels of IL-4 and IL-10, and there was no relationship between Th2 cytokines and disease severity (65). In this study, eosinophils were only sporadically found in nasopharyngeal washings and had no relation to disease severity.

The impact of RSV infection on specific aspects of immunity has been extensively investigated, primarily using mouse models, in attempts to identify strategies for vaccine development. Trafficking of lymphocytes to the murine lung is present by day 5 and peaks at day 7 postinoculation, and these cells express both Th1 (IFN-γ, IL-2) and Th2 (IL-4, IL-5) cytokines (83). RSV-induced IFN-γ has been shown to limit viral replication but predispose to greater airway obstruction (84). Prior sensitization to the RSV G protein appears to result in Th2-type inflammation (IL-4, IL-5, IL-13), more severe illness, poorer viral clearance, and an eosinophilic response to subsequent exposure to wild-type RSV in some models (85,86). A recent report suggests that vaccination of mice with either the F or G proteins using so-called gene gun technology may elicit a Th2 cytokine response on subsequent RSV infection (87). Local expression of IL-4 at the time of antigen presentation diminishes the cytolytic activity of primary and memory CD8+, RSV-specific cytolytic responses in vivo (88), suggesting a mechanism by which preexisting Th2-type inflammation, such as that in asthmatic airways, may reduce the efficiency of virus clearance. Furthermore, RSV infection in mice sensitized to allergens enhances total serum IgE levels (89).

Bronchial hyperresponsiveness can be demonstrated in BALB/c mice after RSV infection. This BHR appears to depend on the presence of CD8+ lymphocytes and IL-4 and IL-5, which result in eosinophil influx (90–92). Follow-up studies showed that adoptive transfer of CD8+ cells from RSV-infected mice resulted in increases in BHR, eosinophil influx, and IL-5 production by naive BALB/c mice upon subsequent ovalbumin sensitization (93). Mice vaccinated with formalin-inactivated RSV (but not with a live intranasal vaccine) showed increased BHR and Th2 cytokine production upon subsequent RSV challenge and allergic sensitization (94). Airway eosinophilia and BHR have also been demonstrated in guinea pigs after RSV infection, in association with long-term persistence of RSV in the lung (95).

In summary, RSV infection may affect the lung cytokine network at several levels. RSV exerts direct, proinflammatory effects on production of cytokines and chemokines by epithelial cells and resident phagocytes in the airways. Prior RSV infection may also exacerbate subsequent allergic inflammation and BHR via effects on immune cells, and prior immune responses to RSV may have an impact on subsequent responses to RSV infection or allergic challenge. In many studies, the end result of these interactions is to amplify Th2 type cytokines and BHR, thus promoting asthma-like airway physiology.

C. Parainfluenza Virus

Parainfluenza virus (PIV) is another common respiratory pathogen, and is the most common cause of epidemic croup in children (61). Nasal wash specimens from school-aged children with acute upper respiratory infection due to PIV contained elevated levels of MIP-1α and RANTES (96). However, the majority of investigations of PIV effects on the cytokine network have been done using in vitro or animal models.

A study of the kinetics of cytokine increases in murine PIV-1 (Sendai virus) infection showed that maximal levels of IL-2, IFN-γ, TNF, IL-6, and IL-10 occurred 7–10 days after inoculation of virus (97). Guinea pigs infected with PIV demonstrate increases in BHR and BALF eosinophils, neutrophils, and monocytes, and the eosinophils correlate with quantities of eotaxin (98,99). In the guinea pig model, IL-5 appears to be necessary for PIV-induced BHR but not influx of inflammatory cells (99). PIV-susceptible Brown Norway rats develop persistent BHR associated with bronchiolar fibrosis. This effect appears to be associated with upregulation of TNF-α in pulmonary macrophages; inhibition of TNF-α with a soluble receptor prevented fibrosis but also led to increased mortality and viral replication (100). Thus, cytokine upregulation important for host defense may also lead to lung remodeling and BHR in susceptible hosts.

Numerous studies have documented the direct activation of cells in vitro by PIV. Incubation of PBMC with PIV was found to induce IL-6, IL-8, TNF-α, and IFN-α via tyrosine-kinase-dependent pathways (101). An exhaustive survey of PIV-induced cytokines in PBMC showed increases for MIP-1α, RANTES, TNF-α, IL-6, and IL-8 (102). In a similar study, PIV was also associated with production of the early cytokines IL-1α and β (103). Treatment of PBMC with the Th2-promoting cytokines IL-4 or IL-10 reduced PIV-induced levels of IFN-α (104), an observation of potential relevance for the asthmatic airway. PIV has also been shown to upregulate PBMC production of the IL-2-like cytokine IL-15, and this activity was responsible for activation of NK cells (105). Pirhonen et al. (106) have observed that GM-CSF-differentiated macrophages respond to PIV in vitro by releasing IL-1β and IL-18, whereas undifferentiated monocytes respond much less strongly. In another report of macrophage responses, PIV was associated with upregulation of MIP-1α, RANTES, and IL-8, while influenza virus appeared to induce MCP-1 preferentially (107). Elias et al. (108,109) observed that PIV-3 infection induces production of IL-11 by airway smooth muscle cells in vitro, and IL-11 increased BHR in BALB/c mice.

D. Influenza

Influenza virus is a major cause of epidemic acute respiratory illness in humans, and is also a documented trigger of asthma exacerbation (38). Children with naturally acquired influenza infection have elevated levels of MIP-1α and RANTES in nasopharyngeal secretions (96). Asthmatic adults with influenza had exacerbation of asthma symptoms, and elevated levels of IL-8, ECP, and neutrophils in induced sputum (110). Several investigators have examined the effects of experimental influenza inoculation on nasal cytokines in human volunteers. Hayden et al. (111) found that IL-6 and IFN-α levels peaked in nasal lavage fluid and correlated with symptoms 2 days after inoculation of influenza A, while TNF-α and IL-8 peaked at 3–4 days. Influenza virus shedding was associated with increases in the cytokines IL-6, IL-8, IL-10, TNF-α, IFN-γ, MCP-1, and MIP-1α in nasal secretions in several other human studies (112–114). Experimental influenza infection in animal models confirms that similar cytokine changes occur in nasal-associated lymphoid tissue and BALF (115–117).

A number of recent reports have examined the direct cytokine-inducing effect of influenza virus on relevant target cells. Human bronchial epithelial cell lines and primary cultures have shown induction of IL-6, IL-8, and RANTES after in vitro exposure to influenza A (118–120). This effect may be cell culture-system-specific, since epithelial chemokine induction was not observed in another study (63). The mechanism for influenza-induced epithelial RANTES production appears to involve reactive oxygen species acting as second messengers for a cascade involving activation of p38 mitogen-activated protein (MAP) kinase, c-Jun N-terminal kinase (JNK), and NF-κB (121,122). Among leukocytes, monocytes and macrophages appear to be susceptible to influenza infection directly. Macrophages and dendritic cells have produced TNF-α, IL-1, IL-6, IFN-α/β, MIP-1α, and RANTES after influenza infection, and differentiation from monocyte to macrophage may be required for this effect (106, 123,124). Of note is that supernatants from influenza-infected macrophages have rapidly induced IFN-γ in T lymphocytes, suggesting a pathway for amplification of Th 1 immunity (125). Influenza-exposed PBMC produce IL-15, which upregulates NK activity in uninfected PBMC (105), suggesting another mechanism for virus-induced immune responses.

The effects of influenza on the cytokine network as it pertains to immunity have also been investigated. CCR2(-/-) and CCR5(-/-) mice both exhibit defective clearance of influenza due to delayed T-cell migration, suggesting that virus-induced local production of CC chemokines is important for timely induction of adaptive immunity (126). Mature dendritic cells, when stimulated by influenza antigen, elicit IFN-γ production by CD8+ T cells (127), and memory CD8+ T cells exposed to influenza respond with increased IFN-γ production, further increasing cell-mediated immunity (128).

Several interesting observations may have relevance for the effects of influenza on cytokines in the presence of allergic or asthmatic inflammation. When influenza-infected dendritic cells were exposed to T cells, Th1-type cytokines were produced at low virus doses, whereas at high doses Th2 cytokines (IL-4, IL,-10) were produced (129); this was considered to be due to viral neuraminidase-mediated desialylation of T-cell surface molecules. Tsitoura et al. (130) reported that normal allergen-induced tolerance was abrogated by concurrent infection with influenza virus in mice, leading to BHR and to the production of IL-4, IL-5, IL-13, and allergen-specific IgE. Whether a Th2 or Th1 response was generated depended on the time interval between virus and allergen exposure. Adoptive transfer experiments of influenza hemagglutinin-specific Th1 and Th2 cells suggest that Th2 cells induce dramatic influenza antigen-specific eosinophilia and eotaxin expression, and this is not inhibited by cotransfer of Th1 cells (131). Finally, overexpression of IL-4 by a lung-specific promoter resulted in decreased infiltration of virus-specific CD8+ T cells and delayed viral clearance (132). Thus, the presence of abundant IL-4 in the asthmatic airway may result in prolonged inflammation via delayed virus clearance.

V. Summary

Numerous studies suggest that viral respiratory infection exacerbates asthmatic airway inflammation, airway obstruction, and BHR. Mechanisms by which viral infection induces increased, cytokine-mediated inflammation include direct induction of cytokines by virus infection in resident airway cells including epithelium, macrophages, and dendritic cells, and subsequent effects on adaptive immunity. These pathways are shown schematically in Figures 1–4. These inflammatory changes may lead to BHR either on their own or as a result of their effects on preexisting, asthma-associated inflammation and cytokine abnormalities.

The asthmatic airway may be primed for exaggerated virus-induced inflammation by virtue of increased expression of virus receptors (e.g., ICAM-1) on epithelial cell surfaces, leading to enhanced susceptibility to infection; a cytokine milieu (e.g., increased IL-4 and IL-10) that promotes eosinophilia and delays clearance of virus, prolonging or intensifying the inflammatory stimulus; and direct viral interaction with cytokine-producing cell types (e.g., monocytes, lymphocytes) not normally present in the mucosa at the onset of infection.

In in vitro experiments, specific viral agents appear to have differing effects on cytokine production by various cell types. This may be a clue as to why certain pathogens are more commonly associated with asthma exacerbation than others. For example, viruses with a greater tendency to elicit direct production of C-C chemokines or Th2 cytokines from target cells may invoke an inflammatory response with a greater tendency to cause BHR.

Important questions remain unresolved about the impact of viral infection on cytokine networks in patients with asthma. Except for some recent work with RV, relatively little is currently known about the true susceptibility of the human asthmatic lower airway to viral infection, due to the invasive nature of definitive diagnostic procedures for detecting the pathogens. It is also unclear what the safe limits are for suppression of cytokine responses to viruses. While cytokine "abnormalities" have been identified in asthmatic patients or disease models, the human cytokine network has apparently evolved as a flexible and complex host defense communications system, allowing rapid and specific responses to potentially harmful microbes. Nonspecific anti-inflammatory treatment therefore has the potential disadvantage of disarming important host defense mechanisms. Thus, a better understanding of the specific pathological cytokine pathways in asthmatic airways, as opposed to normal protective pathways, is needed. The answers to these questions will help to determine whether antiviral or anticytokine strategies will ultimately be the most beneficial in the prevention or treatment of virus-induced asthma exacerbations.

Although a great deal of knowledge has been gained regarding cytokine pathways important in the initiation or amplification of acute inflammation, relatively little is known about the mechanisms for its resolution. Such knowledge may be useful in designing further strategies for limiting the adverse effects of virus-induced inflammation in asthmatic patients.

Acknowledgment

The author thanks Dr. David B. Peden for critical review of the manuscript.

References

1. Zhang P, Summer WR, Bagby GJ, Nelson S. Innate immunity and pulmonary host defense. Immunol Rev 2000; 173:39-51.
2. Graziano FM, Cook EB, Stahl JL. Cytokines, chemokines, RANTES, and eotaxin. Allergy Asthma Proc 1999; 20:141–146.

3. Mehrad B, Standiford TJ. Role of cytokines in pulmonary antimicrobial host defense. Immunol Res 1999; 20:15–27.

4. Campbell EJ. Animal models of emphysema: the next generations. J Clin Invest 2000; 106:1445–1446.

5. Lo D, Feng L, Li L, Carson MJ, Crowley M, Pauza M, Nguyen A, Reilly CR. Integrating innate and adaptive immunity in the whole animal. Immunol Rev 1999; 169:225–239.

6. Becker S, Quay J, Soukup J. Cytokine (tumor necrosis factor, IL-6, IL-8) production by respiratory syncytial virus-infected human alveolar macrophages. J Immunol 1991; 147:4307–12.

7. Roitt I. Essential Immunology, 8th ed. Oxford: Blackwell Scientific Publications, 1994.

8. Kon OM, Kay AB. T cells and chronic asthma. Int Arch Allergy Immunol 1999; 118: 133–135.

9. National Asthma Education and Prevention Panel, Expert Panel Report 2. Guidelines for the Diagnosis and Management of Asthma. Washington, DC: National Institutes of Health, July 1997.

10. Laprise C, Laviolette M, Boutet M, Boulet LP. Asymptomatic airway hyperresponsiveness: relationships with airway inflammation and remodeling. Eur Respir J 1999; 14: 63–73.

11. Gibson PG, Saltos N, Borgas T. Airway mast cells and eosinophils correlate with clinical severity and airway hyperresponsiveness in corticosteroid-treated asthma. J Allergy Clin Immunol 2000; 105:752–759.

12. Louis R, Lau LC, Bron AO, Roldaan AC, Radermecker M, Djukanovic R. The relationship between airways inflammation and asthma severity. Am J Respir Crit Care Med 2000; 161:9–16.

13. Rasmussen F, Lambrechtsen J, Siersted HC, Hansen HS, Hansen NC. Increased eosinophil cation protein level in sensitized nonasthmatics is linked to subsequent hyperresponsiveness to methacholine. Int Arch Allergy Immunol 2000; 121:129–136.

14. Holgate ST. Inflammatory and structural changes in the airways of patients with asthma. Respir Med 2000; 94 (Suppl D):S3-S6.

15. Gundel RH, Letts LG, Gleich GJ. Human eosinophil major basic protein induces airway constriction and airway hyperresponsiveness in primates. J Clin Invest 1991; 87: 1470-1473.

16. Gundel RH, Wegner CD, Letts LG. The onset and recovery from airway hyperresponsiveness: relationship with inflammatory cell infiltrates and release of cytotoxic granule proteins. Clin Exp Allergy 1992; 22:303–308

17. Wardlaw A. The eosinophil: new insights into its function in human health and disease. J Pathol 1996; 179:355–357.

18. Alam R, York J, Boyars M, Stafford S, Grant JA, Lee J, Forsythe P, Sim T, Ida N. Increased MCP-1, RANTES, and MIP-1 alpha in bronchoalveolar lavage fluid of allergic asthmatic patients. Am J Respir Crit Care Med 1996; 153:1398–1404.

19. Simson L, Foster PS. Chemokine and cytokine cooperativity: eosinophil migration in the asthmatic response. Immunol Cell Biol 2000; 78:415–422.

20. Sehmi R, Cromwell O, Wardlaw AJ, Moqbel R, Kay AB. Interleukin-8 is a chemoattractant for eosinophils purified from subjects with a blood eosinophilia but not from normal healthy subjects. Clin Exp Allergy 1993; 23:1027–1036.

21. Noah TL, Henderson FW, Henry MM, Peden DB, Devlin RB. Nasal lavage cytokines in normal, allergic, and asthmatic school age children. Am J Resp Crit Care Med 1995; 152:1290–1296.

22. Gleich GJ. Mechanisms of eosinophil-associated inflammation. J Allergy Clin Immunol 2000; 105:651–663.

23. Gruber W, Eber E, Pfleger A, Modl M, Meister I, Weinhandl E, Zach MS. Serum eosinophil cationic protein and bronchial responsiveness in pediatric and adolescent asthma patients. Chest 1999; 116:301–305.

24. Gauvreau GM, Watson RM, O'Byrne PM. Kinetics of allergen-induced airway eosinophilic cytokine production and airway inflammation. Am J Respir Crit Care Med 1999; 160:640–647.

25. Yssel H, Groux H. Characterization of T cell subpopulations involved in the pathogenesis of asthma and allergic diseases. Int Arch Allergy Immunol 2000; 121:10–18.

26. Kobayashi T, Miura T, Haba T, Sato M, Serizawa I, Nagai H, Ishizaka K. An essential role of mast cells in the development of airway hyperresponsiveness in a murine asthma model. J Immunol 2000; 164:3855–3861.

27. Hamelmann E, Takeda K, Schwarze J, Vella AT, Irvin CG, Gelfand EW. Development of eosinophilic airway inflammation and airway hyperresponsiveness requires interleukin-5 but not immunoglobulin E or B lymphocytes. Am J Respir Cell Mol Biol 1999; 21:480–489.

28. Lei XF, Ohkawara MR, Stampfli MR, Gauldie J, Croitoru K, Jordana M, Xing Z. Compartmentalized transgene expression of granulocyte-macrophage colony stimulating factor (GM-CSF) in mouse lung enhances allergic airways inflammation. Clin Exp Immunol 1998; 113:157–165.

29. Dabbagh K, Xiao, Y Smith C, Stepick-Biek P, Kim SG, Lamm WJ, Liggitt DH, Lewis DB. Local blockade of allergic airway hyperreactivity and inflammation by the poxvirus-derived pan-CC-chemokine inhibitor vCC1. J Immunol 2000; 165:3418–3422.

30. Mosmann TR, Coffman RL. Th1 and Th2 cells: Different patterns of lymphokine secretions lead to different functional properties. Ann Rev Immunol 1989; 7:145–173.

31. Makela MJ, Kanehiro A, Borish L, Dakhama A, Loader J, Joetham A, Xing Z, Jordana M, Larsen GL, Gelfand EW. IL-10 is necessary for the expression of airway hyperresponsiveness but not pulmonary inflammation after allergic sensitization. Proc Natl Acad Sci USA 2000; 97:6007–6012.

32. Tsitoura DC, Blumenthal RL, Berry G, Dekruyff RH, Umetsu DT. Mechanisms preventing allergen-induced airways hyperreactivity: role of tolerance and immune dysfunction. J Allergy Clin Immunol 2000; 106:239–246.

33. Lin CC, Lin CY, Ma HY. Pulmonary function changes and increased Th-2 cytokine expression and nuclear factor kB activation in the lung after sensitization and allergen challenge in brown Norway rats. Immunol Lett 2000; 73:57–64.

34. Sur S, Bouchard P, Holbert D, VanScott MR. Mucosal IL-12 inhibits airway reactivity to methacholine and respiratory failure in asthma. Exp Lung Res 2000; 26:477–789.

35. Hogan SP, Foster PS, Tan X, Ramsay AJ. Mucosal IL-12 gene delivery inhibits allergic airways diseased and restores local antiviral immunity. Eur J Immunol 1998; 28:413–423.

36. Erb KJ, LeGros G. The role of Th2 type CD4+ T cells and Th2 type CD8+ T cells in asthma. Immunol Cell Biol 1996; 74:206-208.

37. Herz U, Lumpp U, Da Palma JC, Enssle K, Takatsu K, Schnoy N, Daser A, Kottgen E, Wahn U, Renz H. The relevance of murine animal models to study the development of allergic bronchial asthma. Immunol Cell Biol 1996; 74:209–217.

38. Johnston SL, et al. Community study of role of viral infections in exacerbations of asthma in 9–11 year old children. Br Med J 1995; 310:1225–1228.

39. Johnston SL, et al. The relationship between upper respiratory infections and hospital admissions for asthma: a time-trend analysis. Am J Respir Crit Care Med 1996; 154: 654-660.

40. Gbadero DA, et al. Microbial inciters of acute asthma in urban Nigerian children. Thorax 1995; 50:739–745.

41. Kondo S, et al. Progressive bronchial obstruction during the acute stage of respiratory tract infection in asthmatic children. Chest 1994; 106:100–104.

42. Nicholson KG, et al. Respiratory viruses and exacerbations of asthma in adults. Br Med J 1993; 307:982–986.

43. Teichtahl H, et al. The incidence of respiratory tract infection in adults requiring hospitalization for asthma. Chest 1997; 112:591–596.

44. Johnston SL. Natural and experimental rhinovirus infections of the lower respiratory tract. Am J Respir Crit Care Med 1995; 152:S46–52.

45. Fleming HE, Little FF, Schnurr D, Avila PC, Wong H, Liu J, Yagi S, Boushey HA. Rhinovirus-16 colds in healthy and in asthmatic subjects: similar changes in upper and lower airways. Am J Respir Crit Care Med 1999; 160:100–108.

46. Grunberg K, Timmers MC, Smits HH, de Klerk EP, Dick EC, Spaan WJ, Hiemstra PS, Sterk PJ. Effect of experimental rhinovirus 16 colds on airway hyperresponsiveness to histamine and interleukin-8 in nasal lavage in asthmatic subjects in vivo. Clin Exp Allergy 1997; 27:36–45.

47. Greiff L, Andersson M, Andersson E, Linden M, Myint S, Svensson C, Persson CG. Experimental common cold increases mucosal output of eotaxin in atopic individuals. Allergy 1999; 54:1204–1208.

48. Greiff L, Andersson M, Svensson C, Linden M, Myint S, Persson CG. Allergen challenge-induced acute exudation of IL-8, ECP and alpha2-macroglobulin in human rhinovirus-induced common colds. Eur Respir J 1999; 13:41–47.

49. Jarjour NN, Gern JE, Kelly EA. Swenson CA, Dick CR, Busse WW. The effect of experimental rhinovirus 16 infection on bronchial lavage neutrophils. J Allergy Clin Immunol 2000; 105:1169–1177.

50. Pacifico L, Iacobini M, Viola F, Werner B, Mancuso G, Chiesa C. Chemokine concentrations in nasal washings of infants with rhinovirus illnesses. Clin Infect Dis 2000; 31:834–838.

51. Zhu Z, Tang W, Ray A, Wu Y, Einarsson O, Landry ML, Gwaltney J Jr., Elisa JA. Rhinovirus stimulation of interleukin-6 in vivo and in vitro. Evidence for nuclear factor kappa B-dependent transcriptional activation. J Clin Invest 1996; 97:421-430.

52. Papadopoulos NG, Bates PJ, Bardin PG, Papi A, Leir SH, Fraenkel DJ, Meyer J, Lackie PM, Sanderson G, Holgate ST, Johnston SL. Rhinoviruses infect the lower airways. J Infect Dis 2000; 181:1875–1884.

53. Subauste MC, Jacoby DB, Richards SM, Proud D. Infection of a human respiratory epithelial cell line with rhinovirus. Induction of cytokine release and modulation of susceptibility to infection by cytokine exposure. J Clin Invest 1995; 96:549-557.

54. Terajima M, Yamaya M, Sekizawa K, Okinaga S, Suzuki T, Yamada N, Nakayama K, Ohrui T, Oshima T, Numazaki Y, Sasaki H. Rhinovirus infection of primary cultures of human tracheal epithelium: role of ICAM-1 and IL-1 beta. Am J Physiol 1997; 273: L749–759.

55. Bianco A, Sethi SK, Allen JT, Knight RA, Spiteri MA. Th2 cytokines exert a dominant influence on epithelial cell expression of the major group human rhinovirus receptor, ICAM-1. Eur Respir J 1998; 12:619–626.

56. Schroth MK, Grimm E, Frindt P, Galagan DM, Konno SI, Love R, Gern JE. Rhinovirus replication causes RANTES production in primary bronchial epithelial cells. Am J Respir Cell Mol Biol 1999; 20:1220–1228.

57. Grunstein MM, Hakonarson H, Maskeri N, Chuang S. Autocrine cytokine signaling mediates effects of rhinovirus on airway responsiveness. Am J Physiol Lung Cell Mol Physiol 2000; 278:L1146–1153.

58. Griego SD, Weston CB, Adams JL, Tal-Singer R, Dillon SB. Role of p38 mitogen-activated protein kinase in rhinovirus-induced cytokine production by bronchial epithelial cells. J Immunol 2000; 165:5211–5220.

59. Kim J, Sanders SP, Siekierski, ES, Casolaro V, Proud D. Role of NF-kappa B in cytokine production induced from human airway epithelial cells by rhinovirus infection. J Immunol 2000; 165:3384–3392.

60. Johnston SL, Papi A, Monick MM, Hunninghake GW. Rhinoviruses induce interleukin-8 mRNA and protein production in human monocytes. J Infect Dis 1997; 175: 323–329.

61. Denny FW, Clyde WA. Acute lower respiratory tract infections in nonhospitalized children. J Pediatr 1986; 108:635-646.

62. Sigurs N, Bjarnason R, Sigurbergsson F, Kjellman B. Respiratory syncytial virus bronchiolitis in infancy is an important risk factor for asthma and allergy at age 7. Am J Respir Crir Care Med 2000; 161:1501–1507.

63. Becker S, Reed W, Henderson FW, Noah TL. Respiratory syncytial virus infection of airway epithelial cells causes production of the β-chemokine RANTES. Am J Physiol 1997; 272 (Lung Cell Mol Physiol 16):L512-L520.

64. Abu-Harb M, Bell F, Finn A, Rao WH, Nixon L, Shale D, Everard ML. IL-8 and neutrophil elastase levels in the respiratory tract of infants with RSV bronchiolitis. Eur Respir J 1999; 14:139–143.

65. Brandenburg AH, Kleinjan A, van Het Land B, Moll HA, Timmerman HH, de Swart RL, Neijens HJ, Fokkens W, Osterhaus AD. Type 1-like immune response is found in children with respiratory syncytial virus infection regardless of clinical severity. J Med Virol 2000; 62:267–277.

66. Hull J, Thomson A, Kwiatkowski D. Association of respiratory syncytial virus bronchiolitis with the interleukin 8 gene region in UK families. Thorax 2000; 55:1023–1027.

67. Harrison AM, Bonville CA, Rosenberg HF, Domachowske JB. Respiratory syncytial virus-induced chemokine expression in the lower airways: eosinophil recruitment and degranulation. Am J Respir Crit Care Med 1999; 159:1918–1924.

68. Noah TL, Becker S. Chemokines in nasal secretions of normal adults experimentally infected with respiratory syncytial virus. Clin Immunol 2000; 97:43–49.

69. Rontved CM, Tjornehoj K, Viuff B, Larsen LE, Godson DL, Ronsholt L, Alexandersen S. Increased pulmonary secretion of tumor necrosis factor-alpha in calves experimentally infected with bovine respiratory syncytial virus. Vet Immunol Immunopathol 2000; 76:199–214.

70. Buckingham SC, Bush AJ, Devincenzo JP. Nasal quantity of respiratory syncytial virus correlates with disease severity in hospitalized infants. Pediatr Infect Dis J 2000; 19: 113–117.

71. Becker S, Soukup J: Yankaskas JR. Respiratory syncytial virus infection of human primary nasal and bronchial epithelial cell cultures and bronchoalveolar macrophages. Am J Resp Cell Mol Biol 1992; 6:369–374.

72. Noah, TL, Becker S. Respiratory syncytial virus-induced cytokine production by a

human bronchial epithelial cell line. Am J Physiol Lung Cell Mol Physiol 1993; 265(9): L472-L478.

73. Haeberle HA, Kuziel WA, Dieterich HJ, Casola A, Gatalica Z, Garofalo RP. Inducible expression of inflammatory chemokines in respiratory syncytial virus-infected mice: role of MIP-1alpha in lung pathology. J Virol 2001; 75:878–890.

74. Noah TL, Wortman IA, Hu P-C, Leigh MW, Boucher RC. Cytokine production by human bronchial epithelial cells infected with an adenoviral gene therapy vector or wild-type adenovirus type 5. Am J Respir Cell Mol Biol 1996; 14:417–424.

75. Noah TL, Wortman IA, Becker S. The effect of fluticasone propionate on respiratory syncytial virus-induced chemokine release by a human bronchial epithelial cell line. Immunopharmacology 1998; 39:193–199.

76. Koga T, Sardina E, Tidwell RM, Pelletier M, Look DC, Holtzman MJ. Virus-inducible expression of a host chemokine gene relies on replication-linked mRNA stabilization. Proc Natl Acad Sci USA 1999; 96:5680–5685.

77. Becker S, Soukup JM. Airway epithelial cell-induced activation of monocytes and eosinophils in respiratory syncytial viral infection. Immunobiology 1999; 201:88–106.

78. Thomas LH, Wickremasinghe MI, Sharland M, Friedland JS. Synergistic upregulation of inerleukin-8 secretion from pulmonary epithelial cells by direct and monocyte-dependent effects of respiratory syncytial virus infection. J Virol 2000; 74:8425-8433.

79. Jaovisidha P, Peeples ME, Brees AA, Carpenter LR, Moy JN. Respiratory syncytial virus stimulates neutrophil degranulation and chemokine release. J Immunol 1999; 163:2816–2820.

80. Diaz PV, Calhoun WJ, Hinton KL, Avendano LF, Gaggero A, Simon V, Arrendondo SM, Pinto R, Diaz A. Differential effects of respiratory syncytial virus and adenovirus on mononuclear cell cytokine responses. Am J Respir Crit Care Med 1999; 160:1157-1164.

81. Bont L, Heijnen CJ, Kavelaars A, van Aalderen WM, Brus F, Draaisma JT, Geelen SM, Kimpen JL. Monocyte IL-10 production during respiratory syncytial virus bronchiolitis is associated with recurrent wheezing in a one-year follow-up study. Am J Respir Crit Care Med 2000; 161:1518–1523.

82. Bendelja K, Gagro A, Lokar-Kolbas R, Krsulovic-Hresic V, Drazenovic V, Mlinaric-Galinovic G, Rabatic S. Predominant type-2 response in infants with respiratory syncytial virus (RSV) infection demonstrated by cytokine flow cytometry. Clin Exp Immunol 2000; 121:332–338

83. Tripp RA, Moore D, Anderson LJ. TH(1)- and TH(2)-type cytokine expression by activated T lymphocytes from the lung and spleen during the inflammatory response to respiratory syncytial virus. Cytokine 2000; 12:801–807.

84. van Schaik SM, Obot N, Enhorning G, Hintz K, Gross K, Hancock GE, Stack AM, Welliver RC. Role of interferon gamma in the pathogenesis of primary respiratory syncytial virus infection in BALB/c mice. J Med Virol 2000; 62:257–266.

85. Tripp RA, Moore D, Jones L, Sullender W, Winter J, Anderson LJ. Respiratory syncytial virus G and/or SH protein alters Th1 cytokines, natural killer cells, and neutrophils responding to pulmonary infection in BALB/c mice. J Virol 1999; 73:7009-7107.

86. Johnson TR, Graham BS. Secreted respiratory syncytial virus G glycoprotein induces interleukin-5 (IL-5), IL-13, and eosinophilia by an IL-4-independent mechanism. J Virol 1999; 73:8485–8495.

87. Bembridge GP, Rodriguez N, Garcia-Beato R, Noclson C, Melero JA, Taylor G. Respiratory syncytial virus infection of gene gun vaccinated mice induces Th2-driven pul-

monary eosinophilia even in the absence of sensitization to the fusion (F) or attachment (G) protein. Vaccine 2000; 19:1038–1046.

88. Aung S, Tang YW, Graham BS. Interleukin-4 diminishes CD8(+) respiratory syncytial virus-specific cytotoxic T-lymphocyte activity in vivo. J Virol 1999; 73:8944–8949.

89. Matsuse H, Behera AK, Kumar M, Lockey RF, Mahapatra SS. Differential cytokine mRNA expression in Dermatophagoides farinae allergen-sensitized and respiratory syncytial virus-infected mice. Microbes Infect 2000; 2:753–759.

90. Schwarze J, Cieslewicz G, Hamelmann E, Joetham A, Shultz LD, Lamers MC, Gelfand EW. IL-5 and eosinophils are essential for the development of airway hyperresponsiveness following acute respiratory syncytial virus infection. J Immunol 1999; 162:2997-3004.

91. Schwarze J, Cieslewicz G, Joetham A, Ikemura T, Hamelmann E, Gelfand EW. CD8 T cells are essential in the development of respiratory syncytial virus-induced lung eosinophilia and airway hyperresponsiveness. J Immunol 1999; 162:4207–4211.

92. Schwarze J, Cieslewicz G, Joetham A, Ikemura T, Makela MJ, Dakhama A, Shultz LD, Lamers MC, Gelfand EW. Critical roles for interleukin-4 and interleukin-5 during respiratory syncytial virus infection in the development of airway hyperresponsiveness after airway sensitization. Am J Respir Crit Care Med 2000; 162:380–386.

93. Schwarze J, Makela M, Cieslewicz G, Dakhama A, Lahn M, Ikemura T, Joetham A, Gelfand EW. Transfer of the enhancing effect of respiratory syncytial virus infection on subsequent allergic airway sensitization by T lymphocytes. J Immunol 1999; 163:5729–5734.

94. Peebles RS Jr, Sheller JR, Collins RD, Jarzecka K, Mitchell DB, Graham BS. Respiratory syncytial virus (RSV)-induced airway hyperresponsiveness in allergically sensitized mice is inhibited by live RSV and exacerbated by formalin-inactivated RSV. J Infect Dis 2000; 182:671–677.

95. Bramley AM, Vitalis TZ, Wiggs BR, Hegele RG. Effects of respiratory syncytial virus persistence on airway responsiveness and inflammation in guinea-pigs. Eur Respir J 1999; 14:1061-1067.

96. Bonville CA, Rosenberg HF, Domachowske JB. Macrophage inflammatory protein one alpha and RANTES in nasal secretions during ongoing upper respiratory tract infection. Pediatr Allergy Immunol 1999; 10:39–44.

97. Mo XY, Sarawar SR, Doherty PC. Induction of cytokines in mice with parainfluenza pneumonia. J Virol 1995; 69:1288–1291.

98. Scheerens J, Folkerts G, Van der Linde H, Sterk PJ, Conroy DM, Williams TJ, Nijkamp FP. Eotaxin levels and eosinophils in guinea pig broncho-alveolar lavage fluid are increased at the onset of a viral respiratory infection. Clin Exp Allergy 1999; 29 Suppl 2:74–77.

99. van Oosterhout AJ, van Ark I, Folkerts G, van der Linde HJ, Savelkoul HF, Verheyen AK, Nijkamp FP. Antibody to interleukin-5 inhibits virus-induced airway hyperresponsiveness to histamine in guinea pigs. Am J Respir Crit Care Med 1995; 151:177–183.

100. Uhl EW, Moldawer LL, Busse WW, Jack TJ, Castleman WL. Increased tumor necrosis factor-alpha (TNF-alpha) gene expression in parainfluenza type 1 (Sendai) virus-induced bronchiolar fibrosis. Am J Pathol 1998; 152:513–522.

101. Megyeri K, Au WC, Rosztoczy I, Raj NB, Miller RL, Tomai MA, Pitha PM. Stimulation of interferon and cytokine gene expression by imiquimod and stimulation by Sendai virus utilize similar signal transduction pathways. Mol Cell Biol 1995; 15:2207–2218.

102. Hua J, Liao MJ, Rashidbagi A. Cytokines induced by Sendai virus in human peripheral blood leukocytes. J Leukoc Biol 1996; 60:125–128.

103. Zidovec S, Mazuran R. Sendai virus induces various cytokines in human peripheral blood leukocytes: different susceptibility of cytokine molecules to low pH. Cytokine 1999; 11:140–143.

104. Payvandi F, Amrute S, Fitzgerald-Bocarsly P. and Exogenous and endogenous IL-10 regulate IFN-alpha production by peripheral blood mononuclear cells in response to viral stimulation. J Immunol 1998; 160:5861–5868.

105. Fawaz LM, Charif-Askari E, Menezes J. Up-regulation of NK cytotoxic activity via IL-15 induction by different viruses: a comparative study. J Immunol 1999; 163:4473–4480.

106. Pirhonen J, Sareneva T, Kurimoto M, Julkunen I, Matikainen S. Virus infection activates IL-1 beta and IL-18 production in human macrophages by a caspase1-dependent pathway. J Immunol 1999; 162:7322–7329.

107. Matikainen S, Pirhonen J, Miettinen M, Lehtonen A, Govenius-Vintola C, Saraneva T, Julkunen I. Influenza A and sendai viruses induce differential chemokine gene expression and transcription factor activation in human macrophages. Virology 2000; 276:138–147.

108. Einarsson O, Geba GP, Zhu Z, Landry M, Elisa JA. Interleukin-11: stimulation in vivo and in vitro by respiratory viruses and induction of airways hyperresponsiveness. J Clin Invest 1996; 97:915–924.

109. Elias JA, Wu Y, Zheng T, Panettieri R. Cytokine- and virus-stimulated airway smooth muscle cells produce IL-11 and other IL-6-type cytokines. Am J Physiol 1997; 273: L648–655.

110. Pizzichini MM, Pizzichini E, Efthimiadis A, Chauhan AJ, Johnston SL, Hussack P, Mahony J, Dolovich J, Hargreave FE. Asthma and natural colds. Inflammatory indices in induced sputum: a feasibility study. Am J Respiri Crit Care Med 1998; 158:1178-1184.

111. Hayden FG, Fritz R, Lobo MC, Alvord W, Strober W, Straus SE. Local and systemic cytokine responses during experimental human influenza A virus infection. Relation to symptom formation and host defense. J Clin Invest 1998; 101:643–649.

112. Fritz RS, Hayden FG, Calfee DP, Cass LM, Peng AW, Alvord WG, Strober W, Straus SE. Nasal cytokine and chemokine responses in experimental influenza A virus infection: results of a placebo-controlled trial of intravenous zanamivir treatment. J Infect Dis 1999; 180:586–593.

113. Gentile D, Doyle W, Whiteside T, Fireman P, Hayden FG, Skoner D. Increased interleukin-6 levels in nasal lavage samples following experimental influenza A virus infection. Clin Diagn Lab Immunol 1998; 5:604–608.

114. Skoner DP, Gentile DA, Patel A, Doyle WJ. Evidence for cytokine mediation of disease expression in adults experimentally infected with influenza A virus. J Infect Dis 1999; 180:10–14.

115. Matsuo K, Iwasaki T, Asanuma H, Yoshikawa T, Chen Z, Tsujimoto H, Kurata T, Tamura SS. Cytokine mRNAs in the nasal-associated lymphoid tissue during influenza virus infection and nasal vaccination. Vaccine 2000; 18:1344–1350.

116. van Reeth K, Nauwynck H, Pensaert M. Bronchoalveolar interferon-alpha, tumor necrosis factor-alpha, interleukin-1, and inflammation during acute influenza in pigs: a possible model for humans? J Infect Dis 1998; 177:1076–1079.

117. van Reeth K, Nauwynck H. Proinflammatory cytokines and viral respiratory disease in pigs. Vet Res 2000; 31:187–213.

118. Adachi M, Matsukura S, Tokunaga H, Kokubu F. Expression of cytokines on human bronchial epithelial cells induced by influenza virus A. Int Arch Allergy Immunol 1997; 113:307–311.

119. Kawaguchi M, Kokubu F, Kuga H, Tomita T, Matsukura S, Kadokura M, Adachi M. Expression of eotaxin by normal airway epithelial cells after influenza virus A infection. Int Arch Allergy Immunol 2000; 122 Suppl 1:44–49.

120. Matsukura S, Kokubu F, Kubo H, Tomita T, Tokunaga H, Kadokura M, Yamamoto T, Kuroiwa Y, Ohno T, Suzaki H, Adachi M. Expression of RANTES by normal airway epithelial cells after influenza virus A infection. Am J Respir Cell Mol Biol 1998; 18: 255–264.

121. Kujime K, Hashimoto S, Gon Y, Shimizu K, Horie T. p38 mitogen-activated protein kinase and c-jun-NH2-terminal kinase regulate RANTES production by influenza virus-infected human bronchial epithelial cells. J Immunol 2000; 164:3222–3228.

122. Flory E, Kunz M, Scheller C, Jassoy C, Stauber R, Rapp UR, Ludwig S. Influenza virus-induced NF-kappaB-dependent gene expression is mediated by overexpression of viral proteins and involves oxidative radicals and activation of IkappaB kinase. J Biol Chem 2000; 275:8307–8314.

123. Hofmann P, Sprenger H, Kaufmann A, Bender A, Hasse C, Nain M, Gemsa D. Susceptibility of mononuclear phagocytes to influenza A virus infection and possible role in the antiviral response. J Leukoc Biol 1997; 61:408–414.

124. Bender A, Albert M, Reddy A, Feldman M, Sauter B, Kaplan G, Hellman W, Bhardwaj N. The distinctive features of influenza virus infection of dendritic cells. Immunobiology 1998; 198:552-567.

125. Saraneva T, Matikainen S, Kurimoto M, Julkunen I. Infleunza A virus-induced IFN-alpha/beta and IL-18 synergistically enhance IFN-gene expression in human T cells. J Immunol 1998; 160:6032–6038.

126. Dawson TC, Beck MA, Kuziel WA, Henderson F, Maeda N. Contrasting effects of CCR5 and CCR2 deficiency in the pulmonary inflammatory response to influenza A virus. Am J Pathol 2000; 156:1951–1959.

127. Larsson M, Nessner D, Somersan S, Fonteneau JF, Donahoe SM, Lee M, Dunbar PR, Cerundolo V, Julkunen I, Nixon DF, Bhardwaj N. Requirement of mature dendritic cells for efficient activation of influenza A-specific memory CD8+ T cells. J Immunol 2000; 165:1182–1190.

128. Mbawuike IN, Fujihashi K, DiFabio S, Kawabata S, McGhee JR, Couch RB, Kiyono H. Human interleukin-12 enhances influenza-specific memory CD8+ cytotoxic T lymphocytes. J Infect Dis 1999; 180:1477–1486.

129. Oh S, Eichelberger MC. Polarization of allogeneic T-cell responses by influenza virus-infected dendritic cells. J Virol 2000; 74:7738–7744.

130. Tsitoura DC, Kim S, Dabbagh K, Berry G, Lewis DB, Umetsu DT. Respiratory infection with influenza A virus interferes with the induction of tolerance to aeroallergens. J Immunol 2000; 165:3484–3491.

131. Li 1, Xia Y, Nguyen A, Feng L, Lo D. Th2-induced eotaxin expression and eosinophilia coexist with Th1 responses at the effector stage of lung inflammation. J Immunol 1998; 161:3128-3135.

132. Bot A, Holz A, Christen U, Wolfe T, Temann A, Flavell R, von Herrath M. Local IL-4 expression in the lung reduced pulmonary influenza virus specific secondary cytotoxic T cell responses. Virology 2000; 269:66–77.

133. Baggiolini M, Loetscher P. Chemokines in inflammation and immunity. Immunol Today 2000; 21:418–420.

134. Einarsson O, Geba GP, Zhou Z, Landry ML, Panettieri RA, Trsitram D, Welliver R, Metinko A, Elias JA. Interleukin-11 in respiratory inflammation. Ann NY Acad Soc 1995; 762:89–100.

135. Laberge S, Cruikshank WW, Kornfeld H, Center DM. Histamine-induced secretion of lymphocyte chemoattractant factor from CD8 + T cells is independent of transcription and translation. Evidence for constitutive protein synthesis and storage. J Immunol 1995; 155:2902–2910.

136. Lalani T, Simmons RK, Ahmed AR. Biology of IL-5 in health and disease. Ann Allergy Asthma Immunol 1999; 82:317–333.

137. Micallef MJ et al. Interferon gamma inducing factor enhances T helper 1 cytokine production by stimulated human T cells: synergism with interleukin 12 for interferon-gamma production. Eur J Immunol 1996; 26 (7): 1647–1651.

138. Nelson S, Summer WR. Innate immunity, cytokines, and pulmonary host defense. Infect Dis Clin North Am 1998; 12:555-567.

139. Reynolds HY. Advances in understanding pulmonary host defense mechanisms: dendritic cell function and immunomodulation. Curr Opin Pulmon Med 2000; 6:209–216.

140. Yamaya M, Sekizawa K, Suzuki T, Yamada N, Furukawa M, Ishizuka S, Nakayama K, Terajima M, Numazaki Y, Sasaki H. Infection of human respiratory submucosal glands with rhinovirus: effects on cytokine and ICAM-1 production. Am J Physiol 1999; 277:L362–371.

9

Molecular Mechanisms of Respiratory Virus-Induced Inflammation

ALBERTO PAPI, GAETANO CARAMORI, and CINZIA M. BELLETTATO

University of Ferrara
Ferrara, Italy

IAN ADCOCK and SEBASTIAN L. JOHNSTON

National Heart and Lung Institute
Imperial College
London, England

I. Introduction

Inflammation is a central feature of many lung diseases, including bronchial asthma. Although the specific characteristics of the inflammatory responses and the site of inflammation differ between one disease and another, they always involve recruitment and activation of inflammatory cells and changes in structural cells of the lung. Inflammatory responses are associated with an increased expression of a cascade of proteins that includes cytokines, chemokines, growth factors, enzymes, adhesion molecules, and receptors. In most cases the increased expression of these proteins is the result of enhanced gene transcription: many of the genes are not expressed in normal cells under resting conditions but they are induced in the inflammatory process in a cell-specific manner. Transcription factors regulate the expression of many genes, including inflammatory genes and may play a key role in the pathogenesis of respiratory inflammatory diseases.

Recent clinical studies have suggested a role for viral infections in the natural history of asthma, and particularly in asthma exacerbations. The precise cellular and molecular mechanisms underlying these events are still largely unknown. In this chapter we will review the relationship between respiratory virus infection and the molecular mechanisms involved in the activation of airway inflammation. In particular, we will focus on the available information on the regulation of transcription factors by common viral infections implicated in asthma.

II.   Cells and Molecules Involved in Respiratory Virus-Driven Airway Inflammation

Despite growing clinical evidence for a role of respiratory viral infections in the pathogenesis of asthma, and in particular of asthma exacerbations, the precise mechanisms of respiratory virus-induced airway inflammation are uncertain. Most of the data available relate to rhinovirus (RV) and respiratory syncytial virus (RSV), which are the respiratory viruses that appear to be more frequently involved in virus-induced asthma/ acute wheezing episodes.

A.   Rhinovirus

There is evidence that the major receptor for RV binding to the cell is the intercellular adhesion molecule-1 (ICAM-1) (1–6). Approximately 90% of RV serotypes, including RV14 and RV16, bind to and enter cells using cell surface ICAM-1. Other RV serotypes, including RV1A, are in the minor receptor group. They do not bind ICAM-1 and instead bind the low-density lipoprotein (LDL) receptor and related proteins (7). Using ICAM-1, RV can infect airway epithelial cells, but there is little evidence of productive replication in other airway cells such as monocytes, macrophages, and eosinophils granulocytes.

Blood

Following RV infection there is a decrease in the total number of peripheral lymphocytes and in the ratio of CD4+/CD8+ cells, probably caused by a migration of T cells from the bloodstream into the tissue to cause a local rather than a systemic reaction (8). In addition, RV16 infection causes increased peripheral blood mononuclear cell (PBMC) proliferation and interferon-gamma (but not interleukin-5 [IL-5]) secretion (9).

Upper Airways

The upper respiratory tract ciliated epithelial cells are the primary site of RV infection (10–14). Scattered isolated foci of infected cells between normal epithelium are typical of rhinovirus infections (12–15). However, histological examinations of rhinovirus-infected nasal epithelium showed no obvious changes in morphology or integrity. Rhinoviruses evoke an inflammatory response characterized by vasodilation, increased permeability, and cellular infiltration (16,17). Within 24 h of inoculation, increased neutrophil counts are noted in the nasal mucosa and nasal secretions (17,18). A few days later the recruitment of monocytes that cross the endothelium to become tissue macrophages is observed (17,18). The involvement of lymphocytes is still the subject of controversy.

Cytotoxic damage of infected epithelial cells has been difficult to demonstrate in past studies (17–20), although recent studies have demonstrated cytopathic effects in primary bronchial epithelial cell cultures (21). This raises the possibility that the clinical features of RV infection may result principally from the induction of proinflammatory mediators.

Subjects with experimentally induced or naturally acquired colds have transient increases in concentrations of several mediators including kinins (22,23), cytokines including IL-1β (24), IL-1Ra, IL-6, IL-11, tumor necrosis factor alpha (TNF-α), granulocyte colony-stimulating factor (G-CSF) and granulocyte–macrophage colony-stimulating factor (GM-CSF) (21,25–31), chemokines (IL-8, monocyte inflammatory protein 1α, eotaxin 1 and 2 [30,33,34]) and the cellular mediators myeloperoxidase and major basic protein (30,34) in nasal secretions during symptomatic RV infections. There is a direct correlation between the severity of the common cold symptoms and the concentration of IL-6 and IL-8 in the secretions (35,36). It has also been reported that intranasal challenge of normal subjects with IL-8 produces a symptom complex that in some respects mimics the common cold (37). The changes in nasal lavage neutrophils correlated with both nasal and serum G-CSF (25). During naturally acquired acute upper respiratory tract infection (mainly caused by RV), the virus-induced inflammatory changes within the nose are more prolonged in atopic than in nonatopic subjects (38). This is associated with reduced IL-10 levels in nasal lavage in atopic than in nonatopic subjects during the acute phase of upper respiratory tract infection (38).

Taken together, these data suggest that at the molecular level the virus-induced airway inflammation may be characterized by the same imbalance of proinflammatory and anti-inflammatory cytokine production characteristic of bronchial asthma (39–41).

Lower Airways

In the past it was believed that RVs could not replicate in the lower airways where the temperature is 37°C, preferring cooler temperatures that occur in the nose (42). However differences in RV replication between 33°C and 37°C are minimal, and there may even be strains that prefer the higher temperature, suggesting that temperature itself is not an important factor in relation to upper and lower airway infections with RV (43). Indeed, rhinoviruses, after experimental nasal inoculation, can reach, penetrate, and replicate in the bronchial epithelium of both normal and asthmatic individuals. This supports the hypothesis that rhinoviruses extend into the lower airway and may induce bronchial inflammation that could contribute to virus-induced asthma exacerbation (21,44).

In asthmatics, during naturally occurring (45) and experimentally induced RV infection (46–50), there is increased recruitment of inflammatory cells and expression of inflammatory mediators. Using bronchoscopy and segmental allergen challenge, it was shown that experimental RV infection promoted mast cell release of histamine (51) and the recruitment of eosinophils (52) and lymphocytes (53) to the airways.

In contrast to the rapid changes in blood neutrophils, the increase in bronchoalveolar lavage (BAL) neutrophils is detectable about 4 days after the inoculation.

Moreover, the changes in BAL neutrophils correlate both with nasal and serum G-CSF and there is a positive trend with G-CSF in BAL, suggesting the potential importance of RV-induced generation of G-CSF in the development of neutrophilic bronchial inflammation (28).

At the molecular level RV infection seems to amplify the effects of the allergic inflammation (52). Many data are consistent with the hypothesis that allergen, by enhancing expression of the ICAM-1 on airway epithelial cells, facilitates RV infection in atopic subjects; RV-induced increases in ICAM-1 levels would favor migration and activation of inflammatory cells to the airway, resulting in enhanced atopic inflammation (49, 54).

Indeed IL-4, IL-5, IL-10, and IL-13 produce in vitro an enhancement of ICAM-1 over the expression induced by RV infection itself (55). Interferon-gamma in combination with each Th2-associated cytokine, only slightly reduced, but did not override, the Th2-induced level of ICAM-1 expression on both RV-uninfected and RV-infected airway epithelial cells (55,56). These data suggest that the effects of Th2-associated cytokines on ICAM-1 expression and recovery of infectious rhinovirus are dominant over the effects of the Th1-associated cytokines such as interferon-gamma. Since the airway mucosa in atopic asthma is predominantly infiltrated by Th2 lymphocytes, these results could partially explain both the increased susceptibility to human rhinovirus infection in asthmatic patients and the associated exacerbation of asthma symptoms (55,56). Indeed, increased ICAM-1 expression in bronchial epithelium after RV inoculation in asthmatic patients has been recently described (49). Therefore, rhinoviruses may potentially facilitate both their own bronchial epithelial infection and the leukocyte infiltration that could contribute to the development of rhinovirus-induced asthma exacerbations. These data are supported by the recent demonstration that asthmatic subjects have more severe lower respiratory symptoms and greater falls in peak expiratory flow (PEF) than do normal subjects when infected with rhinovirus (57).

Experimental RV infection of human airway epithelial cell lines and/or primary bronchial epithelial cells also induces proinflammatory mediator production including cytokines such as IL-6 (19,36), IL-8 (58), IL-11 (26), (GM-CSF (59,60), regulated on activation, normal T-cell expressed and secreted [RANTES] (61–63), 5-lipoxygenase (5-LO), 5-LO-activating protein (FLAP) and cyclo-oxygenase (COX) -2 (64,65), endothelin (64), and adhesion molecules (36,66–69). Recent studies have shown that rhinovirus infection upregulates neurokinin receptor 1 (NK-1R) mRNA expression and synergizes with the neuropeptides substance P (SP) and neurokinin A (NK-A) in IL-6 and IL-8 production by human bronchial epithelial cells (70). In contrast, NK2-R and neutral endopeptidase 24–11 (NEP) cell surface expression did not change significantly after rhinovirus infection (70).

RV can induce inducible nitric oxide synthase (NOS2) expression in human primary bronchial epithelial cells in vitro (71–73) and nitric oxide (NO) can reduce RV replication and the induced inflammatory cytokine release by epithelial cells (71–73).

NO may play an important role in host defenses against viruses (73,74). Replication of a wide range of DNA and RNA viruses is inhibited in vitro by the addition of chemical donors of NO by the induction of NOS2. Studies in animal models have shown that inhibitors of NOS can increase viral load and decrease survival, and mice deficient in NOS2 have been reported to be more susceptible to viral infection (74). In vitro studies of RV-infected human bronchial epithelial cells have shown that NO can inhibit virus replication as well as RV-induced production of the proinflammatory cytokines IL-6, IL-8, and GM-CSF (59,60).

B. Respiratory Syncytial Virus

Respiratory syncytial virus (RSV) is a member of the family Paramyxoviridae, subfamily pneumovirus; it is an enveloped RNA virus. It has a negative-sense, nonsegmented, single-stranded RNA genome.

RSV is a major respiratory pathogen and is most common in infants, where it causes a range of illnesses from asymptomatic infection through upper respiratory tract infection, bronchiolitis, and pneumonia.

In addition, during the past two decades, a growing number of studies have clearly established RSV as a severe pathogen in certain adult populations. The elderly, those with underlying cardiopulmonary disease (chronic cardiac failure, chronic obstructive pulmonary disease, bronchial asthma), and immunocompromised patients appear to be at greatest risk of developing severe, even life-threatening, disease (75,76).

In human bronchial epithelial cells RSV colocalize with ICAM-1, and this binding can be inhibited by an antibody to the fusion F protein. These data suggest that RSV interaction with ICAM-1 involves the F protein and facilitates RSV entry and infection of human bronchial epithelial cells (77).

Although RSV can cause severe viral bronchiolitis in infants, in adults RSV infection is usually confined to upper airways. The preferential localization of RSV infection to the upper airways may be partially due to protective immunity, and does not depend on a difference in susceptibility of epithelial cells from upper and lower airways (78).

Since RSV replication is largely restricted to airway epithelial cells, one hypothesis is that inflammatory cell recruitment by the infected cells will start the later immunopathology (79). The effects of RSV on airway inflammation may be therefore partly mediated by sequential production of proinflammatory cytokines in infected airway epithelium.

Upper Airways

During RSV nasal infection in infants, cellular infiltrates in nasopharyngeal washings consisted mainly of neutrophils granulocytes and monocytes. Eosinophils, IgE-positive cells, and tryptase-positive cells were found sporadically (80). The chemokines IL-8, RANTES, MIP-1alpha, and MCP-1, and the cytokine vascular endothelial cell growth factor (VEGF)/vascular permeability factor (VPF) are all increased in nasal secretions in human RSV infection at the time of virus shedding and symptomatic illness (81–84). Production and release of chemokines can be observed as early as 12 h after infection (85). A significant increase of inducible NOS

(NOS2) gene expression was observed in nasopharyngeal exudate cells obtained from infants during the acute phase of RSV bronchiolitis (86).

RSV infection of human nasal epithelial cells stimulated the production of the cytokines IL-8 and RANTES (87) but not of IL-6, GM-CSF, and TNF-alpha (88). In vitro RSV infection seems to increase the expression of intercellular adhesion molecule (ICAM)-1 in nasal epithelial cell cultures (89).

Lower Airways

The clinical similarities between viral bronchiolitis in children and asthma exacerbations in adults has led to the speculation that the two diseases have similar pathogenetic mechanisms at the molecular level.

Respiratory syncytial virus infection induces profound effects on the human bronchial epithelial ciliated cells obtained from surgical samples: ciliostasis, clumping, and loss of cilia from live cells and sloughing of cells (90). In a very recent study the type of inflammatory cells in nasal lavage, bronchoalveolar lavage, and the peripheral blood of infants with RSV bronchiolitis, RSV-bronchiolitis and age-matched controls were compared (91). Neutrophils were the predominant cells present in the upper and lower airway (91). It has been suggested that the edema of RSV-induced bronchiolitis is due, at least in part, to RSV-induced epithelial necrosis. However, recent studies have demonstrated that in vitro RSV infection of respiratory epithelial cells induces an increase in the production of mediators such as VEGF/VPF, that are known to induce blood vessel permeability alterations directly (83).

Several groups have shown that during RSV bronchiolitis eosinophils are recruited to, and degranulate in, the airways (92–96). In vitro RSV seems to activate eosinophils directly (97,98), while airway epithelial cells infected with RSV support an increased adherence of activated eosinophils (99).

RSV-induced bronchiolitis is associated with increased concentrations in respiratory secretions of leukotriene C4 (100) and eosinophil cationic protein (107). Intubated infants with severe RSV bronchiolitis show elevated MIP-1α levels in lower respiratory tract specimens (94).

The concentrations of RANTES, MIP-1α, IL-6, IL-8, and IL-10 are increased in nasal washings and tracheal aspirates from all children with RSV infection compared with control children (101). The expression of selected adhesion molecules and of major histocompatibility complex (MHC) class I and II antigens on A549 cells infected with RSV has been recently investigated (102). RSV infection of A549 cells significantly upregulates the expression of ICAM-1, VCAM-1, and MHC class I and II antigens on these cells (102). RSV infection also alters the expression of E-cadherin on A549 cells, becoming mainly upregulated around or in RSV-induced giant cells (102).

RSV infection of human bronchial and alveolar epithelial cells stimulated the production of the cytokines IL-6 (90,103), IL-8 (90,103,104), IL-11 (105), soluble tumor necrosis factor receptor type I (103), MIP-1α (106), RANTES (90,106) GM-CSF, endothelin-1 (107), but not IL-1β, eotaxin, monocyte chemotactic protein (MCP)-1 MCP-3, macrophage inflammatory protein-1 beta, interferon alpha and gamma, and leukotriene C_4 (81,84,90,108,109). The observation that RSV-infected epithelial cells upregulate and secrete eosinophil chemoattractants supports the hypothesis that eosinophils are recruited to, and participate in, the immunopathogenesis of RSV disease.

In vitro the chemotactic response of both eosinophils and monocytes is inhibited by antibodies to RANTES, but not to MIP-1α, implicating RANTES as the primary chemokine responsible for selectively recruiting eosinophils and monocytes to the site of RSV infection (84,109).

RSV infection of A549 cells induces the NOS2 gene both in vitro and in vivo; this induction may occur rather promptly (86). The NOS2 gene, which is initially induced by RSV infection, may be further enhanced in a paracrine fashion by proinflammatory cytokines released by infection-activated inflammatory cells (86).

RSV infection of human alveolar macrophages stimulated the production of the cytokines IL-1, IL-6, IL-8, and TNF-α (78,110,111). RSV persistence in mouse alveolar macrophages was found to increase phagocytosis, expression of Fc gamma receptors, and the production of IL-1 beta and IL-6, while the biological activity of secreted TNF-α was decreased (112). RSV infection also stimulates human airway smooth muscle cells' IL-11 production (113).

III. Transcription Factors

Transcription factors bind to DNA-regulatory sequences (enhancers and silencers), usually localized in the 5′ upstream region of target genes, modulating gene transcription and resulting in altered protein synthesis and subsequent cellular function. Many transcription factors are common to several cell types (ubiquitous) and may play a general role in the regulation of inflammatory genes, whereas others are cell- or stimulus-specific and may determine the phenotypic characteristics of a cell (114).

Transcription factor activation is complex and may involve multiple intracellular signal transduction pathways, including kinases mitogen-activated protein [MAPKs], Janus kinases [JAKs], and protein kinase C [PKCs], activated by cell-surface receptors. Transcription factors may therefore convert transient environmental signals at the cell surface into long-term changes in gene transcription, thus acting as nuclear messengers. An alternative theory is that some transcription factors may also be directly activated by ligands (such as glucocorticoids and vitamins A and D) (115).

Transcription factors may physically interact with each other, altering transcriptional activity at a site distinct from the consensus sequence for a particular transcription factor. This then allows cross-talk between different signal transduction pathways at the level of gene expression. Indeed, it is often necessary to have coincident activation of several transcription factors in order to have maximal gene expression (115).

Large proteins that bind to the basal transcription apparatus bind many transcription factors and thus act as integrators of gene transcription. These coactivator molecules include CAMP-responsive element binding protein (CREB)-binding protein (CBP), and the related p300, and allow complex interactions among different signaling pathways (115).

DNA is wound around histone proteins to form nucleosomes. CBP and p300 have histone acetylase activity (HAT) that is activated by the binding of transcription factors such as AP-1, NF-κB, and STATs. Acetylation of histone residues results in unwinding of DNA coiled around the histone core, thus opening up the chromatin structure, which allows transcription factors, remodeling agents, and RNA polymerase II to bind more readily, thereby increasing transcription. Histone deacetylation reverses this process and causes gene repression. Deacetylation is controlled by recruitment of histone deacetylases (HDACs) by corepressors molecules [such as steroid receptor coactivator-1 (SRC-1)] to the site of gene induction.

The activation of several nuclear factors has recently been studied in several respiratory diseases. In the next paragraphs we will review the most relevant in vivo and in vitro findings related to respiratory virus infection.

A. Nuclear Factor-κB

Nuclear factor-κB (NF-κB) is a ubiquitous transcription factor that appears to be of particular importance in inflammatory and immune responses. NF-κB was first identified as a regulator of immunoglobulin k light-chain gene expression in murine B lymphocytes, but has subsequently been identified in most cell types (115–117). NF-κB binds to the κB DNA sequence 5'-GGGACTTTCC-3'.

Several different NF-κB proteins have been characterized and belong to the Rel family that share an approximately 300 amino acid region known as the Rel homology domain that contains the DNA-binding elements. The activated form of NF-κB is a heterodimer, which usually consists of two subunits, p65 (Rel A) and p50, although other forms such as Rel (c-Rel, p75), Rel B (p68), p52, and p105 (NF-κB1) may also occur. p50 may be constitutively bound to DNA but requires p65 for transactivational activity (115–117).

In unstimulated cells, NF-κB is localized to the cytoplasm because of binding to inhibitory proteins (IκB), of which several isoforms exist (IκB-α IκB-β, IκB-γ, IκB-δ, IκB-ε) , the most abundant being IκB-α. When the cell is appropriately stimulated, specific IκB kinases phosphorylate IκB, leading to the rapid addition of ubiquitin residues (ubiquitination), which make it a substrate for the proteasome, a multifunctional cellular protease (115-117).

A specific IκB-α kinase complex (IKK) has now been identified and contains at least two interacting subunits. Several signal transduction pathways are involved in the activation of NF-κB and enzymes from the mitogen-activated protein (MAP) kinase pathways may interact at various points in the activation of NF-κB (115–118). Degradation of IκB uncovers nuclear localization signals (NLS) on p65 and p50, so it is rapidly transported to the nucleus where it binds to specific κB recognition elements in the regulatory regions of target genes.

The IκB-α gene itself has several κB sequences in its regulatory region, so that NF-κB induces the synthesis of IκB-α, which enters the nucleus to bind NF-κB and induce its export to the cytoplasm, thus terminating activation. Newly synthesized IκB-α interacts with, and binds to, NF-κB heterodimers within the cytoplasm and to NF-κB bound to κB sites within the nucleus (115–117).

NF-κB is known to regulate the expression of many genes involved in inflammatory and immune responses. Genes induced by NF-κB include those for the proinflammatory cytokines IL-1β, TNF-α, and GM-CSF and the chemokines IL-8, macrophage inflammatory protein (MIP)-1α, macrophage chemotactic protein-1 (MCP-1), regulated on activation, normal T-cell expressed and secreted (RANTES) and eotaxins, which attract inflammatory cells into sites of inflammation. NF-κB also plays an important role in regulating expression of adhesion molecules, such as E-selectin, vascular cell adhesion molecule-1 (VCAM-1) and intercellular adhesion molecule- 1(ICAM-1) that are expressed on endothelial and epithelial cells at inflammatory sites and play a key role in the initial recruitment of inflammatory cells. NF-κB also regulates the expression of inflammatory enzymes, including NOS2, that produces large amounts of nitric oxide (NO) and inducible cyclo-oxygenase (COX-2) that produces prostanoids (115–117).

B. Activator Protein-1

Activator protein-1 (AP-1) consists of either Jun oncoprotein homodimers or of Fos/Jun oncoprotein heterodimers, which are members of the basic leucine zipper (bZIP) transcription family, characterized by a basic leucine-rich area involved with dimerization with other transcription factors. AP-1 was originally described by binding to the TPA (tetradecanoylphorbol-13-acetate) response element (TRE; 5′-TGA(C/G)TCA-3′) and responsible for the transcriptional activation of various genes activated by phorbol esters (such as TPA, also known as PMA) via activation of protein kinase C (PKC) (115).

AP-1 is a collection of related transcription factors belonging to the Jun (c-Jun, Jun B, Jun D) and Fos (c-Fos, Fos B, Fra-1, Fra-2) families that dimerize in various combination through their leucine zipper region. Fos/Jun heterodimers bind with the greatest affinity and are the predominant form of AP-1 in most cells, whereas Jun/Jun homodimers bind with a low affinity. AP-1 proteins may also form functionally distinct dimeric complexes with members of the related bZIP family of activating transcription factor (ATF)/CREB transcription factors.

A recently identified transcriptional coactivator designated Jun-activation domain-binding protein 1 (JAB1) potentiates transactivation by either c-Jun or Jun D. AP-1 transcription factor components are subject to regulation by both phosphorylation and chemical oxidation of specific cysteine residues mapping within the DNA binding domains of Fos and Jun (115).

AP-1 may be activated via PKC and by various cytokines, including IL-1β and TNF-α via several types of protein tyrosine kinase (PTK) and MAP kinase, which themselves activate a cascade of intracellular kinases. Both IL-1β and TNF-α activate TNF-associated factors (TRAF), which subsequently activate MAP kinases. Certain signals lead to activation of kinases that phosphorylate c-Jun, resulting in increased activation. There are several specific JNKs and they may play an important role in the regulation of cellular responsiveness to cytokine signals. Other signals rapidly increase the transcription of the Fos gene, resulting in increased synthesis of Fos protein.

Jun phosphatases counteract the activation of AP-1. Oxidation of Fos and Jun can be reversed by a cellular redox/DNA repair protein designated Ref-1 (redox factor 1).

C. CAAT/Enhancer-Binding Proteins

CAAT/enhancer-binding proteins (C/EBP) are factors important in IL-1, IL-6 (also known for this reason as nuclear factor-IL-6), and lipopolysaccharide (LPS)-dependent signal transduction. They bind to a consensus sequence ATTGCGCAAT, which includes the CAAT box. C/EBP binds DNA through a bipartite structural motif. Two protein chains dimerize through a set of amphipathic α helices termed the leucine zipper. Highly basic protein regions emerge from the zipper to form a linked set of DNA contact surfaces. C/EBP appears to function exclusively in terminally differentiated, growth-arrested cells. These transcription factors are members of the bZIP class of transcription factors and include C/EBPα, C/EBPβ, C/EBPγ, C/EBPδ, C/EBPϵ all of which exhibit similar DNA-binding specificities and affinities compared with C/EBPα. C/EBPβ and C/EBPδ readily form heterodimers with each other as well as with C/EBPα. These transcription factors are activated by pathways that involve PKC and regulate the expression of several inflammatory and immune genes (115). They often cooperate positively with other transcription factors, particularly other bZIP proteins, such as AP-1, but also with NF-κB. Thus, in the regulation of IL-8 gene expression, there is a marked enhancement of transcription when C/EBPβ is activated together with NF-κB, whereas C/EBPβ activation alone has little effect.

Splice isoforms of these transcription factors, which appear to have blocking effects on transcription, have been identified.

D. GATA

The GATA family of transcription factors includes a family of zinc finger domain-containing proteins with six members (GATA1–6) that share a common DNA-binding motif (A/T) GATA (A/G). Differential gene regulation by the GATA family appears to be controlled in part by expression of specific GATA proteins in different cell types and in part by interaction (cross-talk) with other transcription factors. GATA-1 and GATA-2 proteins play a key role in the regulation of hematopoiesis. GATA-3 is important in stimulating the expression of a number of Th2 cell-specific cytokines such as IL-4, IL-5, and IL-13 and in inhibiting the Th1 cytokine IFN-γ. Increased expression of the transcription factor GATA-3 in peripheral venous blood T lymphocytes isolated from asthmatic subjects compared to normals has been recently described (119). GATA-6, independently or cooperatively with thyroid transcription factor-1 (TTF-1), enhances murine surfactant protein (SP)-A transcription.

The transcription factors GATA-3, -4, and- 6 are expressed in bronchial epithelial cells, and expression is similar in asthmatic and normal subjects (119).

IV. Role of Transcription Factors in the Pathogenesis of Bronchial Asthma

A. Transcription Factors May Modulate the Severity of Airway Inflammation in Asthma

Activation of NF-κB leads to the coordinated induction of multiple genes (including cytokines, chemokines, receptors, and adhesion molecules) that are expressed in inflammatory and immune responses (115–117). Many of these genes are induced in inflammatory and structural cells and play an important role in the inflammatory process. Although NF-κB is not the only transcription factor involved in regulation of the expression of these genes, it often appears to have a decisive regulatory role. NF-κB often functions in cooperation with other transcription factors, such as AP-1 and C/EBP families.

NF-κB is activated by many of the stimuli that exacerbate asthmatic inflammation (e.g., allergen exposure, proinflammatory cytokines, oxidants, infections). Indeed, there is evidence of increased activation of NF-κB in bronchial epithelial cells in asthma (120). The role of NF-κB should be seen as an amplifying and perpetuating mechanism that exaggerates the disease-specific inflammatory process through the coordinated activation of multiple inflammatory genes.

AP-1 may be activated by various inflammatory mediators, including TNF-α and IL-1β, acting via intracellular kinase cascades (118). AP-1, like NF-κB regulates many genes of the inflammatory and immune responses that are overexpressed in asthma. Indeed many of these genes require the simultaneous activation of both transcription factors that work together cooperatively. There is evidence for increased expression of c-Fos in bronchial epithelial cells in asthmatic airways (121).

The role of C/EBP in asthma has not yet been defined, but it is likely that activation of this transcription factor by inflammatory signals is an important amplifying mechanism for the expression of inflammatory genes, such as NOS2, Cox-2, and certain chemokines (such as IL-8), which have C/EBP recognition sequences in their gene-regulatory regions. Many of the effects of IL-6 are mediated through activation of C/EBP. An interesting finding is that IL-6 is produced in increased amounts from macrophages of asthmatic patients (122) and release is further enhanced by allergen exposure via low-affinity immunoglobulin (Ig)E receptors (FcεRII) (123).

B. Transcription Factors May Modulate the Differentiation of Th1/Th2 Lymphocytes

Recent data have suggested the involvement of many families of transcription factors in the molecular mechanisms by which Th1 and Th2 cells differentially express the Th1 and Th2 cytokine genes (114). In the differentiation of helper T cells, a change in the configuration of chromatin is postulated to cause the accessibility of specific transcription factors, leading to the preferential production of specific cytokines. Naive T cells display repressed, transcriptionally incompetent chromatin structure over the IFN-γ and IL-4/IL-5/IL-13 genes that is likely to account for their low levels of transcription. A model proposes that differentiation signals derived from primary contact with antigen and polarizing cytokines elicit subset-specific remodeling of genes encoding cytokines and other effector proteins, which is necessary for mature effector function in the differentiated Th1/Th2 cells (124). For instance, the remodeling of the IL-4, IL-5, and IL-13 Th2-cytokine genes requires both STAT6 and stimulation through the T-cell antigen receptor (124). Antigen-induced transcription factors, such as nuclear factor of activated T cells (NFATs), AP-1, and NF-κB, together with STAT6 proteins may initiate Th2-cytokine gene remodeling. Their activation is rapidly terminated in the absence of continued antigenic stimulation (124). Thus STAT6 activation alone is unlikely to be involved in maintaining a transcriptionally active Th2-cytokine gene locus in the differentiated Th2 cells, as shown in stable asthmatics in vivo (125). Stimulation with antigen and Th2-cytokines (such as IL-4 and IL-13) must instead activate a differentiation-specific genetic program that results in the stable induction of transcription factors expressed selectively in the appropriate Th2-cell subset (124). These Th2-cell subset-selective transcription factors are presumed to bind to a specific DNA regulatory sequence, thereby recruiting histone acetyltransferases and chromatin-remodeling enzymes to the appropriate genetic loci. The resulting accessible chromatin configurations are stably inherited and persist in differentiated cells in the absence of active transcription, a molecular mechanism that may underlie T-cell memory (124). For example, for the differentiation of the Th2 cells and the stable transcription of the IL-4/IL-5/IL-13 genes, the concomitant activation of many families of Th2-specific transcription factors such as GATA-3 (119) and c-Maf (126) appears to be important.

V. Respiratory Viruses and Transcription Factors

Several studies have shown that the cells involved in respiratory virus-induced airway inflammation modify their gene regulatory program after virus infection. On the other hand, both the promoter genomic regions and the related transcription factors that regulate inflammatory mediator production are deeply affected by respiratory virus infection. Most of the data published to date on this issue are mainly related to rhinovirus and respiratory syncytial virus infections. More research is required to clarify the molecular events that determine the changes in gene transcription determined by virus infection in target cells.

A. Rhinovirus

To date, the specific molecular mechanisms involved in the production of proinflammatory mediators by bronchial/lung cells after rhinovirus infection are still not fully characterized. However, some studies have examined at the molecular level the transcription factors involved in RV-induced stimulation of proinflammatory cytokines, chemokines, and adhesion molecules from structural cells of the lungs.

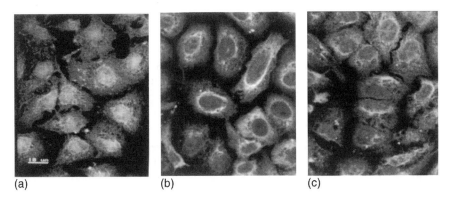

(a)   (b)   (c)

Figure 1   Rhinovirus infection induces NF-κB activation in A549 respiratory epithelial cells. Immunocytochemical staining of A549 cells using an antibody specific for activated protein p65 (major subunit of NF-κB) conjugated to a fluorochrome. NF-κB activation is minimal in uninfected A549 cells (a). Rhinovirus infection for 60 minutes causes cytoplasmic p65 activation (b). After 180 minutes of rhinovirus infection, p65 activation is reduced (c).

It has been recently suggested that early activation of mitogen-activated protein kinase (MAP)p38 kinase by RV infection is a key event in the regulation of RV-induced cytokine transcription, and may provide a new target for inhibition of symptoms and airway inflammation associated with rhinovirus infection (127). Indeed, RV infection of BEAS-2B cells resulted in increased synthesis of cytokines (IL-1, IL-6, G-CSF, and GM-CSF) and CXC chemokines (IL-8, epithelial neutrophil-activating protein-78, and growth-related oncogene-alpha) 24–72 h postinfection (127). RV infection also induced a time- and dose-dependent increase in tyrosine phosphorylation of p38 kinase, which peaked 30 min postinfection and remained elevated for 1 h (127). Treatment of infected cells with SB 239063, a potent inhibitor of p38 kinase, completely inhibited chemokine and cytokine increases. Several transcription factors appear to be activated after rhinovirus infection on a variety of respiratory cells. These proteins include NF-κB (Fig. 1), AP-1, and GATA families.

NF-κB

RV is a potent stimulator of interleukin (IL) -6 and IL-8 production in vitro in human fetal lung fibroblasts and A549 alveolar epithelial type II-like cells. This effect occurs rapidly and is associated with significant increases in IL-6 and IL-8 messenger RNA (mRNA) accumulation and gene transcription (31,36).

RV is also a potent stimulator of IL-6 and IL-8 gene promoter-driven luciferase activity. In the case of IL-6, stimulation is modestly decreased by mutation of the C/EBP binding site while it is abrogated by mutation of the NF-κB binding site in the IL-6 gene promoter (36). RV infection rapidly induces NF-κB-DNA-binding activation, mediated by p65, p50, and p52 NF-κB subunits(36).

In contrast, RV-stimulated IL-8 promoter activation is significantly decreased by mutation of the C/EBP-binding site and abrogated by mutation of the NF-κB-binding site in the IL-8 gene promoter (31). Recent studies conducted on human bronchial epithelial cells have shown, in contrast, that treatment with sulfasalazine and calpain inhibitor I, inhibitors of NF-κB activation, blocks RV-induced formation of NF-κB complexes with oligonucleotides from the promoter of both cytokines, but it does not inhibit mRNA induction for either IL-6 and IL-8 (128).

Binding sites for several transcription factors, including NF-κB, have been identified in the proximal promoter region upstream of the transcription start point in the human factor GM-CSF gene (115).

RV induces the production of GM-CSF in human bronchial epithelial cells (60). Maximal levels of mRNA for GM-CSF were seen 1 h after RV infection. mRNA production is sustained through 24 h and declines by 48 h (60). GM-CSF protein is detectable in cell supernatants by 2 h after infection and reaches maximal concentrations by 24 h, with the most rapid rate of production occurring from 2 to 7 h (60). Treatment with sulfasalazine blocks RV-16-induced formation of NF-κB complexes with oligonucleotides from GM-CSF promoter, and clearly inhibits RV-16 induction of GM-CSF mRNA in the same cells (128).

RV is a potent stimulator of its own receptor ICAM-1 both in A549 cells and in primary human bronchial epithelial cells in vitro (66). This effect is associated with significant increases in ICAM-1 mRNA accumulation and gene transcription (66). RV stimulates ICAM-1 gene promoter activity in a pathway that is critically dependent upon upregulation of NF-κB proteins binding to the -187/-178 NF-κB-binding site on the ICAM-1 gene promoter (66). The protein p65, arranged as homo- or heterodimers, is the principal component of the RV-induced NF-κB binding to the ICAM-1 promoter (Fig. 2) (66).

GATA Proteins

RV also induces VCAM-1 surface expression in A549 cells, 16HBE cells, and normal human bronchial epithelial cells in vitro. This effect is associated with VCAM-1 mRNA accumulation and increased VCAM-1 mRNA transcription (67). RV is also a potent stimulator of VCAM-1 gene promoter, which relies on upregulation of GATA proteins binding to the -254/-251 and -239/-236 GATA binding sites and of NF-κB proteins binding to the -72/-63 and -57/-48 NF-κB-binding sites in the VCAM-1 gene promoter (67).

B. Respiratory Syncytial Virus

RSV-induced cytokine production in airway epithelial cells seems to play an important role in the pathogenesis of RSV respiratory tract infections. Recent studies on RSV–epithelial cell interactions have demonstrated that RSV can act at the molecular level by altering cytokine gene transcription (129–132) or mRNA stability (133).

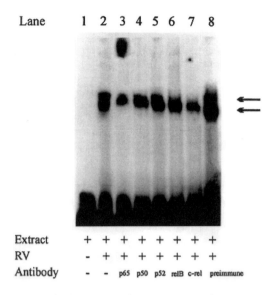

Figure 2 Identification of p65 as the major component of NF-κB proteins binding to -199/-170 ICAM-1 probe after rhinovirus infection of A549 respiratory epithelial cells. Nuclear lysates prepared from 30 min uninfected (lane 1) or rhinovirus 16-infected (lanes 2–8) A549 cells were incubated with radiolabeled -199/-170 ICAM-1 probe in the absence (lanes 1 and 2) or in the presence of antibodies against NF-κB family proteins p65 (lane), p50 (lane 4), p52 (lane 5), Rel-B (lane 6), C-Rel (lane 7), or preimmune serum (lane 8). Only in lane 3 (antibody to p65) was there a clear supershift of both binding complexes associated with a marked reduction in binding at both original sites (arrows), indicating that p65 was a major component of both binding complexes. (Reprinted with permission from Ref. 66.)

Apoptosis

Apoptosis is considered to be a highly efficient defense mechanism against invading viruses, allowing the infected host to dispose of viral proteins and nucleic acids without inducing an inflammatory response. It is therefore not surprising that some viruses have elaborate strategies to evade apoptotic destruction (134).

Despite RSV-infected airway epithelial cells showing an increased expression of apoptosis-associated genes (e.g., interferon regulatory factor 1, interleukin-1β-converting enzyme, and caspase 3) they do not show features typical of apoptosis (135).

After RSV infection, airway epithelial cells also increase their expression of the antiapoptosis gene IEX-1L and this seems to be associated with protection from apoptosis induced by TNF-α (135). Although the 11 RSV proteins do not share homology with any known human proteins involved in apoptotic signaling, they may participate in the *trans* activation of the IEX-1L gene (either directly or indirectly), because active RSV replication is required for IEX-1L gene upregulation. IEX-1L is an apoptosis inhibitor involved in NF-κB-mediated cell survival (136).

RSV-infected airway epithelial cells are a major source of chemokines, and leukocyte recruitment to infected airways epithelium is necessary for RSV clearance from the airways. RSV-infected airway epithelial cells protected from apoptosis may continue to elaborate proinflammatory chemokines, with continued recruitment of cytotoxic virucidal leukocytes thereby facilitating the host response to RSV and its elimination (134).

RSV-infected PBMCs and monocytes isolated from cord blood and adults are protected from apoptosis (137,138). However, the mechanism of protection in this context is unknown.

NF-κB

Interleukin-I, Interleukin-6

RSV-infection of A549 cells results in IL-1 and IL-6 release, and is associated with a net increase in steady-state levels of their mRNA (139). The NF-κB-binding sites in IL-1α, IL-6, and IL-8 promoters are required for RSV-mediated induction of transcription of these promoters (139). Sodium salicylate and aspirin, inhibitors of NF-κB activation, abolished transcriptional induction of all these cytokines by RSV (139).

Interleukin-8

The effects of conditioned medium (CM) from RSV-infected monocytes (RSV-CM) on A549 cell chemokine release have also recently been analyzed (140). RSV-CM stimulates IL-8 secretion from A549 cells within 2 h, and secretion increased over 72 h without affecting cell viability (140). RSV-CM induces degradation of IκBα within 5 min but does not affect IκBβ. RSV-CM activates transient nuclear binding of NF-κB within 1 h, while activation of NF-IL6 is delayed until 8 h but was still detectable at 24 h (140). Promoter-reporter analysis demonstrates that NF-κB binding is the essential transcription factor for IL-8 promoter activity in RSV-CM-activated cells (140). Blocking experiments have revealed that the effects of RSV-CM depend on monocyte-derived IL-1 and that TNF-α is not involved in this network (140). RSV infection of A549 cells produces IκBα proteolysis through a mechanism primarily independent of the proteasome pathway (132).

Interleukin-11

RSV-induced stimulation of IL-11 production by human airway smooth muscle cells is matched by proportionate changes in IL-11 mRNA accumulation (113). RSV infection of A549 cells likewise results in IL-11 induction and a net increase in steady-state level of IL-11 mRNA (139). Nuclear run-on assays show a direct effect of RSV on IL-11 gene transcription (139). Mutational analysis of IL-11 promoter demonstrated the need for two NF-κB-binding regions for RSV-mediated induction of IL-11 promoter activity (139).

ICAM-1

ICAM-1 surface expression is significantly upregulated up to 72 h after RSV infection (141). Cytokine priming with TFN-α, IFN-γ or IL-1α/β induces an enhanced ICAM-1 expression on noninfected as well as on RSV-infected epithelial cells (141).

In contrast, cytokine priming with IL-3, IL-6, GM-CSF, or G-CSF did not lead to a significant increase of ICAM-1 expression on either RSV-infected or noninfected A549 cells up to 72 h of culture time (141). ICAM-1 promoter activation following RSV infection is abolished by site-specific mutation of the NF-κB- or C/EBP- binding sites, suggesting a critical role of the activation of NF-κB and C/EBP in RSV-induced ICAM-1 expression by A549 cells (142).

AP-1

RSV infection of A549 cells results in increased IL-8 gene expression and increased DNA binding of the transcription factors AP-1, NF-κB, and C/EBP. Mutation of the C/EBP DNA-binding site in the regulatory region of the IL-8 gene had minimal effect in the presence of intact binding sites for NF-κB and AP-1. This suggests that AP-1 may be the preferred transcription factor (over C/EBP) for cooperative interaction with NF-κB in RSV-induced IL-8 production (130).

C. Interferon Regulatory Factor

Chemokines (RANTES and MIP-1α)

Although the molecular mechanism(s) by which RANTES and MIP-1α are upregulated following RSV-infection is still under investigation, preliminary studies suggest that they are upregulated via distinct signaling pathways (106).

NF-κB nuclear translocation seems to be a critical step in RSV induction of RANTES secretion from human bronchial epithelial cells (143). The mechanism of RSV-induced RANTES promoter activation in A549 cells has been recently analyzed. Indeed, promoter deletion and mutagenesis experiments indicate that RSV requires the presence of five different *cis* regulatory elements, located in the promoter fragment spanning from −220 to +55 nucleotides, corresponding to NF-κB, C/EBP, Jun/CREB/ATF, and interferon regulatory factor (IRF) binding sites. Although mutations of the NF-κB, C/EBP, and CREB/AP-1-like sites reduce RSV-induced RANTES gene transcription to 50% or less, only mutations affecting IRF binding completely abolish RANTES inducibility (144,145).

The role of reactive oxygen species in RSV-upregulated RANTES gene expression has also been studied in A549 cells (146). The results indicate that RSV infection rapidly induces production of reactive oxygen species, prior to RANTES expression, as measured by oxidation of $2'$, $7'$-dichlorofluorescein (146). Pretreatment of A549 cells with the antioxidant butylated hydroxyanisol (BHA), as well a panel of chemically unrelated antioxidants, blocks RSV-induced RANTES gene expression and protein secretion (146). This effect is mediated through the ability of BHA to inhibit RSV-induced IRF binding to the RANTES promoter interferon-stimulated responsive element, which is critical for inducible RANTES promoter activation. BHA inhibits de novo IRF-1 and -7 gene expression and protein synthesis, and IRF-3 nuclear translocation (146). Together, these data indicate that a redox-sensitive pathway is involved in RSV-induced IRF activation, an event necessary for RANTES gene expression (146).

However, other findings suggest that the increase in RANTES gene transcription is not sufficient for inducible expression and that critical regulatory effects occur at a posttranscriptional level through increased stability of RANTES mRNA (133).

NOS

RSV enhances NOS2 mRNA expression in A549 cells as early as 4 h after RSV infection and this enhancement lasts for several hours. The NOS2 mRNA expression in RSV-infected cells is significantly enhanced also by an exogenous cytokine mixture (IL-1β, TNF-α, and IFN-γ) (86); however, nitric oxide production can be identified only when cytokines are added together with RSV infection (86). RSV infection seems to induces the iNOS gene via the transcription factor IRF-1 (86).

D. Other Viruses and Atypical Bacteria

Influenza A viruses are capable of inducing in airway epithelial cells the expression of a variety of cytokine and proapoptotic genes in infected cells (147). The influenza virus hemagglutinin (HA), matrix protein (M), and nucleoprotein (NP) may act as transcription factors and activate the HIV-1 promoter (147). This process is mediated by oxidants since antioxidants abolish the transactivating ability (147). Expression of different influenza proteins induces activation of NF-κB-dependent gene expression but not transcriptional activation of an AP-1/Ets-dependent promoter, indicating a selectivity for NF-κB transactivation (147). Furthermore, influenza protein expression induces activation of IKK, which is important for the activation of NF-κB (147).

Infection of human monocytes with *influenza A* virus induces a broad range of proinflammatory cytokines and mononuclear cell attracting chemokines before the infected cells undergo apoptosis (148). The underlying mechanisms by which the corresponding genes are transcriptionally initiated after influenza A virus infection are still poorly understood (148). Activation of NF-κB seems to play an important role in the regulation of many proinflammatory cytokine genes, but this cannot be the only mechanism, since several cytokine genes lack NF-κB-binding sites in their promoter regions. In addition, cell-type-specific differential response has been identified: CREB, CCAAT-binding transcription factor/nuclear factor-1 (CTF/NF-1), and NF-κB genes are strongly induced 1–4 h after *influenza A* virus infection in the monocytic cell line Mono Mac 6. In freshly prepared human monocytes no significant change is detectable (148). In infected monocytes, which die by apoptosis, the expression of CREB and CTF is suppressed 8 h after infection (148). This suggests that the long-term regulation of transcription factor gene expression in nonproliferating cells is of minor importance after influenza infection, since in apoptosis-prone cells an immediate availability of transcription factor proteins is required (148).

The activation of transcription factors as a consequence of latent respiratory virus infection has been recently suggested as a possible mechanism for the development of airflow limitation in chronic obstructive pulmonary disease (COPD). Indeed, the inflammatory changes and protease imbalance that occur in patients with COPD are also seen in cigarette smokers without COPD, but to a lesser extent (149). This observation suggests that the accelerated decline in lung function, typical of COPD, may be due to amplification of the normal pulmonary response to irritants, either because of increased production of inflammatory proteins and enzymes or because of defective endogenous anti-inflammatory or antiprotease mechanisms (149). These differences might be explained by polymorphisms in the genes encoding cytokines, proteases, anti-inflammatory proteins, and antiproteases. Another hypothesis is that these differences are due to latent viral infection. The latent adenovirus sequence E1A is more commonly detected in the lungs of patients with COPD than in matched control smokers (150). Transfection of E1A into A549 cells results in increased activation of the transcription factor NF-κB, with consequent increased release of IL-8 in response to LPS and increased expression of ICAM-1, providing a molecular mechanism for the amplification during the inflammatory response (151). In guinea pigs sensitized and challenged with ovalbumin (OA), latent adenoviral infection increased CD8+ cells in the airway wall and CD8+ cells, macrophages, B cells, and CD4+ cells in the lung parenchyma (152). In the presence of both latent adenoviral infection and OA challenge, steroid treatment had no effect on allergen-induced eosinophilia but reduced CD8(+) cells in the airways and CD8(+) cells, CD4(+) cells, and B cells in the parenchyma. These data suggest that the presence of latent adenoviral infection causes OA-induced eosinophilic airway inflammation to become steroid resistant (152).

Besides macrophages and lymphocytes, *Chlamydia pneumoniae* preferentially infects airway epithelial cells. The molecular activation of airway epithelial cells by *Chlamydia pneumoniae* has been recently studied in detail in primary human tracheobronchial epithelial cells (HTBEC) and in the bronchial epithelial cell line BEAS-2B (153). A time-dependent enhanced release of IL-8 and prostaglandin-E (2) and an increased expression of epithelial ICAM-1, followed by subsequent transepithelial migration of neutrophils, have been demonstrated (153). The transepithelial neutrophil migration can be blocked by an anti-ICAM-1 monoclonal antibody (MAb) but not by MAbs against IL-8 (153). In addition, there is an enhanced *C. pneumoniae*-mediated activation of NF-κB within 30–60 min in HTBEC and BEAS-2B, which is followed by increases in mRNA synthesis of IL-8, ICAM-1, and cyclooxygenase-2, with maximal effects occurring 2 h after infection (153). *Chlamydia pneumoniae* infection induces the transcription factors AP-1, NF-IL6, NF-κB, and the glucocorticoid receptor (GR) in human lung epithelial cell lines (HL and Calu3) (154). In vitro infection with *Chlamydia pneumoniae* activates the host's GR, with a kinetic of the cytosol–nucleus translocation of the GR that occurs between 3 and 6 h after infection (154). However, the two epithelial cell lines shows a specific kinetic for GR activation. Functionality of the activated GR was proven by results of luciferase reporter assay (154).

Mycoplasmas are potent macrophage stimulators. The active principles are lipopeptides or lipoproteins with a characteristic N-terminal S-[dihydroxypropyl]-cysteinyl group bearing two ester-bound fatty acids and lacking the amide-bound one common to other bacterial lipoproteins (155). By using synthetic analogs of mycoplasmal lipopeptides, the activation of transcription factor NF-κB has been investigated in the C3H/HeJ mouse-derived DMBM-3 macrophage cell line. Activation of NF-κB by mycoplasmal lipopeptides occurs distinctly earlier than TNF-α liberation, excluding autocrine stimulation by TNF-α (155). As determined by supershift assay, the active NF-κB complex that forms after mycoplasma stimulation consists of the heterodimer p50/p65 (155).

VI. Conclusions

Many studies conducted in the last decade have produced an enormous amount of data on the immunopathogenesis of natural and experimental respiratory virus infections in humans. Most of the studies have been conducted on respiratory epithelial cells, which can be directly infected by respiratory viruses. Respiratory virus infection determines the production of several proinflammatory molecules (such as cytokines, chemokines, and adhesion molecules). Virus repression of anti-inflammatory cytokines and virus activation of neurogenic inflammation are also emerging fields of investigation. Conversely, few studies have been conducted on the molecular mechanisms underlying the proinflammatory derangement induced by respiratory viruses in the airways. Collectively the results of these studies suggest a critical role for several transcription factor families, including the NF-κB, AP-1, and GATA families, in the production of proinflammatory mediators after respiratory virus infection. The relative importance of each transcription factor will be certainly greatly clarified in the next few years, with the growing availability of specific inhibitors such as respirable antisense oligonucleotide (156) capable of blocking activation of a specific transcription factor. Clearly this is an exciting new area of research with promising therapeutic potential. Recent evidence using a specific JNK/AP-1 inhibitor, SP600725, in a mouse model of rheumatoid arthritis exemplifies the potential for these new drugs (156).

Acknowledgments

This work was supported by Associazione per la Ricerca e la Cura dell'Asma (ARCA, Padua, Italy) and by a research grant from GlaxoSmithKline,Verona, Italy.

References

1. Greve JM, Davis G, Meyer AM, Forte CP, Yost SC, Marlor CW, Kamarck ME, McClelland A. The major human rhinovirus receptor is ICAM-1. Cell 1989; 56:839–847.
2. Grunert HP, Wolf KU, Langner KD, et al. Internalization of human rhinovirus 14 into hela and ICAM-1 transfected BHK cells. Med Microbiol Immunol 1997; 186:1–9.
3. Piela-Smith TH, Aneiro L, Korn JH. Binding of human rhinovirus and T cells to intercellular adhesion molecule-1 on human fibroblasts. Discordance between effects of IL-1 and IFN-gamma. J Immunol 1991; 147:1831–1836.
4. Staunton DE, Merluzzi VJ, Rothlein R, Barton R, Marlin SD, Springer TA. A cell

adhesion molecule, ICAM-1, is the major surface receptor for rhinoviruses. Cell 1989; 56:849–853.

5. Staunton DE, Dustin ML, Erickson HP, Springer TA. The arrangement of the immunoglobulin-like domains of ICAM-1 and the binding sites for LFA-1 and rhinovirus. Cell 1990; 61:243–254.

6. Tomassini JE, Graham D, DeWitt CM, Lineberger DW, Rodkey JA, Colonno RJ. cDNA cloning reveals that the major group rhinovirus receptor on HeLa cells is intercellular adhesion molecule 1. Proc Natl Acad Sci USA 1989; 86:4907–4911.

7. Hofer F, Gruenberger M, Kowalski H, Machat H, Huettinger M, Kuechler E, Blaas D. Members of the low density lipoprotein receptor family mediate cell entry of a minor-group common cold virus. Proc Natl Acad Sci USA 1994; 91:1839–1842.

8. Levandowski RA, Ou DW, Jackson GG. Acute-phase decrease of T lymphocyte subsets in rhinovirus infection. J Infect Dis 1986; 153:743–748.

9. Parry DE, Busse WW, Sukow KA, Dick CR, Swenson C, Gern JE. Rhinovirus-induced PBMC responses and outcome of experimental infection in allergic subjects. J Allergy Clin Immunol 2000; 105:692–698.

10. Bardin PG, Johnston SL, Sanderson G, Robinson S, Pickett MA, Fraenkel DJ, Holgate ST. Detection of rhinovirus infection of the nasal mucosa by oligonucleotide in situ hybridization. Am J Respir Cell Mol Biol 1994; 10:2907–2913.

11. Bruce C, Chadwick P, al-Nakib W. Detection of rhinovirus RNA in nasal epithelial cells by in situ hybridization. J Virol Methods 1990; 30:115–125.

12. Arruda E, Boyle TR, Winther B, Pevear DC, Gwaltney JM Jr, Hayden FG. Localization of human rhinovirus replication in the upper respiratory tract by in situ hybridization. J Infect Dis 1995; 171:1329–1333.

13. Turner RB, Hendley JO, Gwaltney JM Jr. Shedding of infected epithelial cells in rhinovirus colds. J Infect Dis 1982; 145:849-853.

14. Turner RB, Winther B, Hendley JO, Mygind N, Gwaltney JM Jr. Sites of virus recovery and antigen detection in epithelial cells during experimental rhinovirus infection. Acta Otolaryngol 1984; (Suppl 413):9–14.

15. Winther B, Gwaltney JM Jr, Mygind N, Turner RB, Hendley JO. Sites of rhinovirus recovery after point inoculation of the upper airway. JAMA 1986; 256:1763–1767.

16. Fraenkel DJ, Bardin PG, Sanderson G, Lampe F, Johnston SL, Holgate ST. Immunohistochemical analysis of nasal biopsies during rhinovirus experimental colds. Am J Respir Crit Care Med 1994; 150:1130–1136.

17. Winther B, Brofeldt S, Christensen B, Mygind N. Light and scanning electron microscopy of nasal biopsy material from patients with naturally acquired common colds. Acta Otolaryngol(Stockholm) 1984; 97:309–318.

18. Winther B, Farr B, Turner RB, Hendley JO, Gwaltney JM, Mygind N. Histopathologic examination and enumeration of polymorphonuclear leukocytes in the nasal mucosa during experimental rhinovirus colds. Acta Otolaryngol(Stockholm) 1984; suppl 413: 19–24.

19. Subauste MC, Jacoby DB, Richards SM, Proud D. Infetion of a human respiratory epithelial cell line with rhinovirus. Induction of cytokine release and modulation of susceptibility to infection by cytokine exposure. J Clin Invest 1995; 96:549–557.

20. Winther B, Gwaltney JM, Hendley JO. Respiratory virus infection of monolayer cultures of human nasal epithelial cells. Am Rev Respir Dis 1990; 141:839–845.

21. Papadopoulos NG, Bates PJ, Bardin PG, Papi A, Leir SH, Fraenkel DJ, Meyer J, Lackie

PM, Sanderson G, Holgate ST, Johnston SL. Rhinovirus infect the lower airways. J Infect Dis 2000; 181:1875–1884.

22. Naclerio RM, Proud D, Lichtenstein LM, Kagey-Sobotka A, Hendley JO, Sorrentino J, Gwaltney JM. Kinins are generated during experimental rhinovirus colds. J Infect Dis 1987; 157:133–142.

23. Proud D, Naclerio RM, Gwaltney JM Jr, Hendley JO. Kinins are generated in nasal secretions during natural rhinovirus colds. J Infect Dis 1990; 161:120–123.

24. Proud D, Gwaltney JM Jr, Hendley JO, Dinarello CA, Gillis S, Schleimer RP. Increased levels of interleukin-1 are detected in nasal secretions of volunteers during experimental rhinovirus colds. J Infect Dis 1994; 169:1007–1013.

25. Gern JE, Vrtis R, Grindle KA, Swenson C, Busse WW. Relationship of upper and lower airway cytokines to outcome of experimental rhinovirus infection. Am J Respir Crit Care Med 2000; 162:2226–2231.

26. Einarsson O, Geba GP, Zhu Z, Landry M, Elias JA. Interleukin-11: stimulation in vivo and in vitro by respiratory viruses and induction of airways hyperresponsiveness. J Clin Invest 1996; 97:915–924.

27. Linden M, Greiff L, Andersson M, et al. Nasal cytokines in common cold and allergic rhinitis. Clin Exp Allergy 1995; 25:166-172.

28. Jarjour NN, Gern JE, Kelly EAB, Swenson CA, Dick CR, Busse WW. The effect of an experimental rhinovirus 16 infection on bronchial lavage neutrophils. J Allergy Clin Immunol 2000; 105:1169–1177.

29. Roseler S, Holtappels G, Wagenmann M, Bachert C. Elevated levels of interleukins IL-1β, IL-6 and IL-8 in naturally acquired viral rhinitis. Eur Arch Otorhinolaryngol 1995; (suppl 252):S61-S66.

30. Teran LM, Johnston SL, Schroder JM, Church MK, Holgate ST. Role of nasal interleukin-8 in neutrophil recruitment and activation in children with virus-induced asthma. Am J Respir Crit Care Med 1997; 155:1362–1366.

31. Zhu Z, Tang W, Gwaltney JM Jr, Wu Y, Elias JA. Rhinovirus stimulation of interleukin-8 in vivo and in vitro: role of NF-κB. Am J Physiol 1997; 273:L814-L824.

32. Yoon HJ, Zhu Z, Gwaltney JM Jr, Elias JA. Rhinovirus regulation of IL-1 receptor antagonist in vivo and in vitro: a potential mechanism of symptom resolution. J Immunol 1999; 162:7461–7469.

33. Papadopoulos NG, Papi A, Meyer J, Stanciu LA, Salvi S, Holgate ST, Johnston SL. Rhinovirus infection up-regulates eotaxin and eotaxin-2 expression in bronchial epithelial cells. Clin Exp Allergy 2001; 31:1060–1066.

34. Teran LM, Seminario MC, Shute JK, Papi A, Compton SJ, Low L, Gleich GJ, Johnston SL. RANTES, macrophage inhibitory protein 1, and the eosinophil product major basic protein are released into upper respiratory secretions during virus-induced asthma exacerbations in children. J Infect Dis 1999; 179:677–681.

35. Turner RB, Weingand KW, Yeh CH, Leedy D. Association between nasal secretion interleukin-8 concentration and symptom severity in experimental rhinovirus colds. Clin Infect Dis 1998; 26:840–846.

36. Zhu Z, Tang W, Wu Y, Einarsson O, Landry ML, Gwaltney JM Jr, Elias JA. Rhinovirus stimulation of interleukin-6 in vivo and in vitro: evidence for nuclear factor kappa B-dependent transcriptional activation. J Clin Invest 1996; 97:421–430.

37. Douglass JA, Dhami D, Gurr CE, Bulpitt M, Shute JK, Howarth PH, Lindley IJ, Church MK, Holgate ST. Influence of interleukin-8 challenge in the nasal mucosa in atopic and nonatopic subjects. Am J Respir Crit Care Med 1994; 150:1108–1113.

38. Corne JM, Lau L, Scott SJ, Davies R, Johnston SL, Howarth PH. The relationship

between atopic status and IL-10 nasal lavage levels in the acute and persistent inflammatory response to upper respiratory tract infection. Am J Respir Crit Care Med 2001; 163:1101–1107.

39. Barnes PJ, Chung KF, Page CO. Inflammatory mediators of asthma: an update. Pharmacol Rev 1998; 50:515–596.
40. Barnes PJ, Lim S. Inhibitory cytokines in asthma. Mol Med Today 1998; 4:452–458.
41. Chung KF, Barnes PJ. Cytokines in asthma. Thorax 1999; 54:825–857.
42. Corne JM, Holgate ST. Mechanisms of virus induced exacerbations of asthma. Thorax 1997; 52:380–389.
43. Papadopoulos NG, Sanderson G, Hunter J, Johnston SL. Rhinoviruses replicate effectively at lower airway temperatures. J Med Virol 1999; 58:100–104.
44. Mosser AG, Brockman-Schneider R, Amineva S, Burchell L, Sedgwick JB, Busse WW, Gern JE. Similar frequency of rhinovirus-infectible cells in upper and lower airway epithelium. J Infect Dis 2002; 185:734–743.
45. Pizzichini MM, Pizzichini E, Efthimidias A, Chauhan AJ, Johnston SL, Hussack P, Mahony J, Dolovich J, Hargreave F. Asthma and natural colds. Inflammatory indices in induced sputum: a feasibility study. Am J Respir Crit Care Med 1998; 158:1178-1184.
46. Grunberg K, Smits HH, Timmers MC, et al. Experimental rhinovirus 16 infection: effects on cell differentials and soluble markers in sputum of asthmatic subjects. Am J Respir Crit Care Med 1997; 156:609–616.
47. Grunberg K, Timmers MC, Smits HH, De Klerk EPA, Dick EC, Spaan WJM, Hiemstra PS, Sterk PJ. Effect of experimental rhinovirus 16 colds on airways hyperresponsiveness to histamine and interleukin-8 in nasal lavage in asthmatic subjects in vivo. Clin Exp Allergy 1997; 27:36–45.
48. Grunberg K, Kuijpers EAP, De Klerk EPA, et al. Effects of experimental rhinovirus 16 (RV16) infection on airway hyperresponsiveness to bradykinin in asthmatic subjects in vivo. Am J Respir Crit Care Med 1997; 155:833–838.
49. Grunberg K, Sharon RF, Hiltermann TJN, Brahim JJ, Dick EC, Sterk PJ, van Krieken HJM. Experimental rhinovirus 16 infection increases intercellular adhesion molecule-1 expression in bronchial epithelium of asthmatics regardless of inhaled steroid treatment. Clin Exp Allergy 2000; 30:1015–1023.
50. de Gouw HWFM, Grunberg K, Schot R, Kroes AC, Dick EC, Sterk PJ. Relationship between exhaled nitric oxide and airway hyperresponsiveness following experimental rhinovirus infection in asthmatic subjects. Eur Respir J 1998; 11:126–132.
51. Calhoun WJ, Swenson CA, Dick EC, Schwartz LB, Lemanske RF Jr, Busse WW. Experimental rhinovirus 16 infection potentiates histamine release after antigen bronchoprovocation in allergic subjects. Am Rev Respir Dis 1991; 144:1267–1273.
52. Calhoun WJ, Dick EC, Schwartz LB, Busse WW. A common cold virus, rhinovirus 16, potentiates airway inflammation after segmental antigen bronchoprovocation in allergic subjects. J Clin Invest 1994; 94:2200–2208.
53. Fraenkel DJ, Bardin PG, Sanderson G, Lampe F, Johnston SL, Holgate ST. Lower airways inflammation during rhinovirus colds in normal and asthmatic subjects. Am J Respir Crit Care Med 1995; 151:879–886.
54. Bianco A, Whiteman SC, Sethi SK, Allen JT, Knight RA, Spiteri MA. Expression of intercellular adhesion molecule-1 (ICAM-1) in nasal epithelial cells of atopic subjects: a mechanism for increased rhinovirus infection? Clin Exp Immunol 2000; 121:339–345.
55. Bianco A, Sethi SK, Allen JT, Knight RA, Spiteri MA. Th2 cytokines exert a dominant

influence on epithelial cell expression of the major group human rhinovirus receptor, ICAM-1. Eur Respir J 1998; 12:619–626.

56. Sethi SK, Bianco A, Allen JT, Knight RA, Spiteri MA. Interferon-gamma (IFN-gamma) down-regulates the rhinovirus-induced expression of intercellular adhesion molecule-1 (ICAM-1) on human airway epithelial cells. Clin Exp Immunol 1997; 110: 362-369.

57. Corne JM, Marshall C, Smith S, Schreiber J, Sanderson G, Holgate ST, Johnston SL. Frequency, severity, and duration of rhinovirus infections in asthmatic and non-asthmatic individuals: a longitudinal cohort study. Lancet 2002; 359:831–834.

58. Cazemier HMAJA, Sterkenburg JA, Manesse-Lazeroms SPG, van Wetering S, Spaan WJM, Sterk PJ, Hiemstra PS. Rhinovirus 16 (RV16) stimulates production and release of the chemokines IL-8 and RANTES in subcultures of human primary bronchial epithelial cells. Eur Respir J 1996; 9(suppl):424S, abstract.

59. Sanders SP, Siekierski ES, Porter JD, Richards SM, Proud D. Nitric oxide inhibits rhinovirus-induced cytokine production and viral replication in a human respiratory epithelial cell line. J Virol 1998; 72:934–942.

60. Sanders SP, Kim J, Connolly KR, Porter JD, Siekierski ES, Proud D. Nitric oxide inhibits rhinovirus-induced granulocyte macrophage colony-stimulating factor production in bronchial epithelial cells. Am J Respir Cell Mol Biol 2001; 24:317–325.

61. Konno S, Grindle KA, Lee WM, Schroth MK, Mosser AG, Brockman-Schneider RA, Busse WW, Gern JE. Interferon-gamma enhances rhinovirus-induced RANTES secretion by airway epithelial cells. Am J Respir Cell Mol Biol 2002; 26:594–601.

62. Schroth MK, Grimm E, Frindt P, Galagan DM, Konno SI, Love R, Gern JE. Rhinovirus replication causes RANTES production in primary bronchial epithelial cells. Am J Respir Cell Mol Biol 1999; 20:1220–1228.

63. Suzuki T, Yamaya M, Sekizawa K, Yamada N, Nakayama K, Ishizuka S, Kamanaka M, Morimoto T, Numazaki Y, Sasaki H. Effects of dexamethasone on rhinovirus infection in cultured human tracheal epithelial cells. Am J Physiol 2000; 278:L560-L571.

64. Behera AK, Kumar M, Matsuse H, Lockey RF, Mohapatra SS. Respiratory syncytial virus induces the expression of 5-lipoxygenase and endothelin-1 in bronchial epithelial cells. Biochem Biophys Res Comm 1998; 251:704–709.

65. Seymour ML, Gilby N, Bardin PG, Fraenkel DJ, Sanderson G, Penrose JF, Holgate ST, Johnston SL, Sampson AP. Rhinovirus infection increases 5-lipoxygenase and cyclooxygenase-2 in bronchial biopsy specimens from nonatopic subjects. J Infect Dis 2002; 185:540–544.

66. Papi A, Johnston SL. Rhinovirus infection induces expression of its own receptor intercellular adhesion molecule 1 (ICAM-1) via increased NF-kappaB-mediated transcription. J Biol Chem 1999; 274:9707–9720.

67. Papi A, Johnston SL. Respiratory epithelial cell expression of VCAM-1 and its upregulation by rhinovirus infection via NF-kB and GATA trancription factors. J Biol Chem 1999; 274:30041-30051.

68. Papi A, Papadopoulos NG, Degitz K, Holgate ST, Johnston SL. Corticosteroids inhibit rhinovirus-induced intercellular adhesion molecule-1 up-regulation and promoter activation on respiratory epithelial cells. J Allergy Clin Immunol 2000; 105:318–326.

69. Yamaya M, Sekizawa K, Suzuki T, Yamada N, Furukawa M, Ishizuka S, Nakayama K, Terajima M, Numazaki Y, Sasaki H. Infection of human respiratory submucosal glands with rhinovirus: effects on cytokine and ICAM-1 production. Am J Physiol 1999; 277:L362-L371.

70. Papadopoulos NG, Papi A, Bossios A, Xatzipsalti M, Stanciu LA, Holgate ST, Johnston SL. Rhinovirus infection upregulates neuropeptide-receptor mRNA expression and synergizes with neuropeptides in cytokine production by bronchial epithelial cells. Am J Respir Crit Care Med 2001; 163:abstract A905.

71. Sanders SP, Siekierski ES, Richards SM, Porter JD, Imani F, Proud D. Rhinovirus infection induces expression of type 2 nitric oxide synthase in human respiratory epithelial cells in vitro and in vivo. J Allergy Clin Immunol 2001; 107:235–243.

72. Sanders SP. Asthma, viruses, and nitric oxide. Proc Soc Exp Biol Med 1999; 220: 123–132.

73. de Gouw HWFM, van Sterkenburg MAJA, van Wetering S, et al. Expression of inducible nitric oxide synthase (iNOS) MRNA in human primary bronchial epithelial cells in vitro: effects of cytokines and rhinovirus-16. Am J Respir Crit Care Med 1998; 157(suppl):A24.

74. Reiss CS, Komatsu T. Does nitric oxide play a critical role in viral infections? J Virol 1998; 72:4547–4551.

75. Falsey AR, Walsh EE. Respiratory syncytial virus infection in adults. Clin Microbiol Rev 2000; 13:371–384.

76. Seemungal T, Harper-Owen R, Bhowmik A, Moric I, Sanderson G, Message S, Maccallum P, Meade TW, Jeffries DJ, Johnston SL, Wedzicha JA. Respiratory viruses, symptoms, and inflammatory markers in acute exacerbations and stable chronic obstructive pulmonary disease. Am J Respir Crit Care Med 2001; 164:1618-1623.

77. Behera AK, Matsuse H, Kumar M, Kong X, Lockey RF, Mohapatra SS. Blocking intercellular adhesion molecule-1 on human epithelial cells decreases respiratory syncytial virus infection. Biochem Biophys Res Commun 2001; 280:188–195.

78. Becker S, Soukup J, Yankaskas JR. Respiratory syncytial virus infection of human primary nasal and bronchial epithelial cell cultures and bronchoalveolar macrophages. Am J Respir Cell Mol Biol 1992; 6:369–374.

79. Becker S, Soukup JM. Airway epithelial cell-induced activation of monocytes and eosinophils in respiratory syncytial viral infection. Immunobiology 1999; 201:88–106.

80. Brandenburg AH, Kleinjan A, van Het Land B, Moll HA, Timmerman HH, de Swart RL, Neijens HJ, Fokkens W, Osterhaus AD. Type 1-like immune response is found in children with respiratory syncytial virus infection regardless of clinical severity. J Med Virol 2000; 62:267–277.

81. Becker S, Reed W, Henderson FW, Noah TL. RSV infection of human airway epithelial cells causes production of the beta-chemokine RANTES. Am J Physiol 1997; 272: L512-L520.

82. Bonville CA, Rosenberg HF, Domachowske JB. Macrophage inflammatory protein-1alpha and RANTES are present in nasal secretions during ongoing upper respiratory tract infection. Pediatr Allergy Immunol 1999; 10:39–44.

83. Lee CG, Yoon HJ, Zhu Z, Link H, Wang Z, Gwaltney JM, Landry M, Elias JA. Respiratory syncytial virus stimulation of vascular endothelial cell growth factor/vascular permeability factor. Am J Respir Cell Mol Biol 2000; 23:662–669.

84. Noah TL, Becker S. Chemokines in nasal secretions of normal adults experimentally infected with respiratory syncytial virus. Clin Immunol 2000; 97:43–49.

85. Domachowske JB, Bonville CA, Rosenberg HF. Gene expression in epithelial cells in response to pneumovirus infection. Respir Res 2001; 2:225–233.

86. Tsutsumi H, Takeuchi R, Ohsaki M, Seki K, Chiba S. Respiratory syncytial virus infection of human respiratory epithelial cells enhances inducible nitric oxide synthase gene expression. J Leukoc Biol 1999; 66:99–104.

87. Saito T, Deskin RW, Casola A, Haeberle H, Olszewska B, Ernst PB, Alam R, Ogra PL, Garofalo R. Respiratory syncytial virus induces selective production of the chemokine RANTES by upper airway epithelial cells. J Infect Dis 1997; 175:497–504.

88. Becker S, Koren HS, Henke DC. Interleukin-8 expression in normal nasal epithelium and its modulation by infection with respiratory syncytial virus and cytokines tumor necrosis factor, interleukin-1 and interleukin-6. Am J Respir Cell Mol Biol 1993; 8: 20–27.

89. Matsuzaki Z, Okamoto Y, Sarashina N, Ito E, Togawa K, Saito I. Induction of intercellular adhesion molecule-1 in human nasal epithelial cells during respiratory syncytial virus infection. Immunology 1996; 88:565–568.

90. Tristram DA, Hicks W Jr, Hard R. Respiratory syncytial virus and human bronchial epithelium. Arch Otolaryngol 1998; 124:777–783.

91. Smith P, Wang SZ, Dowling K, Forsyth K. Leucocyte populations in respiratory syncytial virus-induced bronchiolitis. J Paediatr Child Health 2001; 37:146–151.

92. Colocho Zelaya EA, Orvell C, Strannegard O. Eosinophil cationic protein in nasopharyngeal secretions and serum of infants infected with respiratory syncytial virus. Pediatr Allergy Immunol 1994; 5:100–106.

93. Garofalo R, Kimpen JLL, Welliver RC, Ogra PL. Eosinophil degranulation in the respiratory tract during naturally acquired respiratory syncytial virus infection. J Pediatr 1992; 120:28-32.

94. Harrison AM, Bonville CA, Rosenber HF, Domachowske JB. Respiratory syncytial virus-induced chemokine expression in the lower airways: eosinophil recruitment and degranulation. Am J Respir Crit Care Med 1999; 159:1918–1924.

95. Openshaw PJ. Immunity and immunopathology to respiratory syncytial virus. The mouse model. Am J Respir Crit Care Med 1995; 152:59–62.

96. Sigurs N, Bjarnason R, Sigurbergsson F, Kjellman B, Bjorksten B. Asthma and immunoglobulin E antibodies after respiratory syncytial virus bronchiolitis: a prospective cohort study with matched controls. Pediatrics 1995; 95:500–505.

97. Kimpen JLL, Garofalo R, Welliver RC, Ogra PL. Activation of human eosinophils in vitro by respiratory syncytial virus. Pediatr Res 1992; 32:160–164.

98. Kimpen JLL, Garofalo R, Welliver RC, Fujihara K, Ogra PL. An ultrastructural study of the interaction of human eosinophils with respiratory syncytial virus. Pediatr Allergy Immunol 1996; 7:48–53.

99. Stark JM, Godding V, Sedgwick JB, Busse WW. Respiratory syncytial virus infection enhances neutrophil and eosinophil adhesion to cultured respiratory epithelial cells. Roles of CD18 and intercellular adhesion molecule-1. J Immunol 1996; 156:4774-4782.

100. Volvovitz B, Welliver RC, De Castro G, Krystofik DA, Ogra PL. The release of leukotrienes in the respiratory tract during infection with respiratory syncytial virus: role in obstructive airway disease. Pediatr Res 1988; 24:504–507.

101. Sheeran P, Jafri H, Carubelli C, Saavedra J, Johnson C, Krisher K, Sanchez PJ, Ramilo O. Elevated cytokine concentrations in the nasopharyngeal and tracheal secretions of children with respiratory syncytial virus disease. Pediatr Infect Dis J 1999; 18:115–122.

102. Wang SZ, Hallsworth PG, Dowling KD, Alpers JH, Bowden JJ, Forsyth KD. Adhesion molecule expression on epithelial cells infected with respiratory syncytial virus. Eur Respir J 2000; 15:358–366.

103. Arnold R, Humbert B, Werchau H, Gallati H, Konig W. Interleukin-8, interleukin-6, and soluble tumour necrosis factor receptor type I release from a human pulmonary

epithelial cell line (A549) exposed to respiratory syncytial virus. Immunology 1994; 82:126–133.

104. Fiedler MA, Wernke-Dollries K, Stark JM. Respiratory syncytial virus increases IL-8 gene expression and protein release in A549 cells. Am J Physiol 1995; 269:L865-L872.

105. Elias JA, Zheng T, Einarsson O, Landry M, Trow T, Rebert N, Panuska J. Epithelial interleukin-11: regulation by cytokines, respiratory syncytial virus and retinoic acid. J Biol Chem 1994; 269:22261–22268.

106. Domachowske JB, Dyer KD, Rosenberg HF. Multiple signaling pathways are involved in respiratory syncytial virus induced chemokine expression. Clin Infect Dis 1997; 25: 390.

107. Samransamruajkit R, Gollapudi S, Kim CH, Gupta S, Nussbaum E. Modulation of endothelin-1 expression in pulmonary epithelial cell line (A549) after exposure to RSV. Int J Mol Med 2000; 6:101–105.

108. Noah TL, Wortman IA, Becker S. The effect of fluticasone propionate on respiratory syncytial virus-induced chemokine release by a human bronchial epithelial cell line. Immunopharmacology 1998; 39:193–199.

109. Becker S, Soukup JM. Effect of nitrogen dioxide on respiratory viral infection in airway epithelial cells. Environ Res 1999; 81:159–166.

110. Becker S, Quay J, Soukup J. Cytokine (tumor necrosis factor, IL-6, and IL-8) production by respiratory syncytial virus-infected human alveolar macrophages. J Immunol 1991; 147:4307–4312.

111. Soukup J, Koren HS, Becker S. Ozone effect on respiratory syncytial virus infectivity and cytokine production by human alveolar macrophages. Environ Res 1993; 60:178–186.

112. Guerrero-Plata A, Ortega E, Gomez B. Persistence of respiratory syncytial virus in macrophages alters phagocytosis and pro-inflammatory cytokine production. Viral Immunol 2001; 14:19–30.

113. Elias JA, Wu Y, Zheng T, Panettieri R. Cytokine- and virus-stimulated airway smooth muscle cells produce IL-11 and other IL-6-type cytokines. Am J Physiol 1997; 273: L648-L655.

114. Adcock I, Caramori G. Therapies acting on transcription: overview. In: Hansel TT, Barnes PJ, eds. New Drugs for Asthma, Allergy and COPD. Progress in Respiratory Research, vol 31. Basel: Karger Publishers, 2001; 328–331.

115. Barnes PJ, Adcock IM. Transcription factors and asthma. Eur Respir J 1998; 12:221–234.

116. Barnes PJ, Karin M. Nuclear factor-κB: a pivotal transcription factor in chronic inflammatory diseases. N Engl J Med 1997; 336:1066–1071.

117. Barnes PJ, Adcock IM. NF-κB: a pivotal role in asthma and a new target for therapy. Trends Pharmacol Sci 1997; 18:46–50.

118. Karin M. Mitogen-activated protein kinase cascades as regulators of stress responses. Ann NY Acad Sci 1998; 851:139-146.

119. Caramori G, Lim S, Ito K, Tomita K, Oates T, Jazwari E, Chung KF, Barnes PJ, Adcock IM. GATA transcription factors expression in T cells, monocytes and bronchial biopsies of normal and asthmatic subjects. Eur Respir J 2001; 18: 18:466-473.

120. Hart LA, Krishnan VL, Adcock IM, Barnes PJ, Chung KF. Activation and localization of transcription factor nuclear factor-κB in asthma. Am J Respir Crit Care Med 1998; 158:1585-1592.

121. Demoly P, Chanez P, Pujol JL, Gauthier-Rouviere C, Michel FB, Godard P, Bousquet J. Fos immunoreactivity assessment on human normal and pathological bronchial biopsies. Respir Med 1995; 89:329–335.

122. Gosset P, Tsicopoulos A, Wallaert B, Vannimenus C, Joseph M, Tonnel AB, Capron A. Increased secretion of tumor necrosis factor alpha and interleukin-6 by alveolar macrophages consecutive to the development of the late asthmatic reaction. J Allergy Clin Immunol 1991; 88:561–571.

123. Gosset P, Tsicopoulos A, Wallaert B, Joseph M, Capron A, Tonnel AB. Tumor necrosis factor alpha and interleukin-6 production by human mononuclear phagocytes from allergic asthmatics after IgE-dependent stimulation. Am Rev Respir Dis 1992; 146: 768–774.

124. Agarwal S, Viola JPB, Rao A. Chromatin-based regulatory mechanisms governing cytokine gene transcription. J Allergy Clin Immunol 1999; 103:990–999.

125. Caramori G, Lim S, Tomita K, Ito K, Oates T, Chung K, Barnes PJ, Adcock IM. STAT6 expression in T-cells subsets, alveolar macrophages and bronchial biopsies from normal and asthmatic subjects. Eur Respir J 2000; 16(suppl 31):162s, abstract P1188.

126. Ho I-C, Hodge MR, Rooney JW, Glimcher LH. The proto-oncogene c-maf is responsible for tissue-specific expression of interleukin-4. Cell 1996; 85:973–983.

127. Griego SD, Weston CB, Adams JL, Tal-Singer R, Dillon SB. Role of p38 mitogen-activated protein kinase in rhinovirus-induced cytokine production by bronchial epithelial cells. J Immunol 2000; 165:5211–5220.

128. Kim J, Sanders SP, Siekierski ES, Casolaro V, Proud D. Role of NF-kappa B in cytokine production induced from human airway epithelial cells by rhinovirus infection. J Immunol 2000; 165:3384–3392.

129. Mastronarde JG, He B, Monick MM, Mukaida N, Matsushima K, Hunninghake GW. Induction of interleukin (IL)-8 gene expression by respiratory syncytial virus involved activation of nuclear factor (NF)-κB and NF-IL-6. J Infect Dis 1996; 174:262–267.

130. Mastronarde JG, Monick MM, Mukaida N, Matsushima K, Hunninghake GW. Activator protein-1 is the preferred transcription factor for cooperative interaction with nuclear factor-kB in respiratory syncytial virus-induced interleukin-8 gene expression in airway epithelium. J Infect Dis 1998; 177:1275–1281.

131. Jamaluddin M, Garofalo R, Ogra PL, Brasier AR. Inducible translational regulation of the NF-IL6 transcription factor by respiratory syncytial virus infection in pulmonary epithelial cells. J Virol 1996; 70:1554–1563.

132. Jamaluddin M, Casola A, Garofalo RP, Han Y, Elliott T, Ogra PL, Brasier AR. The major component of IκB proteolysis occurs independently of the proteasome pathway in respiratory syncytial virus- infected pulmonary epithelial cells. J Virol 1998; 72: 4849–4857.

133. Koga T, Sardina E, Tidwell RM, Pelletier M, Look DC, Hotzman MJ. Virus-inducible expression of a host chemokine gene relies on replication-linked mRNA stabilization. Proc Natl Acad Sci USA 1999; 96:5680–5685.

134. Domachowske JB, Bonville CA, Mortelliti AJ, Colella CB, Kim U, Rosenberg HF. Respiratory syncytial virus infection induces expression of the anti-apoptosis gene IEX-1L in human respiratory epithelial cells. J Infect Dis 2000; 181:824–830.

135. Takeuchi R, Tsutsumi H, Osaki M, Haseyama K, Mizue N, Chiba S. Respiratory syncytial virus infection of human alveolar epithelial cells enhances interferon regulatory factor 1 and interleukin-1α-converting enzyme gene expression but does not cause apoptosis. J Virol 1998; 72:4498–4502.

136. Wu MX, Ao Z, Prasad KV, Wu R, Schlossman SF. IEX-1L, an apoptosis inhibitor involved in NF-kappaB-mediated cell survival. Science 1998; 281:998–1001.
137. Krilov LR, McClosky TW, Harkness SH, Pahwa VS. Responses of monocytes in peripheral blood mononuclear leukocytes (PBMLs) exposed to respiratory syncytial virus (RSV) in vitro. Pediatr Res 1998; 43:868 abstract).
138. Pontrelli L, Krilov L, McKloskey T, Harkness S. TUNEL assay and immunophenotyping to quantify apoptosis in cord and adult blood samples exposed to respiratory syncytial virus (RSV). Clin Infect Dis 1998; 27:977A (abstract).
139. Bitko V, Velazquez A, Yang L, Yang YC, Barik S. Transcriptional induction of multiple cytokines by human respiratory syncytial virus requires activation of NF-kappaB and is inhibited by sodium salicylate and aspirin. Virology 1997; 232:369–378.
140. Thomas LH, Wickremasinghe MI, Sharland M, Friedland JS. Synergistic upregulation of interleukin-8 secretion from pulmonary epithelial cells by direct and monocyte-dependent effects of respiratory syncytial virus infection. J Virol 2000; 74:8425–8433.
141. Arnold R, Konig W. ICAM-1 expression and low-molecular-weight G-protein activation of human bronchial epithelial cells (A549) infected with RSV. J Leukoc Biol 1996; 60:766–771.
142. Chini BA, Fiedler MA, Milligan L, Hopkins T, Stark JM. Essential roles of NF-κB and C/EBP in the regulation of intercellular adhesion molecule-1 after respiratory syncytial virus infection of human respiratory epithelial cell cultures. J Virol 1998; 72: 1623–1626.
143. Thomas LH, Friedland JS, Sharland M, Becker S. Respiratory syncytial virus-induced RANTES production from human bronchial epithelial cells is dependent on nuclear factor-kappa B nuclear binding and is inhibited by adenovirus-mediated expression of inhibitor of kappa B alpha. J Immunol 1998; 161:1007–1016.
144. Casola A, Garofalo RP, Jamaluddin M, Vlahopoulos S, Brasier AR. Requirement of a novel upstream response element in respiratory syncytial virus-induced IL-8 gene expression. J Immunol 2000; 164:5944–5951.
145. Casola A, Garofalo RP, Haeberle H, Elliott TF, Lin R, Jamaluddin M, Brasier AR. Multiple cis regulatory elements control RANTES promoter activity in alveolar epithelial cells infected with respiratory syncytial virus. J Virol 2001; 75:6428-6439.
146. Casola A, Burger N, Liu T, Jamaluddin M, Brasier AR, Garofalo RP. Oxidant tone regulates rantes gene expression in airway epithelial cells infected with respiratory syncytial virus. Role in viral-induced interferon regulatory factor activation. J Biol Chem 2001; 276:19715–19722.
147. Flory E, Kunz M, Scheller C, Jassoy C, Stauber R, Rapp UR, Ludwig S. Influenza virus-induced NF-kappaB-dependent gene expression is mediated by overexpression of viral proteins and involves oxidative radicals and activation of IkappaB kinase. J Biol Chem 2000; 275:8307–8314.
148. Bussfeld D, Bacher M, Moritz A, Gemsa D, Sprenger H. Expression of transcription factor genes after influenza A virus infection. Immunobiology 1997; 198:291–298.
149. Barnes PJ. Chronic obstructive pulmonary disease. N Engl J Med 2000; 343:269–280.
150. Matsuse T, Hayashi S, Kuwano K, Keunecke H, Jefferies WA, Hogg JC. Latent adenoviral infection in the pathogenesis of chronic airway obstruction. Am Rev Respir Dis 1992; 146:177-184.
151. Keicho N, Higashimoto Y, Bondy GP, Elliott WM, Hogg JC, Hayashi S. Endotoxin-specific NF-κB activation in pulmonary epithelial cells harboring adenovirus E1A. Am J Physiol 1999; 277:L523-L532.
152. Yamada K, Elliott WM, Hayashi S, Brattsand R, Roberts C, Vitalis TZ, Hogg JC.

Latent adenoviral infection modifies the steroid response in allergic lung inflammation. J Allergy Clin Immunol 2000; 106:844–851.

153. Jahn HU, Krull M, Wuppermann FN, Klucken AC, Rosseau S, Seybold J, Hegemann JH, Jantos CA, Suttorp N. Infection and activation of airway epithelial cells by Chlamydia pneumoniae. J Infect Dis 2000; 182:1678–1687.

154. Gencay M, Tamm M, Rudiger JJ, Black J, Puolakkainen M, Glanville A, Roth M. Chlamydia pneumoniae activates the glucocorticoid receptor in human lung epithelial cells. Am J Respir Crit Care Med 2001; 163(suppl):A673.

155. Sacht G, Marten A, Deiters U, Sussmuth R, Jung G, Wingender E, Muhlradt PF. Activation of nuclear factor-kappaB in macrophages by mycoplasmal lipopeptides. Eur J Immunol 1998; 28:4207–4212.

156. Tanaka M, Nyce JW. Respirable antisense oligonucleotides: a new drug class for respiratory disease. Respir Res 2001 2:5-9.

157. Han Z, Boyle DL, Chang L, Bennett B, Karin M, Yang L, Manning AM, Firestein GS. c-Jun N-terminal kinase is required for metalloproteinase expression and joint destruction in inflammatory arthritis. J Clin Invest 2001; 108:73–81.

10

Nitric Oxide and Other Inflammatory Mediators

RICHARD B. R. MUIJSERS, FRANS P. NIJKAMP, and GERT FOLKERTS

University of Utrecht
Utrecht, The Netherlands

I. Introduction

The free radical nitric oxide is an important mediator of many biological processes. The molecule appears to be a two-edged sword. Besides the agent's role as a paracrine messenger, nitric-oxide-derived oxidants are important weapons against invading pathogens. Likewise, the role of nitric oxide in the airways is ambiguous. Besides its role as a bronchodilator, nitric oxide and derivatives have been hypothesized to play a role in the pathophysiology of asthma via their putative damaging effects on the airways. This may be enhanced by a nitrosative response to respiratory tract infections, since both the infectious agent and the host may suffer from the consequent nitrosative stress. Respiratory infections may also compromise the beneficial (bronchodilatory) effects of nitric oxide. In the following paragraphs an overview of the role of nitric oxide and derivatives in the pathophysiology of asthma will be given, after which the effects of respiratory infection in this context will be discussed.

II. Toxic Molecules

The main function of the immune system is the defense of the host organism against infectious agents. Phagocytic cells such as macrophages and neutrophils play an essential role in antimicrobial responses, because these cells can release large amounts of highly toxic molecules; reactive nitrogen species (RNS) and reactive oxygen species (ROS). In addition to these inflammatory cells, evidence exists that noninflammatory cells including airway epithelium also release these reactive molecules.

Besides their beneficial effects in host defense mechanisms, reactive nitrogen species and reactive oxygen species also have detrimental effects on the host itself, since these molecules can be as toxic to host cells as they are to micro-organisms. The effects on host tissues may be especially evident in inflammatory diseases without the involvement of an intrinsically harmful pathogen, as in allergic and autoimmune disease; and in infections in which a nitrosative response does not help to eliminate the infectious agent.

Reactive oxygen species are mainly derived from superoxide (O_2^{*-}, whereas reactive nitrogen species formation largely starts at the synthesis of nitric oxide (NO). The formation and properties of these two important precursors are discussed below.

A. Nitric Oxide

The free radical nitric oxide is well recognized as a mediator in a wide range of biological processes (1,2). With a molecular weight of 30 g/mol nitric oxide is one of the smallest molecular mediators in biology. The diatomic molecule can be formed in a variety of cells by the conversion of L-arginine to L-citrulline by nitric oxide synthase (NOS) (3).

Three isoforms of NOS exist, each with a distinct function. The isoforms can roughly be classified into two classes: constitutive and inducible NOS. Neuronal NOS (nNOS or NOS1) and endothelial NOS (eNOS or NOS3) are constitutively expressed, and inducible NOS (iNOS or NOS2) expression is upregulated during inflammation (1). nNOS and eNOS activity is dependent on calcium, whereas iNOS activity is independent of calcium fluxes. nNOS-derived nitric oxide is thought to be involved in neurotransmission (4,5). eNOS is important for the relaxation of vascular smooth muscle and is therefore involved in the regulation of blood pressure (6). The inducible form, iNOS, is the main source of nitric oxide involved in inflammatory responses and pathogen killing. Expression of iNOS in macrophages in response to inflammatory mediators leads to the production of high amounts of nitric oxide (1,7–9). Studies performed in iNOS knockout mice clearly demonstrate an essential role for nitric oxide in immune responses to particular micro-organisms (10,11).

Hence, nitric oxide has two faces in biology. In relatively low concentrations nitric oxide is a paracrine messenger, whereas high concentrations of nitric oxide, released in an inflammatory context, have detrimental effects putatively via the formation of reactive nitrogen species (12). Beneficial or deleterious effects of nitric oxide are dependent not only on the concentration but also on the biological microenvironment in which nitric oxide is released (13). The detrimental properties of nitric oxide not only occur when released from inducible NOS, but also when produced by the constitutive isoforms of the enzyme, for example, during ischemia–reperfusion injury (14).

B. Superoxide

The free radical superoxide is released during the respiratory burst of granulocytes and macrophages by NADPH oxidase activity, in response to several stimuli (15). Alternative sources of superoxide are the auto-oxidation of hemoglobin, myoglobin, and cytochrome c. Furthermore, enzymes such as xanthine oxidase, aldehyde oxidase, and a variety of flavin dehydrogenases are a source of superoxide. Superoxide is therefore released by virtually all aerobic cells (16). It is interesting that nNOS can produce both NO and superoxide, when L-arginine concentrations are relatively low (17). Like nitric oxide, superoxide release during the respiratory burst of phagocytes is essential for the killing of invading pathogens (18).

C. Superoxide and Nitric Oxide Interact

Because nitric oxide and superoxide are free radicals (and therefore highly reactive), both molecules rapidly react with many different molecules in a biological environment. Of particular interest is the interaction between both molecules and their reactive downstream metabolites. In many metabolic routes nitric oxide and superoxide are released simultaneously, which is a likely event during inflammatory responses. For example, efficient killing of *Salmonella* by murine macrophages is dependent on both NADPH-oxidase-derived superoxide and iNOS-derived nitric oxide (18). Many of the products formed by the interaction of superoxide and nitric oxide are even more reactive than their precursors. The following paragraphs provide a brief summary of metabolic routes that superoxide and nitric oxide can follow once released in vivo.

Peroxynitrite

The most direct interaction between nitric oxide and superoxide is their rapid isostoichometric reaction to form the potent oxidant peroxynitrite (19,20). The rate constant of this reaction is near the diffusion-controlled limit (4–7×10^9 $M^{-1}S^{-1}$) (20,21). The half-life of peroxynitrite at 37°C and pH 7.4 is approximately 1 s. (22,23). (For review, see Ref. 23.) The reaction of peroxynitrite with carbon dioxide is the most important route for peroxynitrite in biological environments, when carbon dioxide is relatively abundant (24). The exact biochemical fate of peroxynitrite in biological systems, however, is very complex and not yet completely clear (13).

Although peroxynitrite is able to nitrate tyrosine residues (25), the detection of 3-nitrotyrosine does not provide indisputable evidence for peroxynitrite formation, since there are alternative pathways leading to 3-nitrotyrosine formation (26). This is discussed in detail below.

Other Reactive Nitrogen Species

In addition to the direct interaction of superoxide and nitric oxide forming peroxynitrite, many other reactive nitrogen species emanate from the interaction between

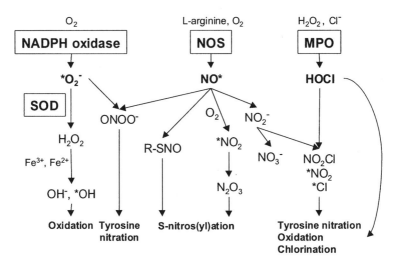

Figure 1 Schematic overview of reactive nitrogen and oxygen species metabolism by inflammatory cells. (Modified from Ref. 27.) NOS: nitric oxide synthase, MPO: myeloperoxidase, SOD: superoxide dismutase. See text for details.

nitric oxide and superoxide. Besides peroxynitrite formation, nitric-oxide-derived nitrite can be utilized in the myeloperoxidase pathway leading to NO_2Cl and NO_2*. An overview of the metabolic routes of reactive nitrogen species is given in Figure 1.

III.   What Can We Measure In Vivo?

As described above, many reactive species originate from the precursors nitric oxide and superoxide. Due to their complex chemistry and often short half-lives, the exact metabolic fate of reactive nitrogen species in vivo remains dubious. Furthermore, it is almost impossible to pinpoint a given effect in vivo to a specific reactive nitrogen intermediate. Nonetheless, some stable end products of reactive nitrogen species are detected in bodily fluids and tissues. First, nitrite and nitrate can be detected in plasma (28,29). Furthermore, 3-nitrotyrosine residues can be detected in tissue samples, using immunohistochemistry (30), but also in biological fluids (31). Moreover, nitric oxide can be measured in the exhaled air of asthmatic patients (32,33) and is thought to reflect the inflammatory state of the airways (34). Nonetheless, it is often difficult to interpret results from these techniques, since there is a high risk of artifacts. Nitrite and nitrate levels in plasma, for example, can reflect dietary intake rather than nitric oxide metabolism in vivo (35). Moreover, nitric oxide is also formed enzyme-independently from nitrite under acidic conditions (36). Hunt et al. recently showed that the pH in the airways dramatically drops during an acute asthma attack, which facilitates the conversion of nitrite to nitric oxide. Hence, increased nitric oxide concentrations in the exhaled air of asthmatic patients may reflect nitrite conversion rather than NOS activity (37).

IV. Reactive Nitrogen Species Make a Difference

The effects of reactive nitrogen species, once formed in vivo, on tissues, cells, and biomolecules are diverse. Important targets of reactive nitrogen species in proteins are tyrosine residues (38), thiols (39), and heme groups (9). Furthermore, reactive nitrogen species alter lipid oxidation pathways (40), cause DNA damage (41), and inhibit mitochondrial respiration (42). For detailed information about reactive nitrogen species mediated changes in biomolecules, the reader is referred to an extended review by Eiserich et al. (43). Despite the fact that the exact mechanisms by which reactive nitrogen species affect the function of biological tissues remain unclear, many studies indicate that reactive nitrogen species are able to compromise cell function. Exposure of cells to reactive nitrogen species leads to both apoptosis and necrosis dependent on the severity of cell damage (44). Again, these detrimental effects may affect both an invading pathogen and the (infected) host.

An important, commonly used, marker of nitrosative stress is the formation of 3-nitrotyrosine residues. Although 3-nitrotyrosine is widely used as a specific marker of peroxynitrite formation, it is now clear that more pathways leading to the formation of 3-nitrotyrosine exist in vivo (26). 3-Nitrotyrosine is readily formed by a nitric-oxide-independent process mediated by myeloperoxidase, with hydrogen peroxide and the nitric oxide metabolite nitrite as substrates (26,45). Moreover, eosinophil peroxidase is an even stronger promoter of 3-nitrotyrosine formation via this pathway (46). At present, the relative contribution of these peroxidase-mediated pathways and peroxynitrite to in vivo 3-nitrotyrosine formation is a subject of debate (25,43).

V. Reactive Nitrogen Species Are a Promising Therapeutic Target

Because of the detrimental effects of reactive nitrogen species on host tissues, protection against these compounds is a promising therapeutic target in inflammatory diseases (47). This can be achieved by scavenging reactive nitrogen species by antioxidants, by limiting nitric oxide synthesis, or by limiting superoxide formation. A disadvantage of limiting reactive nitrogen species formation is of course a compromised defense against invading microorganisms. Moreover, nonspecific NOS inhibition may lead to a compromised function of nitric oxide as a paracrine messenger, which could result in hypertension (48). The successful use of NOS inhibition is therefore dependent on the isoform of NOS involved, and on the selectivity of the inhibitor used. Nonetheless, limiting superoxide production by NADPH oxidase is of particular interest since superoxide release is also required for the formation of many reactive nitrogen species and inhibition of NADPH oxidase should not compromise other nitric oxide functions.

VI. Human Mononuclear Phagocytes Do Not Release High Amounts of Nitric Oxide In Vitro

In contrast to murine macrophages, human mononuclear phagocytes do not release high amounts of nitric oxide in vitro, despite the presence of iNOS (49,50). At present, it is unclear whether the lack of high-output nitric oxide synthesis is an in vitro artifact. A vast number of human disease states are nevertheless associated with increased iNOS expression in mononuclear phagocytes and consequent nitric oxide production (50).

Other NOS-independent pathways leading to the formation of reactive nitrogen species may be of importance in human phagocytes. First, the low pH in phagolysosomes could lead to the conversion of nitrite to nitric oxide in phagocytes (51). Further, the formation of nitrating reactive nitrogen species is readily catalyzed by myeloperoxidase from nitrite and hydrogen peroxide (26). Therefore, iNOS-derived nitric oxide as such may not be a crucial feature of human inflammatory cells in their nitrosative response to invading micro-organisms. As a consequence, limiting nitric oxide synthesis by specific iNOS inhibitors to protect host tissues from nitrosative stress may be a futile strategy in human inflammatory disease.

Important differences appear to exist between human and murine inflammatory cells with regard to NOS-dependent reactive nitrogen species release, which cannot be explained by the limited availability of the NOS substrate L-arginine. Despite low iNOS activity in human mononuclear cells, reactive nitrogen species are readily formed by human monocytes (52) and human neutrophils (26), with nitrite instead of nitric oxide as a precursor.

VII. Two Faces of Nitric Oxide in the Airways

Reactive nitrogen species, which are readily formed during inflammatory responses, have beneficial as well as detrimental effects on biological tissues. Likewise, the role of nitric oxide and its metabolites in the airways is ambiguous. On the one hand, eNOS or nNOS-derived nitric oxide counteracts agonist-induced bronchoconstriction (53,54). Furthermore, NO and NO donors relax human airway smooth muscle in vitro, presumably via the activation of guanylate cyclase and associated increase in cGMP (55). The concentration of nitric oxide in the exhaled air is decreased after acute bronchoconstriction, suggesting a bronchoprotective role for nitric oxide (56). An extended review of the bronchodilatory effects of nitric oxide is provided elsewhere (54). In contrast, the molecule is implicated in the pathobiology of asthma, by way of putatively nitric-oxide-derived reactive nitrogen species (30,38,57,58).

VIII. Reactive Nitrogen Species Are Formed During Allergic Asthma

It is evident that reactive nitrogen species are readily formed during allergic airway disease. First, 3-nitrotyrosine formation is increased in the airways of asthmatic patients (30). Furthermore, the concentration of nitric oxide in the exhaled air of asthmatic patients is increased (32–34), while anti-inflammatory therapy such as inhaled corticosteroids is able to reduce it (59). The concentration of nitric oxide in the exhaled air is thought to reflect the inflammatory state of the airways (59). Nonetheless, low doses of inhaled steroids decrease nitric oxide concentrations in the exhaled air while preventing airway hyperresponsiveness requires higher doses of steroids (60). Last, inflammatory cells isolated from the airways of asthmatic patients after segmental allergen challenge release more superoxide than those from control subjects (61). Despite the fact that reactive nitrogen species are formed during allergic airway disease, their exact role in the pathobiology of asthma remains enigmatic.

IX. Nitric Oxide and T-Cell Differentiation

Besides the involvement of reactive nitrogen species in the development of airway hyperresponsiveness, a number of studies report a putative role for nitric oxide as a mediator of T cell response (62). Nitric oxide can skew the Th1/Th2 balance into the direction of a Th2-response (63). Moreover, exogenously applied nitric oxide decreases IL-4, IL-5, and IFN-γ production by human T lymphocytes in vitro (64). The inhibition of IL-4 and IL-5 production was dependent on cGMP, whereas the decreased IFN-γ production was more persistent and was dependent on additional mechanisms, presumably at the transcriptional level. Formation of reactive nitrogen species could therefore promote allergic responses through T cells.

X. Reactive Nitrogen Species and Allergic Airway Disease

A. Linking Allergen Exposure to Increased Reactive Nitrogen Species Formation

Upregulation of iNOS has been reported in the airway epithelium and inflammatory cells in asthmatic airways (30,65,66) and after allergen challenge in rats (67). Moreover, iNOS expression (68) and activity (68,69) are increased in the lungs of allergen-challenged mice. Last, allergen challenge results in increased levels of nitrate in the plasma, which is not so in iNOS knockout mice (70). iNOS expression in human cells is inhibited by corticosteroids (30,71,72). This is of importance since inhaled corticosteroids prevent both iNOS expression in the airways (30) and increased concentrations of nitric oxide in exhaled air (73) of asthmatic patients. Increased reactive nitrogen species formation during allergic airway inflammation therefore seems to be dependent on iNOS.

The cellular and molecular mechanisms leading to increased nitric oxide synthesis and reactive nitrogen species formation upon allergen challenge are currently incompletely understood. In asthmatic subjects, iNOS protein is upregulated in the airway epithelium due to transcriptional regulation (66,74). IFN-γ is likely to play an important role in the induction of iNOS during asthma, since the cytokine is essential for iNOS expression in human airway epithelial cells in vitro (71,75,76). Furthermore, the concentration of IFN-γ is increased in the epithelial lining fluid of asthmatics (66). Hence, the Th1 cytokine IFN-γ could be the link between allergic airway inflammation and iNOS in humans. The development of allergen-induced hyperresponsiveness in a murine model of allergic asthma is dependent on IFN-γ (77). Therefore, IFN-γ could also be the cytokine responsible for iNOS induction during allergic airway inflammation in mice. A large population of the T lymphocytes present in the airways after allergen challenge is non-antigen-specific and releases IFN-γ (78). Indeed, thoracic lymph node cells from ovalbumin-challenged animals release increased amounts of IFN-γ independently of in vitro ovalbumin stimulation (77).

In contrast to human asthmatic airways, the airway epithelium of mice does not express iNOS during allergic airway inflammation (68). Alveolar macrophages are a likely source of iNOS-dependent nitric oxide production in mice, since allergen-induced inflammatory infiltrates show iNOS expression (68). IFN-γ induces high-output nitric oxide synthesis by murine macrophages in vitro (79). Moreover iNOS expression is increased in machophages after allergen challenge in rats (67).

Another possible mechanism leading to enhanced nitric oxide and reactive nitrogen species release is the activation of the low-affinity IgE receptor (CD23). Stimulation of CD23 on human mononuclear phagocytes enhances iNOS expression and nitric oxide release (80,81). CD23 is also expressed on human airway epithelial cells (82). It is unclear whether CD23 contributes to the expression of iNOS in asthmatic airways (30).

Calhoun et al. previously, showed increased superoxide production by alveolar macrophages from asthmatic patients after segmental allergen challenge (61). Moreover, blood monocytes and neutrophils from asthmatic patients release more superoxide in vitro upon stimulation than those from healthy controls (83,84). In addition to these inflammatory cells, alveolar type II cells (85) and the endothelium of the pulmonary vasculature (86) express NADPH oxidase. Moreover, administration of superoxide dismutase to allergen-challenged guinea pigs prevents the development of airway hyperresponsiveness (87). Therefore, increased superoxide production during allergic airway inflammation is likely to contribute to the nitrosative stress and consequent damage to the airways via the interaction between reactive oxygen and nitrogen species.

In addition, IFN-γ is an important regulator of NADPH oxidase activity and expression in both human and murine phagocytes (83,88), and reactive nitrogen species formation upon IFN-γ/LPS stimulation is dependent on NADPH oxidase (89). Therefore, IFN-γ could be the connection between allergic airway inflammation and both superoxide and nitric oxide release, and consequently reactive nitrogen species. It is tempting to speculate that the formation of reactive nitrogen species during allergic airway inflammation is dependent on a Th1-like response rather than on a Th2 response.

B. Reactive Nitrogen Species and Inflammatory Cell Migration

Data by Feder et al. using the specific iNOS inhibitor L-NIL (90) suggest that iNOS-derived nitric oxide does not contribute to the extravasation and subsequent migration of eosinophils into the airways of mice. In contrast, the selective NOS inhibitors S-ethylisourea and AMT administered during the challenge phase do prevent both eosinophil and neutrophil influx into the airways (68). Moreover, nonspecific NOS inhibition by L-NMMA or eNOS inhibition by L-NAME results in decreased airway eosinophilia after allergen challenge in mice, rats, and guinea pigs, suggesting that eNOS-derived nitric oxide, presumably released by the endothelium of the pulmonary vasculature, is involved in the extravasation of eosinophils (68,90–92). In contrast, knocking out either nNOS or eNOS does not change allergen-induced airway eosinophilia (69), whereas conflicting evidence has been found for iNOS knockouts. In one study no change in airway eosinophilia was observed (69), while in the other airway eosinophilia was decreased in iNOS knockouts (70). In the latter study, increased production of IFN-γ was put forward as an explanation for the decreased eosinophilia. Hofstra et al. showed that IFN-γ has a dual role in allergic airway disease. Endogenous IFN-γ is essential for the development of allergic airway inflammation, whereas administration of excess IFN-γ can inhibit the influx of eosinophils into the airway lumen (93). An overview of the results of different NOS inhibitor and NOS knockout studies on eosinophil recruitment in vivo in various species is given in Table 1. It is clear that further research is required to evaluate the relative contribution of the three NOS isoforms to the extravasation and migration of inflammatory cells during allergic airway inflammation.

Taken together, it is clear that the role of nitric oxide in allergic airway inflammation is, to say the least, enigmatic. Further research is required to elucidate the effects of nitric oxide on inflammatory cell migration and on T-helper cell responses. The effect of nitric oxide on these phenomena seems to be dependent on time, context, and concentration. It is suggested that the in vivo methods available (i.e., systemic NOS inhibition or knocking out NOS isoforms) are too unrefined to investigate the ambiguous and complex effects of nitric oxide on the development of allergic airway inflammation.

C. Reactive Nitrogen Species and Allergen-Induced Airway Hyperresponsiveness

Table 1 provides an overview of the effects of different nitric oxide synthase inhibitors on allergen-induced hyperresponsiveness in vivo in different species as described in literature. As mentioned previously, the effects of the inhibitors are dependent on their relative selectivity towards the three NOS isoforms. Although more or less selective inhibitors are available, even a selective inhibitor will inhibit the other isoforms at high concentrations. The iNOS inhibitor aminoguanidine, for example, is only 10–100 times more potent against iNOS than against eNOS (100).

Table 1 Overview of the Effects of NOS Inhibition or NOS Knockout on Allergen-Induced Airway Hyperresponsiveness and Eosinophil Influx in Different Species In Vivo Compared to Control or Wild-Type Mice as Described in the Literature

Species	Inhibitor	Target[a]	AHR	Eosinophils	Reference
Guinea pig	L-NAME	eNOS		ND	94
	L-NAME	eNOS			92
	AG	iNOS		ND	92
Rat	L-NAME	eNOS		=	95
	L-NAME	eNOS	ND		91
	L-NMMA	NS			95
	AG	iNOS	=		95
	SMLT	nNOS	=		95
	SD3651	iNOS		=	96
Mouse	L-NMMA	NS	ND		90
	L-NIL	iNOS	ND	=	90
	AMT	iNOS	ND		68
	EIT	NS	ND		68
	L-NAME	eNOS	ND		90
	L-NAME	eNOS	ND		68
	AG	iNOS	ND		90
	1400W	iNOS		=	97
Mouse	KO[b]	iNOS	=		70
knockouts	KO[b]	iNOS	=	=	69
	KO[b]	eNOS	=	=	69
	KO[b]	nNOS		=	69
	KO[b]	eNOS+nNOS		=	69

[a] NOS isoform to which the inhibitor is relatively selective.
[b] Knockout mice.
AHR, airway hyperresponsiveness; eosinophil, number of eosinophils in the bronchoalveolar lavage fluid; =, unaltered; ND, not determined; L-NAME; NG-nitro-L-arginine methyl ester; L-NMMA; NG-monomethyl-L-arginine; EIT, S-ethylisothiourea; AMT, 2-amino-5,6-dihydro-6-methyl-4H-1,3-thiazine; AG, aminoguanidine; L-NIL,L-N6-(1-iminoethyl)lysine; SMLT; S-methyl-L-thiocitrulline; 1400W, N-(3-(Aminomethyl)-benzyl) acetamidine; NS, nonspecific.

Since eNOS or nNOS-derived nitric oxide counteracts agonist-induced bronchoconstriction, (53), inhibition of these enzymes may enhance airway hyperresponsiveness (101,102). On the other hand, iNOS inhibition putatively protects against the detrimental effects of high-output nitric oxide release, thereby preventing the development of airway hyperresponsiveness. Hence, nonspecific nitric oxide synthase inhibition may antagonize the detrimental as well as the beneficial effects of nitric oxide. This nonspecificity may largely account for the conflicting data summarized in Table 1.

1400W is a highly selective, tightly binding iNOS inhibitor, which is about 1000-fold selective for iNOS compared with eNOS (99). Hence, the fact that 1400W inhibited allergen-induced airway hyperresponsiveness (97) strongly suggests that iNOS-derived nitric oxide release plays a causative role in the airway changes leading to hyperresponsiveness after allergen exposure in mice. Similar results were obtained in rats using the novel selective iNOS inhibitor SD3651 (96).

iNOS knockout studies so far have not shown a role for iNOS-derived nitric oxide in the development of airway hyperresponsiveness in mice. Xiong et al. reported inhibition of allergic airway inflammation in iNOS knockouts, but unaltered development of airway hyperresponsiveness (70), whereas De Sanctis et al. reported that knocking out the NOS2 gene affects neither allergic inflammation nor airway hyperresponsiveness (69). The fact that the production of IFN-γ by lung cells from iNOS knockout mice is increased is a likely explanation for the discrepancy between iNOS knockout and inhibitor studies. High levels of IFN-γ have been demonstrated to inhibit the development of allergen-induced airway hyperresponsiveness in mice (93). Therefore, the effects of knocking out iNOS on allergic airway disease might stretch further than just an abolishment of nitric oxide synthesis (103), such as, for example, an enhanced release of IFN-γ (70). Likewise, the NOS-inhibitor studies have the important drawbacks that the selectivity of the inhibitors is hard to demonstrate, and that it is impossible to block nitric oxide synthesis in vivo completely and continuously. Hence, it is impossible to draw strong conclusions about the NOS isoform involved in the development of airway hyperresponsiveness in mice. Despite the iNOS knockout results, many other studies strongly suggest a role for iNOS in humans, rats, guinea pigs, and mice, as mentioned above.

The NADPH oxidase inhibitor apocynin completely inhibits allergen-induced hyperresponsiveness in mice (97). This suggests that the development of allergen-induced hyperresponsiveness is dependent on superoxide formation as well as on nitric oxide release. Since reactive nitrogen species release by murine macrophages is dependent on both superoxide and nitric oxide (89), these data suggest that during allergic airway disease, superoxide release enhances the detrimental effects of nitric oxide and vice versa. It is therefore hypothesized that the development of allergen-induced hyperresponsiveness is dependent on the simultaneous release and consequent interaction of nitric oxide and superoxide. Thus, limiting superoxide release by apocynin may be the preferable strategy to limit the release of reactive nitrogen species, since there is no risk of inhibiting to bronchoprotective effects of nitric oxide on the airways.

D. A Puzzling Role for Neuronal Nitric Oxide Synthase in Hyperresponsiveness

Allergen-induced airway hyperresponsiveness is completely abolished in nNOS knockout mice (69). The mechanism by which nNOS could be involved in airway hyperresponsiveness, however, is unclear. nNOS is directly involved in the relaxation of airway smooth muscle by counteracting neuronal cholinergic responses (55,104,105). Moreover, nNOS is expressed in human airway smooth muscle cells and has been suggested to play an antiproliferative role (106).

IFN-γ inhibits nNOS expression in human astrocytoma cells (107) and in rat rectum, spleen, brain, and stomach as confirmed by Western blots (108). Hence, IFN-γ may not only promote the detrimental effects of nitric oxide by iNOS induction but may also compromise the bronchorelaxing function of nNOS.

Similarly to iNOS, nNOS could be of importance because of the detrimental effects of high-output nitric oxide synthesis and consequent reactive nitrogen species formation. Again, further research is required to elucidate whether such high-output nitric oxide synthesis by nNOS can occur in vivo.

Two independent studies show that variations in the nNOS gene are associated with human asthma (109,110), whereas such variations are not found for either iNOS or eNOS. The functional consequences of these variations, however, are unknown.

E. Mechanism of Reactive Nitrogen Species-Induced Airway Hyperresponsiveness

At present, one can only speculate how reactive nitrogen species, once released in the airways, contribute to airway hyperresponsiveness. A likely target for reactive nitrogen species is the airway epithelium, which has two important functions in controlling airway responsiveness. First, the epithelium forms a physical barrier protecting the airway interstitium against contractile agents; second, it is an important source of bronchorelaxant compounds (54). In asthmatic subjects epithelial shedding and damage have been reported (111), which also occur in mice after allergen challenge (112).

It is tempting to speculate that reactive nitrogen species contribute to epithelial damage during allergic airway inflammation, considering the numerous detrimental effects of the compounds on cells (43). In fact, reactive nitrogen species cause pulmonary cell death in vitro (113,114). Moreover, iNOS-mediated damage to the airway epithelium contributes to airway hyperresponsiveness in guinea pigs (115). Besides cytotoxic effects, reactive nitrogen species are likely to induce more subtle changes in the epithelium, such as, for example, changes in cyclo-oxygenase activity (116) and eNOS inhibition (117). Metalloproteases are activated by reactive nitrogen species (118,119); the consequent degradation of (extra)cellular proteins may further contribute to airway damage.

Kotsonis et al. showed that reactive nitrogen species are potent inhibitors of nNOS (120), which is an important source of nitric oxide involved in bronchorelaxation (55,104,105). Superoxide formation could also contribute to airway hyperresponsiveness by scavenging the bronchorelaxant nitric oxide, as shown in guinea pigs by De Boer et al. (121).

Human asthmatic airways show clear staining for 3-nitrotyrosine and iNOS in the airway epithelium (30), indicating that, in humans, the airway epithelium is exposed to nitrosative stress from inside the cells. In mice, however, allergen challenge does not induce iNOS (68) and 3-nitrotyrosine (97) staining in the airway epithelium. Hence, other sources of reactive nitrogen species may be of importance in mice, such as, for example, alveolar macrophages.

XI. Respiratory Tract Infections and Nitric Oxide

During a respiratory infection, NO may be important in three different ways, dependent on the situation. First, the enhanced NO synthesis and consequent reactive nitrogen species aggravate lung pathology because of the detrimental effects of these molecules on the host. Second, NO helps to eliminate the invading pathogen, thereby limiting the detrimental effects of infection. Last, a respiratory infection can compromise the bronchorelaxant effects of NO, which potentially promotes the development of airway hyperresponsiveness.

Although many respiratory infections lead to an enhanced nitric oxide synthesis and consequent release of reactive nitrogen species, this is not always beneficial for the disease outcome. In cases where nitric oxide release does not effectively inhibit the replication of the infectious agent involved, the negative effect of the nitrosative stress on the host may be particularly evident. In such cases, limiting NO synthesis may help to promote a positive disease outcome. This has been demonstrated in HSV-1-induced pneumonia in mice. Treatment of infected mice with a NOS inhibitor resulted in suppression of pneumonia, despite increased viral loads in the airways (122). Comparable results were obtained in mice infected with influenza virus (123). Finally, administration of a NOS inhibitor increased the survival rate of mice infected with *Streptococcus pneumoniae* (124).

A role for NO in host defense has been most strongly implicated in infections with intracellular pathogens including *Leishmania*, *Mycobacteria*, and *Salmonella* (9). Furthermore, iNOS knockout mice show an increased susceptibility to *Chlamydia pneumoniae* (125). In addition, nitric oxide plays a role in the defense against viruses (126). Experimental infection with influenza virus and rhinovirus increases exhaled NO levels in humans (127–129). In fact, increased nitric oxide levels in the exhaled air after rhinovirus infection are inversely correlated with worsening of airway hyperresponsiveness (128), which suggests a protective role for nitric oxide in exacerbations of asthma. Indeed, nitric oxide donors have been shown to inhibit rhinovirus replication in human epithelial cells in vitro (130). The mechanism by which NO or derivatives affect virus replication are not completely clear at present (126). Inhibition of RNA or protein synthesis and of DNA replication have been put forward as likely mechanisms (126). Moreover, nitrosylation of viral structural proteins may affect viral function (126).

The increased responsiveness of guinea pig tracheas after in vivo parainfluenza-3 virus infection is due to a decreased NO production (131). This suggests that viral infection impairs the bronchodilatory function of NO in guinea pig airways, presumably via a limited availability of the NOS substrate L-arginine.

XII. Summary

In conclusion, it appears that NO plays an important role in the pathophysiology of asthma. NO-derived reactive nitrogen species are readily formed during allergic airway inflammation and may have detrimental effects on airway function. In contrast to these detrimental effects, endogenously released NO also has a bronchoprotective role, because it is able to antagonize agonist-induced bronchoconstriction.

Infection of the airways is likely to affect both these pathways. Many respiratory infections induce the release of high amounts of nitric oxide, which in some cases helps to clear the invading pathogen, and in some cases aggravates the situation because of the putative detrimental effects on the host. On the other hand, a respiratory infection and the consequent immunological response may compromise the bronchoprotective effects of nitric oxide.

These phenomena open interesting new therapeutic approaches for the treatment of asthma exacerbations due to respiratory infections. A successful therapeutic approach, however, is dependent on the infectious agent involved. Dependent on the situation, either enhancement or limitation of NO synthesis may be required.

References

1. Moncada S, Palmer RMJ, Higgs EA. Nitric oxide: physiology, pathophysiology and pharmacology. Pharmacol Rev 1991; 43:109–142.
2. Gaston B, Drazen JM, Loscalzo J, Stamler JS. The biology of nitrogen oxides in the airways. Am J Respir Crit Care Med 1994; 149:538–551.
3. Moncada S, Palmer RMJ, Higgs EA. Biosynthesis of nitric oxide from L-arginine: a pathway for the regulation of cell function and communication. Biochem Pharmacol 1989; 38:1709–1715.
4. Kuriyama K, Ohkuma S. Role of nitric oxide in central synaptic transmission: effects on neurotransmitter release. Jpn J Pharmacol 1995; 69:1–8.
5. Snyder SH, Bredt DS. Nitric oxide as a neuronal messenger. TiPS 1991; 12:125–128.
6. Nathan CF. Nitric oxide as a secretory product of mammalian cells. FASEB J 1992; 6:3051–3064.
7. Rees DD, Cellek S, Palmer RMJ, Moncada S. Dexamethasone prevents the induction of a nitric oxide synthase and the associated effects on vascular tone: an insight into endotoxin shock. Biochem Biophys Res Commun 1990; 173:541–547.
8. Fang FC. Mechanisms of nitric oxide-related antimicrobial activity. J Clin Invest 1997; 99:2818–2825.
9. Fang FC. Perspectives series: host/pathogen interactions. Mechanisms of nitric oxide-related antimicrobial activity. J Clin Invest 1997; 99:2818–2825.
10. MacMicking JD, Nathan C, Hom G, Chartrain N, Fletcher DS, Trumbauer M, Stevens K, Xie QW, Sokol K, Hutchinson N. Altered responses to bacterial infection and endotoxic shock in mice lacking inducible nitric oxide synthase [published erratum appears in Cell 1995 Jun 30;81(7):following 1170]. Cell 1995; 81:641–650.
11. Wei XQ, Charles IG, Smith A, Ure J, Feng GJ, Huang FP, Xu D, Muller W. Altered immune responses in mice lacking inducible nitric-oxide synthase. Nature 1995; 375: 408–411.
12. Beckman JS, Koppenol WH. Nitric oxide, superoxide, and peroxynitrite: the good, the bad, and the ugly. Am J Physiol 1996; 40:C1424-C1437.
13. Muijsers RBR, Folkerts G, Henricks PAJ, Sadeghi-Hashjin G, Nijkamp FP. Peroxynitrite: a two-faced metabolite of nitric oxide. Life Sci 1997; 60:1833–1845.

14. Samdani AF, Dawson TM, Dawson VL. Nitric oxide synthase in models of focal ischemia. Stroke 1997; 28:1283–1288.

15. Babior BM. Oxygen dependent microbial killing by phagocytes. N Engl J Med 1978; 298:659–688.

16. McCord JM, Fridovch I. The utility of superoxide dismutase in studying free radical reactions. J Biol Chem 1969; 244:6056–6063.

17. Xia Y, Dawson VL, Dawson TM, Snyder SH, Zweier JL. Nitric oxide synthase generates superoxide and nitric oxide in arginine-depleted cells leading to peroxynitrite-mediated cellular injury. Proc Natl Acad Sci USA 1996; 93:6770–6774.

18. Mastroeni P, Vazquez-Torres A, Fang FC, Xu Y, Khan S, Hormaeche CE, Dougan G. Antimicrobial actions of the NADPH phagocyte oxidase and inducible nitric oxide synthase in experimental salmonellosis. II. Effects on microbial proliferation and host survival in vivo. J Exp Med 2000; 192:237–248.

19. Blough NV, Zafiriou OC. Reaction of superoxide with nitric oxide to form peroxynitrite in alkaline aqueous solution. Inorg Chem 1985; 24:3502–3504.

20. Huie RE, Padmaja S. The reaction of no with superoxide. Free Radic Res Commun 1993; 18:195–199.

21. Goldstein S, Czapski G. The reaction of NO with O_2^-- and HO_2: a pulse radiolysis study. Free Radic Biol Med 1995; 19:505–510.

22. Beckman JS, Beckman TW, Chen J, Marshall PA, Freeman BA. Apparent hydroxyl radical production by peroxynitrite: implications for endothelial injury from nitric oxide and superoxide. Proc Natl Acad of Sci USA 1990; 87:1620–1624.

23. Pryor WA, Squadrito GL. The chemistry of peroxynitrite: a product from the reaction of nitric oxide with superoxide. Am J Physiol 1995; 268:L699-L722.

24. Uppu RM, Squadrito GL, Pryor WA. Acceleration of peroxynitrite oxidations by carbon dioxide. Arch Biochem Biophys 1996; 327:335–343.

25. Reiter CD, Teng RJ, Beckman JS. Superoxide reacts with nitric oxide to nitrate tyrosine at physiological pH via peroxynitrite. J Biol Chem 2000; 275:32461–32466.

26. Eiserich JP, Hristova M, Cross CE, Jones AD, Freeman BA, Halliwell B, Van der Vliet A. Formation of nitric oxide-derived inflammatory oxidants by myeloperoxidase in neutrophils. Nature 1998; 391:393–397.

27. Bogdan C, Rollinghoff M, Diefenbach A. Reactive oxygen and reactive nitrogen intermediates in innate and specific immunity. Curr Opin Immunol 2000; 12:64–76.

28. Ochoa JB, Udekwu AO, Billiar TR, Curran RD, Cerra FB, Simmons RL, Peitzman AB. Nitrogen oxide levels in patients after trauma and during sepsis. Ann Surg 1991; 214:621–626.

29. Kelm M. Nitric oxide metabolism and breakdown. Biochim Biophys Acta 1999; 1411: 273–289.

30. Saleh D, Ernst P, Lim S, Barnes PJ, Giaid A. Increased formation of the potent oxidant peroxynitrite in the airways of asthmatic patients is associated with induction of nitric oxide synthase: effect of inhaled glucocorticoid. FASEB J 1998; 12:929–937.

31. Ohshima H, Celan I, Chazotte L, Pignatelli B, Mower HF. Analysis of 3-nitrotyrosine in biological fluids and protein hydrolyzates by high-performance liquid chromatography using a postseparation, on-line reduction column and electrochemical detection: results with various nitrating agents. Nitric Oxide 1999; 3:132–141.

32. Dupont LJ, Rochette F, Demedts MG, Verleden GM. Exhaled nitric oxide correlates with airway hyperresponsiveness in steroid-naive patients with mild asthma. Am J Respir Crit Care Med 1998; 157:894–898.

33. Massaro AF, Mehta S, Lilly CM, Kobzik L, Reilly JJ, Drazen JM. Elevated nitric oxide concentrations in isolated lower airway gas of asthmatic subjects. Am J Respir Crit Care Med 1996; 153:1510–1514.
34. ten Hacken NH, van der Vaart H, van der Mark TW, Koeter GH, Postma DS. Exhaled nitric oxide is higher both at day and night in subjects with nocturnal asthma. Am J Respir Crit Care Med 1998; 158:902–907.
35. Ahren C, Jungersten L, Sandberg T. Plasma nitrate as an index of nitric oxide formation in patients with acute infectious diseases. Scand J Infect Dis 1999; 31:405–407.
36. Zweier JL, Samouilov A, Kuppusamy P. Non-enzymatic nitric oxide synthesis in biological systems. Biochim Biophys Acta 1999; 1411:250–262.
37. Hunt JF, Fang K, Malik R, Snyder A, Malhotra N, Platts-Mills TA, Gaston B. Endogenous airway acidification. Implications for asthma pathophysiology. Am J Respir Crit Care Med 2000; 161:694–699.
38. Van der Vliet A, Eiserich JP, Shigenaga MK, Cross CE. Reactive nitrogen species and tyrosine nitration in the respiratory tract: epiphenomena or a pathobiologic mechanism of disease? Am J Respir Crit Care Med 1999; 160:1–9.
39. Gaston B. Nitric oxide and thiol groups. Biochim Biophys Acta 1999; 1411:323–333.
40. O'Donnell VB, Eiserich JP, Bloodsworth A, Chumley PH, Kirk M, Barnes S, Darley-Usmar VM, Freeman BA. Nitration of unsaturated fatty acids by nitric oxide-derived reactive species. Methods Enzymol 1999; 301:454–470.
41. Zingarelli B, Oconnor M, Wong H, Salzman AL, Szabo C. Peroxynitrite-mediated DNA strand breakage activates poly-adenosine diphosphate ribosyl synthetase and causes cellular energy depletion in macrophages stimulated with bacterial lipopolysaccharide. J Immunol 1996; 156:350–358.
42. Packer MA, Murphy MP. Peroxynitrite formed by simultaneous nitric oxide and superoxide generation causes cyclosporin-A-sensitive mitochondrial calcium efflux and depolarization. Eur J Biochem 1985; 234:231–239.
43. Eiserich JP, Patel RP, O'Donnell VB. Pathophysiology of nitric oxide and related species: free radical reactions and modification of biomolecules. Mol Aspects Med 1998; 19:221–357.
44. Murphy MP. Nitric oxide and cell death. Biochim Biophys Acta 1999; 1411:401–414.
45. Kettle AJ, van Dalen CJ, Winterbourn CC. Peroxynitrite and myeloperoxidase leave the same footprint in protein nitration. Redox Rep 1997; 3:257–258.
46. Wu W, Chen Y, Hazen SL. Eosinophil peroxidase nitrates protein tyrosyl residues. Implications for oxidative damage by nitrating intermediates in eosinophilic inflammatory disorders. J Biol Chem 1999; 274:25933–25944.
47. Hobbs AJ, Higgs A, Moncada S. Inhibition of nitric oxide synthase as a potential therapeutic target. Annu Rev Pharmacol Toxicol 1999; 39:191–220.
48. Swislocki A, Eason T, Kaysen GA. Oral administration of the nitric oxide biosynthesis inhibitor, N-nitro- L-arginine methyl ester (L-NAME), causes hypertension, but not glucose intolerance or insulin resistance, in rats. Am J Hypertens 1995; 8:1009–1014.
49. Weinberg JB, Misukonis MA, Shami PJ, Mason SN, Sauls DL, Dittman WA, Wood ER, Smith GK, McDonald B, Bachus KE. Human mononuclear phagocyte inducible nitric oxide synthase (iNOS): analysis of iNOS mRNA, iNOS protein, biopterin, and nitric oxide production by blood monocytes and peritoneal macrophages. Blood 1995; 86:1184–1195.
50. Weinberg JB. Nitric oxide production and nitric oxide synthase type 2 expression by human mononuclear phagocytes: a review. Mol Med 1998; 4:557–591.

51. Harvey BH. Acid-dependent dismutation of nitrogen oxides may be a critical source of nitric oxide in human macrophages. Med Hypotheses 2000; 54:829–831.

52. Hazen SL, Zhang R, Shen Z, Wu W, Podrez EA, MacPherson JC, Schmitt D, Mitra SN, Mukhopadhyay C, Chen Y, Cohen PA, Hoff HF, Abu-Soud HM. Formation of nitric oxide-derived oxidants by myeloperoxidase in monocytes: pathways for mono-cyte-mediated protein nitration and lipid peroxidation In vivo. Circ Res 1999; 85:950–958.

53. Lei YH, Barnes PJ, Rogers DF. Regulation of NANC neural bronchoconstriction in vivo in the guinea- pig: involvement of nitric oxide, vasoactive intestinal peptide and soluble guanylyl cyclase. Br J Pharmacol 1993; 108:228–235.

54. Folkerts G, Nijkamp FP. Airway epithelium: more than just a barrier! Trends Pharmacol Sci 1998; 19:334–341.

55. Ward JK, Barnes PJ, Springall DR, Abelli L, Tadjkarimi S, Yacoub MH, Polak JM, Belvisi MG. Distribution of human i-NANC bronchodilator and nitric oxide-immuno-reactive nerves. Am J Respir Cell Mol Biol 1995; 13:175–184.

56. de Gouw HW, Hendriks J, Woltman AM, Twiss IM, Sterk PJ. Exhaled nitric oxide (NO) is reduced shortly after bronchoconstriction to direct and indirect stimuli in asthma. Am J Respir Crit Care Med 1998; 158:315–319.

57. Barnes PJ, Liew FY. Nitric oxide and asthmatic inflammation. Immunol Today 1995; 16:128–130.

58. Barnes PJ. NO or no NO in asthma? Thorax 1996; 51:218–229.

59. Kharitonov SA, Yates DH, Barnes PJ. Inhaled glucocorticoids decrease nitric oxide in exhaled air of asthmatic patients. Am J Respir Crit Care Med 1996; 153:454–457.

60. Jatakanon A, Kharitonov S, Lim S, Barnes PJ. Effect of differing doses of inhaled budesonide on markers of airway inflammation in patients with mild asthma. Thorax 1999; 54:108–114.

61. Calhoun WJ, Reed HE, Moest DR, Stevens CA. Enhanced superoxide production by alveolar macrophages and air-space cells, airway inflammation, and alveolar macro-phage density changes after segmental antigen bronchoprovocation in allergic subjects. Am Rev Respir Dis 1992; 145:317–325.

62. Liew FY. Regulation of lymphocyte functions by nitric oxide. Curr. Opin. Immunol 1995; 7:396–399.

63. Chang RH, Feng MH, Liu WH, Lai MZ. Nitric oxide increased interleukin-4 expression in T lymphocytes. Immunology 1997; 90:364–369.

64. Roozendaal R, Vellenga E, Postma DS, De Monchy JG, Kauffman HF. Nitric oxide selectively decreases interferon-gamma expression by activated human T lymphocytes via a cGMP-independent mechanism. Immunology 1999; 98:393–399.

65. Hamid Q, Springall DR, Riveros-Moreno V, Chanez P, Howarth P, Redington A, Bousquet J, Godard P, Holgate S, Polak JM. Induction of nitric oxide synthase in asthma. Lancet 1993; 342:1510–1513.

66. Guo FH, Comhair SA, Zheng S, Dweik RA, Eissa NT, Thomassen MJ, Calhoun W, Erzurum SC. Molecular mechanisms of increased nitric oxide (NO) in asthma: evidence for transcriptional and post-translational regulation of NO synthesis. J Immunol 2000; 164:5970–5980.

67. Liu SF, Haddad EB, Adcock I, Salmon M, Koto H, Gilbey T, Barnes PJ, Chung KF. Inducible nitric oxide synthase after sensitization and allergen challenge of Brown Norway rat lung. Br J Pharmacol 1997; 121:1241–1246.

68. Trifilieff A, Fujitani Y, Mentz F, Dugas B, Fuentes M, Bertrand C. Inducible nitric oxide synthase inhibitors suppress airway inflammation in mice through down-regulation of chemokine expression. J Immunol 2000; 165:1526–1533.

69. De Sanctis GT, MacLean JA, Hamada K, Mehta S, Scott JA, Jiao A, Yandava CN, Kobzik L, Wolyniec WW, Fabian AJ, Venugopal CS, Grasemann H, Huang PL, Drazen JM. Contribution of nitric oxide synthases 1, 2, and 3 to airway hyperresponsiveness and inflammation in a murine model of asthma. J Exp Med 1999; 189:1621–1630.

70. Xiong Y, Karupiah G, Hogan SP, Foster PS, Ramsay AJ. Inhibition of allergic airway inflammation in mice lacking nitric oxide synthase 2. J Immunol 1999; 162:445–452.

71. Robbins RA, Barnes PJ, Springall DR, Warren JB, Kwon OJ, Buttery LD, Wilson AJ, Geller DA, Polak JM. Expression of inducible nitric oxide in human lung epithelial cells. Biochem Biophys Res Commun 1994; 203:209–218.

72. Walker G, Pfeilschifter J, Kunz D. Mechanisms of suppression of inducible nitric-oxide synthase (iNOS) expression in interferon (IFN)-gamma-stimulated RAW 264.7 cells by dexamethasone. Evidence for glucocorticoid-induced degradation of iNOS protein by calpain as a key step in post-transcriptional regulation. J Biol Chem 1997; 272:16679–16687.

73. Kharitonov SA, Yates DH, Chung KF, Barnes PJ. Changes in the dose of inhaled steroid affect exhaled nitric oxide levels in asthmatic patients. Eur Respir J 1996; 19: 196–201.

74. Guo FH, De-Raeve HR, Rice TW, Stuehr DJ, Thunnissen FB, Erzurum SC. Continuous nitric oxide synthesis by inducible nitric oxide synthase in normal human airway epithelium in vivo. Proc Natl Acad Sci USA 1995; 92:7809–7813.

75. Guo FH, Uetani K, Haque SJ, Williams BR, Dweik RA, Thunnissen FB, Calhoun W, Erzurum SC. Interferon gamma and interleukin 4 stimulate prolonged expression of inducible nitric oxide synthase in human airway epithelium through synthesis of soluble mediators [published erratum appears in J Clin Invest 1997; 100(5):1322]. J Clin Invest 1997; 100:829–838.

76. Punjabi CJ, Laskin JD, Pendino KJ, Goller NL, Durham SK, Laskin DL. Production of nitric oxide by rat type II pneumocytes: increased expression of inducible nitric oxide synthase following inhalation of a pulmonary irritant. Am J Respir Cell Mol Biol 1994; 11:165–172.

77. Hessel EM, Van Oosterhout AJ, Van Ark I, Van Esch B, Hofman G, Van Loveren H, Savelkoul HF, Nijkamp FP. Development of airway hyperresponsiveness is dependent on interferon- gamma and independent of eosinophil infiltration. Am J Respir Cell Mol Biol 1997; 16:325–334.

78. Ying S, Durham SR, Corrigan CJ, Hamid Q, Kay AB. Phenotype of cells expressing mRNA for TH2-type (interleukin 4 and interleukin 5) and TH1-type (interleukin 2 and interferon gamma) cytokines in bronchoalveolar lavage and bronchial biopsies from atopic asthmatic and normal control subjects. Am J Respir Cell Mol Biol 1995; 12: 477–487.

79. Muijsers R, Folkerts G, Van-Den-Worm E, Beukelman C, Postma D, Nijkamp F. Inhibition of peroxynitrite formation by apocynin in a murine macrophage cell-line. Br J Pharmacol 1998; 123:41P.

80. Kolb JP, Paul-Eugene N, Damais C, Yamaoka K, Drapier JC, Dugas B. Interleukin-4 stimulates cGMP production by IFN-gamma-activated human monocytes. Involvement of the nitric oxide synthase pathway. J Biol Chem 1994; 269:9811–9816.

81. Kolb JP, Paul-Eugene DN, Yamaoka K, Mossalayi MD, Dugas B. Role of CD23 in NO production by human monocytic cells. Res Immunol 1995; 146:684–689.

82. Atsuta J, Sterbinsky SA, Plitt J, Schwiebert LM, Bochner BS, Schleimer RP. Phenotyping and cytokine regulation of the BEAS-2B human bronchial epithelial cell: demonstration of inducible expression of the adhesion molecules VCAM-1 and ICAM-1. Am J Respir Cell Mol Biol 1997; 17:571–582.

83. Demoly P, Damon M, Michel FB, Godard P. IFN-gamma activates superoxide anion production in blood monocytes from allergic asthmatic patients. Ann Allergy Asthma Immunol 1995; 75:162–166.

84. Joseph BZ, Routes JM, Borish L. Activities of superoxide dismutases and NADPH oxidase in neutrophils obtained from asthmatic and normal donors. Inflammation 1993; 17:361–370.

85. van Klaveren RJ, Roelant C, Boogaerts M, Demedts M, Nemery B. Involvement of an NAD(P)H oxidase-like enzyme in superoxide anion and hydrogen peroxide generation by rat type II cells. Thorax 1997, 52:465–471.

86. Al-Mehdi AB, Zhao G, Dodia C, Tozawa K, Costa K, Muzykantov V, Ross C, Blecha F, Dinauer M, Fisher AB. Endothelial NADPH oxidase as the source of oxidants in lungs exposed to ischemia or high K+. Circ Res 1998; 83:730–737.

87. Ikuta N, Sugiyama S, Takagi K, Satake T, Ozawa T. Implication of oxygen radicals on airway hyperresponsiveness after ovalbumin challenge in guinea pigs. Am Rev Respir Dis 1992; 145:561–565.

88. Rottenberg ME, Gigliotti Rothfuchs A, Gigliotti D, Ceausu M, Une C, Levitsky V, Wigzell H. Regulation and role of IFN-gamma in the innate resistance to infection with Chlamydia pneumoniae. J Immunol 2000; 164:4812–4818.

89. Muijsers RBR, Van Den Worm E, Folkerts G, Beukelman CJ, Koster AS, Postma DS, Nijkamp FP. Apocynin inhibits peroxynitrite formation by murine macrophages. Br J Pharmacol 2000; 130:932–936.

90. Feder LS, Stelts D, Chapman RW, Manfra D, Crawley Y, Jones H, Minnicozzi M, Fernandez X, Paster T, Egan RW, Kreutner W, Kung TT. Role of nitric oxide on eosinophilic lung inflammation in allergic mice. Am J Respir Cell Mol Biol 1997; 17: 436–442.

91. Ferreira HH, Bevilacqua E, Gagioti SM, De Luca IM, Zanardo RC, Teixeira CE, Sannomiya P, Antunes E, De Nucci G. Nitric oxide modulates eosinophil infiltration in antigen-induced airway inflammation in rats. Eur J Pharmacol 1998; 358:253–259.

92. Iijima H, Uchida Y, Endo T, Xiang A, Shirato M, Nomura A, Hasegawa S. Role of endogenous nitric oxide in allergen-induced airway responses in guinea-pigs. Br J Pharmacol 1998; 124:1019–1028.

93. Hofstra CL, Van Ark I, Hofman G, Nijkamp FP, Jardieu PM, Van Oosterhout AJ. Differential effects of endogenous and exogenous interferon-gamma on immunoglobulin E, cellular infiltration, and airway responsiveness in a murine model of allergic asthma. Am J Respir Cell Mol Biol 1998; 19:826–835.

94. Mehta S, Lilly CM, Rollenhagen JE, Haley KJ, Asano K, Drazen JM. Acute and chronic effects of allergic airway inflammation on pulmonary nitric oxide production. Am J Physiol 1997; 272:L124–131.

95. Tulic MK, Wale JL, Holt PG, Sly PD. Differential effects of nitric oxide synthase inhibitors in an in vivo allergic rat model. Eur Respir J 2000; 15:870–877.

96. Eynott PR, Hanazawa P, Tomita K, Caramori G, Donnelly LE, Adcock IM, Kharitonov SA, Barnes PJ, Chung KF. The effects of selective inhibitor of inducible NO synthase

in a Brown-Norway rat model of allergic asthma. Am J Respir Crit Care Med 2000; 161:A919.

97.   Muijsers RBR, Van Ark I, Folkerts G, Van Oosterhout AJM, Koster AS, Postma DS, Nijkamp FP. Inhibitors of both NADPH-oxidase and nitric oxide synthase prevent airway hyperresponsivenss but not allergic inflammation in a murine model of asthma. Am J Respir Crit Care Med 2000; 161:A746.

98.   Southan GJ, Szabo C. Selective pharmacological inhibition of distinct nitric oxide synthase isoforms. Biochem Pharmacol 1996; 51:383–394.

99.   Garvey EP, Oplinger JA, Furfine ES, Kiff RJ, Laszlo F, Whittle BJ, Knowles RG. 1400W is a slow, tight binding, and highly selective inhibitor of inducible nitric-oxide synthase in vitro and in vivo. J Biol Chem 1997; 272:4959–4963.

100. Misko TP, Moore WM, Kasten TP, Nickols GA, Corbett JA, Tilton RG, McDaniel ML, Williamson JR, Currie MG. Selective inhibition of the inducible nitric oxide synthase by aminoguanidine. Eur J Pharmacol 1993; 233:119–125.

101. Schuiling M, Zuidhof AB, Bonouvrie MA, Venema N, Zaagsma J, Meurs H. Role of nitric oxide in the development and partial reversal of allergen-induced airway hyperreactivity in conscious, unrestrained guinea-pigs. Br J Pharmacol 1998; 123:1450–1456.

102. Nijkamp FP, van-der-Linde HJ, Folkerts G. Nitric oxide synthesis inhibitors induce airway hyperresponsiveness in the guinea pig in vivo and in vitro. Role of the epithelium. Am Rev Respir Dis 1993; 148:727–734.

103. Mashimo H, Goyal RK. Lessons from genetically engineered animal models. IV. Nitric oxide synthase gene knockout mice. Am J Physiol 1999; 277:G745–750.

104. Kakuyama M, Ahluwalia A, Rodrigo J, Vallance P. Cholinergic contraction is altered in nNOS knockouts. Cooperative modulation of neural bronchoconstriction by nnos and cox. Am J Respir Crit Care Med 1999; 160:2072–2078.

105. Ward JK, Belvisi MG, Fox AJ, Miura M, Tadjkarimi S, Yacoub MH, Barnes PJ. Modulation of cholinergic neural bronchoconstriction by endogenous nitric oxide and vasoactive intestinal peptide in human airways in vitro. J Clin Invests 1993; 92:736–742.

106. Patel HJ, Belvisi MG, Donnelly LE, Yacoub MH, Chung KF, Mitchell JA. Constitutive expressions of type I NOS in human airway smooth muscle cells: evidence for an antiproliferative role. FASEB J 1999; 13:1810–1816.

107. Colasanti M, Persichini T, Cavalieri E, Fabrizi C, Mariotto S, Menegazzi M, Lauro GM, Suzuki H. Rapid inactivation of NOS-I by lipopolysaccharide plus interferon-gamma- induced tyrosine phosphorylation. J Biol Chem 1999; 274:9915–9917.

108. Bandyopadhyay A, Chakder S, Rattan S. Regulation of inducible and neuronal nitric oxide synthase gene expression by interferon-gamma and VIP. Am J Physiol 1997; 272:C1790–1797.

109. Gao PS, Kawada H, Kasamatsu T, Mao XQ, Roberts MH, Miyamoto Y, Yoshimura M, Saitoh Y, Yasue H, Nakao K, Adra CN, Kun JF, Moro-oka S, Inoko H, Ho LP, Shirakawa T, Hopkin JM. Variants of NOS1, NOS2, and NOS3 genes in asthmatics. Biochem Biophys Res Commun 2000; 267:761–763.

110. Grasemann H, Yandava CN, Drazen JM. Neuronal NO synthase (NOS1) is a major candidate gene for asthma. Clin Exp Allergy 1999; 29 Suppl 4:39–41.

111. Jeffery P. Structural alterations and inflammation of bronchi in asthma. Int J Clin Pract Suppl 1998; 96:5–14.

112. Garlisi CG, Falcone A, Hey JA, Paster TM, Fernandez X, Rizzo CA, Minnicozzi M, Jones H, Billah MM, Egan RW, Umland SP. Airway eosinophils, T cells, Th2-type cytokine mRNA, and hyperreactivity in response to aerosol challenge of allergic mice

with previously established pulmonary inflammation. Am J Respir Cell Mol Biol 1997; 17:642–651.

113. Gow AJ, Thom SR, Ischiropoulos H. Nitric oxide and peroxynitrite-mediated pulmonary cell death. Am J Physiol 1998; 274:L112-L118.

114. Kampf C, Relova AJ, Sandler S, Roomans GM. Effects of TNF-alpha, IFN-gamma and IL-beta on normal human bronchial epithelial cells. Eur Respir J 1999; 14:84–91.

115. Schuiling M, Meurs H, Zuidhof AB, Venema N, Zaagsma J. Dual action of iNOS-derived nitric oxide in allergen-induced airway hyperreactivity in conscious, unrestrained guinea pigs. Am J Respir Crit Care Med 1998; 158:1442–1449.

116. Watkins DN, Garlepp MJ, Thompson PJ. Regulation of the inducible cyclo-oxygenase pathway in human cultured airway epithelial (A549) cells by nitric oxide. Br J Pharmacol 1997; 121:1482–1488.

117. Sheehy AM, Burson MA, Black SM. Nitric oxide exposure inhibits endothelial NOS activity but not gene expression: a role for superoxide. Am J Physiol 1998; 274:L833–841.

118. Maeda H, Okamoto T, Akaike T. Human matrix metalloprotease activation by insults of bacterial infection involving proteases and free radicals. Biol Chem 1998; 379:193–200.

119. Murrell GA, Jang D, Williams RJ. Nitric oxide activates metalloprotease enzymes in articular cartilage. Biochem Biophys Res Commun 1995; 206:15–21.

120. Kotsonis P, Frey A, Frohlich LG, Hofmann H, Reif A, Wink DA, Feelisch M, Schmidt HH. Autoinhibition of neuronal nitric oxide synthase: distinct effects of reactive nitrogen and oxygen species on enzyme activity. Biochem J 1999; 340:745–752.

121. De Boer J, Pouw FM, Zaagsma J, Meurs H. Effects of endogenous superoxide anion and nitric oxide on cholinergic constriction of normal and hyperreactive guinea pig airways. Am J Respir Crit Care Med 1998; 158:1784–1789.

122. Adler H, Beland JL, Del-Pan NC, Kobzik L, Brewer JP, Martin TR, Rimm IJ. Suppression of herpes simplex virus type 1 (HSV-1)-induced pneumonia in mice by inhibition of inducible nitric oxide synthase (iNOS, NOS2). J Exp Med 1997; 185:1533–1540.

123. Akaike T, Noguchi Y, Ijiri S, Setoguchi K, Suga M, Zheng YM, Dietzschold B, Maeda H. Pathogenesis of influenza virus-induced pneumonia: involvement of both nitric oxide and oxygen radicals. Proc Natl Acad Sci USA 1996; 93:2448–2453.

124. Bergeron Y, Ouellet N, Simard M, Olivier M, Bergeron MG. Immunomodulation of pneumococcal pulmonary infection with N(G)- monomethyl-L-arginine. Antimicrob Agents Chemother 1999; 43:2283–2290.

125. Rottenberg ME, Gigliotti Rothfuchs AC, Gigliotti D, Svanholm C, Bandholtz L, Wigzell H. Role of innate and adaptive immunity in the outcome of primary infection with Chlamydia pneumoniae, as analyzed in genetically modified mice. J Immunol 1999; 162:2829–2836.

126. Reiss CS, Komatsu T. Does nitric oxide play a critical role in viral infections? J Virol 1998; 72:4547–4551.

127. Murphy AW, Platts-Mills TA, Lobo M, Hayden F. Respiratory nitric oxide levels in experimental human influenza. Chest 1998; 114:452–456.

128. de Gouw HW, Grunberg K, Schot R, Kroes AC, Dick EC, Sterk PJ. Relationship between exhaled nitric oxide and airway hyperresponsiveness following experimental rhinovirus infection in asthmatic subjects. Eur Respir J 1998; 11:126–132.

129. Kharitonov SA, Yates D, Barnes PJ. Increased nitric oxide in exhaled air of normal human subjects with upper respiratory tract infections. Eur Respir J 1995; 8:295–297.

130. Sanders SP, Siekierski ES, Porter JD, Richards SM, Proud D. Nitric oxide inhibits rhinovirus-induced cytokine production and viral replication in a human respiratory epithelial cell line. J Virol 1998; 72:934–942.

131. Folkerts G, Van der Linde HJ, Nijkamp FP. Virus-induced Airway hyperresponsiveness in guinea pigs is related to a deficiency in nitric-oxide. J Clin Invest 1995; 95: 26–30.

11

Effects of Virus Infection on Airway Neural Control

RICHARD W. COSTELLO

Royal College of Surgeons in Ireland
Dublin, Ireland

I. Introduction

Many of the clinical features of respiratory tract virus infections, including cough, wheeze, and sputum production, are mediated, in part, by the action of airway nerves. Since stimulation of some airway nerves mimics the clinical features of a respiratory tract virus infection, it is not surprising that activation of these nerves is an important pathogenic feature of these infections. The various mechanisms by which viruses activate airway nerves will be discussed in this chapter. In addition to playing a role in mediating the symptoms of virus infection, airway nerves also play an active role in mediating the host's response to a respiratory virus infection. These interactions between the host, exerted through airway nerves, and respiratory viruses will also be discussed. In humans, it is relatively difficult to study airway nerve function in vivo and hence much of the research outlined in this chapter has been performed in animal models. There is a considerable degree of interspecies variability in neural function, in particular in the function of sensory nerves. This variability in nerve function between species adds to the difficulty of translating the results of animal experiments to humans. Thus, in this chapter the results of studies on human subjects have been emphasized.

II. Innervation of the Airways

The airway walls are innervated with a dense network of several types of nerve fibers from the autonomic nervous system. These nerves function in an integrated manner to protect the airways from potentially harmful inhaled compounds. This protection involves an afferent sensory limb that detects chemical or mechanical changes in the airways and an efferent motor limb that responds to stimuli by changes in the respiratory breathing patterns, by contracting the smooth muscle, and by secreting mucus.

The autonomic innervation of the airways is composed of fibers from the vagus nerves and from fibers from the cranial and thoracic sympathetic ganglia (1). These nerves innervate the anterior and posterior pulmonary plexus at the hilum of the lung. From the hilum the nerves divide into two plexi of nerves: a peribronchial plexus and a periarterial plexus. Based on their position relative to the cartilaginous plates, the peribronchial plexus is further classified into two subdivisions called the extrachondrial plexus and the subchondrial plexus. The peribronchial nerve fibers extend throughout the airways to innervate the bronchi and bronchioles but not the alveoli (1–16). Local ganglia through which these nerves relay are located on the posterior aspect of the trachea and major bronchi. From these ganglia, short postganglionic fibers extend to innervate structures within the trachea, bronchi, and bronchioles such as the mucus glands, smooth muscle, and bronchial blood vessels. The periarterial plexus follows the pulmonary arteries, innervating all vessels except the pulmonary capillaries and veins (17,18). Together these nerves provide the afferent sensory and motor efferent innervation of the lungs.

A. Parasympathetic Airway Neural Innervation

The parasympathetic cholinergic nerves in the vagus nerves provide the dominant innervation of the airways. Stimulation of these nerves results in mucus production, bronchoconstriction, and increased mucosal blood flow, which is of particular importance in the upper airway where it leads to nasal blockage and stuffiness. The cell bodies of the parasympathetic nerves lie in the nucleus ambigus and extend through the neck and chest to the trachea and major bronchi where they relay at cholinergic ganglia (19,20). From these ganglia short postganglionic fibers extend to the smooth muscle, glandular tissue, and the bronchial vessels (Fig.1). Administration of acetylcholine or stimulation of the parasympathetic nerves causes the airway smooth muscle to contract (21), the glandular tissue to secrete mucus (22,23), and the bronchial circulation to dilate (24,25). In the airways the parasympathetic nerves exert their influence by releasing acetylcholine onto nicotinic receptors on the cholinergic ganglia and onto muscarinic receptors. Muscarinic receptors are found on many structures in the lung; most of these are directly innervated by branches from the parasympathetic nerves.

Muscarinic Receptors in the Airways

In 1914, work done by Henry Dale, for which he was later awarded the Nobel Prize for Medicine and Physiology, identified that acetylcholine activated two groups of

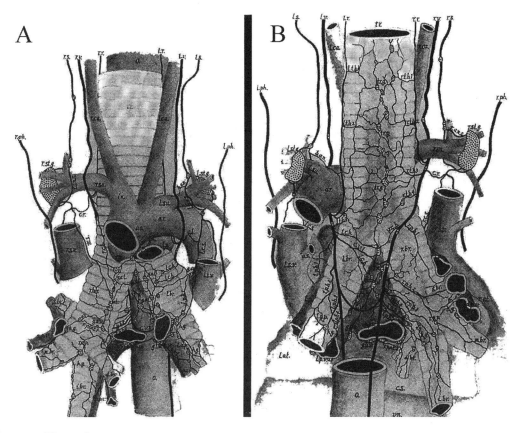

Figure 1 Anterior (A) and posterior (B) aspects of the trachea, bronchi, and great vessels of the mouse. The left (lv) and the right vagus (rv) as well as the left and right recurrent (rr and lr) and superior laryngeal nerves (rs, ls) branches, outlined in black, were demonstrated using the technique of silver staining. The ganglia are interspersed along the posterior wall of the trachea and along the anterior and posterior walls of the bronchi. The densest innervation of the lung is at the hilum. (From Ref. 187.)

receptors that were also activated separately either by muscarine or by nicotine (26). It was subsequently shown by the use of selective muscarinic receptor antagonists that there were four different muscarinic receptor subtypes. Bonner and colleagues screened a rat and human cDNA library and reported the genetic and protein sequences of four human muscarinic receptors and a fifth receptor for which a ligand has yet to be identified (27,28). All of these receptors share the common characteristics of being seven transmembrane domain G-protein linked receptors (29,30). There are considerable structural similarities among the five receptors, in particular their transmembrane folding structure. However, the third intracellular loop is different among the receptors and this allows each receptor to be linked to different intracellular signal transduction systems (31).

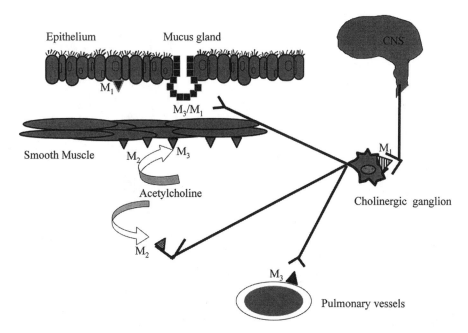

Figure 2 Distribution of muscarinic receptors within human airways. Muscarinic M_1 receptors are also found in high concentrations in the lung periphery and on airway epithelial cells, where they receive no direct innervation. M_3 muscarinic receptors are also found on various inflammatory cells including macrophages.

Distribution and Muscarinic Receptors in the Lungs

Autoradiographic imaging and ligand binding studies have established that M_1, M_2, and M_3 muscarinic receptors are found in the airways of all species studied including humans (32–36). The distribution and function of each of these three muscarinic receptor subtypes will be discussed below and are shown in Figure 2.

Muscarinic M_1 Receptors

M_1 muscarinic receptors make up more than 50% of all muscarinic receptors found in human airways (37). They are found in the peripheral airways in high abundance, although most of them do not appear to be innervated by parasympathetic nerves. Studies have shown that epithelial cells possess the ability to make acetylcholine and thus there may be a local non-neuronal action of acetylcholine exerted by these cells (38). Non-parasympathetic nerve innervated M_1 muscarinic receptors are found on nasal epithelial cells, where they play a role in controlling ciliary beat frequency, release of epithelial neutrophil and monocyte chemoattractants, and possibly also in the regulation of communication between cells (39–42). M_1 muscarinic receptors, along with neutrophil elastase, play a role in the release of the anti-inflammatory agent secretory leukocyte protease inhibitor from submucosal glandular tissue (43). M_1 muscarinic receptors are also located on human pulmonary vein endothelial cells and are responsible for vagally mediated relaxation of these vessels (44,45). M_1 muscarinic receptors are also located on postganglionic cholinergic nerves at cholinergic ganglia. Under normal circumstances the function of M_1 muscarinic receptors within cholinergic ganglia is to play a role in facilitating neurotransmission. Experimental studies have shown that the principal function of these ganglia associated M_1 muscarinic receptors is in the regulation of airway tone rather than mediating bronchoconstrictor responses (46). Thus, although widely distributed in the airways, these receptors do not appear to play a pivotal role in the control of airway function.

Muscarinic M_2 Receptors

In the lungs, muscarinic receptors are located on postganglionic parasympathetic nerve fibers and on airway smooth muscle cells. M_2 muscarinic receptors are coupled to a pertussis toxin-sensitive G-protein, Gi, stimulation of which leads to an inhibition of the enzyme adenylate cyclase (29). Neuronal M_2 muscarinic receptors exert control over the release of acetylcholine from parasympathetic nerves (47–49). In in vitro studies on human tissue as well as in in vivo studies in animals it has been shown that stimulation of M_2 muscarinic receptors with agonists such as pilocarpine inhibits vagally induced bronchoconstriction by as much as 70% (47,50,51). Conversely, blockade of these receptors potentiates the release of acetylcholine by as much as fivefold and increases vagally induced bronchoconstriction by a similar amount. Thus, neuronal M_2 muscarinic receptors provide an important inhibitory control over the release of acetylcholine and subsequently over the magnitude of vagally induced bronchoconstriction.

M_2 muscarinic receptors on the airway smooth muscle make up the majority of all smooth muscle muscarinic receptors in humans. Stimulation of airway smooth muscle M_2 muscarinic receptors functionally promotes the contractile effects of M_3 muscarinic receptors by inhibiting β-adrenoreceptor-induced increases in adenylate cyclase (52,53). Thus, acute dysfunction of M_2 muscarinic receptors on either the smooth muscle or parasympathetic nerves leads to enhanced vagally induced bronchoconstriction. In contrast to these acute effects, recent studies have indicated that chronic agonist stimulation of these receptors leads to enhanced adenylate cyclase activity (54). Thus, in contrast to the acute situation, chronic stimulation of M_2 muscarinic receptors on airway smooth muscle promotes relaxation, in particular following β-adrenoreceptor stimulation. Further studies will be required to investigate whether a similar process occurs, in vivo, in humans.

Muscarinic M_3 Receptors

M_3 muscarinic receptors are found on airway muscle in the pulmonary vasculature, on mucus glands, and on some inflammatory cells found in the airways. Stimulation of M_3 muscarinic receptors leads to smooth muscle contraction (55) and mucus production (56). Thus, stimulation of M_3 muscarinic receptors by acetylcholine leads to a number of effects that mimic the clinical symptoms of a virus infection.

B. Sympathetic Airway Neural Innervation

The cell bodies of the sympathetic nerves arise in the brainstem; branches of these nerves leave the CNS via the thoracic and cervical spinal cord. Preganglionic sympathetic nerve fibers relay at ganglia in the thoracic and sympathetic prevertebral ganglia. Postganglionic fibers enter the lung within the peribronchial and periarterial plexus (19). The majority of these fibers innervate the airway cholinergic ganglia and pulmonary arteries and arterioles. Several studies have shown that the adrenergic innervation of the rest of the lung, and in particular of the airway smooth muscle, is relatively sparse (3,16,57,58). The principal neurotransmitter released from these nerves is norepinephrine and this acts by binding to adrenoreceptors.

Studies using sympathomimetic agonists have shown that there are two main types of adrenoreceptors termed α and β. Both subtypes of adrenoreceptor are further classified into α_{1-2} and β_{1-3} subtypes based on agonist selectivity. In humans submucosal blood vessels, in particular in the upper airway, are well innervated with noradrenergic nerves (59–62). Stimulation of these nerves constricts these blood vessels, which in turn leads to changes in airflow and the heat exchange functions of the nose. Bronchial submucosal gland cells contain α and β adrenoreceptors, stimulation of these receptors leads to mucus production. Thus, in theory, adrenoreceptor agonists which are widely used in the management of obstructive airways diseases such as asthma may lead to mucus plugging of the airways. In practice, however, this effect is overshadowed by the effect of both α_2- and β_2-adrenoreceptors located on postsynaptic nerve terminals. Stimulation of these postsynaptic adrenoreceptors prevents the release of acetylcholine from cholinergic nerves and of norepinephrine from noradrenergic nerves. These inhibitory effects on neurotransmitter release appear to be the dominant effect of adrenoreceptors in the airways (63,64). Airway and vascular smooth muscle contains an abundance of β_2-adrenoreceptors and a relatively small number of stimulatory α_1-adrenoreceptors (65-70). The function of airway smooth muscle-associated β_2-adrenoreceptors is bronchodilation. Since this tissue has a relatively sparse innervation, the principal endogenous agonist of these receptors, in vivo, is epinephrine, which is released into the circulation from the adrenal glands.

C. Afferent Nerves in the Airways

The majority of the nerves innervating the airways are carried in the vagus nerves and within the vagus 80% of nerves are sensory afferents (71). Airway afferent nerves have been classified into several types of different so-called sensory receptors. The term receptor refers to the original sense of the word: something that is sensed rather than the pharmacological definition of a receptor (i.e., a membrane-bound protein). Afferent nerves have been organized into myelinated slowly adapting receptors (SAR), rapidly adapting receptors (RAR) and nonmyelinated C-fiber receptors. C-fiber receptor are usually classified as pulmonary or bronchial, based on their accessibility to stimulants (e.g., phenyl diguanide, capsaicin, and histamine) injected into the pulmonary and bronchial circulation, (72). Vagal afferent sensory nerve fibers from the lungs and airways travel to cell bodies in the nodose and jugular ganglia and from these ganglia fibers pass to the nucleus tractus solitarius in the medulla (73,74). The stimuli to these receptors are shown in Table 1. Stimulation of all receptor subgroups has a profound influence on breathing and airway tone, which leads to either bronchodilation or bronchoconstriction as well as alterations in breathing pattern, cough, changes in local blood flow, and changes in mucus production.

In addition to relaying afferent signals, stimulation of some sensory nerves also leads to local reflex efferent responses. These efferent responses cannot be inhibited with pharmacological inhibition of cholinergic or sympathetic nerves and so the nerves mediating these efferent responses are called non-adrenergic non-cholinergic (NANC) nerves. Most of the observations concerning the effects of NANC nerves have been made in rodent species, with some supporting studies from human subjects.

Stimulation of NANC nerves occurs by chemical stimulation of pulmonary and bronchial C-fibers and some rapidly acting mechanoreceptors. This stimulation leads to the release of a variety of neurotransmitters including neuropeptides, purines, monoamines, and nitric oxide (75,76). Functional studies have shown that, depending on the nature of the stimulus, there are two types of opposing effects of this neurotransmitter system: an excitatory bronchoconstriction and an inhibitory

Table 1 Stimuli to C Fiber Receptors, RARs, and SARs

	Pulmonary C-fibers	Bronchial C-fibers	RARs	SARs
Mechanical	Inflation	Inflation Foreign bodies	Inflation Deflation Dust Mucus Foreign bodies	Inflation
Chemical	Irritant gases Cigarette smoke Capsaicin Volatile anesthetics	Irritant gases Capsaicin	Irritant gases Cigarette smoke Capsaicin Volatile anesthetics	
Mediator	Acetylcholine Histamine Serotonin Prostaglandins Bradykinin Substance P	Histamine Serotonin Prostaglandins Bradykinin	Acetylcholine Histamine Serotonin Prostaglandins Bradykinin Substance P	

Not all neurons in the ganglia respond in a consistent fashion; the result reported is the most typical response. Some of the heterogeneity reflects the different types of species studied.

bronchodilation may be seen. Thus, NANC nerves are often referred to as exerting excitatory (eNANC) or inhibitory (iNANC) effects.

The principal eNANC neurotransmitters are substance P and calcitonin gene-related peptide (CRGP). Substance P and CRGP are frequently colocalized within individual nerves and within ganglia (77–79). In the airways of animals such as guinea pigs and rats there is an extensive innervation by these nerves of epithelial cells, glandular cells, smooth muscle cells, and ganglia (77–79). However, in humans these nerves are less abundant and, in particular, there does not appear to be a significant innervation of airway smooth muscle by these nerves (80). Release of these neurotransmitters from eNANC nerves leads to contraction of the airway smooth muscle, dilation of pulmonary and bronchial blood vessels, mucus production, as well as recruitment and activation of inflammatory cells (81–86). These effects are mediated by stimulation of neurokinin receptors. Based on the potency of the agonist substance P, three subtypes of neurokinin receptor have been identified and these are termed (NK_{1-3}) (87). These receptors are found on mucus glands (both NK_{1-2}), bronchial blood vessels (both NK_{1-2}), inflammatory cells such as eosinophils and macrophages, sensory nerves (NK_1), and airway smooth muscle (NK_1) (81,88–91). Thus, although these structures are not directly innervated by eNANC nerves they may be influenced by locally produced neuropeptides including, possibly, non-neuronally derived neuropeptides. The principal iNANC effects (dilation of the airway and vascular smooth muscle) are mediated by vasoactive intestinal peptide (VIP) and nitric oxide (NO) (92,93).

III. Effect of Respiratory Tract Virus Infections on Nerve Function and Neurotransmitter Receptors

A. Effect of Respiratory Tract Virus Infections on Adrenergic Nerve Function

Several studies have noted that there are impaired bronchodilator responses to β-adrenoreceptor stimulation following a respiratory viral infection. For example, compared with noninfected cells the inhibitory effect of β-agonists on zymosan-induced granulocyte degranulation is impaired in rhinovirus-infected cells (94). In vitro studies have shown an impaired dilator response to β-adrenoreceptor stimulation of antigen-contracted airway smooth muscle in virus-infected animals (95). A mechanism for these changes has recently been proposed by Hakonarson and colleagues, who have suggested that the altered responsiveness of these receptors reflects a virus-induced change in expression and function of the Gi protein $Gi\alpha_3$ (96). This change in Gi protein function leads to impaired cAMP accumulation, which directly inhibits the key intracellular event that follows β-adrenoreceptor stimulation. In addition to the effect on the smooth muscle, this virus-induced impaired β-adrenoreceptor function may also have an indirect effect by influencing the activity of cholinergic nerves through inhibitory β-adrenoreceptors on the cholinergic nerves.

A significant limitation of these studies is that there is little evidence that direct viral infection of airway smooth muscle occurs in vitro (97). Notwithstanding this limitation, impaired responses to β-adrenoreceptor stimulation may contribute to the bronchoconstriction associated with a respiratory tract virus infection, in a number of indirect ways. For example, virus infections are associated with increased levels of the cytokines TNF-α and IL-1β, both of which may directly impair β-adrenoreceptor function in a similar manner (98–100). Perhaps more important than contributing to the bronchoconstriction associated with a respiratory virus infection is the effect of adrenoreceptor dysfunction on the response to treatment during these infections, which may be impaired (101).

B. Effect of Respiratory Tract Virus Infection on Cholinergic Nerve Function

There is evidence that increased vagally mediated activity occurs in the lungs, in humans, during a virus infection. For example, studies by Laitinen and colleagues have demonstrated an increase in bronchial reactivity in subjects with normal lung function during influenza A infection (102). In these studies it was shown that during an experimentally induced influenza A infection there was an increase in the sensitivity of the airways to the histamine in both asthmatic and normal individuals. Empey and colleagues investigated subjects with a naturally acquired virus infection and demonstrated a role for the cholinergic nervous system in the development of hyperresponsiveness to histamine. The authors reported that an inhaled anticholinergic agent protected against this virus-induced hyperresponsiveness (103). Similar studies by Aquilina and colleagues showed that in a cohort of healthy individuals a viral infection of the upper airway resulted in an increased vagally mediated bronchial reactivity to either histamine or exercise in cold air (104). This effect lasted for at least 6 weeks in a significant number of the infected individuals. Thus, respiratory tract virus infections lead to changes in airway function that may persist for some time after the infection has symptomatically cleared. Since these initial studies were performed, several investigations have been undertaken to establish the cause of this virus-induced increase in vagally mediated hyperreactivity. Most of these studies have investigated the effect of virus infections on changes in muscarinic receptor function and are outlined below.

Effect of Respiratory Virus Infection on the Function of Pulmonary M_1 Muscarinic Receptors

It is uncertain whether the function of M_1 muscarinic receptors is altered in patients during a viral infection. However an in vitro study has shown that respiratory syncytial virus infection of the human alveolar epithelial cell line A549 cells leads to an increase in M_1 muscarinic receptor expression (105). Although neither the mechanism nor the clinical significance of this effect has yet been determined one may expect this to lead to bronchospasm and increased mucus production. On the other hand, a recent report has indicated that, in humans, M_1 muscarinic receptors are also located on mucosal mast cells where they function as autoreceptors limiting histamine release from these cells (106). Thus, on these cells M_1 muscarinic receptors may play a protective role, limiting histamine release and so enhanced expression during a viral infection may be protective. In short, little is known of the function of M_1 muscarinic receptors during a respiratory tract virus infection, although the available data suggest that receptor expression may be enhanced by some viruses and that this, in theory, may contribute to the increased mucus production and bronchospasm seen under these circumstances.

Effect of Respiratory Virus Infection on the Function of Pulmonary Neuronal M_2 Muscarinic Receptors

In animal models, in vivo, a respiratory tract infection with viruses such as Sendai virus is associated with loss of function of pulmonary neuronal M_2 muscarinic receptors. This was first demonstrated in anesthetized, paralyzed, and ventilated guinea pigs (107). In these studies it was shown that the M_2 muscarinic receptor agonist pilocarpine induced a dose-dependent inhibition of vagally induced bronchoconstriction in control animals. However, in virus-infected animals pilocarpine had no inhibitory effect on vagally induced contraction of the airways smooth muscle, indicating loss of function of M_2 muscarinic receptors. In subsequent experiments it has been shown that there is loss of function of M_2 muscarinic receptors in rats (108). Loss of neuronal M_2 muscarinic receptor function has the same effect as blocking these receptors with antagonists; it leads to a potentiation of vagally induced bronchoconstriction (109). Since many of the compounds associated with hyperreactivity stimulate the vagus nerves this suggests that M_2 receptor dysfunction is an important mechanism of virus-induced vagal hyperreactivity.

Respiratory tract virus infections appear to induce loss of function of M_2 muscarinic receptors by a number of different mechanisms. In part, the loss of M_2 muscarinic receptor function is inflammatory cell-mediated since virus-induced receptor dysfunction can be prevented by depletion of lung inflammatory cells with cyclophosphamide, a compound that inhibits cell proliferation (110). In these studies it was shown that pretreatment with cyclophosphamide depletes lung granulocytes and lymphocytes and that there was a correlation between the severity of infection and M_2 receptor dysfunction. These data suggest that receptor dysfunction could either be induced directly by a severe infection, or if there was a less severe infection, by an indirect inflammatory cell-mediated effect.

Further studies have shown that it is possible that certain viruses, such as parainfluenza virus, may directly affect M_2 muscarinic receptors. Muscarinic receptors contain a core of sialic acid residues at the binding site for acetylcholine (111). Ligand-binding studies have shown that removal of these glycoproteins from the receptor with compounds such as neuraminidase prevents the binding of acetylcholine, which inhibits normal receptor function (112). Viruses, such as parainfluenza, as well as inflammatory cells such as macrophages express the enzyme neuraminidase (113). Thus, during a respiratory tract virus infection by parainfluenza or other neuraminidase enzyme expressing virus infections, M_2 receptors may become dysfunctional by this mechanism (114).

Viral infections of the respiratory tract can also influence parasympathetic nerves by directly decreasing expression of M_2 muscarinic receptors. Several factors are known to influence the gene expression of M_2 receptors: corticosteroids; growth factors such a leukemia inhibitory factor; and interferon gamma, which acts in an inhibitory manner (115–120). Increased levels of the latter cytokine are a feature of acute respiratory tract infections (116). Thus, loss of neuronal M_2 receptor function during a viral infection can be the result of either decreased M_2 receptor expression or decreased agonist binding to the receptor.

In antigen-challenged guinea pigs there is loss of function of neuronal M_2 muscarinic receptors, and vagally mediated hyperreactivity. Histological studies have shown that after antigen challenge of sensitized animals eosinophils localize to airway nerves in guinea pigs and rats (109,121–124). In these animals eosinophils are found around and inside nerve bundles, parasympathetic ganglia, and along nerve fibers in the smooth muscle of the lungs in antigen-challenged animals (Figure 3). Inhibiting activation or the localization of eosinophils to nerves prevents antigen-induced loss of M_2 muscarinic receptor function (125,126). In contrast, few eosino-

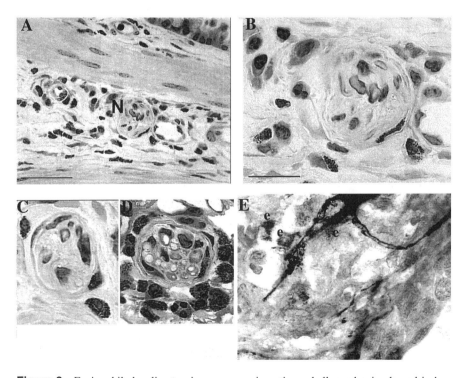

Figure 3 Eosinophils localize to airway nerves in antigen-challenged animals and in humans during acute episodes of asthma. (A,B) A cross-section of airway from an antigen-challenged guinea pig is shown. The epithelium (left) is distorted and displaced,which is a typical feature in asthma. Eosinophils are seen in particular to localize to an airway nerve bundle (N). In these animals eosinophils are frequently seen to penetrate inside the epineurium of airway nerves (C,D). Eosinophils (e) are also frequently seen in association with airway nerves in subjects with asthma during acute, fatal episodes of asthma (E).

phils are associated with nerves in virus-infected animals and inhibiting eosinophils with an antibody to eosinophil major basic protein (MBP) does not prevent virus-induced loss of M_2 receptor function (127). However, in contrast in animals that have been antigen-sensitized respiratory tract virus infections are associated with significant recruitment of eosinophils to nerves; inhibiting eosinophils prevents virus-associated loss of M_2 receptor function, (127). These data suggest that in antigen-sensitized animals the immune response to a respiratory tract virus infection is altered. One potential mechanism for this observation is that antigen-specific T lymphocytes, which are found in increased numbers following allergen sensitization, influence the virus-responding CD_8 lymphocytes to produce IL-5 and other eosinophil-associated cytokines (128).

There is evidence that neuronal M_2 receptors are not functioning normally in some humans with asthma, in particular those with chronic and moderately severe asthma. Two separate studies demonstrated that muscarinic agonists inhibit reflex-induced bronchoconstriction in control, nonasthmatic subjects, but do not prevent reflex-induced bronchoconstriction in the asthmatic subjects (129,130). This failure of muscarinic agonists to limit a vagally mediated reflex bronchoconstriction indicates that there is loss of M_2 muscarinic receptor function. In subjects with mild asthma there is normal M_2 receptor function, but during acute exacerbations there is loss of M_2 receptor function (131,132). For example, subjects with mild asthma have functional M_2 muscarinic receptors while they are clinically stable. This was shown by the ability of the muscarinic receptor agonist pilocarpine to inhibit a reflex-induced vagally mediated bronchoconstriction. However, when these subjects were retested during a naturally acquired viral infection they had experienced increased hyperreactivity and also loss of M_2 receptor function (132).

The studies outlined above demonstrate that neuronal M_2 muscarinic receptors inhibit the release of acetylcholine from parasympathetic nerves. During a respiratory tract virus infection these receptors become dysfunctional and this is due to a number of mechanisms, including reduced gene expression, reduced ligand binding affinity, and (in allergic individuals) antagonism of the receptors by eosinophil MBP. Some preliminary data in patients with asthma indicate that during virus infections there is a similar loss of M_2 receptor function. Whether M_2 muscarinic receptor dysfunction directly contributes to hyperreactivity in human asthmatics and whether it is mediated by activation of eosinophils remains to be tested.

Effect of Respiratory Virus Infection on the Function of M_3 Muscarinic Receptor Function

It is surprising that there has been very little experimental investigation on the number, function, and intracellular receptor coupling of M_3 muscarinic receptors during respiratory tract virus infections. Studies in virus-infected animals have shown no correlation between the in vivo hyperreactivity and the in vitro response to the same compound. For example, in control and virus-infected animals there is no difference in the bronchoconstriction induced in response to intravenous muscarinic agonists (107,127,133,134). This suggests that virus-induced hyperreactivity is not due directly to an abnormality in smooth muscle. In other studies it has been shown that, in contrast to their effects on M_2 muscarinic receptors, neither eosinophil MBP nor neuraminidase affects these receptors (114,135). These data suggest that there is probably no change in the function of M_3 receptors on the smooth muscle during a respiratory tract infection.

C. Effects of Respiratory Virus Infections on Sensory Nerve Function

Direct physiological studies of the function of sensory nerves during virus infections have not been undertaken. This is because studies of this kind are usually performed under circumstances in which an individual nerve serves as it own control, and is studied before and after the application of a stimulus. Since a viral infection takes time to develop pathogenic signs, it is impossible to perform these types of studies during an infection. However, studies have modeled the conditions associated with virus infections such as hyperpnea and the release of chemical mediators from epithelial and inflammatory cells. These studies have focused on factors such as leukotrienes, prostaglandins or kinins, and histamine as changes in the local production or metabolism of these factors occur during viral infections (136,137). These compounds have all been shown to have a wide variety of effects on some or all three sensory nerve receptor types (Table 1, Fig. 4). Thus, changes in the firing threshold of the sensory nerves in the upper airways, in particular, probably occur during virus infections. The activation of sensory nerve receptors during a virus infection leads to enhanced reflex parasympathetic nerve activation, cough, and neurogenic inflammation.

Effect of Respiratory Tract Virus Infections on Reflex Vagally Mediated Responses

Empey and colleagues showed that in subjects with a naturally acquired virus infection there was increased sensory nerve reactivity as demonstrated by increased contractile "responses" to citric acid aerosol. This could be inhibited with atropine, indicating that the apparent increase in sensory nerve activity was due to a cholinergic mechanism (138). In guinea pigs infected with parainfluenza virus, pretreatment with the neurotoxin capsaicin to deplete C-fiber nerves was shown to prevent virus-induced reflex vagal hyperreactivity (139). A mechanism by which virus activation of sensory nerves leads to reflex, vagally mediated hyperreactivity was demonstrated in virally infected guinea pigs. In these studies it was shown that pretreatment with the neurokinin NK_1 receptor antagonist SR10348 inhibited hyperreactivity by protecting M_2 receptor function. It is likely that the tachykinin NK_1 receptor antagonist exerted this effect by preventing activation of macrophages and other inflammatory cells, which in turn prevented virus-induced loss of M_2 receptor function (134).

Effect of Respiratory Tract Virus Infections on Cough

There has been little in vivo work performed to establish the mechanism of virus-induced cough. In part this reflects the difficulty involved in performing these types

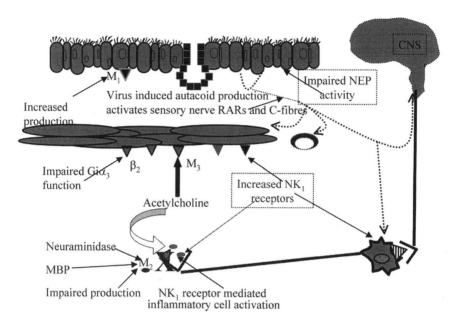

Figure 4 Summary of the multiple mechanisms of virus-induced activation of the airway neural system. Activation of the sensory nerves by locally produced autacoids leads to cough, reflex bronchoconstriction, and neurogenic inflammation. Neurogenic inflammation is increased by both a loss of activity of neutral endopeptidase (NEP), which degrades substance P, and by increased NK_1 receptor expression. Dysfunction of neuronal M_2 muscarinic receptors by a variety of means, including impaired production and the damage induced by neuraminidase, leads to increased vagally induced bronchoconstriction.

of studies as well as the marked interspecies variability in sensory nerve function and the differences between in vivo and in vitro observations (140–142). However, studies have shown that cough is induced by irritant receptors in the laryngeal wall and by RARs in the trachea and bronchial wall. The stimuli to these receptors, as outlined in Table 2, are all known to be increased during viral infections; thus it seems plausible that these nerves mediate virus-induced cough by this mechanism (143). Furthermore, virus infection is associated with denudation of the respiratory epithelium and thus exposure of some sensory nerve receptors. Direct stimulation of C-fibers appears to inhibit coughing, but also indirectly promotes cough by inducing neurogenic inflammation, which activates local RARs, in turn leads to the production of cough (144–146). Studies that may help our understanding of the factors involved and the mechanisms of virus-induced cough, using tachykinin receptor antagonists or other specific autocoid antagonists, have not yet been reported.

Effect of Respiratory Tract Virus Infections on Neurogenic Inflammation

Neurogenic inflammation is mediated by neuropeptides such as substance P, CGRP, and neurokinin A, which are released from unmyelinated C-fibers. Studies have

Table 2 Effects of Autacoids Released During Viral Infections on Some Electrophysiological Properties of Vagal Sensory Neurons

Autacoid	Resting potential	Resistance	After spike hyperpolarization
Serotonin	Depolarize	Decrease	Inhibit
Histamine	Depolarize	Increase	No effect
Bradykinin	Depolarize	Increase	Inhibit
Prostacyclin	Depolarize	Increase	Inhibit
Prostaglandin D_2	Depolarize	Increase	Inhibit
Prostaglandin E_2	Depolarize	Increase	Inhibit
Prostaglandin F_2	No effect	No effect	No effect
Leukotrine C_4	Depolarize	Increase	Inhibit
Nicotine	Depolarize	Decrease	No effect

Not all neurons in the ganglia respond in a consistent fashion; the result reported is the most typical response. Some of the heterogeneity within a ganglion may reflect the different types of neurons represented.

shown that respiratory tract virus infections make the trachea and bronchial mucosa of animals more susceptible to neurogenic inflammation (147–151). For example, infection of experimental animals with viruses such as respiratory syncytial virus (RSV) or Sendai virus leads to increased vascular permeability, increased neutrophil adhesion to postcapillary venules, as well as increased numbers of goblet cells in the nose and large airways (152,153).

The enhanced neurogenic inflammation during a respiratory tract infection can be inhibited by pretreatment with either corticosteroids or by pretreatment with selective neurokinin NK_1 receptor antagonists (154). These data suggest that these compounds may be of benefit if a similar process occurs in vivo in humans. However, to date there have been no reports of studies with these compounds during experimental respiratory tract virus infections. There appear to be several mechanisms involved in the development of respiratory virus-associated neurogenic inflammation. Initial studies indicated that the neurogenic inflammation was due to the loss of function of the enzyme neutral endopeptidase, which neutralizes substance P and other neuropeptides (150,155). Recent studies have also indicated that certain virus infections, such as RSV, directly increase the production of NK_1 receptor, suggesting that the inflammation is due to an increased effectiveness of released neuropeptides (147,148,156). The recent identification of the gene encoding the NK_1 and NK_2 receptor (the preprotachykinin gene) should help to further our understanding the mechanism of virus-associated enhanced NK_1 receptor expression (157).

Respiratory infections have significant chronic effects on airway neural control, in particular in infant animals. For example, in perinatal ferrets infected with human RSV tracheal smooth muscle segments show enhanced cholinergic and eNANC as well as iNANC responses. The balance of these abnormalities favor airway obstruction and hyperreactivity (158). Most significantly, these effects appear to persist for several weeks. In other studies it has been shown that experimental infection of weanling rats with RSV leads to intrapulmonary airway neurogenic edema. This is due to a direct effect of RSV infection on NK_1 receptors leading to increased receptor expression (159). These findings may be of direct clinical significance, since infection with RSV at an early age is considered to be a risk factor for the development of asthma.

IV. Effects of Nerves on the Response to Viral Respiratory Tract Infections

Infection of the respiratory tract by viruses leads to a number of host, neurally mediated, responses aimed at attenuating the effect of the virus infection. As outlined above, virus infections lead to delayed degradation of the neuropeptide substance P and also to increased NK_1 neurokinin receptor expression, leading to persistence of the neuropeptide. In vitro studies have shown that substance P promotes leukocyte adhesion to endothelial, epithelial, and other cells via enhanced expression of adhesion molecules (83,160–162). In addition, this neuropeptide also acts as a leukocyte chemoattractant, promotes leukocyte activation, and delays lymphocyte apoptosis (163–166). Overall, these effects promote inflammation and thus can be seen as an attempt to remove the virus; however, they also lead to local unwanted effects, which cause symptoms such as cough and sputum production. Tachykinins released after virus infection may contribute to longer lasting effects such as airway wall basement membrane thickening through direct activation of fibroblasts and persisting inflammation (167). On the other hand recent, studies have shown that activation of the vagus nerves, by the various mechanisms described above, may lead to attenuated virus-induced release of macrophage-derived inflammatory cytokines, as has been described to occur during bacterial lipopolysaccharide injury (168). The clinical significance of these in vitro observations, which suggest an anti-inflammatory role for the vagus, is not clear.

V. Effect of Treatments on Respiratory Tract Virus Infections

A. Anticholinergic Agents

Nasal application of the anticholinergic agent ipratropium bromide has been demonstrated in clinical studies to be effective in ameliorating rhinorrhea, symptom scores, the frequency of sneezing, and nasal secretion weights associated with an upper respiratory tract infection (169–178). Thus, these data indicate that the principal vagally mediated feature of a virus infection in the upper airway is an increase in nasal blood flow and serous gland secretion. Notwithstanding the evidence that the parasympathetic nerves play a pivotal role in mucus production, treatment with nasal anticholinergic agents during an upper respiratory infection does not limit mucus production, suggesting that other stimuli lead to increases in mucus production during virus infections.

There is considerably less information on the role of anticholinergic agents in the lower airway during respiratory tract infections. Lowry and colleagues showed in a cohort of nonasthmatic individuals that the inhaled quaternary anticholinergic agent oxitropium bromide did not protect against either the small decline in lung function or cough during an acute naturally acquired virus infection in nonasthmatic individuals (179). However, anticholinergic agents may be of benefit in subjects with a persistent cough after a clinical upper respiratory tract infection. For example, in a controlled, double-blind, crossover trial of nonasthmatic nonsmokers it has been shown that inhaled ipratropium bromide (320 µg/per day) produces significantly less day and night-time cough (180). In asthmatics, acute exacerbations in both children and adults are frequently due to virus infections (181,182). These attacks, in particular in children, respond to anticholinergic therapy suggesting that activation of the cholinergic system is an important pathogenic mechanism of virus-induced asthma exacerbations (183,184).

B. Effects of Tachykinin Receptor Antagonists and Neutral Endopeptidase Antagonists in Virus Infections

Several functionally effective nonpeptide-selective tachykinin receptor antagonists have been developed (185,186). As outlined above, a considerable volume of data from in vivo studies in animals suggest that there is a rationale for investigating tachykinin receptor antagonists or neutral endopeptidase agonists in virus infections. However, to date no studies have been reported on the effect of these compounds in humans during a respiratory tract infection.

VI. Summary

There is considerable evidence that virus infections lead to an increase in the vagally mediated effects of bronchoconstriction and mucus production in the airways. In part these abnormalities are due to a defect in the function of the neuronal M_2 muscarinic receptor, due to either a direct effect of the virus on the receptor structure or an indirect effect on receptor expression. Sensory nerves are also activated during virus infections by a number of compounds such as kininis, prostaglandins, and leukotrienes. Activation of these sensory nerves leads to reflex vagally mediated effects as well as to cough and neurogenic inflammation. Neurogenic inflammation, which is a host defense mechanism, may actually worsen symptoms by promoting inflammation. Finally, there is also evidence of impaired function of β-adrenoreceptors, during some respiratory virus infections, which influence the ability of bronchodilator medications. A summary of these mechanisms is shown in Figure 4.

References

1. Richardson JB, Ferguson CC. Neuromuscular structure and function in the airways. Fed Proc 1979; 38:202–208.

2. Verity MA, Bevan JA. Fine structural study of the terminal effecror plexus, neuromuscular and intermuscular relationships in the pulmonary artery. J Anat 1968; 103:49–63.

3. Mann SP. The innervation of mammalian bronchial smooth muscle: the localization of catecholamines and cholinesterases. Histochem J 1971; 3:319–331.

4. Ferguson CC, Richardson JB. A simple technique for the utilization of postmortem tracheal and bronchial tissues for ultrastructural studies. Hum Pathol 1978; 9:463–470.

5. Hammarstrom M, Sjostrand NO. Pathways for excitatory and inhibitory innervation to the guinea-pig tracheal smooth muscle. Experientia 1979; 35:64–65.

6. Jones TR, Kannan MS, Daniel EE. Ultrastructural study of guinea pig tracheal smooth muscle and its innervation. Can J Physiol Pharmacol 1980; 58:974–983.

7. Kannan MS, Daniel EE. Structural and functional study of control of canine tracheal smooth muscle. Am J Physiol 1980; 238:C27–33.

8. Knight DS, Hyman AL, Kadowitz PJ. Innervation of intrapulmonary airway smooth muscle of the dog, monkey and baboon. J Auton Nerv Syst 1981; 3:31–43.

9. Bhatla R, Ferguson CC, Richardson JB. The innervation of smooth muscle in the primary bronchus of the chicken. Can J Physiol Pharmacol 1980; 58:310–315.

10. Andersson RG, Grundstrom N. The excitatory non-cholinergic, non-adrenergic nervous system of the guinea-pig airways. Eur J Respir Dis Suppl 1983; 131:141–157.

11. Pack RJ, Al-Ugaily LH, Widdicombe JG. The innervation of the trachea and extrapulmonary bronchi of the mouse. Cell Tissue Res 1984; 238:61–68.

12. Laitinen A, Partanen M, Hervonen A, Pelto-Huikko M, Laitinen LA. VIP like immunoreactive nerves in human respiratory tract. Light and electron microscopic study. Histochemistry 1985; 82:313–319.

13. Rodriguez-Martinez H, Ekwall H, Ploen L. Ultrastructure and innervation of smooth muscle in the porcine oviduct. Anat Histol Embryol 1985; 14:33–46.

14. Daniel EE, Kannan M, Davis C, Posey-Daniel V. Ultrastructural studies on the neuromuscular control of human tracheal and bronchial muscle. Respir Physiol 1986; 63:109-128.

15. Laitinen A, Partanen M, Hervonen A, Laitinen LA. Electron microscopic study on the innervation of the human lower respiratory tract: evidence of adrenergic nerves. Eur J Respir Dis 1985; 67:209–215.

16. Davis C, Kannan MS. Sympathetic innervation of human tracheal and bronchial smooth muscle. Respir Physiol 1987; 68:53-61.

17. Fillenz M. Innervation of pulmonary and bronchial blood vessels of the dog. J Anat 1970; 106:449–461.

18. Knight DS, Ellison JP, Hibbs RG, Hyman AL, Kadowitz PJ. A light and electron microscopic study of the innervation of pulmonary arteries in the cat. Anat Rec 1981; 201:513–521.

19. Richardson J. Nerve supply to the lungs. Am Rev Respir Dis 1979; 119:785–802.

20. Richardson J. Recent progress in pulmonary innervation. Am Rev Respir Dis 1983; 128:s65–67.

21. Olsen C, Colebatch H, Mebel P, Nadel J, Staub N. Motor control of pulmonary airways studied by nerve stimulation. J Appl Physiol 1965; 20:202–208.

22. Brody JS, Klempfner G, Staum MM, Vidyasagas D, Kuhl DE, Waldhausen JA. Mucociliary clearence after lung denervation and bronchial transection. J Appl Physiol 1972; 32:160–164.

23. Gallagher JT, Kent PW, Passatore M, Phipps RJ, Richardson PS. The composition of tracheal mucus and the nervous control of its secretion in the cat. Proc R Soc Lond 1976; 192:49–76.

24. McCormack DG, Mak JC, Minette P, Barnes PJ. Muscarinic receptor subtypes mediating vasodilation in the pulmonary artery. Eur J Pharmacol 1988; 158:293–297.

25. Coleridge HM, Coleridge JC. Neural regulation of bronchial blood flow. Respir Physiol 1994; 98:1–13.

26. Dale HH. The action of certain esters and ethers of choline and their relation to muscarinie. J Pharmacol Exp Ther 1914; 6:147–190.

27. Bonner TI, Young AC, Brann MR, Buckley NJ. Cloning and expression of the human and rat m5 muscarinic acetylcholine receptor genes. Neuron 1988; 1:403–410.

28. Bonner TI, Buckley NJ, Young AC, Brann MR. Identification of a family of muscarinic acetylcholine receptor genes. Science 1987; 237:527–532.

29. Hulme EC, Kurtenbach E, and Curtis CA. Muscarinic acetylcholine receptors: structure and function. Biochem Soc Trans 1991; 19:133–138.

30. Hulme EC, Curtis CA, Page KM, Jones PG. Agonist activation of muscarinic acetylcholine receptors. Cell Signal 1993; 5:687-694.

31. Buckley NJ, Bonner TI, Buckley CM, Brann MR. Antagonist binding properties of five cloned muscarinic receptors expressed in CHO-K1 cells. Mol Pharmacol 1989; 35:469–476.

32. Haddad EB, Mak JC, Belvisi MG, Nishikawa M, Rousell J, Barnes PJ. Muscarinic and beta-adrenergic receptor expression in peripheral lung from normal and asthmatic patients. Am J Physiol 1996; 270:L947–953.

33. Haddad EB, Mak JC, Hislop A, Haworth SG, Barnes PJ. Characterization of muscarinic receptor subtypes in pig airways: radioligand binding and northern blotting studies. Am J Physiol 1994; 266:L642–648.

34. Mak JC, Baraniuk JN, Barnes PJ. Localization of muscarinic receptor subtype mRNAs in human lung. Am J Respir Cell Mol Biol 1992; 7:344–348.

35. Mak JC, Barnes PJ. Autoradiographic visualization of muscarinic receptor subtypes in human and guinea pig lung. Am Rev Respir Dis 1990; 141:1559–1568.

36. Mak JC, Barnes PJ. Muscarinic receptor subtypes in human and guinea pig lung. Eur J Pharmacol 1989; 164:223–230.

37. Casale TB, Ecklund P. Characterization of muscarinic receptor subtypes on human peripheral lung. J Appl Physiol 1988; 65:594–600.

38. Klapproth H, Reinheimer T, Metzen J, Munch M, Bittinger F, Kirkpatrick CJ, Hohle KD, Schemann M, Racke K, Wessler I. Non-neuronal acetylcholine, a signalling molecule synthezised by surface cells of rat and man. Naunyn Schmiedebergs Arch Pharmacol 1997; 355:515–523.

39. Koyama S, Rennard SI, Robbins RA. Acetylcholine stimulates bronchial epithelial cells to release neutrophil and monocyte chemotactic activity. Am J Physiol 1992; 262:L466–471.

40. Ueda F, Ban K, Ishima T. Irsogladine activates gap-junctional intercellular communication through M1 muscarinic acetylcholine receptor. J Pharmacol Exp Ther 1995; 274:815-819.

41. Yang B, Schlosser RJ, McCaffrey TV. Signal transduction pathways in modulation of ciliary beat frequency by methacholine. Ann Otol Rhinol Laryngol 1997; 106:230–236.

42. Yang B, McCaffrey TV. The roles of muscarinic receptor subtypes in modulation of nasal ciliary action. Rhinology 1996; 34:136–139.

43. Saitoh H, Masuda T, Shimura S, Fushimi T, Shirato K. Secretion and gene expression of secretory leukocyte protease inhibitor by human airway submucosal glands. Am J Physiol Lung Cell Mol Physiol 2001; 280:L79–87.

44. Walch L, Gascard JP, Dulmet E, Brink C, Norel X. Evidence for a M(1) muscarinic receptor on the endothelium of human pulmonary veins. Br J Pharmacol 2000; 130: 73–78.

45. Altiere RJ, Travis DC, Roberts J, Thompson DC. Pharmacological characterization of muscarinic receptors mediating acetylcholine-induced contraction and relaxation in rabbit intrapulmonary arteries. J Pharmacol Exp Ther 1994; 270:269–276.

46. Myers AC, Undem BJ, Weinreich D. Electrophysiological properties of neurons in guinea pig bronchial parasympathetic ganglia. Am J Physiol 1990; 259:L403–409.

47. Fryer AD, Maclagan J. Muscarinic inhibitory receptors in pulmonary parasympathetic nerves in the guinea-pig. Br J Pharmacol 1984; 83:973–978.

48. Blaber LC, Fryer AD, Maclagan J. Neuronal muscarinic receptors attenuate vagally-induced contraction of feline bronchial smooth muscle. Br J Pharmacol 1985; 86:723–728.

49. Patel HJ, Barnes PJ, Takahashi T, Tadjkarimi S, Yacoub MH, Belvisi MG. Evidence for prejunctional muscarinic autoreceptors in human and guinea pig trachea. Am J Respir Crit Care Med 1995; 152:872–878.

50. Minette PA, Barnes PJ. Prejunctional inhibitory muscarinic receptors on cholinergic nerves in human and guinea pig airways. J Appl Physiol 1988; 64:2532–2537.

51. Minette PA, Lammers JW, Dixon CM, McCusker MT, Barnes PJ. A muscarinic agonist inhibits reflex bronchoconstriction in normal but not in asthmatic subjects. J Appl Physiol 1989; 67:2461-2465.

52. Sankary RM, Jones CA, Madison JM, Brown JK. Muscarinic cholinergic inhibition of cyclic AMP accumulation in airway smooth muscle. Role of a pertussis toxin-sensitive protein. Am Rev Respir Dis 1988; 138:145–150.

53. Fernandes LB, Fryer AD, Hirshman CA. M2 muscarinic receptors inhibit isoproterenol-induced relaxation of canine airway smooth muscle. J Pharmacol Exp Ther 1992; 262:119–126.

54. Billington CK, Hall IP, Mundell SJ, Parent JL, Panettieri RA Jr, Benovic JL, Penn RB. Inflammatory and contractile agents sensitize specific adenylyl cyclase isoforms in human airway smooth muscle. Am J Respir Cell Mol Biol 1999; 21:597–606.

55. Roffel AF, Elzinga CRS, Zaagsma J. Muscarinic M_3 receptors mediate contraction of human central and peripheral airway smooth muscle. Pulm Pharmacol 1990; 3:47–51.

56. Ramnarine SI, Haddad EB, Khawaja AM, Mak JC, Rogers DF. On muscarinic control of neurogenic mucus secretion in ferret trachea. J Physiol 1996; 494:577–586.

57. Partanen M, Laitinen A, Hervonen A, Toivanen M, Laitinen LA. Catecholamine-and acetylcholinesterase-containing nerves in human lower respiratory tract. Histochemistry 1982; 76:175-188.

58. Pack RJ, Richardson PS. The aminergic innervation of the human bronchus: a light and electron microscopic study. J Anat 1984; 138:493–502.

59. Baraniuk JN, Castellino S, Lundgren JD, Goff J, Mullol J, Merida M, Shelhamer JH, Kaliner MA. Neuropeptide Y (NPY) in human nasal mucosa. Am J Respir Cell Mol Biol 1990; 3:165–173.

60. Baraniuk JN, Kowalski ML, Kaliner MA. Relationships between permeable vessels, nerves, and mast cells in rat cutaneous neurogenic inflammation. J Appl Physiol 1990; 68:2305–2311.

61. Baraniuk JN. Neural control of human nasal secretion. Pulm Pharmacol 1991; 4:20–31.

62. Chen Y, Getchell TV, Sparks DL, Getchell ML. Patterns of adrenergic and peptidergic innervation in human olfactory mucosa: age-related trends. J Comp Neurol 1993; 334: 104–116.

63. Bergendal A, Linden A, Lotvall J, Skoogh BE, Lofdahl CG.Different effects of salmeterol, formoterol and salbutamol on cholinergic responses in the ferret trachea. Br J Pharmacol 1995; 114:1478–1482.

64. Skoogh BE, Ullman A. Modulation of cholinergic neurotransmission to the airways. Am Rev Respir Dis 1991; 143:1427–1428.

65. Xue QF, Maurer R, Engel G. Selective distribution of beta- and alpha 1-adrenoceptors in rat lung visualized by autoradiography. Arch Int Pharmacodyn Ther 1983; 266:308–314.

66. Carstairs JR, Nimmo AJ, Barnes PJ. Autoradiographic localisation of beta-adrenoceptors in human lung. Eur J Pharmacol 1984; 103:189–190.

67. Carstairs JR, Nimmo AJ, Barnes PJ. Autoradiographic visualization of beta-adrenoceptor subtypes in human lung. Am Rev Respir Dis 1985; 132:541–547.

68. Spina D, Rigby PJ, Paterson JW, Goldie RG. Autoradiographic localization of beta-adrenoceptors in asthmatic human lung. Am Rev Respir Dis 1989; 140:1410–1415.

69. Spina D, Rigby PJ, Paterson JW, Goldie RG. Alpha 1-adrenoceptor function and autoradiographic distribution in human asthmatic lung. Br J Pharmacol 1989; 97:701–708.

70. Henry PJ, Rigby PJ, Goldie RG. Distribution of beta 1- and beta 2-adrenoceptors in mouse trachea and lung: a quantitative autoradiographic study. Br J Pharmacol 1990; 99:136–144.

71. Agostini E, Chinnock JE, DeBurgh Daly M, Murray JG. Functional and histological studies of the vagus nerves and its branches to the heart, lungs and abdominal viscera in the cat. J Physiol 1957; 135:182–205.

72. Widdicombe J. The neural reflexes in the airways: Eur J Respir Dis Suppl 1986; 144: 133.

73. Kummer W, Fischer A, Kurkowski R, Heym C. The sensory and sympathetic innervation of guinea-pig lung and trachea as studied by retrograde neuronal tracing and double-labelling immunohistochemistry. Neuroscience 1992; 49:715–737.

74. Springall DR, Cadieux A, Oliveira H, Su H, Royston D, Polak JM. Retrograde tracing shows that CGRP-immunoreactive nerves of rat trachea and lung originate from vagal and dorsal root ganglia. J Auton Nerv Syst 1987; 20:155–166.

75. Widdicombe JG. Autonomic regulation. i-NANC/e-NANC. Am J Respir Crit Care Med 1998; 158:S171–175.

76. Bennett MR. Non-adrenergic non-cholinergic (NANC) transmission to smooth muscle: 35 years on. Prog Neurobiol 1997; 52:159–195.

77. Nishi Y, Kitamura N, Otani M, Hondo E, Taguchi K, Yamada J. Distribution of capsaicin-sensitive substance P- and calcitonin gene-related peptide-immunoreactive nerves in bovine respiratory tract. Anat Anz 2000; 182:319–326.

78. Cadieux A, Monast NP, Pomerleau F, Fournier A, and Lanoue C. Bronchoprotector properties of calcitonin gene-related peptide in guinea pig and human airways. Effect of pulmonary inflammation. Am J Respir Crit Care Med 1999; 159:235–243.

79. Chanez P, Springall D, Vignola AM, Moradoghi-Hattvani A, Polak JM, Godard P, Bousquet J. Bronchial mucosal immunoreactivity of sensory neuropeptides in severe airway diseases. Am J Respir Crit Care Med 1998; 158:985–990.

80. Howarth PH, Springall DR, Redington AE, Djukanovic R, Holgate ST, Polak JM.

Neuropeptide-containing nerves in endobronchial biopsies from asthmatic and non-asthmatic subjects. Am J Respir Cell Mol Biol 1995; 13:288–296.

81.   Joos GF, Germonpre PR, Pauwels RA. Role of tachykinins in asthma. Allergy 2000; 55:321–337.

82.   Keith IM. The role of endogenous lung neuropeptides in regulation of the pulmonary circulation. Physiol Res 2000; 49:519–537.

83.   Joos GF, Pauwels RA. Pro-inflammatory effects of substance P: new perspectives for the treatment of airway diseases? Trends Pharmacol Sci 2000; 21:131–133.

84.   Reynolds PN, Holmes MD, Scicchitano R. Role of tachykinins in bronchial hyper-responsiveness. Clin Exp Pharmacol Physiol 1997; 24:273–280.

85.   Lundberg JM. Tachykinins, sensory nerves, and asthma—an overview. Can J Physiol Pharmacol 1995; 73:908–914.

86.   Maggi CA, Giachetti A, Dey RD, Said SI. Neuropeptides as regulators of airway function: vasoactive intestinal peptide and the tachykinins. Physiol Rev 1995; 75:277–322.

87.   Maggi CA. Tachykinins as peripheral modulators of primary afferent nerves and visceral sensitivity. Pharmacol Res 1997; 36:153–169.

88.   Dunzendorfer S, Wiedermann CJ. Neuropeptide-induced chemotaxis of eosinophils in pulmonary diseases. Ann Med 2000; 32:429–439.

89.   Chu HW, Kraft M, Krause JE, Rex MD, Martin RJ. Substance P and its receptor neurokinin 1 expression in asthmatic airways. J Allergy Clin Immunol 2000; 106:713–722.

90.   Mapp CE, Miotto D, Braccioni F, Saetta M, Turato G, Maestrelli P, Krause JE, Karpit-skiy V, Boyd N, Geppetti P, Fabbri LM. The distribution of neurokinin-1 and neuroki-nin-2 receptors in human central airways. Am J Respir Crit Care Med 2000; 161:207–215.

91.   Rizzo CA, Valentine AF, Egan RW, Kreutner W, Hey JA. NK(2)-receptor mediated contraction in monkey, guinea-pig and human airway smooth muscle. Neuropeptides 1999; 33:27–34.

92.   Bellinger DL, Lorton D, Brouxhon S, Felten S, Felten DL. The significance of vaso-active intestinal polypeptide (VIP) in immunomodulation. Adv Neuroimmunol 1996; 6:5–27.

93.   Lammers JW, Barnes PJ, Chung KF. Nonadrenergic, noncholinergic airway inhibitory nerves. Eur Respir J 1992; 5:239–246.

94.   Busse WW, Anderson CL, Dick EC, Warshauer D. Reduced granulocyte response to isoproterenol, histamine, and prostaglandin E1 after in vitro incubation with Rhino-virus 16. Am Rev Respir Dis 1980; 122:641–646.

95.   Buckner CK, Clayton DE, Ain-Shoka AA, Busse WW, Dick EC, Shult P. Parainflu-enza 3 infection blocks the ability of a beta adrenergic receptor agonist to inhibit anti-gen-induced contraction of guinea pig isolated airway smooth muscle. J Clin Invest 1981; 67:376–384.

96.   Hakonarson H, Maskeri N, Carter C, Hodinka RL, Campbell D, and Grunstein MM. Mechanism of rhinovirus-induced changes in airway smooth muscle responsiveness. J Clin Invest 1998; 102:1732–1741.

97.   Castleman WL, Lav JC, Dubovi EJ, Slauson DO. Experimental bovine respiratory syncytial virus infection in conventional calves: light microscopic lesions, microbiol-ogy, and studies on lavaged lung cells. Am J Vet Res 1985; 46:547–553.

98.   Laporte JD, Moore PE, Panettieri RA, Moeller W, Heyder J, Shore SA. Prostanoids mediate IL-1beta-induced beta-adrenergic hyporesponsiveness in human airway smooth muscle cells. Am J Physiol 1998; 275:L491–501.

99. Shore SA, Laporte J, Hall IP, Hardy E, Panettieri RA Jr. Effect of IL-1 beta on responses of cultured human airway smooth muscle cells to bronchodilator agonists. Am J Respir Cell Mol Biol 1997; 16:702–712.

100. Emala CW, Kuhl J, Hungerford CL, Hirshman CA. TNF-alpha inhibits isoproterenol-stimulated adenylyl cyclase activity in cultured airway smooth muscle cells. Am J Physiol 1997; 272:L644-650.

101. Reddel H, Ware S, Marks G, Salome C, Jenkins C, Woolcock A. Differences between asthma exacerbations and poor asthma control. Lancet 1999; 353:364–369.

102. Laitinen LA, and Kava T. Bronchial reactivity following uncomplicated influenza A infection in healthy subjects and in asthmatic patients. Eur J Respir Dis Suppl 1980; 106:51–58.

103. Empey DW, Laitinen LA, Jacobs L, Gold WM, Nadel JA. Mechanisms of bronchial hyperreactivity in normal subjects after upper respiratory tract infection. Am Rev Respir Dis 1976; 113:131–139.

104. Aquilina AT, Hall WJ, Douglas RG, Utell MJ. Airway reactivity in subjects with viral upper respiratory tract infections: the effects of exercise and cold air. Am Rev Respir Dis 1980; 122:3–10.

105. Tsutsumi H, Ohsaki M, Seki K, Chiba S. Respiratory syncytial virus infection of human respiratory epithelial cells enhances both muscarinic and beta2-adrenergic receptor gene expression. Acta Virol 1999; 43:267–270.

106. Reinheimer T, Mohlig T, Zimmermann S, Hohle KD, Wessler I. Muscarinic control of histamine release from airways. Inhibitory M1-receptors in human bronchi but absence in rat trachea. Am J Respir Crit Care Med 2000; 162:534–538.

107. Fryer AD, Jacoby DB. Parainfluenza virus infection damages inhibitory M2 muscarinic receptors on pulmonary parasympathetic nerves in the guinea-pig. Br J Pharmacol 1991; 102:267–271.

108. Sorkness R, Clough JJ, Castleman WL, Lemanske RF, Jr. Virus-induced airway obstruction and parasympathetic hyperresponsiveness in adult rats. Am J Respir Crit Care Med 1994;150:28–34.

109. Costello RW, Evans CM, Yost BL, Belmonte KE, Gleich GJ, Jacoby DB, Fryer AD. Antigen-induced hyperreactivity to histamine: role of the vagus nerves and eosinophils. Am J Physiol 1999; 276:L709–714.

110. Fryer AD, Yarkony KA, Jacoby DB. The effect of leukocyte depletion on pulmonary M2 muscarinic receptor function in parainfluenza virus-infected guinea-pigs. Br J Pharmacol 1994; 112:588–594.

111. Gies J-P, Landry Y. Sialic acid is selectively involved in the interaction of agonists with M2 muscarinic acetylcholine receptors. Biochem Biophys Res Commun 1988; 150:673–680.

112. Jacoby DB, Fryer AD. Interaction of viral infections with muscarinic receptors. Clin Exp Allergy 1999;29:59–64.

113. Aymard-Henry M, Coleman MT, Dowdle WR, Laver WG, Schild GC, Webster RG. Influenzavirus neuraminidase and neuraminidase-inhibition test procedures. Bull WHO 1973; 48:199–202.

114. Fryer AD, el-Fakahany EE, Jacoby DB. Parainfluenza virus type 1 reduces the affinity of agonists for muscarinic receptors in guinea-pig lung and heart. Eur J Pharmacol 1990; 181:51–58.

115. Nadler LS, Rosoff ML, Hamilton SE, Kalaydjian AE, McKinnon LA, Nathanson NM. Molecular analysis of the regulation of muscarinic receptor expression and function. Life Sci 1999; 64:375–379

116. Jacoby DB, Xiao HQ, Lee NH, Chan-Li Y, Fryer AD. Virus- and interferon-induced loss of inhibitory M2 muscarinic receptor function and gene expression in cultured airway parasympathetic neurons. J Clin Invest 1998; 102:242–248.

117. Rousell J, Haddad el B, Lindsay MA, Barnes PJ. Regulation of M2 muscarinic receptor gene expression by platelet-derived growth factor: involvement of extracellular signal-regulated protein kinases in the down-regulation process. Mol Pharmacol 1997; 52: 966–973.

118. Barnes PJ, Haddad EB, Rousell J. Regulation of muscarinic M2 receptors. Life Sci 1997; 60:1015–1021.

119. Haddad EB, Rousell J, Lindsay MA, Barnes PJ. Synergy between tumor necrosis factor alpha and interleukin 1beta in inducing transcriptional down-regulation of muscarinic M2 receptor gene expression. Involvement of protein-kinase A and ceramide pathways. J Biol Chem 1996; 271:32586–32592.

120. Rosoff ML, Wei J, Nathanson NM. Isolation and characterization of the chicken m2 acetylcholine receptor promoter region: induction of gene transcription by leukemia inhibitory factor and ciliary neurotrophic factor. Proc Natl Acad Sci USA 1996; 93: 14889–14894.

121. Costello RW, Schofield BH, Kephart GM, Gleich GJ, Jacoby DB, Fryer AD. Localization of eosinophils to airway nerves and effect on neuronal M2 muscarinic receptor function. Am J Physiol 1997; 273:L93–103.

122. Costello RW, Jacoby DB, Fryer AD. Pulmonary neuronal M2 muscarinic receptor function in asthma and animal models of hyperreactivity. Thorax 1998; 53:613–616.

123. Costello RW, Fryer AD, Belmonte KE, Jacoby DB. Effects of tachykinin NK1 receptor antagonists on vagal hyperreactivity and neuronal M2 muscarinic receptor function in antigen challenged guinea-pigs. Br J Pharmacol 1998; 124:267–276.

124. Costello RW, Jacoby DB, Gleich GJ, Fryer AD. Eosinophils and airway nerves in asthma. Histol Histopathol 2000; 15:861-868.

125. Fryer AD, Costello RW, Yost BL, Lobb RR, Tedder TF, Steeber DA, Bochner BS. Antibody to VLA-4, but not to L-selectin, protects neuronal M2 muscarinic receptors in antigen-challenged guinea pig airways. J Clin Invest 1997; 99:2036–2044.

126. Evans CM, Fryer AD, Jacoby DB, Gleich GJ, Costello RW. Pretreatment with antibody to eosinophil major basic protein prevents hyperresponsiveness by protecting neuronal M2 muscarinic receptors in antigen-challenged guinea pigs. J Clin Invest 1997; 100: 2254–2262.

127. Adamko DJ, Yost BL, Gleich GJ, Fryer AD, Jacoby DB. Ovalbumin sensitization changes the inflammatory response to subsequent parainfluenza infection. Eosinophils mediate airway hyperresponsiveness, m(2) muscarinic receptor dysfunction, and anti-viral effects. J Exp Med 1999; 190:1465–1478.

128. Coyle AJ, Erard F, Bertrand C, Walti S, Pircher H, Le Gros G. Virus-specific CD8+ cells can switch to interleukin 5 production and induce airway eosinophilia. J Exp Med 1995; 181:1229–1233.

129. Ayala LE, Ahmed T. Is there loss of a protective muscarinic receptor in asthma? Chest 1989; 96:1285–1291.

130. Minette PJ, Lammers JWJ, Dixon CMS, McCusker MT, Barnes PJ. A muscarinic agonist inhibits reflex bronchoconstriction in normal but not asthmatic subjects. J Appl Physiol 1989; 67:2461-2465.

131. Okayama M, Shen T, Midorikawa J, Lin JT, Inoue H, Takishima T, Shirato K. Effect of pilocarpine on propranolol-induced bronchoconstriction in asthma. Am J Respir Crit Care Med 1994; 149:76–80.

132. Keen HG, Hurst V, Jack S, Warbuton CJ, Pearson MG, Calverley PMA, Costello RW. Loss of function of pulmonary neuronal M2 muscarinic receptors in subjects with mild bronchial hyperreactivity during a respiratory tract viral infection. Eur Respir J 1998; 12:149S.

133. Kahn RM, Okanlami OA, Jacoby DB, Fryer AD. Viral infection induces dependence of neuronal M2 muscarinic receptors on cyclooxygenase in guinea pig lung. J Clin Invest 1996; 98:299-307.

134. Jacoby DB, Yost-BL, Elwood T, Fryer AD. Effects of neurokinin receptor antagonists in virus-infected airways. Am J Physiol Lung Cell Mol Physiol 2000; 279:L59–65.

135. Jacoby DB, Gleich GJ, Fryer AD. Human eosinophil major basic protein is an endogenous allosteric antagonist at the inhibitory muscarinic M2 receptor. J Clin Invest 1993; 91:1314-1318.

136. Fox AJ, Lalloo UG, Belvisi MG, Bernareggi M, Chung KF, Barnes PJ. Bradykinin-evoked sensitization of airway sensory nerves: a mechanism for ACE-inhibitor cough. Nat Med 1996; 2:814-817.

137. Nakazawa H, Sekizawa K, Morikawa M, Yamauchi K, Satoh M, Maeyama K, Watanabe T, Sasaki H. Viral respiratory infection causes airway hyperresponsiveness and decreases histamine N-methyltransferase activity in guinea pigs. Am J Respir Crit Care Med 1994; 149:1180–1185.

138. Empey DW. Effect of airway infections on bronchial reactivity. Eur J Respir Dis Suppl 1983; 128:366–368.

139. Saban R, Dick EC, Fishleder RI, Buckner CK. Enhancement by parainfluenza 3 infection of contractile responses to substance P and capsaicin in airway smooth muscle from the guinea pig. Am Rev Respir Dis 1987; 136:586–591.

140. Kohrogi H, Graf PD, Sekizawa K, Borson DB, Nadel JA. Neutral endopeptidase inhibitors potentiate substance P- and capsaicin-induced cough in awake guinea pigs. J Clin Invest 1988; 82:2063–2068.

141. Fox AJ, Barnes PJ, Urban L, Dray A. An in vitro study of the properties of single vagal afferents innervating guinea-pig airways. J Physiol 1993; 469:21–35.

142. Widdicombe JG. Sensory neurophysiology of the cough reflex. J Allergy Clin Immunol 1996; 98:S84–90.

143. Gwaltney JM Jr. Rhinovirus infection of the normal human airway. Am J Respir Crit Care Med 1995; 152:S36–39.

144. Widdicombe JG. Airway receptors. Respir Physiol 2001; 125:3–15.

145. Widdicombe JG. Advances in understanding and treatment of cough. Monaldi Arch Chest Dis 1999; 54:275–279.

146. Widdicombe JG. Afferent receptors in the airways and cough. Respir Physiol 1998; 114:5–15.

147. King KA, Hu C, Rodriguez MM, Romaguera R, Jiang X, Piedimonte G. Exaggerated neurogenic inflammation and substance P receptor upregulation in RSV-infected weanling rats. Am J Respir Cell Mol Biol 2001; 24:101–107.

148. Piedimonte G, King KA, Holmgren NL, Bertrand PJ, Rodriguez MM, Hirsch RL. A humanized monoclonal antibody against respiratory syncytial virus (palivizumab) inhibits RSV-induced neurogenic-mediated inflammation in rat airways. Pediatr Res 2000; 47:351–356.

149. Piedimonte G, Nadel JA, Umeno E, McDonald DM. Sendai virus infection potentiates neurogenic inflammation in the rat trachea. J Appl Physiol 1990; 68:754–760

150. Borson DB, Brokaw JJ, Sekizawa K, McDonald DM, Nadel JA. Neutral endopeptidase

and neurogenic inflammation in rats with respiratory infections. J Appl Physiol 1989; 66:2653–2658.

151. McDonald DM. Respiratory tract infections increase susceptibility to neurogenic inflammation in the rat trachea. Am Rev Respir Dis 1988; 137:1432–1440.

152. Cao T, Pinter E, Al-Rashed S, Gerard N, Hoult JR, Brain SD. Neurokinin-1 receptor agonists are involved in mediating neutrophil accumulation in the inflamed, but not normal, cutaneous microvasculature: an in vivo study using neurokinin-1 receptor knockout mice. J Immunol 2000; 164:5424–5429.

153. Elwood W, Sun J, Barnes PJ, Giembycz MA, Chung KF. Inhibition of allergen-induced lung eosinophilia by type-III and combined type III- and IV-selective phosphodiesterase inhibitors in brown-Norway rats. Inflamm Res 1995; 44:83–86.

154. Borson DB, Gruenert DC. Glucocorticoids induce neutral endopeptidase in transformed human tracheal epithelial cells. Am J Physiol 1991; 260:L83–89.

155. Dusser DJ, Jacoby DB, Djokic TD, Rubinstein I, Borson DB, Nadel JA. Virus induces airway hyperresponsiveness to tachykinins: role of neutral endopeptidase. J Appl Physiol 1989; 67:1504–1511.

156. Piedimonte G, Rodriguez MM, King KA, McLean S, Jiang X. Respiratory syncytial virus upregulates expression of the substance P receptor in rat lungs. Am J Physiol 1999; 277:L831-840.

157. Qian J, Yehia G, Molina C, Fernandes A, Donnelly R, Anjaria D, Gascon P, Rameshwar P. Cloning of human preprotachykinin-I promoter and the role of cyclic adenosine 5′-monophosphate response elements in its expression by IL-1 and stem cell factor. J Immunol 2001; 166:2553–2561.

158: Colasurdo GN, Hemming VG, Prince GA, Gelfand AS, Loader JE, Larsen GL. Human respiratory syncytial virus produces prolonged alterations of neural control in airways of developing ferrets. Am J Respir Crit Care Med 1998; 157:1506–1511.

159. Colasurdo GN, Hemming VG, Prince GA, Loader JE, Graves JP, Larsen GL. Human respiratory syncytial virus affects nonadrenergic noncholinergic inhibition in cotton rat airways. Am J Physiol 1995; 268:L1006–1011.

160. Quinlan KL, Naik SM, Cannon G, Armstrong CA, Bunnett NW, Ansel JC, Caughman SW. Substance P activates coincident NF-AT- and NF-kappa B-dependent adhesion molecule gene expression in microvascular endothelial cells through intracellular calcium mobilization. J Immunol 1999; 163:5656–5665.

161. Quinlan KL, Song IS, Naik SM, Letran EL, Olerud JE, Bunnett NW, Armstrong CA, Caughman SW, Ansel JC. VCAM-1 expression on human dermal microvascular endothelial cells is directly and specifically up-regulated by substance P. J Immunol 1999; 162:1656–1661.

162. Levite M, Cahalon L, Hershkoviz R, Steinman L, Lider O. Neuropeptides, via specific receptors, regulate T cell adhesion to fibronectin. J Immunol 1998; 160:993–1000.

163. Dimri R, Sharabi Y, Shoham J. Specific inhibition of glucocorticoid-induced thymocyte apoptosis by substance P. J Immunol 2000; 164:2479–2486.

164. Lecci A, Giuliani S, Tramontana M, Carini F, Maggi CA. Peripheral actions of tachykinins. Neuropeptides 2000; 34:303-313.

165. Hood VC, Cruwys SC, Urban L, Kidd BL. Differential role of neurokinin receptors in human lymphocyte and monocyte chemotaxis. Regul Pept 2000; 96:17–21.

166. Koyama S, Sato E, Nomura H, Kubo K, Nagai S, Izumi T. Acetylcholine and substance P stimulate bronchial epithelial cells to release eosinophil chemotactic activity. J Appl Physiol 1998; 84:1528–1534.

167. Harrison NK, Dawes KE, Kwon OJ, Barnes PJ, Laurent GJ, Chung KF. Effects of neuropeptides on human lung fibroblast proliferation and chemotaxis. Am J Physiol 1995; 268:L278–283.

168. Borovikova LV, Ivanova S, Zhang M, Yang H, Botchkina GI, Watkins LR, Wang H, Abumrad N, Eaton JW, Tracey KJ. Vagus nerve stimulation attenuates the systemic inflammatory response to endotoxin. Nature 2000; 405:458–462.

169. Borum P, Olsen L, Winther B, Mygind N. Ipratropium nasal spray: a new treatment for rhinorrhea in the common cold. Am Rev Respir Dis 1981; 123:418–420.

170. Gaffey MJ, Gwaltney JM Jr, Dressler WE, Sorrentino JV, Hayden FG. Intranasally administered atropine methonitrate treatment of experimental rhinovirus colds. Am Rev Respir Dis 1987; 135:241–242.

171. Gaffey MJ, Hayden FG, Boyd JC, Gwaltney JM. Ipratropium bromide treatment of experimental rhinovirus infection. Antimicrob Agents Chemother 1988; 32:1644–1647.

172. Dockhorn R, Grossman J, Posner M, Zinny M, Tinkleman D. A double-blind, placebo-controlled study of the safety and efficacy of ipratropium bromide nasal spray versus placebo in patients with the common cold. J Allergy Clin Immunol 1992; 90:1076-1082.

173. Gwaltney JM Jr. Combined antiviral and antimediator treatment of rhinovirus colds. J Infect Dis 1992; 166:776–782.

174. Doyle WJ, Riker DK, McBride TP, Hayden FG, Hendley JO, Swarts JD, Gwaltney JM. Therapeutic effects of an anticholinergic-sympathomimetic combination in induced rhinovirus colds. Ann Otol Rhinol Laryngol 1993; 102:521–527.

175. Diamond L, Dockhorn RJ, Grossman J, Kisicki JC, Posner M, Zinny MA, Koker P, Korts D, Wecker MT. A dose-response study of the efficacy and safety of ipratropium bromide nasal spray in the treatment of the common cold. J Allergy Clin Immunol 1995; 95:1139–1146.

176. Wood CC, Fireman P, Grossman J, Wecker M, MacGregor T. Product characteristics and pharmacokinetics of intranasal ipratropium bromide. J Allergy Clin Immunol 1995; 95:1111-1116.

177. Hayden FG, Diamond L, Wood PB, Korts DC, Wecker MT. Effectiveness and safety of intranasal ipratropium bromide in common colds. A randomized, double-blind, placebo-controlled trial. Ann Intern Med 1996; 125:89–97.

178. Ostberg B, Winther B, Borum P, Mygind N. Common cold and high-dose ipratropium bromide: use of anticholinergic medication as an indicator of reflex-mediated hypersecretion. Rhinology 1997; 35:58–62.

179. Lowry R, Wood A, Higenbottam T. The effect of anticholinergic bronchodilator therapy on cough during upper respiratory tract infections. Br J Clin Pharmacol 1994; 37: 187-191.

180. Holmes PW, Barter CE, Pierce RJ. Chronic persistent cough: use of ipratropium bromide in undiagnosed cases following upper respiratory tract infection. Respir Med 1992; 86:425–429.

181. Nicholson KG, Kent J, Ireland DC. Respiratory viruses and exacerbations of asthma in adults. Br Med J 1993; 307:982-986.

182. Johnston SL, Pattemore PK, Sanderson G, Smith S, Lampe F, Josephs L, Symington P, O'Toole S, Myint SH, Tyrrell DA, et al. Community study of role of viral infections in exacerbations of asthma in 9–11 year old children. Br Med J 1995; 310:1225-1229.

183. Rodrigo G, Rodrigo C, Burschtin O. A meta-analysis of the effects of ipratropium bromide in adults with acute asthma. Am J Med 1999;107:363–370.
184. Qureshi F, Pestian J, Davis P, Zaritsky A. Effect of nebulized ipratropium on the hospitalization rates of children with asthma. N Engl J Med 1998; 339:1030–1035.
185. Lowe JA, 3rd. Nonpeptide tachykinin antagonists: medicinal chemistry and molecular biology. Med Res Rev 1996; 16:527–545.
186. Joos GF, Kips JC, Peleman RA, Pauwels RA. Tachykinin antagonists and the airways. Arch Int Pharmacodyn Ther 1995; 329:205–219.
187. Honjin R. On the nerve supply of the lung of the mouse with special reference to the structure of the peripheral vegative and nervous system. J Comp Neurol 1956;105: 587.

12

Animal Models of Viral Respiratory Infections

ROSEMARY J. BOYTON and PETER J. M. OPENSHAW

Imperial College London
London, England

I. Introduction

The gas exchange function of the lung and vast mucosal surface area together make this site a prime portal of entry for infection. Among the pathogens that may enter and cause respiratory infections are viruses such as influenza, parainfluenza, respiratory syncytial virus (RSV), rhinoviruses, and adenoviruses. Much of the research on the host–pathogen interaction during these infections has necessarily been done in animal models, particularly mouse. The central issues have been the elucidation of those immune mechanisms that may be particularly involved in rapid viral clearance, on the one hand, or with exacerbated lung pathology on the other. These concerns bear directly on the design of rational vaccines that will be effective but safe. In this chapter we review some of the evidence generated from animal models that select out the protective from the pathogenic mechanisms in respiratory virus infections, and discuss the related issue of whether viral infections or the responses to them are involved in the development of asthma. Understanding of the molecular pathogenesis of asthma is still in its infancy. For example, it is now clear that multiple genes are involved, but the identity of only a few of these candidates is known. One clear starting point is that susceptibility is associated with the balance of Th1 and Th2 cytokines in the lung. As discussed below, a major driving force for the cytokine milieu in the lung comes from viral infection. Furthermore, many of the lessons learnt from studying T-lymphocyte–cytokine responses during viral infection are pertinent to the analysis of asthma and the design of immumodulatory therapies.

II. Protective Mechanisms

The analysis of viral immunity in animal experimental models has clearly offered many advantages to research in this field: the ability to look at experimentally induced disease, to investigate the protective effects of cellular and antibody mechanisms, and to look at manipulation of the immune response using transgenic or gene-knockout approaches. However, an important caveat is that these studies entail the study of human pathogens in a species that is not the natural host. Thus, while basic mechanisms of, for example, influenza virus immunity and clearance can be studied in inbred mice, most models are, unlike the clinical picture, severe and lethal. For some viruses such as human immunodeficiency virus (HIV) and human T-lymphotrophic virus 1 (HTLV1), the cellular receptors for viral entry are absent in mice, so that infection can only be achieved in transgenic mice that have been engineered to express the human viral receptors.

The immune response has the potential to oppose respiratory viral infection in several different ways. Indeed, one of the lessons from experimental models of infection is that there is redundancy of immune mechanisms: several different, overlaid responses appear to duplicate any particular role in host defense. The specific immune response can be classified into humoral and cellular mechanisms. In a previously exposed individual, an initial barrier to infection is from specific antiviral antibodies, both mucosal IgA and systemic IgG. Since the antibody response tends to target the outer, exposed proteins of viruses and these tend to be the more variable virus products, the humoral response offers poor protection against heterologous virus infection. However, they do offer protection from secondary challenge by the homologous strain. The antibodies have the ability to neutralize virus by direct binding to input virions, as well as opsonizing for phagocytic uptake and priming for lysis of infected cells through antibody-dependent cellular cytotoxicity (ADCC). One of the most rapid cellular responses is that of natural killer (NK) cells. These lymphoid cells originate from the same hematopoietic lineage as T lymphocytes, but have differentiated to express a different set of cellular receptors. They are programmed to kill targets by default unless they receive inhibitory signals from a number of cellular ligands expressed by normal cells that have not been virally infected or transformed. NK cells are also a very rapid source of interferon-γ (IFN-γ). An important aspect IFN-γ function is through the upregulation of other immune effector functions, including the induction of major histocompatibility complex (MHC) molecules. The innate response in the lung also involves the nonimmune interferons, IFN-α and β, which have direct antiviral properties. As discussed in detail below, the action of specific T lymphocytes lies at the heart of the response to these respiratory infections. T lymphocytes are subclassified into CD4 and CD8 cells. The former, sometimes called T-helper cells, are characterized by the production of cytokines that stimulate other cell types, the latter being cytolytic. CD4 cells are further defined on the basis of their patterns of cytokine release as being either Th1 or Th2 (1). The hallmark cytokine of a Th1 response is IFN-γ, produced in the absence of interleukin-4 (IL-4) release. These cells are associated with inflammatory, delayed-type hypersensitivity (DTH) responses leading to macrophage activation. Th2 cells produce IL-4 and IL-5 in the absence of IFN-γ and are associated with a range of effector functions broadly associated with the clearance of extracellular pathogens, including help for antibody responses and the stimulation of basophils and eosinophils. The functional dichotomy between Th1 and Th2 cells is often manifest in preferential immunoglobulin isotype switching, the former response leading to the dominance of IgG2a secretion by B cells, the latter to IgG1 and IgE (2,3).

More recently it has become apparent that Th1 and Th2 populations can be differentiated by their expression of chemokine receptors, and thus their chemotactic responses and trafficking in response to different stimuli. In humans, the Th1 phenotype is associated with the chemokine receptors 3 and 5 (4,5) while the Th2 phenotype is associated with chemokine receptors 3 and 4 (4,6,7). As would be predicted from the fact that the nature of the Th1/Th2 dichotomy lies in their program of cytokine release, other differences between Th1 and Th2 cells are in the critical transcription factors used to drive these programmes of gene expression and in the expression of cytokine receptors (8–14). CD8 cytotoxic cells can be subclassified on the same basis into Tc1 and Tc2. The effects of Th1 and Th2 lymphocytes are manifest in the other cellular populations preferentially expanded at the site of response. In particular, Th2 cells are associated with eosinophilia and Th1 cells with activated monocytes, and sometimes with a neutrophilia.

III. Experimental Infection with Influenza Virus

The infection of inbred laboratory mice, particularly BALB/c mice, with influenza A, serves as a prototypic model for the characterization of respiratory immunity and indeed for viral immunity and T-lymphocyte immune responsiveness in general. Typically, mice have been infected by intranasal administration of live virus, allowing the analysis of lung virus clearance, immunity, and lethality. The inoculation doses used are such that infection is lethal in most experimental animals, and one can begin to ask which cells or molecules are needed to confer protective immunity. The central research questions in this field have developed over time. In terms of vaccinology, early studies investigated the viral epitopes recognized by T cells or antibodies that are required to afford protection that is either specific or crossreactive. As it became possible to clone and propagate specific T cells, there was much in vitro analysis of the specificity and cytotoxic function of anti-influenza T-cell clones. Such studies provided the first cellular reagents for in vivo studies investigating the nature of the cellular responses that would give protection from lethal infection. A recurrent theme from these studies, as in others of lung immunity, is the need to regulate the immune response appropriately to achieve efficient virus clearance without engendering T-cell-mediated inflammatory pathology. A balance must be achieved between the risk of tissue damage from the influenza virus itself, which is cytolytic for host lung epithelial cells (15), and the cytopathic effects of the inflammatory response to the virus. Knockout mice and monoclonal antibodies against specific mediators such as chemokines have allowed further identification of the protective or pathogenic properties of innate and specific mechanisms.

A. Mechanisms of Virus Clearance

Mouse and human T cells against influenza virus were among the first cultured T-cell populations to be studied. In some of the first studies of what were to become known as CD8 cytotoxic T lymphocytes (CTL), it was shown that T cells cultured in the presence of target cells infected in vitro with influenza could specifically lyse the infected targets. This could be measured by labeling the membranes of the infected targets with the radioisotope chromium-51, so that cell lysis would result in release of radioisotope into the culture supernatant. The T cells would only recognize viral products that were presented on targets bearing the same MHC molecules as those of the host cells on which virus was originally encountered. This phenomenon of so-called MHC restriction (for which Rolf Zinkernagel and Peter Doherty received a Nobel prize) was appreciated to be the basic mechanisms by which T-cell receptors survey the difference between self molecules and nonself that has had some molecular change imposed, for example, by viral infection or malignant transformation (16). During the 1970s, Andrew McMichael, Brigitte Askonas, and others had demonstrated the role of human leukocyte antigen (HLA) restriction in the presentation of influenza antigen to human T lymphocytes (17). Using a similar experimental system of cloned cytotoxic T cells and virus-infected target cell lines, Alain Townsend and others subsequently showed that CTL, unlike antibodies, tend to recognize internal, virus-encoded proteins such as influenza nucleoprotein (18). Furthermore, these were shown to be recognized by the CTL in the form of short, peptidic fragments of the viral protein that are broken down by the cell and loaded onto newly synthesized MHC molecules. One consequence of this finding was the experimental advance that the immune response could be studied in a reductionist form by pulsing cells with a synthetic peptide of 8–10 amino acids representing the known T-cell target, rather than having to use whole virus.

However, for investigators focused on the understanding of respiratory disease, an enduring question was which of the cellular immune mechanisms that had been described actually played a role in clearance of the virus from the infected lung. For some mouse models of viral infection, such as lymphochoriomeningitis virus (LCMV) infection, it had been shown that infection with the virus was not in itself lethal, the pathology being mediated rather by the lytic T-cell response to the virus. The pathogenic role of the antiviral immune response in mediating lung tissue damage is evident, to a greater or lesser extent, in all of the lung infection models that have been studied, including influenza. Experiments on the role of T cells in clearance of influenza from the mouse lung demonstrate that CD8 CTL are important, particularly with respect to their production of IFN-γ. The importance of CD8 cells was defined by transfer of protection with T-cell clones, by the finding that the cellular exudate in the lungs of infected mice is dominated by CD8 cells, and by the finding that elimination of CD4 T-helper cells by antibody treatment does not alter clearance of virus from the lung (19). Furthermore, transfer of anti-influenza CTL to nude mice (lacking any endogenous, mature, T and B lymphocytes) completely clears infection from the lung, whereas transfer of neutralizing antibody only diminishes viral shedding for as long as antibody administration is continued (20). In line with the finding that CTL clones often recognize epitopes derived from relatively conserved viral proteins, it was observed that CTL clones generated against one influenza A subtype, but cross-reactively recognizing others, could reduce virus titers and protect mice infected with each of the recognized subtypes (21,22). Although cross-protection against variant influenza subtypes by antibody is more limited due to the great antigenic variation of the cell-surface viral proteins, an important exception is the antibody response to the relatively invariant M2 protein, which is highly protective (23). Thus, studies during the 1980s and early 1990s using murine models of influenza infection demonstrated that a potent cytotoxic response by CD8 cells is a key mechanism for clearing lung infection.

However, many subsequent studies using transgenic and knockout mouse models have shown that many other mechanisms, including the effect of CD4 T-helper cells, can be important and that the CD8 response can itself be pathogenic. Transgenic mice are strains in which a particular gene product, for example a viral protein or a T-cell receptor, is overexpressed in the mouse through incorporation of multiple copies of a transgene DNA construct in the germline following microinjection into the fertilized, single-cell embryo. In knockout strains, a specific mouse gene to be studied, for example, the gene encoding a cytokine receptor, is deleted by homologously recombining with the DNA of embryonic stem (ES) cells, a DNA construct in which the flanking regions of the gene have been retained, but the internal exons have been deleted. In the cells of a proportion of the resulting offspring, one chromosome will bear the nonfunctional disrupted gene, and breeding to homozygosity will yield mice that are completely null for the protein.

Depending on the precise conditions used for influenza infection, some researchers found that MHC class I-null mice, lacking any CD8 T cells, showed the expected impairment in viral resistance (24), while others found no defect, suggesting a redundancy in antiviral defense mechanisms (25). Mice lacking CD8 responses are nevertheless protected through the action of CD4 T-helper cells. This is presumed to be partly through the help offered by these cells to B cells in making a neutralizing antibody response (26). However, a caveat is that when panels of CD4 T-cell clones were tested for the ability to mediate clearance of virus from the lung after transfer to infected hosts, some mediated rapid clearance while others exacerbated symptoms. The differential behavior of the clones was believed to be due to differences in Th1 cytokine profiles (27). The protective potential of neutralizing antibodies is further demonstrated by the finding that transfer of IgG2a antibodies against influenza hemagglutinin can completely clear infection from the lung. B-cell-deficient knockout mice have a 50–100-fold greater susceptibility to lethal type A influenza virus infection than do wild-type mice (28). However, this work demonstrates another aspect of the multilayered immune response to infection: after sublethal doses of influenza, B-cell-deficient mice actually showed increased resistance to viral infection compared with controls. The difference was believed to be accounted for by a compensatory enhancement in T-cell-mediated resistance.

Reductionist experiments in which a particular population of cloned T cells are transferred to an infected host or a particular population has been knocked out have clearly been helpful, yet they can also be misleading. What might be termed a belt and suspenders evolution of the mammalian immune response inevitably means that if the upper layer of antiviral immunity is stripped away, some lower level will assume compensatory importance. Thus, experiments with knockout mice, cell transfers, and antibody depletion sometimes appear to show that CD8 cells without CD4 cells, CD4 cells without CD8 cells, or antibody without either can, to some extent, protect from influenza infection. However, on balance, the experiments from mice and humans with an intact immune response implicate the CD8 CTL response as being necessary and sufficient to cure infection. Support for this comes from the very large clonal populations of anti-influenza CTL that can be detected in humans after infection (29). Accurate estimates for the frequency of T cells with a particular specificity out of the total population have become possible though a relatively new technique, termed tetramer staining. The approach is based on the fact that the ligand for any given, specific, T-cell receptor is a particular combination of antigenic peptide bound to an MHC molecule. Thus, if one could synthesize this combination and label it with a visible fluorochrome, it could be used as a laboratory reagent to visualize and enumerate specific T cells. However, because the affinity of the T-cell receptor for its ligand is very low, a stable interaction cannot easily be detected unless a multivalent reagent is used, thus increasing the avidity. This is usually achieved by attaching four molecules of biotinlylated MHC/peptide to the tetrameric molecule avidin. The avidin is generally labeled with a fluorescent fluorochrome such as the red dye phycoerythrin, which can be visualized using the laser of a flow cytometer. Tetramer analysis has been applied to investigation of the T-cell populations involved in the primary and secondary response to influenza virus in the pneumonic lung. Whereas conventional immunological methods had tended to estimate antigen-specific lymphocytes as one in several thousand of the bulk population, this analysis showed that 15% of bronchoalveolar lavage (BAL) cells in the primary response, rising to greater than 65% of cells in the secondary response, are specific for a single, dominant MHC class I/influenza nucleoprotein peptide combination (30). Most of these cells are producing a strong IFN-γ response. The greater frequency of cells participating in the secondary response several months after initial infection causes more rapid clearance of virus from the lung. The maintenance and recruitment of this enhanced CTL population are dependent on CD4 T-helper cells (31).

Studies in this model and in the mouse parainfluenza Sendai virus model indicate the existence of a population of cells that may be distinct from the classic view of memory cells as a circulating population capable of reactivation with reduced costimulatory requirements. The lung infection studies point to a lingering population of protective lymphocytes that is actually resident in the lung in the very long term after all trace of virus has disappeared, and has the cell surface phenotype of an activated cell rather than the dormant, memory cell (32,33). The ability to quantify the various parameters of the enhanced response in secondary infection has greatly clarified our understanding of this phenomenon. It had not been predicted that, even for a virus like influenza that is entirely cleared following infection and has no persistent or latent state in the host, there is an extremely substantial and long-lived enhancement in the frequency of influenza specific CTL, both in the lungs and in the systemic immune pool (34).

The same tetramer approach has been applied to investigation of immunity to a novel, highly lethal influenza strain. In the summer of 1997, there was concern over what was considered a potential influenza pandemic following characterization of an influenza type A strain that had caused six deaths out of 18 people infected in Hong Kong (35). The cause for alarm was that the influenza strain was found to be a hemagglutinin 5, nucleoprotein 1 (H5N1) isolate. It had been previously thought that H5 influenza viruses were restricted to avian strains and would not be able to infect humans. As would be predicted from this, humans lack protective antibodies specific for H5 epitopes. The strain had earlier been isolated from chicken stocks, having caused the deaths of 4500 chickens on three farms earlier in the year. Doherty and colleagues (36) used tetramers and conventional approaches to investigate the level of protection that might be conferred against a lethal, avian isolate by prior exposure to a normal, H3N2 influenza isolate. Strong protection was conferred by prior exposure to the mammalian, H3N2 isolate, and in this case a large component of it seemed to reside in the antibody response, since Ig-null, immune mice did not show protection. However, tetramer analysis showed the recruitment of a high frequency of influenza nucleoprotein-specific CTL to the lung and these could protect Ig-null mice at lower inoculation doses.

Similarly to other T-cell populations, CD8 CTLs make various different cytokines and mediators. Which are important in resolving influenza infections? The cell lysis program of these cells is generally believed to depend on either of two pathways: the release of perforin causing direct cytotoxicity in targets and Fas/Fas-ligand recognition leading to apoptosis. CTL can also release tumor necrosis factor α (TNF-α) which has a cytotoxic effect on target cells as well as modulating other immune molecules. IFN-γ, the prototypic Th1/Tc1 cytokine, can be made by activated CD8 cells and is strongly correlated with clearance of infection. The role of IFN-γ release has been investigated by several groups, using mice that are null for either IFN-γ or its receptor (37,38). The presence of IFN-γ production by CTL is correlated with effector cell recruitment and with more controlled lung inflammation, giving rise to reduced lung damage (39). However, no absolute dependence on IFN-γ has ever been demonstrated in the primary or secondary immune response to influenza or in heterosubtypic immunity (that is, cross-protection against an influenza virus of a different serotype) (40). Another study compared the effect of knocking out the receptor for IFN-γ with knockouts for the IFN-α/β receptor (that is, lacking the capacity for nonimmune, antiviral interferon responses). In this case it was found that lung virus titers were not significantly different between any of the knockouts and control mice although, in some studies, lung pathology is much exacerbated in the absence of normal interferon pathways (37,38). This again suggested a high level of redundancy in the mechanisms of antiviral protection. In support of this, the IFN-α/β receptor-null mice show a compensatory antibody response with accelerated and enhanced neutralizing antibody production.

B. Mechanisms of Immunopathology

Transgenic mice can be used also to model the immunopathological component of lung damage, removed from the effects of damage caused by influenza virus. Enelow and co-workers created a transgenic model for investigating the role of CD8 cells in inflammatory lung disease (41). In this model influenza hemagglutinin is ectopically expressed in alveolar cells by juxtaposing the gene for this product alongside the promoter normally responsible for directing transcription of the surfactant protein C gene in the lung. When this chimeric transgene is incorporated into the germline DNA of mice, influenza hemagglutinin is constitutively expressed in lung alveolar epithelium. It is then possible to look at the consequences of introducing CTL specific for the immunodominant epitope, amino acids 210–219 from hemagglutinin (41). The result of transferring specific CTL is a dramatic effect on lung structure and function with progressive, lethal injury. Death ensues within 8 days with patchy lung hemorrhage and bronchiolitis. Progressive traffic is seen from the bronchovascular bundles outwards, towards the peribronchiolar interstitium, reflecting the pattern of T-cell trafficking into the lung parenchyma. Oxygen-diffusing capacity is dramatically decreased within 3 days of T-cell transfer and then declines progressively. Lung compliance is also markedly reduced. Indeed, the entire cascade of inflammatory events that results in interstitial pneumonia could be reiterated, in the absence of any infectious agent, by a known, molecular interaction among MHC class I, peptide, and the receptor of a CD8 T cell. It was later demonstrated that pathology in this model is dependent on the release of TNF (42). This appears to act, at least in part, through activation of alveolar cells to release chemokines. Chemokines are a large family of soluble factors that confer tropism on the trafficking of specific cell types bearing the receptors for that chemokine. In this case, alveolar cells secrete the chemokines macrophage chemotactic protein 1 (MCP-1) and macrophage inhibitory protein 1 (MIP-1). Neutralization of the MCP-1 largely inhibited the parenchymal infiltration seen after T-cell transfer.

In summary, the models of lung infection by influenza in inbred, transgenic, and knockout mice have been the prototypic models for understanding lung infection. They emphasize the many layers of immune components that are overlayed to protect against infection and clear the virus. Particular emphasis has been placed on the role of CTL, which, because they tend to recognize the more conserved viral products, often confer heterosubtypic immunity. Neutralizing antibody also plays an important role, but is often directed at subtype-specific epitopes. The outcome of the antiviral response in the lung represents a balance between prevention of tissue damage by the lytic virus itself and the risk of collateral damage from inflammatory cytokines released in the course of the T-cell response. In recent years, the use of influenza tetramers has allowed precise quantification of the primary and secondary response to influenza, demonstrating a pronounced and long-lived enhancement in the frequency of specific T cells after primary infection.

IV. Models of Respiratory Syncytial Virus Infection

Respiratory syncytial virus (RSV) is a common cold virus that causes bronchiolitis in infants and kills about 1 million children per year worldwide (43). Early RSV vaccine trials in children, using formalin-inactivated virus, showed a much enhanced mortality and morbidity in the vaccinated group, emphasizing the critical importance of gaining a detailed understanding of the interplay between viral pathology, the specific T-cell response, and the role of local cytokines (44-47). Since that time, an enormous amount has been learnt about the nature of the response to RSV, offering some possible explanations and solutions for the outcome of the early vaccine trials. The mouse model of RSV lung disease reproduces many aspects of the human disease, in particular, the role of antiviral T cells in both eliminating virus and causing disease (48). As in the influenza models, it was established several years ago that transfer of CD8, class I-restricted CTL is efficient at clearing live virus from the lung but can also lead to the development of acute respiratory disease (49). An earlier source of protective IFN-γ during the antiviral response comes from NK1.1 cells (50). IL-12-activated NK cells have been demonstrated to inhibit eosinophilia without causing illness (51).

An important tool for dissecting the role of different viral products in the immune response has been the ability to express isolated gene products in recombinant vaccinia viruses. An interesting finding from this molecular characterization of the virally encoded proteins has been the ability of different proteins to activate different types of immune response and pathology. Prior sensitization to the attachment protein (G), fusion protein (F), or second matrix (22K) protein (expressed by recombinant vaccinia virus) results in different T cell responses (52–54). Immunization with the 22K protein results in predominantly class I restricted cytolytic CD8$^+$ cells in H-2^d mice, while sensitization with the fusion protein (F) results in a mixture of cytolytic CD8$^+$ cells and Th1 CD4$^+$ cells and the attachment protein (G) results in largely Th2 CD4$^+$ cells in the absence of detectable CD8 cells. These findings have possible implications for the caution needed with respect to subunit vaccines, not only against this virus but also for viral immunology generally. Many strains of RSV infected mice previously sensitized with the G protein demonstrate enhanced disease, lung eosinophilia, and increased weight loss after RSV challenge. IL-4- and IL-5-secreting CD4$^+$ T cells are necessary and sufficient for this response (52). Prior sensitization with the F protein results in a T-cell infiltrate and weight loss, but without eosinophil recruitment (53).

Experiments in which immunization with the G protein have leads to pathogenic eosinophilia, illness, and death on rechallenge with RSV, have been regarded models for the pathology induced in the course of the 1960s vaccine trials. The response to the G protein appears, at least in H-2^d mice, to be largely focused on one epitope: amino acids 185–193. There is a degree of focus also in the responding

CD4 T-cell population, since the response becomes dominated by clones of T cells characterized by the use of a particular gene family in assembly of the T-cell receptor: Vβ14 (54). These mouse model studies allow the opportunity to use substituted peptides, varied amino acid by amino acid, to identify those residues making contact with the T-cell receptor. This raises the possibility of designing antagonist peptide vaccines, as has been attempted in murine and human autoimmune diseases, able to drive T cells into planned, alternative programs of cytokine release, so modifying pathogenesis (55,56).

As in humans, there is a genetic contribution from the host, determining aspects of the nature of the specific immune response, the efficiency of virus clearance, and the propensity to develop tissue damage. Inbred mouse strains that differ, either only at the MHC or only in the other genes outside the MHC, or both, can be compared. Furthermore, there is the possibility of conducting back-cross experiments to look at dominance and to start to map additional disease susceptibility loci. Mouse strains have been compared with respect to susceptibility to disease following conventional RSV infection, or following initial infection with the glycoprotein G vaccinia recombinant virus. A starting point for this analysis is the observation in commonly used mouse strains that there are differences in the pattern of RSV infection: the BALB/c and DBA/2 strains develop very pronounced airway pathology, while C57BL/6 mice have a much milder response (57,58). The response of C57BL/6 (but not DBA/2 mice) to infection is characterized by a rapid IFN-γ response, followed by a later peak in IL-12 (59). Conversely, the susceptible DBA/2 and BALB/c strains show a follow-on increase in IL-13 release, not seen in C57BL/6 mice, correlating with the development of AHR and mucus production (60). These findings suggest that part of the genetic difference in disease susceptibility lies in the balance between the IL-12-driven Th1 response and the Th2, IL-13 response that controls it: Th2 "overshoot" leading to tissue damage. Evidence for this comes from the ability of neutralizing anti-IL-13 antibody to protect from lung disease. Further light is shed on this from studies on the genetics of the pathogenic, Th2-driven, eosinophilic response to the G protein (61). H-2^d strains showed the susceptibility-associated eosinophilia, irrespective of other background genes. This may reflect preferential presentation of an immunodominant G protein 185–193 epitope by the H2-E^d class II molecule within this MHC haplotype (54). No mouse strains with an H-2^k MHC showed eosinophilia, while H-2^b strains gave variable results. However, across all of the mouse strains, the presence or absence of eosinophilia had no bearing on clearance of virus, emphasizing the distinction between mechanisms involved in the antiviral response (mainly antibody and CTL) and those involved in causing tissue damage. A possible clue to control of the response comes from the observation that development of the eosinophilic response is often associated with reduced CD8 numbers among BAL. This may suggest an interplay between IFN-γ-secreting CD8 cells and the pathogenic, CD4, Th2 response. This was investigated by in vivo depletion of C57BL/6 mice (which do not develop eosinophilia after sensitization to G) with anti-CD8 or anti-IFN-γ antibodies (62). Loss of CD8 cells or IFN-γ converted the phenotype to an eosiniphilia, as seen in the susceptible strains. Such findings suggest that vaccines designed to enhance CD8 recognition might avoid disease caused by Th2 cells. However, the studies are in contrast to other work, utilizing both primary infection and challenge with wild-type RSV, in which CD8 depletion was associated with amelioration of AHR and eosinophilia, indicating support for development of a Th2 environment from these cells (63). Taken together, the work suggests that while CD8 cells clearly perform a protective, antiviral, and immunoregulatory role during the clearance of RSV, they can also, in certain circumstances, contribute to pathology, as had been predicted by early T-cell transfer studies (49).

If we assume that the CD8 CTL response is predominantly protective, one means of preferentially stimulating these cells would be to immunize with the F glycoprotein. The response to RSV F protein involves CTL and antibody, but not Th1 or Th2 cells (64). The frequency and function of CTL against the immunodominant F antigen, amino acids 85–93, were investigated using tetramer staining. It has been proposed, however, that these cells may be defective with respect to effector function, since cells from the lung show lower than expected expression of IFN-γ and lack the surface phenotype of terminally differentiated effectors (65).

An alternative approach to the manipulation of protective relative to pathogenic T-cell responses is to engineer a virus that lacks the pathogenic epitope. When the CD4 T-cell epitope of G protein for BALB/c mice was mapped using RSV frameshift mutants and recombinant vaccinia viruses expressing partial or mutant G proteins, it was narrowed down to an epitope within amino acids 193–203. Recombinant virus lacking this epitope induced protection without weight loss or eosinophilia, while virus containing only this epitope induced illness without protection (66). Other manipulations capable of shifting the Th1/Th2 balance and so influencing the balance between protection and lung damage include the use of enterotoxin-based mucosal adjuvants (67) or prior infection with a virus such as influenza (68).

V. The Antiviral Response: Implications for Delivery of Gene Therapy

The prospects of gene therapy targeted to the lung have raised new issues of viral immunity in the lung. Many diseases have gene therapy trials in prospect, notably the transfer of wild-type cystic fibrosis transmembrane conductance regulator (CFTR) to the lung of cystic fibrosis patients to restore normal chloride channel function. The technical challenge in gene therapy is to create a delivery system that will be safe for the patient, while ensuring that the new gene reaches the target tissue and can be expressed there, in the long term, at an appropriate level to restore function (69). Many of the first-generation gene therapy vectors have been based on modified adenovirus constructs lacking E1. Thus, if the CFTR gene or another construct is to survive in the lung, the requirement is the opposite of that in normal models of virus research: to establish how to evade all immunity in the lung so that the virus can survive and continue to be expressed (70). Although CFTR therapy has, to date, been the major target for gene therapy in the lung, there are many other possibilities for modulating gene expression in the lung during disease. Based on the observation that TGF-β plays an important role in lung fibrosis, experiments have been under-taken in the bleomycin fibrosis mouse model to look at gene therapy for the expres-sion of Smad7, an antagonist of TGF-β signaling (71). In a disease involving dysreg-ulated local cytokine production such as asthma, there may be the prospect of gene therapy with Thl cytokines to reset the cytokine balance. An example of this is the construction of a replication-deficient adenovirus construct containing IL-18 for tri-als in reversal of airway hyperreactivity (AHR) in the mouse model of ovalbumin-induced asthma (72). It was found that treatment of ovalbumin-sensitized mice with the gene therapy construct reduced allergen-specific IL-4 production, airway eosino-philia, mucus production, and AHR. The treatment was also effective in mice with established AHR. Indeed, there have been many attempts in mouse models to use adenoviral vectors for the manipulation of the lung cytokine environment, including the use of intrapulmonary TNF to reverse sepsis-induced suppression of lung immu-nity (73). Caution will be needed in the translation of corrective cytokine gene ther-apy to the clinical setting because of the risk of an irreversible overshoot, which may, for example, convert a so-called Th2 asthmatic lung into a Thl sarcoid lung.

If adenovirus-based gene therapy is to be effective, a number of manipulations may have to be undertaken. The first possibility is to identify the regions of the virus or inserted sequence that are immunogenic and determine whether they can be mutated or removed. The second is to characterize the specific immune response to the virus and inserted gene and identify treatments capable of suppressing these responses to the gene therapy construct. Studies aimed at modeling the lung T-cell response to adenovirus vectors show that CD8 CTL responses as well as CD4 Thl and Th2 responses are rapidly induced in the lung (74). CTL responses in particular seem to be responsible for the rapid elimination of the viral construct from mouse lungs (75). Furthermore, the formation of IgA antiviral antibodies contributes to a block in gene transfer that occurs following a second administration of virus. Be-cause the generation of an IgA response is dependent on help from Th2 CD4 cells, one group reasoned that the inhibitors might be prevented by coadministration of a Thl cytokine such as IL-12. By administering recombinant IL-12 into the airway at the same time as the recombinant virus, it was found that the formation of neu-tralizing antibody was diminished, allowing for efficient readministration of virus (76), although this approach has clear dangers in humans. Another approach for modulating the local cytokine environment at the time of transduction with the ret-roviral construct rests on the fact that the viral IL-l0 homolog sequences possess only a subset of human IL-10's properties, notably the suppression of cytokine syn-thesis by Thl clones (77). It was found that constructs containing viral IL-10 showed greatly prolonged expression in the lung and suppressed acute inflammatory re-sponses in the lung to intratracheal administration of adenovirus. More conventional methods of immunosuppression have also been used in the context gene therapy, including therapy with the nondepleting antihuman CD4 monoclonal antibody Clenoliximab (78) and with CTLA4Ig (79).

Thus, for the development of gene therapy in the lung with viral vectors, the antiviral immune response that would normally clear virus rapidly from the lung along with the gene product of interest constitutes a significant challenge. A number of strategies to overcome this problem have been investigated, including infection under the cover of cytokines and other forms of immunosuppression. It remains to be seen whether the newer gene therapy vectors such as the Filovirus-pseudotyped lentiviral vector will confer strong gene expression while attracting less attention from the immune response.

VI. Lessons for Susceptibility to Asthma

Clinical and epidemiological analysis of the relationship between childhood infections and susceptibility to asthma have inevitably yielded complex and often inconclusive results. Infection with certain viruses during infancy has been implicated as having a potential role in initiation of an asthmatic phenotype (80). However, with most infections passing largely undetected and the lymphocyte and lung tissues essentially inaccessible, the problems inherent in translating these observations into a mechanistic model in human pediatric patients are self-evident.

The murine models of viral infection of the type described above, in which there is a very detailed understanding of the nature of the infection, its clearance, and the associated cytokine microenvironment, offer a potential avenue for investigating the relationship between viral infection and atopy. It is possible to investigate susceptibility to experimentally induced asthma against this background of viral immunity. Most commonly, this involves analysis of the influence of prior infection on the induction of an asthmatic response in the inhaled ovalbumin model or a related model such as sensitization with cockroach antigen. It will be clear from the above that many different NK cell, Th1, Th2, and CTL T-cell populations may contribute to the antiviral response in the lung. As a generalization, the clearance of virus will often have been associated, initially at least, with the release of IFN-γ from CTL, and thus the creation of a local environment permissive for Th1 generation, but inhibitory for Th2 responses. In many viral infections, IL-12, the major Th1-promoting cytokine, is associated with clearance of virus and recovery (81). It is thus paradoxical that childhood infections with RSV are an independent risk factor for the development of asthma, a Th2-associated phenotype (82). Analysis of RSV infection in the mouse models is illuminating with respect to possible underlying causes for this effect. The IL-12 response to RSV infection has been compared between the BALB/c and DBA/2 strains on the one hand, which show overt airway pathology in response to infection, and the C57BL/6 strain, which show a more favorable response (59). Infection of the C57BL/6 strain causes a strong IL-12 response not evident in the other strains. Neutralization of this IL-12 switches the phenotype of the C57BL/6 strain, so that they start to show pronounced AHR, mucus production, IL-13 release, eosinophilia, and tissue damage, similarly to the susceptible mouse strains. The implication from these and other similar studies is that in inbred mice, as in children, an unfavorable outcome of RSV infection may be the consequence of an inappropriately Th2-biased immune response (60,83,84).

Tekkanat and colleagues examined the development of AHR in the context of the local cytokine response during the clearance of RSV from the mouse lung.

As shown by others, there is initially a high IFN-γ response, presumed to be important for clearance of infection. This is followed by a large peak of IL-13 release (60). Furthermore, treatment with a neutralizing anti-IL-13 antibody caused an early increase in pulmonary IL-12 and reduced virus in the lungs. This again implied that, in this model, IL-13 was downregulating a Th1 antiviral pathway. ALthough less is known about the role of IL-13 in the immune response than about the related Th2 cytokine, IL-4, a highly informative model for pulmonary effects of IL-13 has been produced by ectopic overexpression of an IL-13 transgene on a lung-specific promoter (85). Mice in which IL-13 expression is artificially expressed in the respiratory epithelium by exploiting the gene targeting of the Clara cell 10 kDa promoter show a profound phenotype: they have tissue inflammation, mucus hyperproduction, goblet cell hyperplasia, subepithelial airway fibrosis, Charcot-Leyden-like crystal deposition, airways obstruction, and AHR. Thus, many of the aspects of an unfavorable infection with RSV can be reiterated simply by creating a highly Th2 environment. Detailed descriptions of the influence of this Th2 environment on development of allergic hyperresponsiveness are covered in other chapters of this volume. The regulatory burst of Th2-predisposing IL-13 release and accompanying increase in AHR induced by RSV infection are associated with increased AHR and eosinophil and neutrophil influx into the lung on challenge with ovalbumin (83). Similar studies have looked at the effect of RSV preinfection on models of cockroach allergen or dust mite *Dermatophagoides farinae* allergen challenge (86,87). Viral infection in these models can be associated with a significant increase in AHR, enhanced peribronchial inflammation, and augmented IgE and MIPlα. In the cockroach allergen model, this enhanced disease phenotype was largely abolished by treatment with neutralizing anti-IL-13.

In summary, experiments in murine models of viral infection can provide important clues to the possible mechanisms underlying susceptibility to asthma. In the case of RSV preinfection models, the evidence indicates a synergistic contribution to induction of the asthmatic phenotype through enhanced AHR and inflammation and generation of a Th2-promoting environment, particularly through IL-13.

VII. Concluding Remarks

Research using murine models of human viral infection comes with the caveat that disease is often being studied outside the natural host and that, as a consequence, patterns of disease pathology may differ from the clinical picture seen in humans. Most important is that human disease occurs in genetically diverse individuals with complex antigenic and infective histories leading to variable immunopathogenesis, only now being appreciated using studies of genetically diverse mouse strains. However, these mouse models have allowed us to understand many of the basic rules about the interaction between protective and pathogenic immune mechanisms, and much has been learnt about the relative contributions of CTL cells and CD4 Th1 and Th2 populations. Based on information about the components of the immune response typically associated with clearance of virus on the one hand or with lung damage on the other, it is possible to start designing highly specific vaccines, capable of inducing only the desired nonpathogenic, protective immune response. Furthermore, animal models can be used to discover possible links between virus-induced lung changes and susceptibility to reactive airways disease, which can be (to various degrees) sought in studies of human asthma.

References

1. Mosmann TR, Cherwinski H, Bond MW, Giedlin MA, Coffman RL. Two types of murine helper T cell clone. I. Definition according to profiles of lymphokine activities and secreted proteins. J Immunol 1986; 136:2348–2354.
2. Mosmann TR, Sad S. The expanding universe of T cell subsets: Th1, Th2 and more. Immunol Today 1996; 17:138–146.
3. Abbas AK, Murphy KM, Sher A. Functional diversity of helper T lymphocytes. Nature 1996; 383:787–793.
4. Bonecchi R, Bianchi G, Bordignon PP, D'Ambrosio D, Lang R, Borsatti A, Sozzani S, Allavena P, Gray PA, Mantovani A. Differential expression of chemokine receptors and chemotacyic responsiveness of type 1 helper cells (Th1s) and Th2s. J Exp Med 1998; 187:129–134.
5. Loetscher P, Uguccioni M, Bordoli L, Baggiolini M, Moser B, Chizzolini C, Dayer J M. CCR5 is characteristic of Th1 lymphocytes. Nature 1998; 391:244–345.
6. Sallusto F, Mackay CR, Lanzavecchia A. Selective expression of the exotaxin receptor CCR3 by human T helper 2 cells. Science 1997; 277:2005–2007.
7. Sallusto F, Lenig D, Mackay CR, Lanzavecchia A. Flexible programs of chemokine receptor expression on human polarized T helper 1 and 2 lymphocytes. J Exp Med 1998; 187:875–883.
8. Zheng W, Flavell RA. The transcription factor GATA-3 is necessary and sufficient for Th2 cytokine gene expression in CD4 T cells. Cell 1997; 89:587–596.
9. Szabo SJ, Kin ST, Costa GL, Zhang X, Fathman CG, Glimcher LH. A novel transcription factor, T-bet, directs Th1 lineage commitment. Cell 2000; 100:655–665.
10. Ho IC, Hodge MR, Rooney JW, Glincher LH. The proto-oncogene c-maf is responsible for tissue specific expression of interleukin-4. Cell 1996; 85:973–983.
11. Coyle AJ, Lloyd C, Tian J, Nguyen T, Erikkson C, Wang L, Ottoson P, Persson P, Delaney T, Lehar S. Crucial role of the interleukin 1 receptor family member T1/ST2 in T helper cell type 2-mediated lung mucosal immune responses. J Exp Med 1999; 190:895–902.
12. Lohning M, Stroehmann A, Coyle A J, Grogan J L, Lin S, Gutierrez R J, Levinson D, Radbruch A, Kamradt T. T1/ST2 is preferentially expressed on murine Th2 cells, independent of interleukin 4, interleukin 5, and interleukin 10, and important for Th2 effector function. Proc Natl Acad Sci USA 1998; 95:6930-6935.
13. Xu D, Chan W L, Leung B P, Hunter D, Schulz K, Carter R W, McInnes I B, Robinson J H, Liew F Y. Selective expression and functions of interleukin 18 receptor on T helper (Th) type 1 but not Th2 cells. J Exp Med 1998;188:1485–1492.
14. Xu D, Chan WL, Leung BP, Huang F, Wheeler R, Piedrafita D, Robinson JH, Liew FY. Selective expression of a stable cell surface molecule on type 2 but not type 1 helper T cells. J Exp Med 1998; 187:787–794.
15. Ada GL, Jones PD. The immune response to influenza infection. Curr Top Microbiol Immunol 1986; 128:1–54.

16. Zinkernagel RM, Doherty PC. MHC restricted cytotoxic T cells: studies on the biological role of polymorphic major transplantation antigens determining T cell restriction specificity, function and responsiveness. Adv Immunol 1979; 27:51–177.

17. McMichael AJ, Ting A, Zweerink HJ, Askonas B. HLA restriction of cell mediated lysis of influenza virus infected human cells. Nature 1977; 270:524–526.

18. Townsend AR, Goch FM, Davey J. Cytotoxic T cells recognize fragments of the influenza nucleoprotein. Cell 1985; 42:457-467.

19. Allan W, Tabi Z, Clearly A, Doherty PC. Cellular events to the lymph node and lung of mice with influenza: consequences of depleting CD4$^+$ T cells. J Immunol 1990; 144: 3980-3986.

20. Bender BS, Small PA. Influenza: pathogenesis and host defense. Semin Respir Infect 1992; 7:38–45.

21. Zweerink HJ, Coutneidge SA, Skehel JJ, Crumpton MJ, Askonas BA. Cytotoxic T cells kill influenza virus but do not distinguish between serologically distinct type A viruses. Nature 1977; 267:354–356.

22. Kuwano K, Scott M, Young JF, Ennis FA. Active immunisation against virus infections due to antigenic drift by induction of crossreactive cytotoxic T lymphocytes. J Exp Med 1989; 169:1361-1371.

23. Neirynck S, Deroo T, Saelens X, Vanlanschoot P, Jou WM, Fiers W. A universal influenza A vaccine based on the extracellular domain of the M2 protein. Nat Med 1999; 5:1157-1163.

24. Bender BS, Croghan T, Zhang L, Small PA. Transgenic mice lacking class I major histocompatibility complex-restricted T cells have delayed viral clearance and increased mortality after influenza virus challenge. J Exp Med 1992; 175:1143–1145.

25. Eichelberger M, Allan W, Zijlstra M, Jaenisch R, Doherty PC. Clearance of influenza virus respiratory infection in mice lacking class I major histocompatibility complex restricted CD8$^+$ T cells. J Exp Med 1991; 174:875–880.

26. Gerhard W, Mozdzanowska K, Furchner M, Washko G, Maise K. Role of the B cell response in recovery of mice from primary influenza virus infection. Immunol Rev 1997; 159:95–103.

27. Taylor PM, Esquivel F, Askonas BA. Murine CD4$^+$ T cell clones vary in function in vitro and in influenza infection in vivo. Int Immunol 1990; 2:323–328.

28. Graham MB, Braciale TJ. Resistance to and recovery from lethal influenza virus infection in B lymphocyte deficient mice. J Exp Med 1997; 186:2063–2068.

29. Altman JD, Moss PAH, Goulder PJR, Barouch DH, McHeyzer-Williams MG, Bell JI, McMichael AJ, Davis MM. Phenotypic analysis of antigen specific T lymphocytes. Science 1996; 274:94–96.

30. Flynn KJ, Belz GT, Altman JD, Woodland R, Doherty PC. Virus specific CD8$^+$ cells in primary and secondary pneumonia. Immunity 1998; 8:683–691.

31. Riberdy JM, Christensen JP, Branum K, Doherty PC. Diminished primary and secondary influenza virus specific CD8$^+$ T cell responses in CD4 depleted Ig-/- mice. J Virol 2000; 74:9762–9765.

32. Hogan RJ, Usherwood EJ, Zhong W, Roberts AD, Dutton RW, Harmsen AG, Woodland DL. Activated antigen specific CD8$^+$ T cells persist in the lungs following recovery from respiratory virus infections. J Immunol 2001; 166:1813-1822.

33. Hogan RJ, Zhong W, Usherwood EJ, Cookenham T, Roberts AD, Woodland DL. Protection from respiratory virus infections can be mediated by antigen specific CD4$^+$ T cells that persist in the lungs. J Exp Med 2001; 193:981–986.

34. Doherty PC, Christensen JP. Accessing complexity: the dynamics of virus specific T cell responses. Annu Rev Immunol 2000; 18:561–592.
35. Cohen J. The flu pandemic that might have been. Science 1997; 277:1600–1601.
36. Riberdy JM, Flynn KJ, Stech J, Webster RG, Altman JD, Doherty PC. Protection against a lethal avian influenza A virus in a mammalian system. J Virol 1999; 73:1453–1459.
37. Durbin JE, Fernandez-Sesma A, Lee C, Rao T, Frey AB, Moran TM, Vukmanovic S, Garcia-Sastre A, Levy DE. Type I IFN modulates innate and specific antiviral immunity. J Immunol 2000; 164:4220-4228.
38. Price GE, Gaszewska-Masterlarz A, Moskophidis D. The role of alpha/beta interferons in development of immunity to influenza A virus in mice. J Virol 2000; 74:3996–4003.
39. Wiley JA, Cerwenka A, Harkema JR, Dutton RW, Harmsen AG. Production of interferon gamma by influenza haemagglutiinin specific CD8 effector T cells influences the development of pulmonary immunopathology. Am J Pathol 2001; 158:119–130.
40. Nguyen HH, van Ginkel FW, Vu HL, Novak MJ, McGhee JR, Mestecky J. Gamma interferon is not required for mucosal cytotoxic T lymphocyte responses or heterosubtypic immunity to influenza A virus infection in mice. J Virol 2000; 74:5495-5501.
41. Enelow RI, Mohammed AZ, Stoler MH, Liu AN, Young JS, Lou Y, Braciale TJ. Structural and functional consequences of alveolar cell recognition by CD8$^+$ T lymphocytes in experimental lung disease. J Clin Invest 1998; 102:1653–1661.
42. Zhao MQ, Stoler MH, Liu AN, Wei B, Soguero C, Hahn YS, Enelow RI. A lveolar epithelial cell chemokine expression triggered by antigen specific cytolytic CD8$^+$ T cell recognition. J Clin Invest 2000; 106:R49-R58.
43. Simoes EA. Respiratory syncytial virus and subsequent lower respiratory tract infections in developing countries: a new twist to an old virus. J Pediatr 1999; 135:657–666.
44. Kapikian AZ, Mitchell RH, Chanock RM, Shvedoff RA, Stewart CE. An epidemiologic study of altered reactivity to respiratory syncytial (RS) virus infection in children previously vaccinated with inactivated RS virus vaccine. Am J Epidemiol 1969; 89:405-421.
45. Chin J, Magoffin LA, Shearer, JH, Schieble JH, Lennette EH. Field evaluation of a respiratory syncytial virus vaccine and trivalent parainfluenza virus vaccine in a pediatric population. Am J Epidemiol 1969; 89:449–463.
46. Kim HW, Canchola, CD, Brandt G, Pyles G, Chanock RM, Jensen K, Parrott RH. Respiratory syncytial virus disease in infants despite prior administration of antigenic inactivated vaccine. Am J Epidemiol 1969; 89:422–434.
47. Fulginiti, VA, Eller JJ, Sieber JW, Joyner W, Minamitani M, Meiklejohn G. Respiratory virus immunization. I. A field trial of two inactivated respiratory virus vaccine: an aqueous trivalent parainfluenza virus vaccine and an alum-precipitated respiratory syncytial virus vaccine. Am J Epidemiol 1969; 89:436–448.
48. Openshaw PJM. Immunity and immunopathology to respiratory syncytial virus. The mouse model. Am J Respir Crit Care Med 1995; 152:S59–62.
49. Cannon MJ, Openshaw PJ, Askonas BA. Cytotoxic T cells clear virus but augment lung pathology in mice infected with respiratory syncytial virus. J Exp Med 1988; 168:1163–1169.
50. Hussell T, Openshaw PJ. Intracellular IFN gamma expression in natural killer cells precedes lung CD8$^+$ recruitment during respiratory syncytial virus infection. J Gen Virol 1998; 79:2593–2601.
51. Hussell T, Openshaw PJM. IL-12 activated NK cells reduce lung eosinophillia to the

attachment protein of respiratory syncytial virus but do not enhance the severity of illness in CD8 T cell immunodeficient conditions. J Immunol 2000; 165:7109-7115.

52. Alwan WH, Kozlowska WJW, Openshaw PJM. Distinct types of lung disease caused by the functional subsets of antiviral T cells. J Exp Med 1994; 179:81–89.

53. Alwan WH, Openshaw PJM. Distinct patterns of T and B cell immunity to respiratory syncytial virus induced by individual viral proteins. Vaccine 1993; 11:431–437.

54. Varga SM, Wissinger EL, Braciale TJ. The attachment (G) glycoprotein of respiratory syncytial virus contains a single immunodominant epitope that elicits both Th1 and Th2 CD4$^+$ T cell responses. J Immunol 2000; 165:6487-6495.

55. Nicholson LB, Greer JM, Sobel RA, Lees MB, Kuchroo VK. An altered peptide ligand mediates immune deviation and prevents autoimmune encephalomyelitis. Immunity 1995; 3:397–405.

56. Kappos L, Comi G, Panitch H, Oger J, Antel J, Conlon P, Steinman L. Induction of a non-encephalitogenic type 2 T helper-cell autoimmune response in multiple sclerosis after administration of an altered peptide ligand in a placebo-controlled, randomized phase II trial. The altered peptide ligand in relapsing MS study group. Nat Med 2000; 6:1176–1182.

57. Byrd LG, Prince GA. Animal models of respiratory syncytial virus infection. Clin Infect Dis 1997; 25:1363–1368.

58. van Schaik SM, Enhorning G, Vargas I, Welliver RC. Respiratory syncytial virus affects pulmonary function in BALB/c mice. J Infect Dis 1998; 177:269–276.

59. Tekkanat KK, Maasssab H, Berlin AA, Lincoln PM, Evanoff HL, Kaplan MH, Lukas NW. Role of interleukin 12 and STAT 4 in the regulation of airway inflammation and hyperreactivity in respiratory syncytial virus infection. Am J Pathol 2001; 159:631-638.

60. Tekkanat KK, Maassab HF, Cho DS, Lai JJ, John A, Berlin A, Kaplan MH, Lukacs NW. IL-13 induced airway hyperreactivity during respiratory syncytial virus infection in STAT6 dependent. J Immunol 2001; 166:3542–3548.

61. Hussell T, Georgiou A, Sparer TE, Matthews S, Pala P, Openshaw PJM. Host genetic determinants of vaccine induced eosinophilia during respiratory syncytial virus infection. J Immunol 1998; 161:6215–6222.

62. Hussell T, Baldwin CJ, O'Garra A, Openshaw PJ. CD8$^+$ T cells control Th2 driven pathology during pulmonary respiratory syncytial virus infection. Eur J Immunol 1997; 27:3341–3349.

63. Schwarze J, Cieslewicz G, Joetham A, Ikemura T, Hamelmann E, Gelfand EW. CD8 T cells are essential in the development of respiratory syncytial virus-induced lung eosinophilia and airway hyperresponsiveness. J Immunol 1999; 162:4207–4211.

64. Pemberton RM, Cannon MJ, Openshaw PJ, Ball LA, Wertz GW Askonas BA. Cytotoxic T cell specificity for respiratory syncytial virus proteins: fusion protein is an important target antigen. J Gen Virol 1987; 68:2177–2182.

65. Chang J, Srikiatkhachorn A, Braciale TJ. Visualization and chracterization of respiratory syncytial virus F-specific CD8$^+$ T cells during experimental virus infection. J Immunol 2001; 167:4254–4260.

66. Sparer TE, Matthews S, Hussell T, Rae AJ, Garcia-Barreno B, Melero JA, Openshaw PJM. Eliminating a region of respiratory syncytial virus attachment protein allows induction of protective immunity without vaccine-enhanced lung eosinophilia. J Exp Med 1998; 187:1921–1926.

67. Simmons CP, Hussell T, Sparer T, Walzl G, Openshaw PJM, Dougan G. Mucosal delivery of a respiratory syncytial virus CTL peptide with enterotoxin based adjuvants elicits

protective immunopathogenic, and immunoregulatory antiviral CD8$^+$ T cell responses. J Immunol 2001; 166:1106–1113.

68. Walzl G, Tafuro S, Moss P, Openshaw PJM, Hussell T. Influenza virus lung infection protects from respiratory syncytial virus induced immunopathology. J Exp Med 2000; 192:1317–1326.

69. Alton EW, Geddes DM. Prospects for respiratory gene therapy. Br J Hosp Med 1997; 58:47–49

70. Flotte T R, Laube BL. Gene therapy in cystic fibrosis. Chest 2001; 120:124S-131S.

71. Nakao A, Fuji M, Matsumura R, Kumano K, Saitio Y, Miyazono K, Iwamoto I. Transient gene transfer and expression of Smad7 prevents bleomycin-induced lung fibrosis in mice. J Clin Invest 1999; 104:5–11.

72. Walter DM, Wong CP, DeKruyff RH, Berry GJ, Levy S, Umetsu DT. IL-l8 gene transfer by adenovirus prevents the development of and reverses established allergen-induced airway hyperreactivity. J Immunol 2001; 166:6392–6398.

73. Chen GH, Reddy RC, Newstead MW, Tateda K, Kyasapura BL, Standiford P. Intrapulmonary TNF gene therapy reverses sepsis-induced suppression of lung antibacterial host defense. J Immunol 2000; 165:6496–6503.

74. van Ginkel FW, McGhee J R, Liu C, Simecka JW, Yamamoto M, Frizzell RA, Sorscher EJ, Kiyono H, Pascual DW. Adenoviral gene delivery elicits distinct pulmonary-associated T helper cell responses to the vector and its transgene. J Immunol 1997; 159:685–693.

75. Yang Y, SU Q, Wilson JM. Role of viral antigens in destructive cellular immune responses to adenovirus vector-transduced cells in mouse lung. J Virol 1996; 70:7209–7212.

76. Yang Y, Trinchieri G, Wilson JM. Recombinant IL-12 prevents formation of blocking IgA antibodies to recombinant adenovirus and allows repeated gene therapy to mouse lung. Nat Med 1995; 1:887–889.

77. Minter RM, Ferry MA, Rectenwald JE, Bahjat FR, Oberholzer A, Oberholzer C, La Face D, Tsai V, Ahmed CM, Hutchins B, Copeland EM 3rd, Ginsberg HS, Moldawer LL. Extended lung expression and increased tissue localization of viral IL-10 with adenoviral gene therapy. Proc Natl Acad Sci USA 2001; 98:277-282

78. Chirmule N, Truneh A, Haecker SE, Tazelaar J, Gao G, Raper SE, Hughes JV, Wilson JM. Repeated administration of adenoviral vectors in lungs of human CD4 transgenic mice treated with a non-depleting CD4 antibody. J Immunol 1999; 163:448–455.

79. Joos K, Turka LA, Wilson JM. Blunting of immune responses to adenoviral vectors in mouse liver and lung with CTLA-4Ig. Gene Ther 1998; 5:309–319.

80. Gern JE, Lemanske RF Jr, Busse WW. Early life origins of asthma. J Clin Invest 1999; 104:837–843.

81. Haraguchi S, Day NK, Nelson RP, Emmanuel P, Duplantier JE, Christondoulou CS, Good RA. Interleukin 12 deficiency associated with recurrent infections. Proc Natl Acad Sci USA 1998; 95:13125-13129.

82. Johnston SL. Influence of viral and bacterial respiratory infections on exacerbations and symptom severity in childhood asthma. Pediatr Pulmonol Suppl 1997; 16:88–89.

83. Schwarze J, Hammelmann E, Bradley KL, Takeda K, Gelfand EW. Respiratory syncytial virus infection results in airway hyperresponsiveness and enhanced airway sensitization to allergen. J Clin Invest 1997; 100:226–233

84. Roman M, Calhoun WJ, Hinton KL, Avendano LF, Simon V, Escobar AM, Gaggero A, Diaz PV. Respiratory syncytial virus infection in infants is associated with predominant Th2-like response. Am J Crit Care Med 1997; 156:190–195

85. Zhu Z, Homer RJ, Wang Z, Chen Q, Geba GP, Wang J, Zhang Y, Elias JA. Pulonary expression of interleukin 13 causes inflammation, mucus hypersecretion, subepithelial fibrosis, physiologic abnormalities, and eotaxin production. J Clin Invest 1999; 103: 779–788.

86. Lukacs NW, Tekkanat KK, Berlin A, Hogaboam CM, Miller A, Evanoff H, Lincoln P, Maassab H. Respiratory syncytial virus predisposes mice to augmented allergic airway responses via IL-13 mediated mechanisms. J Immunol 2001; 167:1060–1065.

87. Matsuse H, Behera AK, Kumar M, Rabb H, Lockey RF, Mohapatra SS. Recurrent respiratory syncytial virus infections in allergen sensitized mice lead to persistent airway inflammation and hyperresponsiveness. J Immunol 2000; 164:6583–6592.

13

Modulation of Immune Responses to Virus Infection in the Lung

TRACY HUSSELL, IAN HUMPHREYS, and GERHARD WALZL

Imperial College London
London, England

I. Introduction

The induction of immunity and pathology during viral infection of the lung depends on a number of factors. These include one or more of the following: the age of the host, the presence of an efficient immune system, host genetic makeup, the presence of coinfecting pathogens, underlying congenital abnormalities and maternal antibody, and the extent of previous infections. In this chapter we review a number of these variables in relation to the immunopathology induced by viral infection of the lung and the subsequent development of asthma and atopy

A. The Lung as a Mucosal Organ

To understand why problems arise in the lung during infection we first need to appreciate how the lung maintains homeostasis in an immunocompetent individual. The lung is an integral part of mucosal-associated lymphoid tissue (MALT). Such MALT structures separate the external environment from the body's interior at most sites by a single layer of epithelium. Mucosal surfaces are constantly bombarded with antigenic material. The induction of immune responses to all foreign particles we eat and breathe would be inappropriate. Large inflammatory reactions in delicate sites such as the lung would likewise lead to bystander tissue damage and a state of immunological exhaustion. The mucosal tissues (including the respiratory, gastrointestinal, and urogenital tracts and the ducts of all exocrine glands) have therefore evolved a specialized immune network that seeks to exclude, eliminate, or tolerate antigen rather than reacting to it. One of the hallmarks of mucosal immunity is the selective production of dimeric immunoglobulin A (IgA). The joining chain present in dimeric IgA selectively binds to secretory component on the basolateral surface of mucosal epithelium. IgA is then actively transported through the epithelium and secreted into the lumen where complexes with antigen form. This effectively prevents the absorption of antigen by a process called immune exclusion. IgA therefore functions to exclude antigens from the body without causing overt inflammation. IgA is particularly appropriate for mucosal surfaces since it is more resistant to degradation by luminal proteases than other antibody isotypes and it does not fix complement. The impact of this mechanism on antigen control at mucosal surfaces is highlighted by the recurrent lung infections that occur in patients with a selective IgA deficiency. It can be difficult to diagnose such a deficiency because induction of other antibody isotypes such as pentameric IgM often compensate. For example, IgA-deficient mice seem equally efficient at controlling sublethal influenza virus infection via the production of other antibody isotypes (1). Dimeric IgA can also complex antigen within the submucosa itself and transport it into the lumen of the lung or gut via the secretory component: joining chain interaction. Even agents that infect the mucosal epithelium can be mopped up during the transition of IgA through the epithelial cell (2).

B. T-Cell Subsets at Mucosal Sites

The predominance of IgA at mucosal surfaces is explained by the production of Th2 cytokines such as IL-4, IL-5, IL-6, and IL-10 by resident T cells, which promote humoral immunity. Th2 cells have been isolated at high frequency from mucosal tissues (3) and there is a clear predominance of Th2 cytokine mRNA at various sites in the gut (4). The Th2 cytokine IL-4 is also a differentiation factor for transforming growth factor beta (TGF-β) -secreting Th3 cells (5) and TGF-β with IL-6 together induce the expression of IgA on the B cell surface (6).

TGF-β and IL-10 are essential regulatory cytokines at mucosal surfaces. Without these, uncontrolled inflammatory reactions would lead to bystander tissue damage. The role of CD4+ T cells producing the immunoregulatory cytokines IL-10 and/or TGF-β has been extensively examined in the gut. Naive CD4+ T cells expressing high levels of CD45RB (CD45RB[high]) cause symptoms reminiscent of inflammatory bowel disease (IBD) after adoptive transfer into mice lacking a functional immune system (SCID mice) (7–10). Cotransfer of activated or memory CD4+ CD45RB[low] T cells prevents this inflammatory condition. Recent evidence suggests that both CD45RB[high] and CD45RB[lo] CD4+ T cells can in fact induce IBD, but the kinetics vary (11). A consistent observation is that the regulation of these inflammatory reactions depends on IL-10 and/or TGF-β (12). For example, IL-10 knockout mice develop IBD via responses to normal enteric antigens, which can be prevented by IL-10 reconstitution (13). Suppression of CD4+ T-cell-mediated diabetes and autoimmune myelitis likewise occurs when cells producing TGF-β are transferred from orally tolerized mice (14,15). These regulatory T cells (often termed T-regulatory 1 [Tr1] or Th3 cells) can even suppress immune responses to other antigens in the same environment. Transfer of ovalbumin-specific regulatory T cells (producing IL-10) inhibits IBD induced by CD4+ CD45RB^high cells. These Tr1 cells, which do not respond very well to costimulation through CD3 and CD28, are also evident in humans (16).

IL-10 is produced by many different cell subsets including T and B cells, macrophages, monocytes, and keratinocytes. It functions predominantly as an anti-inflammatory cytokine inhibiting the protein synthesis of other cytokines, chemo-kines, and enzymes such as inducible nitric oxide synthetase (iNOS). IL-10 also inhibits the accessory functions of antigen-presenting cells by reducing expression of major histocompatibility complex (MHC) II and B7 costimulatory molecules and is therefore important for maintaining homeostasis and tolerance (for a review see 17). IL-10 is also reported to inhibit indirectly the development of T cells producing interferon (IFN)-γ (Th1 cells) by downregulating the production of IL-12 from mac-rophages and dendritic cells (18). Certain infectious agents have utilized the anti-inflammatory activity of IL-10 to subvert host responses. Epstein-Barr virus, for example, encodes an IL-10 homolog whereas respiratory syncytial virus infection of macrophages elicits IL-10, which may account for the lack of effective immune memory to this virus (19).

The role of cells (in particular CD4+ and CD8+ T cells) producing immuno-regulatory cytokines such as IL-10 in regulating immune responses in the lung has been relatively ignored. Primary lung infection with respiratory syncytial virus (RSV) and influenza induces a mild illness with CD8+ and CD4+ T-cell infiltration. The CD4+ T cells assume a Th1 phenotype producing IFN-γ and no IL-4 or IL-5. Using the technique of intracellular cytokine staining and flow cytometry, we have observed CD4+ and CD8+ T cells producing high levels of IL-10 during these primary lung infections (see Fig. 1). The majority of this IL-10 is coexpressed in cells that also produce IFN-γ (20). Whether these cells possess a regulatory function is currently under investigation.

C. Induction of Tolerance in the Mucosae

It is precisely this immunosuppressive environment that has made mucosal sites potentially attractive for the development of tolerance to a number of different anti-gens. Oral tolerance is essential to prevent inflammatory reactions at mucosal sur-faces and is the immunological mechanism by which the mucosal immune system maintains unresponsiveness to antigens that might otherwise induce untoward im-mune responses. The selective inactivation of T-cell subsets occurs via clonal dele-tion, clonal anergy, and the induction of suppressor cells depending on the dose of antigen administered. Tolerance of B cells is less well defined since the reduction in antibody may simply represent reduced T-cell help. Inactivation of T-cell re-sponses to antigen via oral tolerance is currently being exploited in the treatment of allergy and asthma.

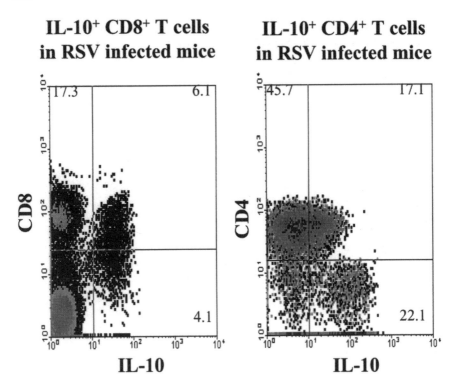

Figure 1   The expression of IL-10 in CD4 and CD8+ T cells during lung RSV infection of mice. Mice were intranasally infected with respiratory syncytial virus and 4 days later bronchoalveolar fluid removed by lavage. The cells were stimulated for 4 h in the presence of PMA, ionomycin, and brefeldin A. After incubation with quantum red conjugated antibodies to murine CD4 or CD8 on ice for 30 min, cells were washed and fixed with 2% formaldehyde. Cells were then permeabilized with 0.5% saponin to allow entry of fluorochrome-conjugated antibody specific for murine IL-10 and fluorescence quantified on a flow cytometer collecting data on 40,000 lymphocytes. IL-10 in CD8+ (left panel) and CD4+ (right panel) T cells is shown in the upper right hand quadrant.

Despite the best efforts of evolution, untoward inflammatory reactions are common at mucosal sites and the lung is no exception. Inflammation of the lung is one of the most prevalent causes of hospitalization worldwide. Of the 50.5 million deaths worldwide in 1990, lower respiratory tract infections accounted for 4.3 million and was only beaten in prevalence by cerebrovascular disease (4.4 million) and ischemic heart disease (6.3 million) (21). The development of asthma relies on a breakdown in mechanisms designed to prevent damaging responses at mucosal sites. Inappropriate recruitment of T cells, production of inflammatory rather than immunoregulatory cytokines, and the induction of complement-fixing antibodies create an environment that is damaging to the host and may be fatal. This whole cascade often begins with the type of T-cell response induced after infection.

II. Mechanisms for Inflammation in the Lung

Development of appropriate immune responses to infection is crucial for the clearance of the pathogen and for the prevention of associated pathology. The differentiation of CD4+ T cells into those with a Th1 or Th2 cytokine phenotype has been extensively studied in many systems.

Th1 cells produce predominantly IFN-γ, promote cell-mediated immunity, and induce IgG2a antibody isotype switching in antigen-activated B cells. Th2 cells, on the other hand produce IL-4, IL-5, and IL-13, promote humoral immunity, and induce IgG1 antibody isotype switching in mice. The cytokines produced during an infection determine the phenotype of associated pathology. Production of excess IFN-γ is associated with delayed-type hypersensitivity reactions whereas IL-5 promotes the activation, survival, and recruitment of eosinophils. One important criterion in the development of vaccines is to induce the most effective form of immunity while trying to avoid the associated immunopathological sequelae.

There are many mechanisms by which the CD4+ T-cell phenotype can be altered. The production of cytokine from one Th subset reciprocally inhibits the other. It is important to remember that cells other than CD4+ T cells produce Th1 and Th2 cytokines. For example, mast cells and eosinophils produce IL-5, NK and CD8+ T cells are potent sources of IFN-γ, and macrophages and dendritic cells (DC) produce IL-12 and IL-10. Studies have even labeled dendritic cells, CD8+ T cells, and NK cells according to the Th1/Th2 classification such that we now have DC1/DC2, Tc1/Tc2, and NK1/NK2, respectively (the list is growing). However, in this complex picture a clear message does emerge. Any immune cell can differentiate into any phenotype depending on the cytokine environment, which in turn depends on the nature and dose of the antigen.

The development of immunity and pathology in the murine model of RSV infection depends on the protein used to sensitize the mice. Dermal sensitization with the attachment protein (G) of RSV induces lung eosinophilia after intranasal challenge with whole virus (22–24). If CD4+ T cells are depleted (25) or the immunodominant CD4+ T-cell epitope removed (26), then eosinophilia does not occur. The development of eosinophilia to RSV infection critically depends on the level of IFN-γ present. Administration of recombinant IL-12 prevents eosinophilia in G-protein-primed mice by inducing excess IFN-γ production by NK and CD8+ T cells (27,28). Depletion of IL-4 and IL-5 likewise abrogates G-protein-induced lung eosinophilia (29). One popular concept is that allergy and asthma depend on CD4+ T cells secreting type 2 cytokines. In the RSV murine model the development of eosinophilia seems to depend more on the *absence* of a CD8+ T-cell response than on a simple dominance of Th2 cells. This conclusion has been determined as follows:

1. Not all G-protein-primed mouse strains develop lung eosinophilia after intranasal RSV challenge. C57BL/6 mice, for example, are resistant even though they can be infected equally well with RSV. If CD8+ T cells are removed with specific antibody or by TAP-1, CD8, or β2 microglobulin gene deletions from C57BL/6 mice they develop eosinophilic responses

to G (30). This suggests that CD8+ T-cell responses in C57BL/6 mice are preventing eosinophilia to the G protein.

2. The second matrix (M2) protein of RSV contains an immunodominant H-2D-restricted CD8+ T-cell epitope. If this epitope is inserted into the G protein and this construct used to sensitize BALB/c mice lung, eosinophilia is not evident after RSV challenge, this again suggests that induction of CD8+ T-cell responses can prevent eosinophilia (31).

3. If M2-specific CD8+ T-cell lines are transferred into a naive BALB/c mouse, which is then sensitized with the G protein, eosinophilia does not develop after RSV challenge (22).

4. The fusion protein of RSV induces both CD4+ and CD8+ T-cell responses in BALB/c mice. The CD4+ T cells assume a Th1 phenotype and no eosinophilia is evident during RSV challenge. Vigorous eosinophilia does occur, however, if CD8+ T cells are depleted with specific antibody during fusion protein priming (25).

NK cells are an additional source of IFN-γ. Kos and Engleman (32) have shown that NK cells are required for CD8+ T cells to mature into effector cells. Studies in the RSV murine model suggest that they may assist in CD8+ T-cell activation. During a primary RSV infection, NK cytotoxic activity and IFN-γ secretion peak early on days 2–4 when CD4+ and CD8+ T-cell recruitment occurs (33). The IFN-γ from both NK and CD8+ T cells induces CD4+ Th1 cells. In the absence of CD8+ T cells, mild lung eosinophilia is evident during a primary RSV infection; NK cell-derived IFN-γ alone does not appear to drive CD4 Th1 cells. If IL-12 is administered, IFN-γ production by NK cells increases. In the absence of CD8+ T cells, IL-12 administration still prevents the development of eosinophilia, which suggests that IL-12 can act on another cell type. By additionally removing NK cells we have shown that the reduction of eosinophilia by IL-12 requires the presence of CD8+ T cells or NK cells. This effect critically relies on IFN-γ since its removal causes eosinophilia (34). NK cells can therefore only influence CD4+ T cell phenotype if additionally activated by IL-12.

All of these studies suggest that patients who develop Th2 reactions to virus infection or allergen may do so because CD8+ T cells are deficient. Studies to assess NK and CD8+ T-cell responses in asthmatic and allergic patients are therefore essential. Allergens in general are nonreplicating soluble proteins that will predominantly be processed through a MHC class II pathway and therefore predominantly induce CD4+ T cells. Without the cytokine input from CD8+ T cells, Th2 cells secreting IL-4 and IL-5 will develop. This is also supported by data collected during the disastrous RSV vaccine trials in the 1960s. Formalin-inactivated (FI) RSV was administered to children in four parallel trials. On subsequent natural RSV infection more of the vaccinated subjects experienced severe lower respiratory tract complications leading to hospitalization and even death than did controls (35). Postmortem studies indicated peripheral and lung eosinophilia in some patients. Formalin-inactivated RSV is effectively a dead particulate antigen and would be presented predominantly through an MHC class II pathway. Considering the CD8+ T-cell

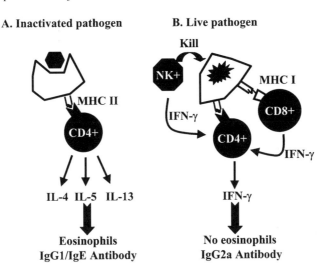

Figure 2 Immune responses depend on the nature of the antigen. (A) Dead particulate antigen such as inactivated vaccine preparations will be engulfed by antigen-presenting cells. Such antigen does not replicate within the cell and will therefore be processed and presented through the MHC class II pathway. CD4+ T cells will be activated and will secrete type 2 cytokines (IL-4, IL-5, and IL-13). The uptake of particulate antigen does not modulate MHC class I and so NK cells will not be activated. The lack of IFN-γ from CD8+ T cells and NK cells means that the Th2 cytokine nature of the CD4+ T cell is not regulated. Eosinophilia will result and antibody production is driven towards IgG1 and IgE. (B) A live pathogen will infect and replicate within the antigen-presenting cell. Proteins will therefore be processed via MHC class I and II. Activated CD8+ T cells secrete IFN-γ, which skews CD4+ T-cell responses to a Th1 cytokine phenotype. During some viral infections MHC class I is downregulated, which signals NK cells to lyse the infected cell. NK cell activation also results in IFN-γ secretion. This, combined with IFN-γ from CD8+ T cells, inhibits the development of eosinophilia and induces IgG2a antibody isotype switching in B cells. It should be noted that inactivated and live pathogens may also be taken up by functional distinct antigen-presenting cells. A live infection may also induce different inflammatory cytokine release from the APC compared to inactivated pathogens.

depletion experiments described above, one would expect eosinophilia to develop. These vaccine trials are supported by the extensive data obtained with FI-RSV in the BALB/c murine model. Mice primed with FI-RSV develop pulmonary eosino-philia after intranasal RSV challenge. As in mice primed with the G protein, this effect depends on CD4+ T cells secreting IL-4 and IL-5 (for example, see Refs. 36–38). Figure 2 summarizes the interaction among different cell subsets.

III. Strategies to Prevent Eosinophilic Reactions in the Lung

Based on this knowledge of how eosinophilic responses are induced in the inflamed lung, several therapeutic strategies to prevent it are apparent. Eosinophilia could theoretically be prevented by depleting cell subsets responsible for eosinophil recruitment, by skewing the immune response towards a Th1 cytokine phenotype or by administering antigenic material in a manner that allows presentation through an MHC class I pathway. Attempts have proved successful in animal models, although the transition to the equivalent illness in humans has been hampered mostly due to the cost of providing such immunological reagents on a large scale.

A. Specific Depletion of T-Helper-Cell Subsets

The selective depletion of Th1 or Th2 cells would provide a novel therapeutic strategy but requires the identification of stable markers associated with these CD4+ T-cell subsets. To date, the Th1 phenotype in humans or mice is associated with chemokine receptors (CCR) 1,3, and 5 (39,40) and IL-18 receptor (41) expression. The Th2 phenotype, on the other hand, preferentially upregulates the transcription factors c-maf (42) and GATA-3 (43), the CCR 3 and 4 (39,44,45), and the orphan receptor T1/ST2 (46-50). Resting murine Th2 cells constitutively express the energy-dependent multidrug resistance protein transmembrane pump, whereas expression on Th1 and Th2 cells is equal after antigenic stimulation (51;52). Recent studies have revealed a novel G-protein-coupled leukocyte chemoattractant receptor family member that is expressed on activated human Th2 but not Th1 cells (designated CRTH2 for chemoattractant receptor-homologous molecule expressed on Th2 cells). Allergen-induced proliferation of peripheral blood mononuclear cells (PBMCs) is significantly reduced by antibody-mediated depletion of CRTH2 cells (53).

We have recently investigated the role of T1/ST2-expressing cells in the murine model of RSV infection. T1/ST2 is an IL-1 receptor family member originally identified in murine fibroblasts (54,55) and via alternative 3' processing generates a long and short mRNA. The short mRNA (preferentially expressed in embryonic tissues, mammary tumors, and induced in fibroblasts) encodes a secreted protein that is heavily glycosylated. The long mRNA is restricted to the lung and hematopoietic organs and encodes a membrane spanning protein (56–58). Eliminating T1/ST2 using antibody or fusion proteins partially inhibits Th2 differentiation and allergic airway inflammation (46,48,50). Previous studies have shown that T1/ST2 is preferentially expressed on T cells that predominantly produce IL-4, IL-5, or IL-10 but not IFN-γ or IL-2 (50). In addition, expression colocalizes with the Th2-induced granulomatous lung disease during *S. mansoni* infection (49) and in vitro studies demonstrate upregulation of T1/ST2 under Th2 polarizing conditions (46). Eosinophilic responses are induced in BALB/c mice when given ovalbumin (OVA) by inhalation. This occurs via the induction of ovalbumin-specific CD4+ T cells secreting IL-4 and IL-5. When OVA-specific cells are adoptively transferred into naive mice, T1/ST2 depletion abrogates Th2 cytokine secretion into the lung lavage but does not significantly alter IFN-γ. Mediastinal lymph node cells from T1/ST2 knockout mice also produce less IL-4 and IL-5 and increased IFN-γ in response to *S. mansoni* eggs (59).

However, two recent studies using independently derived gene depleted mice show conflicting data regarding the specificity of T1/ST2 for Th2 cells (60). One group reported that T1/ST2-deficient animals failed to show decreased Th2 cytokine or immunoglobulin production in response to *Nippostrongylus braziliensis* infection or allergen-induced airway inflammation (60). An independently derived T1/ST2 knockout model, however, shows that basal immunological functions are not affected but Th2 cytokine responses are impaired in a fashion similar to that seen in depletion studies. The findings in the latter study suggest that this molecule plays an important role in the early events of Th2 development since primary but not secondary granuloma formation in response to *S. mansoni* was of decreased magnitude (61). Because T1/ST2 is not only expressed on CD4+ T cells but also on mast cells and fibroblasts (62), the knockout mice may not only reflect T-helper cell phenotype modulation but also harbor other developmental changes.

CD4+ T cells expressing T1/ST2 are evident during G-protein-induced eosinophilic pulmonary inflammation but are reduced by treatment with IL-12. T1/ST2 depletion abrogates lung eosinophilia, inflammatory cell recruitment, and weight loss only in those mice undergoing a Th2-driven immune response to RSV. Administration of antibodies to T1/ST2 has no effect in mice undergoing Th1 immune responses in this model (62a). These data support the concept that T1/ST2 is a specific marker of Th2 cells. The selective depletion of Th2 cells in children hospitalized with RSV-induced bronchiolitis may therefore provide a novel therapeutic strategy that would prevent the later development of allergy and atopy.

B. Cytokine Depletion During Lung Infection

The development of allergic and asthmatic responses in the lung critically depends on the cytokines produced by incoming T cells. Allergy is associated with the production of IL-4 and IL-5, which have multiple effects on the immune system. IL-5 is an antiapoptotic and maturation factor for eosinophils and stimulates their release from the bone marrow. Depletion of Th2 cytokines is therefore being considered as a therapeutic strategy in many systems. In an elegant study by Karras et al. (63) administration of an antisense oligonucleotide specifically inhibited IL-5 expression and reduced, lung eosinophilia and airway hyperresponsiveness during ovalbumin challenge. A similar effect is observed in a murine model of allergic peritonitis and corresponds with a decrease in IL-5 protein levels. When C57BL/6 mice are sensitized with ovalbumin and challenged with the same protein, intranasally enhanced IL-5 production and eosinophilia are observed in the lung. This does not occur, however, in IL-4 and IL-5 gene knockout mice. Airway hyperresponsiveness to metacholine is likewise only increased in immunocompetent animals. This effect in IL-4 knockout mice can be restored by reconstitution with recombinant IL-5 (64).

Previous studies have associated most viral infections with the induction of CD8+ T cells and CD4+ T cells secreting type 1 cytokines. When examined in finer detail, however, mRNA transcripts and protein for multiple cytokines are evident. The variability in the cytokines detected by different groups depends in part on the technique used to quantify them. For example, there is a tendency to detect more cytokines by analyzing mRNA than can be detected by enzyme-linked immunosorbent assay (ELISA) protein analysis on cell supernatants. Intracellular cytokine staining likewise requires an in vitro stimulation step with either antigen or phorbol 12-myristate 13-acetate (PMA) and ionomycin. The cytokine protein detected using this method may therefore not reflect the level that would actually have been secreted in vivo. Analysis of cytokine-producing cells by enzyme-linked immunosorbent spot assay (ELISPOT) with or without prior limiting dilution suffers from the fact that cells at the end of their useful life may have contributed significantly in vivo but would not be detected in in vitro assays. Several techniques are therefore usually employed.

During a primary RSV infection in mice, IFN-γ is the predominant cytokine present. However, protein and mRNA transcripts for IL-10 are also observed (20). Although other cytokines have been demonstrated during a primary RSV infection, the cells producing IL-2 and IFN-γ express higher levels of IgG2+IgM than those producing IL-4 or IL-5. This suggests that cells producing Th1 cytokines are more activated and indicates a predominant Th1 cytokine response (65). This is similar to that reported by Sarawar et al.: during influenza virus infection many cytokines are observed by in situ hybridization (66). It appears that many cell types contribute to this cytokine environment since depletion of both CD4 and CD8+ T cells reduces, but does not completely eliminate IL-2, IL-4, and IFN-γ expression. A similar heterogeneous cytokine profile is also apparent in cells from the draining mediastinal lymph nodes of influenza-infected mice. When secondarily stimulated in vitro, analysis of culture supernatants showed minimal IL-4, IL-5, and tumor necrosis factor (TNF) protein, but prominent IL-2, IL-10, and IFN-γ (67). In both the mediastinal lymph node and the influenza virus-infected lung, mRNA for IFN-γ and tumor necrosis factor are commonly found in CD8+ T cells whereas IL- 4 and IL-10 mRNA are more prevalent in CD4+ T cells. IL-2, IL-4, and IFN-γ can also be seen in gamma/delta T cells recovered from the inflammatory exudate (68). A heterogeneous cytokine profile is also observed in the nasal-associated lymphoid tissue (NALT) at early time points after influenza infection. The cytokines induced, however, depend on the formulation of the influenza virus itself since intranasal administration of inactivated influenza vaccine induces a Th2-dominated profile (strong IL-4 and weak IFN-γ) whereas live virus infection induces high levels of IFN-γ (69).

We have previously reported that IFN-γ depletion in C57BL/6 mice results in the development of lung eosinophilia during a primary RSV infection and in G-protein-primed animals subsequently challenged with RSV (30). Mice deficient in IFN-γ via gene disruption likewise display enhanced production of influenza-specific IgG1, IL-4, and IL-5 compared to wild-type littermate controls (70). During the primary response to influenza vaccination in young mice, anti-IFN-γ stimulates IgG1 and IgE but inhibits IgG2a, IgG2b, and IgG3, indicative of a skewing toward a Th2 cytokine phenotype (71).

Depletion of IL-4 in mice primed with formalin-inactivated RSV and then challenged intranasally with whole virus reduces bronchoalveolar but not perivascular eosinophilia and cell recruitment. Although depletion of IL-10 alone has no effect, a complete inhibition of pathology is observed when anti-IL-10 and anti-IL-4 are administered together (72). The precise role of IL-10 is somewhat unclear. It is included in the long list of cytokines supposedly produced by Th2 cells but also has profound immunoregulatory activities. Ovalbumin administration into the lungs of IL-10-deficient mice does not result in airway hyperresponsiveness but eosinophilic pulmonary inflammation is present (73). IL-10 gene transfer into the lungs of ovalbumin-sensitized mice likewise prevents mononuclear cell, eosinophil, and neutrophil migration in the alveolar spaces after ovalbumin challenge. Expression of IL-10 is associated with reduced IL-4 and IL-5 levels in lung lavage fluid but does not impede the expansion of CD4+ or CD8+ T cells. However, Yang et al. (74) showed that IL-5 production, eosinophilia, and mucus production are reduced in ovalbumin-sensitized and challenged IL-10 gene knockout mice, whereas IFN-γ and IL-12 levels are increased. Further studies are necessary to reconcile these conflicting results.

These studies reveal an important role for IL-10 but it is not clear whether it is acting as an immunoregulatory cytokine or whether its absence specifically prevents Th2 CD4+ T-cell development. During immune responses to intravenously injected *Schistosoma mansoni* eggs, immunocompetent mice mount a Th2 cytokine response. IL-10-deficient mice, however, display a mixed Th1/Th2 phenotype with reduced pulmonary granuloma formation. What is surprising is that IL-4-deficient mice do not mount a polarized Th1 type response, whereas IL-4 and IL-10 doubly deficient mice do. Even more striking is that IL-10 and IL-12 doubly deficient mice mount a polarized Th2 cytokine response (75). In a separate study, addition of recombinant IL-10 to virus-stimulated mediastinal lymph node cells from influenza-infected mice decreased IFN-γ production, while addition of anti-IL-10 had the opposite effect (67). It appears that the effect of IL-10 is complex and can influence both Th1 and Th2 immune responses. Further studies are required to clarify what is obviously an important role for IL-10 in pulmonary immune responses.

In the BALB/c murine model, RSV infection can enhance allergic sensitization and airway hyperresponsiveness. Immune responses to inhaled ovalbumin are enhanced when administered during the acute phase of RSV replication. This is presumably a consequence of enhanced antigen uptake by the damaged respiratory mucosa. The mechanisms are not entirely clear but increased IL-5 production in recruited T cells is evident (76). This phenomenon has been studied in more depth by Gelfand's group (77). Anti-IL-5 treatment during RSV infection effectively reduces eosinophil recruitment to the lung and airway hyperresponsiveness during a subsequent ovalbumin challenge. A similar effect was observed in IL-4 and IL-5 gene knockout mice, an effect that could be reversed by administration of recombinant IL-5. Allergen exposure of IFN-γ-deficient mice also increases airway hyperresponsiveness, which is enhanced by prior exposure to RSV.

Interleukin-13 also critically regulates asthmatic responses in the lung (78). IL-13 binds the alpha chain of the IL-4 receptor and shares similar signaling pathways with IL-4. Two independent studies published at the same time in *Science* (79) showed that administration of a soluble portion of the IL-4 receptor specific to IL-13 (IL-13α2-IgGFc) 24 h prior to intratracheal allergen challenge prevented airway hyperresponsiveness and mucus production. IL-13 administration to naive mice, on the other hand, enhanced airway hyperresponsiveness and eosinophil recruitment to the lung. In addition administration of IL-13 or IL-4 to nonimmunized mice lacking T cells induced an asthmalike state that depends on the IL-4 receptor alpha chain (79). When Th2 cell culture supernatants are given intranasally to mice potent induction of eotaxin and recruitment of eosinophils are observed. Selective depletion of cytokines from the culture supernatant reveals IL-13 as the most effective cytokine in the induction of eotaxin (80). It is interesting to note that linkage analysis maps susceptibility to asthma in humans to chromosome position 5q25–31. This region contains the genes for both IL-4 and IL-13 (81). Asthma in humans is also linked to two mutations in the alpha chain of the IL-4 receptor (82). In some models additional IL-13 depletion is essential to eliminate lung eosinophilia, whereas in others IL-4 absence alone is enough. For example, lung eosinophilic responses to an inhalational ovalbumin challenge are reduced in IL-4 knockout mice. However, unless IL-13 is also depleted in these IL-4 knockout mice, mild eosinophilia still occurs after inhalational challenge (83). The cytokine requirement for the generation of eosinophilic pathology appears to depend on the site of initial allergen encounter. Using a pulmonary granuloma model induced with *Schistosoma mansoni* eggs, lung eosinophilia, IgE, and IL-5 production are only abolished in the combined absence of both IL-4 and IL-13 (84). Finally, overexpression of IL-13 in the lung induces an inflammatory response around both small and large airways and significant eosinophilia (85). The role of IL-13 in the development of eosinophilia therefore warrants further investigation in other models.

C. Cytokine Administration During Lung Viral Infection

Instead of manipulating the pathological phenotype by depleting cytokines, a number of studies have administered the recombinant cytokine during lung viral infection. As mentioned above, IL-12 administration during RSV G-protein sensitization prevents the eosinophilic response after intranasal RSV challenge. Although eosinophilia is reduced, illness assessed by monitoring weight loss and degree of cachexia is markedly enhanced. This introduces an important point that must be considered when using agents that skew immunity in humans. Although induction of eosinophilia is undesirable, severely skewing immunity to the opposite phenotype may be even worse. The key is therefore **balance**. A balanced immune response will prevent eosinophilia and minimize immunopathology, whereas a skewed immune response will lead to bystander tissue damage. At mucosal sites Th2 immunity has evolved to combat tissue damage precisely. We will therefore have to consider the consequences of inducing potent Th1 or CD8+ T cell immunity carefully before applying the results of mouse studies to humans.

It is interesting to note that recombinant IL-12 administered at the time of immunization with a formalin-inactivated (FI) alum-precipitated RSV preparation reduces eosinophilia but does not result in enhanced pathology after intranasal RSV infection. IL-12 treatment during FI-RSV vaccination increases IFN-γ mRNA in the lungs, IgG2a, and IL-12 p40 mRNA expression (28). The contrast between this study and when IL-12 is administered during sensitization to the G protein expressed in a vaccinia virus construct probably reflects the nature of the priming antigen (replicating vaccinia expressing the G protein compared to particulate FI-RSV). Similar pathological responses to IL-12 treatment have been demonstrated during influenza virus infection of mice. Administration of 1000 ng IL-12 on days −1 to +4 of influenza infection by intraperitoneal injection resulted in a 75% reduction in body weight. Control-treated mice started to recover by day 5 whereas recovery in IL-12-treated animals was delayed until day 9. In this study IL-12 treatment had no beneficial effect on virus clearance, antibody titers, or secondary cytotoxic T lymphocyte (CTL) activity. Even though IFN-γ protein levels are enhanced, pathology and inflammation are exacerbated by IL-12 treatment (27). Enhanced pathology is probably mediated by elevated TNF levels, which is supported by our own studies showing elimination of illness and weight loss during RSV-induced Th1 and Th2 responses by TNF depletion (85a).

The effect of IL-12 on immunopathology seems to depend on the nature of the coadministered infectious agent. When mice are infected with inactivated influenza, a Th2 cytokine immune response occurs. If IL-12 and anti-IL-4 are administered at the same time, the response is skewed towards a Th1 response with no obvious pathological effects (86). This may simply reflect different levels of cytokine production to live vs. dead virus. Live virus will itself enhance IL-12 and TNF production, whereas inactivated virus may not. When recombinant IL-12 is coadministered with live virus, the additive effect may tip the balance towards pathology. IFN-γ and especially TNF may reach levels at which they spill over into the systemic circulation causing thymic atrophy, increased glucocorticoid secretion, cachexia, and weight loss. IL-12 may therefore be beneficial in diverting Th2 responses to inactivated vaccines towards a Th1 phenotype but can prove lethal when administered during live viral infections. This hypothesis is supported by the effect of administering IL-12 with an influenza subunit vaccine in neonatal mice. When treated with both within 24 h of birth, elevated splenic IFN-γ, IL-10, and IL-15 mRNA levels are observed. Enhanced cytokine production, elevated IgG2a antibody, and increased virus clearance is also apparent when mice are rechallenged later in life compared to mice given the subunit vaccine alone at birth (87).

This study does not report any untoward side effects, which may again be due to the particulate rather than an infectious nature of the antigen. Administration of IL-12 with the fusion protein of RSV in alum or phosphate buffered saline (PBS) likewise accelerates virus clearance, increases IgG2a, IFN-γ, and cytotoxic activity but decreases IgE without drastically altering illness during subsequent challenge. These effects depend on IL-12 coformulation with alum. Although a Th1 cytokine response is indicated in this study, extensive lung eosinophilia is still apparent in mice given the RSV fusion or attachment protein in alum or FI-RSV, whether coformulated with IL-12 or not (88). The 190–289 amino acid sequence of the RSV fusion protein expressed in insect cells partially protects BALB/c mice from an intranasal challenge but induces a Th2 cytokine response. Administration of 10 ng IL-12 at the same time reduces IL-4 and IL-5 secretion and an inflammatory infiltrate occurs. IL-12 treatment in this setting does not appear to enhance immunopathology nor does it improve virus clearance from the lung (89). Bypassing the requirement for IL-12 by intranasal administration of plasmids expressing IFN-γ cDNA decreases viral replication, epithelial cell damage, and inflammatory infiltrate into the lung without causing overt illness (90). The difference between plasmid IFN-γ and recombinant IL-12 treatment may involve the levels of IFN-γ produced by the two treatment strategies. A more detailed comparison is required before any further conclusions can be drawn.

With the advent of reverse genetics an exciting variety of recombinant RSV strains is appearing in the scientific literature. One such recombinant RSV encoding murine IFN-γ has been constructed in the laboratories of Peter Collins. This recombinant, although replicating less efficiently than wild-type RSV, elevates IFN-γ and IL-12 mRNA in the lung and completely protects mice from an intranasal RSV challenge (91). Such recombinant virus strains are appealing to future vaccine strategies, since they appear to incorporate effectively attenuation, replication, and immunogenicity without inducing overt pathology.

Both treatment with IL-12 and induction of Th2 cytokines have a detrimental effect. Treatment of mice with IL-4 during A/PR/8/34 influenza virus infection significantly delays virus clearance and suppresses cytotoxic T cells. The same effect on virus clearance is seen when influenza-specific cells are secondarily stimulated in vitro in the presence of IL-4 and then adoptively transferred into syngeneic recipients, which are then infected with homologous virus. Mice that receive cells cultured in the presence of IL-4 clear the virus more slowly than those given cells cultured in the absence of IL-4 (92). The explanation for delayed virus clearance in this study probably reflects the immunological function of the cytokines involved. IL-4 predominantly promotes B-cell responses and antibody isotype switching whereas type 1 cytokines, such as IFN-γ, induce cell-mediated immunity and CTL and NK activation. The activation of cell-mediated immunity is more appropriate during infection with noncytopathic viruses since they predominantly replicate within cells without causing cell lysis and are therefore inaccessible to antibody. This concept is highlighted in a study by Graham et al. (24) who skewed influenza-virus-specific CD4+ T-cell responses in vitro towards a Th1 or Th2 cytokine profile and then transferred them into syngeneic recipients that were then intranasally infected with homologous virus. Those with a Th1 cytokine profile are cytolytic in vitro and protect mice against a subsequent virus challenge, whereas cells with a Th2 phenotype are noncytolytic and induce pulmonary eosinophilia without viral clearance.

Bot and colleagues reported a similar effect in transgenic mice that express IL-4 under the control of a lung-specific promoter (93). CD4+ and CD8+ T-cell recruitment to the lung is unaffected by the presence of the transgene during a primary influenza lung infection. CD8+ T cells are, however, significantly impaired during recall responses to a homologous virus challenge and delayed virus clearance occurs. The fact that virus clearance is only delayed is attributed to the increase in virus-specific antibody in IL-4 transgenic mice.

The inhibitory effect of IL-4 on virus-specific CD8+ T cells appears controversial. Aung and colleagues (94) constructed a recombinant vaccinia virus expressing the immunodominant CD8+ T-cell epitope for RSV with or without the gene for IL-4. Mice infected with vaccinia expressing the RSV epitope and IL-4 display less CTL activity than mice infected with vaccinia containing the epitope alone. In addition, reduced intracellular IFN-γ is apparent when cells are stimulated with specific peptide. Tang and Graham (29) showed that depletion of IL-4 during formalin-inactivated RSV vaccination of mice increases CTL activity and IFN-γ while reducing weight loss, illness, and virus replication. Geraldine Taylor's group, on the other hand, constructed a vaccinia recombinant containing the fusion protein and the genes for IL-2, IFN-γ, or IL-4. CTL activity to the fusion protein was unaffected if the vaccinia additionally contained IL-4, whereas insertion of genes for IL-2 and IFN-γ significantly reduced CTL activity. This differential effect is explained by the altered kinetics of vaccinia virus clearance. Insertion of genes for IL-2 or IFN-γ enhances, whereas insertion of the IL-4 gene delays, vaccinia clearance (95). The differences between these two studies may reflect the nature of the RSV protein or peptide and the point of insertion of cytokine genes into vaccinia virus.

IV. Protective Role of Infections in the Establishment of Th2-Mediated Illnesses

The effect of exposure to one organism on the pathogenesis of subsequent unrelated infections may have major biological consequence. We have recently published a series of studies showing that influenza virus infection of the lung protects from immunopathology caused by RSV (96). BALB/c mice sensitized to the G protein of RSV develop pulmonary eosinophilia after intranasal RSV challenge. Mice treated in this way also lose weight, become cachexic, have reduced mobility, and display ruffled fur. This enhanced illness is not observed, however, if the mice have previously recovered from an influenza virus infection. The possible mechanisms for alleviation of eosinophilia and illness include specific cross-reactivity in RSV T and B cell epitopes by influenza-primed cells, bystander activation of influenza-specific cells, so-called immunological imprinting skewing towards a Th1 phenotype, and remodeling of the lung by the first infection.

It has been estimated that each naive CD4+ and CD8+ T cell may react with up to 1 million peptides (97). Indeed cross-reactive memory cytotoxic T-cell recognition of heterologous viruses has previously been described (98). Prior infections can alter the hierarchy of immunodominant epitopes recognized by CD8+ T cells during a subsequent unrelated infection (99). Although this mechanism of protection cannot be totally excluded, we did not observe cross-reactivity between influenza and RSV in CD4+ and CD8+ T-cell responses. Nor did we observe any evidence of lung-remodeling by the first infection. Matrix metalloproteinase activity had returned to baseline before the G protein priming and RSV infection. There is likewise no increase in vascularity or basement membrane thickness.

We believe that the beneficial effect of infection history in the RSV infection model is explained by a combination of the second and third points noted above. Sensitive reagents are now available to detect the movement of antigen-specific T cells. One of these techniques involves MHC tetramer technology. Four MHC class I chains loaded with a peptide recognized by CD8+ T cells are joined via a biotin molecule. This construct can be used as a surface stain to locate CD8+ T cells that bind to that epitope. Binding of the tetramer is then detected using fluorochrome-conjugated avidin and the whole interaction is visualized on a flow cytometer. Using such MHC tetramers loaded with the immunodominant CD8 epitope from influenza, we have shown that influenza-specific CD8+ T cells return to the lung during a subsequent RSV challenge. In the context of a heterologous viral infection, these influenza-specific CD8+ T cells are activated and induced to secrete IFN-γ. We believe it is the contribution of IFN-γ from these unrelated influenza-specific CD8+ T cells that adds to an environment inhibitory to eosinophils.

We also observed that prior RSV exposure prevented eosinophilia in mice subsequently infected with the G protein and challenged with RSV. The first RSV exposure will induce CD4+Th1 and CD8+ T-cell responses to many viral proteins (20). These effectively override the G protein eosinophilic response by rapidly proliferating to the same proteins during the final RSV challenge. Mechanisms associated with protection from eosinophilia by prior RSV or influenza exposure are summarized in Figure 3. The reduction of weight loss and cachexia by prior infection is interesting. Most of the pathology associated with viral infection of the lung arises due to the recruitment of an enhanced inflammatory infiltrate, which obstructs the airways and causes bystander tissue damage. When mice are previously infected with influenza virus, a reduced pulmonary infiltrate occurs. The location of the infiltrate also changes: only perivascular and not additional peribronchiolar consolidation is evident. This reduction of inflammation by prior infection may therefore explain the lack of illness in G-primed RSV-challenged mice previously exposed to influenza virus or RSV.

The important influence of infection history on the development of asthma and atopy is also highlighted by studies on family size. The presence of older siblings appears to protect younger children against the development of atopy (100–102), which may be linked to cross-infections between children in the same household (103). Nonwheezing lower respiratory tract illnesses in the first 3 years of life are associated with lower IgE levels, lower skin test reactivity, and increased IFN-γ production from mononuclear cells in later life (104). The surveys by von Mutius *et al.* soon after the unification of East and West Germany show a higher frequency of respiratory symptoms (suggesting more respiratory infections) but a lower prevalence of asthma in East German children (105). Shirakawa show that strong tuberculin responders in a Bacillus Calmette–Guérin (BCG)-vaccinated population are one-half to one-third as likely as nonresponders to have asthma symptoms and remission of asthma symptoms in strong responders is more likely during childhood (106). In addition to respiratory infections, measles (107,108) and hepatitis A (109) have been linked to protection from atopic illness. Measles vaccination, on the other hand, is not protective. Antibiotic use during the first 2 years of life may be associated with an increased prevalence of atopy, emphasizing the importance of microbial exposure in the normal development of the immune system.

What are the proposed immunological mechanisms for the protective effect of infections in the development of atopic disease? Atopy is related to the expression of allergen-specific responses with production of Th2 cytokines such as IL-4 and IL-5, which promote IgE production and eosinophilia (110). In normal individuals the T-cell system is biased to a T-helper 1 phenotype with production of IFN-γ and inhibition of Th2 cells. Pregnancy is associated with a strong skewing toward a Th2 cytokine pattern, enabling the survival of the placenta and fetus. Development of a balanced Th1/Th2 immune phenotype is determined genetically and modified by environmental factors. One environmental factor of importance may be the microbial gut flora and changes in its composition by altered lifestyle and diet, including changes in breastfeeding, and even antibiotic use (111). Leukocyte surface markers change markedly from the fetal to adult life. Neonates have the highest leukocyte counts and highest counts of all T-cell subsets, and the percentage of CD2+, CD3+, CD4+, and CD8+ increases significantly from fetus to adult. B-cell absolute and relative counts are highest in the fetus and decrease in adulthood, which reflects a move from a Th2 to a Th1 cytokine environment (112). This movement may be a consequence of antigen exposure.

Intrauterine T-cell priming takes place and fetally derived allergen-reactive T cells exhibiting a Th2 phenotype exist (113). Prescott et al. have demonstrated the persistence during infancy of these fetal allergen-specific Th2 responses with a decreased capacity to produce IFN-γ in atopic neonates (114). Strong IL-4 and IL-13 responses and reduced production of IL-12 and IFN-γ has been observed in young mice and infants (115). Environmental factors such as microbial agents may exert their effects during early life and aid in the maturation of the adaptive immune response into a Th1-dependent system. The critical period in humans during which immunomodulation by intense systemic infections is postulated to have a lasting effect is the first 2 years of life. Romagnani (116) suggests that the rising prevalence of atopy is related to a reduction in childhood infections like tuberculosis with a resultant reduced production of cytokines antagonistic to Th2 cell differentiation. Some animal studies have supported this concept of immune modulation by microorganisms. Erb et al. (117) found that allergen-induced airway eosinophilia in mice was suppressed by prior BCG infection, which was dependent on the ability of the animals to produce IFN-γ. Wang and Rook also show that the established allergic response to ovalbumin in mice is inhibited by killed *Mycobacterium vaccae* (118).

The importance of intestinal bacterial flora is highlighted in a study by Sudo et al. Oral administration of OVA in germ-free mice failed to induce Th1 responses upon subsequent systemic challenge with OVA, but instead a Th2-mediated response was present. In animals with intact intestinal flora, such oral tolerance induction suppresses both Th1 and Th2 responses. Reconstitution of intestinal flora in germ-free mice restored the Th2-downregulation by oral tolerance induction only if performed in the neonate (119).

The immunological basis of the hygiene hypothesis can be summarized as follows. Allergen-specific T cells exhibiting a Th2 phenotype exist in genetically predisposed individuals. Macrophages and dendritic cells are induced to produce cytokines that favor a type 1 phenotype by immunomodulatory micro-organisms such as intracellular bacteria (e.g., *Mycobacteria*) and viruses (e.g., measles). The resultant high IFN-γ level provides the environment for the differentiation of antigen-specific CD4+ T cells into Th1 cells and CD8+ T cells into Tc1 cells with

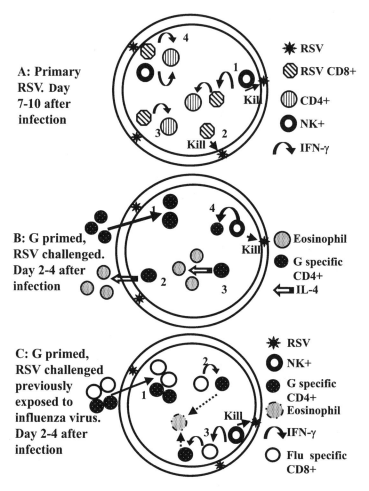

Figure 3 The influence of differential cell recruitment on the development of eosinophilia. The illustrations represent the events inside the airways of RSV infected hosts schematically. (A) During a primary RSV infection, cell recruitment to the lung peaks on days 7–10. NK cells are activated locally and lyse virus-infected bronchoalveolar epithelial cells. NK cells also produce IFN-γ, which contributes to CD8+ T-cell activation. CD8+ T cells in turn also produce IFN-γ, which promotes the development of CD4+ Th1 cells (1). CD8+ T cells also lyse virus-infected epithelial cells (2). IFN-γ produced by CD8+ T cells in the absence of NK cell stimuli may drive the development of a Th1 phenotype (3). The production of IFN-γ from CD8+ T cells and NK cells independently drives an environment conducive to Th1 development (4). (B) In mice previously sensitized with the attachment protein (G) of RSV, CD4+ T cells are recruited to the lung at early time points during the RSV challenge (1). These respond quickly to the G protein in the challenge virus before the primary response to other viral proteins takes effect. In the absence of IFN-γ production by CD8+ T cells, a Th2 phenotype develops that recruits eosinophils to the lung (2). Th2 cytokines promote the activation, survival, and differentiation of eosinophils (3). There is a lack of NK cells and NK-cell-derived IFN-γ to act on CD4+ T cells in this model. Unlike a primary infection,

even higher IFN-γ production. In the absence of such early stimuli, the Th2-biased immature immune system persists and the allergen-specific responses become established to express an atopic phenotype

Not all studies, however, support the protective influence of infections (113). A high prevalence of asthma is not restricted to developed communities but exists also in poor African cities and among low-income minority groups in the United States (120). These communities are unlikely to have experienced a drop in microbial exposure and the hygiene hypothesis can hardly apply here. Other factors such as pollution and levels of allergen exposure may now come into play and it should be noted that the increase in asthma in nondeveloped countries might be the result of other parasitic infections that induce a strong Th2 cytokine response.

V. Causative Role for Infections in the Pathogenesis of Asthma

Viruses are now considered the most important triggers for acute exacerbation of established asthma (121). Altered cytokine responses in asthmatic subjects, reflected in prolonged eosinophil accumulation in the lungs following viral infection (122) and enhanced penetration of inhaled allergens during virus-induced lung inflammation (76), are the most likely mechanisms.

However, some evidence for an additional causal role of viruses in the establishment of asthma exists. Infants hospitalized with RSV bronchiolitis have a higher chance of being diagnosed with asthma or wheezing in the ensuing years (123–125). Respiratory symptoms may persist for several years in children after RSV bronchiolitis (126) and histamine responsiveness demonstrates hyperreactivity 10 years or more after the event (127). Although these studies may point to a causal link between RSV bronchiolitis and asthma, the possibility of a genetic predisposition to both asthma and bronchiolitis cannot be ruled out.

The causal link between viral bronchiolitis and asthma is supported by results of animal studies. Brown Norway rats, although genetically predisposed, develop chronic, episodic, and reversible airway obstruction after viral bronchiolitis (128) and display a predominant CD4+ T-cell response with reduced IFN-γ production, leading to airway remodeling with persistent inflammation, fibrosis, and deposition of extracellular matrix material. Exposure to the major surface glycoprotein G of RSV in certain mouse strains (30) leads to Th2 cell predominance with airway eosin-

---

Figure 3 (cont.)   G-protein-primed mice therefore develop Th2-driven pulmonary eosinophilia during RSV challenge. (C) If mice have previously been exposed to influenza virus prior to G protein priming, Th2-driven pulmonary eosinophilia does not occur during RSV challenge. Both G-specific CD4+ T cells and influenza-specific CD8+ T cells return to the lung during the RSV challenge (1). This environment activates influenza-specific CD8+ T cells causing IFN-γ production, which promotes the development of a Th1 phenotype in the G-specific CD4+ T cells (2). NK cells, responding to RSV-infected epithelial cells, additionally activate influenza-specific CD8+ T cells, which in turn promotes Th1 development. The reduction of IL-4 and IL-5 and the increase in IFN-γ mean that eosinophils are not recruited or maintained (3).

ophilia, which is in contrast to the usual Th1 response seen in most primary viral infections. This response is linked to the inability of the G protein to stimulate CD8+ T cells (22), emphasizing the important noncytolytic role of CD8+ cells. CD8+ T cells also exhibit type 1 and type 2 cytokine production patterns (Tc1 and Tc2) and may have an important role in determining CD4 phenotypes (129).

Concurrent exposures to respiratory viruses and allergens have been reported that could lead to the establishment of asthma. In children presenting to an emergency room with acute airway obstruction, the combination of both atopy and concurrent viral illness is a greater risk factor than any one of these factors alone (130). In individuals with allergic rhinitis, experimental rhinovirus-16 inoculation alters their response to allergen bronchoprovocation to favor the development of the late-phase response (131). This suggests that viruses may induce the development of an asthmatic phenotype under specific conditions. Again, animal studies support this concept. Uninfected mice develop no IgE antibody against inhaled antigen (ovalbumin), but during acute influenza infection sensitization does take place (132). Alone neither influenza A virus nor ovalbumin causes changes in serum IgE or airway responsiveness to inhaled metacholine, but both are increased when antigen exposure coincides with influenza infection (133). O'Donnell observed acute systemic illness in response to cutaneous ovalbumin administration in mice exposed to concurrent RSV infection and nebulized ovalbumin but not in animals exposed to either of these insults alone (76). The ability of viral infections to promote or exacerbate allergic responses may simply reflect the extensive tissue damage at affected sites. We mentioned, when describing how mucosal tissues prevent inflammatory reactions, that immune exclusion promoted by secretory IgA was one of the most important mechanisms. This can hardly function in the context of a lung infection in which the epithelial barrier is severely compromised. Viral inflammation may be associated with allergy simply because it allows inhaled antigen to penetrate the barrier of the respiratory mucosa, promoting sensitization.

Immune responses in chronic *Chlamydia pneumoniae* infection in asthmatics could suggest a role for *Chlamydia* in the pathogenesis of asthma (134). Cunningham et al. investigated 108 children with asthma and found a tendency to remain PCR positive for *Chlamydia* in those with frequent acute episodes, suggesting chronic infection. Previous chlamydial exposure has also been demonstrated in 34.8% of patients with severe chronic asthma (135). Other studies (136) provide no evidence of chlamydial disease in asthmatics. Evidence of *Mycoplasma pneumoniae* infection has been found in the lower airways of stable asthmatics with greater frequency than in control subjects, suggesting a pathogenic role (137). In all studies showing an association between infection and asthma, it is possible that an existing asthmatic state is not conducive to pathogen clearance. There are many conflicting findings and the issues require further investigation. As with the RSV data, a genetic predisposition to both asthma and these infections cannot be ruled out.

The mechanisms by which viral and other infections during early life could affect later development of lung disease include virus chronicity, persistence, or latency; permanent changes to local anatomy; impaired lung growth; local foothold for other acute or chronic infections; immunological tolerance; and establishment of local immunological mood (138). The sensitization to aeroallergens during respiratory infections can be added to this list.

VI. Summary

In the majority of cases the lung effectively maintains homeostasis using regulatory mechanisms that limit inflammatory responses to infection in the lung. It is clear that a number of mechanisms divert this so-called ignorant state into an inflammatory environment. The sequence of events required to mature the lung environment in the newborn is an area of intense investigation. As our immune system has co-evolved with pathogens, it is reasonable to assume that signals from the environment are necessary for the successful maturation of immunity. Our immune system learns to manage infections in a manner appropriate to the affected site. Infection of the blood could effectively transport the invading pathogen throughout the body and may, in evolutionary terms, provide a more alarming signal to the immune system. Immunological alarm at delicate mucosal surfaces, on the other hand, may do more harm than good. Scientists are now using immunological reagents to redress the balance between immunity and ignorance. In the future we may need to design vaccines that signal the immune system in a similar manner to the original pathogen. This will provide appropriate immunity to that pathogen and enable our immune system to mature. Using the formalin-inactivated RSV vaccine trials as an example, it is possible that particulate antigens processed predominantly via an MHC class II pathway are not appropriate signals to an immune system that eradicates such viruses using CD8+ T and NK cells. The use of live attenuated RSV strains as vaccines therefore holds much promise for the future.

Acknowledgments

Tracy Hussell is supported by an MRC career establishment grant (G0000077), Gerhard Walzl by a National Asthma Campaign project grant (00/07), and Ian Humphreys by a Biochemistry Departmental bursary.

References

1. Mbawuike IN, Pacheco S, Acuna CL, Switzer KC, Zhang Y, Harriman GR. Mucosal immunity to influenza without IgA: an IgA knockout mouse model. J Immunol 1999; 162:2530–2537.
2. Mostov KE. Transepithelial transport of immunoglobulins. Annu Rev Immunol 1994; 12:63–84.
3. Xu AJ, Kiyono H, Jackson RJ, Staats HF, Fujihashi K, Burrows PD, Elson CO, Pillai S, McGhee JR. Helper T cell subsets for immunoglobulin A responses: oral immunization with tetanus toxoid and cholera toxin as adjuvant selectively induces Th2 cells in mucosa associated tissues. J Exp Med 1993; 178:1309–1320.

4. Bao S, Goldstone S, Husband AJ. Localization of IFN-gamma and IL-6 mRNA in murine intestine by in situ hybridization. Immunology 1993; 80:666–670.

5. Inobe J, Slavin AJ, Komagata Y, Chen Y, Liu L, Weiner HL. IL-4 is a differentiation factor for transforming growth factor-beta secreting Th3 cells and oral administration of IL-4 enhances oral tolerance in experimental allergic encephalomyelitis. Eur J Immunol 1998; 28:2780–2790.

6. Goodrich ME, McGee DW. Preferential enhancement of B cell IgA secretion by intestinal epithelial cell-derived cytokines and interleukin-2. Immunol Invest 1999; 28:67–75.

7. Powrie F, Correa OR, Mauze S, Coffman RL. Regulatory interactions between CD45RBhigh and CD45RBlow CD4+ T cells are important for the balance between protective and pathogenic cell-mediated immunity. J Exp Med 1994; 179:589–600.

8. Morrissey PJ, Charrier K, Braddy S, Liggitt D, Watson JD. CD4+ T cells that express high levels of CD45RB induce wasting disease when transferred into congenic severe combined immunodeficient mice. Disease development is prevented by cotransfer of purified CD4+ T cells. J Exp Med 1993; 178:237-244.

9. Powrie F, Leach MW, Mauze S, Menon S, Caddle LB, Coffman RL. Inhibition of Th1 responses prevents inflammatory bowel disease in scid mice reconstituted with CD45RBhi CD4+ T cells. Immunity 1994; 1:553–562.

10. Aranda R, Sydora BC, McAllister PL, Binder SW, Yang HY, Targan SR, Kronenberg M. Analysis of intestinal lymphocytes in mouse colitis mediated by transfer of CD4+, CD45RBhigh T cells to SCID recipients. J Immunol 1997; 158:3464–3473.

11. Claesson MH, Bregenholt S, Bonhagen K, Thoma S, Moller P, Grusby MJ, Leithauser F, Nissen MH, Reimann J. Colitis-inducing potency of CD4+ T cells in immunodeficient, adoptive hosts depends on their state of activation, IL-12 responsiveness, and CD45RB surface phenotype. J Immunol 1999; 162:3702–3710.

12. Powrie F, Carlino J, Leach MW, Mauze S, Coffman RL. A critical role for transforming growth factor-beta but not interleukin 4 in the suppression of T helper type 1-mediated colitis by CD45RB(low) CD4+ T cells. J Exp Med 1996; 183:2669-2674.

13. Kuhn R, Lohler J, Rennick D, Rajewsky K, Muller W. Interleukin-l0-deficient mice develop chronic enterocolitis. Cell 1993; 75:263–274

14. Chen Y, Kuchroo VK, Inobe J, Hafler DA, Weiner HL. Regulatory T cell clones induced by oral tolerance: suppression of autoimmune encephalomyelitis. Science 1994; 265:1237–1240.

15. Han HS, Jun HS, Utsugi T, Yoon JW. A new type of CD4+ suppressor T cell completely prevents spontaneous autoimmune diabetes and recurrent diabetes in syngeneic islet-transplanted NOD mice. J Autoimmun 1996; 9:331–339.

16. Groux H, O'Garra A, Bigler M, Rouleau M, Antonenko S, de VJ, Roncarolo MG. A CD4+ T-cell subset inhibits antigen-specific T-cell responses and prevents colitis. Nature 1997; 389:737-742.

17. De Vries JE. Immunosuppressive and anti-inflammatory properties of interleukin 10. Ann Med 1995; 27:537–541.

18. Fiorentino DF, Zlotnik A, Vieira P, Mosmann TR, Howard M, Moore KW, O'Garra A. IL-10 acts on the antigen-presenting cell to inhibit cytokine production by Th 1 cells. J Immunol 1991; 146:3444–3451.

19. Panuska JR, Merolla R, Rebert NA, Hoffmann SP, Tsivitse P, Cirino NM, Silverman RH, Rankin JA. Respiratory syncytial virus induces interleukin-10 by human alveolar macrophages—suppression of early cytokine production and implications for incomplete immunity. J Clin Invest 1995; 96:2445–2453.

20. Hussell T, Spender LC, Georgiou A, O'Garra A, Openshaw PJM. Th1 and Th2 cytokine induction in pulmonary T-cells during infection with respiratory syncytial virus. J Gen Virol 1996; 77:2447–2455.

21. Murray CJ, Lopez AD. Mortality by cause for eight regions of the world: Global Burden of Disease Study. Lancet 1997; 349:1269–1276.

22. Alwan WH, Kozlowska WJ, Openshaw PJM. Distinct types of lung disease caused by functional subsets of antiviral T cells. J Exp Med 1994; 179:81–89.

23. Openshaw PJM, Clarke SL, Record FM. Pulmonary eosinophilic response to respiratory syncytial virus infection in mice sensitized to the major surface glycoprotein G. Internat Immunol 1992; 4:493–500.

24. Graham MB, Braciale VL, Braciale TJ. Influenza virus-specific CD4+ T helper type 2 T lymphocytes do not promote recovery from experimental virus infection. J Exp Med 1994; 180:1273–1282.

25. Hussell T, Baldwin CJ, O'Garra A, Openshaw PJM. CD8+ T-cells control Th2-driven pathology during pulmonary respiratory syncytial virus infection. Eur J Immunol 1997; 27:3341–3349.

26. Sparer TE, Matthews S, Hussell T, Rae AJ, Garcia BB, Melero JA, Openshaw PJ. Eliminating a region of respiratory syncytial virus attachment protein allows induction of protective immunity without vaccine-enhanced lung eosinophilia. J Exp Med 1998; 187:1921–1926.

27. Hussell T, Khan U, Openshaw PJM. IL-12 treatment attenuates Th2 and B cell responses but does not improve vaccine-enhanced lung illness. J Immunol 1997; 159: 328–334.

28. Tang YW, Graham BS. Interleukin-12 treatment during immunization elicits a T helper cell type 1-like immune response in mice challenged with respiratory syncytial virus and improves vaccine immunogenicity. J Infect Dis 1995; 172:734–738.

29. Tang YW, Graham BS. Anti-IL-4 treatment at immunization modulates cytokine expression, reduces illness, and increases cytotoxic T lymphocyte activity in mice challenged with respiratory syncytial virus. J Clin Invest 1994; 94:1953–1958.

30. Hussell T, Georgiou A, Sparer TE, Matthews S, Pala P, Openshaw PJM. Host genetic determinants of vaccine-induced eosinophilia during respiratory syncytial virus infection. J Immunol 1998; 161:6215–6222.

31. Srikiatkhachorn A, Braciale TJ. Virus specific CD8+ T lymphocytes downregulate T helper cell type 2 cytokine secretion and pulmonary eosinophilia during experimental murine respiratory syncytial virus Infection. J Exp Med 1997; 186:421–432.

32. Kos FJ, Engleman EG. Requirement for natural killer cells in the induction of cytotoxic T cells. J Immunol 1995; 155:578-584.

33. Hussell T, Openshaw PJM. Intracellular interferon-gamma expression in natural killer cells precedes lung CD8+ T cell recruitment during respiratory syncytial virus infection. J Gen Virol 1998; 79:2593–2601.

34. Hussell T, Openshaw PJ. IL-12-activated NK cells reduce lung eosinophilia to the attachment protein of respiratory syncytial virus but do not enhance the severity of illness in CD8 T cell-immunodeficient conditions. J Immunol 2000; 165:7109-7115.

35. McIntosh K, Fishaut JM. Immunopathologic mechanisms in lower respiratory tract disease of infants due to respiratory syncytial virus. Prog Med Virol 1980; 26:94–118.

36. Graham BS, Henderson GS, Tang YW, Lu X, Neuzil KM, Colley DG. Priming immunization determines T helper cytokine mRNA expression patterns in lungs of mice challenged with respiratory syncytial virus. J Immunol 1993; 151:2032–2040.

37. Graham BS. Immunological determinants of disease caused by respiratory syncytial virus. Trends Microbiol 1996; 4:290–293.

38. Waris ME, Tsou C, Erdman DD, Zaki SR, Anderson LJ. Respiratory syncytial virus infection in BALB/c mice previously immunized with formalin-inactivated virus induces enhanced pulmonary inflammatory response with a predominant Th2-like cytokine pattern. J Virol 1996; 70:2852–2860.

39. Bonecchi R, Bianchi G, Bordignon PP, D'Ambrosio D, Lang R, Borsatti A, Sozzani S, Allavena P, Gray PA, Mantovani A, Sinigaglia F. Differential expression of chemokine receptors and chemotactic responsiveness of type 1 T helper cells (Th1s) and Th2s. J Exp Med 1998; 187:129–134.

40. Loetscher P, Uguccioni M, Bordoli L, Baggiolini M, Moser B, Chizzolini C, Dayer JM. CCR5 is characteristic of Th1 lymphocytes. Nature (London) 1998; 391:344–345.

41. Xu D, Chan WL, Leung BP, Hunter D, Schulz K, Carter RW, McInnes IB, Robinson JH, Liew FY. Selective expression and functions of interleukin 18 receptor on T helper (Th) type 1 but not Th2 cells. J Exp Med 1998; 188:1485–1492.

42. Ho IC, Hodge MR, Rooney JW, Glimcher LH. The proto-oncogene c-maf is responsible for tissue-specific expression of interleukin-4. Cell 1996; 85:973–983.

43. Zheng W, Flavell RA. The transcription factor GATA-3 is necessary and sufficient for Th2 cytokine gene expression in CD4 T cells. Cell 1997; 89:587–596.

44. Sallusto F, Lenig D, Mackay CR, Lanzavecchia A. Flexible programs of chemokine receptor expression on human polarized T helper 1 and 2 lymphocytes. J Exp Med 1998; 187:875–883.

45. Sallusto F, Mackay CR, Lanzavecchia A. Selective expression of the eotaxin receptor CCR3 by human T helper 2 cells. Science 1997; 277:2005–2007.

46. Coyle AJ, Lloyd C, Tian J, Nguyen T, Erikkson C, Wang L, Ottoson P, Persson P, Delaney T, Lehar S, Lin S, Poisson L, Meisel C, Kamradt T, Bjerke T, Levinson D, Gutierrez RJ. Crucial role of the interleukin 1 receptor family member T1/ST2 in T helper cell type 2-mediated lung mucosal immune responses. J Exp Med 1999; 190: 895–902.

47. Kropf P, Schopf LR, Chung CL, Xu D, Liew FY, Sypek JP, Muller I. Expression of Th2 cytokines and the stable Th2 marker ST2L in the absence of IL-4 during Leishmania major infection. Eur J Immunol 1999; 29:3621–3628.

48. Xu D, Chan WL, Leung BP, Huang F, Wheeler R, Piedrafita D, Robinson JH, Liew FY. Selective expression of a stable cell surface molecule on type 2 but not type 1 helper T cells. J Exp Med 1998; 187:787–794.

49. Lohning M, Grogan JL, Coyle AJ, Yazdanbakhsh M, Meisel C, Gutierrez RJ, Radbruch A, Kamradt T. T1/ST2 expression is enhanced on CD4+ T cells from schistosome egg-induced granulomas: analysis of Th cell cytokine coexpression ex vivo. J Immunol 1999; 162:3882–3889.

50. Lohning M, Stroehmann A, Coyle AJ, Grogan JL, Lin S, Gutierrez RJ, Levinson D, Radbruch A, Kamradt T. T1/ST2 is preferentially expressed on murine Th2 cells, independent of interleukin 4, interleukin 5, and interleukin 10, and important for Th2 effector function. Proc Natl Acad Sci USA 1998; 95:6930-6935.

51. Lohoff M, Prechtl S, Sommer F, Roellinghoff M, Schmitt E, Gradehandt G, Rohwer P, Stride BD, Cole SP, Deeley RG. A multidrug-resistance protein (MRP)-like transmembrane pump is highly expressed by resting murine T helper (Th) 2, but not Th1 cells, and is induced to equal expression levels in Th1 and Th2 cells after antigenic stimulation in vivo. J Clin Invest 1998; 101:703–710.

52. Prechtl S, Roellinghoff M, Scheper R, Cole SP, Deeley RG, Lohoff M. The multidrug resistance protein 1: a functionally important activation marker for marine Th1 cells. J Immunol 2000; 164:754–761.

53. Nagata K, Tanaka K, Ogawa K, Kemmotsu K, Imai T, Yoshie O, Abe H, Tada K, Nakamura M, Sugamura K, Takano S. Selective expression of a novel surface molecule by human Th2 cells in vivo. J Immunol 1999; 162:1278–1286.

54. Rossler U, Andres AC, Reichmann E, Schmahl W, Werenskiold AK. T1, an immunoglobulin superfamily member, is expressed in H-ras-dependent epithelial tumours of mammary cells. Oncogene 1993; 8:609–617.

55. Klemenz R, Hoffmann S, Werenskiold AK. Serum- and oncoprotein-mediated induction of a gene with sequence similarity to the gene encoding carcinoembryonic antigen. Proc Natl Acad Sci USA 1989; 86:5708–5712.

56. Yanagisawa K, Takagi T, Tsukamoto T, Tetsuka T, Tominaga S. Presence of a novel primary response gene ST2L, encoding a product highly similar to the interleukin 1 receptor type 1. FEBS Lett 1993; 318:83–87.

57. Rossler U, Thomassen E, Hultner L, Baier S, Danescu J, Werenskiold AK. Secreted and membrane-bound isoforms of T1, an orphan receptor related to IL-1-binding proteins, are differently expressed in vivo. Dev Biol 1995; 168:86–97.

58. Bergers G, Reikerstorfer A, Braselmann S, Graninger P, Busslinger M. Alternative promoter usage of the Fos-responsive gene Fit-1 generates mRNA isoforms coding for either secreted or membrane-bound proteins related to the IL-1 receptor. EMBO J 1994; 13:1176–1188.

59. Esolen LM, Ward BJ, Moench TR, Griffin DE. Infection of monocytes during measles. J Infect Dis 1993; 168:47–52.

60. Hoshino K, Kashiwamura S, Kuribayashi K, Kodama T, Tsujimura T, Nakanishi K, Matsuyama T, Takeda K, Akira S. The absence of IL-1R-related T1/ST2 does not affect T helper cell type 2 development and its effector function. J Exp Med 1999; 190:1541–1547.

61. Townsend MJ, Fallon PG, Matthews DJ, Jolin HE, McKenzie ANJ. T1/ST2-deficient mice demonstrate the importance of T1/ST2 in developing primary T helper cell type 2 responses. J Exp Med 2000; 191:1069–1075.

62. Gachter T, Werenskiold AK, Klemenz R. Transcription of the interleukin-1 receptor-related T1 gene is initiated at different promoters in mast cells and fibroblasts. J Biol Chem 1996; 271:124–129.

62a. Walzl G, Matthews S, et al. Inhibition of T_1/ST_2 during respiratory syncytial virus infection prevents T helper cells (TH2) but not TH1-driven immunopathology. J Exp Med 2001; 193:785–792.

63. Karras JG, McGraw K, McKay RA, Cooper SR, Lemer D, Lu T, Walker C, Dean NM, Monia BP. Inhibition of antigen-induced eosinophilia and late phase airway hyperresponsiveness by an IL-5 antisense oligonucleotide in mouse models of asthma. J Immunol 2000; 164:5409–5415.

64. Hamelmann E, Takeda K, Haczku A, Cieslewicz G, Shultz L, Hamid Q, Xing Z, Gauldie J, Gelfand EW. Interleukin (IL)-5 but not immunoglobulin E reconstitutes airway inflammation and airway hyperresponsiveness in IL-4-deficient mice. Am J Respir Cell Mol Biol 2000; 23:327–334.

65. Tripp RA, Moore D, Anderson LJ. TH(1)- and TH(2)-type cytokine expression by activated T lymphocytes from the lung and spleen during the inflammatory response to respiratory syncytial virus. Cytokine 2000; 12:801–807.

66. Sarawar SR, Carding SR, Allan W, McMickle A, Fujihashi K, Kiyono H, McGhee JR, Doherty PC. Cytokine profiles of bronchoalveolar lavage cells from mice with influenza pneumonia: consequences of CD4+ and CD8+ T cell depletion. Reg Immunol. 1993; 5:142–150.

67. Sarawar SR, Doherty PC. Concurrent production of interleukin-2, interleukin-10, and gamma interferon in the regional lymph nodes of mice with influenza pneumonia. J Virol 1994; 68:3112–3119.

68. Carding SR, Allan W, McMickle A, Doherty PC. Activation of cytokine genes in T-cells during primary and secondary murine influenza pneumonia. J Exp Med 1993; 177:475–482.

69. Matsuo K, Iwasaki T, Asanuma H, Yoshikawa T, Chen Z, Tsujimoto H, Kurata T, Tamura SS. Cytokine mRNAs in the nasal-associated lymphoid tissue during influenza virus infection and nasal vaccination. Vaccine 2000; 18:1344–1350.

70. Graham MB, Dalton DK, Giltinan D, Braciale VL, Stewart TA, Braciale TJ. Response to influenza infection in mice with a targeted disruption in the interferon gamma gene. J Exp Med 1993; 178:1725–1732.

71. Dobber R, Tielemans M, Nagelkerken L. The in vivo effects of neutralizing antibodies against IFN-gamma, IL-4, or IL-10 on the humoral immune response in young and aged mice. Cell Immunol 1995; 160:185–192.

72. Connors M, Giese NA, Kulkarni AB, Firestone C-Y, Morse HC III, Murphy BR. Enhanced pulmonary histopathology induced by respiratory syncytial virus (RSV) challenge of formalin-inactivated RSV-immunized BALB/c mice is abrogated by depletion of interleukin- 4 (IL-4) and IL-10. J Virol 1994; 68:5321-5325.

73. Makela MJ, Kanehiro A, Borish L, Dakhama A, Loader J, Joetham A, Xing Z, Jordana M, Larsen GL, Gelfand EW. IL-10 is necessary for the expression of airway hyperresponsiveness but not pulmonary inflammation after allergic sensitization. Proc Natl Acad Sci USA 2000; 97:6007–6012.

74. Yang X, Wang S, Fan Y, Han X. IL-10 deficiency prevents IL-5 overproduction and eosinophilic inflammation in a murine model of asthma-like reaction. Eur J Immunol 2000; 30:382–391.

75. Hoffmann KF, James SL, Cheever AW, Wynn TA. Studies with double cytokine-deficient mice reveal that highly polarized Th1- and Th2-type cytokine and antibody responses contribute equally to vaccine-induced immunity to Schistosoma mansoni. J Immunol 1999; 163:927–938.

76. O'Donnell DR, Openshaw PJM. Anaphylactic sensitisation to aeroantigen during respiratory virus infection. Clin Exp Allergy 1998; 28:1501–1508.

77. Schwarze J, Cieslewicz G, Joetham A, Ikemura T, Makela MJ, Dakhama A, Shultz LD, Lamers MC, Gelfand EW. Critical roles for interleukin-4 and interleukin-5 during respiratory syncytial virus infection in the development of airway hyperresponsiveness after airway sensitization. Am J Respir Crit Care Med 2000; 162:380–386.

78. Wills-Karp M, Luyimbazi J, Xu X, Schofield B, Neben TY, Karp CL, Donaldson DD. Interleukin-13: central mediator of allergic asthma. Science 1998; 282:2258–2261.

79. Grunig G, Warnock M, Wakil AE, Venkayya R, Brombacher F, Rennick DM, Sheppard D, Mohrs M, Donaldson DD, Locksley RM, Corry DB. Requirement for IL-13 independently of IL-4 in experimental asthma. Science 1998; 282:2261–2263.

80. Li L, Xia Y, Nguyen A, Lai YH, Feng L, Mosmann TR, Lo D. Effects of Th2 cytokines on chemokine expression in the lung: IL-13 potently induces eotaxin expression by airway epithelial cells. J Immunol 1999; 162:2477–2487.

81. Postma DS, Bleecker ER, Amelung PJ, Holroyd KJ, Xu J, Panhuysen CI, Meyers DA, Levitt RC. Genetic susceptibility to asthma—bronchial hyperresponsiveness coinherited with a major gene for atopy. N Engl J Med 1995; 333:894–900.

82. Mitsuyasu H, Izuhara K, Mao XQ, Gao PS, Arinobu Y, Enomoto T, Kawai M, Sasaki S, Dake Y, Hamasaki N, Shirakawa T, Hopkin JM. Ile50Val variant of IL4R alpha upregulates IgE synthesis and associates with atopic asthma. Nat Genet 1998; 19:119–120.

83. Herrick CA, MacLeod H, Glusac E, Tigelaar RE, Bottomly K. Th2 responses induced by epicutaneous or inhalational protein exposure are differentially dependent on IL-4. J Clin Invest 2000; 105:765–775.

84. McKenzie GJ, Fallon PG, Emson CL, Grencis RK, McKenzie AN. Simultaneous disruption of interleukin (IL)-4 and IL-13 defines individual roles in T helper cell type 2-mediated responses. J Exp Med 1999; 189:1565–1572.

85. Zhu Z, Homer RJ, Wang Z, Chen Q, Geba GP, Wang J, Zhang Y, Elias JA. Pulmonary expression of interleukin-13 causes inflammation, mucus hypersecretion, subepithelial fibrosis, physiologic abnormalities, and eotaxin production. J Clin Invest 1999; 103: 779–788.

85a. Hussell T, Pennycook A, Openshaw PJM. Inhibition of tumor necrosis factor reduces the severity of virus-specific immunopathology. Eur J Immunol 2001; 31:2566–2573.

86. Moran TM, Park H, Fernandez SA, Schulman JL. Th2 responses to inactivated influenza virus can be converted to Th1 responses and facilitate recovery from heterosubtypic virus infection. J Infect Dis 1999; 180:579–585.

87. Arulanandam BP, Mittler JN, Lee WT, O'Toole M, Metzger DW. Neonatal administration of IL-12 enhances the protective efficacy of antiviral vaccines. J Immunol 2000; 164:3698–3704.

88. Hancock GE, Smith JD, Heers KM. The immunogenicity of subunit vaccines for respiratory syncytial virus after co-formulation with aluminum hydroxide adjuvant and recombinant interleukin-12. Viral Immunol 2000; 13:57–72.

89. Werle B, Fromantin C, Alexandre A, Kohli E, Pothier P. Dose-dependent effects of IL-12 treatment to immune response induced after immunization with a recombinant respiratory syncytial virus (RSV) fusion protein fragment. Vaccine 1999; 17:2983–2990.

90. Tripp RA, Jones L, Anderson LJ, Brown MP. CD40 ligand (CD154) enhances the Th1 and antibody responses to respiratory syncytial virus in the BALB/c mouse. J Immunol 2000; 164:5913-5921.

91. Bukreyev A, Whitehead SS, Bukreyeva N, Murphy BR, Collins PL. Interferon gamma expressed by a recombinant respiratory syncytial virus attenuates virus replication in mice without compromising immunogenicity. Proc Natl Acad Sci USA 1999; 96: 2367–2372.

92. Moran TM, Isobe H, Fernandez SA, Schulman JL. Interleukin-4 causes delayed virus clearance in influenza virus-infected mice. J Virol 1996; 70:5230–5235.

93. Bot A, Holz A, Christen U, Wolfe T, Temann A, Flavell R, von HM. Local IL-4 expression in the lung reduces pulmonary influenza-virus-specific secondary cytotoxic T cell responses. Virology 2000; 269:66–77.

94. Aung S, Tang YW, Graham BS. Interleukin-4 diminishes CD8(+) respiratory syncytial virus-specific cytotoxic T-lymphocyte activity in vivo. J Virol 1999; 73:8944–8949.

95. Bembridge GP, Lopez JA, Cook R, Melero JA, Taylor G. Recombinant vaccinia virus

coexpressing the F protein of respiratory syncytial virus (RSV) and interleukin-4 (IL-4) does not inhibit the development of RSV-specific memory cytotoxic T lymphocytes, whereas priming is diminished in the presence of high levels of IL-2 or gamma interferon. J Virol 1998; 72:4080-4087.

96. Walzl G, Tafuro S, Moss P, Openshaw PJ, Hussell T. Influenza virus lung infection protects from respiratory syncytial virus-induced immunopathology. J Exp Med 2000; 192:1317–1326.

97. Mason D. A very high level of crossreactivity is an essential feature of the T-cell receptor. Immunol Today 1998; 19:395–404.

98. Selin LK, Nahill SR, Welsh RM. Cross-reactivities in memory cytotoxic T lymphocyte recognition of heterologous viruses. J Exp Med 1994; 179:1933–1943.

99. Selin LK, Vergilis K, Welsh RM, Nahill SR. Reduction of otherwise remarkably stable virus-specific cytotoxic T lymphocyte memory by heterologous viral infections. J Exp Med 1996; 183:2489–2499.

100. Butland BK, Strachan DP, Lewis S, Bynner J, Butler N, Britton J. Investigation into the increase in hay fever and eczema at age 16 observed between the 1958 and 1970 British birth cohorts. Br Med J 1997; 315:717–721.

101. Strachan DP, Griffiths JM, Anderson HR. Allergic sensitization and position in the sibship: a national study of young British adults. Thorax 1994; 49:1053.

102. Strachan DP, Taylor EM, Carpenter RG. Family structure, neonatal infection, and hay fever in adolescence. Arch Dis Child 1996; 74:422–426.

103. Strachan DP. Is allergic disease programmed in early life? Clin Exp Allergy 1994; 24:603–605.

104. Martinez FD, Stern DA, Wright AL, Taussig LM, Halonen M. Association of non-wheezing lower respiratory tract illnesses in early life with persistently diminished serum IgE levels. Thorax 1995; 50:1067–1072.

105. von Mutius E, Martinez FD, Fritzsch C, Nicolai T, Roell G, Thiemann HH. Prevalence of asthma and atopy in two areas of West and East Germany. Am J Respir Crit Care Med 1994; 149:358–364.

106. Shirakawa T, Enomoto T, Shimazu S, Hopkin JM. The inverse association between tuberculin responses and atopic disorder. Science 1997; 275:77–79.

107. Shaheen SO, Aaby P, Hall AJ, Barker DJ, Heyes CB, Shiell AW, Goudiaby A. Measles and atopy in Guinea-Bissau. Lancet 1996; 347:1792–1796.

108. Bodner C, Godden D, Seaton A. Family size, childhood infections and atopic diseases. The Aberdeen WHEASE Group. Thorax 1998; 53:28–32.

109. Matricardi PM, Rosmini F, Ferrigno L, Nisini R, Rapicetta M, Chionne P, Stroffolini T, Pasquini P, D'Amelio R. Cross sectional retrospective study of prevalence of atopy among Italian military students with antibodies against hepatitis A virus. Br Med J 1997; 314:999–1003.

110. Romagnani S. Induction of TH1 and TH2 responses: a key role for the 'natural' immune response? Immunol Today 1992; 13:379–381.

111. Bjorksten B. The intrauterine and postnatal environments. J Allergy Clin Immunol 1999; 104:1119–1127.

112. Schultz C, Reiss I, Bucsky P, Gopel W, Gembruch U, Ziesenitz S, Gortner L. Maturational changes of lymphocyte surface antigens in human blood: comparison between fetuses, neonates and adults. Biol Neonate 2000; 78:77–82.

113. Prescott SL, Macaubas C, Holt BJ, Smallacombe TB, Loh R, Sly PD, Holt PG. Transplacental priming of the human immune system to environmental allergens: universal

skewing of initial T cell responses toward the Th2 cytokine profile. J Immunol 1998; 160:4730–4737.

114. Prescott SL, Macaubas C, Smallacombe T, Holt BJ, Sly PD, Holt PG. Development of allergen-specific T-cell memory in atopic and normal children. Lancet 1999; 353: 196–200.

115. Siegrist CA. Vaccination in the neonatal period and early infancy. Int Rev Immunol 2000; 19:195–219.

116. Romagnani S. Regulation of the development of type 2 T-helper cells in allergy. Curr Opin Immunol 1994; 6:838–846.

117. Erb KJ, Holloway JW, Sobeck A, Moll H, Le Gros G. Infection of mice with Mycobacterium bovis–bacillus Calmette-Guerin (BCG) suppresses allergen-induced airway eosinophilia. J Exp Med 1998; 187:561–569.

118. Wang CC, Rook GA. Inhibition of an established allergic response to ovalbumin in BALB/c mice by killed Mycobacterium vaccae. Immunology 1998; 93:307–313.

119. Sudo N, Sawamura S, Tanaka K, Aiba Y, Kubo C, Koga Y. The requirement of intestinal bacterial flora for the development of an IgE production system fully susceptible to oral tolerance induction. J Immunol 1997; 159:1739–1745.

120. Schenker MB, Gold EB, Lopez RL, Beaumont JJ. Asthma mortality in California, 1960–1989. Demographic patterns and occupational associations. Am Rev Respir Dis 1993; 147:1454-1460.

121. Bardin PG, Johnston SL, Pattemore PK. Viruses as precipitants of asthma symptoms. II. Physiology and mechanisms. Clin Exp Allergy 1992; 22:809–822.

122. Teran LM, Johnston SL, Schroder JM, Church MK, Holgate ST. Role of nasal interleukin-8 in neutrophil recruitment and activation in children with virus-induced asthma. Am J Respir Crit Care Med 1997; 155:1362–1366.

123. Sigurs N, Bjarnason R, Sigurbergsson F, Kjellman B, Bjorksten B. Asthma and immunoglobulin E antibodies after respiratory syncytial virus bronchiolitis: a prospective cohort study with matched controls. Pediatrics 1995; 95:500–505.

124. Sly PD, Hibbert ME. Childhood asthma following hospitalization with acute viral bronchiolitis in infancy. Pediatr Pulmonol 1989; 7:153–158.

125. Murray M, Webb MS, O'Callaghan C, Swarbrick AS, Milner AD. Respiratory status and allergy after bronchiolitis. Arch Dis Child 1992; 67:482–487.

126. Connochie KM Roghmann KJ. Wheezing at 8 and 13 years: changing importance of bronchiolitis and passive smoking. Pediatr Pulmonol 1989; 6:138–146.

127. Pullan CR Hey EN. Wheezing, asthma, and pulmonary dysfunction 10 years after infection with respiratory syncytial virus in infancy. Br Med J 1982; 284:1665–1669.

128. Kumar A, Sorkness RL, Kaplan MR, Lemanske RF, Jr. Chronic, episodic, reversible airway obstruction after viral bronchiolitis in rats. Am J Respir Crit Care Med 1997; 155:130–134.

129. Mosmann TR, Sad S. The expanding universe of T-cell subsets: Th1, Th2 and more. Immunol Today 1996; 17(3):138–146.

130. Duff AL, Pomeranz ES, Gelber LE, Price GW, Farris H, Hayden FG, Platts MT, Heymann PW. Risk factors for acute wheezing in infants and children: viruses, passive smoke, and IgE antibodies to inhalant allergens. Pediatrics 1993; 92:535–540.

131. Calhoun WJ, Swenson CA, Dick EC, Schwartz LB, Lemanske-RF J, Busse WW. Experimental rhinovirus 16 infection potentiates histamine release after antigen bronchoprovocation in allergic subjects. Am Rev Respir Dis 1991; 144:1267–1273.

132. Sakamoto M, Ida S, Takishima T. Effect of influenza virus infection on allergic sensitization to aerosolized ovalbumin in mice. J Immunol 1984; 132:2614–2617.

133. Suzuki S, Suzuki Y, Yamamoto N, Matsumoto Y, Shirai A, Okubo T. Influenza A virus infection increases IgE production and airway responsiveness in aerosolized antigen-exposed mice. J Allergy Clin Immunol 1998; 102:732–740.

134. Cunningham AF, Johnston SL, Julious SA, Lampe FC, Ward ME. Chronic Chlamydia pneumoniae infection and asthma exacerbations in children. Eur Respir J 1998; 11: 345–349.

135. Cook PJ, Davies P, Tunnicliffe W, Ayres JG, Honeybourne D, Wise R. Chlamydia pneumoniae and asthma. Thorax 1998; 53:254-259.

136. Larsen FO, Norn S, Mordhorst CH, Skov PS, Milman N, Clementsen P. Chlamydia pneumoniae and possible relationship to asthma. Serum immunoglobulins and histamine release in patients and controls. APMIS 1998; 106:928–934.

137. Kraft M, Cassell GH, Henson JE, Watson H, Williamson J, Marmion BP, Gaydos CA, Martin RJ. Detection of Mycoplasma pneumoniae in the airways of adults with chronic asthma. Am J Respir Crit Care Med 1998; 158:998–1001.

138. Openshaw PJ, Lemanske RF. Respiratory viruses and asthma: can the effects be prevented? Eur Respir J 1998; 27:35s-39s

14

Animal Models of Allergen and Virus-Induced Asthma

JÜRGEN SCHWARZE

National Heart and Lung Institute
Imperial College London
London, England

ERWIN W. GELFAND

National Jewish Medical and Research
  Center
Denver, Colorado, U.S.A.

I. Introduction

In the majority of patients, asthma appears to be mediated by an immune response to allergen resulting in pulmonary inflammation and bronchial or airway hyperreactivity (AHR). Data from clinical studies of asthma patients and animal models of allergic pulmonary inflammation have shown that both T cells and inflammatory cells, especially eosinophils, are essential in the initiation and progression of the lung pathology. Mast cells mediate effector function through binding of allergen-specific immunoglobulin E (IgE), resulting in degranulation and release of numerous mediators, including cytokines and chemokines. On the other hand, IgE-dependent mast cell (and basophil) activities in human disease may be more relevant in the early phase response and less critical for sustaining long-term, chronic inflammation or airway remodeling. In contrast, T lymphocytes and eosinophils play significant roles in the progression of chronic inflammation and changes in airway function.

There is increasing awareness of the complexity of asthma as a syndrome and not a single disease. The heterogeneity of T-cell subsets involved in asthma pathogenesis likely accounts for some of the variability in disease patterns and expression. Although asthma has been described as a T-helper cell 2 (Th2) driven disease based on the distinct expression profile of T-cell derived cytokines, the number of cytokines now implicated further complicates simple modeling of the disease.

Animal models have proven useful and important in identifying components of allergic inflammation in the lung. Nonetheless, human disease differs in many ways that preclude simple extrapolation from animal models to humans. We will focus here primarily on murine models of allergic inflammation and AHR as well as the interplay between lower respiratory tract virus infection and the response to allergen.

II. Murine Models of Allergic Asthma

Murine models have been important in contributing to our understanding of the immune mechanisms involved in the development of asthma. The majority of investigations have focused on allergen- driven models of airway inflammation and AHR. The elicitation of these allergic responses and alterations in airway function can vary depending on the particular protocol used and the methods employed for monitoring airway function.

A. Methods of Allergic Airway Sensitization

Sensitization Exclusively Via the Airways

Several methods of allergic sensitization have been used to induce airway pathology. Allergen exposure without adjuvant exclusively via the airways can result in allergic sensitization with elevated serum levels of allergen-specific IgE and IgG antibodies (1) and antigen-specific immediate cutaneous reactivity (2). In this approach, mice are exposed to an allergen-containing aerosol for 20 min daily over a period of 10 days. Ovalbumin (OVA), cat, and ragweed have been used as antigens (1,3,4). Allergic sensitization following this protocol was associated with increased responsiveness of tracheal smooth muscle preparations to electrical field stimulation in vitro (1). Only small changes in airway responsiveness were detected in vivo following provocation with methacholine (MCh) unless the sensitization period was followed by a second 10 day period of allergen exposure 20 days later (5). Following such a secondary allergen challenge, AHR to MCh developed. Furthermore, numbers of CD3+ T cells increased in peribronchial lymph nodes (PBLN) up to 10-fold following this method of airway sensitization. On lung histological examination, some degree of edema surrounding the small and medium-sized airways and an increase in numbers of mucus-secreting cells were noticeable, but little influx of inflammatory cells to the airways was detected. Indeed, routine staining of eosinophils and mast cells was noticeably unrevealing.

Passive Sensitization Followed by Airway Challenge

In a different approach, mice were sensitized passively by intravenous injection of OVA-specific monoclonal IgE and IgG1 antibodies on two consecutive days. This resulted consistently in positive immediate cutaneous hypersensitivity reactions to intradermal allergen challenge. On days 3 and 4 after the second injection, mice were exposed to OVA aerosol for 20 min daily. This allergen challenge resulted in AHR, as assessed by electrical field stimulation of tracheal smooth muscle preparations in vitro, and in airway inflammation with increased numbers of macrophages and eosinophils in the bronchoalveolar lavage (BAL), elevated numbers of lymphocytes and eosinophils in total lung cell isolates, peribronchial eosinophilia, and increased eosinophil peroxidase (EPO) activity in BAL fluid (6). Administration of anti-OVA IgG2a or OVA-specific IgG3 or IgE specific for an irrelevant antigen (TNP) followed by airway allergen challenge did not induce airway inflammation or changes in airway responsiveness.

Systemic Sensitization Followed by Airway Challenge

In a more commonly used approach, mice are actively sensitized to an allergen, usually by intraperitoneal injection of the antigen in combination with an adjuvant such as aluminum hydroxide (alum) or Freund's incomplete adjuvant. Many different protocols of active sensitization have been employed, most of them using repeated antigen injections to obtain a high level of sensitization (7–10). Active allergen sensitization is also possible without adjuvant and can be achieved by the intraperitoneal route (11) and by painting the skin with high concentrations of allergen (12). These protocols elicit allergen-specific IgE and IgG antibodies of different subclasses and positive immediate skin reactivity. If sensitization is followed by airway challenge with aerosolized allergen or intranasal allergen instillation, a marked airway inflammatory response develops with influx of CD3 + T lymphocytes, eosinophils, and neutrophils to the airways and AHR to nonspecific bronchoconstrictor provocation.

Regardless of the experimental approach to sensitization, altered airway function is dependent on local allergen challenge of the airways. Allergic sensitization without local allergen exposure does not induce airway pathology or altered airway function (9,12).

B. Monitoring Airway Function and Development of AHR

Electrical Field Stimulation of Tracheal Smooth Muscle Segments

Airway responsiveness in murine models of allergic airway inflammation has been assessed by a range of methods, both in vitro and in vivo. Following initial studies by Martin et al. (13), we developed an in vitro system to assess airway smooth muscle responsiveness. Segments of tracheal smooth muscle were mounted in an organ bath and exposed to electrical field stimulation with increasing frequencies. Muscle contraction was monitored by an isometric force transducer and the electrical frequency inducing half maximal contraction (ES_{50}) was calculated. In mice sensitized via the airways, ES_{50} was significantly lower than in naive mice (1).

Resistance and Dynamic Compliance in Ventilated Mice

Martin et al. introduced in vivo measurements of airway resistance and dynamic compliance in mice (13). Anesthetized, tracheotomized, and intubated animals were ventilated in a body plethysmograph. In addition, thoracotomies of 5×2 mm were performed on each side of the chest so that pleural pressure was equal to body surface pressure. Tidal flows and volumes and transpulmonary pressure were monitored and airway resistance, conductance, and dynamic compliance were calculated by the method of Amdur and Mead (14). Provocation with increasing concentrations of MCh, administered through a cannula in the internal jugular vein, resulted in increases in airway resistance and decreases in dynamic compliance. When applied to models of allergic sensitization, these changes were more pronounced in mice sensitized and challenged via the airways than in controls.

Airway Pressure Time Index and Volume Overflow

Other measures of airway responsiveness have also been described in ventilated mice. Levitt and Mitzner measured time-integrated changes in peak airway pressure following placement of an intratracheal cannula in ventilated mice following anesthesia and relaxation (15). Intravenous acetylcholine challenge resulted in increases in airway pressure and in an increased area under the pressure curve, the airway pressure time index (APTI). In a similar setup, Foster et al. assessed airway responsiveness by measuring respiratory volume overflow at the distal port of a tracheal cannula in ventilated mice (10). Values were expressed as percentage of maximal overflow volume obtained by complete occlusion of the tracheal cannula. Intravenous MCh provocation resulted in increases in overflow volumes in mice following sensitization and allergen challenge.

Noninvasive Body Plethysmography

Additional methods of lung function testing in nonanesthetized, spontaneously breathing mice have been described. Vijayaraghavan et al. used a two-chamber plethysmograph in which they monitored air flow, tidal volumes, and the timing of respiration separately in a head chamber and in a body chamber. In addition, transpulmonary pressure was assessed using a catheter-tip pressure transducer placed in the pleural cavity of the mouse. Lung resistance and dynamic compliance were calculated from these measurements (16). This system was developed for toxicology studies, but has since also been used in murine models of asthma.

Barometric whole-body plethysmography in mice following allergic sensitization and airway challenge has also been evaluated (9). In this system, a conscious, unrestrained mouse is placed in a single plethysmograph chamber. Pressure differences between this main chamber and a reference chamber are recorded. The resulting box pressure curve, which is caused by volume changes during the respiratory cycle of the animal, is used to calculate tidal volumes, pause, and enhanced pause (Penh), a value that correlates closely to lung resistance (9). Following provocation with increasing concentrations of aerosolized MCh in the plethysmograph, Penh increases. In mice sensitized and challenged with allergen, this increase exceeds changes in Penh in nonsensitized mice.

Methods of Provocation

In the systems described above, nonspecific airway provocation with acetylcholine, a neuromuscular transmitter of airway smooth muscle, or with the stable analogue, MCh, has primarily been used (9,13,15). Other substances used for nonspecific provocation include serotonin (17,18) and propranolol (13,16). Two routes of administration are commonly used: intravenous injection or aerosol inhalation of the bronchoconstrictor. The latter seems to allow better differentiation between mice with allergen- or virus-induced airway hyperreactivity and normal controls, and it corresponds to bronchial provocation tests in humans. Furthermore, allergen-specific provocation has also been used in mice (19). Following inhalation of OVA aerosol, increased airway responsiveness can be detected in mice sensitized and challenged with the allergen. Both a transient early-phase response that arises within minutes and a late-phase response with a peak at around 6 h after allergen exposure are induced, paralleling observations in human asthmatics following allergen inhalation (20). In the assessment of airway responsiveness, marked strain differences in cholinergic reactivity have to be taken into account. Although some inbred strains of mice like AJ mice are extremely responsive to MCh provocation, others (SJL or C3H mice) exhibit little responsiveness. This responsiveness is under genetic control (21). Airway responsiveness of the two strains most commonly used in murine asthma models, BALB/c and C57/BL6 mice, are of comparable magnitude when tracheal smooth muscle responses are compared but differ significantly in response to MCh administration (22).

C. Immune Mechanisms of Allergen-Induced Airway Inflammation and AHR

Murine models of allergen sensitization and challenge have enabled researchers to delineate the immunological basis for the development of allergen-induced airway inflammation and altered airway responsiveness. Active sensitization to allergen results in the production of allergen-specific IgE and IgG antibodies. Allergen exposure via the airways in sensitized mice induces airway inflammation with the influx of eosinophils, neutrophils, and lymphocytes; increased local cytokine production; increased mucus production; and the development of AHR following provocation. The relative contributions of allergen-specific IgE, mast cells, T cells, cytokines, and eosinophils in the development of AHR have been investigated in numerous models.

IgE and Mast Cells

Following passive sensitization and allergen challenge or following active sensitization exclusively via the airways, allergen-specific IgE appears critical for the development of AHR. These sensitization protocols only induce mild airway inflammation with a limited influx of eosinophils (6,23). Allergen sensitization to OVA via the airways in mice genetically deficient in B cells resulted in airway eosinophilia similar to normal controls, but not in AHR (24). Administration of anti-OVA IgE in these B-cell-deficient mice during sensitization restored AHR, indicating that anti-OVA IgE was essential to the development of AHR in this model. T-cell responses to allergen and the influx of eosinophils to the airways were unaffected by the lack of B cells and absence of allergen-specific IgE. It is assumed that the absence of specific IgE prevented the development of AHR, not because of impaired T-cell activation or impaired eosinophil recruitment but secondary to the lack of mast cell activation. This notion is supported by the observation that responses to allergen-specific IgE are mediated through the high-affinity IgE receptor (FcεR1). In contrast to mice deficient in CD23 (25) (the low-affinity IgE receptor), mice deficient in FcεR1 do not develop AHR following passive sensitization and allergen challenge (26). In addition, allergen-specific IgE, while not required for T-cell activation, may amplify the development of AHR by enhancing T-cell responses to allergen (27).

In contrast, following active sensitization to allergen with adjuvant and subsequent airway challenge, which induces airway inflammation with a more robust influx of eosinophils, allergen-specific IgE is not required for the development of AHR. Both sensitization of B-cell-deficient mice (26) and sensitization of mast-cell-deficient mice (28) in this way resulted in airway inflammation, eosinophil activation, and AHR to the same extent as in sensitized control mice. Treatment of actively sensitized mice with a nonanaphylactic anti-IgE antibody before the allergen challenge significantly reduced levels of allergen-specific IgE without affecting cytokine production by PBLN cells, eosinophil accumulation, or AHR (29). However, anti-IgE treatment eliminated IgE-mediated allergic responses such as allergen-mediated mast cell activation in vitro and systemic and cutaneous anaphylaxis after allergen injection.

Cumulatively, these data indicate that AHR can develop independently of allergen-specific IgE if the sensitization induces pronounced airway eosinophilia. Following allergic sensitization with limited influx of eosinophils to the airways, allergen-specific IgE is involved in the development of AHR, likely through activation and degranulation of mast cells and through enhanced activation of T cells and possibly eosinophils.

T Cells

T cells are recruited to the airways following sensitization and airway allergen challenge. They play a pivotal role in the development of eosinophilic airway inflammation, mucus hypersecretion, and AHR. Following sensitization to OVA exclusively via the airways, allergen-specific Vβ8.1 and Vβ8.2 T-cell subsets expand that stimulate anti-OVA IgE and IgG1 production by allergen-primed B cells (3,30). Transfer of these T cells induced an anti-OVA IgE response, immediate cutaneous hypersensitivity, and AHR in nonsensitized recipients (3). This demonstrates that allergen-reactive T cells can induce both allergen-specific antibody production and AHR. To dissect further the role of T cells in the development of allergen-driven AHR, T-cell-deficient, athymic nude mice were passively sensitized with anti-OVA IgE. Upon cutaneous OVA challenge, immediate cutaneous hypersensitivity developed, but airway allergen challenge did not induce influx of eosinophils nor AHR (31). Reconstitution of nude mice with either T cells or IL-5 prior to passive sensitization restored the capacity for development of lung eosinophilia and AHR. These observations indicate that T cells, although not necessary for IgE-mediated immediate hypersensitivity reactions, are required for the development of allergen-induced eosinophilic airway inflammation and AHR.

CD4+ T Cells

To delineate the contribution of CD4+ and CD8+ T-cell subsets to allergen-induced airway pathology, depletion and transfer studies have been performed. Antibody-mediated depletion of CD4+ T cells prior to allergen challenge in sensitized mice prevented both AHR and influx of eosinophils to the airways (32). Transfer of OVA-specific, IL-4 and IL-5-producing CD4+ T cells from sensitized animals to mice genetically deficient in IL-5 resulted in airway eosinophilia and AHR following OVA challenge via the airways. In contrast, transfer of OVA-specific CD4-negative T cells that produced IFN-γ and no IL-4 or IL-5 upon in vitro stimulation did not induce these responses following allergen exposure (33). In a different model, transfer of CD4+ T cells alone to mice that lack both T and B cells restored allergen-induced airway inflammation and AHR in these animals, which were otherwise unable to develop these responses to allergic sensitization and allergen challenge (34). These observations demonstrate that CD4+ T cells capable of Th2 cytokine production are necessary not only for allergic sensitization but also for the development of airway inflammation and AHR induced by allergen challenge via the airways.

Studies by Cohn et al. focused on the role of CD4+ T cells in allergen-induced mucus hypersecretion. In their model, allergen-specific CD4+ Th1 and Th2 cells, generated from OVA T-cell receptor transgenic mice, were adoptively transferred into nonsensitized mice that were subsequently challenged with OVA via the airways. Transfer of OVA-Th2 cells resulted in eosinophilic airway inflammation and increased mucus production, whereas transfer of OVA-Th1 cells had no such effect (35). Cotransfer of OVA-Th1 cells with OVA-Th2 cells induced a significant reduction in mucus production and airway eosinophilia (36). To delineate the roles of IL-4, IL-5 and IFN-γ in the regulation of mucus secretion, the following experiments were performed. OVA-Th2 cells from genetically IL-4-deficient mice (IL-4 -/-) were transferred into wild-type mice. This resulted in mucus hypersecretion if recruitment of these cells to the lung was induced by TNF-α. Without TNF-α, IL4 -/- Th2 cells did not migrate to the lung (35). Transfer of IL-4 -/- Th2 cells to mice deficient in the IL-4 receptor α chain had no effect on mucus production, indicating that signaling through the IL-4 receptor α chain, a molecule shared by the receptors for IL-4 and IL-13, is essential for mucus hypersecretion (37). Transfer of Th-2 cells from mice deficient in IL-5 (IL-5 -/-) to IL-5 -/- mice induced mucus hypersecretion in the absence of eosinophils (37). This demonstrated that neither IL-5 nor eosinophils are directly involved in upregulating mucus production. Transfer of OVA-Th1 cells to mice deficient in the IFN-γ receptor also induced increased mucus staining in the airways, suggesting that IFN-γ signaling is essential for the inhibitory effects of Th1 cells on mucus production (36). When interpreted cumulatively, these data demonstrate a critical role for CD4+ T cells in the regulation of mucus production. Their enhancing effects are dependent on signaling through the IL-4 receptor α chain following binding by IL-13 or IL-4, their inhibitory effects are mediated through IFN-γ signaling, downstream of the effects of Th2 cytokines.

CD8+ T Cells

The role of CD8+ T cells in the development of allergen-induced eosinophilic airway inflammation and AHR remains controversial. Depletion of CD8+ T cells with anti-CD8+ antibody prior to allergen sensitization exclusively via the airways (without adjuvant) prevented the development of AHR and significantly reduced IL-5 production and airway eosinophilia (23). Allergen-specific IgE production was enhanced by this treatment. On the other hand, transfer experiments demonstrated suppressive effects of CD8 T cells with inhibition of allergen-specific IgE production and suppression of AHR, associated with IFN-γ production by these cells (38). These data taken cumulatively suggest a complex role of CD8+ T cells in allergic sensitization of the airways probably involving different CD8+ T cell subsets. On the one hand, IFN-γ-producing CD8+ T cells inhibit the development of allergic sensitization and its consequences. On the other hand, in the Th2 cytokine environment of the lung and PBLN during allergic sensitization, CD8+ T cells may develop that are potent producers of IL-5. These cells likely contribute to the development of airway eosinophilia and AHR.

γδ + T Cells

In addition to αβ+ T cells, γδ+ T cells have also been implicated in the development of allergic airway inflammation and AHR. Allergen sensitization and subsequent allergen airway challenge in mice genetically deficient in γδ+ T cells resulted in decreased production of allergen-specific IgE and IgG1 and of IL-5 in the airways, as well as decreased airway eosinophilia compared to wild-type controls (39). Administration of IL-4 to γδ+ T-cell-deficient mice restored the responses to sensitization, indicating that in this model γδ+ T cells modulate and enhance the response of αβ+ T cells to allergen sensitization. In a different model of allergic airway sensitization, the depletion of γδ+ T cells (in knockout mice and following γδ+ T cell depletion by antibody) also resulted in reduced airway eosinophilia, but in enhanced AHR (40).

Allergen exposure of the airways without prior systemic sensitization also induced AHR in these mice lacking γδ+ T cells. These findings imply that γδT cells have a role in the maintenance of normal airway tone, independently of allergic sensitization and of αβ+ T cells, as demonstrated in αβ+ T-cell-deficient mice that exhibited increased AHR following γδ+ T-cell depletion.

Cytokines

Airway challenge of sensitized mice is associated with increases in the production of a number of Th2- cytokines including IL-4, IL-5, and IL-13 (41,42), but increases in airway levels of the Th-1 cytokine IFN-γ have also been detected (43,44).

Interleukin-4

IL-4, a cytokine secreted by Th2 cells, plays a pivotal role in allergic sensitization. IL-4 is critical for IgE isotype switching (45) and it induces Th2-cell development and proliferation (46). Its role in the development of airway inflammation and AHR following airway allergen challenge in sensitized mice has been investigated using IL-4 depletion by antibody and in IL-4 deficient animals. Depletion of IL-4 prior to allergen challenge, following sensitization in the presence of IL-4, did not alter eosinophil influx to the airways or AHR (8,47). On the other hand, blockade of the IL-4 receptor by antibody before allergen challenge prevented airway eosinophilia, goblet cell hyperplasia, and the development of AHR (44). These apparently conflicting results indicate that IL-4 may not be essential for the development of airway eosinophilia and AHR in previously sensitized hosts. The effects of IL-4 receptor blockade were possibly due, at least in part, to the simultaneous inhibition of IL-13 signaling through the IL-4 receptor α-chain. In contrast, the absence of IL-4 during the period of initial allergen sensitization has profound effects on the sequelae following allergen challenge. Hogan et al. reported diminished airway eosinophilia but unaltered development of AHR following sensitization and allergen challenge in genetically IL-4 deficient mice (BALB/c) (48), while we observed a loss of AHR in addition to reduced airway eosinophilia in similar experiments in C57BL/6 mice (49). Depletion of IL-4 during allergen sensitization had no effects on airway inflammation and AHR following allergen challenge in one study (50) while it resulted in suppression of AHR in another (47). These findings suggest that the protocol for sensitization as well as the strain of mouse may determine the role of IL-4 during the sensitization phase in the development of airway inflammation and AHR following allergen challenge. A major role for IL-4 is the expansion of allergen-specific Th2 cells, which have been demonstrated to be sufficient for the induction of eosinophilic airway inflammation and AHR upon allergen challenge, even if they themselves are genetically deficient in IL-4 (51).

Interleukin-13

IL-13 is a Th2 cytokine closely related functionally to IL-4 and signals through a receptor complex that shares the IL-4 receptor α-chain. Blockade of the IL-13 receptor by a soluble IL-13 α2–IgG Fc fusion protein prior to allergen challenge in sensitized mice reduced AHR in two studies (52,53). The effects of IL-13 receptor blockade on airway inflammation nonetheless differed in these two studies: Wills-Karp et al. found no effect on the influx of lymphocytes and eosinophils, (53) while Grünig et al. reported suppression of eosinophil accumulation and mucus production with no effect on the influx of neutrophils (52). Administration of IL-13 to naïve mice induced a transient influx of eosinophils, increased mucus production, and the development of AHR (53). Total serum IgE was also elevated. Selective overexpression of IL-13 in Clara cells had similar consequences: increased inflammation with mononuclear cells, eosinophils, and macrophages; epithelial and mucous cell hyperplasia and mucus hypersecretion; subepithelial fibrosis; enhanced eotaxin production; and increased baseline resistance and AHR (54). Administration of IL-13 to RAG 1-deficient mice, which lack both T and B lymphocytes, also induced airway eosinophilia, goblet cell hyperplasia, and AHR (52). Administration of IL-13 to mice genetically deficient in the IL-4 receptor α-chain had no effect (52). A recent study in IL-13-deficient mice demonstrated that allergen sensitization and challenge in these animals resulted in eosinophil influx to the airways and AHR, that was higher than in wild-type mice (55). Mucus production was, however, inhibited. Depletion of either IL-4 or IL-5 in these IL-13 knockout mice prevented the development of airway eosinophilia and AHR. In normal controls, depletion of IL-4 only reduced AHR and depletion of IL-5 had no effect on AHR. The role of IL-13 is somewhat complex but appears to exert its effects in concert with IL-4 and IL-5, which themselves seem to be sufficient for the induction of AHR if IL-13 is absent during ontogenesis. IL-13 may even serve to limit excessive IL-4-driven immune responses (55). An excess of IL-13 exerts proinflammatory effects on the airways, resulting in increased eotaxin release, increased mucus production, subepithelial fibrosis, and the development of elevated baseline resistance and AHR. These effects are not dependent on T or B lymphocytes, they may be mediated by eotaxin (56), and they require signaling through the IL-4 receptor α chain of the IL-13 receptor.

Activation of the IL-4 receptor transduces signals leading to activation of STAT 6, which has been demonstrated to be essential for the development of Th2 cells (57,58). Not surprisingly, mice genetically deficient in this signaling molecule do not develop a Th2 immune response, airway eosinophilia, mucus hypersecretion, or AHR following allergen sensitization and challenge (59,60). This indicates that the STAT 6 pathway is essential for the induction of an allergic/asthmatic phenotype through IL-4 and IL-13. An interesting finding is that administration of IL-5 to sensitized STAT 6-deficient mice prior to allergen challenge restored airway eosinophilia and AHR (59), suggesting that, in the absence of STAT6, there is little or no activation of the IL-5-dependent pathway for induction of AHR. IL-5 dependent triggering of eosinophilia itself is independent of STAT 6 signaling.

Interleukin-5

IL-5 is an essential cytokine for proliferation, maturation, activation and survival of eosinophils (61,62). It has been the focus of numerous investigations in murine and other animal models of allergen-driven airway inflammation and AHR. In these models, airway eosinophilia and AHR following allergic sensitization have been closely associated with increases in IL-5 production in the airways and PBLN. In virtually all of these models, the absence of IL-5, in mice genetically deficient (IL5-/-) or following anti-IL-5 antibody treatment, there is inhibition of eosinophil accumulation in the airways (8,10,29,47,63). In sensitized IL5-/- mice, intramuscular IL-5 gene transfer, which increases IL-5 serum levels, also restores eosinophilic airway inflammation and induces bone marrow and blood eosinophilia following allergen challenge (64). In contrast, local IL-5 gene transfer by intranasal application, which induced substantial IL-5 production in the airways, did not restore airway eosinophilia. These findings indicate that availability of IL-5 in the bone marrow is essential for eosinophil mobilization from this organ as a prerequisite for the influx of eosinophils to the airways following allergen challenge. Basal IL-5 production by bone marrow stromal cells (65) and allergen-induced increases in bone marrow IL-5 production by T cells (66) has been demonstrated.

The role of IL-5 and of eosinophils in the development of increased airway responsiveness is controversial since conflicting results have been obtained in different models. In the majority of models used in our laboratory, following both exclusive sensitization via the airways and systemic sensitization followed by airway challenges, anti-IL-5 antibody treatment prevented the development of AHR and the influx of eosinophils to the airways (29,63). In IL5-/- mice parallel results were obtained (10,49). Other investigators have reported a dissociation of airway eosinophilia and AHR. In these models, administration of anti-IL-5 antibody resulted in a reduction of airway eosinophilia but the development of AHR was unaffected (8,47). In these studies, the bronchoconstrictor was generally administered intravenously rather than by inhalation. In the model reported by Hessel et al. it was interesting that reduced AHR was detected in sensitized and saline challenged mice following anti-IL-5 treatment (8). When interpreted cumulatively, the data support the notion that IL-5 contributes to the development of AHR probably through effects on eosinophils. A model of virus-induced AHR suggests that IL-5 alone, in the absence of eosinophils and lymphocytes following anti-VLA-4 treatment, is not sufficient for the development of AHR (67). Whether eosinophils are indeed the effector cells of AHR remains unproven. In the absence of IL-4 and IL-13-induced STAT 6 signaling, IL-5 is sufficient for the development of airway eosinophilia and AHR (59). Depending on the sensitization protocol and the strain of mouse used, an IL-5-driven pathway leading to increased airway responsiveness may be dominant. In other models, IL-4 and IL-13 may be more important and possibly sufficient for the induction of AHR.

Interleukin-10

IL-10 was originally described as a factor inhibiting Th1 cytokine production (68), but IL-10 is also capable of downregulating IL-4 and IL-5 production by Th2 cell clones (69). Due to its immune suppressive effects it has been proposed as a potential therapy for allergic inflammation and asthma. The first study of allergen-induced airway inflammation and AHR in mice genetically deficient in IL-10 (IL-10 -/-) supported this concept (70). IL-10 -/- mice developed enhanced airway inflammation with increases in eosinophilia and in the levels of IL-5 and IFN-γ in BAL fluid following sensitization and challenge with *Aspergillus fumigatus*. In vitro, restimulated lung cells from IL-10 -/- mice produced more IL-4, IL-5 and IFN-γ than wild-type controls. Airway responsiveness was elevated in nonsensitized IL-10 -/- mice, but it was not different from controls following sensitization and challenge. Conflicting results were obtained if OVA was used as an allergen in IL-10 -/- mice. Yang et al. reported a reduction in airway eosinophilia, mucus production, and IL-5 secretion in the airways of these animals, associated with reduced IL-5 production in vitro and increases in production of IFN-γ and IL-12 (71). Production of IL-4 and serum levels of IgE were unaffected by the absence of IL-10. These authors conclude that endogenous IL-10 is critical in promoting rather than suppressing pulmonary eosinophilic inflammation and mucus production. In addition, they argued that IL-10 may play a particular role in the development of IL-5-secreting Th2 cells.

Findings from the model reported by Makela et al. extend these observations (72). Sensitization and challenge with OVA resulted in reduced but still robust airway eosinophilia and an increased influx of neutrophils to the lung in IL-10 -/- mice. In these animals, development of AHR was abolished but could be restored by reconstitution with IL-10. Simultaneous treatment with anti-IL-5 antibody prevented both airway eosinophilia and AHR. These data suggest that IL-10 may not only be involved in the regulation of eosinophilic inflammation but also appears to modulate airway function by mechanisms downstream of eosinophilic inflammation. A recent report of the effects of IL-10 administration during challenge with ragweed further strengthens this hypothesis. Production of IL-4, IL-5 and IFN-γ was suppressed and airway eosinophilia was reduced by this treatment (73) as had been previously demonstrated in other models (74,75). An important finding was that AHR was enhanced by administration of IL-10 (73). When interpreted cumulatively, these data demonstrate that IL-10 is capable of inhibiting both Th1 and Th2 cytokine responses in vitro. In vivo, in models of allergic airway disease, the role of IL-10 is complex. Exogenous IL-10 inhibits allergen-induced airway eosinophilia and the production of IL-4, IL-5 and IFN-γ. Depending on the model used, endogenous IL-10 may be involved in both limitation of cytokine production and airway inflammation or enhancement of IL-5 production and eosinophil recruitment to the airways. Furthermore, IL-10 seems to have an effect on airway function per se, promoting the development of AHR through mechanisms downstream of the inflammatory cascade.

Interleukin-9

IL-9, a pleiotropic cytokine produced by Th2 cells, has been associated by gene-mapping studies with susceptibility to asthma (76). Studies in several murine models support the notion that IL-9 plays a pivotal role in asthma development. Transgenic mice that overexpress IL-9 in the lung developed pulmonary infiltrates consisting primarily of eosinophils and lymphocytes (77). Numbers of intraepithelial mast cells were elevated and epithelial hypertrophy, increased subepithelial collagen deposition and intracellular mucus accumulation were observed. In addition, these animals developed AHR to MCh (77) and also to challenge with *Aspergillus fumigatus* (78). Total serum IgE was elevated (78). Similar findings resulted from intratracheal administration of IL-9 in naïve mice (79). Increases in airway eosinophil influx may be mediated by upregulation of IL-5 receptor α chain expression (79) and by increased production of CC-chemokines, which was demonstrated in vivo in allergen-challenged IL-9 transgenic mice and in vitro following treatment of epithelial cell cultures with recombinant IL-9 (80). IL-9 also upregulates MUC 2 and MUC 5AC gene expression and periodic acid–Schiff PAS staining in airway epithelial cells in vivo and in vitro, implying a direct role for IL-9 in inducing mucus production (81). Mast cells are a potent source of IL-9 following stimulation by IgE–antigen complexes (82). IL-9 production by mast cells was further enhanced in the presence of IL-10, which stabilized mRNA and increased transcription of the IL-9 promotor.

These data suggest that IL-9 has a critical role in the initiation of airway inflammation following allergen exposure. Secreted by mast cells upon allergen-IgE cross-linking, IL-9 induces CC-chemokine production and mucin gene expression in airway epithelial cells, which results in recruitment of eosinophils and lymphocytes to the airways, mucus hypersecretion, and AHR.

Interferon-γ, Interleukin-12, and Interleukin-18

Th1 cytokines IFN-γ and IL-12 can suppress the development of Th2 cells in vitro and restore the balance or inhibit Th2 cell-dominated immune responses in vivo. In models of allergic airway disease both exogenous IFN-γ and IL-12 are effective in reducing allergen-specific IgE, eosinophilic infiltration of the airways, and AHR (11,83,84). Endogenous IL-12 seems to be essential in limiting allergen-induced Th2 responses leading to AHR. Treatment with anti- IL-12 induced AHR and Th2 cytokine production, while decreasing IFN-γ production in C3H mice, which are otherwise resistant to allergic airway disease (85).

In some models of allergic sensitization, increases in IFN-γ concentrations in the airways along with increased Th2 cytokines were observed following allergen challenge (43,44). Hessel et al. studied the role of the cytokines IL-4, IL-5, IFN-γ, and TNF-α in airway inflammation and AHR in a model of intense sensitization (seven intraperitoneal injections of OVA with alum, followed by eight OVA aerosol challenges 4 weeks later). Antibodies against these cytokines were administered prior to allergen challenge. Anti-IFN-γ prevented the development of AHR but did not alter eosinophilic airway inflammation. All of the other antibodies did not have significant effects on AHR (8). In a more recent study from the same laboratory, airway eosinophilia was reduced in mice genetically deficient in IFN-γ (IFN-γ -/-) following sensitization and challenge (86). These data indicate that endogenous IFN-γ may contribute to the development of airway eosinophilia and AHR in some models.

The role of IL-18 has recently become a focus of research. IL-18 is an IFN-γ-inducing cytokine secreted by macrophages that acts synergistically with IL-12 (87). This synergism could also be demonstrated in a model of allergen sensitization and challenge. Although treatment with either IL-12 or IL-18 alone had no effect, combined treatment abolished antigen-specific Th2 cells, airway eosinophilia, and AHR in this model (88). Inhibitory effects on allergic airway inflammation were confirmed in mice genetically deficient in IL-18 (89). These animals developed increased airway eosinophilia and lung damage following allergen sensitization and challenge. Reconstitution with IL-18 reduced eosinophil influx and lung damage and was associated with reduced IL-4 levels, little change in production of IFN-γ and IL-5, and increases in expression of Fas-ligand and apoptosis. Two recent reports suggest that IL-18 may also contribute to allergic airway inflammation. Kumano et al. observed increased airway eosinophilia following administration of IL-18 prior to OVA challenge in sensitized mice (90).This treatment did not affect AHR and was associated with increased production of IFN-γ and TNF-α. Levels of IL-5 were unchanged. Wild et al. reported in a model of sensitization and challenge with ragweed that systemic administration of IL-18 during the challenge period inhibited airway eosinophilia and increased IFN-γ expression in the lung (91). In contrast, IL-18 treatment during the sensitization phase resulted in increased eosinophil recruitment and an increase in IL-5 and IFN-γ. Furthermore, intrapulmonary IL-18 facilitated sensitization to ragweed via the airways, inducing Th2 cytokine expression, IgE production, airway eosinophilia, and increased mucus secretion. The suppressive effects of IL-18 on airway eosinophilia were dependent on IFN-γ, as was demonstrated in IFN-γ-/-mice, in which no reduction of airway eosinophilia occurred following IL-18 treatment.

Taken together, these findings indicate that endogenous IFN-γ may contribute to the development of allergic sensitization, eosinophilic airway inflammation, and AHR in some situations despite its capacity to inhibit allergic inflammation and AHR if administered exogenously. A proinflammatory role for IFN-γ may be particularly significant in models of very intense or chronic allergen exposure. The IFN-γ -inducing cytokines IL-12 and IL-18 have different effects on allergic airway disease. IL-12 seems to be an inhibitor of allergic responses, but the role of IL-18 is more complex. IL-18 can promote allergic sensitization and its consequences if administered during primary allergen exposure, but is also capable of reducing allergic airway inflammation if given during allergen challenge in sensitized animals.

Conclusion

Murine models of asthma have contributed significantly to our understanding of the immune mechanisms involved in the development of allergen-induced airway inflammation, mucus hypersecretion, and AHR. In interpreting the results of these models, it has to be appreciated that different models may reflect different aspects of allergic airway disease. Mast cell activation by allergen-specific IgE is essential for the early-phase obstructive responses following allergen challenge, and mast cells appear to be involved in the earliest phases of induction of airway inflammation. Release of IL-9 from mast cells may induce increased CC-chemokine production, which promotes further recruitment of inflammatory cells, primarily T cells and eosinophils. T lymphocytes, especially CD4+ T cells, are pivotal in this inflammatory response. By secreting IL-4 and IL-13 they promote differentiation, recruitment, and proliferation of Th2 lymphocytes. These cells are essential for the development of mucus hypersecretion and AHR. The role of CD8+ T cells in allergic airway disease remains controversial. These cells produce IFN-γ, a Th1 cytokine, and inhibit Th2 responses. In the Th2 cytokine milieu of allergic inflammation, IL-5-producing CD8 + T cell subsets may develop and become critical for the recruitment of eosinophils and the development of AHR. γδ+ T cells can modulate the responses of αβ+ T cells to allergen sensitization. In addition, they seem to have a role in maintaining normal airway tone, thus inhibiting the development of AHR.

Eosinophils are recruited to the airways in large numbers following allergen challenge. Their migration from the bone marrow to the lung is dependent on the presence of IL-5. The association of eosinophils with AHR in many models as well as the results of IL-5 depletion have supported the notion that they are the critical effector cells of AHR. In other models of IL-5 depletion, a dissociation of eosinophilia and AHR occurs, demonstrating that pathways not involving IL-5 and eosino-phils may also result in AHR. One such pathway is the signaling cascade through the IL-4 receptor α chain and STAT-6, which is activated by IL-4 and IL-13 and results in mucus hypersecretion and AHR. Depending on the model used, the relative roles of these alternative pathways may vary.

Other Th2 cytokines promoting allergen-induced obstructive airway disease include IL-9 and IL-10. In addition to promoting inflammatory cell recruitment, IL-9 directly upregulates mucus production. IL-10, a cytokine capable of inhibiting both Th1 and Th2 cytokine responses, may also enhance IL-5 production and eosinophil recruitment to the airways. IL-10 also seems to promote the development of AHR through mechanisms downstream of airway inflammation. Th1 cytokines are gener-ally thought to inhibit Th2 immune responses and exogenous IFN-γ, IL-12, and IL-18 can suppress allergic inflammation and its consequences. Endogenous IFN-γ may contribute to airway eosinophilia and AHR, especially in models of very intense and prolonged allergen sensitization. IL-18, if present during allergen sensitization can promote allergic inflammation and the development of AHR.

The importance of any of these pathways in the pathogenesis of human disease awaits proof-of-concept testing. With increasing availability of such reagents for use in clinical trials, the applicability of animal model data to human asthma will become more or less apparent.

III. Murine Models of Virus-Induced Airway Hyperresponsiveness

A. Epidemiology of Viral Respiratory Infections, Sensitization to Aeroallergens, and Asthma Development

Asthma in childhood is associated in most cases with sensitization to inhaled aller-gens and with allergic airway inflammation. The onset of asthma has been associated with viral lower respiratory tract infections (92). Furthermore, acute viral respiratory infections can trigger wheezing and exacerbations of asthma in children and adults (93,94). Indeed, 80% of wheezing episodes in school-aged children have been asso-ciated with viral respiratory tract infections most often with rhinovirus infection (95). In infants and toddlers under the age of 2 years, the most frequent virus isolated during wheezing episodes was respiratory syncytial virus (RSV) (96,97). Epidemio-logical evidence suggests that respiratory viruses, especially RSV, may not only trigger asthma exacerbations but also contribute to or facilitate allergic sensitization to aeroallergens and subsequently to the development of asthma. Frick and col-leagues (98) observed a coincidence of respiratory infections and the onset of aller-gic sensitization to aeroallergens in infants with a positive family history of allergy. In these children, allergic sensitization could be first detected 1–2 months following a viral respiratory tract infection. A close link between RSV-induced bronchiolitis and development of asthma has been recognized in several studies (99–104). In a recent prospective cohort study with matched controls, Sigurs and colleagues (105) identified RSV bronchiolitis in infancy as the most important risk factor for the subsequent development of asthma and sensitization to common allergens by the age of 3 years. This risk increased further if there was a family history of asthma or atopy. A follow-up report showed that by the age of 7 years, allergic sensitization and asthma were still more prevalent in the group of children who had had RSV brochiolitis in the first year of life than in the controls (106). A number of other studies, however, did not find an association between RSV bronchiolitis and allergic sensitization (100,104,107). A recent quantitative metanalysis of studies investigating associations of RSV disease in infants with development of asthma in childhood confirmed an increased risk of recurrent wheezing during the first 5 years of life, but not thereafter (108). An association of RSV infection with a personal or family history of atopy was not detected. Due to the heterogeneity of the studies analyzed, the relationship between RSV infection and allergic sensitization, as assessed by results of skin prick test, could not be evaluated. In addition, this metanalysis did not include the 7-year follow up by Sigurs et al. and did not take into account that only the studies by this group were based on a prospectively controlled longitudinal cohort. All of the other studies used retrospective control groups. One criticism of these epidemiological studies has been their selection of children with RSV disease severe enough to require hospitalization. Selection of this small minority of RSV-infected children constitutes a bias that likely selects for a predisposition to severe RSV disease, such as atopy. A study by Stein et al. (109) that utilizes the large birth cohort from the Tucson children's respiratory study group did not have this selection bias. In this study, less severe RSV infection during the first 3 years of life was found to be a transient risk factor for wheezing at age 6, but it did not persist at age 13. RSV infection was not associated with an increased risk for allergic sensitization in this population. Despite some inconsistency in the conclusions, it appears that RSV infection can facilitate or enhance allergic sensitization and the development of allergic airway disease, at least in some patients.

To investigate some of the underlying immunological mechanisms involved in the interplay among lower respiratory tract infections with respiratory viruses, allergic airway sensitization, and the development of obstructive airway disease and asthma, a number of animal models have been utilized.

B. Immune Mechanisms of Airway Inflammation and AHR in Models of Acute Respiratory Virus Infections

Respiratory viruses initially infect the respiratory epithelium of the upper airways but the infection can spread to the lower airways. This has long been recognized for RSV infections. Following RSV bronchiolitis, viral antigen can be detected in bronchioles on pathological examination (110). Rodent and other animal models also show evidence of lower airway infection (111-113). These viral infections trigger an inflammatory response in the airways. In guinea pigs, infection with parainfluenza virus (PIV) type 3 results in the influx of macrophages, monocytes, lymphocytes, and eosinophils (114). This inflammatory response is associated with increased airway reactivity to histamine and acetylcholine in vitro (115) and with AHR to MCh in vivo (116). Infection with RSV in guinea pigs yields similar results (113,117).

In a model we have used, mice were infected intranasally with RSV; after 4 days, infection in the lungs could be demonstrated by plaque-forming assays of whole lung homogenates. On day 6 postinfection airway responsiveness to nonspecific provocation with inhaled MCh was assessed by barometric body plethysmography. RSV infection, but not sham infection or ultraviolet (UV) inactivated RSV, resulted in transient AHR, which persisted for about 15 days. By day 21 after the initial RSV infection, airway responsiveness to inhaled MCh returned to baseline. Numbers of lung neutrophils and eosinophils were increased significantly 6 days after RSV infection. RSV-induced airway inflammation and AHR were associated with an increase in the production of IFN-γ and a decrease in IL-4 production in cultures of mononuclear cells from PBLN. IL-5 concentrations did not differ significantly between the groups (118).

Clinical observations have implicated a role for eosinophils in virus-induced obstructive airway disease. RSV bronchiolitis has been associated with increased levels of eosinophilic cationic protein in nasal secretions and with increased numbers of peripheral blood eosinophils (119 120). In addition, activation of eosinophils by RSV in vitro has been demonstrated (121). To define the role of eosinophils in our model of RSV-induced AHR, mice were treated with anti-IL-5 antibody (TRFK-5) during acute infection. This treatment prevented the increase in numbers of eosinophils, but not of neutrophils, and resulted in a failure of development of AHR. The increases in IFN-γ production were not affected by anti-IL-5 (118). Suppression of virus-induced AHR by anti-IL-5 antibody treatment has previously been reported in a guinea pig model of PIV III infection (122). Our findings were corroborated in experiments with mice genetically deficient in IL-5 (67). These mice did not develop AHR or lung eosinophilia following RSV infection, while wild-type controls clearly did. Treatment of the deficient mice with exogenous IL-5 during infection fully restored the responses to RSV infection. To understand further the roles of IL-5 and eosinophils, an antibody to the alpha-4 integrin subunit of the very late antigen (VLA)-4, an adhesion molecule expressed on eosinophils and other circulating leukocytes, except neutrophils, was utilized (123,124). Anti-VLA-4 antibody inhibits recruitment of eosinophils and leukocytes to the lungs in models of allergic airway inflammation (125,126). Treatment of IL-5-deficient mice that were reconstituted with IL-5 with anti-VLA-4 during RSV infection prevented both eosinophil migration to the lung and development of AHR (67). This suggested that both IL-5 and eosinophils were critical in the development of AHR during RSV infection. In addition, these data demonstrate that IL-5, while necessary for the recruitment of eosinophils to the lung, and probably for their activation, does not directly induce AHR.

Studies in IL-4 or IFN-γ-deficient mice demonstrated that neither cytokine was essential for the development of airway inflammation and AHR during acute RSV infection (67). Acute RSV infection in either strain of mice resulted in an influx of eosinophils and neutrophils to the lungs and in the development of AHR. Eosinophilia and AHR in IFN-γ-deficient mice exceeded the responses to RSV infection in wild-type controls, indicating that IFN-γ may have a protective role against virus-induced development of eosinophilic inflammation and AHR.

Furthermore, the model of acute RSV infection was used to define regulatory cells involved in the development of airway disease. T lymphocytes are recruited to the airways in viral-induced asthma exacerbations (127,128). The CD8+ T-cell subset plays a pivotal role in immune responses to viral infections (129,130). CD8+ T cells have also been demonstrated to be critical for the development of allergen-induced AHR (23). To assess the role of T cells in virus-induced airway inflammation and AHR, mice were depleted of either CD4+ or CD8+ T cells just prior to infection. Depletion of CD4+ T cells reduced the development of AHR but did not alter the influx of eosinophils and neutrophils into the lung. In contrast, depletion of CD8+ T cells prevented both the influx of eosinophils and neutrophils and the development of AHR (131). Administration of exogenous IL-5 during RSV infection in mice depleted of CD8+ T cells restored lung eosinophilia and AHR, but not lung neutrophilia. IL-5 treatment in noninfected mice was without effect. In addition, following RSV infection, increased levels of IFN-γ and of IL-5 were detected in bronchoalveolar lavage fluid. In mice depleted of CD8+ T cells, no increase in either cytokine was detected (131). These data demonstrate that while CD8+ but not CD4+ T cells are essential for the influx of inflammatory cells to the airways, both T-cell subsets are critical in the development of AHR in acute RSV infection. This suggests that in addition to the CD8+ T-cell-dependent eosinophilic inflammatory response, a second CD4+ T-cell dependent pathway plays a role in the development of AHR. Taking into account the critical role for IL-5 in this model, it seems likely that CD8+ T cells capable of IL-5 production are essential in inducing the eosinophilic component of airway inflammation and the development of AHR. Such noncytotoxic, IL-5-producing CD8+ T cells have been demonstrated during viral infection and as inducing lung eosinophilia (132,133). The nature of the influence of CD4+ T cells on the development of virus-induced AHR remains to be determined. As in allergen-induced AHR, IL-13 (as well as IL-4) could be an important CD4+ T-cell-derived mediator of AHR following respiratory virus infections.

C. Models of Virus-Induced Enhancement of Allergic Sensitization

Since the 1980s, researchers have studied the effects of infection with respiratory viruses on allergic sensitization to inhaled antigens. Initially, the focus was on allergen-specific antibodies. Sakamoto and colleagues (134) infected mice with influenza virus at dosages high enough to result in bronchopneumonia. Following infection, these mice were sensitized to OVA aerosol complexed with alum and OVA-specific IgE levels were titrated by passive cutaneous anaphylaxis. Influenza infection prior to sensitization resulted in elevated OVA-IgE levels provided that the OVA aerosol exposure occurred during the acute infection phase on days 2–6 postinfection. Sensitization 14 days postinfection was not enhanced in this model. More recent studies confirmed these observations using parallel models extended by an additional allergen challenge 3–4 weeks after primary sensitization (135,136). Yamamoto and colleagues (136) reported a transient increase in airway dendritic cells from days 2 to 5 of influenza infection. In mice exposed to OVA aerosol at the time of infection, the increase in dendritic cells persisted for up to 5 weeks and was associated with high MHC II expression by these cells. The authors concluded that recruitment of dendritic cells as professional antigen-presenting cells to the airways during influenza infection may have contributed to enhanced sensitization to aeroallergens.

Holt and colleagues (137) studied the effects of influenza infection in a model of tolerance induction. If mice were exposed to OVA-aerosol prior to intraperitoneal sensitization with OVA and alum, reduced levels of OVA-IgE and increased levels of OVA-IgG were detected. This phenomenon was interpreted as development of tolerance. Influenza infection at the time of OVA-aerosol exposure prevented this development of tolerance, resulting in increased levels of OVA–IgE following subsequent intraperitoneal sensitization. Parallel findings were reported recently by Tsitoura and colleagues (138). The effects of influenza infection were assessed in a model of tolerance induction by intranasal application of OVA prior to intraperitoneal sensitization, which in turn was followed by an intranasal OVA challenge. Influenza infection at the same time as the initial OVA application prevented development of tolerance, resulting in increased OVA-specific T-cell proliferation, increased OVA-IgE levels, and increased Th2 cytokine production. When influenza infection did not coincide with the initial allergen exposure, but preceded it by 15 or 30 days, tolerance was still prevented as demonstrated by the lack of inhibition of OVA-induced T-cell proliferation. However, under these conditions sensitization was associated with a strong Th1 immune response with reduced production of IL-4, IL-5, and IL-13 and increased production of IFN-γ upon restimulation with antigen. This Th1 response suppressed the production of OVA-IgE but resulted in enhanced OVA-IgG2a serum levels. These findings suggest that infection with influenza prevents development of tolerance and enhances IgE-mediated allergic sensitization if infection and sensitization coincide. If infection precedes primary allergen exposure, a non-allergic Th1-driven sensitization is promoted.

Leibowitz et al. (139) and Freihorst et al. (140) studied the virus primarily implicated in promotion of allergic sensitization via the airways and in asthma development in children. They determined in a murine model the impact of infection with RSV on sensitization to inhaled allergens (ragweed and OVA) during acute infection. In both sets of experiments, RSV infection resulted in increased levels of allergen-specific antibodies in serum (IgE, IgG) and in bronchoalveolar lavage (BAL) fluid (IgA, IgG). In a recent publication by O'Donell and colleagues (141), induction of anaphylactic antibodies by respiratory viral infections was reported. Following infection with influenza or RSV and concomitant sensitization to OVA aerosol, but not after sensitization without infection, a large proportion of mice collapsed upon subsequent cutaneous challenge with the antigen. In mice susceptible to features of anaphylaxis, OVA-specific IgG1 was detected. This class of antibodies, which is known to mediate anaphylaxis in mice (142), was not detected in mice that failed to react to cutaneous antigen challenge.

In guinea pig models of PIV 3 and RSV infection studied by Riedel et al. (143) and by Dakhama et al. (144), this ability of respiratory viruses to increase production of allergen-specific antibodies was confirmed. In both sets of studies, sensitization was begun during acute infection when an increased permeability of the respiratory mucosa was demonstrated by Riedel et al. (26). Serum levels of horseradish peroxidase were increased following inhalation of horseradish peroxidase in acutely infected mice compared to noninfected animals. The investigators suggested that the increased permeability of the airway mucosa may be an important factor for virus-induced enhancement of sensitization via the airways.

These studies and additional data from a rat model of influenza infection (145) and a bovine model of RSV infection (146) demonstrate that viral lower respiratory tract infections can enhance allergic sensitization to inhaled antigens and can prevent tolerization that may be induced by allergen exposure via the airways in the absence of infection. Among the mechanisms involved, increased permeability of the airway mucosa to allergens and the recruitment of dendritic cells to the airway epithelium during acute infection may be important, facilitating sensitization through increased antigen uptake and more effective antigen presentation. Effects of respiratory viruses on sensitization appear to be dependent on timing, due to changes in the quality of immune responses during the course of infection. As a result, infection with a given respiratory virus can result in either promotion or inhibition of allergic sensitization.

D. Models of Airway Inflammation and Airway Hyperresponsiveness Following Respiratory Virus Infection and Airway Allergen Exposure

In addition to allergen-specific immunoglobulins as markers of sensitization, the consequences of virus-induced allergic airway sensitization have become a major focus of research. Airway inflammation and airway responsiveness to bronchoprovocation, both of which are features of bronchial asthma, were first monitored in guinea pig models of virus infection with allergen sensitization (143,147). Following infection with PIV 3 or RSV, enhanced sensitization to OVA was associated with increased airway inflammation, marked eosinophilia, and AHR to allergen challenge and to nonspecific provocation with MCh (143,144). Kudlacz and colleagues (147) in contrast, did not find any consequences of enhanced sensitization following infection with PIV 3. On the contrary, in their model PIV 3 infection prior to sensitization to OVA prevented increases in histamine release, numbers of leukocytes in BAL fluid, and MCh-induced dyspnea, which were observed in noninfected sensitized guinea pigs. The discrepancy between these observations and the findings reported by Riedel et al. (143,144) may be due to the fact that Kudlacz et al. used 10-fold higher amounts of PIV 3 for infection, possibly inducing a long-lasting and significant Th1 response that may have modified the initial sensitization response. It is unfortunate that allergen-specific antibodies, as parameters of sensitization, were not monitored in this study.

In mice, enhanced sensitization to aeroallergens following respiratory virus infection was also associated with increased airway inflammation and AHR. Suzuki et al. (135) and Yamamoto et al. (136) sensitized mice to OVA during the acute phase of influenza infection and challenged them with the allergen 2–3 weeks after primary sensitization. In both studies, this resulted in increased OVA-IgE levels, increased airway inflammation, and AHR compared to sensitization in the absence of infection or infection without sensitization. The composition of inflammatory cells was assessed in BAL fluid. Both groups observed a predominant increase in CD8+ T cells following sensitization in infected mice. In addition, Yamamoto et al. also reported increases in CD4+ T cells, eosinophils, and macrophages.

E. Murine Model of RSV Infection and Subsequent Allergic Airway Sensitization

We have investigated a model of RSV infection and subsequent allergic sensitization to OVA via the airways in mice. Our approach differed from previously established models in that sensitization was begun after the acute phase of infection and resolution of the consequences of acute respiratory virus disease, that is, on days 11–21 or 21–30 postinfection. Following RSV infection in mice, maximal viral replication occurs on day 4 and maximal inflammatory changes and AHR can be detected on days 6–8. By day 21 postinfection, airway inflammation and AHR completely resolve. Exposure to OVA-aerosol on 10 consecutive days alone resulted in sensitization as indicated by OVA-specific IgE and IgG1 antibodies, but these mice did not develop altered airway responses to inhaled MCh. Acute RSV infection prior to sensitization did not affect serum levels of allergen-specific antibodies (118). This is in contrast to the models discussed above in which exposure to allergen was begun during the acute phase of infection and resulted in increased allergen-specific antibody production.

Following RSV infection and subsequent exposure to allergen, airway responsiveness to nonspecific provocation with inhaled MCh was assessed by barometric body plethysmography, monitoring so-called enhanced pause; a calculated value that correlates with airway resistance (9). Twenty-four hours later, lungs and PBLN, the regional lymph nodes of the lung, were harvested. Lung cells were isolated by collagenase digestion and inflammatory cells were identified under light microscopy. Mononuclear cells from PBLN were cultured and concentrations of the cytokines IFN-γ, IL-4, and IL-5 were measured in supernates by enzyme-linked immunosorbent assay (ELISA). RSV infection, but not sham infection or administration of UV-inactivated virus, prior to sensitization resulted in lung eosinophilia and neutrophilia and in the development of AHR to inhaled MCh. These effects of RSV infection on subsequent exposure to allergen were associated with a decrease in IFN-γ and an increase in IL-4 production in cultures of mononuclear cells from PBLN. IL-5 concentrations did not change significantly (118).

Cytokines

Due to the pivotal role of IL-5 in the development of airway eosinophilia and AHR both in allergic sensitization (10,29,63) and in acute RSV infection (67), we sought to delineate the role of IL-5 in RSV-induced effects on allergic airway sensitization. To do so, both anti-IL-5 antibody treatment and mice genetically deficient in IL-5 were studied. Treatment with anti-IL-5 antibody during the allergen sensitization phase prevented eosinophil influx to the lungs and development of AHR (118). This was in keeping with the effects of anti-IL-5 treatment reported in models of allergen-induced airway inflammation and AHR (10,29,63). Anti-IL-5 treatment during the

RSV infection phase alone significantly reduced lung eosinophilia and AHR following subsequent allergen exposure in the presence of IL-5 (148). Mice genetically deficient in IL-5 failed to develop lung eosinophilia and AHR following RSV infection and allergen sensitization. Both were restored by administration of exogenous IL-5 during acute infection. In contrast, reconstitution with IL-5 only during the allergen sensitization phase did not restore AHR, despite inducing significant lung eosinophilia (148). These data illustrate that the presence of IL-5 and possibly of eosinophils during the acute infection phase is critical, if not essential, to the development of lung eosinophilia and AHR following subsequent allergen sensitization via the airways.

To delineate further the mechanisms involved, the role of IL-4 and IFN-γ in this model was studied utilizing mice deficient in either of these cytokines. Mice deficient in IL-4 did not develop lung eosinophilia or AHR following RSV infection and sensitization. The absence of IL-4 was compensated for by administration of IL-5, indicating that the availability of IL-4 may be essential for IL-5 production, at least sufficient for the development of RSV-induced effects on airway sensitization (148). IFN-γ did not appear to contribute to the effects of RSV infection on allergen sensitization. On the contrary, mice deficient in IFN-γ developed increased lung eosinophilia and AHR, exceeding the effects of RSV infection and sensitization in wild-type controls (148).

T Lymphocytes

To define the role of T cells as possible regulatory cells in RSV infection and allergen sensitization we utilized two approaches: depletion of T cells during RSV infection and sensitization, and adoptive transfer of T cells isolated from the PBLN of RSV-infected mice and transferred (intravenously) to naive mice prior to allergen sensitization via the airways. Treatment of mice with anti-CD8 antibody resulted in almost complete depletion of CD8+ T cells (> 96%) (149). This prevented influx of neutrophils and eosinophils to the lungs and the development of AHR. Depletion of CD4+ T cells was also almost complete during RSV infection (> 98%) but could not be sustained during the allergen sensitization phase (72% depletion). While resulting in a reduction in lung eosinophilia and AHR, CD4+ T-cell depletion did not prevent the consequences of RSV infection on allergen sensitization. Adoptive transfer of CD3+ T cells, harvested from PBLN 14 days postinfection, resulted in eosinophil influx to the lungs and development of AHR associated with an increase in IL-5 production in noninfected recipients following allergen sensitization. In contrast, no such effects were observed following transfer of T cells from noninfected mice or following transfer of T cells from RSV-infected animals without subsequent allergen sensitization. Furthermore, the effects of RSV infection on allergen sensitization could also be transferred by CD8+ T cells isolated from PBLN. Transfer of isolated CD4+ T cells, in contrast, did not result in influx of eosinophils and AHR following allergen sensitization (149). These observations indicate that T cells, in particular CD8+ T cells, appear to be critical in mediating the effects of RSV infection on subsequent exposure of the airways to allergen. A possibility is that IL-5-producing

CD8+ T cells (Tc2) play a pivotal role in this interaction in contrast to the cytotoxic, IFN-γ producing CD8+ T cells (Tc1), which dominate the acute response to viral infection. This former CD8+Tc2 cell subset may expand and become more dominant after the acute phase of RSV infection has resolved, thus favoring eosinophilic airway inflammation and the development of AHR in response to sensitization via the airways.

Similar studies from a number of laboratories demonstrate that enhanced sensitization to allergen following respiratory virus infections can be associated with increases in airway inflammation and airway responsiveness (132,134–141). In addition, RSV infection appears capable of enhancing the consequences of subsequent allergen sensitization independently of increasing levels of allergen-specific antibodies. The effects of RSV infection and also of infections with other respiratory viruses on allergic airway sensitization are likely mediated and regulated by T cells and, under certain conditions, CD8+ T cells. An interesting finding is that CD8+ T cells were also pivotal in the development of AHR in both acute RSV infection (131) and allergic sensitization (23). Furthermore, the presence of IL-5 during acute RSV infection appeared essential for eosinophil influx into the airways and for the development of AHR following subsequent allergen sensitization. In light of these observations, it appears that RSV infection can prime and induce differentiation of a subset of CD8+ T cells to produce IL-5 both during acute infection and following subsequent allergen exposure. This results in increased levels of IL-5 in the airways, favoring the development of eosinophilic inflammatory responses. The eosinophils in turn appear to be critical effector cells of the development of AHR, both in acute RSV infection and following subsequent allergic sensitization. An extension of these studies is that IL-4 in the lung milieu is essential for this induction of CD8+ T cells to differentiate into IL-5 producers.

F. Models of Respiratory Virus Infections in Animals with Established Allergic Airway Inflammation

The corollary to the issue of whether virus infection affects the response to allergen is whether allergic individuals suffer more severe virus-induced disease than nonallergic individuals. This issue and the question of effects of respiratory virus infection on established allergic airway sensitization have been addressed by only a few studies in animal models. In these studies, the impact of respiratory virus infections on the development of airway inflammation and AHR in animals already sensitized to allergen has been investigated.

Robinson et al. (150) studied the effects of RSV infection in guinea pigs previously sensitized to OVA via the airways, by monitoring airway responsiveness to acetylcholine and airway inflammation. Both sensitization alone and RSV infection alone resulted in AHR and airway inflammation with epithelial necrosis, airway wall edema, mononuclear and granulocyte infiltrates, bronchoalveolar lymphoid tissue hyperplasia, and goblet cell metaplasia. RSV infection in allergic animals further increased AHR and airway inflammation, especially promoting airway epithelial cell necrosis. The authors concluded that prior sensitization potentiated the physiological and structural changes associated with RSV infection and posited that an established allergic diathesis may increase the severity of RSV infection in children.

Peebles and colleagues (151) utilized a mouse model of intraperitoneal sensitization to OVA with alum followed by OVA aerosol challenge to assess the effects of RSV infection during the challenge phase. Monitoring airway responsiveness to MCh at weekly intervals, they observed that RSV infection prolonged AHR. Eight days postinfection, MCh provocation resulted in AHR to the same degree in sensitized and challenged mice with or without RSV infection. However, on day 15 postinfection AHR was still present in mice that had been infected with RSV, but not in the mice sensitized and challenged without infection. This prolongation of AHR was associated with an increase in numbers of lymphocytes in the BAL fluid on day 15. Eosinophils were the predominant cell type in the BAL fluid, but their numbers did not differ between RSV infected and noninfected animals. In addition, on histological examination, increased alveolar and interstitial inflammation and increased mucus production were noted in the mice infected with RSV. Prior allergen sensitization did not have an impact on the virus load as determined by plaque assays from lung homogenates 4 days postinfection.

A study recently reported by Matsuse et al. (152) focused on the effects of recurrent RSV infection in mice sensitized to *Dermatophagoides farinae* (Df). Following intraperitoneal sensitization (together with alum), mice were challenged intranasally with the allergen 2, 6, and 14 weeks after sensitization. The day following each 3 day challenge period, mice were infected with RSV or were sham infected. Controls were neither sensitized nor challenged and only infected with RSV or sham infected. Following each challenge period, airway responsiveness to MCh was measured by barometric body plethysmography. Primary RSV infection resulted in increased airway responsiveness in nonsensitized mice and lasted for 10 days. In these animals, the duration of AHR was shortened after the second RSV infection and was no longer detectable following tertiary infection. In contrast, RSV infection in mice sensitized to Df resulted in AHR that increased in duration following the secondary infection and was even more pronounced after tertiary infection. The magnitude of airway responsiveness in these mice exceeded the levels measured in animals sensitized without infection or infected without sensitization. The enhancement of AHR in mice sensitized and infected with RSV was associated with increased airway inflammation, with bronchial exudates composed of mononuclear cells and eosinophils as well as massive tissue eosinophilia. RSV infection also resulted in increased levels of MIP-1α in the lungs of Df-sensitized mice and in a Th2 cytokine shift, with increased production of IL-4 and IL-5 and a decrease in production of IFN-γ by anti-CD3 stimulated thoracic lymph node mononuclear cells. Increased levels of total serum IgE, but no changes in allergen-specific IgE or IgG1, were detectable. Measurements of RSV antigen by ELISA in lung homogenates revealed an increased virus load in sensitized compared to nonsensitized mice following tertiary infection. These observations suggest that recurrent RSV infections augment the synthesis of Th2 cytokines, total IgE, and MIP-1α following allergen sensitization, thus inducing persistent and increased airway inflammation and AHR. In the absence of sensitization, the effects of RSV infection were attenuated following subsequent reinfection.

These three studies indicate that there are consequences of respiratory virus infection in previously sensitized mice that lead to enhanced airway inflammation and increased AHR that can persist for long periods of time. Factors involved in such potentiation in allergic hosts could be increased production of chemokines in response to infection, increased recruitment of T lymphocytes, possibly Th2 lymphocytes, resulting in increased production of Th2 cytokines such as IL-4, IL-5, IL-9, and IL-13. These changes support an inflammatory response dominated by eosinophils as well as the development of persistent AHR. Less effective clearance of virus during an immune response with a Th2 bias may also be contributory to the changes seen. These findings in rodent models identify immune mechanisms that may also be of importance in humans and that allergic airway inflammation may indeed predispose to more severe obstructive airway disease following respiratory virus infections.

G. Conclusion

Not only can respiratory virus infections trigger exacerbations of asthma, but severe virus infection of the lower airways may also contribute to allergic sensitization to aeroallergens and to the development of asthma. On the other hand, atopy or allergic airway sensitization may predispose to more severe virus-induced airway disease.

A variety of animal models demonstrate that respiratory virus infections can not only acutely induce lower airway inflammation and AHR but also enhance sensitization to inhaled allergens and result in increased levels of antigen-specific antibodies. Enhanced allergic airway sensitization can result in increased airway inflammation and in the extent of airway hyperresponsiveness, both of which are features of bronchial asthma. In addition, respiratory viruses appear capable of enhancing the consequences of subsequent allergen sensitization independently of increasing levels of allergen-specific antibodies. Mechanisms involved in enhanced sensitization could be the increased permeability of the airway mucosa to allergens and the recruitment of dendritic cells to the respiratory epithelium during acute respiratory virus infection. Factors involved in augmenting the consequences of allergic airway sensitization appear to be T cells, including CD8+ T cells, as regulators, IL-5 as a pivotal cytokine required for the development of eosinophilic airway inflammation, and eosinophils themselves as likely effector cells of increased airway responsiveness. Furthermore, models of respiratory virus infection in animals previously sensitized to aeroallergens indicate that the immune responses to allergen sensitization and infection interact resulting in increases in inflammation and responsiveness of the airways.

These animal models support the hypothesis that respiratory virus infection can promote allergic sensitization via the airways and the development of asthma. In addition, they identify potential mechanisms for these interactions. Variables include the timing of allergen exposure and infection, on the one hand, leading to a protective Th1 response and inhibition of allergic sensitization; while on the other hand, a Th2 response and aggravation of allergen-induced responses may be seen. The models discussed further indicate that allergic airway sensitization and inflammation may predispose to more severe disease following respiratory virus infections.

Acknowledgments

The authors thank E. Hamelmann, K. Takeda, G. Cieslewicz, M. Makela. A. Dakhama, M. Lahn, T. Ikemura, L.D. Shultz, and M.C. Lamers for their collaboration and K.L. Bradley and A. Joetham for technical support.

This work was supported by grants HL-61005 and HL-36577 (to E.W.G.) from the National Institutes of Health, Grant Schw 597/1-1 from Deutsche Forschungsgemeinschaft, and Grant 01GC9802 (to J.S.) from Bundesministerium für Bildung und Forschung.

References

1. Larsen GL, Renz H, Loader JE, Bradley KL, Gelfand EW. Airway response to electrical field stimulation in sensitized inbred mice. Passive transfer of increased responsiveness with peribronchial lymph nodes. J Clin Invest 1992; 89:747–752.

2. Saloga J, Renz H, Lack G, Bradley KL, Greenstein JL, Larsen G, Gelfand EW. Development and transfer of immediate cutaneous hypersensitivity in mice exposed to aerosolized antigen. J Clin Invest 1993; 91:133–140.

3. Renz H, Saloga J, Bradley KL, Loader JE, Greenstein JL, Larsen G, Gelfand EW. Specific V beta T cell subsets mediate the immediate hypersensitivity response to ragweed allergen. J Immunol 1993; 151:1907–1917.

4. Oshiba A, Hamelmann E, Bradley KL, Loader JE, Renz H, Larsen GL, Gelfand EW. Pretreatment with allergen prevents immediate hypersensitivity and airway hyperresponsiveness. Am J Respir Crit Care Med 1996; 153:102–109.

5. Renz H, Smith HR, Henson JE, Ray BS, Irvin CG, Gelfand EW. Aerosolized antigen exposure without adjuvant causes increased IgE production and increased airway responsiveness in the mouse. J Allergy Clin Immunol 1992; 89:1127–1138.

6. Oshiba A, Hamelmann E, Takeda K, Bradley KL, Loader JE, Larsen GL, Gelfand EW. Passive transfer of immediate hypersensitivity and airway hyperresponsiveness by allergen-specific immunoglobulin (Ig) E and IgG1 in mice. J Clin Invest 1996; 97:1398–1408.

7. Kung TT, Jones H, Adams III GK, Umland SP, Kreutner W, Egan RW, Chapman RW, Watnick AS. Characterization of a murine model of allergic pulmonary inflammation. Int Arch Allergy Immunol 1994; 105:83–90.

8. Hessel EM, Van Oosterhout AJ, Van Ark I, Van Esch B, Hofman G, Van Loveren H, Savelkoul HF, Nijkamp FP. Development of airway hyperresponsiveness is dependent on interferon- gamma and independent of eosinophil infiltration. Am J Respir Cell Mol Biol 1997; 16:325–334.

9. Hamelmann E, Schwarze J, Takeda K, Oshiba A, Larsen GL, Irvin CG, Gelfand EW. Noninvasive measurement of airway responsiveness in allergic mice using barometric plethysmography. Am J Respir Crit Care Med 1997; 156:766–775.

10. Foster PS, Hogan SP, Ramsay AJ, Matthaei KI, Young IG. Interleukin 5 deficiency abolishes eosinophilia, airways hyperreactivity, and lung damage in a mouse asthma model. J Exp Med 1996; 183:195–201.

11. Schwarze J, Hamelmann E, Cieslewicz G, Tomkinson A, Joetham A, Bradley K, Gelfand EW. Local treatment with IL-12 is an effective inhibitor of airway hyperresponsiveness and lung eosinophilia after airway challenge in sensitized mice. J Allergy Clin Immunol 1998; 102:86–93.

12. Saloga J, Renz H, Larsen GL, Gelfand EW. Increased airways responsiveness in mice depends on local challenge with antigen. Am J Respir Crit Care Med 1994; 149:65–70.
13. Martin TR, Gerard NP, Galli SJ, Drazen JM. Pulmonary responses to bronchoconstrictor agonists in the mouse. J Appl Physiol 1988; 64:2318–2323.
14. Amdur MO, Mead J. Mechanics of respiration in unanesthetized guinea pigs. Am J Physiol 1958; 192:364–368.
15. Levitt RC, Mitzner W. Expression of airway hyperreactivity to acetylcholine as a simple autosomal recessive trait in mice. FASEB J 1988; 2:2605–2608.
16. Vijayaraghavan R, Schaper M, Thompson R, Stock MF, Alarie Y. Characteristic modifications of the breathing pattern of mice to evaluate the effects of airborne chemicals on the respiratory tract. Arch Toxicol 1993; 67:478–490.
17. Levitt RC, Mitzner W. Autosomal recessive inheritance of airway hyperreactivity to 5-hydroxytryptamine. J Appl Physiol 1989; 67:1125–1132.
18. Brusselle G, Kips J, Joos G, Bluethmann H, Pauwels R. Allergen-induced airway inflammation and bronchial responsiveness in wild-type and interleukin-4-deficient mice. Am J Respir Cell Mol Biol 1995; 12:254–259.
19. Cieslewicz G, Tomkinson A, Adler A, Duez C, Schwarze J, Takeda K, Larson KA, Lee JJ, Irvin CG , Gelfand EW. The late, but not early, asthmatic response is dependent on IL-5 and correlates with eosinophil infiltration. J Clin Invest 1999; 104:301–308.
20. Cockcroft DW, Ruffin RE, Dolovich J, Hargreave FE. Allergen-induced increase in non-allergic bronchial reactivity. Clin Allergy 1977; 7:503–513.
21. Levitt RC, Mitzner W, Kleeberger SR. A genetic approach to the study of lung physiology: understanding biological variability in airway responsiveness. Am J Physiol 1990; 258:L157–164.
22. Takeda A, Haczku A, Lee JJ, Irvin GC, Gelfand EW. Strain dependence of airway hyperresponsiveness reflects differences in eosinophil localization in the lung. Am J Physiol 2001; in press
23. Hamelmann E, Oshiba A, Paluh J, Bradley K, Loader J, Potter TA, Larsen GL, Gelfand EW. Requirement for CD8+ T cells in the development of airway hyperresponsiveness in a marine model of airway sensitization. J Exp Med 1996; 183:1719–1729.
24. Hamelmann E, Vella AT, Oshiba A, Kappler JW, Marrack P, Gelfand EW. Allergic airway sensitization induces T cell activation but not airway hyperresponsiveness in B cell-deficient mice. Proc Natl Acad Sci USA 1997; 94:1350–1355.
25. Haczku A, Takeda K, Hamelmann E, Oshiba A, Loader J, Joetham A, Irvin C, Kikutani H, Gelfand EW. CD23 deficient mice develop allergic airway hyperresponsiveness following sensitization with ovalbumin. Am J Respir Crit Care Med 1997; 156:1945–1955.
26. Hamelmann E, Tadeda K, Oshiba A, Gelfand EW. Role of IgE in the development of allergic airway inflammation and airway hyperresponsiveness—a murine model. Allergy 1999; 54:297–305.
27. Oshiba A, Hamelmann E, Haczku A, Takeda K, Conrad DH, Kikutani H, Gelfand EW. Modulation of antigen-induced B and T cell responses by antigen-specific IgE antibodies. J Immunol 1997; 159:4056–4063.
28. Takeda K, Hamelmann E, Joetham A, Schultz LD, Larsen GL, Irvin CG, Gelfand EW. Development of eosinophilic airway inflammation and airway hyperresponsiveness in mast cell-deficient mice. J Exp Med 1997; 186:449–454.
29. Hamelmann E, Cieslewicz G, Schwarze J, Ishizuka T, Joetham A, Heusser C, Gelfand EW. Anti-interleukin 5 but not anti-IgE prevents airway inflammation and airway hyperresponsiveness. Am J Respir Crit Care Med 1999; 160:934–941.

30. Renz H, Bradley K, Saloga J, Loader J, Larsen GL, Gelfand EW. T cells expressing specific V beta elements regulate immunoglobulin E production and airways responsiveness in vivo. J Exp Med 1993; 177:1175–1180.

31. Hamelmann E, Oshiba A, Schwarze J, Bradley K, Loader J, Larsen GL, Gelfand EW. Allergen specific IgE and IL-5 are essential for the development of airway hyperresponsiveness. Am J Respir Cell Mol Biol 1997; 16:674–682.

32. Gavett SH, Chen X, Finkelman F, Wills-Karp M. Depletion of murine CD4+ T lymphocytes prevents antigen-induced airway hyperreactivity and pulmonary eosinophilia. Am J Respir Cell Mol Biol 1994; 10:587–593.

33. Hogan SP, Koskinen A, Matthaei KI, Young IG, Foster PS. Interleukin-5-producing CD4+ T cells play a pivotal role in aeroallergen-induced eosinophilia, bronchial hyperreactivity, and lung damage in mice. Am J Respir Crit Care Med 1998; 157:210-218.

34. Corry DB, Grunig G, Hadeiba H, Kurup VP, Warnock ML, Sheppard D, Rennick DM, Locksley RM. Requirements for allergen-induced airway hyperreactivity in T and B cell-deficient mice. Mol Med 1998; 4:344–355.

35. Cohn L, Homer RJ, Marinov A, Rankin J, Bottomly K. Induction of airway mucus production by T helper 2 (Th2) cells: a critical role for interleukin 4 in cell recruitment but not mucus production. J Exp Med 1997; 186:1737–1747.

36. Cohn L, Homer RJ, Niu N, Bottomly K. T helper 1 cells and interferon gamma regulate allergic airway inflammation and mucus production. J Exp Med 1999; 190:1309–1318.

37. Cohn L, Homer RJ, MacLeod H, Mohrs M, Brombacher F, Bottomly K. Th2-induced airway mucus production is dependent on IL-4R alpha, but not on eosinophils. J Immunol 1999; 162:6178-6183.

38. Renz H, Lack G, Saloga J, Schwinzer R, Bradley K, Loader J, Kupfer A, Larsen GL, Gelfand EW. Inhibition of IgE production and normalization of airways responsiveness by sensitized CD8 T cells in a mouse model of allergen- induced sensitization. J Immunol 1994; 152:351–360.

39. Zuany-Amorim C, Ruffie C, Haile S, Vargaftig BB, Pereira P, Pretolani M. Requirement for gamma delta T cells in allergic airway inflammation. Science 1998; 280: 1265–1267.

40. Lahn M, Kanehiro A, Takeda K, Joetham A, Schwarze J, Kohler G, O'Brien R, Gelfand EW, Born W, Kanehio A. Negative regulation of airway responsiveness that is dependent on gammadelta T cells and independent of alphabeta T cells. Nat Med 1999; 5:1150-1156.

41. Ohkawara Y, Lei XF, Stampfli MR, Marshall JS, Xing Z, Jordana M. Cytokine and eosinophil responses in the lung, peripheral blood, and bone marrow compartments in a murine model of allergen-induced airways inflammation. Am J Respir Cell Mol Biol 1997; 16:510–520.

42. Serebrisky D, Teper AA, Huang CK, Lee SY, Zhang TF, Schofield BH, Kattan M, Sampson HA, Li XM. CpG oligodeoxynucleotides can reverse Th2-associated allergic airway responses and alter the B7.1/B7.2 expression in a murine model of asthma. J Immunol 2000; 165:5906–5912.

43. Yu CK, Yang BC, Lee SC, Wang JY, Hsiue TR, Lei HY. Dermatophagoides-farinae-induced pulmonary eosinophilic inflammation in mice. Int Arch Allergy Immunol 1997; 112:73-82.

44. Gavett SH, O'Hearn DJ, Karp CL, Patel EA, Schofield BH, Finkelman FD, Wills-Karp M. Interleukin-4 receptor blockade prevents airway responses induced by antigen challenge in mice. Am J Physiol 1997; 272:L253–261.

45. Lebman DA, Coffman RL. Interleukin 4 causes isotype switching to IgE in T cell-stimulated clonal B cell cultures. J Exp Med 1988; 168:853–862.

46. Swain SL, Weinberg AD, English M, Huston G. IL-4 directs the development of Th2-like helper effectors. J Immunol 1990; 145:3796–3806.

47. Corry DB, Folkesson HG, Warnock ML, Erle DJ, Matthay MA, Wiener-Kronish JP, Locksley RM. Interleukin 4, but not interleukin 5 or eosinophils, is required in a murine model of acute airway hyperreactivity. J Exp Med 1996; 183:109–117.

48. Hogan SP, Mould A, Kikutani H, Ramsay AJ, Foster PS. Aeroallergen-induced eosino-philic inflammation, lung damage, and airways hyperreactivity in mice can occur inde-pendently of IL-4 and allergen-specific immunoglobulins. J Clin Invest 1997; 99: 1329–1339.

49. Hamelmann E, Takeda K, Haczku A, Cieslewicz G, Shultz L, Hamid Q, Xing Z, Gaul-die J, Gelfand EW. Interleukin (IL)-5 but not immunoglobulin E reconstitutes airway inflammation and airway hyperresponsiveness in IL-4-deficient mice. Am J Respir Cell Mol Biol 2000; 23:327–334.

50. Nagai H, Maeda Y, Tanaka H. The effect of anti-IL-4 monoclonal antibody, rapamycin and interferon- gamma on airway hyperreactivity to acetylcholine in mice. Clin Exp Allergy 1997; 27:218–224.

51. Cohn L, Tepper JS, Bottomly K. IL-4-independent induction of airway hyperrespon-siveness by Th2, but not Th1, cells. J Immunol 1998; 161:3813–3816.

52. Grunig G, Warnock M, Wakil AE, Venkayya R, Brombacher F, Rennick DM, Shep-pard D, Mohrs M, Donaldson DD, Locksley RM, Corry DB. Requirement for IL-13 independently of IL-4 in experimental asthma. Science 1998; 282:2261–2263.

53. Wills-Karp M, Luyimbazi J, Xu X, Schofield B, Neben TY, Karp CL, Donaldson DD. Interleukin-13: central mediator of allergic asthma. Science 1998; 282:2258–2261.

54. Zhu Z, Homer RJ, Wang Z, Chen Q, Geba GP, Wang J, Zhang Y, Elias JA. Pulmonary expression of interleukin-13 causes inflammation, mucus hypersecretion, subepithelial fibrosis, physiologic abnormalities, and eotaxin production. J Clin Invest 1999; 103: 779–788.

55. Webb DC, McKenzie AN, Koskinen AM, Yang M, Mattes J, Foster PS. Integrated signals between IL-13, IL-4, and IL-5 regulate airways hyperreactivity. J Immunol 2000; 165:108–113.

56. Li L, Xia Y, Nguyen A, Lai YH, Feng L, Mosmann TR, Lo D. Effects of Th2 cytokines on chemokine expression in the lung: IL-13 potently induces eotaxin expression by airway epithelial cells. J Immunol 1999; 162:2477–2487.

57. Kaplan MH, Schindler U, Smiley ST, Grusby MJ. Stat6 is required for mediating responses to IL-4 and for development of Th2 cells. Immunity 1996; 4:313–319.

58. Shimoda K, van Deursen J, Sangster MY, Sarawar SR, Carson RT, Tripp RA, Chu C, Quelle FW, Nosaka T, Vignali DA, Doherty PC, Grosveld G, Paul WE, Ihle JN. Lack of IL-4-induced Th2 response and IgE class switching in mice with disrupted Stat6 gene. Nature 1996; 380:630–633.

59. Tomkinson A, Kanehiro A, Rabinovitch N, Joetham A, Cieslewicz G, Gelfand EW. The failure of STAT6-deficient mice to develop airway eosinophilia and airway hyper-responsiveness is overcome by interleukin-5. Am J Respir Crit Care Med 1999; 160: 1283–1291.

60. Miyata S, Matsuyama T, Kodama T, Nishioka Y, Kuribayashi K, Takeda K, Akira S, Sugita M. STAT6 deficiency in a mouse model of allergen-induced airways inflamma-tion abolishes eosinophilia but induces infiltration of CD8+ T cells. Clin Exp Allergy 1999; 29:114–123.

61. Lopez AF, Sanderson CJ, Gamble JR, Campbell HD, Young IG, Vadas MA. Recombinant human interleukin 5 is a selective activator of human eosinophil function. J Exp Med 1988; 167:219-224.

62. Yamaguchi Y, Hayashi Y, Sugama Y, Miura Y, Kasahara T, Kitamura S, Torisu M, Mita S, Tominaga A, Takatsu K. Highly purified murine interleukin 5 (IL-5) stimulates eosinophil function and prolongs in vitro survival. IL-5 as an eosinophil chemotactic factor. J Exp Med 1988; 167:1737–1742.

63. Hamelmann E, Oshiba A, Loader J, Larsen GL, Gleich G, Lee J, Gelfand EW. Antiinterleukin-5 antibody prevents airway hyperresponsiveness in a murine model of airway sensitization. Am J Respir Crit Care Med 1997; 155:819–825.

64. Wang J, Palmer K, Lotvall J, Milan S, Lei XF, Matthaei KI, Gauldie J, Inman MD, Jordana M, Xing Z. Circulating, but not local lung, IL-5 is required for the development of antigen-induced airways eosinophilia. J Clin Invest 1998; 102:1132–1141.

65. Hogan MB, Piktel D, Landreth KS. IL-5 production by bone marrow stromal cells: implications for eosinophilia associated with asthma. J Allergy Clin Immunol 2000; 106:329–336.

66. Minshall EM, Schleimer R, Cameron L, Minnicozzi M, Egan RW, Gutierrez-Ramos JC, Eidelman DH, Hamid Q. Interleukin-5 expression in the bone marrow of sensitized Balb/c mice after allergen challenge. Am J Respir Crit Care Med 1998; 158:951-957.

67. Schwarze J, Cieslewicz G, Hamelmann E, Joetham A, Shultz LD, Lamers MC, Gelfand EW. IL-5 and eosinophils are essential for the development of airway hyperresponsiveness following acute respiratory syncytial virus infection. J Immunol 1999; 162:2997-3004.

68. Fiorentino DF, Bond MW, Mosmann TR. Two types of mouse T helper cell. IV. Th2 clones secrete a factor that inhibits cytokine production by Th1 clones. J Exp Med 1989; 170:2081-2095.

69. Borish L. IL-10: evolving concepts. J Allergy Clin Immunol 1998; 101:293–297.

70. Grunig G, Corry DB, Leach MW, Seymour BW, Kurup VP, Rennick DM. Interleukin-10 is a natural suppressor of cytokine production and inflammation in a murine model of allergic bronchopulmonary aspergillosis. J Exp Med 1997; 185:1089–1099.

71. Yang X, Wang S, Fan Y, Han X. IL-10 deficiency prevents IL-5 overproduction and eosinophilic inflammation in a murine model of asthma-like reaction. Eur J Immunol 2000; 30:382–391.

72. Makela MJ, Kanehiro A, Borish L, Dakhama A, Loader J, Joetham A, Xing Z, Jordana M, Larsen GL, Gelfand EW. IL-10 is necessary for the expression of airway hyperresponsiveness but not pulmonary inflammation after allergic sensitization. Proc Natl Acad Sci USA 2000; 97:6007–6012.

73. van Scott MR, Justice JP, Bradfield JF, Enright E, Sigounas A, Sur S. IL-10 reduces Th2 cytokine production and eosinophilia but augments airway reactivity in allergic mice. Am J Physiol Lung Cell Mol Physiol 2000; 278:L667–674.

74. Fiorentino DF, Zlotnik A, Mosmann TR, Howard M, O'Garra A. IL-10 inhibits cytokine production by activated macrophages. J Immunol 1991; 147:3815–3822.

75. Zuany-Amorim C, Haile S, Leduc D, Dumarey C, Huerre M, Vargaftig BB, Pretolani M. Interleukin-10 inhibits antigen-induced cellular recruitment into the airways of sensitized mice. J Clin Invest 1995; 95:2644–2651

76. Nicolaides NC, Holroyd KJ, Ewart SL, Eleff SM, Kiser MB, Dragwa CR, Sullivan CD, Grasso L, Zhang LY, Messler CJ, Zhou T, Kleeberger SR, Buetow KH, Levitt RC. Interleukin 9: a candidate gene for asthma. Proc Natl Acad Sci USA 1997; 94: 13175–13180.

77. Temann UA, Geba GP, Rankin JA, Flavell RA. Expression of interleukin 9 in the lungs of transgenic mice causes airway inflammation, mast cell hyperplasia, and bronchial hyperresponsiveness. J Exp Med 1998; 188:1307–1320.

78. McLane MP, Haczku A, van de Rijn M, Weiss C, Ferrante V, MacDonald D, Renauld JC, Nicolaides NC, Holroyd KJ, Levitt RC. Interleukin-9 promotes allergen-induced eosinophilic inflammation and airway hyperresponsiveness in transgenic mice. Am J Respir Cell Mol Biol 1998; 19:713–720.

79. Levitt RC, McLane MP, MacDonald D, Ferrante V, Weiss C, Zhou T, Holroyd KJ, Nicolaides NC. IL-9 pathway in asthma: new therapeutic targets for allergic inflammatory disorders. J Allergy Clin Immunol 1999; 103:S485–491.

80. Dong Q, Louahed J, Vink A, Sullivan CD, Messler CJ, Zhou Y, Haczku A, Huaux F, Arras M, Holroyd KJ, Renauld JC, Levitt RC, Nicolaides NC. IL-9 induces chemokine expression in lung epithelial cells and baseline airway eosinophilia in transgenic mice. Eur J Immunol 1999; 29:2130–2139.

81. Louahed J, Toda M, Jen J, Hamid Q, Renauld JC, Levitt RC, Nicolaides NC. Interleukin-9 upregulates mucus expression in the airways. Am J Respir Cell Mol Biol 2000; 22:649–656.

82. Stassen M, Arnold M, Hultner L, Muller C, Neudorfl C, Reineke T, Schmitt E. Murine bone-marrow derived mast cells as potent producers of IL-9: costimulatory function of IL-10 and kit ligand in the presence of IL-1. J Immunol 2000; 164:5549–5555.

83. Gavett SH, O'Hearn DJ, Li X, Huang SK, Finkelman FD, Wills-Karp M. Interleukin 12 inhibits antigen-induced airway hyperresponsiveness, inflammation, and Th2 cytokine expression in mice. J Exp Med 1995; 182:1527–1536.

84. Lack G, Renz H, Saloga J, Bradley KL, Loader J, Leung DY, Larsen G, Gelfand EW. Nebulized but not parenteral IFN-gamma decreases IgE production and normalizes airways function in a murine model of allergen sensitization. J Immunol 1994; 152: 2546-2554.

85. Keane-Myers A, Wysocka M, Trinchieri G, Wills-Karp M. Resistance to antigen-induced airway hyperresponsiveness requires endogenous production of IL-12. J Immunol 1998; 161:919–926.

86. Hofstra CL, Van Ark I, Hofman G, Nijkamp FP, Jardieu PM, Van Oosterhout AJ. Differential effects of endogenous and exogenous interferon-gamma on immunoglobulin E, cellular infiltration, and airway responsiveness in a murine model of allergic asthma. Am J Respir Cell Mol Biol 1998; 19:826–835.

87. Okamura H, Tsutsi H, Komatsu T, Yutsudo M, Hakura A, Tanimoto T, Torigoe K, Okura T, Nukada Y, Hattori K, et al. Cloning of a new cytokine that induces IFN-gamma production by T cells. Nature 1995; 378:88–91.

88. Hofstra CL, Van Ark I, Hofman G, Kool M, Nijkamp FP, Van Oosterhout AJ. Prevention of Th2-like cell responses by coadministration of IL-12 and IL-18 is associated with inhibition of antigen-induced airway hyperresponsiveness, eosinophilia, and serum IgE levels. J Immunol 1998; 161:5054–5060.

89. Kodama T, Matsuyama T, Kuribayashi K, Nishioka Y, Sugita M, Akira S, Nakanishi K, Okamura H. IL-18 deficiency selectively enhances allergen-induced eosinophilia in mice. J Allergy Clin Immunol 2000; 105:45–53.

90. Kumano K, Nakao A, Nakajima H, Hayashi F, Kurimoto M, Okamura H, Saito Y, Iwamoto I. Interleukin-18 enhances antigen-induced eosinophil recruitment into the mouse airways. Am J Respir Crit Care Med 1999; 160:873–878.

91. Wild JS, Sigounas A, Sur N, Siddiqui MS, Alam R, Kurimoto M, Sur S. IFN-gamma-inducing factor (IL-18) increases allergic sensitization, serum IgE, Th2 cytokines, and

airway eosinophilia in a mouse model of allergic asthma. J Immunol 2000; 164:2701-2710.

92. Busse WW. Respiratory infections: their role in airway responsiveness and the patho-genesis of asthma. J Allergy Clin Immunol 1990; 85:671–683.

93. Cypcar D, Stark J, Lemanske RF, Jr. The impact of respiratory infections on asthma. Pediatr Clin North Am 1992; 39:1259–1276.

94. Nicholson KG, Kent J, Ireland DC. Respiratory viruses and exacerbations of asthma in adults. Br Med J 1993; 307:982–986.

95. Johnston SL, Pattemore PK, Sanderson G, Smith S, Lampe F, Josephs L, Symington P, O'Toole S, Myint SH, Tyrrell DA, et al. Community study of role of viral infections in exacerbations of asthma in 9–11 year old children. Br Med J 1995; 310:1225-1229.

96. McIntosh K, Ellis EF, Hoffman LS, Lybass TG, Eller JJ, Fulginiti VA. The association of viral and bacterial respiratory infections with exacerbations of wheezing in young asthmatic children. J Pediatr 1973; 82:578–590.

97. Johnston SL. The role of viral and atypical bacterial pathogens in asthma pathogenesis. Pediatr Pulmonol Suppl 1999; 18:141–143.

98. Frick OL, German DF, Mills J. Development of allergy in children. I. Association with virus infections. J Allergy Clin Immunol 1979; 63:228–241.

99. Eisen A, Bacal H. The relationship of acute bronchiolitis to bronchial asthma. Pediat-rics 1963; 31:859.

100. Sims DG, Downham MA, Gardner PS, Webb JK, Weightman D. Study of 8-year-old children with a history of respiratory syncytial virus bronchiolitis in infancy. Br Med J 1978; 1:11-14,

101. Webb MS, Henry RL, Milner AD, Stokes GM, Swarbrick AS. Continuing respiratory problems three and a half years after acute viral bronchiolitis. Arch Dis Child 1985; 60:1064–1067.

102. Sly PD, Hibbert ME. Childhood asthma following hospitalization with acute viral bronchiolitis in infancy. Pediatr Pulmonol 1989; 7:153–158.

103. Sporik R, Holgate ST, Cogswell JJ. Natural history of asthma in childhood—a birth cohort study. Arch Dis Child 1991; 66:1050–1053.

104. Murray M, Webb MS, O'Callaghan C, Swarbrick AS, Milner AD. Respiratory status and allergy after bronchiolitis. Arch Dis Child 1992; 67:482–487.

105. Sigurs N, Bjarnason R, Sigurbergsson F, Kjellman B, Bjorksten B. Asthma and immu-noglobulin E antibodies after respiratory syncytial virus bronchiolitis: a prospective cohort study with matched controls. Pediatrics 1995; 95:500–505.

106. Sigurs N, Bjarnason R, Sigurbergsson F, Kjellman B. Respiratory syncytial virus bron-chiolitis in infancy is an important risk factor for asthma and allergy at age 7. Am J Respir Crit Care Med 2000; 161:1501–1507.

107. Pullan CR, Hey EN. Wheezing, asthma, and pulmonary dysfunction 10 years after infection with respiratory syncytial virus in infancy. Br Med J 1982; 284:1665–1669.

108. Kneyber MCJ, Steyerberg EW, de Groot R, Moll HA. Long-term effects of respiratory syncytial virus (RSV) bronchiolitis in infants and young children: a quantitative re-view. Acta Paediatr 2000; 89:654–660.

109. Stein RT, Sherrill D, Morgan WJ, Holberg CJ, Halonen M, Taussig LM, Wright AL, Martinez FD. Respiratory syncytial virus in early life and risk of wheeze and allergy by age 13 years. Lancet 1999; 354:541–545.

110. Neilson KA, Yunis EJ. Demonstration of respiratory syncytial virus in an autopsy series. Pediatr Pathol 1990; 10:491–502.

111. Prince GA, Horswood RL, Berndt J, Suffin SC, Chanock RM. Respiratory syncytial virus infection in inbred mice. Infect Immun 1979; 26:764–766.

112. Kakuk TJ, Soike K, Brideau RJ, Zaya RM, Cole SL, Zhang JY, Roberts ED, Wells PA, Wathen MW. A human respiratory syncytial virus (RSV) primate model of enhanced pulmonary pathology induced with a formalin-inactivated RSV vaccine but not a recombinant FG subunit vaccine. J Infect Dis 1993; 167:553–561.

113. Hegele RG, Robinson PJ, Gonzalez S, Hogg JC. Production of acute bronchiolitis in guinea-pigs by human respiratory syncytial virus. Eur Respir J 1993; 6:1324–1331.

114. Folkerts G, Van Esch B, Janssen M, Nijkamp FP. Virus-induced airway hyperresponsiveness in guinea pigs in vivo: study of broncho-alveolar cell number and activity. Eur J Pharmacol 1992; 228:219–227.

115. Folkerts G, Verheyen A, Nijkamp FP. Viral infection in guinea pigs induces a sustained non-specific airway hyperresponsiveness and morphological changes of the respiratory tract. Eur J Pharmacol 1992; 228:121–130.

116. Kudlacz EM, Shatzer SA, Farrell AM, Baugh LE. Parainfluenza virus type 3 induced alterations in tachykinin NK1 receptors, substance P levels and respiratory functions in guinea pig airways. Eur J Pharmacol 1994; 270:291–300.

117. Robinson PJ, Hegele RG, Schellenberg RR. Increased airway reactivity in human RSV bronchiolitis in the guinea pig is not due to increased wall thickness. Pediatr Pulmonol 1996; 22:248-254.

118. Schwarze J, Hamelmann E, Bradley KL, Takeda K, Gelfand EW. Respiratory syncytial virus infection results in airway hyperresponsiveness and enhanced airway sensitization to allergen. J Clin Invest 1997; 100:226–233.

119. Garofalo R, Kimpen JL, Welliver RC, Ogra PL. Eosinophil degranulation in the respiratory tract during naturally acquired respiratory syncytial virus infection. J Pediatr 1992; 120:28-32.

120. Garofalo R, Dorris A, Ahlstedt S, Welliver RC. Peripheral blood eosinophil counts and eosinophil cationic protein content of respiratory secretions in bronchiolitis: relationship to severity of disease. Pediatr Allergy Immunol 1994; 5:111–117.

121. Kimpen JL, Garofalo R, Welliver RC, Ogra PL. Activation of human eosinophils in vitro by respiratory syncytial virus. Pediatr Res 1992; 32:160–164.

122. van Oosterhout AJ, van Ark I, Folkerts G, van der Linde HJ, Savelkoul HF, Verheyen AK, Nijkamp FP. Antibody to interleukin-5 inhibits virus-induced airway hyperresponsiveness to histamine in guinea pigs Am J Respir Crit Care Med 1995; 151:177–183.

123. Berlin C, Berg EL, Briskin MJ, Andrew DP, Kilshaw PJ, Holzmann B, Weissman IL, Hamann A, Butcher EC. Alpha 4 beta 7 integrin mediates lymphocyte binding to the mucosal vascular addressin MAdCAM-1. Cell 1993; 74:185–185.

124. Carlos TM, Harlan JM. Leukocyte-endothelial adhesion molecules. Blood 1994; 84:2068–2101.

125. Nakajima H, Sano H, Nishimura T, Yoshida S, Iwamoto I. Role of vascular cell adhesion molecule 1/very late activation antigen 4 and intercellular adhesion molecule one/lymphocyte function-associated antigen 1 interactions in antigen-induced eosinophil and T cell recruitment into the tissue. J Exp Med 1994; 179:1145–1154.

126. Henderson WR, Jr., Chi EY, Albert RK, Chu SJ, Lamm WJ, Rochon Y, Jonas M, Christie PE, Harlan JM. Blockade of CD49d (alpha4 integrin) on intrapulmonary but not circulating leukocytes inhibits airway inflammation and hyperresponsiveness in a mouse model of asthma. J Clin Invest 1997; 100:3083–3092.

127. Walker C, Bode E, Boer L, Hansel TT, Blaser K, Virchow JC, Jr. Allergic and nonaller-

gic asthmatics have distinct patterns of T-cell activation and cytokine production in peripheral blood and bronchoalveolar lavage. Am Rev Respir Dis 1992; 146:109–115.

128. Gonzalez MC, Diaz P, Galleguillos FR, Ancic P, Cromwell O, Kay AB. Allergen-induced recruitment of bronchoalveolar helper (OKT4) and suppressor (OKT8) T-cells in asthma. Relative increases in OKT8 cells in single early responders compared with those in late-phase responders. Am Rev Respir Dis 1987; 136:600-604.

129. Lukacher AE, Braciale VL, Braciale TJ. In vivo effector function of influenza virus-specific cytotoxic T lymphocyte clones is highly specific. J Exp Med 1984; 160:814–826.

130. Doherty PC, Allan W, Eichelberger M, Carding SR. Roles of alpha beta and gamma delta T cell subsets in viral immunity. Annu Rev Immunol 1992; 10:123–151.

131. Schwarze J, Cieslewicz G, Joetham A, Ikemura T, Hamelmann E, Gelfand EW. CD8 T cells are essential in the development of respiratory syncytial virus-induced lung eosinophilia and airway hyperresponsiveness. J Immunol 1999; 162:4207–4211.

132. Coyle AJ, Erard F, Bertrand C, Walti S, Pircher H, Le Gros G. Virus-specific CD8+ cells can switch to interleukin 5 production and induce airway eosinophilia. J Exp Med 1995; 181:1229–1233.

133. Erard F, Wild MT, Garcia-Sanz JA, Le Gros G. Switch of CD8 T cells to noncytolytic CD8-CD4-cells that make TH2 cytokines and help B cells. Science 1993; 260:1802–1805.

134. Sakamoto M, Ida S, Takishima T. Effect of influenza virus infection on allergic sensitization to aerosolized ovalbumin in mice. J Immunol 1984; 132:2614–2617.

135. Suzuki S, Suzuki Y, Yamamoto N, Matsumoto Y, Shirai A, Okubo T. Influenza A virus infection increases IgE production and airway responsiveness in aerosolized antigen-exposed mice. J Allergy Clin Immunol 1998; 102:732–740.

136. Yamamoto N, Suzuki S, Shirai A, Suzuki M, Nakazawa M, Nagashima Y, Okubo T. Dendritic cells are associated with augmentation of antigen sensitization by influenza A virus infection in mice. Eur J Immunol 2000; 30:316–326.

137. Holt PG, Vines J, Bilyk N. Effect of influenza virus infection on allergic sensitization to inhaled antigen in mice. Int Arch Allergy Appl Immunol 1988; 86:121–123.

138. Tsitoura DC, Kim S, Dabbagh K, Berry G, Lewis DB, Umetsu DT. Respiratory infection with influenza A virus interferes with the induction of tolerance to aeroallergens. J Immunol 2000; 165:3484–3491.

139. Leibovitz E, Freihorst J, Piedra PA, Ogra PL. Modulation of systemic and mucosal immune responses to inhaled ragweed antigen in experimentally induced infection with respiratory syncytial virus implication in virally induced allergy. Int Arch Allergy Appl Immunol 1988; 86:112–116.

140. Freihorst J, Piedra PA, Okamoto Y, Ogra PL. Effect of respiratory syncytial virus infection on the uptake of and immune response to other inhaled antigens. Proc Soc Exp Biol Med 1988; 188:191–197.

141. O'Donnell DR, Openshaw PJ. Anaphylactic sensitization to aeroantigen during respiratory virus infection. Clin Exp Allergy 1998; 28:1501–1508

142. Miyajima I, Dombrowicz D, Martin TR, Ravetch JV, Kinet JP, Galli SJ. Systemic anaphylaxis in the mouse can be mediated largely through IgG1 and Fc gammaRIII. Assessment of the cardiopulmonary changes, mast cell degranulation, and death associated with active or IgE- or IgG1-dependent passive anaphylaxis. J Clin Invest 1997; 99:901–914.

143. Riedel F, Krause A, Slenczka W, Rieger CH. Parainfluenza-3-virus infection enhances allergic sensitization in the guinea-pig. Clin Exp Allergy 1996; 26:603–609.

144. Dakhama A, Bramley AM, Chan NG, McKay KO, Schellenberg RR, Hegele RG. Effect of respiratory syncytial virus on subsequent allergic sensitization to ovalbumin in guinea-pigs. Eur Respir J 1999; 13:976–982.

145. Lebrec H, Sarlo K, Burleson GR. Effect of influenza virus infection on ovalbumin-specific IgE responses to inhaled antigen in the rat. J Toxicol Environ Health 1996; 49:619–630.

146. Gershwin LJ, Himes SR, Dungworth DL, Giri SN, Friebertshauser KE, Camacho M. Effect of bovine respiratory syncytial virus infection on hypersensitivity to inhaled Micropolyspora faeni. Int Arch Allergy Immunol 1994; 104:79-91.

147. Kudlacz EM, Knippenberg RW. Parainfluenza virus type-3 infection attenuates the respiratory effects of antigen challenge in sensitized guinea pigs. Inflamm Res 1995; 44:105–110.

148. Schwarze J, Cieslewicz G, Joetham A, Ikemura T, Makela MJ, Dakhama A, Shultz LD, Lamers MC, Gelfand EW. Critical roles for interleukin-4 and interleukin-5 during respiratory syncytial virus infection in the development of airway hyperresponsiveness after airway sensitization. Am J Respir Crit Care Med 2000; 162:380–386.

149. Schwarze J, Makela M, Cieslewicz G, Dakhama A, Lahn M, Ikemura T, Joetham A, Gelfand EW. Transfer of the enhancing effect of respiratory syncytial virus infection on subsequent allergic airway sensitization by T lymphocytes. J Immunol 1999; 163: 5729–5734.

150. Robinson PJ, Hegele RG, Schellenberg RR. Allergic sensitization increases airway reactivity in guinea pigs with respiratory syncytial virus bronchiolitis. J Allergy Clin Immunol 1997; 100:492–498.

151. Peebles RS Jr, Sheller JR, Johnson JE, Mitchell DB, Graham BS. Respiratory syncytial virus infection prolongs methacholine-induced airway hyperresponsiveness in ovalbumin-sensitized mice. J Med Virol 1999; 57:186–192.

152. Matsuse H, Behera AK, Kumar M, Rabb H, Lockey RF, Mohapatra SS. Recurrent respiratory syncytial virus infections in allergen-sensitized mice lead to persistent airway inflammation and hyperresponsiveness. J Immunol 2000; 164:6583–6592.

15

Origin of Respiratory Virus-Induced Chronic Airway Dysfunction

Exploring Genetic, Developmental, and Environmental Factors in a Rat Model of the Asthmatic Phenotype

LOUIS A. ROSENTHAL, RONALD L. SORKNESS, and ROBERT F. LEMANSKE, Jr.

University of Wisconsin
Madison, Wisconsin, U.S.A.

I. Introduction

Despite recent advances, a detailed understanding of the origins of asthma remains elusive. Various lines of evidence suggest that genetic, environmental, and developmental factors contribute to the inception of asthma, but the complex interplay of these factors is only beginning to be elucidated. One central issue in the study of asthma is the role that acute environmental insults to the airways play in the eventual development of chronic airway physiological abnormalities. Animal models of chronic airway dysfunction can serve as important investigative tools with respect to these issues because they permit control and manipulation of genetic and developmental factors through the use of defined animal strains evaluated at specific stages of development. Furthermore, the nature of the environmental insult, for example, a respiratory virus, is known, and the animals can be exposed to it in a specific and controlled manner. In this chapter, we discuss the potential roles of cytokine dysregulation and respiratory viral infection in the development of childhood asthma, and describe the use of a rat model of virus-induced chronic airway dysfunction to study the interactions of these two recognized risk factors.

II. Origins of Asthma: Important Questions

For many individuals with asthma, the development of the asthmatic phenotype has its roots in early life. Genetic (atopy), environmental (allergens, viruses), and developmental (age) factors have been implicated in asthma pathogenesis in the first decade of life, but their relative importance either alone, or in combination, has yet to be fully established. Indeed, at present, a number of important questions remain unanswered. Does dysregulation in cytokine production, which may already be present at birth (1), influence the immunological response to respiratory viral infections, leading to more severe disease (i.e., bronchiolitis)? Do respiratory viral infections promote the development of cytokine dysregulation, thereby increasing the risk of developing atopy (2)? Do imprinted patterns of cytokine secretion interact with respiratory virus-induced bronchiolitis at a critical time, leading to the development of the asthmatic phenotype (3)? Answering these questions and establishing the relationship of these factors to the inception of asthma will be critical for designing therapeutic strategies to prevent the development of asthma in children.

III. Rat Model of Respiratory Virus–Induced Chronic Airway Dysfunction

The heterogenous nature of asthma with its range of disease severity, numerous environmental triggering factors (viruses, allergens, and irritants), fluctuations with age, and variable response to therapeutic intervention has presented challenges to investigators attempting to use animal models to gain insight into basic pathogenic mechanisms. Allergen challenge models have been widely used to evaluate both the immediate (minutes) and late response (hours) to allergen challenge in order to gain insight into possible links between allergen-induced airway inflammation and alterations in pulmonary physiology (resistance, compliance, conductance, response to methacholine bronchoprovocation) (4). A number of models have been developed that evaluate immunological, biological, and physiological responses to viral respiratory infections as well (5–31). Although these and other animal models have provided considerable insight into the asthmatic phenotype by studying factors that play a role in the acute changes following exposure to either allergen or virus, they have not been designed to study comprehensively the variables that contribute to the chronic, as opposed to acute, features of this disease, including chronic airway inflammation; airway fibrosis and remodeling; and chronic, episodic, reversible obstruction. A model incorporating these chronic abnormalities as well as providing a means to study any observed structure–function relationships longitudinally would be able to address the important questions mentioned above and complement the studies performed in models designed to examine the more acute processes related to asthma.

To address this need, we have extensively studied virus-induced airway dysfunction using parainfluenza type 1 (Sendai) virus infection in rats as a model for the inception of childhood asthma (32–42). Sendai virus is a naturally occurring rodent strain of parainfluenza type 1 virus that causes acute respiratory illness in rats by infecting airway epithelium and initiating an inflammatory response. We have characterized the virus-associated changes in airway physiology, both during the acute viral illness and after recovery from viral illness, in different ages and strains of rats. Our observations, in conjunction with the studies of airway morphology and histology in the laboratory of a collaborator, Dr. William Castleman, have revealed chronic postviral airway abnormalities in rats that have multiple features in common with human asthma. The features of this so-called asthma-like phenotype include histopathological changes consistent with airway remodeling (subepithelial fibrosis, an increased deposition of extracellular matrix material, and mast cell hyperplasia) (37). Correlative physiological alterations include chronic (over weeks) episodic increases in airway resistance that can be significantly attenuated following corticosteroid treatment and methacholine hyperresponsiveness (36–38). The development of these airway changes is influenced both by the age (neonatal vs. weanling vs. adult) and strain [Brown Norway (BN)(high IgE producers, so-called atopic strain) vs. Fischer 344 (F344) (low IgE producers, so-called nonatopic strain)] of the rat (37). In the susceptible BN rat, we have noted that functional abnormalities (increases in pulmonary resistance and hyperresponsiveness to methacholine) were most strongly associated with bronchiolar mural thickening and fibrosis as well as with recruitment of inflammatory cells, including macrophages, mast cells, lymphocytes, and eosinophils, into the bronchiolar wall. It should be noted that many of these changes have been reported in human asthma (43–45). Most important, however, is that completed and continuing experiments strongly support the concept suggested by human observations that two factors, an imbalance in cytokine responses and a viral lower respiratory tract infection, are needed to interact at a critical developmental time to enhance the likelihood that asthma will develop during childhood.

IV. Factors Influencing the Expression of Asthma

A. What Is the Role of Viral Infections in Producing Airway Dysfunction Early in Life?

Studies in Humans

Acute viral infections have been demonstrated to be temporally associated with a number of important clinical consequences (46), including the development of wheezing-associated illnesses in infants and small children (47–53); initiating acute exacerbations of asthma both in children and adults (47,50,54,55); and inducing short- and long-term alterations in airway physiology, including increasing airway responsiveness (56) and creating abnormalities in airflow (57), lung volumes (58,59), and gas exchange (60). In addition, there is evidence to suggest that certain viral infections, especially respiratory syncytial virus (RSV) infections, may contribute to the inception of childhood asthma in the first decade of life (61,62). Despite continued interest in the role of viral infections in inducing both acute and chronic airway dysfunction, the precise mechanisms by which viral illnesses produce these pathophysiological manifestations in the susceptible host remain unknown, indicating the importance of continued investigation into potential pathogenic mechanisms in both human subjects and animal models.

In patients with established asthma, viral upper respiratory tract infections have been documented to play a significant role in producing acute exacerbations of airway obstruction (47,50,63). In infants, infection with RSV has received much attention because of its predilection to produce a pattern of symptoms termed bronchiolitis, which parallels many of the features of childhood and adult asthma (64). During 1980–1996, rates of hospitalization of infants with bronchiolitis increased substantially, as did the proportion of total and lower respiratory tract hospitalizations associated with bronchiolitis (65); RSV causes about 70% of these episodes. Ironically, despite these statistics, it is estimated that by age 1 and 2 years, 50–65% and nearly 100% of children will have been infected with this virus, respectively (66). Children aged 3–6 months are most prone to develop lower respiratory tract symptoms, suggesting that a developmental component (e.g., lung and/or immunological maturation) may be an important factor related to outcomes (66). Although some controversy exists regarding the relevance of antecedent RSV infections and the development of recurrent wheezing (67), long-term prospective studies of large numbers of children have convincingly demonstrated that this particular infection is a significant independent risk factor for the development of asthma in the first decade of life (2,62). It remains to be established, however, how RSV infections produce these outcomes due to the fact that virtually all children have been infected with this virus before their second birthday. Some of the factors evaluated include the immune response (both innate and adaptive) to the virus (68–71) and host-related differences [gender, lung size, passive smoke exposure(61)] that may predispose an infant or child to lower airway physiological alterations as a consequence of RSV infection. Finally, the severity of the lower airway involvement (i.e., the development of bronchiolitis) may also influence the emergence of both asthma and allergic sensitization (2).

Studies Defining a Chronic Postviral Asthma-Like Phenotype in BN Rats

After exposure to an aerosol containing active Sendai virus, rats develop an acute bronchiolitis and interstitial pneumonia with a neutrophilic infiltrate by day 3 and an influx of lymphocytes at about days 5–7. Epithelial cell lysis, appearance of antiviral serum antibody, and disappearance of virus occur 5–10 days after inoculation (Fig. 1) (72–74). In adult rats, abnormalities in airway physiology, including airway obstruction and airway hyperresponsiveness, develop during the acute viral illness and persist for a few weeks after clearance of the virus and the acute infiltration of inflammatory cells from the airways (35). However, in contrast to rats infected as adults, in which airways normalize within 8 weeks of infection, BN rats infected during the first month of life (weanling period) may instead develop chronic morphological, histological and physiological abnormalities of the airways that persist for weeks (an asthma-like phenotype) (Fig. 1).

This single respiratory viral infection in rats during the first month of life may result in airway abnormalities that persist into adulthood. In the lungs from

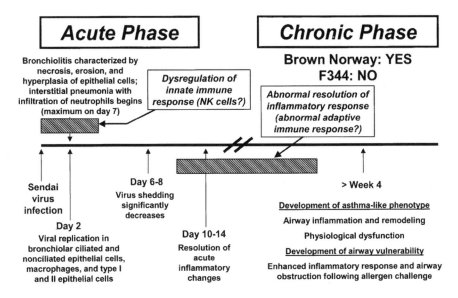

Figure 1 Development of an asthma-like phenotype following Sendai virus infection of BN, but not F344, weanling rats.

postbronchiolitis rats, terminal bronchioles have thickened walls due to increased extracellular matrix and collagen deposition, and increased numbers of mast cells, macrophages, and lymphoid aggregates; lung homogenates reveal increases in eosinophils (32,33,37,72,74,75). Airway obstruction can be detected as increased pulmonary resistance and decreased dynamic compliance in susceptible postbronchiolitis rats at times measured between 4 and 18 weeks after infection (32,34,36–38).

A longitudinal study involving six sets measurements in each rat between 11 and 18 weeks postinfection has revealed that airway obstruction has an episodic pattern, with the majority of postbronchiolitis rats having elevated pulmonary resistance during at least one of the six measurement times, but none having obstruction consistently over the repeated evaluations (38). Rats with elevated pulmonary resistance exhibit a reversible component when treated with bronchodilator, and also normalize their pulmonary resistance after a 3-day course of systemic glucocorticoid treatment (36,38). The steroid effect is transient, however, with airway obstruction returning within 1–3 weeks after the last glucocorticoid dose (38). The postbronchiolitis rats also have increased airway responsiveness to challenge with aerosolized methacholine (33,34,37).

We have also recently proposed tentative evidence that postbronchiolitis airways in BN rats may have an increased vulnerability to allergen exposure. In these preliminary studies, postviral, *Alternaria*-sensitized BN rats, when challenged with a low dosage of aerosolized *Alternaria* antigen that produced only mild airway inflammation and no airway obstruction in uninfected, *Alternaria*-sensitized BN rats, exhibited enhanced airway inflammation and airway obstruction compared with postviral rats not exposed to *Alternaria* antigen (76). These results suggest that post-bronchiolitis BN rats may have an increased susceptibility to allergen-induced exacerbations of chronic airway dysfunction. The presence, in postviral BN rats, of airways with increased vulnerability to allergen exposure would be consistent with a novel paradigm, recently developed by Holgate and colleagues, that implicates airway vulnerability as a critical factor in human asthma pathogenesis (77).

Thus, analogous to human asthma, the postbronchiolitis rats exhibit chronic, episodic airway obstruction that is reversible with glucocorticoid treatment (and relapses after cessation of treatment), chronic airway hyperresponsiveness, chronic airway inflammation that may involve mast cells and eosinophils, and chronic thickening of bronchiolar walls with collagen deposition at the basement membrane. This rat model is unique among animal models of asthma in that the airway abnormalities are chronic rather than transient, the initiating perturbation is an infection with a naturally occurring pathogen, and the experiments are controllable with respect to age, gender, environment, and genetic background.

B. What Is the Role of Atopy?

Cytokines and Atopy: Human Observations

Based on original work in rodents (78), lymphocyte cytokine elaboration has been organized into a Th1 [interferon (IFN)-γ, interleukin (IL)-2], and Th2 (IL-4, IL-5, IL-10, IL-13) pattern of response. This paradigm has received criticism for its simplicity in terms of the overall immune cytokine network (79), yet many groups have considered it as a useful starting point in unraveling the pathogenesis of allergic inflammation (80). The Th2 pattern of response has been found in tissue samples obtained at sites of allergic or parasitic inflammation, while the Th1 response has been more associated with delayed hypersensitivity and responses to virus infections and intracellular microorganisms. Th1- and Th2-type responses appear to be reciprocally regulated.

The extensive contribution of cytokines to the pathophysiology of asthmatic airway inflammation has received intense interest over the past decade (81–83). An intriguing related aspect of this research has been the observation that cytokine imbalance, or dysregulation, may play a role in the inception, development, and/or clinical expression of both allergic diseases and asthma. Aberrations in Th1 and Th2 cytokine production have been the most intensely studied. In this regard, at birth, most children have in-vitro-stimulated mononuclear cell Th1/Th2 cytokine profiles skewed in a Th2 direction (84). In children who are destined to be at increased risk of developing allergic diseases and/or asthma, a further diminution in cord blood mononuclear cell generation of IFN-γ (85,86) and IL-13 (87) has been noted, and the capacity of these children to generate normal IFN-γ responses lags behind a nonatopic control population as well (84,88,89). Mechanisms considered to contribute to these observations include both a diminished production of, and response to, IL-12 (90,91) and a posttranslational defect in IFN-γ secretion (92).

If defects in cytokine production contribute significantly to the development of atopic diseases, including asthma, one would expect that these defects should persist over time and be associated mechanistically with the clinical manifestations of various atopic phenotypes. As indicated above, investigators have demonstrated diminished secretion of IFN-γ from mononuclear cells in children and adults (91), some of which can be correlated with asthma disease severity (91). However, some groups have found increased levels of IFN-γ in bronchoalveolar lavage (BAL) fluid obtained from asthmatic children (93) and increased intracellular cytokine levels of IL-4 and IFN-γ from peripheral blood cells in asthmatic patients, but decreased levels of IFN-γ in atopic nonasthmatic patients (94). These latter observations have raised questions as to the specificity of these findings to asthma vs. atopy (or both), but have also suggested the possibility that if cytokine dysregulation contributes to disease, it may do so only at a critical time point in the overall development of the immune system. Also, it is important to note that imbalances in Th1/Th2 cytokine production have been observed in nonasthmatic patients (85,95). Thus, any observed aberrant findings may be more of a marker for atopy than for asthma. Although this type of cytokine profile may be a risk factor associated with the development of asthma, some other factor appears to be necessary to "push" a given individual toward the asthmatic phenotype. This second factor may be the development of a viral lower respiratory tract infection during a critical time of lung and/or immunological development.

Cytokines and Atopy: Animal Models

To determine the potential relationship of any of these observed defects in cytokine production to pathophysiological outcomes, studies in animal models have been performed. In a murine model of virus infection and allergic sensitization, IFN-γ was found to protect against the development of airway hyperresponsiveness if airway allergen exposure occurred weeks following influenza infection (96). Similar results have been noted by other groups not only on airway hyperresponsiveness but also on the development of pulmonary eosinophilia, mucus hypersecretion, and IgE production (97–99). In work described in more detail below, we have noted that IFN-γ treatment of genetically susceptible BN rats (Th2 skewed) immediately prior to and 1 week following Sendai virus inoculation prevents the development of a chronic asthmatic phenotype (41). Since these developments can be induced during the weanling but not adult period of life in this animal model, these results lend further support to the concept that cytokine dysregulation may only need to be present at a critical time in the development of the immune system in order to influence responses to various environmental factors such as viral infections.

Cytokines and Atopy: Influences of Genetic Background

After initial studies in outbred CD (Sprague-Dawley-derived) rats, three inbred strains were tested to determine if differences in genetic background might contribute to the likelihood of developing the chronic postbronchiolitis asthma-like phenotype. BN, F344, and Lewis inbred strains were compared in their responses to acute viral illness at an early age, based on previous reports of individual sensitivities to inflammatory challenges. (BN rats are known to be so-called atopic analogs, with eosinophilic and high IgE responses to allergen exposure. F344 and Lewis rats are both less sensitive to allergen, but are more likely to develop chronic pulmonary infections with *Mycoplasma pulmonis* and chronic arthritis, respectively.) After inoculation with Sendai virus, BN rats are the most sensitive and F344 rats the least sensitive: the BN rats have a larger neutrophil infiltration during the acute infection, larger numbers of bronchiolar mast cells and eosinophils after the infection, and a longer persistence of macrophage and lymphocyte-rich bronchiolar aggregates (37,75,100). BN and F344 rat strains differ also in their T-lymphocyte responses during acute viral illness: the BN rats have proportionally more CD4+ cells, and the F344 rats have more CD8+ cells identified by immunocytochemical studies of lung sections (101). A comparison of the responses of BN and F344 weanling rats to Sendai virus infection is summarized in Figure 1. Weanling rats from both strains experience the acute phase of the infection and develop bronchiolitis, but the strains differ markedly with respect to the resolution of the viral bronchiolitis. Postviral BN rats develop a chronic asthma-like phenotype characterized by airway inflammation, airway wall remodeling, airway hyperresponsiveness, and episodic, reversible airway obstruction (37). In contrast, this chronic phase is absent in the postviral F344 rats, who resolve the effects of the viral bronchiolitis and have normal airways (37).

We reasoned that strain-related differences in the innate and adaptive immune responses to acute viral infection and the subsequent development of a virus-induced asthma-like phenotype in rats may be caused by qualitative or quantitative differences in the cytokine response to viral infection, and/or changes in the pattern of cytokine responses induced by the infection. We therefore have begun to investigate virus-related expression of cytokines in order to understand the reasons why the postviral asthma-like phenotype develops in one rat strain and not in another.

During acute respiratory viral infection of weanlings, lung tissue from BN rats had lower amounts of mRNA for IFN-γ and higher amounts of IL-4 mRNA than that of F344 rats (101), suggesting a difference in the Th1 and Th2 cytokine responses of these two rat strains to viral infection. BN weanling rats, compared with F344 weanlings, also had significantly reduced peak levels of IFN-γ protein in their BAL fluid on day 5 after Sendai virus inoculation (Fig. 2) (102). Moreover, we have recently shown, in a preliminary study, that IL-13 levels in BAL fluid, although initially higher in postviral F344 rats, are persistently elevated in postviral BN rats for a prolonged period of time during which the F344 rats have undetectable levels (103). The mRNA for a profibrotic cytokine, transforming growth factor-β1, was more abundant, and remained elevated for more days, in the lung tissue of Sendai virus-infected BN rats than in F344 rats, consistent with the propensity of BN rats to develop postviral bronchiolar fibrosis (37).

In Vivo Studies Evaluating IFN-γ Expression

Based on data regarding IFN-γ dysregulation as a potential contributor to the inception of asthma (104), we designed experiments to characterize these potential relationships in more detail. We first completed an in vivo interventional study to determine the effect of intermittent enrichment of IFN-γ in the airways of young BN rats during viral illness (41). Weanling BN rats were exposed to an aerosol containing

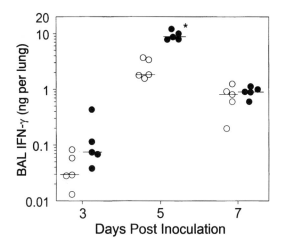

Figure 2 IFN-γ levels in BAL fluid from Sendai virus-infected BN and F344 weanling rats. BN and F344 rats were inoculated as weanlings with aerosolized Sendai virus. BAL fluid was harvested from the lungs of BN (○) and F344 (●) rats at the indicated times postinoculation (or from uninfected control rats) and then concentrated to a final volume of 1 ml. IFN-γ levels were measured by ELISA. Data represent values from individual rats of each strain. Bars indicate medians. BAL fluid from uninfected weanlings of each strain (n = 5) contained no detectable IFN-γ.* Significant difference (p < 0.01; Mann-Whitney test) between BN and F344 responses. (Adapted from Ref. 102.)

either phosphate-buffered saline (PBS) or recombinant rat IFN-γ from 2 days prior to inoculation with Sendai virus through postinoculation day 7. Lungs from each experimental group were obtained for viral titers during the first week, and for morphological/histological examination at 4 weeks postinoculation; physiological studies were conducted in the remaining rats at 8–10 weeks postinoculation. The IFN-γ treatment did not change Sendai virus replication, but there were significant treatment effects on the development of postviral bronchiolar fibrosis and bronchiolar inflammation, and on the development of postviral abnormalities in pulmonary physiology (41). Compared with the uninfected control group, postviral rats that had been treated with PBS had significant bronchiolar fibrosis and inflammation. The levels of bronchiolar fibrosis and inflammation in postviral rats that had been treated with IFN-γ were not significantly different from those of the uninfected control group (Fig. 3). PBS-treated postviral rats likewise exhibited pulmonary abnormalities characterized by elevated resistance and decreased dynamic compliance compared with uninfected rats, whereas measurements of resistance and dynamic compliance in the IFN-γ-treated postviral rats did not significantly differ from those of uninfected rats (Fig. 4). Therefore, this therapeutic intervention with aerosolized IFN-γ prevented the development of the postbronchiolitis airway sequelae the BN rats. These results indicate that the processes that produce the postviral asthma-like phenotype in BN rats are initiated, and may be modified, during the first week after infection. Furthermore, the presence of IFN-γ in the airways during the acute infec-

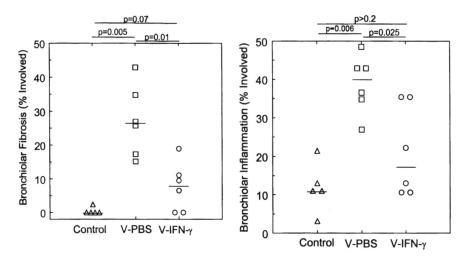

Figure 3 Bronchiolar fibrosis and inflammation at 4 weeks after inoculation. Postviral rats from the PBS-treated group (V-PBS) had significantly greater bronchiolar fibrosis and inflammation than both uninfected control and IFN-γ-treated postviral (V-IFN-γ) groups. The p values for pairwise group comparisons are above each plot. Each symbol represents one rat; bars indicate group medians. (Adapted from Ref. 41.)

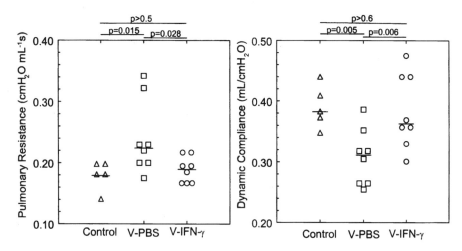

Figure 4 Pulmonary resistance and dynamic compliance at 8–10 weeks after inoculation. Postviral rats from the PBS-treated group (V-PBS) had significantly greater resistance and reduced dynamic compliance than both uninfected control and IFN-γ-treated postviral (V-IFN-γ) groups. The p values for pairwise group comparisons are above each plot. Each symbol represents the average of two measurements in one rat; bars indicate group medians. (Adapted from Ref. 41.)

tion is by itself sufficient to attenuate the development of the asthma-like phenotype, consistent with the idea that a relative deficiency in IFN-γ production may predispose the BN rat to the asthma-like phenotype. Finally, the postviral asthma-like phenotype is not invariably linked with differences in viral titers or viral clearance. Thus, in both humans and in this rat model, dysregulation in the production, release, and/or metabolism of IFN-γ appear to be playing a significant role in the development of the asthmatic phenotype.

In Vitro Studies Evaluating IFN-γ Expression

These in vivo results launched a series of in vitro experiments to permit a more comprehensive evaluation of potential mechanisms underlying these findings. These experiments are currently progressing from unfractionated spleen cells, to purified spleen cell populations, to unfractionated lung mononuclear cells, to purified lung cell populations. We first evaluated the response of splenocytes from uninfected weanling rats to Sendai virus or IL-12, a potent inducer of IFN-γ, and found that BN splenocytes produced significantly less IFN-γ following incubation for 24 h with either virus or IL-12 than did F344 splenocytes (102). Because splenocytes contain a number of different cell populations capable of producing IFN-γ (NK cells and CD8+ and CD4+ T cells), we have been investigating whether these various populations differ numerically between strains, and/or if individual cell populations differ in their individual ability to produce IFN-γ. Since NK cells are an important source of IFN-y during early innate host responses to viral infection (105), we first analyzed this cell population. Using flow cytometry, we determined that the frequency of NK cells in the spleens of weanling rats was significantly lower in the BN than in the F344 strain (102). We next purified the splenic NK cells from uninfected weanling BN and F344 rats by magnetic cell sorting and characterized their cytokine secretion profiles. NK cells obtained from BN weanling rats produced significantly less IFN-γ in response to IL-12 than did NK cells from F344 weanlings (Fig. 5) (102). We believe that NK cells are the primary IFN-γ-producing cells in the unfractionated splenocyte cultures because of experiments in which depletion of NK cells abrogated the ability of splenocytes to produce IFN-γ in response to either Sendai virus or IL-12 (unpublished observations, 2001). Recently, we have also found that Sendai virus induces IL-12 production in 24 h splenocyte cultures, and that splenocytes from BN weanlings produce significantly less IL-12 in response to Sendai virus than do those from F344 weanlings (unpublished observations). Therefore, a number of factors contribute to the reduced ability of splenocytes from BN weanlings to produce IFN-γ in response to Sendai virus or IL-12, including the reduced capacity of BN NK cells to produce IFN-γ in response to IL-12, the reduced frequency of NK cells in the BN spleens, and the reduced production of IL-12 by BN splenocytes in response to Sendai virus.

The mechanisms responsible for the reduced capacity of NK cells from BN weanlings, compared with those from F344 weanlings, to produce IFN-γ are still unclear. However, it is intriguing that we have identified two subpopulations of splenic NK cells based on the relative level of expression of the NK cell marker NKR-P1A as measured by flow cytometry: NKR-P1A+[bright] and NKR-P1A+[dim] cells

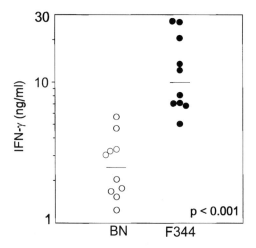

Figure 5 Comparison of the ability of NK cells from BN and F344 weanling rats to secrete IFN-γ in response to stimulation with IL-12. NK (NKR-P1A+ CD3−) cells were isolated from spleens of BN and F344 weanlings by magnetic cell sorting. BN (○) and F344 (•) NK cells were incubated for 24 h in the presence of IL-12 (2 ng/ml), and IFN-γ levels were measured in the supernatant fluids by ELISA. Data represent the means of triplicate cultures from 10 independent experiments comparing the responses of BN and F344 NK cells. Bars indicate medians. A Mann-Whitney test was used to compare the BN and F344 responses. Supernatant fluids from NK cells cultured in the absence of IL-12 contained no detectable IFN-γ. (Adapted from Ref. 102.)

(Fig. 6) (102). We consistently found a significantly higher percentage of NKR-P1A+ bright cells in F344 NK cell isolates than in BN isolates (102). This observation could contribute to the observed strain differences in IFN-γ production if NKR-P1A+ bright cells are more capable of secreting IFN-γ than are NKR-P1A+ dim cells. In fact, we have obtained preliminary evidence that increased levels of NKR-P1A expression are significantly correlated with an increased capacity to produce IFN-γ (106).

The target organ for Sendai virus infection in our model is the lung. In our studies, therefore, we are now focusing on the innate responses of lung mononuclear cells from weanling rats. Our preliminary studies indicate that the reduced ability of splenocytes and purified splenic NK cells from weanling BN rats to produce IFN-γ is consistent with data derived from experiments with lung mononuclear cells and purified lung NK cells. That is, lung mononuclear cells and lung NK cells from weanling BN rats, compared with those from F344 weanlings, also appear to have a reduced capacity to produce IFN-γ, validating the results obtained with spleen cells (107).

We have also embarked on studies comparing the ability of CD8+ and CD4+ T cells in BN and F344 weanling rats to produce IFN-γ because these cells may also be important sources of IFN-γ, particularly during the adaptive immune response to Sendai virus infection. In preliminary studies, strain differences in cell proliferation

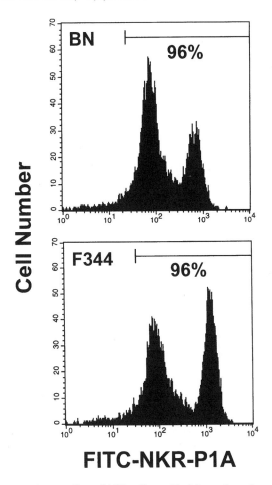

Figure 6 Flow cytometry profiles of NK cells purified from the spleens of weanling BN and F344 rats. NK (NKR-P1A+ CD3-) cells were isolated from spleens of BN and F344 weanlings by magnetic cell sorting. The intensity of staining of the BN (upper histogram) and F344 (lower histogram) cells with fluorescein isothiocyanate (FITC)-conjugated anti-NKR-P1A was determined using a flow cytometer. Splenocytes stained with a control FITC-labeled antibody were used to set the gates, and the percentage of positive cells (96%) is indicated. Two subpopulations of NK cells were consistently isolated: an NKR-P1A+[bright] and an NKR-P1A+[dim] population. (From Ref. 102.)

and IFN-γ production were also demonstrable in purified populations of splenic CD8+ T cells in response to in vitro stimulation with either immobilized antibodies to CD3 or CD3 plus CD28; CD8+ T cells from BN weanlings had significantly lower levels of proliferation and IFN-γ production than did CD8+ T cells from F344 weanlings (108). In contrast, splenic CD4+ T cells from BN and F344 weanling rats exhibited comparable levels of proliferation and IFN-γ production in response to stimulation with either immobilized antibodies to CD3 or CD3 plus CD28, suggesting that any strain differences in T-cell function may be specific to CD8+ T cells (108). Thus, strain differencces in IFN-γ production may involve both quantitative and qualitative mechanisms.

IFN-γ Dysregulation: A Developmental Component

In addition to strain (genetic) differences in both in vivo and in vitro responses following Sendai virus exposure, this animal model demonstrates developmental differences as well; BN rats develop the asthma-like phenotype when infected as weanlings but not as adults. To evaluate immune response differences (primarily focusing on differences in IFN-γ production) in relationship to age (development), a number of experiments have been conducted. Our preliminary data indicate that purified splenic NK cells obtained from weanling BN rats produce significantly less IFN-γ in response to IL-12 stimulation than do splenic NK cells from adult BN rats (109). We also have preliminary data indicating that the ratio of NKR-P1A+^{bright} to NKR-P1A+^{dim} cells was greater in BN adults than in BN weanlings, suggesting a developmentally regulated difference in NK cell subpopulations (109). As mentioned above, NK cells from F344 weanlings, compared with those from BN weanlings, also have an increased ratio of NKR-P1A+^{bright} to NKR-P1A+^{dim} cells, indicating the possibility that the strain-dependent differences in IFN-γ production by NK cells may reflect, at least in part, differences in the kinetics of NK cell ontogeny between the strains.

Effects of Immunomodulation on the Asthma-Like Phenotype in BN Rats

In addition to the above interventional study with IFN-γ, we have completed trials with other immunomodulator drugs, dexamethasone and imiquimod, testing the effects of each drug given during the first week of viral illness on the development of the postviral asthma-like phenotype in BN rats, and also the effects of each drug given after week 8 on the postviral airway obstruction. Dexamethasone was given by daily injection for a week, starting with the day of inoculation with Sendai virus, to weanling BN rats. Viral titers were measured in the lungs of some of the rats on day 7, and the remaining rats were evaluated for pulmonary physiology at weeks 9–12. Dexamethasone-treated rats had viral titers about 2 logs higher than the saline-treated group at day 7, but all rats recovered from the viral illness. At weeks 9–12, infected rats from both the dexamethasone and saline-treated groups had postviral airway obstruction, with no significant differences between the treatment groups with respect to pulmonary physiology. Thus, the glucocorticoid treatment compromised viral clearance but did not prevent the development of the postviral asthma-like phenotype (110). In an analogous study, imiquimod, an inducer of IFN-α production (along with smaller amounts of tumor necrosis factor-α and other related cytokines), was administered the day prior to inoculation and again on postinoculation days 3 and 7 in weanling BN rats. Despite slightly lower viral titers and fewer inflammatory cells in the BAL fluid during the first week after inoculation in the imiquimod-treated group, there was no difference in postviral airway obstruction between the imiquimod- and placebo-treated groups at 8–10 weeks (111).

Both imiquimod and dexamethasone were tested for effects on existing postviral airway obstruction as well. Both drugs had anti-inflammatory effects on the airways: lung sections from dexamethasone-treated rats had fewer bronchiolar inflammatory cells, and BAL fluid from imiquimod-treated rats showed a marked decrease in eosinophils. Pulmonary resistance also decreased significantly after treatment with either drug (36,38), although further monitoring of dexamethasone-treated rats revealed a return to pretreatment levels of resistance within 2–3 weeks (38). Thus, the chronic airway obstruction of the asthma-like phenotype appears to have an inflammatory component that is suppressed, but not eliminated, by a brief course of anti-inflammatory drug treatment.

Structure–Function Correlates in Rats Following Virus-Induced Airway Dysfunction

Qualitative and quantitative associations among histological/morphological and physiological changes that develop after viral infection at an early age may provide valuable insights to the underlying causative mechanisms. Our earlier studies in outbred CD strain rats infected with Sendai virus at 5 days of age revealed differences from uninfected controls with respect to alveolar dysplasia, bronchiolar wall thickening, and increased numbers of mast cells and eosinophils (32,33,73,74,112). Later comparisons of viral effects in sensitive BN rats and nonsensitive F344 rats revealed bronchiolar wall thickening and increased mast cells in BN rats, which had abnormal airway physiology, but no significant differences in bronchiolar wall thickness or mast cells in F344 rats, which also had no postviral physiological abnormalities (37). In contrast, the F344 rats were more sensitive than the BN rats to neonatal viral illness with respect to developing alveolar dysplasia (37); thus, the alveolar dysplasia does not appear to be a necessary feature for the postviral asthma-like phenotype. Subsequent studies in rats infected as 3–4-week-old weanlings, which have more fully developed alveoli and do not develop alveolar dysplasia (37), confirmed that the postviral asthma-like phenotype would develop independently of the presence of alveolar dysplasia.

In addition to comparing group responses of different strains, we have begun to examine associations between structure and function within a single inbred strain. Our study of BN rats 8–9 weeks after neonatal Sendai virus infection or inoculation with sterile vehicle revealed a significant correlation between the measures of airway obstruction and the bronchiolar mast cell density (36). This same study demonstrated that glucocorticoid treatment markedly depleted bronchiolar mast cells and reversed airway obstruction (36). However, there were significant differences between dexamethasone-treated rats of the postviral and uninfected groups with respect to dynamic lung compliance, which likely represented the physiological effects of bronchiolar fibrosis in the postviral group (36). We have developed techniques to measure lung volumes and elastic properties of the lungs (35). We have recently adapted these techniques for use in longitudinal studies, which will enable us to assess the physiological effects of airway fibrosis more precisely.

Airway wall thickening is believed to contribute to airway obstruction by ex-

aggerating the airway-narrowing effects of neural inputs or of inflammatory mediators (113,114), and it is possible that postviral changes in the bronchiolar extracellular matrix of BN rats may interact with other more variable bronchoconstrictor
mechanisms to create the episodic elevations in pulmonary resistance observed in the
postviral asthma-like phenotype. Inflammatory mediators also might contribute to episodic airway obstruction. In addition to the single-point correlates with bronchiolar
mast cells mentioned previously, we have conducted studies to evaluate correlates
between pulmonary physiology and inflammatory cells obtained via BAL in BN rats
studied repeatedly over several weeks. We developed techniques that allowed segmental BAL in rats without injury to their lungs, and we obtained paired measurements of
lung mechanics and BAL cell differential counts over a 4-week period of time (115).
We found that BN rats, known to have a prevalence of eosinophilic pulmonary inflammation within a group, also have spontaneous fluctuations in the proportion of
eosinophils in their BAL over time. Using analysis of covariance techniques to test
whether the percentage of eosinophils was associated with changes in lung mechanics
in individual rats of the postviral and uninfected groups, we found that the percentage
of eosinophils was a significant covariate for both resistance and dynamic compliance.
However, the association was present in the uninfected rats as well as the postviral rats,
the magnitude of the percentage of eosinophils effect was small, and the fluctuations in
the percentage of eosinophils did not predict the larger variations in lung mechanics
present in the postviral rats (116). Fluctuations of the other cell types in the BAL
had no relationship with changes in lung mechanics (116). Thus, how the interactions
among airway wall extracellular matrix, airway inflammatory processes, and airway
neural inputs result in episodic airway obstruction remains to be determined.

V. Summary

The data accumulated from this rat model have revealed that the development of
the asthma-like phenotype is dependent on three factors: cytokine dysregulation in
the susceptible strain (BN) characterized by a preferential Th2-like response, the
age of the animal (implying that certain aspects of pulmonary and/or immune system
developmental stages influence various outcomes), and the presence of a lower respiratory tract viral infection. These data, coupled with similar observations in humans,
suggest the following so-called two-hit hypothesis (summarized in Fig. 7). The development of the persistent wheezing phenotype in children, or childhood asthma,
requires the presence of at least two factors: first, dysregulation of cytokine responses at birth reflected by a diminished production of IFN-γ (genetic factor); and
second, the development of a clinically significant lower respiratory tract viral infection (primarily RSV bronchiolitis) (environmental factor) at a critical time point in
lung development.

Cytokine dysregulation (the evidence in both humans and our animal model
would suggest that aberrations in IFN-γ production are most likely involved) present
at birth is influential in determining the host response to viral infections. For example, if an infection occurs with a particular virus (i.e., RSV) at a critical time period

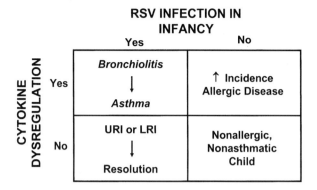

Figure 7 A so-called two-hit hypothesis for the inception of childhood asthma. The development of the persistent wheezing phenotype in children, or childhood asthma, requires at least two factors: dysregulation of cytokine responses at birth (genetic factor), and the development of a clinically significant lower respiratory tract viral infection (primarily RSV bronchiolitis: environmental factor) at a critical time in lung development.

(i.e., infancy), the combination of cytokine dysregulation and RSV infection may have a significant chance of producing the clinical phenotype of bronchiolitis and, over time, the development of the persistent wheezing phenotype or asthma. In contrast, infants and children who have demonstrable cytokine dysregulation but do not develop an infantile RSV infection have an increased probability to develop allergic disease, including asthma, which may have its initial presentation in later childhood or adolescence. In children with normal cytokine regulatory patterns, RSV infections can produce both upper and lower respiratory tract illnesses (the latter being more common in premature infants or in term infants with diminished pulmonary function at birth), but the wheezing and coughing associated with these infections resolve over time.

To establish and advance our knowledge about these very important relationships, experiments must be designed to answer the following questions. Is IFN-γ dysregulated in persistent wheezers or asthmatic children? If so, how early in life can these abnormalities be demonstrated? At birth? Following infection? As the child encounters his or her environment for various periods of time? Is IFN-γ the only cytokine that can be linked with such outcomes, or are other cytokines also relevant? If IFN-γ regulation can be shown to be causally linked with various outcomes, what is the mechanism of the defect (abnormal response due to decreased IL-12 production or diminished responses to IL-12?)? How closely do any demonstrable abnormalities in cytokine responses or regulation track with the development of antigen-specific IgE-antibody production or clinically apparent allergic disease such as atopic dermatitis, allergic rhinitis, and/or asthma? The BN rat model of virus-induced airway dysfunction described herein incorporates many, if not all, of the factors, which appear to be critical to the development of asthma in the first decade of life. Continued investigations using this model should provide information that will contribute significantly to our understanding of the relative influences that genetic and environmental risk factors have on the development of childhood asthma.

Acknowledgments

This work was supported by National Institutes of Health Grants AI-34891, HL-56396, and 1RO1HL61879–01

References

1. Prescott SL, Holt PG. Abnormalities in cord blood mononuclear cytokine production as a predictor of later atopic disease in childhood. Clin Exp Allergy 1998; 28:1313–1316.

2. Sigurs N, Bjarnason R, Sigurbergsson F, Kjellman B. Respiratory syncytial virus bronchiolitis in infancy is an important risk factor for asthma and allergy at age 7. Am J Respir Crit Care Med 2000; 161:1501–1507.

3. Renzi PM, Turgeon JP, Marcotte JE, Drblik SP, Bérubé D, Gagnon MF, Spier S. Reduced inteferon-γ production in infants with bronchiolitis and asthma. Am J Respir Crit Care Med 1999; 159:1417–1422.

4. Lemanske RF, Jr., Kaliner MA. Late phase allergic reactions. In: Middleton E Jr, Reed CE, Ellis EF, Adkinson NF Jr, Yunginger JW, Busse WW, eds. Allergy: Principles and Practice. St. Louis, MO: Mosby-Year Book, 1993:320–361.

5. Allan W, Carding SR, Eichelberger M, Doherty PC. Analyzing the distribution of cells expressing mRNA for T-cell receptor gamma and delta chains in a virus-induced inflammatory process. Cell Immunol 1992; 143:55–65.

6. Allan WZ, Tabi Z, Cleary A, Doherty PC. Cellular events in the lymph node and lung of mice with influenza: consequences of depleting CD4+ T cells. J Immunol 1990; 144:3980-3986.

7. Alwan WH, Kozlowska WJ, Openshaw PJ. Distinct types of lung disease caused by functional subsets of antiviral T cells. J Exp Med 1994; 179:81–89.

8. Borson DB, Brokaw JJ, Sekizawa K, Mcdonald DM, Nadel JA. Neutral endopeptidase and neurogenic inflammation in rats with respiratory infections. J Appl Physiol 1989; 66:2653–2658.

9. Buckner CK, Songsiridej V, Dick EC, Busse WW. In vivo and in vitro studies on the use of the guinea pig as a model for virus-provoked airway hyperreactivity. Am Rev Respir Dis 1985; 132:305-310.

10. Coyle AJ, Erard F, Bertrand C, Walti S, Pircher H, Le Gros G. Virus-specific CD8+ cells can switch to interleukin 5 production and induce airway eosinophilia. J Exp Med 1995; 181:1229–1233.

11. Doherty PC. Immune responses to viruses. In: Rich RR, Fleisher TA, Schwartz BD, Shearer WT, Strober W, eds. Clinical Immunology. Principles and Practice. St. Louis: Mosby-Year Book, 1996:535–549.

12. Dusser DJ, Jacoby DB, Djokic TD, Rubinstein I, Borson DB, Nadel JA. Virus induces airway hyperresponsiveness to tachykinins: role of neutral endopeptidase. J Appl Physiol 1989; 67:1504–1511.

13. Einarsson O, Geba GP, Zhu Z, Landry M, Elias JA. Interleukin-11: stimulation in vivo and in vitro by respiratory viruses and induction of airways hyperresponsiveness. J Clin Invest 1996; 4:915–924.

14. Einarsson O, Geba GP, Panuska JR, Zhu Z, Landry M, Elias JA. Asthma-associated viruses specifically induce lung stromal cells to produce interleukin-11, a mediator of airways hyperreactivity. Chest 1995; 107:132S-133S.

15. Elias JA, Zheng T, Einarsson O, Landry M, Trow T, Rebert N, Panuska JR. Epithelial interleukin-11. Regulation by cytokines, respiratory syncytial virus, and retinoic acid. J Biol Chem 1994; 269:22261–22268.

16. Folkerts G, Verheyen A, Janssen M, Nijkamp FP. Virus-induced airway hyperresponsiveness in the guinea pig can be transferred by bronchoalveolar cells. J Allergy Clin Immunol 1992; 90:364–372.

17. Hennet T, Ziltener HJ, Frei K, Peterhans E. A kinetic study of immune mediators in the lungs of mice infected with influenza-A virus. J Immunol 1992; 149:932–939.

18. Hou S, Doherty PC. Partitioning of responder CD8$^+$ T cells in lymph node and lung of mice and Sendai virus pneumonia by LECAM-1 and CD45RB phenotype. J Immunol 1993; 150:5494–5500.

19. Jacoby DB, Tamaoki J, Borson DB, Nadel JA. Influenza infection causes airway hyperresponsiveness by decreasing enkephalinase. J Appl Physiol 1988; 64:2653–2658.

20. Lemen RJ, Quan SF, Witten ML, Sobonya RE, Ray CG, Grad R. Canine parainfluenza type 2 bronchiolitis increases histamine responsiveness in beagle puppies. Am Rev Respir Dis 1990; 141:199–207.

21. Mcdonald DM. Respiratory tract infections increase susceptibility to neurogenic inflammation in the rat trachea. Am Rev Respir Dis 1988; 137:1432–1440.

22. Piedimonte G, Nadel JA, Umeno E, Mcdonald DM. Sendai virus infection potentiates neurogenic inflammation in the rat trachea. J Appl Physiol 1990; 68:754–760.

23. Saban R, Dick EC, Fishleder RI, Buckner CK. Enhancement by parainfluenza 3 infection of contractile responses to substance P and capsaicin in airway smooth muscle from the guinea pig. Am Rev Respir Dis 1987; 136:586–591.

24. Sarawar SR, Sangster M, Coffman RL, Doherty PC. Administration of anti-IFN-gamma antibody to β$_2$-microglobulin-deficient mice delays influenza virus clearance but does not switch the response to a T helper cell 2 phenotype. J Immunol 1994; 153: 1246–1253.

25. Scherle PA, Palladino G, Gerhard W. Mice can recover from pulmonary influenza virus infection in the absence of class I-restricted cytotoxic T cells. J Immunol 1992; 148:212–217.

26. Tang Y-W, Graham BS. Anti-IL-4 treatment at immunization modulates cytokine expression, reduces illness, and increases cytotoxic T lymphocyte activity in mice challenged with respiratory syncytial virus. J Clin Invest 1994; 94:1953–1958.

27. Yamawaki I, Geppetti P, Bertrand C, Chan B, Massion P, Piedimonte G, Nadel JA. Viral infection potentiates the increase in airway blood flow produced by substance P. J Appl Physiol 1995; 79:398–404.

28. Sorkness R, Johns K, Castleman WL, Lemanske RF, Jr. Late pulmonary allergic responses in actively but not passively IgE-sensitized rats. J Appl Physiol 1990; 69: 1012–1021.

29. Johns K, Sorkness R, Graziano F, Castleman W, Lemanske RF Jr. Contribution of upper airways to antigen-induced late airway obstructive responses in guinea pigs. Am Rev Respir Dis 1990; 142:138–142.

30. Sorkness R, Blythe S, Lemanske RF Jr. Pulmonary antigen challenge in rats passively sensitized with a monoclonal IgE antibody induces immediate but not late change in airway mechanics. Am Rev Respir Dis 1988; 138:1152–1156.

31. Blythe S, England D, Esser B, Junk P, Lemanske RF Jr. IgE antibody mediates inflammation of rat lung: histologic and bronchoalveolar lavage assessment. Am Rev Respir Dis 1986; 134:1246–1251.

32. Castleman WL, Sorkness RL, Lemanske RF Jr, Grasee G, Suyemoto MM. Neonatal

viral bronchiolitis and pneumonia induce bronchiolar hypoplasia and alveolar dysplasia in rats. Lab Invest 1988; 59:387–396.

33. Castleman WL, Sorkness RL, Lemanske RF, Jr., McAllister PK. Viral bronchiolitis during early life induces increased numbers of bronchiolar mast cells and airway hyperresponsiveness. Am J Pathol 1990; 137:821–831.

34. Sorkness R, Lemanske RF, Jr., Castleman WL. Persistent airway hyperresponsiveness after neonatal viral bronchiolitis in rats. J Appl Physiol 1991; 70:375–383.

35. Sorkness R, Clough JJ, Castleman WL, Lemanske RF, Jr. Virus-induced airway obstruction and parasympathetic hyperresponsiveness in adult rats. Am J Respir Crit Care Med 1994; 150:28–34.

36. Sheth KK, Sorkness RL, Clough JJ, McAllister PK, Castleman WL, Lemanske RF Jr. Reversal of persistent postbronchiolitis abnormalities with dexamethasone in rats. J Appl Physiol 1994; 76:333–338.

37. Uhl EW, Castleman WL, Sorkness RL, Busse WW, Lemanske RF Jr., McAllister PK. Parainfluenza virus-induced persistence of airway inflammation, fibrosis, and dysfunction associated with TGF-β1 expression in Brown Norway rats. Am J Respir Crit Care Med 1996; 154:1834–1842.

38. Kumar A, Sorkness R, Kaplan MR, Castleman WL, Lemanske RF Jr. Chronic, episodic, reversible airway obstruction after viral bronchiolitis in rats. Am J Respir Crit Care Med 1997; 155:130-134.

39. Stokes JR, Sorkness RL, Kaplan MR, Castleman WL, Tomai MA, Miller RL, Lemanske RF Jr. Attenuation of virus-induced airway dysfunction in rats treated with imiquimod. Eur Respir J 1998; 11:324–329.

40. Sorkness R, Lemanske RF Jr. Attenuation of airway hyperresponsiveness during acute viral infection using the 21-aminosteroid U-83836E in rats. Pulm Pharmacol 1996; 9: 219–222.

41. Sorkness RL, Castleman WL, Kumar A, Kaplan MR, Lemanske RF Jr. Prevention of chronic post-bronchiolitis airway sequelae with interferon-γ treatment in rats. Am J Respir Crit Care Med 1999; 160:705–710.

42. Sorkness RL, Mehta H, Kaplan MR, Miyasaka M, Hefle SL, Lemanske RF Jr. Effect of ICAM-1 blockade on lung inflammation and physiology during acute viral bronchiolitis in rats. Pediatr Res 2000; 47:819–824.

43. Lemanske RF Jr. Mechanisms of airway inflammation. Chest 1992; 101:372S-377S.

44. McFadden ER Jr, Gilbert IA. Asthma. N Engl J Med 1992; 327:1928–1937.

45. Calhoun WJ, Liu MC. Bronchoalveolar lavage and bronchial biopsy in asthma. In: Busse WW, Holgate ST, eds. Asthma and Rhinitis. Boston: Blackwell Scientific Publications, 1995:130-144.

46. Cypcar D, Stark J, Lemanske RF, Jr. The impact of respiratory infections on asthma. In: Stempel DA, Szefler SJ, eds. The Pediatric Clinics of North America. Philadelphia: WB Saunders, 1992:1259–1276.

47. Johnston SL, Pattemore PK, Sanderson G, Smith S, Lampe F, Josephs L, Symington P, O'Toole S, Myint SH, Tyrrell DA, Holgate ST. Role of virus infections in children with recurrent wheeze or cough. Thorax 1993; 48:1055.

48. Minor TE, Baker JW, Dick EC, DeMeo AN, Ouellette JJ, Cohen M, Reed CE. Greater frequency of viral respiratory infections in asthmatic children as compared with their nonasthmatic siblings. J Pediatr 1974; 85:472–477.

49. Minor TE, Dick EC, DeMeo AN, Ouellette JJ, Cohen M, Reed CE. Viruses as precipitants of asthmatic attacks in children. JAMA 1974; 227:292–298.

50. Johnston SL, Pattemore PK, Sanderson G, Smith S, Lampe F, Josephs L, Symington

P, O'Toole S, Myint SH, Tyrrell DAJ, Holgate ST. Community study of role of viral infections in exacerbations of asthma in 9–11 year old children. Br Med J 1995; 310: 1225-1228.

51. Henderson FW, Clyde WA Jr, Collier AM, Denny FW, Senior RJ, Sheaffer CI, Conley WG, Christian RM. The etiologic and epidemiologic spectrum of bronchiolitis in pediatric practice. J Pediatr 1979; 95:183–190.

52. Carlsen KH, Orstavik I, Leegaard J, Hoeg H. Respiratory virus infections and aeroallergens in acute bronchial asthma. Arch Dis Child 1984; 59:310–315.

53. Mertsola J, Ziegler T, Ruuskanen O, Vanto T, Koivikko A, Halonen P. Recurrent wheezy bronchitis and viral respiratory infections. Arch Dis Child 1991; 66:124–129.

54. Nicholson KG, Kent J, Hammersley V, Cancio E. Risk factors for lower respiratory complications of rhinovirus infections in elderly people living in the community: prospective cohort study. Br Med J 1996; 313:1119–1123.

55. Rylander E, Eriksson M, Pershagen G, Nordvall L, Ehrnst A, Ziegler T. Wheezing bronchitis in children. Incidence, viral infections, and other risk factors in a defined population. Pediatr Allergy Immunol 1996; 7:6–11.

56. Empey DW, Laitinen LA, Jacobs L, Gold WM, Nadel JA. Mechanisms of bronchial hyperreactivity in normal subjects after upper respiratory tract infection. Am Rev Respir Dis 1976; 113:131–139.

57. Grünberg K, Timmers MC, de Klerk EPA, Dick EC, Sterk PJ. Experimental rhinovirus 16 infection causes variable airway obstruction in subjects with atopic asthma. Am J Respir Crit Care Med 1999; 160:1375–1380.

58. Wohl MEB, Stigol L, Mead J. Resistance of the total respiratory system in healthy infants with bronchiolitis. Pediatrics 1969; 43:495–509.

59. Stokes GM, Milner AD, Hodges IGC, Groggins RC. Lung function abnormalities after acute bronchiolitis. J Pediatr 1981; 98:871–874.

60. Hall CB, Hall WJ, Gala CL, MaGill FB, Leddy JP. Long-term prospective study of children after respiratory syncytial virus infection. J Pediatr 1984; 105:358–364.

61. Martinez FD, Wright AL, Taussig LM, Holberg CJ, Halonen M, Morgan WJ, Group Health Medical Associates. Asthma and wheezing in the first six years of life. N Engl J Med 1995; 332:133-138.

62. Stein RT, Sherrill D, Morgan WJ, Holberg CJ, Halonen M, Taussig LM, Wright AL, Martinez FD. Respiratory syncytial virus in early life and risk of wheeze and allergy by age 13 years. Lancet 1999; 354:541–545.

63. Johnston SL, Pattemore PK, Sanderson G, Smith S, Campbell MJ, Josephs LK, Cunningham A, Robinson SB, Myint SH, Ward ME, Tyrrell DAJ, Holgate ST. The relationship between upper respiratory infections and hospital admissions for asthma: a time-trend analysis. Am J Respir Crit Care Med 1996; 154:654-660.

64. Landau LI. Bronchiolitis and asthma: are they related? Thorax 1994; 49:293–296.

65. Shay DK, Holman RC, Newman RD, Liu LL, Stout JW, Anderson LJ. Bronchiolitis-associated hospitalizations among US children, 1980–1996. JAMA 1999; 282:1440–1446.

66. Openshaw PJ. Immunological mechanisms in respiratory syncytial virus disease. Springer Semin Immunopathol 1995; 17:187–201.

67. Reijonen TM, Kotaniemi-Syrjänen A, Korhonen K, Korppi M. Predictors of asthma three years after hospital admission for wheezing in infancy. Pediatrics 2000; 106: 1406–1412.

68. Bendelja K, Gagro A, Bace A, Lokar-Kolbas R, Krsulovic-Hresic V, Drazenovic V, Mlinaric-Galinovic G, Rabatic S. Predominant type-2 response in infants with respira-

tory syncytial virus (RSV) infection demonstrated by cytokine flow cytometry. Clin Exp Allergy 2000; 121:332–338.

69. Bont L, Heijnen CJ, Kavelaars A, Van Aalderen WMC, Brus F, Draaisma JTM, Geelen SM, Kimpen JLL. Monocyte IL-10 production during respiratory syncytial virus bronchiolitis is associated with recurrent wheezing in a one-year follow-up study. Am J Respir Crit Care Med 2000; 161:1518–1523.

70. Domachowske JB, Rosenberg HF. Respiratory syncytial virus infection: Immune response, immunopathogenesis, and treatment. Clin Microbiol Rev 1999; 12:298–309.

71. Hall CB. Respiratory syncytial virus: a continuing culprit and conundrum. J Pediatr 1999; 135:S2-S7.

72. Sorden SD, Castleman WL. Virus-induced increases in bronchiolar mast cells in BN rats are associated with both local mast cell proliferation and increases in blood mast cell precursors. Lab Invest 1995; 73:197–204.

73. Castleman WL, Brundage-Anguish LJ, Kreitzer L, Neunschwander SB. Pathogenesis of bronchiolitis and pneumonia induced in neonatal and weanling rats by parainfluenza (Sendai) virus. Am J Pathol 1987; 129:277–286.

74. Castleman WL, Owens SB, Brundage-Anguish LJ. Acute and persistent alterations in pulmonary inflammatory cells and airway mast cells induced by Sendai virus infection in neonatal rats. Vet Pathol 1989; 26:18–25.

75. Sorden SD, Castleman WL. Virus-induced increases in airway mast cells in Brown Norway rats are associated with enhanced pulmonary viral replication and persisting lymphocytic infiltration. Exp Lung Res 1995; 21:197–213.

76. Sorkness RL, Tuffaha A, Lemanske RF Jr. Exacerbation of chronic airway dysfunction by low-level alternaria antigen exposure in post-bronchiolitis rats. Am J Respir Crit Care Med 163, A290. 2001 (abstract).

77. Holgate ST, Lackie P, Wilson S, Roche W, Davies D. Bronchial epithelium as a key regulator of airway allergen sensitization and remodeling in asthma. Am J Respir Crit Care Med 2001; 163: A290 (abstr).

78. Mossmann TR, Chrewinski H, Bond MW, Giedlin MA, Coffman RL. Two types of murine helper T cell clones. I. Definition according to profiles of lymphokine activities and secreted proteins. J Immunol 1986; 136:2348–2354.

79. Holtzman MJ, Sampath D, Castro M, Look DC, Jayaraman S. The one-two of T helper cells: does interferon-gamma knock out the TH2 hypothesis for asthma? Am J Respir Crit Care Med 1996; 14:316–318.

80. Umetsu DT, DeKruyff RH. TH1 and TH2 CD4$^+$ cells in human allergic diseases. J Allergy Clin Immunol 1997; 100:1-6.

81. Chung KF, Barnes PJ. Cytokines in asthma. Thorax 1999; 54:825–857.

82. Donovan CE, Finn PW. Immune mechanisms of childhood asthma. Thorax 1999; 54: 938–946.

83. Drazen JM, Arm JP, Austen KF. Sorting out the cytokines of asthma. J Exp Med 1996; 183:1–5.

84. Prescott SL, Macaubas C, Holt BJ, Smallacombe TB, Loh R, Sly PD, Holt PG. Transplacental priming of the human immune system to environmental allergens: universal skewing of initial T cell responses toward the Th2 cytokine profile. J Immunol 1998; 160:4730–4737.

85. Tang MLK, Kemp AS, Thorburn J, Hill DJ. Reduced interferon-gamma secretion in neonates and subsequent atopy. Lancet 1994; 344:983–985.

86. Matsui E, Kaneko H, Teramoto T, Fukao T, Inoue R, Kasahara K, Takemura M, Seishima M, Kondo N. Reduced IFNgamma production in response to IL-12 stimulation

and/or reduced IL-12 production in atopic patients. Clin Exp Allergy 2000; 30:1250–1256.

87. Williams TJ, Jones CA, Miles EA, Warner JO, Warner JA. Fetal and neonatal IL-13 production during pregnancy and at birth and subsequent development of atopic symptoms. J Allergy Clin Immunol 2000; 105:951–959.

88. Martinez FD, Stern DA, Wright AL, Holberg CJ, Taussig LM, Halonen M. Association of interleukin-2 and interferon-gamma production by blood mononuclear cells in infancy with parental allergy skin tests and with subsequent development of atopy. J Allergy Clin Immunol 1995; 96:652–660.

89. Hoekstra MO, Hoekstra Y, De Reus D, Rutger B, Gerritsen J, Kauffman HF. Interleukin-4, interferon-gamma and interleukin-5 in peripheral blood of children with moderate asthma. Clin Exp Allergy 1997; 27:1254–1260.

90. Chou CC, Huang MS, Hsieh KH, Chiang BL. Reduced IL-12 level correlates with decreased IFN-gamma secreting T cells but not natural killer cell activity in asthmatic children. Ann Allergy Asthma Immunol 1999; 82:479–484.

91. van der Pouw Kraan TCTM, Boeije LCM, de Groot ER, Stapel SO, Snijders A, Kapsenberg ML, van der Zee JS, Aarden LA. Reduced production of IL-12 and IL-12-dependent IFN-γ release in patients with allergic asthma. J Immunol 1997; 158:5560–5565.

92. Koning H, Neijens HJ, Baert MR, Oranje AP, Savelkoul HF. T cell subsets and cytokines in allergic and non-allergic children. I. Analysis of IL-4, IFN-gamma and IL-13 mRNA expression and protein production. Cytokine 1997; 9:416–426.

93. Marguet C, Jouen-Boedes F, Dean TP, Warner JO. Bronchoalveolar cell profiles in children with asthma, infantile wheeze, chronic cough, or cystic fibrosis. Am J Respir Crit Care Med 1999; 159:1533–1540.

94. Magnan AO, Mély LG, Camilla CA, Badier MM, Montero-Julian FA, Guillot CM, Casano BB, Prato SJ, Fert V, Bongrand P, Vervloet D. Assessment of the Th1/Th2 paradigm in whole blood in atopy and asthma. Increased IFN-γ-producing CD8+ T cells in asthma. Am J Respir Crit Care Med 2000; 161:1790-1796.

95. Lagier B, Pons N, Rivier A, Chanal I, Chanez P, Bousquet J, Pene J. Seasonal variations of interleukin-4 and interferon-gamma release by peripheral blood mononuclear cells from atopic subjects stimulated by polyclonal activators. J Allergy Clin Immunol 1995; 96:932–940.

96. Tsitoura DC, Kim S, Dabbagh K, Berry G, Lewis DB, Umetsu DT. Respiratory infection with influenza A virus interferes with the induction of tolerance to aeroallergens. J Immunol 2000; 165:3484–3491.

97. Hessel EM, Van Oosterhout AJM, Van Ark I, Van Esch B, Hofman G, Van Loveren H, Savelkoul HFJ, Nijkamp FP. Development of airway hyperresponsiveness is dependent on interferon-gamma and independent of eosinophil infiltration. Am J Respir Cell Mol Biol 1997; 16:325–334.

98. Cohn L, Homer RJ, Niu N, Bottomly K. T helper 1 cells and interferon gamma regulate allergic airway inflammation and mucus production. J Exp Med 1999; 190:1309–1318.

99. Dow SW, Schwarze J, Heath TD, Potter TA, Gelfand EW. Systemic and local interferon gamma gene delivery to the lungs for treatment of allergen-induced airway hyperresponsiveness in mice. Hum Gene Ther 1999; 10:1905–1914.

100. Sorden SD, Castleman WL. Brown Norway rats are high responders to bronchiolitis, pneumonia, and bronchiolar mastocytosis induced by parainfluenza virus. Exp Lung Res 1991; 17:1025–1045.

101. Castleman WL, Busse WW, Sorden SD, Dukes KR. Hyperresponsiveness of BN rats

to virus induced persistent lung dysfunction is associated with delayed viral clearance, high IL-4 and IL-5 response, and low CD8 cell and gamma-interferon response. Am J Respir Crit Care Med 1996; 153:A866. (abstract)

102. Mikus LD, Rosenthal LA, Sorkness RL, Lemanske RF, Jr. Reduced interferon-γ secretion by natural killer cells from rats susceptible to postviral chronic airway dysfunction. Am J Respir Cell Mol Biol 2001; 24:74–82.

103. Mikus LD, Rosenthal LA, Sorkness RL, Lemanske RF, Jr. Persistent IL-13 in BAL fluid is associated with post-viral chronic airway dysfunction. J Allergy Clin Immunol 2001; 107:S226 (abstract).

104. Halonen M, Martinez FD. A deficient capacity to produce interferon-gamma: is it a risk for asthma and allergies? Clin Exp Allergy 1997; 27:1234–1236.

105. Biron CA, Nguyen KB, Pien GC, Cousens LP, Salazar-Mather TP. Natural killer cells in antiviral defense: Function and regulation by innate cytokines. Ann Rev Immunol 1999; 17:189-220.

106. Mikus LD, Rosenthal LA, Tuffaha AS, Sorkness RL, Lemanske RF Jr. Reduced IFN-γ production is associated with differential expression of NK cell subpopulations. Am J Respir Crit Care Med 2001; 163:A522 (abstract).

107. Tuffaha A, Rosenthal LA, Mikus LD, Sorkness RL, Lemanske RF, Jr. Reduced interferon-γ production by lung mononuclear cells in rats susceptible to virus-induced airway dysfunction. J Allergy Clin Immunol 2001; 107:S228 (abstract).

108. Rosenthal LA, Mikus LD, Sorkness RL, Lemanske RF Jr. Reduced activation of CD8+, but not CD4+, T cells is associated with susceptibility to the development of a post-viral asthmatic phenotype. J Allergy Clin Immunol 2001; 107: S43 (abstract).

109. Mikus LD, Rosenthal LA, Sorkness RL, Lemanske RF Jr. Age-dependent regulation of interferon-γ production by natural killer cells from rats susceptible to the development of a post-viral asthma-like phenotype. Am J Respir Crit Care Med 2000; 161: A898 (abstract).

110. Kumar A, Sorkness R, Kaplan MR, Castleman WL, Lemanske RF Jr. Effects of dexamethasone administered during acute viral bronchiolitis in Brown Norway rats. J Allergy Clin Immunol 1996; 97:243 (abstract).

111. Varner AE, Sorkness RL, Kumar A, Kaplan MR, Miller R, Tomai M, Castleman WL, Lemanske RF Jr. Effects of imiquimod on post-viral asthma-like syndrome in BN rats. J Allergy Clin Immunol 1997; 99:S127 (abstract).

112. Castleman WL. Alterations in pulmonary ultrastructure and morphometric parameters induced by parainfluenza (Sendai) virus in rats during postnatal growth. Am J Pathol 1984; 114:322-335.

113. Wiggs BR, Bosken C, Pare PD, James A, Hogg JC. A model of airway narrowing in asthma and in chronic obstructive pulmonary disease. Am Rev Respir Dis 1992; 145: 1251–1258.

114. James AL, Pare PD, Hogg JC. The mechanics of airway narrowing in asthma. Am Rev Respir Dis 1989; 139:242–246.

115. Varner AE, Sorkness RL, Kumar A, Kaplan MR, Lemanske RF, Jr. Serial segmental bronchoalveolar lavage in individual rats. J Appl Physiol 1999; 87:1230–1233.

116. Sorkness R, Varner A, Kumar A, Kaplan M, Lemanske R Jr. Correlates between BAL inflammatory cells and pulmonary physiology in individual BN rats over time. Am J Respir Crit Care Med 1997; 155:A65 (abstract).

16

Human Experimental Models of Virus Infection and Asthma

PHILIP G. BARDIN

Monash Medical Centre and University
Melbourne, Australia

GWENDOLYN SANDERSON

Imperial College London
London, England

I. Introduction

Vaccination against smallpox and the eradication of the disease still stands as monumental achievements. In addition to its direct benefits in the prevention of a lethal disease, the method employed directed the thinking of later investigators to the use of volunteers in medical research. It is now more than 200 years since Jenner conducted his first experiments with vaccination. In recent years experimental viral disease programs in volunteers have been extended and refined, yielding many advances in knowledge of the epidemiology, transmission, and clinical manifestations of such diseases.

Kruze in Leipzig, to verify the proposal that the common cold was caused by filterable agents, performed the first studies of human experimental virus infection in 1914. In Britain, a Medical Research Council working group began studies in 1946 at the Harvard Hospital, Salisbury, providing space for 24 volunteers under good conditions of isolation and observation. A significant achievement of this program was the elucidation of methods of cultivation of rhinovirus (RV). Other early studies did not use volunteer isolation methods, but studied volunteers (after inoculation) in the community, which made it possible to include relatively large numbers of subjects. More recent work has used volunteer studies to examine the role of viruses in allergic disease and asthma. In these investigations subjects were evaluated in groups and physiological responses to viral infections were measured. A few detailed studies employing newer research techniques such as flexible fiberoptic bronchoscopy (FFB), mucosal biopsy, and immunohistochemistry have been performed. Although difficult, it remains a necessity to study mechanisms that relate virus-associated pathophysiology to cellular and immunological events, both in normal and atopic and asthmatic individuals. Furthermore, differences in the clinical expression of viral illness in these groups may provide clues to the operative mechanisms and provide a window for observation and investigation of such aspects not readily yielded by studies in normal volunteers.

Experimental infection has several advantages over naturally occurring infections when investigating the mechanisms of virus-induced asthma:

Known single agent with same inoculum in each subject reduces variability in data due to the agents themselves.
Known timing of sampling relative to initial infection and onset of symptoms reduces variability.
Homogeneous study group reduces variability in host responses.
Ability to sample more invasively under controlled conditions.
Ability to intervene prospectively with preventive and therapeutic agents.

Experimental infection studies that have been performed in the last 30 years employed RV, respiratory syncytial virus (RVS), and influenza A. The investigations were primarily done to improve understanding of the disease process and to assess the benefits of pharmaceutical agents (1–4). Important aspects of the pathogenesis of infection were revealed by such studies. Treatment with novel compounds such as the neuraminidase inhibitors (for example, oseltamivir, zanamivir) was demonstrated to be of considerable benefit. It remains of interest to know whether immune and tissue inflammatory responses in allergic and asthmatic patients are similar to changes in normal individuals; further studies are needed to assess this aspect.

Safety aspects and ethical considerations are naturally of prime importance and comprehensive safety testing of inocula must be performed prior to use in studies. These have recently been updated and now include many new recommendations, including screening of donors from whom nasal washes are obtained. In this chapter we review methodological and safety considerations during experimental infection, clinical and functional measurements, and bronchoscopic observations during such infections. Studies of RV will be outlined because this is the predominant type of viral infection used to date to study experimental associations with atopy and asthma, and because it has been demonstrated to be associated with exacerbations of asthma.

II. Preparation of Validated Inocula

Experimental viral disease studies in volunteers have been particularly useful in human RV infection, which is the most frequent cause of the common cold. Recent epidemiological studies have suggested that RV may be associated with the majority of exacerbations of asthma (5). Interest has consequently been focused on this particular group of viruses, and has prompted several recent human volunteer studies to examine this observation in more depth. Moreover, experimental RV cold studies in atopic individuals have demonstrated new late asthmatic reactions to allergen provocation in association with infection (6), underscoring the value of examining in vivo responses to viral disease. Rhinovirus serotype 16 infection has consistently induced changes in airway reactivity in volunteers; it is one of more than 100 rhinovirus serotypes causing the majority of common colds in the community.

Early (7,8) and more recent (9,10) human volunteer studies of RV colds have clarified many aspects of virus transmission, infectivity, serological responses, and immunity in normal subjects. Studies used safety-tested inocula prepared in-house using guidelines detailed in 1964 (11). Some workers used tissue culture fluids containing virus, while in others the virus used was obtained as a nasal washing from a volunteer or group of volunteers living in isolation. The methods used for safety testing at that time reflected current knowledge and practice and have developed greatly over the subsequent 40 years. Updated recommendations were recently suggested in a consensus report (12).

As a part of a larger program of investigation, our own studies in this area have recently employed these guidelines with modifications for the preparation of an inoculum. We compared changes in airway responsiveness (AR) in a validated and a new inoculum to seek additional evidence that virus–host interactions were preserved. These investigations demonstrate important principles in the preparation of inoculum and the overall design of experimental human studies of viral infection.

A. Design of Studies

Studies using experimental infection have generally been designed to evaluate patients prior to, during, and after recovery from infection (3,4,6,13,14). Subject numbers have varied widely but most studies included 15–30 patients. The use of so-called placebo mock inoculation has also varied given that patients can generally serve as their own controls for comparisons of various measurements. In studies that investigated the benefits of therapeutic agents, randomized controlled trials have been conducted (3,15).

An outline of a series of studies conducted in nonsmoking, clinically healthy volunteers is shown in Figure 1. This entailed various study-related procedures and aspects that will be discussed later. Volunteers did not have neutralizing antibody to RV 16 in their serum. A microneutralization test was used as previously detailed (14) and a negative test result required total absence of antibody. A validated inoculum of RV 16 was used in the first subjects, and a newly prepared inoculum was used in the subsequent volunteers.

Subjects were studied in three phases, having established absence of neutralizing antibody to RV 16 4 weeks prior to inoculation. In phase 1, baseline observations were conducted 14 days prior to viral inoculation and included symptom scores, obtaining serum for neutralizing antibody (again), and nasal washing for viral culture. In phase 2, subjects were isolated for 7 days during the experimental RV 16 infection. After a repeat of baseline tests, inoculation was performed and subjects

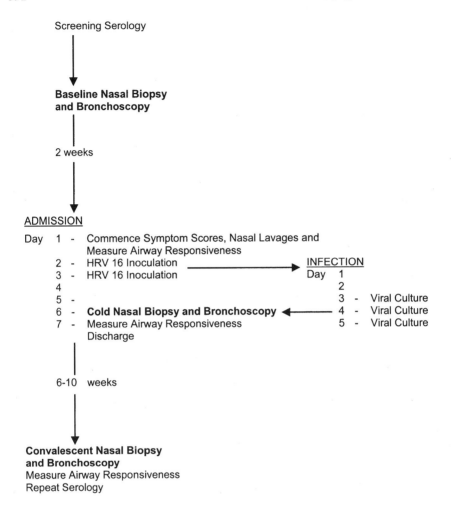

Screening Serology

**Baseline Nasal Biopsy
and Bronchoscopy**

2 weeks

ADMISSION

| Day | 1 | - | Commence Symptom Scores, Nasal Lavages and
Measure Airway Responsiveness |
	2	-	HRV 16 Inoculation ————————→ INFECTION
	3	-	HRV 16 Inoculation Day 1
	4		2
	5	-	3 - Viral Culture
	6	-	**Cold Nasal Biopsy and Bronchoscopy** ←——— 4 - Viral Culture
	7	-	Measure Airway Responsiveness 5 - Viral Culture
Discharge

6-10 weeks

**Convalescent Nasal Biopsy
and Bronchoscopy**
Measure Airway Responsiveness
Repeat Serology

Figure 1 Example of a study protocol for experimental RV studies (also incorporating various investigative procedures used in our studies). Neutralizing antibody to RV16 was measured 6–8 weeks prior to study to assess previous infection. Volunteers were isolated for 7 days during the study period.

then had daily nasal washes for 7 days, assessment of symptoms (16), and various procedures that constituted part of overall study protocols. In phase 3, investigations were repeated after 8–10 weeks (Fig. 1).

All subjects completed a validated questionnaire daily for 2 weeks prior to, during, and for 8–10 weeks after RV 16 infection. Nasal inoculation with virus was performed using RV16 suspension by spraying the virus ($10^3 \mathrm{TCID}_{50}$ in a volume of 0.5 mL) into each nostril using an atomizer (Fig. 2) and an equal amount as

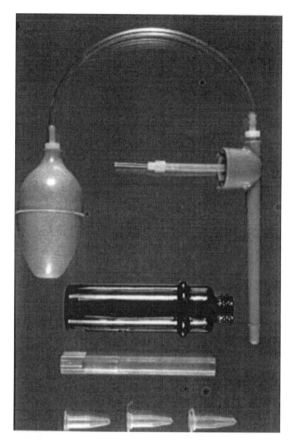

Figure 2 Atomizer used to inoculate volunteers. After inoculum was placed inside the atomizer, pressure on the bulb produced a fine spray that was directed into the nose. An RV16 dose of approximately $10^3 TCID_{50}$ was given.

droplets using a disposable pipette. Clinical illness was considered present if a volunteer had a minimum cumulative symptom score of 14 over a 4-day period, and had a subjective impression that he or she had a cold, or if rhinorrhea was present on at least 3 of the 5 days of observation (16). Positive infection was established by at least one identified viral isolate or a fourfold rise in titer of neutralizing antibody in some cases. Measurement of AR employing histamine bronchoprovocation was undertaken at baseline, on day 5 after infection, and at 8–10 weeks using a standard bronchial provocation technique (17).

Other investigators have used similar study designs and protocols (3–6,13–15,18). The inclusion of a placebo group has increased the power and ability of studies to differentiate between RV and other factors (for example, the effects of allergen) (15,18).

B. Safety Testing and Validation

Viral shedding was evaluated in the first volunteers, and subjects were chosen who had consistently produced high levels of RV16 in nasal washes. In addition, they did not belong to any high-risk groups for human immunodeficiency virus (HIV) infection (19). The nasal washes were divided into two pools and both pools examined for the presence of viral and other pathogens.

Virological, Bacterial, and Fungal Screening

Cultures

The two pools were filtered separately (Nalgene filters). Filtered inoculum [pool 1 (P1) and pool 2 (P2)] was divided into aliquots for subsequent use and vials of both pools were separated for screening. Inocula were cultured and passaged twice on HEp-2 cells (for respiratory syncytial virus and coxsackievirus B) and after neutralization with RV16 antiserum on MRC-5 (for adenoviruses, rhinoviruses, echoviruses, and some coxsackievirus A). Finally, P1 and P2 were cultured on LLC-MK$_2$ cells, which were subsequently stained and observed for influenza or parainfluenza viruses. Inocula were also observed for growth of *Haemophilus influenzae, Streptococcus pneumoniae*, and other bacteria using standard culture techniques. Fungi were not isolated on culture media, and no viruses were isolated and no bacterial growth was found.

Animal Inoculation

Three litters of suckling mice were inoculated intracerebrally (20 µl), intraperitoneally (50 µL), and subcutaneously (30 µL) within 24 h of birth. The mice were then monitored daily for 2 weeks for any signs of group A or B coxsackievirus infection, manifested by paralysis. The three litters of suckling mice survived 2 weeks and were healthy with no signs of paralysis.

Screening for Mycoplasma Pneumoniae

Tubes of Oxoid mycoplasma broth were inoculated (with a positive clinical sample as control) and incubated at 37°C for growth of *Mycoplasma pneumoniae* over a period of 3 months. *M. pneumoniae* was only demonstrated in the medium inoculated with a positive control sample. A sensitive polymerase chain reaction (PCR) (20) was used to exclude further the presence of *M. pneumoniae*. A reference preparation of M. pneumoniae was obtained and a dilution series was included as a positive control. Sensitivity of the PCR for *M. pneumoniae* detection was 10–50 organisms as reported previously (20), and PCR product of the expected number of base pairs was detected in positive controls, confirming the absence of PCR inhibitors.

Donor Serology

Serum was obtained from the seven subjects who contributed to the pools at the following times: 2 weeks prior to experimental colds and 6 weeks after RV16 colds. The following infections were sought employing serological techniques: *Legionella pneumophilia, M. pneumoniae,* psittacosis, Q fever, influenza A and B, respiratory syncytial virus, adenovirus, mumps virus, measles virus, cytomegalovirus, herpes simplex virus, varicella zoster, hepatitis B antigen, hepatitis C, *Treponema pallidum,* and HIV antibody. All this testing gave negative results (with three exceptions), and no rises in serum antibody to any of the pathogens tested were detected. For the three exceptions, low-level (four fold) rises in titer were noted to measles, adenovirus, and cytomegalovirus but patients had no indications of clinical infection and no abnormality of biochemical parameters (such as liver function measurements) was noted. Tests for HIV were repeated after 6–8 months and were negative.

Other Tests

Skin tests for tuberculosis with a purified protein derivative (PPD) were performed and a chest radiograph was obtained in volunteers 1–2 months after their RV16 cold. No abnormalities were noted on chest radiographs obtained from volunteers. Weakly positive PPD reactions were observed in three out of seven subjects, all of whom had received bacillus Calmette-Guérin (BCG) vaccination as children.

C. Physiological Responses to Experimental RV Infection

Overall more than 50 volunteers were screened for the presence of serum-neutralizing antibodies as part of the series of studies; 52% had antibodies present and 28% were unsuitable for other reasons such as smoking, unreliable attendance, and psychiatric illness. A clinical cold developed in 84% of subjects (21/25) inoculated as evaluated by symptom scores (16). Those who had low symptom scores (<14) all had positive viral cultures or significant rises ($>4\times$) in neutralizing antibodies. In comparing cold symptom scores in the two inoculum groups, no significant differences were noted (median scores 18 and 17.5, respectively). Nasal wash albumin levels have been shown to reflect accurately the severity of a cold (21), and in our studies revealed no differences between the two inoculation groups.

No differences were noted in other variables between the first subjects (validated inoculum) and the last subjects (new inoculum) entered into the study. The two inocula elicited similar antibody rises after infection. Significant increases in AR were noted both in the validated and new inoculum groups of volunteers. Median provocative concentration of histamine causing a 20% reduction in forced expiratory volume in 1 s $(FEV_1)(PC_{20})$ was 23.7 mg/mL before the cold and 14.3 mg/mL during the cold in the validated inoculum group. Values were 32.0 and 16.8 mg/mL, respectively, for the new inoculum group. Comparison of the degree of change in AR in each inoculum group did not reveal any difference.

In summary, the inocula were compared in two groups: an initial group of volunteers (validated inoculum) and a subsequent group of subjects (new inoculum). The clinical severity of the colds as measured by symptom scores was identical, as was viral shedding assessed by cytopathic effect (CPE) scores. Finally, the new inoculum induced significant increases in AR of a degree similar to the initial preparation.

D. Observations and Recommendations

Over the past four decades, large numbers of volunteers have been safely infected with respiratory viruses, particularly RV (3-6,13–15,18). In recent years, a number of new transmissible infectious agents have been discovered and there have been technological advances, which have improved methods for their detection in inoculum. Recommendations for safety testing have been published (12), concentrating on inocula prepared in cell culture (usually human embryonic lung cells) but they are now outdated and should be revised. Our studies have followed these guidelines in general, but additional investigations were performed based on new information.

The period between initial evaluation and retesting for HIV antibody status was set at 6 months because this has been judged to be an adequate length of time to identify persons infected but who had not yet developed antibody. However, the advent of sensitive assays to detect the virus itself makes it possible to screen volunteers accurately prior to study. None of the volunteers belonged to any of the recognized high-risk groups (19) and it is prudent for individuals in this group not to be considered for studies in which nasal secretions may be used later to produce inocula.

Because *M. pneumoniae* can be present in airway secretions and culture may be insensitive, a PCR yielding high detection sensitivity should be used. The presence of PCR inhibitors in nasal washes can be excluded using a reference strain of the organism as a positive control. Culture of *M. tuberculosis* is recommended in geographical areas with a high prevalence. Although testing for corona virus was not performed, PCR is recommended to exclude another important cause of common colds. Finally, the presence of particles such as prions should be considered in nasal secretions following nasal leakage of such proteins present in plasma. Their presence should be excluded using recently available methods of detection (22,23).

In conclusion, all new inocula should be assessed broadly employing the methods as described with updated versions since tests are always being introduced and refined. The safety and infectious assessments are of crucial importance and should be augmented by modern techniques for detection of viruses and infectious proteins. Validation of physiological responses is difficult but should be done using changes in symptom scores, seroconversion, AR, nasal and sputum cells, and cytokines to compare responses in new to validated inocula. Future development of recombinant virus inoculum may circumvent many of the recent safety concerns but will still require host response validation.

III. Experimental RV Infection in Normal and Atopic Subjects: Can Allergies Augment or Protect Against the Effects of RV Colds?

Although viral diseases are prevalent, the pathogenesis of symptoms and their relationship to atopic diseases such as asthma are not yet fully understood. Some investigators have suggested that atopic individuals may be more sensitive to the effects of viral infections as reflected by augmented airway responsiveness and the induction of late reactions in asthmatics (6). Atopic subjects may intrinsically be more prone to develop severe cold symptoms including chest symptoms. Human experimental disease has been a valuable tool to investigate this issue and our own and another recent study have examined whether clinical expression of rhinoviral colds is modulated by the allergic status of an individual (14,18). This section details aspects of this relationship that were investigated employing experimental RV infection.

A. Design of Studies and Measurements

Our studies examined nonsmoking nonatopic volunteers and nonsmoking atopic subjects who had no measurable antibody to RV16 in their serum at initial screening. Subjects were studied in three phases as detailed previously. Measurement of neutralizing antibodies was undertaken on serum (obtained 1–2 months prior to inoculation) from all volunteers before admission to the study (screening) as well as on the day prior to inoculation with RV16, day 3 of experimental disease, and finally 8–10 weeks later.

Skin-prick tests were performed using a panel of five common allergens with histamine used as a positive control and atopic individuals were defined as those with at least two positive tests to the allergens used. IgE was measured using a double-antibody solid-phase enzyme-linked immunosorbent assay (ELISA). All subjects completed a validated questionnaire (16) daily for 2 weeks prior to, during, and for 8–10 weeks after RV16 infection as described. Because a recent report had suggested that cold symptoms are influenced by alcohol intake (24), all subjects were contacted and their intake at the time quantified as the average number of drinks per day.

B. Patients and Response to Infection

Overall a definite clinical cold developed in 73% (16/22) of subjects as assessed by symptom scores. Subjects with scores below 14 were all normal individuals. However, these subjects all had either positive viral shedding and cultures or significant rises in neutralizing antibody to RV 16. All atopic volunteers had clinical colds based on symptom scores calculated after baseline rhinitic symptoms had been subtracted. Comparison of scores obtained from normal and atopic volunteers was not significantly different, partly as a result of a few very high scores in the normal volunteers.

Serological tests were performed 1–3 months before actual inoculation to screen subjects for admission into the study. Repeat baseline serology on the day before inoculation yielded unexpected results. In the normal group 44% of volunteers had developed an increase in antibody up to 1:8 dilution and in the atopic volunteers this had occurred in 50% of individuals. Taking this preinoculation antibody into account, a marked difference was noted between normal and atopic individuals in their symptomatic responses to infection. Normal volunteers with detectable antibody present tended to have mild symptoms as well as attenuated development of neutralizing antibody. This contrasted with atopic individuals, who

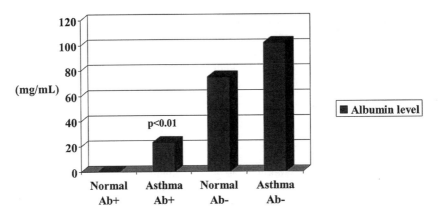

Figure 3 Changes in nasal albumin levels in normal and asthmatic individuals during RV experimental RV infections. There was an incremental increase in nasal albumin in the groups depending on whether they were asthmatic and whether neutralizing antibody to RV16 was present. This finding demonstrates the amplified tissue responses to RV present in asthmatics; an observation also supported by differences in symptom scores. Ab, neutralizing antibody. (Data from Ref. 14.)

had high cold symptom scores in spite of the presence of preinoculation antibody and small or absent serum antibody responses. The trend was for normal persons to have mild to severe symptoms whereas atopic individuals tended to all have severe symptoms irrespective of preinoculation neutralizing antibody status. Levels of IgE were not correlated with symptom scores, viral CPE scores, or serological responses.

Nasal albumin levels were similar in normal and atopic persons overall. With neutralizing antibody present in normal persons, nasal wash albumin was unchanged: but when preinoculation antibody was absent, they had an increase in nasal albumin. Contrasting results were obtained in the atopic group. Irrespective of neutralizing antibody, atopic individuals still developed significant cold symptoms in combination with increases in nasal albumin levels. There was a graded increase in nasal albumin changes associated with a cold, being lowest in normal antibody-positive individuals and highest in atopic antibody-negative subjects, again suggesting increased sensitivity (Fig. 3).

Studies by Avila and co-workers (18) compared the severity of RV16 experimental colds in 2 groups of 10 subjects with allergic rhinitis. Groups received three nasal allergen challenges or placebo a week before nasal inoculation with RV16. Subjects kept symptom diaries and had nasal lavages on days 2, 4, 7, 10, 15, and 30 after inoculation.

The two groups developed equal rates of infection (90%) as well as similar cold symptom scores in the allergen- and placebo-treated groups. Unexpectedly, there was a significant delay in the onset of cold symptoms in the allergen group. The duration of symptoms was also shorter. Cellular profiles in nasal lavage fluid were similar and an inverse correlation between the percentage of eosinophils in nasal lavage fluid before inoculation and severity of cold symptoms was noted. It was surprising that nasal allergic inflammation induced before RV16 infection failed to worsen the severity of cold symptoms and appeared to protect against the effects of RV colds.

C. Interpretation of Differences in Severity of RV Colds

There is general agreement that complications of viral respiratory infections are more likely in allergic and asthmatic patients (25–27). This raises the possibility that allergic inflammation amplifies the consequences of RV infection and the likelihood of exacerbated asthma.

We have found in volunteers that atopic individuals, in contrast to normal volunteers, tended to have more severe cold symptoms as well as greater increases in nasal albumin levels during RV colds. These studies suggested that the presence or absence of neutralizing antibody is the primary determinant of the host's clinical response to a RV cold. This overrides the effects of atopy and conceals its influence in any comparisons because of the relative severity of disease in normal antibody-negative individuals. However, when these antibody-negative normal and atopic groups are excluded from analysis, the increased sensitivity of atopic subjects (compared with normal individuals) becomes apparent. Prospectively designed studies are required to confirm these observations.

Atopic individuals may therefore exhibit an increased sensitivity to the consequences of a common cold, prompting the suggestion that allergic tissues were primed by the existing allergic disease (27). Although the mediators involved in cold symptoms are not defined, it can be speculated that the quantities of various cytokines (for example interleukin-8 [IL-8], granulocyte–macrophage colony-stimulating factor [GM-CSF], granulocyte CSF [G-CSF]) as well as inflammatory mediators (leukotrienes, kinins) may be increased in atopic tissues, causing more severe symptoms when released. Kinins are potent vasoactive peptides identified in nasal secretions during colds; they cause vasodilation and increased vascular permeability, and are probably generated in the nose during a cold (19). Additionally, because intercellular adhesion molecule-1 (ICAM-1) is the cellular receptor for the major group of RVs and may be upregulated in allergic inflammation, atopic individuals may be predisposed to higher rates of RV infection. This may then lead to even further increases in ICAM-1 accompanied by the nasal recruitment of mediator cells able to amplify existing inflammation.

In contrast, the results of studies by Avila and co-workers suggest a possible protective effect of allergy and seem to be at odds with our own and other studies. However, a number of methodological issues need to considered. Studies performed by others and us were conducted in normal and atopic individuals, whereas Avila and co-workers compared two groups of subjects who were both atopic; the studies are thus not directly comparable (6,14,18). It may be that the presence of allergic disease alone and not necessarily a recent allergen exposure increases the risk for virus-induced airway symptoms, hyperresponsiveness, and exacerbated asthma. Moreover, nasal antigen challenge before virus inoculation does not replicate natural exposure to allergen in which the dose is smaller but exposure more persistent. With high-dose allergen challenge there is an initial proinflammatory response that is gradually counterbalanced by IL-10, and other mediators with anti-inflammatory actions (for example, nitric oxide) may suppress RV infectivity. If this latter scenario was to take place after repeated allergen challenges, the inflammatory response to allergen would gradually downregulate and the effects of a RV infection would be blunted.

IV. Pulmonary Function, Bronchoscopy, and Induced Sputum in Human Experimental Models of Virus Infection

Flexible fiberoptic bronchoscopy (FFB), bronchoalveolar lavage (BAL), and endobronchial biopsies have been useful research tools in many pulmonary diseases and also asthma (29).

First performed in 1985 in asthmatic patients during RV infection (10), the technique has recently been used to examine lower airway infection during experimental infections.

Although changes in AR have been fairly well documented during experimental virus infection, changes in pulmonary function measurements have been difficult to detect. To an extent, the validity of human experimental infection models is dependent on the generation and documentation of changes in peak expiratory flow (PEF) and forced expiratory volume in 1 s (FEV_1) similar to that found in previous longitudinal studies in children and adults. It is feasible that RV infection induces transient decreases in PEF, possibly in the period after clinical cold symptoms have regressed and that this accompanies changes in AR. One way to study this possibility is to use experimental RV infection and to perform PEF measurements during and after the study period in normal, atopic, and asthmatic subjects. Our studies have used these methods during experimental infection to assess the lower airway effects of RV colds. Studies by Grunberg and co-workers have performed similar assessments and measured FEV_1 for the first 10 days using a microspirometer (1).

A. Bronchoscopic Observations

Subjects were again studied in three phases (Fig 1). Following RV16 inoculation, fiberoptic bronchoscopy was performed. Bronchoscopy, BAL, and biopsy were performed in a research bronchoscopy suite specifically dedicated to experimental studies of airway disease. Having adopted a strict protocol to ensure safety and comfort (29), more than 600 of these procedures have been performed by some centers in normal and asthmatic volunteers.

All volunteers who participated completed the studies including convalescent assessments and FFB. Chest symptoms, mostly cough, were noted in 80% of subjects but no exacerbations of wheezing were observed in asthmatics. All invasive research procedures, FFB in particular, were well tolerated. Few (8%) volunteers reported lethargy and a slight fever the day after bronchoscopy performed during their cold, and one subject had an episode of moderate pleuritic pain that resolved spontaneously within 36 h. In asthmatic subjects with a cold, bronchoscopy was well tolerated and oximetry and FEV$_1$ remained unchanged during and after the procedure, except for one asthmatic patient who had a transient decrease of 30% from baseline FEV$_1$ postbronchoscopy.

Macroscopic mucosal appearances observed during FFB were noticeably altered with a cold, particularly in the upper airways and trachea. In addition to irritability and increased mucus secretion during instrumentation, generalized redness and erythema were observed in the throat and larynx. Marked redness was also seen in the trachea in most subjects but changes were variable beyond the carina. Some subjects (and normal individuals in particular) appeared to have only minimal macroscopic evidence of mucosal inflammation more peripherally, although blotchy areas of redness could be observed in the larger airways. Observational images thus suggested spread of RV infection to the trachea in addition to upper airway involvement, but more peripheral spread appears uncertain and was not invariably and uniformly signified by the appearance of the endobronchial mucosa. These subjective observations are in some respects similar to the findings of an earlier bronchoscopic study in which RV was identified in tracheal cultures (10).

B. PEF and FEV$_1$ Measurements

PEF was measured with a mini-Wright peak flowmeter. Patients recorded the highest of three values on diary cards for at least 2 weeks prior to inoculation and for 8–10 weeks thereafter. Significant decreases in PEF were defined as 2 or more days at or below the 10th centile for morning PEF recording for that subject, preceded by a day above the median and followed by 2 days at or above the median.

PEF measurements were analyzed by charting morning values over the period of study. Thirty percent of subjects had significant decreases in PEF during or within 10 days of the start of their RV16 cold. A representative example from a subject with significant reductions in PEF is shown in Figure 4. It could not be determined if episodes were related to atopic or asthmatic status because of small subject numbers. However, measurements of FEV$_1$ were not significantly reduced with no significant changes in normal, atopic, and atopic asthmatic subjects.

Grunberg and co-workers (1) found similar changes at an earlier stage with a minimum in FEV$_1$ measured 2 days after inoculation. In the RV16 group the lowest FEV$_1$ correlated with cold score, asthma score, and changes in AR. Volunteers were allowed to live at home and were presumably exposed to an array of household and environmental allergens, which may have played an important role as a cofactor to elicit the changes observed in FEV$_1$.

C. Induced Sputum and Endobronchial Biopsy

Noninvasive sampling of the lower airway has recently been achieved using sputum induced after inhalation of hypertonic saline. The technique has now been used in several studies (both natural and experimental RV infections) to assess lower airway inflammation caused by RV (30–32). Studies by Grunberg and Gern and their co-workers have examined differential cell counts, IL-8, IL-6, G-CSF, IFN-γ – IL-5

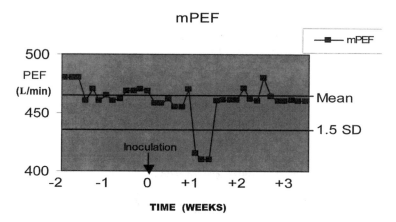

Figure 4 Changes in PEF observed after experimental RV16 infection in a volunteer. Significant reductions occurred 4–6 days after inoculation and showed a pattern similar to changes in PEF observed in outpatient studies of asthma exacerbations. (From Ref. 14.)

ratios, as well eosinophil cationic protein (ECP) levels in sputum (31,32). The results have provided evidence that RV cause augmented airway inflammation coupled to changes in AR.

Studies of induced sputum during experimental RV16 have highlighted the possible important role of neutrophils in airway events (31). Elevated numbers of both upper and lower airway neutrophils were detected that correlated with levels of IL-8 and G-CSF. The pattern of Th1- and Th2-like cytokine responses as indicated by changes in sputum IFN-γ mRNA and IL-5 mRNA was also assessed. RV infection increased both IFN-γ and IL-5, indicating activation of both types of cytokines. Ratios between the cytokine mRNAs (IFN-γ/IL-5) were inversely related to cold symptom scores and time to viral clearance. It suggests that the balance of responses may help to determine the outcome of common cold infections and that the individual's immune response, rather than atopic status per se, is important in this process. These studies again underlined the value and utility of experimental infections; our understanding of pathological processes will be dependent on future studies employing this methodology.

Endobronchial sampling by means of tissue biopsies has also been used to examine the lower-airway consequences of RV infection (25, 33, 35). These studies have revealed that inflammatory cells infiltrate the airway mucosa during infections and that lymphocytes appear to be the predominant cells present. There was also an excess of eosinophils in asthmatic subjects and they appear to be resident for at least 6 weeks after infection. We have recently used endobronchial tissue obtained during experimental infection to confirm spread of RV to the lower airway (35). Future work in this area is required to give a more comprehensive picture of lower airway tissue events during RV infections.

D. Summary

Some doubt existed as to whether a good number of suitable volunteers could be recruited for an arduous study, involving isolation, a cold, and two or three FFBs. Surprisingly, recruitment was relatively easy in the normal and atopic nonasthmatic groups. After a thorough explanation and some clarification, the majority of prospective volunteers were prepared to help and none of the volunteers terminated their involvement prematurely.

Only volunteers who were well motivated and who appeared to possess stable personalities were included: these factors may have contributed significantly to success. Recruitment of asthmatic volunteers was more difficult, chiefly because they represent a relatively small group that may have had reservations about this type of study. Although a formal evaluation of the tolerability of the various investigations and procedures was not done, overall assessment revealed that no serious problems were encountered. Bronchoscopy performed in mild asthmatic subjects during the cold appeared to be safe and O_2 saturation and FEV_1 results were generally unchanged.

The validity of experimental RV disease to serve as a model of wild-type infections in the community and of asthma exacerbations has been questioned. One possible way to link exacerbations and experimental infections was to demonstrate exacerbations using accepted PEF criteria. Such observations are not representative of real life but rather a model of it given that it would be ethically unjustified to induce real exacerbations. Significant decreases in PEF were demonstrated in up to one-third of our adult volunteers. Reductions in PEF were similar to changes detected in association with community-acquired RV colds (5,34). Most other experimental studies have not reported the results of longitudinal PEF data and may have missed changes that occurred after volunteers had recovered from the acute infection. The studies outlined suggest that experimental infection with RV16 may induce significant and measurable lower airway changes in respiratory physiology and function that accompany mucosal cellular and other changes in the bronchial tree. This favors a causative role for RV colds in asthma exacerbations and is in keeping with the concept of RV-induced worsening of airway inflammation.

V. Conclusion

Human experimental models of virus infections have been important tools to study the transmission, symptoms, and disease expression of viral respiratory diseases. Early studies (not experimental infection studies) led to the discovery of RV and coronaviruses and made it possible to clarify virus transmission and infectivity as well as to identify susceptibility factors in the human host. Subsequent experimental infection studies have helped to clarify many aspects of the disease pathogenesis and will contribute to future advances. Safety of inoculum is of paramount importance. Through the development of protocols for safety testing it has been possible to produce appropriate material for use in human studies.

In recent years the close association between viral respiratory infections and atopic and allergic diseases such as asthma has been increasingly recognized after Johnston and co-workers demonstrated the important role of RV in asthma exacerbations (5). Studies over the last 10 years have examined the lower airway effects of RV infection in more depth and demonstrated amplified responses in atopic and allergic individuals. Procedures such as bronchoscopy and bronchoalveolar lavage were introduced and found to be well tolerated and valuable, yielding important information on in vivo events during viral infection. Using careful studies of tissue obtained during experimental RV infections in combination with other methods, our recent studies have demonstrated lower airway infection by RV (35). Future studies will examine mechanisms by which lower airway responses to viruses may be mediated in susceptible individuals.

Future use of human experimental models of virus infection will be valuable to continue the study of various aspects of infectivity and host response and to clarify interactions with atopic disease. It will be of crucial importance to elucidate the molecular and immunological mechanisms by which symptoms are caused and airway function becomes altered. Future innovative use of experimental human infections will help to advance our understanding and knowledge of viral infections and the complex interactions between the virus and its host.

References

1. Grunberg K, Timmers MC, de Klerk EP, Dick EC, Sterk PJ. Experimental rhinovirus infection causes variable airway obstruction in subjects with atopic asthma. Am J Respir Crit Care Med 1999; 160: 1375–1380.
2. Mills J, Van Kirk JE, Wright PF, Chanock RM. Experimental respiratory syncytial virus infection in adults. Possible mechanisms of resistance to infection and illness. J Immunol 1971; 107: 123–130.
3. Hayden FG, Treanor JJ, Fritz RS, Lobo M, Betts RF, Miller M, Kinnersley N, Mills RG, Ward P, Straus SE. Use of the oral neuramidase inhibitor oseltamivir in experimental human influenza. JAMA 1999; 282:1240–1246.
4. Skoner DP, Doyle WJ, Seroky J, Fireman P. Lower airway responses to influenza A virus in healthy allergic and nonallergic subjects. Am J Respir Crit Care Med 1996; 154: 661-664.
5. Johnston SL, Pattemore PK, Sanderson G, Smith S, Lampe F, Joseph L, Symington P, O'Toole S, Myint SH, Tyrrell DA, Holgate ST. Community study of role of viral infections in exacerbations of asthma in 9–11 year old children. Br Med J 1995; 310: 1225-1229.
6. Lemanske RF, Dick EC Swenson CA, Vrts RF, Busse WW. Rhinovirus upper respiratory tract infection increases airway reactivity and late asthmatic reactions. J Clin Invest 1989; 83: 1–10.
7. Couch RB, Cate TR, Douglas GR, Gerone PJ, Knight V. Effect of route of inoculation on experimental respiratory viral disease in volunteers and evidence for airborne transmission. Bacteriol Rev 1966; 30: 517–529.
8. Mufson MA, Ludwig WM, James HD, Gauld LW, Rourke JA. Effect of neutralising antibody on experimental RV infection. JAMA 1963; 186: 578–584.

9. Meschievitz CK, Schultz SB, Dick EC. A model for obtaining predictable natural transmission of rhinovirus in human volunteers. J Infect Dis 1984; 150: 195–201.

10. Halperin SA, Eggleston PA, Beasley P, Suratt PM, Henley JO, Gröschel DHM. Exacerbations of asthma in adults during experimental rhinovirus infection. Am Rev Respir Dis 1985; 132: 976–980.

11. Knight V. The use of volunteers in medical virology. Progr Med Virol 1964; 6: 1–26.

12. Gwaltney JM, Hendley O, Hayden FG, McIntosh K, Hollinger FB, Melnick JL. Updated recommendations for safety-testing of viral inocula used in volunteer experiments of rhinovirus colds. Progr Med Virol 1992; 39: 256–263.

13. Grünberg K, Timmers MC, Smiths HH, De Klerk PA, Dick EC, Spaan WJM. Effect of experimental rhinovirus 16 colds on airway hyperresponsiveness to histamine and interleukin-8 in nasal lavage in asthmatic subjects in vivo. Clin Exp Allergy 1997; 27: 36–45.

14. Bardin PG, Fraenkel DJ, Sanderson G, Dorward M, Lau LCK, Johnston SL, Holgate ST. Amplified rhinovirus colds in atopic subjects. Clin Exp Allergy 1994; 24: 457–464.

15. Grunberg K, Sharon RF, Sont JK, In'T Veen CCM, Van Schadewyk WA, De Klerk EPA, Dick CR, Van Krieken JM, Sterk PJ. Rhinovirus-induced airway inflammation in asthma. Effect of treatment with inhaled corticosteroids before and during experimental infection. Am J Resp Crit Care Med 2001; 164: 1816-1822.

16. Dowling HF, Jackson GC, Inouye T. Transmission of the experimental common cold in volunteers II. The effect of certain host factors upon susceptibility. J Lab Clin Med 1957; 50: 516-525.

17. Townley RJ, Hopp RJ. Inhalation methods for the study of airway responsiveness. J Allergy Clin Immunol 1987; 80: 111-124.

18. Avila PC, Abisheganaden JA, Wong H, Liu J, Yagi S, Schnurr D, Kishiyama JL, Boushey HA. Effects of allergic inflammation of the nasal mucosa on the severity of rhinovirus 16 cold. J Allergy Clin Immunol 2000; 105: 923–932.

19. Bird AG, Gore SM, Burns SM, Duggie JG. Study of infection with HIV and related risk factors in young offenders' institution. Br Med J 1993; 307: 228–231.

20. Narita M, Matsuzono Y, Togashi T, Kajii M. DNA diagnosis of central nervous system infection with *Mycoplasma pneumoniae*. Pediatrics 1992; 90: 250–253.

21. Naclerio RM, Proud D, Lichtenstein LM, Kagey-Sobotka A, Hendley JO, Sorrentino J. Kinins are generated during experimental rhinovirus colds. J Infect Dis 1988; 157: 133-142.

22. MacGregor I. Prion protein and developments in its detection. Transfusion Med 2001; 11: 3–14.

23. Prusiner SB. Shattuck lecture—neurodegenerative diseases and prions. N Engl J Med 2001; 344: 1516–1526.

24. Cohen S, Tyrrell DAJ, Russell MAH, Jarvis MJ, Smith AP. Smoking, alcohol consumption and susceptibility to the common cold. Am J Public Health 1993; 83: 1277–1283.

25. Sterk PJ. Virus-induced airway hyperresponsiveness in man. Eur Respir J 1993; 6: 894–902.

26. Corne JM, Holgate ST. Mechanisms of virus induced exacerbations of asthma. Thorax 1997; 52: 380–389.

27. Folkerts G, Busse WW, Nikander K, Sorkness R, Gern JE. Virus-induced airway hyperresponsiveness and asthma. Am J Respir Cell Mol Biol 1998; 157:1708–1720.

28. Bardin PG, Johnston SL, Pattemore PK. Viruses as precipitants of asthma symptoms: II. Physiology and mechanisms. Clin Exp Allergy 1992; 22: 809–822.

29. Djukanovic R, Wilson JW, Lai CKW, Holgate ST Howarth PH. The safety aspects of

fiberoptic bronchoscopy, bronchoalveolar lavage, and endobronchial biopsy in asthma. Am Rev Respir Dis 1991; 143: 772–777.

30. Pizzichini MM, Pizzichini E, Eftimiadis A, Chauhan AJ, Johnston SL, Hussack P, Mahony J, Dolovich J, Hargreave FE. Asthma and natural colds. Inflammatory indices in induced sputum: a feasibility study. Am J Respir Crit Care Med 1998; 158: 1178-1184.

31. Gern JE, Vrtis R, Grindle KA, Swenson CA, Busse WW. Relationship of upper and lower airway cytokines to outcome of experimental rhinovirus infection. Am J Respir Crit Care Med 2000; 162: 2226–2231.

32. Grunberg K, Smits HH, Timmers MC, de Klerk EPA, Radbout JE, Dolhain M, Dick EC, Hiemstra PS, Sterk PJ. Experimental rhinovirus 16 infection: effects on cell differentials and soluble markers in sputum in asthmatic subjects. Am J Respir Crit Care Med 1997; 156: 609–616.

33. Fraenkel DJ, Bardin PG, Sanderson G, Lampe F, Johnston SL, Holgate ST. Lower airways inflammation during rhinovirus infections in normal and asthmatic subjects. Am J Resp Crit Care Med 1995; 151: 879–886.

34. Nicholson KG, Kent J, Ireland DC. Respiratory viruses and exacerbations of asthma in adults. Br Med J 1993; 307: 982-986.

35. Papadopoulos NG, Bates PJ, Bardin PG, Papi A, Leir SH, Fraenkel DJ, Meyer J, Lackie PM, Sanderson G, Holgate ST, Johnston SL. Rhinoviruses infect the lower airways. J Infect Dis 2000; 181: 1875–1884.

17

The Interactions of Virus Infection and Allergy

G. DANIEL BROOKS, JAMES E. GERN, and WILLIAM W. BUSSE

University of Wisconsin
Madison, Wisconsin, U.S.A.

I. Introduction

Respiratory viruses, particularly rhinoviruses (RV), are the most common cause of asthma exacerbations. Approximately 80% of asthma exacerbations in school-aged children and about 50% of exacerbations in adults have been associated with viral infections, of which rhinovirus is the most common (1,2). Although these events are common, the mechanisms by which a respiratory infection exacerbates asthma are not fully understood. Many studies have been conducted in humans, animals, and respiratory cell cultures to evaluate the interactions of viral infection with the allergic response. This review addresses two observations that stem from these experiments. First, there are distinct features of the immune response to viral infection in atopic individuals, and evidence for an interaction between allergic and virus-induced inflammation. Second, individuals with atopic disease may have different lower airway and immune responses to viral infection than normal individuals, and these differences may contribute to the viral effects on airway function.

II. Effects of Experimental Rhinovirus Infections on Allergic Responses

Experimental viral respiratory infections have provided an effective research tool to determine the effects of respiratory illnesses on allergen-induced changes in pulmonary physiology. For example, when atopic patients with asthma are challenged with a sufficient dose of inhaled allergen, they develop acute airflow obstruction. After this initial decline, the forced expiratory volume in 1 s (FEV_1) gradually improves. Some patients, however, have a second fall in FEV_1 that occurs 4–6 h later, termed the late asthmatic response (see Fig. 1). The late asthmatic response has been proposed as a model to study allergic inflammation. Based on this premise, we investigated the relationship between rhinovirus infections and the airway response to an inhaled allergen challenge (3). Four weeks prior to inoculation with rhinovirus type 16 (RV 16), 10 allergic subjects underwent an allergen challenge to establish baseline values. All of the subjects had an immediate decrease in their pulmonary function after the inhalation of allergen, but only one subject had a late-phase response. One month later, the subjects were inoculated with RV 16. All 10 were infected by RV 16, as demonstrated both by symptoms and rhinovirus recovery in the nasal washings. Forty-eight hours into the infection, the subjects demonstrated an increase in airway responsiveness to inhaled histamine. In addition, 8 of the 10 subjects now had a late-phase response to the allergen challenge. Four weeks later, the allergen challenge was repeated. The increased frequency of a late asthmatic response was still present. Using a similar protocol in eight volunteers with allergic rhinitis, parallel changes in lung function occurred (4). Methacholine, histamine,

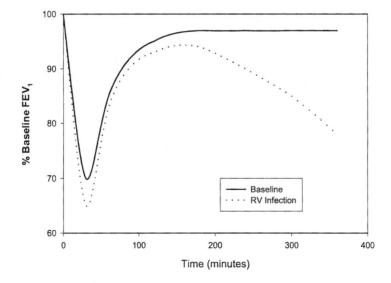

Figure 1 Effects of RV infection on allergen-induced airway responses (see text).

and antigen responsiveness all increased during viral infection. In summary, infection with rhinovirus increased the intensity of the early-phase pulmonary response to allergen and caused the appearance of a late-phase response. These findings suggest that viral infections can enhance the inflammatory response to inhaled allergen and that these infections promote allergic inflammation and thus the likelihood for increased asthma.

Another research technique, bronchoscopy with segmental antigen challenge, has also been used in combination with experimental RV 16 infection to determine whether virus infection amplifies allergen-induced cellular inflammation in the airways (5). During a segmental antigen challenge, a bronchoscope is introduced into the airway, and bronchial segments are identified. Saline is delivered into one segment, to act as a control, and antigen is introduced into a different segment. Bronchoalveolar lavage (BAL) is performed at the time of challenge (immediate response) and 48 h later (late response). Seven subjects with allergic rhinitis and five normal subjects were tested by segmental antigen challenge 1 month before RV 16 inoculation, during the acute infection, and 1 month postinfection. In allergic subjects, but not controls, enhanced histamine release to allergen challenge occurred during the experimental cold and was still present 1 month after the infection. Moreover, airway eosinophil recruitment following instilled antigen was increased in the late response during the cold.

A number of conclusions can be drawn from these experiments. First, RV infection changes the nature of the allergic airway response to inhaled antigen. During and after a cold, allergic subjects are more likely to generate an inflammatory response as indicated by the increased frequency of late-phase allergic reactions. Second, the changes in allergic responses are seen at a number of levels. Mast cell mediator release is enhanced as measured by greater histamine release to antigen at the time of the cold. In addition, the late allergic reaction is characterized by enhanced eosinophil recruitment to the lungs. The greater intensity of eosinophil recruitment during the cold may explain the greater frequency of the late-phase response to inhaled antigen. Finally, the enhanced allergic reaction is present for weeks after the cold. Collectively, these findings indicate that a rhinovirus respiratory infection can enhance and promote the allergic reaction to allergen. If similar effects occur during a natural cold, it is possible that asthma severity is increased.

III. Effects of Atopy on Outcomes of Experimental RV Infection

A. Lower Airway Responses

To compare airway responsiveness in normal subjects and those with allergic rhinitis (6), 18 subjects with allergic rhinitis and 13 normal volunteers were experimentally infected with RV 16. Baseline spirometry and histamine challenge were performed before inoculation and again 2 days after inoculation, at the time of an acute cold. The presence of allergy did not have a statistically significant effect on cold symptom scores or RV replication. However, during acute infection, the allergic subjects had

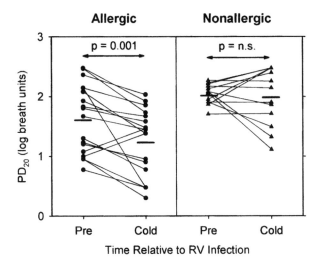

Figure 2 Effect of allergy on RV 16–induced changes in lower airway histamine responsiveness. Subjects were grouped according to the presence or absence of allergy, and histamine PD_{20} was plotted pre-cold (pre), and 2 days following RV 16 inoculation (cold). Heavy horizontal lines represent group mean data. (From Ref. 6.)

a significant increase in histamine responsiveness, whereas the normal subjects, as a group, did not have a significant change in this parameter of lung function (see Fig. 2).

Although these studies detect a consistent difference between normal and allergic subjects, other studies of RV 16 infection have had more variable results. For example, Fraenkel et al. (7) also found that RV 16 infection led to a significant increase in histamine responsiveness in asthmatic but not normal volunteers. However, Fleming and colleagues (8) were unable to show a change in methacholine responsiveness either in allergic or nonallergic subjects. In addition, experimental inoculation with other serotypes (RV 2, RV EL, and RV 39) did not consistently cause an increase in airway responsiveness in allergic subjects or controls (9,10). The difference in results among these RV studies is not readily apparent but could be secondary to variability in strain virulence, the inoculating dose or method, or measurement of histamine vs. methacholine responsiveness. It is also possible that individual subject differences exist.

B. Upper Airway Responses

Although upper airway responses to a viral infection differ from lower airway responses, there are practical advantages to the study of the nasal responses to infection. Several investigators have evaluated upper airway responses in allergic individuals; differences between allergic and nonallergic patients have been small. For example, Bardin and colleagues (11) infected 5 atopic nonasthmatic subjects, 6 atopic asthmatic subjects, and 11 normal individuals with RV 16. The difference in symptom scores between the groups was minimal; there was, however, an unexpected finding: several subjects in each group had positive RV 16 titers on the day of inoculation. The normal individuals with positive antibody titers developed mild symptoms, if any, whereas the atopic individuals, even with positive RV 16 titers, developed symptoms similar to antibody-negative individuals. This could indicate that atopic subjects have an enhanced susceptibility to infection, even with the presence of neutralizing antibodies.

Others have not found significant differences in upper airway response. Fleming and colleagues (8) examined nasal cytokine responses in atopic and nonatopic individuals. They found minimal differences in the responses of eosinophils, neutrophils, IL-6, and IL-8 between the two groups. Doyle and colleagues (12) compared atopic and nonatopic subjects inoculated with RV 39. They found little or no difference between groups in cold symptoms, T-cell responses, or nasal histamine challenges (13,14). Thus, experimental infections have demonstrated only small differences in the upper airway responses of allergic compared to nonallergic individuals.

IV. Allergic Mechanisms During Viral Infection

A. Histamine Responsiveness

Experimental RV 16 infections in humans have generally caused a change in airway responsiveness to inhaled histamine during infections (3,6,7). In contrast, experimental rhinovirus infections have had a variable effect on methacholine responsiveness (8,15). This raises the question of whether histamine-dependent mechanisms are more susceptible to virus effects or work through different mechanisms. Histamine contracts the airway directly by its effect on airway smooth muscle and indirectly through reflex responses. Methacholine, in contrast, acts only on airway smooth muscle. This difference suggests that indirect effects, possibly vagally mediated responses, are more likely to be affected by virus than a direct action on airway smooth muscle. This relationship also suggests a plausible mechanism by which chronic allergen exposure may induce histamine release and thus increase virus-induced asthma symptoms in allergic individuals.

More recent studies have focused on cytokine responses to virus instead of histamine or IgE-initiated responses. However, studies of at least one cytokine, IL-8, still indicate a possible interaction with histamine. IL-8 levels change during the immune response to virus both in allergic and nonallergic individuals, and correlate with clinical symptoms, histamine responsiveness, and viral shedding during experimental RV 16 infections (16,17). Douglass and colleagues (18) examined the upper respiratory effects of topical recombinant IL-8 on allergic and nonallergic subjects. IL-8 alone had little effect on symptoms or neutrophil infiltration in either group. However, if intranasal histamine was applied to the nasal mucosa prior to IL-8 challenge, neutrophilic airway secretions increased, as did symptoms of nasal congestion and nasal pain. In addition, a few atopics had a marked influx of eosinophils. The histamine appeared to have a priming effect on the nasal mucosa, favoring recruitment of granulocytes. Despite the small sample size, this study suggests that virus-induced cytokines might have increased effects in the presence of allergic inflammation, specifically histamine.

B. Granulocytic Inflammation

Both neutrophils and eosinophils serve as effector cells for immune reactions and probably play a role in host defense against viral respiratory infections as well as causing inflammation. Neutrophil counts in the peripheral blood increase during the acute phase of a RV infection (19,20). Grunberg and colleagues found that peripheral blood neutrophil counts correlated with symptoms and changes in airway hyperresponsiveness during experimental RV 16 infection (16).

During RV infection, there may be greater eosinophil recruitment to the airways of allergic individuals. Fraenkel and colleagues infected 11 normal and 6 atopic asthmatic subjects with RV 16 (7). Fiberoptic bronchoscopy was performed 2 weeks prior to inoculation, 4 days after inoculation, and again 6–10 weeks later. Submucosal lymphocytes and eosinophils were increased 4 days after infection in both groups. The lymphocytes returned to normal levels after infection. However, the eosinophils remained elevated for 6–10 weeks in the asthmatic group, but not in the normal group. This prolonged tissue eosinophilia may be due to changes in allergen responsiveness in the setting of natural allergen exposure. We have also seen persistent eosinophil recruitment to the airway after RV 16 infection and allergen challenge (5).

RV may also activate eosinophils. Levels of eosinophilic cationic protein (ECP) are thought to serve as a marker for eosinophil activation. Grunberg and colleagues (21) measured sputum ECP levels during RV 16 infection of subjects with mild asthma. The increase in ECP correlated with airway responsiveness to inhaled histamine, suggesting that eosinophils may contribute to this effect on the airway. Other investigators have discovered the presence of eosinophilic granule proteins in the nasal secretions of wheezing children with rhinovirus or RSV (22,23), suggesting that respiratory viruses may activate these cells to cause airway obstruction.

Animal models also support the importance of eosinophilic inflammation in airway hyperresponsiveness in viral infections. IL-5 is a potent activator of eosinophils, and antibodies against IL-5 (anti-IL-5) have been used in several experiments to explore the role of eosinophils in virus-induced airway hyperresponsiveness. Van Oosterhout et al. (24) found anti-IL-5 prevented an increase in airway responsiveness in guinea pigs infected with parainfluenza. Schwarze and colleagues (25) found that the RSV-induced hyperresponsiveness and concomitant eosinophil infiltration into the lung could be blocked by anti-IL-5. Furthermore, mice deficient in IL-5 were protected against RSV-induced hyperresponsiveness (26). Eosinophil infiltration could also be prevented with antibody against very late antigen-4, suggesting an effect on eosinophil migration. Thus, in human and animal studies there is evidence that respiratory viruses promote eosinophil recruitment and changes in airway responsiveness (26).

C. Th1 Versus Th2 Responses to Viral Infections

T cells have an important role in directing both allergic and virus-induced immune responses. T-helper cells can be categorized as either type 1 (Th1) or type 2 (Th2) based on their patterns of cytokine secretion. Allergens typically stimulate a Th2-like response with increased production of IL-4, IL-5, and IL-13. IL-4 and IL-13 stimulate the production of IgE, while IL-5 is involved in eosinophil production, recruitment, and activation. In contrast, many viral infections stimulate a Th1-like response with increased production of IFN-γ. IFN-γ plays an important role in immune defense through activation of macrophages, cytotoxic T cells, and natural killer cells. The Th1 and Th2 processes often inhibit one another, which may be an important consideration in the interaction of virus and allergic inflammation. For example, allergen-induced secretion of IL-4 could inhibit IFN-γ secretion, and, theoretically, alter the course of infection. In RSV-infected mice, a monoclonal antibody against IL-4 increased cytotoxic T-cell activity, decreased viral replication, and reduced the severity of the respiratory infection (27).

Animal models of RSV infection also point to mechanisms for the induction of a Th2 response. Alwan et al. have found that RSV attachment protein G can induce a Th2 type of response (28). Furthermore, if mice are given protein G-specific T cells, followed by RSV infection, there is more eosinophilia and more severe lung disease (29). Based on experiments like these, some have speculated that RSV may induce a Th2 response, which then contributes to the development of bronchiolitis and subsequent wheezing.

Many investigators have tried to determine whether Th2 cytokine profiles with naturally acquired RSV infections are associated with more severe disease; however, this is controversial. For example, Roman et al. (30) measured IL-4 and interferon gamma levels from phytohemagglutinin stimulated peripheral blood mononuclear cells (PBMCs) from infants hospitalized with RSV lower respiratory illness and healthy controls. An increase in the IL-4/IFN-γ ratio was found in infants infected with RSV. However, changes in these ratios were secondary to a reduction in interferon gamma, whereas the absolute level of IL-4 was actually reduced. Aberle et al. (31) measured IFN-γ mRNA in PBMCs of infants with RSV lower respiratory illness. Infants with an increase in IFN-γ mRNA did not require oxygen. In contrast, infants with no increase in IFN-γ mRNA did require oxygen, suggesting that IFN-γ responses may be important to control the infectious response, and that the degree to which IFN-γ is generated may reflect the immune responsiveness in some patients.

In contrast to these findings, two studies have suggested that a Th2 response is associated with milder RSV infections. Van Schaik et al. (32) found higher IFN-γ/IL-4 ratios in nasopharyngeal secretions or children with bronchiolitis than in those with isolated upper respiratory infection. Furthermore, Bendelja et al. (33) found that the percentage of IL-4 producing CD 4[+] and CD 8[+] lymphocytes in peripheral blood was higher in the infants with milder RSV infections. Additional information is needed to sort out the relationship among T-cell responses, Th1 and Th2 cytokine production, and the severity of RSV infection.

There are data to suggest that the character of the mononuclear response during the acute infection is an indication of the risk of subsequent wheezing. For example, Renzi et al. (34) measured IFN-γ production from IL-2-stimulated peripheral blood mononuclear cells obtained from infants with bronchiolitis. Reduced IFN-γ responses during infection and 5 months later were associated with a diagnosis of probable asthma that was made two years later. Studies are now underway to determine whether mononuclear cell responses measured before RSV infection can predict the outcome of the infection (35).

Virus-specific Th2 cells have rarely been isolated from humans during acute infection; however, indirect evidence exists that these cells are present. The generation of IgE specific to RSV and parainfluenza infection has been detected in some children (36,37). The ability of specific viral antigens to cause a Th2 type of response has also been evaluated. Jackson and Scott (38) developed T-cell lines with peripheral blood samples from adults with serological evidence of a prior RSV infection. T cells specific to protein F or live RSV secreted a Th1 cytokine pattern, whereas T cells specific for protein G or fixed RSV secreted a Th2 cytokine pattern. The relevance of these findings during an infection with live virus is not clear, although there are obvious implications for vaccine development. Rhinovirus-specific T-cell clones have also been isolated from the peripheral blood of human subjects, but the patterns of cytokine secretion were most consistent with a predominant Th1 response (39). All 29 clones isolated from a rhinovirus-infected individual secreted primarily IFN-γ when incubated with rhinovirus, although some of these clones also released small amounts of IL-4 and/or IL-5.

The conversion of viral protein specific T-cell subsets to a Th2 profile by allergen exposure has been demonstrated in an animal model. Coyle and colleagues (40) have found that virus-specific CD 8[+] cells can switch to IL-5 production if exposed to IL-4 or ovalbumin in mice. They developed transgenic mice having a large portion of CD 8[+] cells that express MHC specific for a peptide from lymphocytic choriomeningitis virus (LCMV). The mice were sensitized with ovalbumin or placebo, and LCMV peptide was then delivered intranasally. Lung T cells were obtained 72 h later and restimulated with LCMV peptide in vitro. The mice exposed to ovalbumin secreted more IL-5 but less interferon than controls. In a second series of experiments, LCMV-specific CD 8[+] cells were incubated with viral peptide and IL-4. The cells had the same response as in the ovalbumin-sensitized mice, demonstrating the creation of a Th2 subset. This observation shows that, under the appropriate conditions, virus-specific T cells may be driven toward a Th2 phenotype by a subsequent allergen sensitization, and thus suggests a potential mechanism for production of virus-specific IgE.

D.   Intracellular Adhesion Molecule-1 and Rhinovirus

Intracellular adhesion molecule-1 (ICAM-1) is important for T-cell, neutrophil, and eosinophil recruitment to the lung (41,42). ICAM-1 expression is increased in the bronchial mucosa of asthmatic patients and increases even further after allergen challenge (43,44). In the nasal mucosa of patients with allergic rhinitis, ICAM-1 has a greater expression than in nonallergic patients, and its expression is even higher during their allergy season (45). Despite this increased expression of ICAM-1 in allergic inflammation, it is unknown whether this causes, or even contributes to, the development of allergic rhinitis, asthma, asthma exacerbations, or susceptibility for a cold.

For 90% of the rhinovirus subtypes, ICAM-1 is the receptor for virus attachment and entry into cells (46,47). In addition, experimental infection of bronchial and pulmonary epithelial cell lines with RV 16 upregulates ICAM-1 (48), suggesting two possible interactions between the virus and allergic inflammation. First, because atopic patients have increased expression of rhinovirus receptors (ICAM-1), they may have increased susceptibility to infection. Second, because rhinovirus infection can induce more ICAM-1, infection may lead to an increase in infectious and allergic inflammation.

Bianco and colleagues (49) used an in vitro model to investigate the hypothesis that increased expression of ICAM-1 in atopic patients enhances patient susceptibility to rhinovirus infection. In an earlier study (50), they had infected epithelial cell cultures in vitro with RV 14 to examine the effects of various cytokines on RV-induced ICAM-1. Tumor necrosis factor α and IL-8 both enhance ICAM-1 expression. However, IFN-γ decreases ICAM-1 expression in infected epithelial cell cultures while increasing ICAM-1 expression in uninfected cell cultures. In a second set of experiments, the effect of allergic cytokines on rhinovirus-induced ICAM-1 expression was evaluated (49). Bronchial epithelial cells were cultured with varying concentrations of IL-4, IL-5, IL-10, and IL-13 for 24 h and then infected with RV 16. Incubation with IL-4, IL-5, or IL-13 prior to infection increases the expression of ICAM-1 more than infection alone. About twice as many cells were infected in the group that had been incubated with the Th2 cytokines, suggesting that the allergic cytokines may increase epithelial cell susceptibility to rhinovirus infection. Furthermore, viral replication was significantly higher in epithelial cells that had been incubated in the Th2 cytokines. Thus, incubating epithelial cell lines with Th2 cytokines in vitro supports the hypothesis that allergic inflammation increases susceptibility to rhinovirus.

A second hypothesis suggests that by upregulating epithelial cell ICAM-1 expression, respiratory viruses promote the binding of inflammatory cells to the epithelium, and thereby enhance epithelial cell damage. Rhinovirus, respiratory syncytial virus, parainfluenza virus, and adenovirus can all increase expression of ICAM-1 in respiratory cells or cell lines (42,51–53). The importance of ICAM-1 expression to airway inflammation is supported by a study of parainfluenza-induced bronchiolitis in rats (54). Administering an anti-ICAM-1-blocking antibody to virus-infected rats caused a small but significant decrease in the effects of the virus on methacholine responsiveness.

Glucocorticoids reduce expression of ICAM-1 in cell lines, probably through transcriptional repression of the ICAM-1 gene; this may not apply to primary bronchial tissue (55). Six weeks of inhaled beclomethasone did not decrease expression of ICAM-1 in bronchial biopsy specimens (56), even though topical glucocorticoid therapy of other clinical conditions has resulted in decreased levels of ICAM-1

(57,58). However, the question of whether glucocorticoids can alter the induction of ICAM-1 by respiratory viruses is slightly different and has been addressed in two in vitro studies. Papi and colleagues (59) found that corticosteroid treatment inhibits ICAM-1 mRNA induction during RV 16 infection of cultured bronchial epithelial cells. Corticosteroid treatment also inhibits the induction of ICAM-1 during RV 14 infection of tracheal epithelial cells (60).

Finally, Grunberg and colleagues (53) evaluated whether inhaled corticosteroid treatment could prevent the ICAM-1 induction by rhinovirus. Twenty-five atopic asthmatic subjects were randomly assigned to receive either placebo or budesonide (800 μg twice daily for 2 weeks). Bronchoscopy with bronchial biopsy was performed 2 days before and 6 days after inoculation with either RV 16 or placebo. ICAM-1 expression increased after infection, but budesonide did not significantly affect its expression either before or after rhinovirus infection.

In summary, RV infection can induce ICAM-1 and this effect is greater in the presence of Th2 cytokines. Allergic individuals, with greater Th2 cytokine production, may provide more ICAM-1 sites for RV binding and therefore have an enhanced susceptibility.

E. Allergic Sensitization in Animal Models of Viral Infection

Experiments in animal models have evaluated whether viral infections augment allergic inflammation (see Table 1). Allergic sensitization of animals usually involves short-term exposure to relatively high concentrations of airborne allergens. O'Donnell and Openshaw (61) studied the effects of a RSV or influenza A infection on allergic sensitization in mice. The mice were inoculated with RSV, influenza, or placebo, and then underwent allergic sensitization. Nebulized ovalbumin was given to the mice for 20 min every day for 10 days. The mice were then given subcutaneous ovalbumin 5 days later. Mice that had been infected with RSV or influenza had anaphylaxis to ovalbumin, while the uninfected mice did not. O'Donnell and Openshaw's experiment suggest that a respiratory virus infection can act as an adjuvant during allergic sensitization. The mechanism of these effects was not defined in these experiments.

Several other investigators have also studied the effects of viral infections on allergen specific IgE production. Sakamoto and colleagues (62) evaluated the sensitization of mice to a single dose of inhaled ovalbumin with alum adjuvant at

Table 1 Effects of Respiratory Virus Infection in Animal Models of Allergen Sensitization

Laboratory parameters	Physiological observations
↑Allergen-specific IgE production	↑Airway responsiveness
↑Th2 cytokine production	Promotes anaphylaxis
↑Pulmonary eosinophils	

various times after infection with influenza. Sensitization occurred if allergen exposure was within 2–6 days of virus inoculation. Leibovitz and colleagues (63) infected mice with RSV and then exposed them to inhaled ragweed antigen in alum adjuvant. The infected animals had a small increase (10–25%) in ragweed-specific IgE, IgG, and IgA responses.

These observations have been extended to allergen sensitization of the lung. Schwarze and colleagues (25) evaluated the relationship among ovalbumin sensitization, methacholine responsiveness, and experimental RSV infection in mice. Mice exposed to nebulized ovalbumin sensitization did not develop changes in airway hyperresponsiveness. However, if the mice were inoculated with RSV prior to ovalbumin exposure, there was a significant increase in airway responsiveness. Sensitization was associated both with neutrophilic and eosinophilic inflammation of the lungs. Noninfectious UV-irradiated virus did not cause this effect. Administration of anti-IL-5 monoclonal antibodies prevented eosinophilic inflammation and the increase in airway responsiveness in the mice, but not the neutrophilic inflammation. These findings suggest that IL-5 generation, possibly as a response to the RSV virus, caused the changes in inflammation and airway responsiveness. Neither IgG_1 nor IgE to ovalbumin was increased. Suzuki et al. (64) also developed a protocol for sensitizing mice with aerosol exposures to ovalbumin: mice infected with influenza developed increased airway responsiveness and ovalbumin-specific IgE.

Several investigators have developed tolerance-inducing procedures to inhibit allergen sensitization. Viral infections appear to mitigate the induction of tolerance. For example, Holt and colleagues (65) demonstrated that influenza interferes with tolerance to allergic sensitization. Normally, administration of inhaled ovalbumin to mice for 5 days reduced sensitization to ovalbumin. This immune tolerance did not develop if the inhaled ovalbumin was given during an acute influenza infection. More recently, Tsitoura et al. (66) assessed the effects of influenza on allergen tolerance. Although their experimental approach was different than that of Holt et al., they also found that an influenza infection prevented antigen tolerance.

To define the possible mechanisms by which respiratory viruses promote allergic sensitization, investigators have evaluated production of Th2 cytokines (61,66). Schwarze et al. (67) suggest that the effects of virus infection on allergen sensitization are mediated by T cells. To test this possibility, T cells were transferred from RSV-infected mice into RSV-naïve mice, which were then sensitized to ovalbumin. The RSV-infected mice had increased IL-5 production, pulmonary eosinophils, sensitization to ovalbumin, and airway responsiveness to methacholine compared to control mice. The effect was greatest with transfer of CD 8^+ cells.

V. Could Allergic Inflammation Be Protective Against Viral Infections?

Most of the research performed thus far has focused on mechanisms by which viral infections interact with allergen exposure to increase airway inflammation and allergen sensitization. To extend this possibility, and to evaluate the possibility that acute allergic processes promote the development of a cold, Avila et al. (68) identified subjects with allergic rhinitis and gave them either placebo or allergen nasal challenges prior to RV 16 inoculation. It was surprising that the subjects who were acutely exposed to allergen immediately prior to virus inoculation had a decrease in the time to onset of symptoms and duration of symptoms. There was also a delay in the time to the peak generation of IL-6 and IL-8. These findings suggest that, under conditions of acute allergic inflammation, the response to RV can be diminished.

One explanation for the unexpected results of Avila et al. (68) could be a negative feedback regulation of the immune response. Most immune responses begin with multiple positive feedback mechanisms, which are often downregulated by modulating factors that are in response to the acute reaction. Some of these mechanisms are likely to exist in allergic inflammation. For example, IL-10, a cytokine involved in immune downregulation, increases during the late phase of an allergen challenge (69). If the symptoms of a cold are secondary to the immune response, as has been proposed, then this compensatory, anti-inflammatory response to the allergen challenge may protect against symptoms (70).

Another possibility is that allergic inflammation may actually have antiviral activity. In the experiments by Avila and colleagues (68), there were fewer symptoms in subjects who had more nasal eosinophils. Eosinophils have been shown to bind rhinovirus and activate virus-specific T cells (71). In addition, the large cytoplasmic granules of eosinophils contain two ribonucleases, eosinophil cationic protein and eosinophil derived neurotoxin, both of which have direct antiviral activity against RSV (72,73). Furthermore, the role of eosinophils in viral immunity has also been examined in an animal model. Adamko et al. (74) have shown that allergic sensitization of guinea pigs with ovalbumin can alter parainfluenza-induced airway hyperresponsiveness. The sensitized animals had more eosinophils in lavage fluid and an 80% reduction in the viral content of the lung. Anti-IL-5 antibodies caused a considerable reduction in eosinophils and a marked increase in viral recovery from the lung.

A third mechanism of protection involves nitric oxide production (68). Nitric oxide levels increase in allergic rhinitis (75–77). More recently, Sanders et al. (78) have shown that nitric oxide inhibits rhinovirus replication and cytokine production in a human epithelial cell line. Thus, the increased presence of nitric oxide from the allergen challenge could have inhibited viral replication.

VI. Other Host Factors That Modify Outcomes of RV Infections: IFN-γ

Respiratory symptoms after experimental infection with a single lot of RV have had a great individual variability despite the standardization of inoculation methods and doses (3,12). The quantity of virus shed after these experimental infections also varies between individuals, even when no neutralizing antibody can be detected (4,6). We studied the relationship between in vitro T-cell responses to RV 16 and

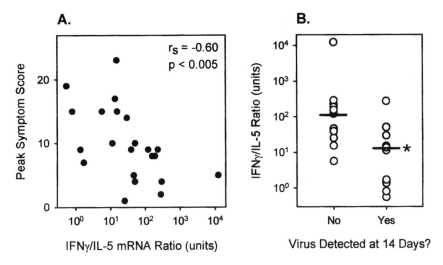

Figure 3   Association of the IFN-γ/IL-5 mRNA ratio to outcomes of the respiratory infection. The IFN-γ/IL-5 mRNA ratios were calculated during the acute cold (48 h after inoculation) for each individual. These ratios were (A) compared to the peak symptom score during the acute cold, and (B) grouped according to viral clearance at 14 days after inoculation with RV 16. (From Ref. 17.)

the development of symptoms and viral shedding after experimental infection (79). Twenty-two seronegative subjects with either allergic rhinitis or asthma were inoculated with RV 16. Peripheral blood mononuclear cells were obtained prior to inoculation to determine lymphocyte proliferation and RV-induced IFN-γ production.

   In subjects with vigorous generation of IFN-γ, there was a decrease in viral shedding. Induced sputum samples were also obtained during the acute infection to measure interferon gamma and IL-5 mRNA (17). The ratio of interferon gamma to IL-5 messenger RNA in the sputum was inversely related to both the peak symptom score and the length of time in which viral RNA was detectable in sputum (see Fig. 3). That is, a greater Th1 response was associated with fewer cold symptoms and a more rapid viral clearance. Both of these studies suggest that the character of cytokine responses of an individual subject can affect outcomes of viral infections.

VII.   Conclusions

Experimental inoculation of humans shows that respiratory viruses increase inhaled histamine responsiveness, allergen-induced airway responsiveness, the likelihood for late-phase asthmatic reactions, and eosinophilic inflammation. These findings are supported by animal studies, which also suggest that respiratory viruses augment IgE allergen sensitization and eosinophilic airway responses. In general, there is convincing evidence that viral respiratory infections increase allergic inflammation.

However, further study has begun to explore the relationships among host, virus, and allergen that determine the outcome of infection. Experiments both in humans and animals suggest that specific host immune responses may determine the outcome of viral infections, and more specifically that IFN-γ may be an important factor in this interaction. Are these responses different in atopic and nonatopic individuals? Are Th2 responses also important in host defenses against viruses? Do individuals have specific immune responses that can determine both their response to viruses and their risk of atopic disease? These are questions to be answered in the next generation of experiments.

References

1. Johnston SL, Pattemore PK, Sanderson G, Smith S, Lampe F, Josephs L, Symington P, O'Toole S, Myint SH, Tyrrell DA. Community study of role viral infections in exacerbations of asthma in 9-11 year old children. Br Med J 1995; 310(6989):1225–1229.

2. Nicholson KG, Kent J, Ireland DC. Respiratory viruses and exacerbations of asthma in adults. Br Med J 1993; 307(6910):982–986.

3. Lemanske RF, Jr., Dick EC, Swenson CA, Vrtis RF, Busse WW. Rhinovirus upper respiratory infection increases airway hyperreactivity and late asthmatic reactions. J Clin Invest 1989; 83(1):1–10.

4. Calhoun WJ, Swenson CA, Dick EC, Schwartz LB, Lemanske RF Jr, Busse WW. Experimental rhinovirus 16 infection potentiates histamine release after antigen bronchoprovocation in allergic subjects. Am Rev Respir Dis 1991; 144(6):1267–1273.

5. Calhoun WJ, Dick EC, Schwartz LB, Busse WW. A common cold virus, rhinovirus 16, potentiates airway inflammation after segmental antigen bronchoprovocation in allergic subjects. J Clin Invest 1994; 94(6):2200–2208.

6. Gern JE, Calhoun W, Swenson C, Shen G, Busse WW. Rhinovirus infection preferentially increases lower airway responsiveness in allergic subjects. Am J Respir Crit Care Med 1997; 155(6):1872–1876.

7. Fraenkel DJ, Bardin PG, Sanderson G, Lampe F, Johnston SL, Holgate ST. Lower airways inflammation during rhinovirus colds in normal and in asthmatic subjects. Am J Respir Crit Care Med 1995; 151(3 Pt 1):879–886.

8. Fleming HE, Little FF, Schnurr D, Avila PC, Wong H, Liu J, Yagi S, Boushey HA. Rhinovirus-16 colds in healthy and in asthmatic subjects: similar changes in upper and lower airways. Am J Respir Crit Care Med 1999; 160(1):100–108.

9. Summers QA, Higgins PG, Barrow IG, Tyrrell DA, Holgate ST. Bronchial reactivity to histamine and bradykinin is unchanged after rhinovirus infection in normal subjects. Eur Respir J 1992; 5(3):313–317.

10. Skoner DP, Doyle WJ, Seroky J, Van Deusen MA, Fireman P. Lower airway responses to rhinovirus 39 in healthy allergic and nonallergic subjects. Eur Respir J 1996; 9(7): 1402–1406.

11. Bardin PG, Fraenkel DJ, Sanderson G, Dorward M, Lau LC, Johnston SL, Holgate ST. Amplified rhinovirus colds in atopic subjects. Clin Exp Allergy 1994; 24(5):457–464.

12. Doyle WJ, Skoner DP, Fireman P, Seroky JT, Green I, Ruben F, Kardatzke DR, Gwaltney JM. Rhinovirus 39 infection in allergic and nonallergic subjects. J Allergy Clin Immunol 1992; 89(5):968–978.

13. Doyle WJ, Skoner DP, Seroky JT, Fireman P, Gwaltney JM. Effect of experimental rhinovirus 39 infection on the nasal response to histamine and cold air challenges in allergic and nonallergic subjects. J Allergy Clin Immunol 1994; 93(2):534–542.

14. Skoner DP, Whiteside TL, Wilson JW, Doyle WJ, Herberman RB, Fireman P. Effect of rhinovirus 39 infection on cellular immune parameters in allergic and nonallergic subjects. J Allergy Clin Immunol 1993; 92(5):732–743.

15. Cheung D, Dick EC, Timmers MC, de Klerk EP, Spaan WJ, Sterk PJ. Rhinovirus inhalation causes long-lasting excessive airway narrowing in response to methacholine in asthmatic subjects in vivo. Am J Respir Crit Care Med 1995; 152(5 Pt 1):1490–1496.

16. Grunberg K, Timmers MC, Smits HH, de Klerk EP, Dick EC, Spaan WJ, Hiemstra PS, Sterk PJ. Effect of experimental rhinovirus 16 colds on airway hyperresponsiveness to histamine and interleukin-8 in nasal lavage in asthmatic subjects in vivo. Clin Exp Allergy 1997; 27(1):36–45.

17. Gern JE, Vrtis R, Grindle KA, Swenson C, Busse WW. Relationship of upper and lower airway cytokines to outcome of experimental rhinovirus infection. Am J Respir Crit Care Med 2000; 162(6):2226–2231.

18. Douglass JA, Dhami D, Gurr CE, Bulpitt M, Shute JK, Howarth PH, Lindley IJ, Church MK, Holgate ST. Influence of interleukin-8 challenge in the nasal mucosa in atopic and nonatopic subjects. Am J Respir Crit Care Med 1994; 150(4):1108–1113.

19. Turner RB. The role of neutrophils in the pathogenesis of rhinovirus infections. Pediatr Infect Dis J 1990; 9(11):832–835.

20. Levandowski RA, Weaver CW, Jackson GG. Nasal-secretion leukocyte populations determined by flow cytometry during acute rhinovirus infection. J Med Virol 1988; 25(4):423–432.

21. Grunberg K, Smits HH, Timmers MC, de Klerk EP, Dolhain RJ, Dick EC, Hiemstra PS, Sterk PJ. Experimental rhinovirus 16 infection. Effects on cell differentials and soluble markers in sputum in asthmatic subjects. Am J Respir Crit Care Med 1997; 156 (2 Pt 1):609–616.

22. Rakes GP, Arruda E, Ingram JM, Hoover GE, Zambrano JC, Hayden FG, Platts-Mills TA, Heymann PW. Rhinovirus and respiratory syncytial virus in wheezing children requiring emergency care. IgE and eosinophil analyses. Am J Respir Crit Care Med 1999; 159(3):785–790.

23. Garofalo R, Kimpen JL, Welliver RC, Ogra PL. Eosinophil degranulation in the respiratory tract during naturally acquired respiratory syncytial virus infection. J Pediatr 1992; 120(1):28–32.

24. van Oosterhout AJ, van Ark I, Folkerts G, van der Linde HJ, Savelkoul HF, Verheyen AK, Nijkamp FP. Antibody to interleukin-5 inhibits virus-induced airway hyperresponsiveness to histamine in guinea pigs. Am J Respir Crit Care Med 1995; 151(1):177–183.

25. Schwarze J, Hamelmann E, Bradley KL, Takeda K, Gelfand EW. Respiratory syncytial virus infection results in airway hyperresponsiveness and enhanced airway sensitization to allergen. J Clin Invest 1997; 100(1):226–233.

26. Schwarze J, Cieslewicz G, Hamelmann E, Joetham A, Shultz LD, Lamers MC, Gelfand EW. IL-5 and eosinophils are essential for the development of airway hyperresponsiveness following acute respiratory syncytial virus infection. J Immunol 1999; 162(5):2997–3004.

27. Tang YW, Graham BS. Anti-IL-4 treatment at immunization modulates cytokine expression, reduces illness, and increases cytotoxic T lymphocyte activity in mice challenged with respiratory syncytial virus. J Clin Invest 1994; 94(5):1953–1958.

28. Alwan WH, Record FM, Openshaw PJ. Phenotypic and functional characterization of T cell lines specific for individual respiratory syncytial virus proteins. J Immunol 1993; 150(12):5211–5218.

29. Alwan WH, Kozlowska WJ, Openshaw PJ. Distinct types of lung disease caused by functional subsets of antiviral T cells. J Exp Med 1994; 179(1):81–89.

30. Roman M, Calhoun WJ, Hinton KL, Avendano LF, Simon V, Escobar AM, Gaggero A, Diaz PV. Respiratory syncytial virus infection in infants is associated with predominant Th-2-like response. Am J Respir Crit Care Med 1997; 156(1):190–195.

31. Aberle JH, Aberle SW, Dworzak MN, Mandl CW, Rebhandl W, Vollnhofer G, Kundi M, Popow-Kraupp T. Reduced interferon-gamma expression in peripheral blood mononuclear cells of infants with severe respiratory syncytial virus disease. Am J Respir Crit Care Med 1999; 160(4):1263–1268.

32. van Schaik SM, Tristram DA, Nagpal IS, Hintz KM, Welliver RC, Welliver RC. Increased production of IFN-gamma and cysteinyl leukotrienes in virus-induced wheezing. J Allergy Clin Immunol 1999; 103(4):630–636.

33. Bendelja K, Gagro A, Bace A, Lokar-Kolbas R, Krsulovic-Hresic V, Drazenovic V, Mlinaric-Galinovic G, Rabatic S. Predominant type-2 response in infants with respiratory syncytial virus (RSV) infection demonstrated by cytokine flow cytometry. Clin Exp Immunol 2000; 121(2):332–338.

34. Renzi PM, Turgeon JP, Marcotte JE, Drblik SP, Berube D, Gagnon MF, Spier S. Reduced interferon-gamma production in infants with bronchiolitis and asthma. Am J Respir Crit Care Med 1999; 159(5 Pt 1):1417–1422.

35. Brooks GD, Anklam KS, Roberg KA, Mikus LD, Rosenthal LA, Zeng L, et al. Reduced newborn mononuclear cell production of interleukin-5 (IL-5) and interleukin-13 (IL-13) is associated with wheezing in the first year of life. J Allergy Clin Immunol 2001; 107, S65.

36. Welliver RC, Wong DT, Sun M, Middleton E, Vaughan RS, Ogra PL. The development of respiratory syncytial virus-specific IgE and the release of histamine in nasopharyngeal secretions after infection. N Engl J Med 1981; 305(15):841–846.

37. Welliver RC, Wong DT, Middleton E, Sun M, McCarthy N, Ogra PL. Role of parainfluenza virus-specific IgE in pathogenesis of croup and wheezing subsequent to infection. J Pediatr 1982; 101(6):889–896.

38. Jackson M, Scott R. Different patterns of cytokine induction in cultures of respiratory syncytial (RS) virus-specific human TH cell lines following stimulation with RS virus and RS virus proteins. J Med Virol 1996; 49(3):161–169.

39. Gern JE, Dick EC, Kelly EA, Vrtis R, Klein B. Rhinovirus-specific T cells recognize both shared and serotype-restricted viral epitopes. J Infect Dis 1997; 175(5):1108–1114.

40. Coyle AJ, Erard F, Bertrand C, Walti S, Pircher H, Le Gros G. Virus-specific CD8+ cells can switch to interleukin 5 production and induce airway eosinophilia. J Exp Med 1995; 181(3):1229–1233.

41. Bochner BS. Road signs guiding leukocytes along the inflammation superhighway. J Allergy Clin Immunol 2000; 106(5 Pt 1):817–828.

42. Stark JM, Godding V, Sedgwick JB, Busse WW. Respiratory syncytial virus infection enhances neutrophil and eosinophil adhesion to cultured respiratory epithelial cells. Roles of CD18 and intercellular adhesion molecule-1. J Immunol 1996; 156(12):4774–4782.

43. Bentley AM, Durham SR, Robinson DS, Menz G, Storz C, Cromwell O, Kay AB, Wardlaw AJ. Expression of endothelial and leukocyte adhesion molecules: intercellular

adhesion molecule-1, E-selectin, and vascular cell adhesion molecule-1 in the bronchial mucosa in steady-state and allergen-induced asthma. J Allergy Clin Immunol 1993; 92(6):857–868.

44. Manolitsas ND, Trigg CJ, McAulay AE, Wang JH, Jordan SE, D'Ardenne AJ, Davies RJ. The expression of intercellular adhesion molecule-1 and the beta 1-integrins in asthma. Eur Respir J 1994; 7(8):1439–1444.

45. Bianco A, Whiteman SC, Sethi SK, Allen JT, Knight RA, Spiteri MA. Expression of intercellular adhesion molecule-1 (ICAM-1) in nasal epithelial cells of atopic subjects: a mechanism for increased rhinovirus infection? Clin Exp Immunol 2000; 121(2):339–345.

46. Staunton DE, Merluzzi VJ, Rothlein R, Barton R, Marlin SD, Springer TA. A cell adhesion molecule, ICAM-1, is the major surface receptor for rhinoviruses. Cell 1989; 56(5):849–853.

47. Greve JM, Davis G, Meyer AM, Forte CP, Yost SC, Marlor CW, Kamarck ME, McClelland A. The major human rhinovirus receptor is ICAM-1. Cell 1989; 56(5):839–847.

48. Papi A, Johnston SL. Rhinovirus infection induces expression of its own receptor intercellular adhesion molecule 1 (ICAM-1) via increased NF-kappaB-mediated transcription. J Biol Chem 1999; 274(14):9707–9720.

49. Bianco A, Sethi SK, Allen JT, Knight RA, Spiteri MA. Th2 cytokines exert a dominant influence on epithelial cell expression of the major group human rhinovirus receptor, ICAM-1. Eur Respir J 1998; 12(3):619–626.

50. Sethi SK, Bianco A, Allen JT, Knight RA, Spiteri MA. Interferon-gamma (IFN-gamma) down-regulates the rhinovirus-induced expression of intercellular adhesion molecule-1 (ICAM-1) on human airway epithelial cells. Clin Exp Immunol 1997; 110(3):362–369.

51. Tosi MF, Stark JM, Hamedani A, Smith CW, Gruenert DC, Huang YT. Intercellular adhesion molecule-1 (ICAM-1)-dependent and ICAM-1-independent adhesive interactions between polymorphonuclear leukocytes and human airway epithelial cells infected with parainfluenza virus type 2. J Immunol 1992; 149(10):3345–3349.

52. Stark JM, Amin RS, Trapnell BC. Infection of A549 cells with a recombinant adenovirus vector induces ICAM-1 expression and increased CD-18-dependent adhesion of activated neutrophils. Hum Gene Ther 1996; 7(14):1669–1681.

53. Grunberg K, Sharon RF, Hiltermann TJ, Brahim JJ, Dick EC, Sterk PJ, Van Krieken JH. Experimental rhinovirus 16 infection increases intercellular adhesion molecule-1 expression in bronchial epithelium of asthmatics regardless of inhaled steroid treatment. Clin Exp Allergy 2000; 30(7):1015–1023.

54. Sorkness RL, Mehta H, Kaplan MR, Miyasaka M, Hefle SL, Lemanske RF Jr. Effect of ICAM-1 blockade on lung inflammation and physiology during acute viral bronchiolitis in rats. Pediatr Res 2000; 47(6):819–824.

55. Liden J, Rafter I, Truss M, Gustafsson JA, Okret S. Glucocorticoid effects on NF-kappaB binding in the transcription of the ICAM-1 gene. Biochem Biophys Res Commun 2000; 273(3):1008–1014.

56. Montefort S, Roche WR, Howarth PH, Djukanovic R, Gratziou C, Carroll M, Smith L, Britten KM, Haskard D, Lee TH. Intercellular adhesion molecule-1 (ICAM-1) and endothelial leucocyte adhesion molecule-1 (ELAM-1) expression in the bronchial mucosa of normal and asthmatic subjects. Eur Respir J 1992; 5(7):815–823.

57. Tingsgaard PK, Larsen PL, Bock T, Lange VG, Tos M. Expression of intercellular adhesion molecule-1 on the vascular endothelium in nasal polyps before, during and after topical glucocorticoid treatment. Acta Otolaryngol 1998; 118(3):404–408.

58. Berti E, Cerri A, Marzano AV, Richelda R, Bianchi B, Caputo R. Mometasone furoate decreases adhesion molecule expression in psoriasis. Eur J Dermatol 1998; 8(6):421–426.

59. Papi A, Papadopoulos NG, Degitz K, Holgate ST, Johnston SL. Corticosteroids inhibit rhinovirus-induced intercellular adhesion molecule-1 up-regulation and promoter activation on respiratory epithelial cells. J Allergy Clin Immunol 2000; 105(2 Pt 1):318–326.

60. Suzuki T, Yamaya M, Sekizawa K, Yamada N, Nakayama K, Ishizuka S, Kamanaka M, Morimoto T, Numazaki Y, Sasaki H. Effects of dexamethasone on rhinovirus infection in cultured human tracheal epithelial cells. Am J Physiol Lung Cell Mol Physiol 2000; 278(3):L560–L571.

61. O'Donnell DR, Openshaw PJ. Anaphylactic sensitization to aeroantigen during respiratory virus infection. Clin Exp Allergy 1998; 28(12):1501–1508.

62. Sakamoto M, Ida S, Takishima T. Effect of influenza virus infection on allergic sensitization to aerosolized ovalbumin in mice. J Immunol 1984; 132(5):2614–2617.

63. Leibovitz E, Freihorst J, Piedra PA, Ogra PL. Modulation of systemic and mucosal immune responses to inhaled ragweed antigen in experimentally induced infection with respiratory syncytial virus implication in virally induced allergy. Int Arch Allergy Appl Immunol 1988; 86(1):112–116.

64. Suzuki S, Suzuki Y, Yamamoto N, Matsumoto Y, Shirai A, Okubo T. Influenza A virus infection increases IgE production and airway responsiveness in aerosolized antigen-exposed mice. J Allergy Clin Immunol 1998; 102(5):732–740.

65. Holt PG, Vines J, Bilyk N. Effect of influenza virus infection on allergic sensitization to inhaled antigen in mice. Int Arch Allergy Appl Immunol 1988; 86(1):121–123.

66. Tsitoura DC, Kim S, Dabbagh K, Berry G, Lewis DB, Umetsu DT. Respiratory infection with influenza A virus interferes with the induction of tolerance to aeroallergens. J Immunol 2000; 165(6):3484–3491.

67. Schwarze J, Makela M, Cieslewicz G, Dakhama A, Lahn M, Ikemura T, Joetham A, Gelfand EW. Transfer of the enhancing effect of respiratory syncytial virus infection on subsequent allergic airway sensitization by T lymphocytes. J Immunol 1999; 163(10):5729–5734.

68. Avila PC, Abisheganaden JA, Wong H, Liu J, Yagi S, Schnurr D, Kishiyama JL, Boushey HA. Effects of allergic inflammation of the nasal mucosa on the severity of rhinovirus 16 cold. J Allergy Clin Immunol 2000; 105(5):923–932.

69. Lim S, John M, Seybold J, Taylor D, Witt C, Barnes PJ, Chung KF. Increased interleukin-10 and macrophage inflammatory protein-1 alpha release from blood monocytes ex vivo during late-phase response to allergen in asthma. Allergy 2000; 55(5):489–495.

70. Busse WW, Gern JE. Do allergies protect against the effects of a rhinovirus cold? J Allergy Clin Immunol 2000; 105(5):889–891.

71. Handzel ZT, Busse WW, Sedgwick JB, Vrtis R, Lee WM, Kelly EA, Gern JE. Eosinophils bind rhinovirus and activate virus-specific T cells. J Immunol 1998; 160(3):1279–1284.

72. Domachowske JB, Dyer KD, Adams AG, Leto TL, Rosenberg HF. Eosinophil cationic protein/RNase 3 is another RNase A-family ribonuclease with direct antiviral activity. Nucleic Acids Res 1998; 26(14):3358–3363.

73. Domachowske JB, Dyer KD, Bonville CA, Rosenberg HF. Recombinant human eosinophil-derived neurotoxin/RNase 2 functions as an effective antiviral agent against respiratory syncytial virus. J Infect Dis 1998; 177(6):1458–1464.

74. Adamko DJ, Yost BL, Gleich GJ, Fryer AD, Jacoby DB. Ovalbumin sensitization

changes the inflammatory response to subsequent parainfluenza infection. Eosinophils mediate airway hyperresponsiveness, m(2) muscarinic receptor dysfunction, and antiviral effects. J Exp Med 1999; 190(10):1465–1478.

75. Martin U, Bryden K, Devoy M, Howarth P. Increased levels of exhaled nitric oxide during nasal and oral breathing in subjects with seasonal rhinitis. J Allergy Clin Immunol 1996; 97(3):768–772.

76. Garrelds IM, van Amsterdam JG, Graaf-in't VC, Gerth vW, Zijlstra FJ. Nitric oxide metabolites in nasal lavage fluid of patients with house dust mite allergy. Thorax 1995; 50(3):275–279.

77. Kharitonov SA, O'Connor BJ, Evans DJ, Barnes PJ. Allergen-induced late asthmatic reactions are associated with elevation of exhaled nitric oxide. Am J Respir Crit Care Med 1995; 151(6):1894–1899.

78. Sanders SP, Siekierski ES, Porter JD, Richards SM, Proud D. Nitric oxide inhibits rhinovirus-induced cytokine production and viral replication in a human respiratory epithelial cell line. J Virol 1998; 72(2):934–942.

79. Parry DE, Busse WW, Sukow KA, Dick CR, Swenson C, Gern JE. Rhinovirus-induced PBMC responses and outcome of experimental infection in allergic subjects. J Allergy Clin Immunol 2000; 105(4):692–698.

18

Virus-Induced Wheeze in Young Children
A Separate Disease?

MICHAEL SILVERMAN, JONATHAN GRIGG, and MIKE McKEAN

University of Leicester
Leicester, England

I. Wheezing

A. A Brief History of Wheeze

The last 40 years have seen great changes in the attitudes of clinicians and scientists to wheezing disorders in general, and in particular to asthma. Central to the arguments has been the response of the airways to viral infections of the respiratory tract, particularly in childhood. In the 1960s, astute clinicians in primary or secondary care settings were aware of a disorder variously called wheezy bronchitis, infant wheeze, or recurrent bronchiolitis, which affected very young children and whose clinical hallmark was recurrent wheezing in association with respiratory tract infection (RTI) (1). It was common and often severe in the first years of life, but its prognosis was good and it appeared clinically distinct from (atopic) asthma. Indeed, it was stated that a diagnosis of asthma should not be made in infancy.

However, with the term "bronchitis" came the reflex response of many medical practitioners to prescribe ineffective and costly antibiotic therapy. The advent of safe and effective inhaled therapy for asthma around 1970 led to a campaign to eliminate terms such as wheezy bronchitis and to label young wheezers as asthmatic. The aim was to discourage antibiotic prescribing and to encourage the use of short-term β_2 agonists and subsequently inhaled corticosteroids. All of the disorders whose common clinical feature was wheezing were henceforth to be called asthma. Given the functional definition of asthma proposed by the Ciba Symposium of 1958—that asthma is a disorder characterized by short-term variations in intrathoracic airway caliber—this was reasonable (2).

However, in the 1980s the definition of asthma was usurped by those who believed that allergy (atopy) and bronchial hyperresponsiveness (BHR) were essential features of asthma (3). The 1990s brought advances in cell biology and techniques of bronchial biopsy, revealing inflammation and so-called remodeling in the airways of mainly young, atopic, male, mildly asthmatic volunteers. The T-helper 1 and T-helper 2 lymphocyte (TH_1/TH_2) paradigm of allergy emerged and often seemed to be used to explain asthma too, denying both the evidence of epidemiology, that allergy and asthma are not coterminous, and the existence of some distinctive varieties of asthma such as aspirin-sensitive disease and non-IgE-mediated occupational asthma. The objective seemed to be to fit all forms of wheezing disease into this model of atopic inflammation with BHR.

Even acute infantile bronchiolitis was forced into the model on the spurious evidence that it was often followed by recurrent wheeze and must therefore be a cause of asthma. In fact, in terms of risk factors, pathology, immunobiology, and natural history, acute respiratory syncytial virus-positive infantile bronchiolitis is now generally accepted to be distinct from later atopic childhood asthma. This example of poor science (imputing cause from clinical association) underpins much of the effort to force wheezing disorders of young children into the atopic asthmatic model.

The last few years have seen this reductionist, exclusive approach superseded by a more inclusive view of asthma. It is fashionable to refer to asthma as a complex disease, which implies both its unpredictability and the likelihood that its clinical features may be the outcome of widely differing processes (5). For instance, the simplistic TH_1/TH_2 paradigm does not explain the dissociation between the production of specific IgE and end-organ sensitivity to an allergen, highlighted by the recent studies of helminth infection in children (6,7). Under the asthma umbrella, separate diseases (so-called phenotypes) can be identified. Each represents a consistent but distinctive cluster of features, encompassing clinical features (although variable airway obstruction, whether measured or implied, is common to all), therapeutic responses, natural history and epidemiology, immunopathology, and genetic basis. We will review the evidence that, along with some other clearly defined phenotypes of asthma, viral episodic wheeze has the characteristics of a distinctive disease, albeit within the spectrum of asthma (defined as variable intrathoracic airway caliber). In doing so, we will acknowledge that our forbears got it right: recurrent wheezy bronchitis, or episodic (or exclusive) viral wheeze (VW) does exist in children (and possibly in adults too).

In this chapter, we will first discuss some of the hurdles to be overcome in studying wheezing disorders in young children. We will then critically review the clinical and experimental evidence that viral wheeze is a disorder separate from other forms of asthma.

B. The Nature of Wheeze

Asthma phenotypes are (almost) all characterized by the presence of wheeze, a symptom recognized by patients (or their carers) or a sign detected by auscultation by health professionals. The term wheeze is widely used in English-speaking countries but poorly understood by lay people and, to a lesser extent, by professionals (8,9). Its interpretation in questionnaires, especially in indirect translation, into languages other than English has been questioned. To complicate matters, in clinical airway obstruction, wheeze is usually accompanied by other symptoms: cough (dry or moist), rattly breathing (especially in very young children), chest tightness (in those old enough to describe the sensation), and breathlessness. These may be mistakenly reported as wheeze (9,10). In a severe airway obstruction, wheeze may be absent (the "silent chest"). Thus, the symptom that defines asthma and related disorders in young children, usually in the absence of any other supporting evidence, is inherently unreliable.

Health professionals are poor at differentiating wheeze from other transmitted noises such as rattles, stridor, or glottic noises (8). Often, crackles accompany acute viral episodes of wheeze (including acute bronchiolitis). In children with episodic symptoms, wheeze is far more often reported to health professionals than detected by them. As a counsel of perfection, the minimum requirement for research into wheezing disorders in young children should be the detection of wheeze by a doctor or nurse, in order to avoid misclassification. This exacting standard has been used in one very influential cohort study (11).

Wheeze is not specific. Its physiological basis is in the dissipation of energy by vibration of the airway walls at a site of flow-limitation during exhalation (8). Flow limitation occurs in airways of different sizes (generations) during forced expiration, dependent on two important local properties of the airways: cross-sectional area (and therefore flow resistance) and airway wall compliance (and therefore collapsibility under an adverse transmural pressure gradient).

Airway cross-sectional area may be reduced by:

- intraluminal obstruction (by mucus, for example)
- airway smooth muscle contraction
- airway wall thickening (sometimes called remodeling)
- extraluminal factors such as uncoupling the airways from the surrounding lung tissues, thereby unloading the airway smooth muscle

Airway wall compliance may be affected by:

- primary developmental or secondary inflammatory remodeling of structural airway components (cartilage, matrix proteins, etc.)
- functional properties of airway smooth muscle (such as intrinsic tone)
- loss of interdependence of airways and lung parenchyma

The polyphonic wheeze of asthma and related disorders is the sum of the effects of widespread, variable flow limitation in airways of different sizes and locations, which are the result of a number of possible pathophysiological mechanisms. Monophonic wheeze, by contrast, is due to the fluttering of a single (normally large) airway in relation to a localized airway problem (such as a foreign body, tumor, or zone of bronchomalacia).

C. Does Wheeze Equate with Airway Obstruction?

The association between the presence of wheeze during tidal or forced expiration and the level of airway obstruction in adults is poor, possibly because of the difficulty in quantifying wheeze and because of great differences between individuals (8). A better relationship exists between wheeze and bronchodilator response, indirectly implying that wheeze indicates airway obstruction. In young children during bronchial challenge, some have found by auscultation that wheeze occurs as the forced expiratory volume in 1s (FEV_1) falls by about 20% (i.e., PC_{20} = PC_{wheeze}) (12,13). Others found wheeze to be an insensitive indicator of airway obstruction (14). Nevertheless, in young children in whom lung function measurements for clinical purposes have been impossible until recently (15,16), wheeze is used clinically as an indication of airway obstruction and (in the absence of other disorders) variable wheeze is the prime (and often the only) clinical marker of asthma. Virus-induced wheeze therefore suffers from the same basic diagnostic problems as asthma in general in young children.

D. Problems in Studying Airway Disease in Young Children

The Spectrum of Viral Lower Respiratory Tract Illness

Because the respiratory system has a limited repertoire of clinical features, we only recognize a few clinical syndromes (Fig. 1). We may not detect important differences (between bacterial and viral pharyngitis, for example). Moreover, syndromes usually exhibit a large degree of overlap. For instance, an infant with bronchiolitis may have clinical features of rhinitis, tracheobronchitis, and pneumonitis; many adults with acute rhinitis also complain of productive cough (bronchitis).

There are only a few close associations between virus type and clinical syndrome, such as adenovirus and acute viral pneumonia; parainfluenza and acute laryngobronchitis (croup); RSV and acute infantile bronchiolitis. On the whole, however, the syndromes are not specific. This is particularly the case for acute wheezing

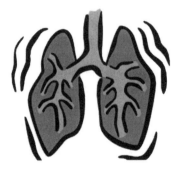

- rhinitis (HRV, HCV, RSV)
- pharyngitis (several)
- laryngitis (Paraflu)
- tracheobronchitis (Flu A)
- wheeze or asthma (HRV, HCV, etc.)
- bronchiolitis (RSV, adenovirus)
- pneumonitis (RSV, adenovirus)

Figure 1 Acute respiratory infection: spectrum of clinically defined syndromes and their viral causes. HRV, human rhinovirus; HCV, human coronavirus; Paraflu, parainfluenza; Flu A, influenza A; RSV, respiratory syncytial virus.

episodes (whether or nor in the context of atopic asthma); a wide range of viruses may produce a similar clinical picture. Conversely, active infections often occur without symptoms. This suggests that in the formula:

Virus infection + Host responsiveness → Acute wheezy episode

the predominant determinant of outcome is the nature of the host response rather than the specificity of the viral infection. The nature of the "host responsiveness" may be critical in differentiating VW from other forms of asthma.

Patterns of Airway Disease in Children

It is a matter of simple logic that the patterns of airway obstruction seen in wheezing disorders and asthma can be resolved into three components (Fig. 2):

- acute episodes (Fig. 2a)
- variable day-to-day (or interval) features (with or without acute episodes) (Fig. 2b)
- fixed (irreversible) or persistent airway obstruction (with or without variability + acute episodes) (Fig. 2c).

Any set of symptoms or lung function measurements can be analyzed in terms of these three components, but is there a functional basis for this classification and is it clinically useful? We will show that there is a particular group of children who suffer from repeated and often severe episodes of wheeze (Fig. 2a) in association with viral RTI, and who, unlike other chronic asthmatics, have few or no symptoms between episodes (Fig. 2b).

Even in subjects with atopic asthma, it is now clear that from a physiological, immunological, and therapeutic point of view, acute severe episodes, most of which occur in association with viral RTI, are different from the sort of day-to-day symptoms of the intervals between episodes (17,18).

(a) acute episodes   (b) variability   (c) fixed obstructive element

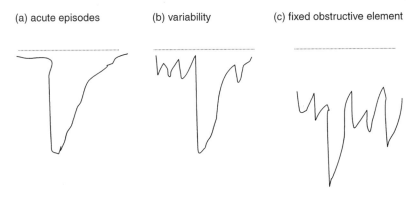

Figure 2   Patterns of symptoms or lung function in wheezing disorders.

Clinical Measurement

The hurdles to clinical measurement, for diagnostic, mechanistic, or therapeutic purposes are especially high in young children (19,20). This means that much of the evidence in support of specific asthma phenotypes has been based on clinical observation, supported by noninvasive measurements, and clinical epidemiology, rather than on cellular or physiological measurement. A few ingenious opportunistic studies, such as bronchoalveolar lavage (BAL) during incidental general anesthesia have contributed enormously (21). Bronchial mucosal biopsy data are slowly becoming available (22). Older children can be studied in greater detail. Cross-sectional designs as well as careful, longitudinal clinical observations have contributed to the evidence.

E. Viral Diagnosis

Apart from acute infantile bronchiolitis, there is relatively little direct evidence of the viral etiology of acute lower respiratory tract (LRT) wheezing illnesses or exacerbations of asthma in very young children (23–26), although the circumstantial clinical evidence is overwhelming. In strict terms, concomitant viral diagnosis is essential in order to justify the separate existence of viral wheeze. Without comprehensive viral diagnosis, the results can become distorted. For instance, the diagnostic toolkit used in the Tucson Cohort Project did not include rhinovirus and may therefore have given a distorted impression of the importance of RSV in VW (27).

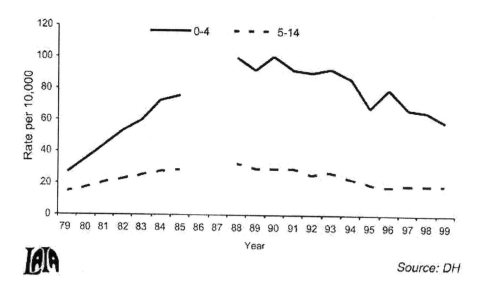

Figure 3 The health service burden of viral respiratory infections in young children. (Data from Lung & Asthma Information Agency, with permission.)

F. Measuring the Burden of Viral LRT Illness in Young Children

In temperate zones, the lower respiratory tract effects of viral RTIs present a huge, seasonal public health burden (Fig. 3). Much of this burden is due to episodes of virus-induced wheeze, cough, and exacerbations of atopic asthma. In secondary care, respiratory syncytial virus (RSV) infection probably accounts for a high proportion of admissions, even beyond the peak age for acute viral bronchiolitis: infants under 6 months.

The prevalence of viral wheeze in young children is high (Table 1). There is widespread reliance on inhalation therapy, with 26% of under 5s in the United Kingdom receiving inhaled therapy for wheezing disorders in 1998 (31). A conservative estimate of the healthcare costs of all wheezing disorders in under 5s for the United Kingdom in 2000 gave a figure of £91 million ($145 million) for a total population of 61 million, representing 0.25% of total National Health Service costs (33).

Given the extent of the public health burden, it is surprising how little research has been carried out into the nature and management of early childhood wheezing disorders.

G. A Separate Condition?

Defining diseases is more than butterfly collecting: it has vital clinical benefits. If viral wheeze differs from atopic asthma as clearly as does type I from type II diabetes, then the case will be self-evident. To make the case presupposes other well-characterized conditions from which it can be differentiated.

- quantitative or qualitative differences in a number of key features (Fig. 4)
- clinically important distinctive therapeutic or prognostic features
- ultimately, genetic differences

Table 1 Estimates of the Population Prevalence of Wheeze, and Virus-Induced Wheeze in Children

Source of data (Ref.)	Age group (year)	Prevalence (%) Any wheeze	Viral wheeze
Aberdeen, UK 1969 (28)	Schoolchildren	11.4	6.6
Leicester, UK 1990 (30)	Under 5	14	9
Tucson, AZ, USA, 1995 (11)[b]	Under 3	34	20[a]
Southampton, UK, 1997 (29)	7–9		3.3[c]
Leicester, UK, 1988 (31)	Under 5	29	19
Manchester, UK, 2001 (32)[d]	1st year of life	31	25

[a] Reported as "transient" wheeze: present before age 3, but not at age 6.
[b] Cumulative prevalence.
[c] ≥ five episodes (one ≥ 3 days) in last year.
[d] Estimated.

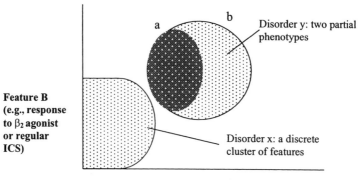

Figure 4 Diseases and wheeze phenotypes. The population of wheezy children might be classified as belonging to disorder x or y on the basis of clustering of features A and B. Disorder y can be considered to exhibit two partial phenotypes (a and b) on the basis of feature A alone.

We will show that there are discrete differences between viral wheeze and other asthma phenotypes, for a range of characteristics (Table 2). The major alternative phenotypes that will be considered are viral exacerbations of atopic asthma, intrinsic asthma, and chronic obstructive pulmonary disease (COPD). We will also review the evidence that other disorders that may be considered discrete, such as acute viral bronchiolitis and postbronchiolitic wheeze, fall within the spectrum of virus-induced wheeze.

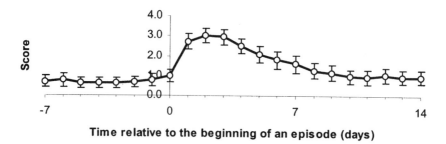

Figure 5 The pattern of acute virus-induced wheeze compiled for symptom diaries of preschool children with a history of viral wheeze. (From Ref. 34.)

Table 2 Clinical Characteristics for Which
Evidence Exists That Virus-Induced Wheeze Is
a Separate Condition (reviewed in this chapter)

Clinical features
- Description of the condition
- Natural history
- Clinical physiology
- Therapeutic responses

Epidemiology
- Risk factors and associations

Pathogenesis
- Immunopathology: host–virus interaction
- Airway physiology
- Genetic basis

Experimental models
- Human
- Animal

II. Clinical Features

A. Presenting Features

The sequence of events in an episode of viral wheeze is typically as follows:

- a cold (acute rhinitis), mild febrile illness or sore throat
- within 1–2 days (or occasionally preceding upper respiratory tract [URT] symptoms by up to a day or so), onset of LRT symptoms: wheeze, dyspnea, and cough, which may be dry, rattly, or wet
- worsening symptoms over 1–2 days followed by gradual resolution over 7–14 days (Fig. 5)
- a period of variable duration with few or no symptoms, until the next episode

There are individual differences in the severity of symptoms (from the mildest to severe respiratory distress), duration of symptoms (from hours to weeks), the duration of intervals between episodes (so that frequent seasonal viral infections may cause almost continuous symptoms), and the frequency of episodes. For some children, the first episode of viral wheeze occurs in the first months of life, in association with RSV, and may be called acute infantile bronchiolitis. Whether bronchiolitis should be considered a cause of recurrent viral wheeze or whether acute bronchiolitis and VW are manifestations of the same disorder is discussed later. Since only about 2% of infants are diagnosed with acute viral bronchiolitis, but (at any time) up to 25% of preschool children report current wheeze only with colds (Table 1), most viral wheeze is unrelated to acute infantile bronchiolitis. Conversely, most infants who are symptomatic with RSV infection simply suffer a wheezy spell and do not receive a diagnosis of acute viral bronchiolitis (27).

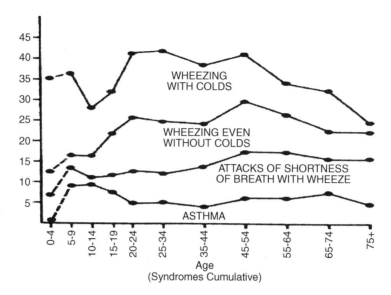

Figure 6 Cumulative population prevalence of wheezing disorders, showing the dominance of wheeze only with colds in the youngest age groups but its continued occurrence at all ages. (From Ref. 40.)

In preschool children, the acute episodes have been described from daily symptom record charts (Fig. 5) (34). There is a parallel increase in nocturnal wheeze (and croup), daytime wheeze, cough or dyspnea, and daytime limitation of exercise. In schoolchildren it is possible to supplement symptom records with daily peak expiratory flow (PEF) monitoring (35). Both these approaches clearly describe children with discrete episodes on a background of symptom-free intervals of varying duration. The episodes resemble acute exacerbations of asthma in both their severity (which may vary widely) and symptom pattern. The difference between asthma and viral wheeze lies in the intervals between episodes. Asthma is a chronic disease (Fig. 2b, c) on which acute viral episodes (Fig. 2a) are superimposed, whereas in acute viral wheeze there are few or no chronic symptoms (Fig. 2a). It has been possible to identify young children (34,36,37), schoolchildren (38), and young adults (39) with this pattern of disease, for inclusion in research projects.

The peak age group is 1–4 years, but similar albeit milder episodes occur at all ages (Fig. 6) (40). The number of young children in the population who suffer recurrent wheeze only with colds is probably far greater than the total of schoolchildren with asthma.

The natural history of the condition is considered below. Whether episodic viral wheeze is the same condition as what is termed transient wheeze (11) in young children seems likely but remains to be proved.

Physical examination between episodes is usually normal (in the absence of comorbidity). During episodes, there are usually features of acute upper respiratory tract infection (URTI), together with evidence of widespread intrathoracic airway obstruction. The severity of airway obstruction varies from minimal recession and mild end-expiratory wheeze to extreme dyspnea with marked recession, use of accessory muscles of breathing, biphasic wheeze, and hypoxemia. Basal coarse crackles may be heard during episodes.

Hypoxemia (by oximetry) depends on severity and is more frequent in the youngest children. Other investigations are rarely performed in this condition, unless there is deteriorating respiratory distress or respiratory failure, when chest x-ray will usually slow hyperinflation and patchy collapse/consolidation. Arterial blood gas analysis may show type 1 or type 2 respiratory failure.

B. Clinical Physiology

During episodes there is little information on pulmonary function in preschool children with viral wheeze. In schoolchildren studied prospectively at home, acute symptoms are accompanied by changes in PEF indicating acute airway obstruction (Fig. 7) (35). In an adult model of viral wheeze induced by an experimental infection with human coronavirus (HCoV) 229E, symptoms were relatively mild and changes in FEV_1 and PEF were trivial, but there was a marked and progressive increase in bronchial responsiveness (to methacholine), which was independent of allergy and persisted for at least 17 days (when the experiment ended) (Fig. 8) (39).

Between episodes, there may be evidence of abnormal airway function in young children, despite an absence of symptoms. Developmental airway dysfunction

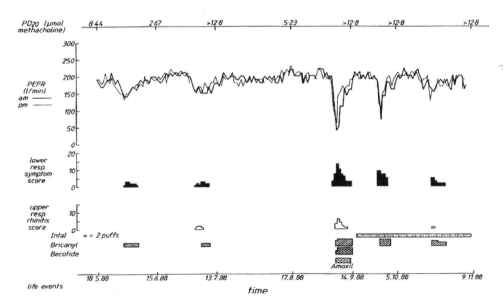

Figure 7 Pattern of symptoms, lung function, and infection over a 6-month period in a nonatopic, recurrently wheezy boy. (From Ref. 35.)

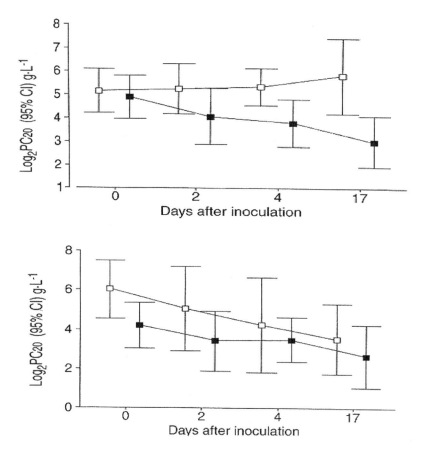

Figure 8 Changes in bronchial responsiveness (PC_{20} methacholine) in a group of young adults following experimental HCoV 229E infection. A progressive fall in PC_{20} occurred in subjects with a history of exclusive viral wheeze (closed squares, top), but not in healthy volunteers and in both atopic and non-atopic (open squares, bottom). (From Ref. 39.)

may precede and therefore possibly predispose to wheezing in general in infants and young children (see later) (41). In young children, abnormalities between episodes include:

- increased airway or respiratory resistance (42)
- abnormal airway wall compliance (43,44)
- diminished maximum expiratory flow (42,44–46)

The few data that exist on schoolchildren and adults with viral wheeze suggest that their lung function is normal between episodes (35,38,39).

Most studies show that bronchial responsiveness does not differ between infants with and without established viral wheeze (42,45,46). This is difficult to reconcile with the evidence that, at least for baby girls, BHR in the neonatal period is a risk factor for subsequent wheezy episodes (46,47). In adults, there is no evidence for BHR during symptom-free intervals, in clear distinction to those with asthma (39). Since BHR is considered by many to be a sine qua non of classic asthma, this is strong evidence that viral wheeze and classic asthma are qualitatively different.

One study reported lower PC_{40} histamine 5 months after acute bronchiolitis in infants who subsequently wheezed (48). This group had not recorded lung function prior to the onset of bronchiolitis, and so cannot exclude the possibility that BHR preceded both the acute bronchiolitis and the subsequent wheeze, as has been shown in the Perth Cohort (49,50).

C. Virology

There are few comprehensive data on the distribution of viruses responsible for acute episodes. This is largely due to the fact that until recently virus identification was based on techniques that relied upon virus culture, a process now known to be insensitive. Recent advances in molecular biology have permitted the sequencing of large parts of the genome of infectious agents, including the common respiratory viruses. This has permitted the development of reverse transcriptase–polymerase chain reaction (RT-PCR) assays that provide sensitive and specific detection. The results of previous epidemiology should therefore be interpreted in the light of this knowledge.

These recent advances in technology have shown us that the most common viruses associated with acute exacerbations of asthma in older children and adults are human rhinovirus (HRV) and HCoV. However, in young children from whom prospective data have been collated, it is often incomplete. The Tucson cohort, for example, did not include any attempt to isolate HRV, and hence concluded that RSV was responsible for most episodes under the age of 3 (27). It is well known that RSV and parainfluenza virus are major causes of wheezing in infancy, but other viruses such as HRV (23,26) and HCoV (24–26) identified with earlier technology are also known to cause wheeze in preschool children. From what is known of respiratory viral epidemiology, it is clear that many virus types are responsible for wheezy episodes in young children and, therefore, that although some seem to be more potent than others, the disease is host- and not virus-specific. There is no virus-specific evidence to support a separate disorder of viral wheeze.

D. Immunology

The immune status of children with viral wheeze, in particular whether or not they are atopic (allergic) and therefore differentiated from children with atopic asthma, is of central importance. The best evidence comes from a cohort of under-5s studied in Leicestershire (UK) (30), which showed that children with transient, mainly viral, wheeze were less likely to be atopic than those with persistent asthma. Evidence from the Tucson cohort is supportive, showing that in contrast to wheezing in school-children, wheeze confined to the first 3 years of life is not (or is even negatively) associated with later evidence of atopic disease, positive skin test responses, or raised IgE (51). In another small study, even in the children of atopic parents wheeze in infancy was unrelated to later atopy or to wheeze or BHR at the age of 11 (52), or asthma at age 22 (53).

The issue of acute infantile bronchiolitis, postbronchiolitic wheeze, allergy, and asthma has been debated for many years. A recent review by one of the early proponents of the relationship between RSV bronchiolitis, allergy, and asthma has concluded that no such association exists (54). Indeed, the cytokine response to acute RSV infection was shown to be inimical to enhanced TH_2 activity in those who wheezed (55).

E. Response to Treatment

Two approaches have been advocated in the treatment of preschool children who wheeze: acute treatment to relieve symptoms during an exacerbation and chronic or prophylactic treatment aiming to reduce the frequency and/or severity of episodes. Inhaled bronchodilators and oral corticosteroids have been used for relief and low-dosage inhaled corticosteroids for attempted prevention. Very few clinical trials have attempted to differentiate between children with VW and those with interval symptoms too. Over the last decade evidence has been published suggesting that children with episodic viral wheeze respond differently from those with chronic (allergic) asthma, although there has been no head-to-head study. Without such a study, the uncertainty will remain.

The key question to be resolved is: In children (of any age) do isolated acute viral episodes (Fig. 2a) respond differently to therapy, in comparison with acute episodes set in a background of chronic, interval symptoms (Fig. 2b)? If so, then the case for viral wheeze as a separate condition will be strengthened.

The statistical techniques necessary to differentiate episodes and interval symptoms in patients with chronic asthma (56,57) are not well developed.

Bronchodilators

β_2-agonists are the main rescue therapy during acute exacerbations of asthma, the majority of which are associated with a virus infection both in childhood and adulthood. It has been assumed that bronchodilators are of benefit in viral wheeze, but the evidence does not fully support this with conflicting results in different age groups.

The response to β_2-agonists in wheezy children under 2 years of age has not been well established. Nevertheless, β_2-agonists remain the most frequently prescribed medication for wheeze in this age group and are the recommended treatment in many international guidelines (58,59). Suggested reasons for perceived lack of efficacy include heterogeneous patient groups, difficulty in the effective administration of the drug to very young children, airway obstruction caused by virus-induced airway inflammation and edema rather than smooth muscle contraction, and developmental abnormality of airway structure or function (60). A Cochrane systematic review identified that 37 studies of β_2-agonists in children under 2 years of age, of which 8 were suitable, randomized controlled trials for review and 6 were suitable for meta-analysis (61). Some of the studies reported minor improvements in symptoms, but without a significant effect on admission rates or duration of hospital stay. Others reported no difference in symptom scores. A marginal (1.6%) improvement in oxygen saturation (SaO_2) was seen, but three studies reported a paradoxical decrease in SaO_2. Three studies have reported a protective effect of β_2-agonists against deterioration of lung function due to histamine challenge in infants. Although this demonstrates the potential to respond, its clinical relevance is uncertain. The review concluded that there was no clear benefit of using β_2-agonists in the management of recurrent wheeze in the first 2 years of life. Since both children with episodic wheeze, predominantly virus-induced, and atopic children with chronic asthma may have been included in these studies, we cannot draw any conclusions about the difference between the two clinical phenotypes. There appears to be an overwhelming effect of age rather than phenotype on β_2 responsiveness.

There is quantitative evidence that β_2-agonists are beneficial in adults with episodic viral wheeze. Godden and colleagues followed up a cohort of 167 children with viral wheeze 25 years later and found that 30% continued wheezing with 12% reporting benefit from inhaled β_2-agonists (62). In an experimental viral infection in adults with a history of episodic viral wheeze, methacholine-induced hyperresponsiveness was relieved by inhaled salbutamol, indirectly implying a beneficial role for this drug (39). Under these circumstances, whether β_2-agonists are as effective in viral episodic wheeze as in acute viral exacerbations of asthma is unclear, but clinical experience shows that their effect in the latter situation is often poor.

Corticosteroids

A systematic review of the use of corticosteroids in viral wheeze published by the Cochrane Collaboration (63) identified only five recent papers on this subject, two assessing low-dosage prophylactic inhaled corticosteroids, one in preschool (36) and the other in schoolaged children (38), and three evaluating episodic high-dosage inhaled corticosteroids in preschool children (37,64,65). Thirty-seven studies were excluded from the review for various reasons including treatment of postbronchiolitic wheeze; treatment of classic asthmatics with persistent symptoms; treatment of recurrent preschool wheezing without a clear description of presence/absence of chronic intercurrent symptoms; and nonrandomized or uncontrolled trials. The lack of attention in the literature to viral wheeze is in itself an important finding of this review, highlighting the denial or poor awareness of this potential phenotype.

As well as reviewing these five studies in detail, outcomes were examined and where possible data merged in a meta-analysis to highlight important findings (Fig. 9). The two studies of prophylactic inhaled corticosteroids (400 µg of beclomethasone or budesonide per day for 4–6 months by metered-dose inhaler/spacer) were parallel in design and did not demonstrate any clear benefit from corticosteroids over placebo in terms of reduction of oral corticosteroid requirement, hospital admission, or other outcomes (36,38). The three studies of episodic high-dosage inhaled

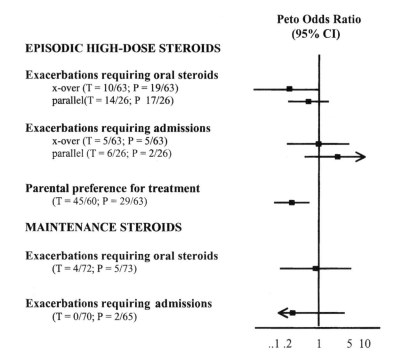

Figure 9 Schematic of odds ratios for episodic and maintenance steroids in those outcomes meta-analyzed in the Cochrane review. Those outcomes where steroids had a favorable effect compared to placebo are to the left of the center line. Numbers in each group are given: T = treatment (i.e., steroids); P = placebo.

corticosteroids (1.6–2.25mg beclomethasone or budesonide per day for 5–10 days by metered-dose inhaler/spacer) included two of crossover and one of parallel design (37,64,65). Active treatment led to a reduction in the requirement for oral corticosteroids during episodes; parents expressed a clear preference for inhaled corticosteroid over placebo. It is arguable whether this form of therapy is preferable to a short oral course of prednisolone from a practical or a pharmacological viewpoint. However, there were no randomized controlled trials of oral corticosteroids specifically in patients with viral wheeze to confirm this. One small study (66) and one that used only historic controls (67) have demonstrated a beneficial effect of oral corticosteroids in young so-called asthmatics, some of whom may have been viral wheezers, whereas a third study found no difference between oral corticosteroids and placebo (68). The review adds weight to the assertion that episodic viral wheeze is a distinct disorder. A lack of chronic inflammation seen in those with viral wheeze compared to atopic asthma may explain the lack of response to maintenance inhaled corticosteroids (see also Fig. 10). It is possible that different mechanisms are responsible for chronic daily asthma symptoms and acute exacerbations (17), but in classic asthma, low-dosage inhaled steroids may ameliorate both types of symptom (57,69).

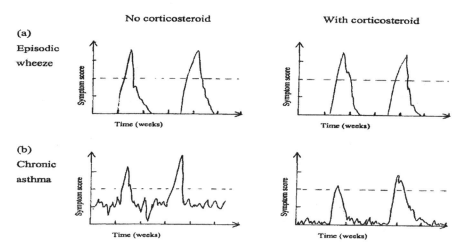

Figure 10 Theoretical explanation of the good response of acute episodes to regular prophylactic inhaled corticosteroids (ICS) in chronic asthma in contrast to exclusive viral wheeze. If only intercurrent (presumed inflammatory) symptoms are amenable to ICS therapy, by reducing the symptom baseline, acute episodes may appear to be reduced to amplitude too, even if their overall amplitude is unaltered.

Evidence regarding the potential benefits of the treatment of viral wheeze is not strong. Most studies have not clearly differentiated those with chronic allergic asthma from those with episodic viral wheeze. Indeed only recently have studies attempted to do so. Response to β_2-agonists is influenced by age. Many young wheezy children, the majority of whom are likely to have viral wheeze, respond poorly if at all. Viral wheezers do seem to gain marginal relief from high-dosage inhaled corticosteroids and possibly from oral corticosteroids, but unlike allergic asthmatic children, they do not respond to low-dosage prophylactic inhaled corticosteroids. Without head-to-head clinical trials, comparing the outcome of acute episodes in viral wheezers and in chronic wheezers with exacerbations, the therapeutic evidence to support splitting rather than lumping these conditions, will remain inconclusive.

F. Impact of Acute Viral Wheeze

Impact on the Family

Only one study has attempted to measure the impact of preschool wheeze on the quality of life (70) and economic burden on families (33). This was in the context of a clinical trial of guided self-management for families of children who attended secondary care because of an acute episode. Over half of the 200 children were reported as wheezing only with colds compared with those who wheezed on other occasions. Families of children wheezing only with colds had significantly better quality of life indices than those with interval symptoms (unpublished analysis).

Although the overall public health of preschool wheeze has been estimated (33), there are no differential data for episodic viral wheeze and multiple chronic wheeze. Based on a recent population survey (31), and assuming similar degrees of severity, about 65% of the overall health burden of preschool wheeze is due to viral episodic wheeze, but these data provide no support for viral wheeze as a separate condition, although they do indicate its importance to public health.

III. Epidemiology and Natural History

A. Definitions

Change in definition with time, as our understanding of disease evolves, has bedeviled epidemiology and is particularly important in the context of wheezing disorders. The definition of viral wheeze and its differentiation from other forms of wheezing is central to attempts to gather epidemiological evidence to support its existence as a separate condition, with an age spectrum, risk factors, and natural history that differentiate viral wheeze from other disorders, in particular atopic asthma (71,72).

By the nature of population studies, in which large numbers of subjects are surveyed, a simple approach to disease definition is needed. Studies of childhood wheeze have employed a range of definitions, mostly derived from work on adults.

Physician-Diagnosed Asthma

Some studies based upon the term "physician-diagnosed asthma" are undermined by lack of any standard definition for the term and by clear bias towards the atopic phenotype (73). Comparing a survey today when asthma refers to the allergic phenotype to a survey 20 years ago, when many physicians believed that all wheezing in infancy and early childhood (with obvious exceptions) be labeled as asthma, is likely to be misleading. The examination of population-based data in which definitions are based on symptoms has proved more useful.

Symptom-Based Epidemiology: "Wheeze" Is Not Always Wheeze

The study of symptoms such as wheeze has the advantage of avoiding doctors' preferences for specific diagnoses. However, even the study of wheeze is plagued by difficulty, as discussed in the Introduction (above). In a recent questionnaire to parents of wheezing children, some thought it a sound such as whistling, squeaking, or rasping; others defined it as a different rate, style, or timbre of breathing; and some thought it was the same as coughing (9). This is an important reminder to those studying and treating wheeze that reported wheeze might not be wheezing after all. Second, if wheeze is a sign or symptom produced by the physical narrowing of the airways, then just as hemiplegia can have several different causes so airway narrowing can be the end result of several different pathological processes. These intrinsic complexities create difficulty when collecting data based solely on patient questionnaires or doctors' interpretation of a symptom or sign.

The approach most widely used in surveys is to collect data on wheeze, assuming that wheeze is equivalent to intrathoracic airway obstruction and therefore that (with obvious exceptions) all conditions that include wheeze fall within the broad definition of asthma. This circumvents the variations and inconsistencies in doctor diagnoses and allows a symptom-based approach. In older subjects, simple physiological measurements such as PEF may be employed to support evidence of variable airway obstruction. It is, however, important not to accept the false assumption that asthma is a single-phenotype disorder. This very basic approach to epidemiological research in asthma has been advocated strongly by Pearce and colleagues (74).

Multicomponent Asthma Phenotypes

In contrast to this simple approach, Woolcock, Peat and colleagues (3) have advocated a more complex definition of asthma for epidemiological purposes: wheeze + allergy + BHR. This very narrow view of asthma, precluding all other possible wheezing phenotypes, is clearly inappropriate in the search for other conditions (phenotypes) that fall within the basic definition of asthma (2). Moreover, in clinical practice adding BHR as a requirement does not improve diagnostic specificity and decreases sensitivity in children (75).

Considering the individual components (so-called partial phenotypes) is critically important in building up evidence for different conditions. Some form of principal component or cluster analysis could be applied to sets of clinical, physiological, and immunological features to justify new syndromes or even separate diseases (Fig. 4).

B. Evidence That Viral Wheeze Is Separate

Natural History

Three major cohort studies of the natural history of early childhood wheeze point clearly to the existence of at least two major phenotypes. One crucial question when considering the evidence is whether there is a feature that could be said to be the sine qua non for viral wheeze and at the same time establish this as an easily identified disorder distinct from allergic asthma.

Cogswell and colleagues demonstrated in Poole (England) that, notwithstanding the importance of early exposure to the dust-mite antigen *Der p*I for the subsequent development of asthma at school age, the odds ratio for atopic asthma was no greater in those children who wheezed in the first 2 years of life than in those who did not (52). Nor, in retrospect, were those children subsequently shown to be atopic at the age of 11 more likely to have wheezed in the first 2 years of life. These data suggested for the first time that wheezing disorders of young children and childhood atopic asthma were completely independent disorders. The conclusions are unchanged after 22 years (53).

The second major epidemiological evidence supporting different phenotypes of childhood wheezing comes from the cohort followed in Tucson, Arizona (11). In this study more than 800 infants have been followed from birth with reports published to their teenage years. At least two different prognostic categories of preschool wheeze with distinctive risk factors have been identified. One group ("persistent wheezers") initially suffered wheeze during viral infections, but wheezing persisted into school age in association with risk factors characteristic of classic, atopic asthma (elevated IgE levels, personal atopy, and family history of asthma). Another group of children ("transient wheezers") also suffered wheeze during viral infections, but were not associated with early markers to atopy. An interesting finding was that the transient wheezers had reduced lung function measured in the first weeks of life (prior to the onset of symptoms) whereas the persistent wheezers did not. The risk of wheeze in the first years, in contrast to school age, was inversely related to atopic status (51) (Fig. 11). This strongly suggests a wheezing condition in young children associated with reduced lung function in infancy, and unrelated (or inversely related) to allergy.

The third piece of evidence comes from a cohort of 2,511 children in Aberdeen, Scotland enrolled at primary school and followed for 25 years (62,76). Three groups were selected based on clinical diagnoses of asthma (defined as recurrent dyspnea, sometimes without a cold, $n = 121$), wheezy bronchitis (wheeze only in the presence of cold, $n = 167$), and healthy controls ($n = 167$). Around 80% in each group were seen 25 years later when both asthmatics and viral wheezers were more likely to have current wheeze than controls (odds ratios [95% confidence inter-

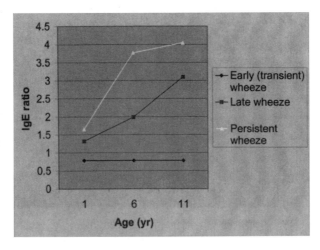

Figure 11 Ratio of IgE in symptomatic groups to IgE in nonwheezers for each age group, from the Tucson cohort (recalculated from data in Ref. 51). Early (transient) wheezers only wheezed under 3 years; persistent wheezers reported wheeze at 3, 6, and 11 year surveys; late wheezers wheezed after 3 years, but not before.

nal CI] of 14.4 [6.9–30.3], 3.8 [1.9–7.6] and 1, respectively). More asthmatics used bronchodilators than viral wheezers and controls (42%, 12%, and 6%, respectively), and more asthmatics took inhaled steroids than did viral wheezers and controls (15%, 3%, 2%, respectively). There was no difference between the viral wheezers and controls in airway responsiveness, but the asthmatics displayed the characteristic hyperresponsiveness to an inhaled challenge. IgE levels in the adults who had had viral wheeze as children was intermediate between the levels of those with a history of asthma and those who were normal as children (76). This was the first study to demonstrate clearly the physiological as well as symptomatic differences between adults with a history of wheezy bronchitis (viral wheeze) and atopic asthma in childhood.

These cohort studies strongly suggest that there are different types of wheezing disorder. They fall short in one key respect: there is no direct evidence to equate transient preschool wheezing with either clinically or microbiologically defined virus-induced wheeze (although the Aberdeen cohort came close to this). Thus, although the evidence is strong, we are short of absolute proof.

The data derived from the follow-up of children in secondary care are likely to be biased by the inclusion of children whose disease is more severe and likely to be multifactorial in cause. For instance, the probability that allergic children are overrepresented among cases of acute infantile bronchiolitis treated in hospital is one explanation for inconsistencies between studies. Hospital-based studies of RSV-positive bronchiolitis tend to show a weak association with allergy during follow-up, whereas the best population-based data show no such long-term effect (27).

Nevertheless, careful analysis of hospitalized children can reveal useful information. For instance, studies by Wilson and colleagues (71,72) showed that in young wheezy children, wheeze only with virus infections was not associated with atopy, but by the age of 5 the distinction between subgroups was blurred. A personal history of atopy and parental asthma (or BHR in the child) were the main risk factors for both attack severity and interval symptoms, but there was no difference in the risk for children with viral episodes or persistent symptoms.

Prevalence

Data on prevalence assume that viral wheeze is a separate condition, and therefore cannot be used to answer the question. However, given its importance, it is worth summarizing. Because few surveys have included a question such as "Does your child wheeze only with a cold and not at other times?" most data must be culled from general surveys of preschool wheeze, making the assumption that so-called transient wheeze is equivalent to viral wheeze. Any estimates must be interpreted in this context.

The prevalence of a wheezing disorder as measured by a cross-sectional population survey may be influenced by the case definition and the method of data collection. In general, past British surveys that enquire about specific diagnoses, such as wheezy bronchitis and asthma, obtain somewhat lower prevalence figures, by as much as one-quarter to one-half, than those that refer to symptoms such as wheeze. Estimates of changes in prevalence over time are difficult to ascertain due to the evolution of diagnostic terms such as "wheezy bronchitis" into "viral wheeze" (71). These complexities limit our understanding of the prevalence of viral wheeze, but by looking at "wheezy bronchitis" and studies of preschool wheeze we can estimate the prevalence of viral wheeze and deduce the resulting burden on society (Table 1).

Although viral wheeze in young children as a specific clinical diagnosis has only been studied prospectively in one cohort (31), the evidence above suggests that it may be very common in young children, with perhaps as many as 20–30% of under-3s having at least one episode. These are children who do not fit the classic asthma phenotype because either they do not report interval symptoms or their asthma is transient, and confined to early childhood. However, it is important to remember that the majority of acute exacerbations of asthma in later childhood are also associated with viral upper respiratory tract infections and hence share a common trigger, if not the same pattern of illness.

Has the prevalence of viral wheeze altered recently? The only direct evidence to support an increase comes from the Leicester cohort (30,31) (Table 1), which showed a doubling of all forms of preschool wheeze and all grades of severity over the 1990s. Assuming that viral wheeze is a nonatopic condition, this implies that a factor other than allergy is responsible for alterations in the prevalence of wheeze. This is supported indirectly by a study of older children, in which an increase in the prevalence of asthma was not explained by changes in the prevalence of atopy (77).

In contrast, repeated questionnaire studies in school children in Aberdeen, Scotland, found that although classic-pattern asthma had increased in prevalence, viral wheeze remained unaltered (78).

Risk Factors

Risk factors provide clues to pathophysiology and thereby suggest interventions to prevent or ameliorate disease. A large amount of information regarding risk factors has been obtained in relation to asthma, but until recently possible phenotypes of childhood wheeze have been lumped together in epidemiological surveys.

Lower Levels of Lung Function

Several groups have shown a relationship between premorbid lung function and subsequent episodes of wheezing in infancy (Table 3). The most consistent finding is reduced maximal expiratory flow at functional residual capacity (FRC) (V_{max} FRC) by the rapid thoracic compression technique (RTC) (41).

Other physiological evidence suggests that the reduction in maximal flow is due to a reduction in airway caliber rather than to altered lung or airway compliance. However, in the absence of tissue samples, the evidence is all indirect. Gender differences in risk between studies have not been adequately explained.

Table 3 Contribution of Fetal Lung Development to Risk of Wheezing in Infancy

Source of data (Ref.)	n^a	Premorbid lung function: the principal factors associated with subsequent wheezing
Tucson, USA 1988 (79)	124	Low $t_{PEF}:t_E$ (boys)
		Low FRC_{He} (girls)
		Low respiratory conductance
Boston, MA, USA 1993 (80)	159	Low V_{max} FRC (girls)
London, UK 1992 (47)	73	Low V_{max} FRC (boys)
		Low PC_{30} histamine (girls)
Perth, Australia 1990 (46)	252	Tidal flow limitation at rest

[a] Number who underwent premorbid lung function tests.
Source: Adapted from Ref. 41.

BHR in the neonatal period was clearly shown in one study to be a (dose-dependent) risk factor for subsequent infant wheeze in girls (47) and in another for the development of classic asthma or reduced lung function (but not for BHR) in childhood many years later (50).

Only one study has provided evidence that premorbid lung function (reduced V_{max} FRC and increased respiratory resistance) is a risk factor for early transient wheeze (which may be equated with virus-induced wheeze), but not for persistent or late-onset (atopy-associated) wheeze (11).

The absence of BHR in wheezy infants (42,45,46) and in teenage children (81) and adults (39,62) shows that enhanced bronchial responsiveness does not occur between episodes of viral wheeze. It is interesting that an experimental infection of adults predisposed to viral wheeze did demonstrate an increase in BHR and methacholine from a normal (symptom-free) baseline during and after the wheezing illness (39) (Fig. 8), but the mechanisms are not yet explained.

Passive Smoking

The evidence that exposure to environmental tobacco smoke (ETS) or passive smoking is strongly associated with wheezing in the first 5 years of life, infantile bronchiolitis, and asthma has recently been reviewed (82). A dose-dependent relationship has been found between the proportion of young children with so-called bronchitis and the number of maternal cigarettes smoked (83,84). The effect may operate prenatally, as demonstrated by its association with reduced airway caliber in the neonates of maternal smokers (79,80) and with bronchial hyperresponsiveness in animal studies (85). A precise relationship between ETS and viral wheeze has not yet been established. The Tucson cohort has demonstrated a twofold increased risk for developing both transient and persistent wheeze in early childhood (79), and so does not provide further evidence to discriminate between them. Maternal smoking was a risk factor for both viral wheeze and so-called multiple wheeze in the Leicester cohort (31).

Air Pollution

There are no specific data on the relationship between other forms of air pollution and viral wheezing, although information can again be deduced from studies of children with so-called bronchitis or wheeze, some of whom are likely to have had viral wheeze. The comparison of children living in Leipzig and Munich, where different pollutants were found (sulfur dioxide and particulates vs. nitrogen dioxide, respectively) demonstrated a higher level of so-called bronchitis in Leipzig (31% vs. 16%) and a higher level of hayfever in Munich (8.6% vs. 2.4%) (86). It is believed that airway inflammation results from certain forms of pollution and perhaps this could predispose a child to wheeze during a viral upper respiratory tract infection. The interaction between chronic exposure to different pollutants, including particulates and ETS, and acute viral infections is an area that requires further study (87,88).

Other Risk Factors

Other studies have compared the risk factors for transient wheeze with persistent or late wheeze, either prospectively (as for the Tucson studies) or retrospectively, as in the Italian SIDRIA study (89). The latter showed an increased risk of transient vs. late-onset wheeze for increased sibling number and daycare attendance in the first 2 years of life (both of which were associated with a reduced risk of late-onset disease) and maternal age over 35. Breastfeeding for over 6 months reduced the risk of transient wheeze, but conversely increased the risk of late-onset wheeze. These results confirm data from Tucson on siblings and daycare (90) (Fig. 12) and

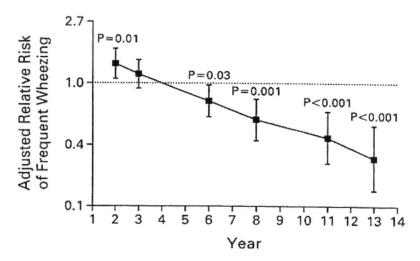

Figure 12 Adjusted odds ratio of wheezing for children with two or more older siblings (compared with zero or one older siblings) at various ages in a single cohort of children. (From Ref. 90.)

Table 4 Risk Factors That Differentiate Viral Wheeze from Wheeze Due to Multiple Triggers in Preschool Children

Risk factors that discriminate		Risk factors that do not discriminate
Maternal asthma and "bronchitis"	↑MW	Paternal asthma
Male gender	↑MW	Other parental atopy
Fossil fuel stove[a]	↑VW	Age
Older siblings[b]	↑MW	Breastfeeding; deprivation index

[a] Only in White families.
[b] Only in South Asian families.
VW, viral wheeze; MW, multiple-trigger wheeze.
Source: Unpublished data from the Leicester Cohort Study.

on breastfeeding (91), and reinforce the evidence that the two patterns of wheeze represent different disorders.

Further detailed analysis of the Leicester cohort (31), which was specifically designed to identify children who only wheeze with a "cold, fever or sore throat," has detected several risk factors that differ between such children and those who wheeze with response to a variety of triggers (classic asthma), and several that do not (Table 4), again providing support for a real difference.

C. Relationship with COPD

Since the discovery by Barker and colleagues of the links among birthweight, respiratory infection in infancy, and COPD in adulthood (92), there has been considerable interest in the long-term outcome of childhood diseases. The observation that children with viral lower respiratory tract illness in the first few years of life have a poorer long-term outcome is not new. It was suggested 50 years ago by Oswald and colleagues in a retrospective study. The evidence that early lung development predetermines lifelong respiratory health was reviewed many years ago (93). However, in a review of a number of databases, Strachan showed that for a number of outcomes, acute chest illness in infants during the winter months (the peak "virus season") was not associated with adverse outcomes (94). Despite the lack of evidence, the concept of viral damage to the developing lung has prompted considerable interest in vaccine research, especially in relation to RSV infection.

The concept of secondary damage is not supported in the data from Tucson, in which transient wheezers have apparently normal lung health (albeit a continuation of their postnatal reduction in airway function) in later childhood (11). If there is a connection between viral wheeze and COPD, it could be in a common risk factor (developmental, genetic or both) for both. The true consequences of viral wheeze for the development of chronic bronchitis will only become clearer when birth cohorts are revisited in late adult life. There are huge funding and data-protection issues to be overcome if such lifelong data are to be gathered.

There are, however, interesting similarities between viral wheeze in childhood and chronic obstructive pulmonary disease in adulthood. Viral upper respiratory tract infections are triggers for both disorders, the inflammatory changes in both are characterized by neutrophilic infiltration of the airways (95–97), and neither seems responsive to inhaled corticosteroids or β_2-agonists.

IV. Immunopathology

A. Introduction

If exclusively VW is an inflammatory condition distinct from classic so-called atopic asthma, VW will not be associated with the TH_2 activation: pulmonary CD4-positive lymphocytes skewed to produce increased interleukin (IL)-5 and IL-4, reduced interferon-γ (IFN-γ), leading via C-C chemokines to tissue eosinophilia and eosinophilic cationic protein (ECP) release (98). An alternative and testable view is that VW represents the mild end of the classic asthma spectrum, and is due to intermittent TH_2-driven inflammation. There is one other possibility: that inflammation in acute viral episodes in both classic atopic asthmatics and in VW is similar but is separate from the pattern of inflammation in chronic atopic asthma in the intervals between episodes.

As discussed elsewhere in this book, acute deteriorations of classic atopic asthma are usually triggered by viral colds. If TH_2 activation is always the driving force behind wheeze in atopic asthma, VW without a TH_2 pattern of bronchial inflammation would be compelling evidence of a separate condition. The ideal experiment would compare pulmonary inflammation in patients with a history of classic atopic asthma with those with a history of VW during an acute attack of wheeze triggered by a cold. The purpose of this section is to discuss whether such evidence exists directly, or indirectly, from observational studies or experimental models.

B. Observational Studies

Studies in Adults

The majority of invasive studies of the lower airway in wheezing adults have not considered that VW could be a separate entity. Bronchial biopsy has, however, defined some important aspects of the inflammation underlying symptoms in classic atopic asthma. First, adult asthma with chronic symptoms (as defined by physicians) is probably a single inflammatory entity, irrespective of the presence of so-called atopy as defined by a positive skin prick test. For example, bronchial eotaxin expression, a hallmark of TH_2-driven inflammation, is increased in both atopic and nonatopic (so-called intrinsic) chronic asthmatics (99,100). Second, the level of symptoms at time of sampling is important. Thus adults with persistent symptoms of atopic asthma have higher numbers of EG2-positive cells (eosinophils) in their bronchi than those with intermittent symptoms (101). Indeed, one-third of adults with so-called intermittent symptoms have tissue eosinophils within the normal range

EOSINOPHILS

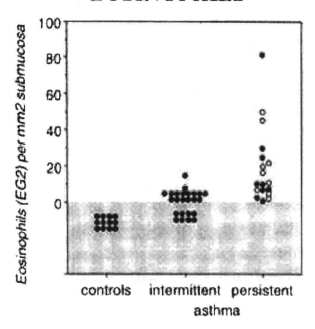

Figure 13 EG2-positive eosinophils in the submucosa from bronchial epithelial biopsies in adults. (From Ref. 101.)

(101) (Fig. 13). These data can be interpreted in two ways. First, TH_2-associated bronchial inflammation is always detectable in atopic asthmatics with active symptoms, but can fall into the normal range during asymptomatic intervals. As an alternative, some adults labeled as asthmatics have in fact VW (notwithstanding some may, like 40% of the population, be allergic by skin prick testing), and in this subgroup bronchial inflammation resolves completely when they are asymptomatic.

VW in Children

Biopsy studies for research in wheezy children are not ethically acceptable. Since the majority of preschool children with acute viral wheeze do not become atopic asthmatics (see above), indirect markers of pulmonary inflammation in young viral wheezers do, however, provide important information about the cellular substrate of VW. Analysis of inflammatory cells in lower airway of preschool and older children with a history of wheeze is now possible using the technique of nonbronchoscopic BAL. In this opportunistic method, lavage is performed via a catheter inserted prior to elective surgery (usually orthopedic or abdominal). The technique is simple. With the head turned to the left, a suction catheter is blindly wedged into the bronchi. Two or three aliquots of 1 ml/kg (up to 20 ml per aliquot) are instilled and rapidly aspirated. In normal healthy children, the resulting leukocyte differential that is very similar to that obtained by fiberoptic BAL (102).

Using nonbronchoscopic BAL, Stevenson and colleagues (21) described the pattern of pulmonary inflammation associated with VW. These children had no family history of atopic disease, and wheezed only with colds. An appropriate symptom-matched group of atopic asthmatic children with extended intervals between attacks and atopic nonasthmatics were also recruited. BAL was performed when the children were asymptomatic, and showed that those with VW did not have an increased percentage of airway eosinophils compared with healthy atopic controls. In contrast, children with atopic asthma with or without prolonged asymptomatic periods had an increased percentage of eosinophils compared with both those with VW (Fig. 14) and normal controls. An absence of persistent TH$_2$ inflammation in the asymptomatic phase of VW has also been reported in a study from Australia. Maclennan et al. (103) recruited children (age 6 months to 12 years) with a history of infrequent wheeze. Although triggers were not specifically recorded at recruitment, the majority of children had VW (Prof. N. Freezer, personal communication). Children with intermittent wheeze had a normal BAL fluid eosinophil differential (compared to healthy controls) and a normal pattern of T-cell markers (HLA DR, IL-2 receptor, CD69, CD28). Furthermore, there was no evidence for TH$_2$-skewed cytokine production by airway CD4 T lymphocytes in the intermittent wheeze group. A clinically more severe group of infantile wheezers has been studied using fiberoptic bronchoscopy.

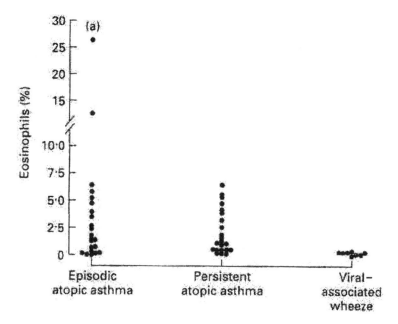

Figure 14 Eosinophil differential count in bronchial lavage fluid from children with different asthma phenotypes. (From Ref. 21.)

Marguet et al. (104) performed fiberoptic BAL on infants (4–46 months) who had at least three successive episodes of wheeze and cough during colds, and compared them with atopic and nonatopic older asthmatics with a history of recurrent wheezing. Although asthmatic children had airway eosinophilia, eosinophils were rare in viral wheezers and healthy controls (Fig. 15). In summary, these data support the argument that VW is not associated with a continuous activation of pulmonary TH$_2$-skewed lymphocytes, but do not address the question of the inflammatory substrate for active wheezing episodes.

Clear proof of a different inflammatory substrate can only come from BAL performed during an acute attack of viral wheeze. The effect of colds per se on the lower respiratory tract of children is an important starting point. We found rhinovirus in the airways of children who had trivial upper respiratory tract symptoms prior to elective surgery. Isolation of a cold virus from the BAL fluid (BALF) was associated with an increased percentage of lymphocytes and neutrophils, but not of eosinophils (105) (Table 5). Thus infection of the pediatric lower respiratory tract with a cold virus and the subsequent inflammation is not sufficient in itself to initiate wheeze. These data are similar to those of Pizzichini et al. (106), who examined induced sputum on adults with naturally acquired colds and found evidence for a profound airway neutrophilia but no increase in eosinophils. No serendipitous BAL study has looked at airway inflammation in acute viral wheeze, since elective surgery is always postponed.

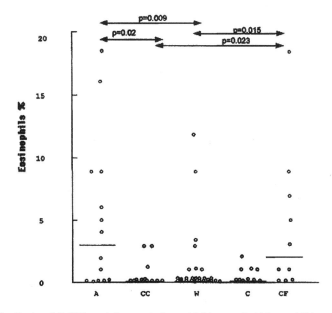

Figure 15 Eosinophil differential count in bronchial lavage fluid from children with a variety of illnesses. A, asthma; CC, chronic cough in infantile wheeze; C, control; CF, cystic fibrosis. (From Ref. 104.)

Table 5 Bronchoalveolar Lavage Fluid Cellularity in Children with Colds Compared with Normal Controls

BALF parameter	Active cold (n = 7)	Controls (n = 7)
Leuk ($\times 10^3$/ml)	210 (180, 890)*	130.0 (100, 190)
AM (%)	60 (25, 73)*	96.0 (95, 97)
AM ($\times 10^3$/ml)	147 (139, 263)	122.0 (95, 184)
Lymph (%)	5 (3.5, 25)*	2.5 (1.6, 3.0)
Lymph ($\times 10^3$/ml)	44 (10, 54)*	3.0 (2.5, 4.4)
Neut (%)	35 (0.3, 72)*	1.0 (0.3, 2.2)
Neut ($\times 10^3$/ml)	64 (0.5, 563)	1.0 (0.6, 2.2)
Eos (%)	0 (0,0)	0 (0,0)
EPI (% nucleated)	2 (1.5, 7.2)	3.0 (1.0, 9.0)

Values are expressed as medians (25th, 75th percentiles).
BALF, bronchoalveolar lavage fluid; Leuk, total leukocytes; AM, alveolar macrophage; Lymph, lymphocytes; Neut, neutrophils; EOS, eosinophils; EPI, ciliated epithelial cells (as a percentage of all nucleated cells).
* $p < 0.05$ compared with controls, Wilcoxon's signed rank test.
Source: Ref. 105.

In contrast, indirect markers of pulmonary inflammation have been used in this age group. These studies need to be treated with more caution since their validity in predicting airway inflammation has rarely been tested. However, the pattern of markers of acute atopic asthma in children is very similar to that of the TH_2-associated activation seen in adults. Thus acutely wheezy children with atopic asthma (viral status unknown) have a pattern of markers characterized by increased serum levels of IL-5, soluble IL-2 receptor (released by activated T cells), ECP, and increased urinary leukotriene E4 (107,108). These markers of TH_2 activation fall as the wheeze resolves, but may still remain elevated above normal during convalescence. The closest information on airway inflammation during virus-triggered so-called classic asthma comes from Norzila et al. (109) who used sputum induction during the acute and convalescent phase in older children (>8 years) admitted with a pre-existing diagnosis of asthma. Although not analyzed separately, 68% of the children studied had acute symptoms triggered by a viral cold. In the acute phase, significant inflammation was present with increased number of sputum eosinophils, neutrophils, and mast cells. Increased sputum ECP, IL-5, and IL-8 (a neutrophil chemoattractant) were also seen. On recovery, there was a significant fall in the number of all inflammatory cells and inflammatory markers. Of particular note is that the inflammatory pattern in the acute phase would be produced by combining the neutrophilic pattern seen in our study of asymptomatic children with trivial colds, with the eosinophil pattern seen in the airways of classic asthmatics during antigen challenge (110). Similar results have recently been found in adults with acute severe asthma. (140).

No similar study has defined the serum TH_2 cytokine profile in symptomatic children with a history of VW, in part because of the ethical considerations. In contrast, measurement of inflammatory markers in the breath is a noninvasive and ethically acceptable. An increased concentration of exhaled nitric oxide (eNO) is now regarded as the hallmark of steroid-naive atopic asthma. Elevated eNO has been reported in asthmatics during an exacerbation (viral status unknown), and after allergen challenge (111). Although elevated eNO also occurs with nonwheezing colds (112), the absence of increased eNO in a group of steroid naïve wheezers would be strong evidence of a different inflammatory pattern. Baraldi et al. (113) collected exhaled nitric oxide (eNO) from infants (9–14 months) with no family history of asthma, during their first episode of viral wheeze. These symptomatic, steroid-naïve first time viral wheezers had eNO levels of 8.3 parts per billion (ppb) similar to normal healthy controls (5.5 ppb). In contrast, children (7–33 months) with a history of recurrent exacerbations and acute wheeze (viral status unknown) had significantly elevated eNO (14.1 ppb), which fell after oral steroid therapy. Ratjen et al. (114) confirmed these observations in a group of 17 infants with acute virus-associated wheeze. Compared to 22 term infants with no respiratory disease, end-tidal NO was reduced in the viral-wheezers. Because of their young age, and lack of follow-up data, none of the acutely wheezing infants would fulfil the strict definition of VW. However, these data are a clear indication that viral-triggered wheeze can occur without an asthmatic pattern of inflammation. Indeed, a population of adults has been defined who wheeze but do not have increased eNO or airway hyperresponsiveness to histamine (115). This group is not considered as having classic asthma, but whether they have VW remains unknown.

Other indirect evidence for an absence of TH_2 activation in pediatric viral wheeze is provided by the mediator profile in nasal lavage. Van Schaik et al. (55) measured the concentrations of IL-4 (TH_2) and IFN-γ (TH_1) in young children during acute episodes of virus-induced wheeze and uncomplicated upper respiratory tract infections. In the wheezing group the concentration of IFN-γ, but not IL-4, was increased, a pattern not compatible with a TH_2-type response.

If TH_2 inflammation is not a feature of VW, what mediators could cause bronchoconstriction? Van Schaik et al. (55) found significantly higher levels of cysteinyl leukotrienes (cystLTs) in the nasal lavage of infants with viral wheeze than in those with an acute cold. In classic asthma, cystLTs, especially LTE_4 released from IgE-activated mast cells, act as potent bronchoconstrictors (116). LTE_4 is the end product of pulmonary cystLT metabolism, and is excreted unchanged in urine when released from the lung. Children with chronic atopic asthma have higher urinary (u)LTE_4 than healthy controls (117), and uLTE_4 increases acutely in atopic asthmatics challenged by aerosolized antigen (118). However, cystLTs can be elevated in conditions not associated with the TH_2 activation such as neonatal lung disease (119). We measured uLTE_4 in children aged between 1 and 5 years admitted to hospital with acute viral wheeze and compared them with children without respiratory disease. uLTE_4 was significantly higher in children with acute viral wheeze than in controls (median [IQR]; 165 [110,285] vs. 125 [82,163] ng/mmol creatinine, p = 0.03), and levels fell into the normal range between the acute and convalescent phase (mean [95% confidence interval] difference, 60 [13,105] ng/mmol creatinine) (120). However, these children are selected for severe disease, and are at increased risk of developing classic asthma as older children. Some may therefore already have pulmonary TH₂ activation. A recent study in nonasthmatic adults has shown leukotriene production during simple rhinovirus infection (141). Such data highlight the difficulty of observational studies. Unless the population has been defined very carefully, assumptions have to be made retrospectively about what has triggered symptoms, and about the previous disease pattern. Unless they are followed up carefully, it may not be possible to describe phenotypic features (such as atopy or BHR) fully.

In summary, there is a group of children with viral wheeze who do not exhibit the features of classic asthma. When studies are combined, they are defined by an absence of airway eosinophilia between episodes, low levels of eNO when wheezy, and increased production of IFN-γ. These data indirectly suggest that viral wheeze can be a separate inflammatory condition, but by no means constitute adequate proof. Furthermore, the (unlikely) possibility that viral wheeze in atopic asthmatics and those with VW is a similar condition separate from chronic asthma has not been addressed by observational studies, and it is very unlikely that any observational study will result in an unbiased group of patients with VW and viral-induced atopic asthma triggered by the same virus. A clear understanding of differences and similarities in inflammatory substrate must therefore come from experimental infections using well-defined study groups, and the assessment of as wide a range as possible of inflammatory cells and mediators.

C. Viral Wheeze Models

Human Models

Experimental models in which laboratory-grown virus is inoculated into the nose of volunteers have long been used to study the effects of so-called common cold viruses. Such models have the advantages of avoiding the heterogeneity of wild-type viruses. They also allow the exact timing of measurements and samples, thus avoiding the noise inherent in wild-type infections when the exact onset and progression of infection may be less easy to establish. The main drawback of such models is the reliance on a virus passaged in cell culture and inoculated into the nose in high titer. It is theoretically possible that the use of a virus that may have been attenuated by laboratory growth and applied in an artificial way to the nose may result in a different illness to that seen in wild infections. However, the many experimental inoculation studies would support the notion that the disease spectrum is similar to that of wild-type infection.

Experimental infections, the majority using human rhinovirus (HRV), have helped to establish the inflammatory response seen in the upper respiratory tract during a cold. This is characterized by neutrophilic infiltration (121–123), although in subjects with allergic rhinitis eosinophils are also found (124,125). Experimental infections have also been used to study changes in airway physiology and inflammation in subjects with allergic asthma. Experimental infections, again predominantly using HRV, have found evidence of inflammation occurring in the lower respiratory tract of asthmatics during the infections. One of the key cells associated with airway inflammation seen in allergic asthma is the eosinophil. Several experimental infections have identified an increase in eosinophils and their products in the lower respiratory tract during the infection (126–128), leading to the widely held belief that the eosinophil is a key cell during asthma exacerbation. An increase in neutrophils and associated chemoattractants such as IL-8 has also been found (126,129). Indeed, there are now many current hypotheses for the pathogenesis of virus-induced asthma exacerbations, including epithelial disruption, airway remodeling, alterations in neural responses, as well as induction of inflammation (130).

In Leicester, we have established an experimental model of adult viral wheeze with the aim of studying the inflammatory mechanisms that underlie VW (39,96). We recruited 24 adults who wheezed only in the presence of common colds (i.e., did not wheeze with exercise, dust or pollen exposure, or animal contact) and 19 healthy controls. Fifteen (60%) viral wheezers and 7 (37%) controls were atopic by skin prick testing. After being infected intranasally with human coronavirus (HCoV) 229E, the second most prevalent of the common cold viruses, 19 of the viral-wheezers and 11 controls developed a cold. Sixteen of the 19 viral wheezers and none of the controls with colds developed lower respiratory tract symptoms (wheeze, shortness of breath, or chest tightness). The viral wheezers were identical to the controls in airway responsiveness at baseline; however, the viral wheezers had a progressive increase in airway responsiveness during the study (Fig. 8). This persisted beyond the symptoms of the illness, which lasted from days 3 to 7 postinoculation. Despite this convincing change in airway responsiveness, the viral wheezers had only minor (3–4%) reductions in FEV_1 and PEF on days with LRT symptoms, a finding seen in experimental infections of allergic asthmatics using HRV (126,127,131–133). The viral wheezers were different from typical allergic asthmatics in their pattern of illness, their lack of use of inhaled corticosteroids, although 14 used occasional β2-agonists, and normal airway responsiveness prior to the infection. Both atopic and nonatopic viral wheezers developed changes in PC_{20} (Fig. 8).

Inflammation was studied in nasal lavages and hypertonic saline-induced sputum collected prior to, during, and after the experimental illness. Viral wheezers had identical nasal and sputum cell counts and levels of IL-8, IFN-γ, tumor necrosis factor α (TNFα), ECP, and LTC_4 to the controls at baseline (96). Small increases in nasal neutrophil counts were seen in both groups with colds during the study, with no significant difference between the two groups. In this respect, both groups behaved much the same as healthy subjects in other experimental infections, although there was no evidence of the eosinophilia that has been described in the nasal samples of those with allergic rhinitis (124). There were no significant changes in nasal cytokines during the study, although there was a trend towards an increase in IL-8 during the symptomatic colds, a finding seen in previous experimental infections (125,129,134). Of note, there was no change in nasal ECP in either atopic or nonatopic viral-wheeze subjects.

A significant increase in the proportion of sputum neutrophils was seen in the viral wheeze group with colds between days 0 and 4 postinoculation, returning towards baseline by day 17, with a reciprocal effect in the proportion of macrophages (96). There was no such effect in the control group. No differences were seen in sputum lymphocytes or eosinophils during the study. Indeed, very low numbers of these cells were present. A significant increase in sputum IL-8 was seen in both viral wheezers and controls with colds on day 4, with levels in both groups returning towards baseline on day 17. There was no difference between groups in IL-8. No significant changes were seen in IFN-γ, TNFα, or LTC$_4$. Of note, there were no significant changes in ECP in the viral wheezers either with or without atopy.

Nasal epithelial disruption, especially ciliary damage and disorganization, was a striking feature of the experimental infection (135) and might explain many of the symptoms.

This is the first experimental infection to study adults with VW. Although their illness was mild, some important information regarding airway physiology and inflammation has been obtained. This model supports the hypothesis that VW is a separate disorder from allergic asthma despite some striking similarities. The clinical history of the illness was distinct with no intercurrent symptoms and no long-term inhaled corticosteroids, although by definition those with VW developed a wheezing illness identical to mild viral exacerbations of asthma with some using inhaled β2-agonists during colds. There was no baseline bronchial hyperresponsiveness, as one would expect in allergic asthma, although subjects developed increased responsiveness during the illness. Finally, the most striking difference was the lack of eosinophilic infiltration into the airways either at baseline or during the infection, as one would expect in allergic asthma. Instead, subjects with VW developed neutrophilic inflammation in both upper and lower respiratory tracts, a feature also seen in viral exacerbations of asthma.

Animal Models

Evidence that viral wheeze is a separate disorder is unlikely to be obtained from animal experiments. Such studies may be used to dissect host–virus interactions in sensitized (so-called allergic) and nonsensitized animals and to determine their modulation by environmental and pharmacological agents.

V. Conclusions

A. Is Virus-Induced Wheeze a Separate Condition?

We have made the case that episodic viral wheeze of (mainly) young children is qualitatively distinct from classic atopic asthma, in the following respects:

- the clinical pattern is different, in particular between episodes (by definition)
- there is no evidence of BHR between episodes
- viral wheeze is independent of atopic allergy
- if it is equivalent to so-called transient early wheeze, the natural history of viral wheeze is distinct
- the immunopathology differs, especially between episodes

- the disorder is not responsive to standard antiasthma therapy (in particular long-term, low-dose inhaled corticosteroids).

Is it simply a form of "intrinsic" asthma? We show that there is no evidence for a localized form of airway allergy, the current hypothesis to explain intrinsic asthma (100), or that BHR is a feature of viral wheeze (except during episodes in the experimental model).

B. Research Agenda

Clinical Research

There are few practicable tools with which to supplement nonspecific clinical features in classifying wheezing disorders of young children. More research is needed into the most fundamental issue: the recognition of symptoms and signs by lay people and professionals. Rather than use the term wheeze, it would be worth exploring a classification in which children with episodic or persistent chestiness are subclassified into clinical syndromes or disorders by applying a range of investigations into their underlying immunopathology, disturbed physiology, and genetics.

Only one cohort has hitherto been studied in an attempt to prospectively investigate the epidemiology of viral wheeze, and to determine whether it is coterminous with transient wheeze (31). Follow-up data from this cohort are awaited but will be vital in helping definitively to answer the question posed in the title. Support for a separate asthma phenotype of viral wheeze will then inform future prenatal (or preconception) cohort studies that will explore fetal developmental and genetic contributions to the disorder.

Until we have direct techniques to biopsy the lower airway in young children with viral wheeze, our understanding of the immunopathology and of the structural basis for viral wheeze will be limited. Ethical constraints are clearly overwhelming.

It is clear that lumping wheezing disorders (or even episodic and interval features within the single disorder atopic asthma) leads to inappropriate therapy. Therapeutic targets must be better defined before appropriate research into mechanisms can be usefully performed, followed by properly targeted clinical trials. Much recent research into the management of wheezy preschool children has produced inconclusive results because viral wheeze, atopic asthma, and possibly other discrete but not as yet ill-defined phenotypes, with potentially different mechanisms and therapeutic responses, have been lumped together in clinical trials. Head-to-head trials should be performed.

Physiological measurement techniques are becoming sufficiently noninvasive and mathematically sophisticated to allow detailed analysis of the functional causes and consequences of viral wheeze (43,44). It will soon be possible to employ these in large numbers of newborn babies to gain further insight into the fetal developmental factors that contribute to disturbed lung function and increased risk of wheeze.

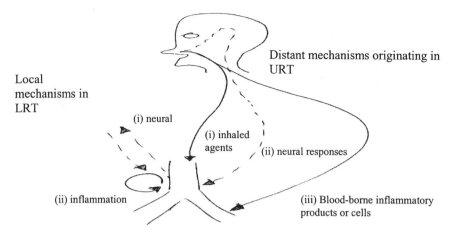

Distant mechanisms originating in URT

Local mechanisms in LRT

(i) neural

(i) inhaled agents

(ii) neural responses

(ii) inflammation

(iii) Blood-borne inflammatory products or cells

Figure 16   A model of viral wheeze.

Host–Virus Interaction

The nature of the host response to a wide variety of virus types is clearly an important research objective. Where is the final common pathway, which could be labeled viral hyperresponsiveness (VHR) by analogy with BHR in classic asthma? A model has been proposed (Fig. 16). The components are all amenable to study, ideally in the context of a human experimental model such as that described by McKean (39). It can be used to answer questions such as:

Is VHR a manifestation of a specific immune response to viral infection of the respiratory tract (analogous to intrinsic asthma)?

What are the separate contributions of upper and lower airway inflammation to this process, given that we now have clear evidence that even human rhinovirus can directly infect the lower airways.

If there is no measurable difference in the immune response to infection between those with and without episodic viral wheeze, does the difference lie in some physiological response to inflammatory products?

If so, can this be mimicked by a bronchial challenge technique?

Is there any evidence of airway remodeling in viral wheeze, given that this has been described in nonatopic individuals (136)?

Can valid indirect techniques to explore the host response to virus infection be developed in adult models and applied to young children?

The issue of viral latency has been raised in the possible relationship between adenovirus and asthma (137). The possibility that this could be an explanation for postbronchiolitic recurrent wheeze should be examined.

Models of Viral Wheeze

Ethical constraints limit experimental studies of young wheezy children to therapeutic trials or preventive interventions. All other research is observational. Further developing adult human volunteer models will be important, although they have many limitations as models of viral wheeze in very young children (age of subjects, mildness of episodes, artificial infection technique, etc.). Most of these limitations also apply to adult models of viral exacerbations of atopic asthma.

Animal models of acute viral RTI are widely available and have shed light on the pathogenesis of RSV-like infections. Their relevance to viral wheeze in young children is doubtful, in particular since we know that in human infants fetal pulmonary development factors put children at risk. This cannot easily be replicated in animal models. If adult models are one step removed from the problem of virus-induced wheeze in children, animal models are several steps further away.

If there are problems describing the ideal features of a human model, virological issues are even more complex. Scores of virus strains can provoke wheeze. In asthma models, not all are equally effective; in fact some reports have been based on studies in which the clinical syndrome under investigation was not apparently produced (138). Viral strains with known propensity to produce the clinical response should be developed, ideally as molecular clones, to avoid genetic drift in clinical samples and laboratory cultures, and to facilitate collaborative research worldwide. A variety of virus types (HRV, HCoV, etc.) should be made available, all produced under vaccine-standard, GMP conditions (to avoid all potentially transmissible agents), and backed up by the necessary molecular toolkits.

There are advantages of molecular clones in parallel, tissue-based research, since key genes can be manipulated in order to explore important viral determinants of particular tissue responses in dissecting out host–virus epithelial interactions.

Genetics

Better case definition together with a better understanding of the immunopathology of VW will be a preliminary to candidate gene studies and genetic epidemiology. There are hints of familial clustering (139). Given the evidence that fetal lung developmental differences explain some of the risk, genes that affect airway development may be a fruitful area of study. The β-adrenoceptor may be one such gene (personal observations).

References

1. Silverman M. Out of the mouths of babes and sucklings: lessons from early childhood asthma. Thorax 1993; 48:1200–1204.
2. Ciba Foundation Guest Symposium. Terminology, definitions and classification of chronic pulmonary emphysema and related conditions. Thorax 1959; 14:286–299.
3. Toelle BG, Peat JK, Salome CM, Mellis CM, Woolcock AJ. Toward a definition of asthma for epidemiology. Am Rev Respir Dis 1992; 146:633–637.

4. Hargreave FE, Ryan G, Thomson NC, O'Byrne PM, Latimer K, Juniper EF, Dolovich J. Bronchial responsiveness to histamine or methacholine in asthma: measurement and clinical significance. J Allergy Clin Immunol 1981; 68:347–355.

5. Silverman M. Introduction. In: Silverman M, ed. Childhood Asthma and Other Wheezing Disorders, 2nd ed. London: Arnold, 2002.

6. van den Biggelaar AH, van Ree R, Rodrigues LC, Lell B, Deelder AM, Kremsner PG, Yazdanbaksh M. Decreased atopy in children infected with schistosoma haematobium: a role for parasite-induced interleukin-10. Lancet 2000; 356:1723–1727.

7. van den Biggelaar AH, Lopuhaa C, van Ree R, van der Zee JS, Jans J, Hoek A, Migombet B, Borrmann S, Luckner D, Kremsner PG, Yazdanbaksh M. The prevalence of parasite infestation and the house dust mite sensitisation in Gabonese schoolchildren. Int Arch Allergy Immunol 2001; 126:231–238.

8. Meslier N, Charbonneau G, Racineux JL. Wheezes. Eur Respir J 1995; 8:1942–1948.

9. Cane RS, Ranganathan SC, McKenzie SA. What do parents of wheezy children understand by "wheeze"? Arch Dis Child 2000; 82:327–332.

10. Elphick HE, Sherlock P, Foxall G, Simpson EJ, Shiell NA, Primhak RA, Everard ML. Survey of respiratory sounds in infants. Arch Dis Child 2001; 84:35–39.

11. Martinez FD, Wright AL, Taussig LM, Holberg CJ, Halonen M, Morgan WJ, The Group Health Medical Associates. Asthma and wheezing in the first six years of life. N Engl J Med 1995; 332:133–138.

12. Noviski N, Cohen L, Springer C, Bar-Yishay E, Avital A, Godfrey S. Bronchial provocation determined by breath sounds compared with lung function. Arch Dis Child 1991; 66:952–955.

13. Sanchez I, Powell RE, Pasterkamp H. Wheezing and airflow obstruction during methacholine challenge in children with cystic fibrosis and in normal children. Am Rev Respir Dis 1993; 147:705-709.

14. Phagoo S, Wilson NM, Silverman M. Evaluation of a new interrupter device for measuring bronchial responsiveness and the response to bronchodilator in 3 year old children. Eur Respir J 1996; 9:1374–1380.

15. Klug B, Bisgaard H. Lung function and short-term outcome in young asthmatic children. Eur Respir J 1999; 14:1185–1189.

16. Bridge PD, McKenzie SA. Airway resistance measured by the interrupter technique: expiration or inspiration, mean or median? Eur Respir J 2001; 17:495–498.

17. Reddel H, Ware S, Marks G, Salome C, Jenkins C, Woolcock A. Differences between asthma exacerbations and poor asthma control. Lancet 1999; 353:364–369.

18. Krawiec ME, Westcott JY, Chu HW, Balzar S, Trudeau JB, Schwartz LB, Wenzel SE. Persistent wheezing in very young children is associated with lower respiratory inflammation. Am J Respir Crit Care Med 2001; 163:1338–1343.

19. Silverman M, Pedersen S. Outcome measures in early childhood asthma and other wheezing disorders. Eur Respir J 1996; 9(Suppl 21):1–49.

20. Silverman M, Pedersen S, Grigg J. Measurement of airway inflammation in children. Am J Respir Crit Care Med 2000; 162 (Part 2):S1.

21. Stevenson EC, Turner G, Heaney LG, Schock BC, Taylor R, Gallagher T, Ennis M, Shields MD. Bronchoalveolar lavage findings suggest two different forms of childhood asthma. Clin Exp Allergy 1997; 27:1027–1035.

22. Bush A, Pohunek P. Brush biopsy and mucosal biopsy. Am J Respir Crit Care Med 2000; 162 (Part 2):S18–S22.

23. Horn ME, Brain E, Gregg I, Inglis JM, Yealland SJ, Taylor P. Respiratory viral infection and wheezy bronchitis in childhood. Thorax 1979; 34:23–28.

24. McIntosh K, Ellis EF, Hoffman LS, Lybass TG, Eller JJ, Fulginiti VA. The association of viral and bacterial respiratory infections with exacerbations of wheezing in young asthmatic children. J Paediatr 1973; 82:578–590.

25. Isaacs D, Flowers D, Clarke JR, Valman HB, MacNaughton MR. Epidemiology of coronavirus respiratory infections. Arch Dis Child 1983; 58:500–503.

26. Mertsola J, Ziegler T, Ruuskanen O, Vanto T, Koivikko A, Halonen P. Recurrent wheezy bronchitis and viral respiratory infections. Arch Dis Child 1991; 66:124–129.

27. Stein RT, Sherrill D, Morgan WJ, Holberg CJ, Halonen M, Taussig LM, Wright AL, Martinez FD. Respiratory syncytial virus in early life and risk of wheeze and allergy by age 13 years. Lancet 1999; 29:541–545.

28. Dawson B, Illsley R, Horobin G, Mitchell R. A survey of childhood asthma in Aberdeen. Lancet 1969; 1:827–830.

29. Clough JB, Holgate ST. Episodes of respiratory morbidity in children with cough and wheeze. Am J Respir Crit Care Med 1994; 150:48–53.

30. Brooke AM, Lambert PC, Burton PR, Clarke C, Luyt DK, Simpson H. The natural history of respiratory symptoms in preschool children. Am J Respir Crit Care Med 1995; 152:1872–1878.

31. Kuehni CE, Davis A, Brooke AM, Silverman M. Are all wheezing disorders in very young (preschool) children increasing in prevalence? Lancet 2001; 357:1821–1825.

32. Custovic A, Simpson BM, Simpson A, Kissen P, Woodcock A; NAC Manchester Asthma and Allergy Study Group. Effect of environmental manipulation in pregnancy and early life on respiratory symptoms and atopy during first year of life: a randomised trial. Lancet 2001; 358:188–193.

33. Stevens C, Turner D, Kuehni C, Couriel J, Silverman M. The economic impact of wheezing and asthma in the under fives. Eur Resp J 2003; 21:in press.

34. Silverman M, Wang M, Taub N. A clinical trial of nasal corticosteroids in young children with viral episodic wheeze. Thorax 2003; 57:in press.

35. Clough JB, Williams JD, Holgate ST. Effect of atopy on the natural history of symptoms, peak expiratory flow, and bronchial responsiveness in 7- and 8-year old children with cough and wheeze. A 12-month longitudinal study [published erratum appears in Am Rev Respir Dis 1992 Aug;146(2)540]. Am Rev Respir Dis 1991; 143:755–760.

36. Wilson N, Sloper K, Silverman M. Effect of continuous treatment with topical corticosteroid on episodic viral wheeze in preschool children. Arch Dis Child 1995; 72:317–320.

37. Wilson NM, Silverman M. Treatment of acute, episodic asthma in preschool children using intermittent high dose inhaled steroids at home. Arch Dis Child 1990; 65:407–410.

38. Doull IJ, Lampe FC, Smith S, Schreiber J, Freezer NJ, Holgate ST. Effect of inhaled corticosteroids on episodes of wheezing associated with viral infection in school age children: randomised double blind placebo controlled trial. Br Med J 1997; 315:858–862.

39. McKean MC, Leech M, Lambert PC, Hewitt C, Myint S, Silverman M. A model of viral wheeze in nonasthmatic adults: symptoms and physiology. Eur Respir J 2001; 18:23–32.

40. Dodge RR, Burrows B. The prevalence and incidence of asthma and asthma-like symptoms in a general population sample. Am Rev Respir Dis 1980; 122:567–575.

41. Dezateux C, Stocks J. Lung development and early origins of childhood respiratory illness. Br Med Bull 1997; 53:40–57.

42. Clarke JR, Reese A, Silverman M. Bronchial responsiveness and lung function in infants with lower respiratory tract illness over the first six months of life. Arch Dis Child 1992; 67:1454-1458.

43. Frey U, Jackson AC, Silverman M. Differences in airway wall compliance as a possible mechanism for wheezing disorders in infants. Eur Respir J 1998; 12:136–142.

44. Frey U, Makkonen K, Wellman T, Beardsmore C, Silverman M. Alterations in airway wall properties in infants with a history of wheezing disorders. Am J Respir Crit Care Med 2000; 161:1825–1829.

45. Stick SM, Arnott J, Turner DJ, Young S, Landau LI, Le Souef PN. Bronchial responsiveness and lung function in recurrently wheezy infants. Am Rev Respir Dis 1991; 144:1012–1015.

46. Young S, Arnott J, O'Keeffe PT, Le Souef PN, Landau LI. The association between early life lung function and wheezing during the first 2 years of life. Eur Respir J 2000; 15:151–157.

47. Clarke JR, Salmon B, Silverman M. Bronchial responsiveness in the neonatal period as a risk factor for wheezing in infancy. Am J Respir Crit Care Med 1995; 151:1434–1440.

48. Renzi PM, Turgeon JP, Marcotte JE, Drblik SP, Berube D, Gagnon MF, Spier S. Reduced interferon-gamma production in infants with bronchiolitis and asthma. Am J Respir Crit Care Med 1999; 159:1417–1422.

49. Young S, O'Keeffe PT, Arnott J, Landau LI. Lung function, airway responsiveness, and respiratory symptoms before and after bronchiolitis. Arch Dis Child 1995; 72:16–24.

50. Palmer LJ, Rye PJ, Gibson NA, Burton PR, Landau LI, Le Souef PN. Airway responsiveness in early infancy predicts asthma, lung function and respiratory symptoms by school age. Am J Respir Crit Care Med 2001; 163:37–42.

51. Sherrill DL, Stein R, Halonen M, Holberg CJ, Wright A, Martinez FD. Total serum IgE and its association with asthma symptoms and allergic sensitisation among children. J Allergy Clin Immunol 1999; 104:28–36.

52. Sporik R, Holgate ST, Platts-Mills TA, Cogswell JJ. Exposure to house-dust mite allergen (Der p I) and the development of asthma in childhood. A prospective study. N Engl J Med 1990; 323:502–507.

53. Rhodes HL, Thomas P, Sporik R, Holgate ST, Cogswell JJ. A birth cohort study of subjects at risk of atopy: twenty-two-year follow-up of wheeze and atopic status. Am J Respir Crit Care Med 2002; 165:176–180.

54. Welliver RC. Immunologic mechanisms of virus-induced wheezing and asthma. J Pediatr 1999; 135:14–20.

55. van Schaik SM, Tristram DA, Nagpal IS, Hintz KM, Welliver RC 2nd, Welliver RC. Increased production of IFN-gamma and cysteinyl leukotrienes in virus-induced wheezing. J Allergy Clin Immunol 1999; 103:630–636.

56. Clough JB, Sly PD. Association between lower respiratory tract symptoms and falls in peak expiratory flow in children. Eur Respir J 1995; 8:718–722.

57. Tattersfield AE, Postma DS, Barnes PJ, Svensson K, Bauer CA, O'Byrne PM, Lofdahl CG, Pauwels RA, Ullmann A. Exacerbations of asthma: a descriptive study of 425 severe exacerbations. The FACET International Study Group. Am J Respir Crit Care Med 1999; 160:594–599.

58. British Thoracic Society. Asthma in children under five years of age. Thorax 1997; 52:S1-9-10s.

59. Anonymous. Guidelines for the diagnosis and management of asthma. Expert Panel Report 2. NIH Publication 97-4051, 1997.

60. Clough JB. Bronchodilators in infancy. Thorax 1993; 48:308.

61. Chavasse R, Bara A, Seddon P, McKean MC. Short acting beta-agonists for recurrent wheeze in children under 2 years of age (Cochrane Review). In: The Cochrane Library. Oxford: Update Software, 2002.

62. Godden DJ, Ross S, Abdalla M, McMurray D, Douglas A, Oldman D, Friend JA, Legge JS, Douglas JG. Outcome of wheeze in childhood. Symptoms and pulmonary function 25 years later. Am J Respir Crit Care Med 1994; 149:106–112.

63. McKean M, Ducharme F. Inhaled steroids for episodic viral wheeze of childhood (Cochrane Review). In: The Cochrane Library, 1. Oxford: Update Software, 2002.

64. Connett G, Lenney W. Prevention of viral induced asthma attacks using inhaled budesonide. Arch Dis Child 1993; 68:85–87.

65. Svedmyr J, Nyberg E, Asbrink-Nilsson E, Hedlin G. Intermittent treatment with inhaled steroids for deterioration of asthma due to upper respiratory tract infections. Acta Paediatr 1995; 84:884–888.

66. Gleeson JG, Loftus BG, Price JF. Placebo controlled trial of systemic corticosteroids in acute childhood asthma. Acta Paediatr Scand 1990; 79:1052–1058.

67. Brunette MG, Lands L, Thibodeau LP. Childhood asthma: prevention of attacks with short-term corticosteroid treatment of upper respiratory tract infection. Pediatrics 1988; 81:624–629.

68. Webb MS, Henry RL, Milner AD. Oral corticosteroids for wheezing attacks under 18 months. Arch Dis Child 1986; 61:15–19.

69. Pauwels RA, Lofdahl CG, Postma DS, Tattersfield AE, O'Byrne P, Barnes PJ, Ullman A. Effect of inhaled formoterol and budesonide on exacerbations of asthma. Formoterol and Corticosteroids Establishing Therapy (FACET) International Study Group. N Engl J Med 1997; 337:1405–1411.

70. Stevens CA, Wesseldine LJ, Couriel JM, Dyer AJ, Osman LM, Silverman M. Parental education and guided self-management of asthma and wheezing in the pre-school child: a randomised controlled trial. Thorax 2002; 57:39–44.

71. Wilson NM, Phagoo SB, Silverman M. Atopy, bronchial responsiveness and symptoms in wheezy 3 year olds. Arch Dis Child 1992; 67:491–495.

72. Wilson NM, Doré CJ, Silverman M. Factors relating to the severity of symptoms at 5 yrs in children with severe wheeze in the first 2 yrs of life. Eur Respir J 1997; 10:346–353.

73. Sibbald B, Kerry S, Strachan DP, Anderson HR. Patient characteristics associated with the labelling of asthma. Fam Pract 1994; 11:127–132.

74. Pekkanen J, Pearce N. Defining asthma in epidemiological studies. Eur Respir J 1999; 14:951–957.

75. Remes ST, Pekkanen J, Remes K, Salonen RO, Korppi M. In search of childhood asthma: questionnaire, tests of bronchial hyperresponsiveness, and clinical evaluation. Thorax 2002; 57:120–126.

76. Ross S, Godden DJ, Abdalla M, McMurray D, Douglas A, Oldman D, Friend JA, Legge JS, Douglas JG. Outcome of wheeze in childhood: the influence of atopy. Eur Respir J 1995; 8:2081–2087.

77. Nystad W, Magnus P, Gulsvik A. Increasing risk of asthma without other atopic diseases in school children: a repeated cross-sectional study after 13 years. Eur J Epidemiol 1998; 14:247–252.

78. Omran M, Russell G. Continuing increase in respiratory symptoms and atopy in Aberdeen schoolchildren. Br Med J 1996; 312:34.

79. Martinez FD, Morgan WJ, Wright AL, Holberg CJ, Taussig LM. Diminished lung function as a predisposing factor for wheezing respiratory illness in infants. N Engl J Med 1988; 319:1112-1117.

80. Tager IB, Hanrahan JP, Tosteson TD, Castile RG, Brown RW, Weiss ST, Speizer FE. Lung function, pre- and postnatal smoke exposure, and wheezing in the first year of life. Am Rev Respir Dis 1993; 147:811-817.

81. Voter KZ, Henry MM, Stewart PW, Henderson FW. Lower respiratory illness in early childhood and lung function and bronchial reactivity in adolescent males. Am Rev Respir Dis 1988; 137:302-307.

82. Cook DG, Strachan DP. Health effects of passive smoking-10: Summary of effects of parental smoking on the respiratory health of children and implications for research. Thorax 1999; 54:357-366.

83. Harlap S, Davies AM. Infant admissions to hospital and maternal smoking. Lancet 1974; 30:529-532.

84. Fergusson DM, Horwood LJ, Shannon FT, Taylor B. Parental smoking and lower respiratory illness in the first three years of life. J Epidemiol Community Health 1981; 35:180-184.

85. Joad JP, Ji C, Kott KS, Bric JM, Pinkerton KE. In utero and postnatal effects of sidestream cigarette smoke exposure on lung function, hyperresponsiveness, and neuroendocrine cells in rats. Toxicol Appl Pharmacol 1995; 132:63-71.

86. von Mutius E, Fritzsh C, Weiland SK, Ross G, Magnussen H. Prevalence of asthma and allergic disorders among children in united Germany: a descriptive comparison. Br Med J 1992; 305:1395-1399.

87. Grigg J. The health effects of fossil fuel derived particles. Arch Dis Child 2002; 86: 79-83.

88. Becker S, Soukup JM. Exposure to urban air particulates alters the macrophage-mediated inflammatory response to respiratory viral infection. J Toxicol Environ Health A 1999; 57:445-457.

89. Rusconi F, Galassi C, Corbo GM, Forastiere F, Biggeri A, Ciccone G, Renzoni E. Risk factors for early, persistent, and late-onset wheezing in young children. SIDRIA Collaborative Group. Am J Respir Crit Care Med 1999; 160:1617-1622.

90. Ball TM, Castro-Rodriguez JA, Griffith KA, Holberg CJ, Martinez FD, Wright AL. Siblings, day-care attendance, and the risk of asthma and wheezing during childhood. N Engl J Med 2000; 343:538-543.

91. Wright AL, Holberg CJ, Taussig LM, Martinez FD. Factors influencing the relation of infant feeding to asthma and recurrent wheeze in childhood. Thorax 2001; 56:192-197.

92. Barker DJ, Godfrey KM, Fall C, Osmond C, Winter PD, Shaheen SO. Relation of birth weight and childhood respiratory infection to adult lung function and death from chronic obstructive airways disease. Br Med J 1991; 303:671-675.

93. Burrows B, Taussig LM. "As the twig is bent, the tree inclines" (perhaps). Am Rev Respir Dis 1980; 122:813-816.

94. Strachan DP, Seagroatt V, Cook DG. Chest illness in infancy and chronic respiratory disease in later life: an analysis by month of birth. Int J Epidemiol 1994; 23:1060-1068.

95. Everard ML, Swarbrick A, Wrightham M, McIntyre J, Dunkley C, James PD, Sewell

HF, Milner AD. Analysis of cells obtained by bronchial lavage of infants with respiratory syncytial virus infection. Arch Dis Child 1994; 71:428–432.

96. McKean M, Hewitt C, Lambert P, Myint S, Silverman M. An adult experimental model of viral wheeze: inflammatory changes in the upper and lower respiratory tract. Clin Exp Allergy 2003; 33: in press.

97. Keatings VM, Barnes PJ. Granulocyte activation markers in induced sputum: comparison between chronic obstructive pulmonary disease, asthma, and normal subjects. Am J Respir Crit Care Med 1997; 155:449–453.

98. Chung KF, Barnes PJ. Cytokines in asthma. Thorax 1999; 54:825–857.

99. Ying S, Meng Q, Zeibecoglou K, Robinson DS, Macfarlane A, Humbert M, et al. Eosinophil chemotactic chemokines (eotaxin, eotaxin-2, RANTES, monocyte chemoattractant protein-3 (MCP-3), and MCP-4), and C-C chemokine receptor 3 expression in bronchial biopsies from atopic and nonatopic (intrinsic) asthmatics. J Immunol 1999; 163:6321–6329.

100. Humbert M, Menz G, Ying S, Corrigan CJ, Robinson DS, Durham SR, Kay AB. The immunopathology of extrinsic (atopic) and intrinsic (non-atopic) asthma: more similarities than differences. Immunol Today 1999; 20:528–533.

101. Vignola AM, Chanez P, Campbell AM, Souques F, Lebel B, Enander I, et al. Airway inflammation in mild intermittent and in persistent asthma. Am J Respir Crit Care Med 1998; 157:403–409.

102. Grigg J, Riedler J. Developmental airway cell biology. The "normal" young child. Am J Respir Crit Care Med 2000; 162:S52–S55.

103. Maclennan C, Hutchinson P, Freezer N, Holdsworth S. Airway inflammation in children with infrequent episodic wheeze. Eur Respir J 2000; 16:S197.

104. Marguet C, Jouen-Boedes F, Dean TP, Warner JO. Bronchoalveolar cell profiles in children with asthma, infantile wheeze, chronic cough, or cystic fibrosis. Am J Respir Crit Care Med 1999; 159:1533–1540.

105. Grigg J, Riedler J, Robertson CF. Bronchoalveolar lavage fluid cellularity and soluble intercellular adhesion molecule-1 in children with colds. Pediatr Pulmonol 1999; 28: 109–116.

106. Pizzichini MM, Pizzichini E, Efthimiadis A, Chauhan AJ, Johnston SL, Hussack P, et al. Asthma and natural colds. Inflammatory indices in induced sputum: a feasibility study. Am J Respir Crit Care Med 1998; 158:1178–1184.

107. El-Radhi AS, Hogg CL, Bungre JK, Bush A, Corrigan CJ. Effect of oral glucocorticoid treatment on serum inflammatory markers in acute asthma. Arch Dis Child 2000; 83: 158–162.

108. Sampson AP, Castling DP, Green CP, Price JF. Persistent increase in plasma and urinary leukotrienes after acute asthma. Arch Dis Child 1995; 73:221–225.

109. Norzila MZ, Fakes K, Henry RL, Simpson J, Gibson PG. Interleukin-8 secretion and neutrophil recruitment accompanies induced sputum eosinophil activation in children with acute asthma. Am J Respir Crit Care Med 2000; 161:769–774.

110. Brown JR, Kleimberg J, Marini M, Sun G, Bellini A, Mattoli S. Kinetics of eotaxin expression and its relationship to eosinophil accumulation and activation in bronchial biopsies and bronchoalveolar lavage (BAL) of asthmatic patients after allergen inhalation. Clin Exp Immunol 1998; 114:137–146.

111. Gibson PG, Norzila MZ, Fakes K, Simpson J, Henry RL. Pattern of airway inflammation and its determinants in children with acute severe asthma. Pediatr Pulmonol 1999; 28:261–270.

112. Kharitonov SA, Yates D, Barnes PJ. Increased nitric oxide in exhaled air of normal human subjects with upper respiratory tract infections. Eur Respir J 1995; 8:295–297.
113. Baraldi E, Dario C, Ongaro R, Scollo M, Azzolin NM, Panza E, et al. Exhaled nitric oxide concentrations during treatment of wheezing exacerbation in infants and young children. Am J Respir Crit Care Med 1999; 159:1284–1288.
114. Ratjen F, Kavuk I, Gartig S, Wiesemann HG, Grasemann H. Airway nitric oxide in infants with acute wheezy bronchitis. Pediatr Allergy Immunol 2000; 11:230–235.
115. Salome CM, Roberts AM, Brown NJ, Dermand J, Marks GB, Woolcock AJ. Exhaled nitric oxide measurements in a population sample of young adults. Am J Respir Crit Care Med 1999; 159:911–916.
116. Gauvreau GM, Parameswaran KN, Watson RM, O'Byrne PM. Inhaled leukotriene E(4), but not leukotriene D(4), increased airway inflammatory cells in subjects with atopic asthma. Am J Respir Crit Care Med 2001; 164:1495–1500.
117. Severien C, Artlich A, Jonas S, Becher G. Urinary excretion of leukotriene E4 and eosinophil protein X in children with atopic asthma. Eur Respir J 2000; 16:588–592.
118. Westcott JY, Smith HR, Wenzel SE, Larsen GL, Thomas RB, Felsien D, et al. Urinary leukotriene E4 in patients with asthma. Effect of airways reactivity and sodium cromoglycate. Am Rev Respir Dis 1991; 143:1322–1328.
119. Sheikh S, Null D, Gentile D, Bimle C, Skoner D, McCoy K, et al. Urinary leukotriene E(4) excretion during the first month of life and subsequent bronchopulmonary dysplasia in premature infants. Chest 2001; 119:1749–1754.
120. Oommen A, Peck K, McGarr C, McNally T, Grigg J. Cysteinyl leukotriene production and eosinophil activation in pre-school viral wheeze. Eur Respir J 2000; 16:485s.
121. Winther B, Farr B, Turner RB, Hendley JO, Gwaltney JM Jr, Mygind N. Histopathologic examination and enumeration of polymorphonuclear leukocytes in the nasal mucosa during experimental rhinovirus colds. Acta Otolaryngol Suppl 1984; 413:19–24.
122. Turner RB. The role of neutrophils in the pathogenesis of rhinovirus infections. Paediatr Infect Dis J 1990; 9:832–835.
123. Levandowski RA, Weaver CW, Jackson GG. Nasal-secretion leukocyte populations determined by flow cytometry during acute rhinovirus infection. J Med Virol 1988; 25:423–432.
124. Beppu T, Ohta N, Gon S, Sakata K, Inamura S, Fukase Y, Kimura Y, Koike Y. Eosinophil and eosinophil cationic protein in allergic rhinitis. Acta Otolaryngol 1994; 511: 221–223.
125. Greiff L, Andersson M, Svensson C, Linden M, Myint S, Persson CG. Allergen challenge-induced acute exudation of IL-8, ECP and alpha2-macroglobulin in human rhinovirus-induced common colds. Eur Respir J 1999; 13:41–47.
126. Grunberg K, Smits HH, Timmers MC, de Klerk EPA, Dolhain EM, Dick EC, Hiemstra PS, Sterk PJ. Experimental rhinovirus 16 infection: effects on cell differentials and soluble markers in sputum in asthmatic subjects. Am J Respir Crit Care Med 1997; 156:609–616.
127. Fraenkel DJ, Bardin PG, Sanderson G, Lampe F, Johnston SL, Holgate ST. Lower airways inflammation during rhinovirus colds in normal and in asthmatic subjects. Am J Respir Crit Care Med 1995; 151:879–886.
128. Bardin PG, Fraenkel DJ, Sanderson G, Lampe F, Holgate ST. Lower airways inflammatory response during rhinovirus colds. Int Arch Allergy Immunol 1995; 107:127–129.
129. Gern JE, Vrtis R, Grindle KA, Swenson C, Busse WW. Relationship of upper and

lower airway cytokines to outcome of experimental rhinovirus infection. Am J Respir Crit Care Med 2000; 162:2226–2231.

130. Message SD, Johnston SL. The immunology of virus infection in asthma. Eur Respir J 2001; 18:1013–1025.

131. Lemanske RF Jr, Dick EC, Swenson CA, Vrtis RF, Busse WW. Rhinovirus upper respiratory infection increases airway hyperreactivity and late asthmatic reactions. J Clin Invest 1989; 83:1–10.

132. Cheung D, Dick EC, Timmers MC, de Klerk EP, Spaan WJ, Sterk PJ. Rhinovirus inhalation causes long-lasting excessive airway narrowing in response to methacholine in asthmatic subjects in vivo. Am J Respir Crit Care Med 1995; 152:1490–1496.

133. Gern JE, Calhoun W, Swenson C, Shen G, Busse WW. Rhinovirus infection preferentially increases lower airway responsiveness in allergic subjects. Am J Respir Crit Care Med 1997; 155:1872–1876.

134. Teran LM, Johnston SL, Schroder JM, Church MK, Holgate ST. Role of nasal interleukin-8 in neutrophil recruitment and activation in children with virus-induced asthma. Am J Respir Crit Care Med 1997; 155:1362–1366.

135. Chilvers MA, McKean M, Rutman A, Myint BS, Silverman M, O'Callaghan C. The effects of coronavirus on human nasal ciliated respiratory epithelium. Eur Respir J 2001; 18:965–970.

136. Karjalainen EM, Laitinen A, Sue-Chu M, Altraja A, Bjermer L, Laitinen LA. Evidence of airway inflammation and remodeling in ski athletes with and without bronchial hyperresponsiveness to methacholine. Am J Respir Crit Care Med 2000; 161:2086–2091.

137. Marin J, Jeler-Kacar D, Levstek V, Macek V. Persistence of viruses in upper respiratory tract of children with asthma. J Infect 2000; 41:69–72.

138. Grunberg K, Sharon RF, Sont JK, In't Veen JC, Van Schadewijk WA, De Klerk EP, Dick CR, Van Krieken JH, Sterk PJ. Rhinovirus-induced airway inflammation in asthma: effect of treatment with inhaled corticosteroids before and during experimental infection. Am J Respir Crit Care Med 2001; 164:1816–1822.

139. Christie GL, Helms PJ, Ross SJ, Godden DJ, Friend JA, Legge JS, Haites NE, Douglas JG. Outcome of children of parents with atopic asthma and transient childhood wheezy bronchitis. Thorax 1997; 52:953–957.

140. Wark PA, Johnston SL, Moric I, Simpson JL, Hensley MJ, Gibson PG. Neutrophil degranulation and cell lysis is associated with clinical severity in virus-induced asthma. Eur Respir J 2002; 19:68–75.

141. Seymour ML, Gilby N, Bardin PG, Fraenkel DJ, Sanderson G, Penrose JF, Holgate ST, Johnston SL, Sampson AP. Rhinovirus infection increases 5-lipoxygenase and cyclooxygenase-2 in bronchial biopsy specimens from nonatopic subjects. J Infect Dis 2002; 185:540–544.

19

Respiratory Virus Infections in Adults and the Elderly

IAIN STEPHENSON and KARL G. NICHOLSON

Leicester Royal Infirmary
Leicester, England

I. Introduction

Despite advances in control of most infectious diseases in the developed world, acute respiratory infections (ARIs), largely caused by viruses with both RNA and DNA genomes, inflict considerable morbidity and mortality among patients with underlying medical conditions and particularly those of advancing years. Acute respiratory viral infections also have an enormous public health and socioeconomic impact on healthy working adults.

The respiratory tract is subject to infection from a large number of pathogens that produce illness ranging in severity from asymptomatic or mild afebrile upper respiratory illness to fulminating pneumonia. Studies of ARIs have revealed that in the region of 200 viruses affect the respiratory tract (Table 1). Some, such as measles and varicella, may cause prominent respiratory symptoms but are recognized more for their systemic manifestations. Others may have respiratory symptoms as infrequent clinical manifestations. Human parvovirus B19, for example, is either asymptomatic or causes systemic illness, but coryza and sore throat have been noted. The presence of B19 DNA in respiratory secretions suggests that respiratory transmission is important. The term "respiratory virus" conventionally refers to those viruses whose predominant manifestations are respiratory. The large number of viruses

Table 1   Viruses Causing Respiratory Syndromes

Virus	Subtypes
RNA viruses	
Picornaviridae	Rhinoviruses (>102 serotypes)
	Enteroviruses
Coronaviridae	Coronaviruses 229E and OC43
Orthomyxoviridae	Influenza
	Type A (currently H1N1, H1N2, & H3N2)
	Type B (with antigenic drift)
	Type C
Paramyxoviridae	Parainfluenza virus types 1–3, 4a, 4b
	Respiratory syncytial virus types A and B
	Measles virus
Metapneumoviridae	Human metapneumovirus
Bunyaviridae	Sin nombre (Four Corners) and related viruses
DNA viruses	
Adenoviridae	Adenoviruses
Herpesviridae	Herpes simplex virus
	Epstein-Barr virus
	Cytomegalovirus
	Varicella zoster virus

that can infect and reinfect the respiratory tract explains the high incidence of community-acquired ARIs. The clinical characteristics of illness associated with these viruses are broadly similar.

II.   Assessing the Burden of Respiratory Virus Infections

It is necessary to attribute the causes and frequency of ARI to specific pathogens to determine priorities for their control. This has been achieved by studies of outbreaks within defined populations such as nursing homes or the immunocompromised; by longitudinal surveillance of communities; by primary-care sentinel surveillance schemes; by studies of hospital admissions; and by other means including analyses of placebo recipients participating in trials of vaccines and antivirals. Mathematical modeling has also been used to correlate deaths with outbreaks of influenza and respiratory syncytial virus. Data from large databases, such as those maintained by health maintenance organizations, provide information on the overall impact of ARI, but these are syndrome-based and are disadvantaged by lack of laboratory diagnoses.

Studies of respiratory viruses have been hampered by the absence of pathognomonic clinical features and by other factors including the large number of human rhinovirus (HRV) serotypes, the fastidious growth of certain HRVs, difficulty in culturing coronaviruses and diagnosing these infections serologically, and by the common use of insensitive complement fixation tests. In addition, the timing and method of collection and transportation of nasopharyngeal specimens in relation to illness, and factors influencing viral shedding (such as prior antibody status due to repeated infection), may contribute to underdiagnosis. Recent developments in molecular biology have permitted the development of polymerase chain reaction (PCR) assays to provide sensitive and specific diagnoses. PCR provides much higher rates of detection of respiratory viruses than culture (1,2). The increased sensitivity of PCR is of particular importance in adults (3) but its increasing application has tended to cause a reduction in virus isolation and culture with resultant loss of antigenic data that is only available from viable virus. PCR was used to detect the newly described human metapneumovirus (4) and has been used on archived or preserved tissue specimens from the time of the 1918 influenza pandemic in an attempt to identify virulence factors (5). Serological diagnosis depends on the detection and rise of serum antibodies, usually by haemagglutination inhibition and neutralization methods. There is increasing interest in the detection of antibodies in other body fluids such as nasal washes and oral fluid as correlates of immune protection (6). This is of particular interest in the field of respiratory viruses, in which mucosal delivery of vaccines is now actively pursued.

A. Community Surveillance

The Tecumseh study, a family-based surveillance study of respiratory illness in Michigan (USA), maintained weekly surveillance of around 1000 individuals or 10% of the community (7). It ran in two phases, covering the periods 1965–1972 and 1976–1981, and examined the characteristics and frequency of respiratory illnesses due to specific pathogens and their relationship to environmental variables. Similar studies were conducted in Seattle (The Seattle Virus Watch) and Houston (The Houston Family Study) in the United States; Port Chalmers in New Zealand; and in the United Kingdom (8–12). The annual number of all respiratory illnesses experienced per year among persons on surveillance in Tecumseh is shown in Table 2. The peak incidence of respiratory illnesses in patients of both genders occurs in the 1–2 year age group with approximately 4.5–5.5 symptomatic acute respiratory illnesses per year. The rate falls during childhood, but increases in young adults, particularly women, before continuing the downward trend to a rate of 1–2.2 illnesses per person per year in those 40 years of age and older (7,13,14).

The increase in young adults, especially women, presumably relates to parenthood and greater exposure to young children. For possibly the same reason, ARls are less common in working women than in women not working outside the home, although differential perceptions of infection as illness might also be important. Observations indicate that schoolchildren are central to the spread of respiratory viruses. For example, rapid rises in influenza virus infection has been noted following return to school after vacations; children have been found to be the main introducers of influenza into families; and during early stages of influenza epidemics, a disproportionate number of cases have been older schoolchildren, with the contribu-

Table 2 Incidence of Respiratory Viruses
in Adult Age Groups During Tecumseh
Studies

Age group (years)	Incidence of respiratory illness per year
15–19	2–2.4
20–24	2.2–2.8
25–29	2.4–2.8
30–39	2.0–2.3
40–49	1.0–1.9
50–59	1.6–1.8
>60	1.2–2.2

Source: From Refs. 7,13,14.

tion of this group dropping during the late stage of epidemics (15–19). Although HRV infection may take place at any time during the year, there appear to be two peaks: one in the autumn and another during spring. It has been postulated that children become infected at school and later transmit infection to their parents and siblings. Although annual HRV infection rates were related to number of children in Seattle families (20,21), the simultaneous occurrence of peaks of respiratory illness among children and adults and adults with and without children suggested that factors other than transmission in schools accounted for the autumn increase (22). The Tecumseh studies reveal an increase in the mean number of respiratory illnesses per person per year with decreasing annual family income from 2.7 in the highest income bracket to 3.8 in the lowest (7). Crowded living conditions and exposure to pollutants such as nitrogen dioxide, cigarette and wood smoke increase the likelihood of exposure or susceptibility to respiratory viruses (16,23–25).

Virus isolation rates in community studies of respiratory illness vary between studies. However, care must be taken in interpreting the data since the older community studies used virus isolation (cell culture systems are unreliable for primary isolation of coronaviruses and certain HRVs) or serology rather than more sensitive tests such as polymerase chain reaction (PCR). Moreover, coronavirus serology was not universally applied and tests for the recently described human meta-pneumovirus were unavailable. Overall, HRVs have been recovered from 16–55% of individuals with acute respiratory illness, coronaviruses from 1–42%, influenza A from 2.3–27%, influenza B from 1.2–26%, RSV from 9–14%, parainfluenza viruses from 0–8.6%, and adenoviruses from 0–6.5% (9,13,21,26–30). Virus isolations in Tecumseh fell with increasing age from 31.3% in children aged 0–4 years to 15.8% in adults 40 years and over (13). These investigators reasoned that the fall was related to decreased shedding secondary to previous infections. Such an age-related decrease in virus shedding may in part explain why the elderly, who interact mostly with other elderly people, have fewer acute respiratory infections.

As evidenced by family studies, studies in the elderly people living in the community (31), studies of elderly people living in residential care (32), and trials of neuraminidase inhibitors in people with influenza-like illness, it is not possible to differentiate respiratory viral infections clinically. Although influenza is typified as a severe acute respiratory illness with systemic features, subclinical or asymptomatic infection has been found consistently in studies that compare antibody titers at the beginning and end of the winter (12,29,33,34). Influenza activity is seasonally limited between the months of November to April, when it emerges abruptly, reaches a peak rapidly over a few weeks, before gradually disappearing over several months (18,35–37). The spread of influenza within age groups varies with each epidemic and can depend on herd immunity to the prevalent strain. For H3N2, pre-existing immunity is often limited because of frequent antigenic changes. Influenza H1N1 and B are more antigenically stable, resulting in higher herd immunity. Comparative studies have revealed type A (H3N2) influenza to produce the most severe illnesses, type A (H1N1) the mildest, with type B intermediate (29,38–40). These clinical data correlate with data on hospitalizations and deaths. In the United States, average seasonal rates of excess pneumonia and influenza (P&I) hospitalization during 26 influenza seasons (1970–1995) were twice as high during A (H3N2) influenza seasons as during A (H1N1)/B seasons (41). During the period 1972–1992, most influenza A (H3N2) seasons were likewise associated with high numbers of excess deaths (23,000–45,000 all-cause excess deaths), whereas most A (H1N1) and B seasons were associated with fewer deaths (0–23,000) (42). Surveillance data covering 1987–1996 from sentinel practices in England, Wales, and The Netherlands found that influenza H3N2 epidemics were associated with highest consultation rates, particularly in the >65 year age group, during which an estimated excess of 2–3% of the practice population are seen over a 4 week period (43).

Viruses isolated during community studies have been categorized according to respiratory syndrome, and severity has been evaluated based on restriction of normal daily activity (44). Overall, HRV infections were most commonly upper respiratory and activity restriction was low. In contrast, influenza A infections were most commonly lower respiratory and they exhibited a high frequency of activity restriction. Illnesses associated with other viruses were intermediate in both syndrome type and level of activity restriction. Further analyses in Tecumseh revealed age-related increases in severity of HRV illness (45). Lower respiratory syndromes occurred in almost two-thirds of people aged 40 years and older, and HRV infections in this group had a median duration three times longer than in schoolchildren and were responsible for twice as many physician consultations.

B. Surveillance in General Practice

Because most respiratory virus activity takes place in the community and affected subjects present to primary care, many countries have developed surveillance networks based around sentinel practices with the primary goal of developing an early warning system for the emergence and spread of influenza. Schemes such as the one coordinated in England and Wales by the Royal College of General Practitioners (RCGP) Research Unit are mostly syndrome based. Variations in the methods em-

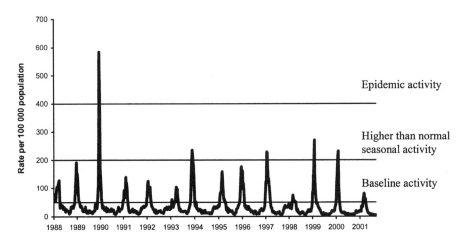

Figure 1   Royal College of General Practitioners consultation rates for influenza-like illnesses 1988–2001 in England and Wales. (Baseline activity: 50 consultations per 100,000 population, normal seasonal activity: 50–200 consultations per 100,000, epidemic activity: 400 consultations per 100,000.)

ployed to produce consultation rates and in the definitions used to monitor illness mean that comparisons between illness rates reported by different schemes must be interpreted with care. However, comparisons from week to week or from year to year within an individual country are considered safe, providing that the population sampled is sufficiently large and representative of the population as a whole. Schemes that incorporate virological surveillance are especially valuable but, even without these, weekly consultation rates for influenza-like illness (ILI) usually correlate extremely well with laboratory reports of influenza, pneumonia and influenza admissions, and all-cause mortality (43,46,47; Fig. 1). Data from sentinel networks of general practitioners provide estimates of excess consultations for respiratory syndromes and their relation to hospital admissions and deaths during outbreaks. The data reveal strong associations between the incidence of ARI and all-cause mortality in the United Kingdom (48,49). By comparing virus isolation data for influenza and RSV with data from clinical surveillance, Fleming and Cross suggested that RSV is an important respiratory pathogen for the elderly in the community. Subsequently, Nicholson studied the role of influenza A and B and RSV on deaths in England and Wales for the period 1975–1990 by regression analysis of aggregated ARI reported by the RCGP scheme, Public Health Laboratory Service (PHLS) laboratory reports, all-cause mortality data, and ambient temperature (50). Although estimated excess mortality associated with influenza was considerable during years without major epidemics, the estimated mortality in England and Wales associated with RSV infection was 60–80% more than that associated with influenza. The modeling also demonstrated that pathogens other than influenza and RSV are involved in winter excess mortality.

Using data collected by the Weekly Returns Service of the RCGP sentinel network of practitioners from 1989 to 1998, Fleming assessed the impact of influenza on hospital admissions for cardiac and respiratory diseases and to deaths (51). An average of 12,554 deaths occurred in England and Wales during influenza epidemics each year. Each year an average of 422,000 extra people consulted physicians and were diagnosed with influenza-like illness during the epidemic among 1.1 million extra people who presented with ARIs. There were 3028 concomitant excess respiratory admissions (England only) in the age group 65–74 years and 6049 who were aged over 75 years. Nguyen Van Tamme attempted to quantify excess hospital admissions in three health districts in England (population circa 1.5 million) due to influenza using regression analysis, while taking into account seasonal variation, temperature, and long-term trends in hospital admissions (52). The regression model explained 41% of the total variation in hospital admissions for P & I, and influenza activity explained 14%. Virological surveillance of influenza-like illness in a subset of practices that report to the RCGP sentinel practices provides further insight into the role of RSV in causing ILI in adults. During the 3 years of surveillance, up to 22% of specimens collected from adults aged ≥45 years were positive for RSV, and more than 45% of specimens were negative for both influenza and RSV (3). The relative proportion of RSV to influenza changed over the season and from year to year. In 1997–1998, RSV-positive samples (114/500, 23%) were greater than influenza-positive samples (80/500, 16%) among 15–64-year-olds. Similar sentinel networks have been set up in a number of countries to monitor community-acquired viral infections due to respiratory viruses.

The UK-based General Practice Research Database provides a further insight into the burden from influenza-like illness (53). The investigators quantified influenza-related physician visits, clinical complications of and risk factors for influenza, and related drug use in all age groups from 1991 to 1996. This study examined 141,293 subjects with ILI and the same number of controls matched for age, gender, calendar time, and practice. The study excluded subjects with cancer of the hemopoeitic system, acquired immunodeficiency sydrome (AIDS), organ transplantation, or exposure to cyclosporine, azothiaprine, or oral steroids. In absolute terms, otherwise healthy adults (15–64 years of age) accounted for the greatest proportion of all influenza-related medical consultations as well as complications. In healthy adults, the rate of respiratory tract complications increased with age from 6.5% in those 15–49 years of age to 9% in the over 65s (Table 3). The incidence of complications increased substantially with pre-existing chronic diseases (Table 4). Death complicated around 1.1% of cases in the healthy elderly (over 65s) and 1.5% of elderly with pre-existing medical conditions. Overall, 59.4% of consultations resulted in the prescription of drugs, with antibiotics being prescribed most commonly (up to 45%). Clearly respiratory viruses responsible for ILI exert an enormous toll in terms of socioeconomic costs, morbidity, and mortality. Cost-of-illness studies have estimated that in 1989 the cost of influenza activity in France was 2.1 billion euro. On the basis of 1997 German Sickness Funds, influenza costs (mainly direct medical and indirect cost attributed to loss of productivity and absenteeism) were 1 billon euro (54).

Table 3 Clinical Complications Reported Within 1 Month of Influenza
Diagnosis Based on Analysis of 141,293 Patients Entered into the UK
General Practice Research Database 1991–1996

Complication	Adults (15–64 years) n = 102,845 (%)	Elderly (>65 years) n = 17,552 (%)
Respiratory tract	7577 (7.4)	1573 (9.0)
Cardiovascular	40 (0.04)	68 (0.4)
Neurological	116 (0.1)	44 (0.3)
Renal	14 (0.01)	17 (0.1)
Otitis media	619 (0.6)	32 (0.2)
Death	49 (0.05)	224 (1.3)

Source: From Ref. 53.

Table 4 Risk of Influenza-Related Complications in Relation to Underlying Disease
from UK General Practice Research Database

Predisposing condition	Complication	No complication	Odds ratio (95% CI)[a]
None	9729	102,865	1.0
Respiratory disease	2036	10,747	1.9 (1.8–2.0)
Cardiovascular disease	515	3731	1.4 (1.3–1.6)
Diabetes mellitus	167	1691	1.1 (0.9–1.3)
Parkinson's disease	23	147	1.6 (1.0–2.5)
Cancer	538	6025	1.0 (0.9–1.1)
Two or more conditions	449	2603	1.8 (1.6–2.0)

[a] 95% confidence limits.
Source: From Ref. 53.

C. Surveillance in Hospital Settings

Surveillance in hospital settings provides useful information on the age-related burden of different respiratory viruses. For example, the impact of acute respiratory disease during influenza A and B epidemics in Houston were studied in seven hospitals containing 40% of locally available beds by Glezen et al. (55). During the peaks of influenza activity in 1982 and 1983, 593 of 1319 (45%) and 518 of 1264 (41%) samples submitted for diagnosis were positive for influenza B and influenza A H3N2 respectively. Table 5 shows the hospitalization rates and visits for ARI during the two epidemic peak periods and summer nadir. The influenza outbreaks were associated with comparable numbers of admissions in the elderly and people aged <65 years who were not in the high-risk categories recommended for influenza vaccination. The importance of RSV in causing community-acquired lower respiratory tract infection has been shown in hospital-based studies. In Ohio, Dowell and colleagues

Table 5 Acute Respiratory Tract Disease During Two Influenza Epidemic Winters and During the Midsummer Nadir in Houston, 1981–1983

No. of visits for acute respiratory disease (rate per 100 persons)

Age (yrs)	Weeks 3–12, 1982	Weeks 22–31, 1982	Weeks 2–11, 1983
20–34	2,829 (10.1)	1012 (3.4)	2686 (8.0)
35–44	999 (13.3)	281 (3.5)	1071 (10.0)
45–54	361 (10.2)	99 (2.6)	410 (8.7)
>55	212 (12.8)	74 (4.2)	175 (7.6)

No. of hospitalizations for acute respiratory disease (rate per 100,000 persons)

Age (yrs)	Weeks 3–12, 1982	Weeks 22–31, 1982	Weeks 2–11, 1983
20–24	60 (2.2)	47 (1.7)	64 (2.3)
25–34	291 (5.5)	100 (1.8)	164 (3.0)
35–44	134 (4.2)	97 (3.0)	154 (4.8)
45–54	174 (7.2)	70 (2.9)	120 (4.8)
55–64	227 (12.7)	110 (6.0)	247 (13.5)
>65	856 (55.0)	254 (15.9)	659 (41.2)

Source: From Ref. 55.

showed that RSV was the fourth most frequently identified cause of hospitalized community acquired pneumonia in 18–59-year-old patients (57). These investigators also examined the role of parainfluenza virus among adults hospitalized for lower respiratory tract infection. During their respective epidemic seasons, PIV-1 was the fourth most common pathogen isolated, behind influenza A (9.8%), *Streptococcus pneumoniae* (3.5%) and *Legionella pneumophilia* (3.2%). During the PIV-3 season, PIV-3 was the fifth most frequent pathogen identified in adults hospitalized with lower respiratory tract illness. However, for each season around 75% of patients had no pathogen identified (58).

D. Virological Surveillance of Placebo Recipients

Studies of placebo recipients participating in trials of influenza vaccines and antivirals provide information on the attack rate of influenza and the incidence of complications, including hospitalizations. In addition, a recent double-blind, placebo-controlled trial of the neuraminidase inhibitor oseltamivir provides an insight into the role of picornaviruses in influenza-like illnesses (defined by temperature 38°C plus one respiratory and one constitutional symptom) of adults (59). From a total of 719 subjects enrolled in the clinical trial within 36 h of the onset of symptoms, 475 (66%) had evidence of recent influenza A or B virus infections based on results of culture and/or serological testing. Of the 244 remaining patients, 36 (15%) had seroconversion for at least one of the common respiratory viruses or atypical pathogens. A reverse transcriptase PCR (RT-PCR) assay for picornavirus was positive in a subset of 15 (19%) of 78 patients with ILI of undetermined cause. Sequence analysis revealed that 14 (93%) had greater homology to HRVs, whereas 1 (7%) was related to enteroviruses. The median total symptom scores and oral temperatures of picorna-virus-positive patients (n = 15) and placebo-treated influenza virus-positive patients (n = 161) were similar over a 3-week period. The authors con-cluded that among the influenza virus-negative cases of this study, HRVs were relatively frequent pathogens associated with important respiratory and systemic symptoms.

E. Military Recruits

In young military recruits, adenoviruses have been identified as a dominant patho-gen. Outbreaks of adenovirus, mainly serotypes 4 and 7, were responsible for in-fecting up to 80% of new military recruits within the first few months of training, a quarter of whom were hospitalized with pneumonia (60–63). Factors including overcrowding, winter training, physical and mental stress, frequent travel, and con-tact with novel strains facilitate transmission (64). Control was achieved following the introduction of live adenovirus types 4 and 7 vaccine to new recruits. Since 1996 when vaccine production stopped, however, there has been a doubling in the number of adenoviral respiratory infections from 3 to 6 cases/1000 recruits/week (65). In addition, explosive outbreaks have re-emerged in military training centers and included sporadic deaths (66,67). Gray documented the presence of adenovirus in throat swabs of 1814 of 3413 (53%) recruits with respiratory illness at four mili-tary training centers; serotypes 4 and 7 accounted for 57% and 25% of isolates, respectively (66).

III. Respiratory Virus Infections in Specific Risk Groups

A. The Elderly

Assessments of the number of respiratory virus infections suffered by elderly people are likely to be underestimates since elderly patients usually present later, are not often investigated virologically, and shed less virus than children. ARI in the elderly are often associated with enhanced morbidity, presumably because of waning physi-ological reserves, age-related declines in immune function, and the effects of con-comitant chronic medical conditions. Although influenza is responsible for consider-able morbidity and mortality in aging populations, RSV, parainfluenza, HRV, and coronavirus are increasingly recognized as causes of serious illness.

Community-Living Elderly

Comparatively few studies have focused on the burden from respiratory virus infec-tions in elderly people living in the community. During the winters of 1992–1993 and 1993–1994, Nicholson and colleagues in Leicester studied the causes and bur-den of ARI in 533 subjects aged 60–90 years of age (31). Infections occurred at a rate of 1.2 episodes per person per annum and were clinically indistinguishable. A pathogen was identified for 43% of 497 episodes for which diagnostic specimens were available; 121 (52%) were HRVs, 59 (26%) were coronaviruses, 22 (9.5%) were influenza A or B, 17 (7%) were RSV, 7 (3%) were parainfluenza viruses, and 3 (1%) were *Chlamydia* species; an adenovirus and *Mycoplasma pneumoniae* caused one infection each. Lower respiratory tract symptoms complicated 65% of upper respiratory infections and increased medical consultations by 2.4-fold. The median duration of the episodes was 15 days. It was longer in those with lower respiratory symptoms (16 days vs. 12 days, p < 0.001), which occurred in 18 of 42 (43%, 95% confidence interval [$CI_{95\%}$] 28–58 coronavirus infections, 54 of 85 (64%, 54–74) HRV infections, 93 of 134 (69%, 61–77) unknown infections, 15 of 19 (79%, 61–97) influenza infections, and 9 of 11 (82%, 59–100) RSV infections (p < 0.02). Medical practitioners reviewed 40% of the episodes and 34% were treated with antibiotics. Overall 3 of the 497 infections led to admission to the hospital and another was fatal. Although influenza and RSV caused considerable individual morbidity, these investigators found that the burden of disease from HRV infections and infections of unknown cause were greater overall. Chronic ill health and smoking independently increased the likelihood of lower respiratory HRV illness. Thus it is probable that considerable morbidity and mortality from regular seasonal infections with HRVs, coronaviruses, and RSV are overshadowed by less regular, readily recognizable epidemics of influenza.

Greenberg, in Houston (TX, USA) studied the role of viruses in elderly people who acted as age-matched controls for patients with chronic obstructive pulmonary disease (COPD) (68). Infections occurred at a rate of 1.4 acute respiratory illnesses per annum, virtually identical to the rate in Leicester. Documented viral infections were common, with picornaviruses, parainfluenza viruses, and coronaviruses being the most frequently identified agents in this heavily influenza-vaccinated cohort. None of 87 ARIs in 55 ambulatory elderly persons (approximately half of whom had coronary artery disease, hypertension, or diabetes mellitus) resulted in hospitalization, but almost one-third of the controls had at least one medical consultation for an ARI.

Falsey and colleagues recruited volunteers at several sites of a day care program for older persons in Rochester, New York (69,70). Although living in the community, many were frail and their mean age was almost 80 years. During the first period of surveillance, January 1992–April 1993, 165 illnesses were documented in 165 day-care participants as well as 113 illnesses among 67 staff members. The rate of ARI among the elderly was 1.3 illnesses per annum, and the most common causes were RSV, influenza A, and coronavirus. The causes of illness in the staff compared to those in the elderly group were similar, but the elderly experienced significantly more cough, dyspnea, and sputum production than did the staff. Pathogen-specific analysis did not show significant differences in syndromes. At baseline, wheezing and crackles were found in 4% and 18%, respectively, compared with 19% wheezing and 57% with crackles when ill. Most patients were managed in the community; however, 6% were admitted to hospital, and 1 in 40 died during their acute illness. Similar to Nicholson's results, patients with coronavirus were frequently dyspneic and had crackles on examination, suggesting that this virus, which is usually mild in children and young adults, may be more serious in older people (31). A second report by Falsey provided data on 522 illnesses that occurred throughout the 44 months of the study and focused on the clinical HRV and coronavirus infections. Although HRV and coronavirus infections have only rarely been found to be the cause of pneumonia in adults, similarly to Nicholson, these investigators found that approximately 50% of illnesses were associated with evidence of lower respiratory tract involvement as defined by the presence of sputum production, shortness of breath, new wheezing, and/or new crackles on examination. Wheezing was found to be equally prevalent in those with chronic lung disease as those without. No deaths occurred, but one individual with HRV infection was hospitalized and treated for congestive heart failure and recovered (70).

A further study by these investigators examined the relative numbers of hospitalizations in persons >65 years old that were associated with RSV infection and compared the clinical manifestations with influenza A infection (71). The study was conducted between November and April during 3 successive years, beginning in 1989, as part of the nationwide Medicare Influenza Vaccine Demonstration Project. The importance of these pathogens is illustrated by the fact that influenza A and B evidently accounted for 14% of admissions by the over 65s with acute cardiopulmonary disease, and that RSV accounted for 10%. As in the United Kingdom, RSV and influenza virus infections occurred simultaneously during each of the study years. RSV illnesses were comparable in severity to influenza, in terms of mean length of stay in hospital (RSV, 16 days vs. influenza, 13 days), admission to the intensive care unit (RSV, 18% vs. influenza, 18%), and requirement for ventilation (RSV, 10% vs. influenza, 9%). Moreover, the discharge diagnoses for patients with RSV were comparable to those for influenza, with high numbers being diagnosed with pneumonia (RSV, 44%; influenza, 33%), exacerbations of chronic bronchitis (RSV, 19%; influenza, 11%), and heart failure (RSV, 20%; influenza, 16%). The mortality rates were also similar (RSV, 10%; influenza, 6%).

In 2001, a new pneumovirus, human meta-pneumovirus (hMVP) was detected in the nasopharyngeal aspirates of 28 Dutch hospitalized children taken over 10 years who presented with ARI exhibiting similar signs and symptoms to those of RSV infection. Seroprevalence data suggested that it is a ubiquitous organism, detected in 100% of children >5 years of age (4). Analysis by PCR and culture of 38 archived clinical specimens in Canada have also identified hMPV. Seventeen of 38 (45%) were from hospitalized patients >65 years presenting with ARI of previously undetermined cause (72). Virological surveillance data during winter 2000–2001 in England and Wales identified hMPV in 9 of 711 (2.5%) of influenza-like illness presentations to sentinel primary care practices and was detected in four people aged 20–64 and 4 aged >65 years. Six of nine (67%) had clinical evidence of lower respiratory tract involvement and four received antibiotic therapy. All made a complete recovery. Phylogenetic analysis suggested the presence of at least two serotypes (73). It remains to be elucidated whether this virus plays a significant clinical role in the burden of hospital admissions in different age groups of the general population.

Institutionalized Elderly

The relatively close contact between frail elderly individuals and their caregivers in residential care readily facilitates transmission of respiratory viruses by droplets, aerosol, and fomites. Outbreaks of ARI, particularly those leading to hospitalization or deaths, have traditionally been ascribed to influenza, but experience during the last two decades indicates that other pathogens are responsible for considerable morbidity.

In a study of ARI in nursing home patients by Nicholson in Leicester, 170 residents experienced 179 episodes (74). Virological testing revealed that respiratory symptoms in the study population were evidently caused mostly by pathogens other than influenza during the influenza period documented nationally. This led the investigators to question the validity of assumptions used by the US Committee on Issues and Priorities for New Vaccine Development in its assessment of the impact of influenza and value of vaccines against the disease. Lower respiratory tract complications developed during 25% of ARIs including 3 of the 12 coronavirus infections, 3 of 9 RSV infections, 2 of 4 adenovirus infections, 1 of 11 HRV infections, but none of 12 influenza A and B infections. Six deaths (3.4%) occurred within 4 weeks of onset of upper respiratory illness. The overall burden from outbreaks of respiratory tract infections in long-term care facilities for older persons can be extremely high. Loeb identified 16 outbreaks involving 480 residents in 5 nursing homes in metropolitan Toronto over 3 years (75). Pneumonia occurred in 72 (15%) of the residents, 58 (12%) required transfer to hospital, and the case fatality rate was 8% (37/480). As noted elsewhere in this chapter, clinical findings were nonspecific and could not be used to differentiate between causal agents.

Although the disease burden of RSV is concentrated in infants and young children, severe outbreaks have been described in elderly patients in hospitals and nursing homes. One outbreak in a psychogeriatric hospital in the English West Midlands affected 17 of 40 (42.5%) residents, of whom one gradually deteriorated and died 1 month later (76). Two of 24 patients in a psychogeriatric unit died during one outbreak reported to the PHLS, and in a geriatric hospital 15 patients were affected, 8 (53%) of whom died (77). In a further outbreak in Devon, 20 of 50 (40%) residents of a residential home were affected and 4 patients died within a week of onset of illness (78). In Missouri (USA) an outbreak in a nursing home affected 15 of 77 (19%) residents, 7 of whom developed pneumonia (79). In Rochester (New York) Mathur described concurrent RSV and influenza A infections in a chronic care geriatric hospital (80). Patients in the 634 beds (in three facilities) were surveyed for febrile ARIs during the period 15 November 1977–15 March 1978. Seventy-one developed acute febrile ARIs. Of 32 patients with a diagnosis, 7 had RSV, 24 had influenza, and 1 had both. A comparison of the clinical features revealed no significant differences in respiratory or constitutional symptoms or signs except coryza, which was more common in the RSV group. None of the patients died, but two of those infected with RSV developed pneumonia. Morales reported 12 RSV infections with 2 deaths among 159 respiratory episodes during a 6 month study of respiratory infections (81). Sorvillo described an outbreak in a Los Angeles County nursing home in which 40 of 101 (40%) residents were affected, 22 (55%) of whom had pneumonia and 8 (20%) died (82). In the winter of 1984–1985, an outbreak of RSV infection occurred among elderly people at the Pasteur Hospital (Poitiers, France). Among all patients, the clinical and serological attack rates were 61% and 75%, respectively. Among the 52 patients with RSV infection, 6 (11.5%) died during the first month, and bronchopneumonia was diagnosed in 22 (42%) subjects with respiratory symptoms. Additional RSV outbreaks in the residential elderly have been described, and although mortality is not universally reported (83,84), the data indicate that RSV is a more important and frequent pathogen in the elderly than previously suspected. Moreover, the data confirm that because simultaneous occurrence of clinically indistinguishable influenza and RSV infections may not be a rare occurrence, virological studies are essential to ensure that antiinfluenza drugs are used appropriately.

Parainfluenza (PIV) types 1 and 2 usually occur in the autumn, but PIV-3 usually appears in the spring or summer following influenza outbreaks. PIV is a common cause of croup and bronchitis in young children, and infection in young healthy adults typically presents as an upper respiratory infection. PIV infections in the elderly have not been well characterized. During 1976–1982, the PHLS Communicable Diseases Surveillance Centre (CDSC) received a total of 5781 laboratory reports of PIV infection. Only 121 (2%) of these infections were in people aged 65 years or older (77). About half of the patients had pneumonia or other lower respiratory tract infections. CDSC reported an outbreak of PIV-1 in geriatric wards in Hull; four men died before specimens were collected, but subsequently 9 of 16 subjects tested were positive. The CDSC report referred to four outbreaks due to PIV-3. Glasgow describes an outbreak due to PIV-3 in a nursing home in Toronto (85). It occurred in late spring, several months after the end of local influenza activity. There were 26 cases among 84 residents. Half the affected residents developed lower respiratory tract illness, but lower respiratory illness occurred significantly more frequently (82%) in the frail elderly than in those who were ambulatory. The mean duration of illness in patients was almost twice as long as in the younger staff. One resident was hospitalized, but none died.

Simultaneous occurrence of PIV and influenza in nursing homes is evidently common and associated with an overall mortality following virus isolation of 4% for PIV 1-4 (70,84,86). Drinka and colleagues conducted virological surveillance in a Wisconsin Veterans Home to focus the timing for influenza A chemoprophylaxis (32). During the 7 years covered by their report, 2652 cultures were performed, and 19% of these revealed a viral pathogen, which included 270 (53%) influenza A, 112 (22%) influenza B, 50 (10%) PIV-1, 18 (4%) PIV 2-4, 25 (5%) RSV, and 32 (6%) HRV infections. PIV was the predominant pathogen in one season and contributed more than 20% of isolates in a further two seasons. Outbreaks of PIV infection in residential care are apparently common in long-term care facilities for older people. During Loeb's 3-year study of five residential facilities, PIV was implicated in 13 of the 16 outbreaks identified prospectively, and in 12 of 30 outbreaks identified by a retrospective audit of surveillance records (75).

Despite extensive investigation of HRV infections in younger age groups, comparatively few prospective studies have been conducted in elderly people, especially those living in residential facilities. Few studies have carried out laboratory tests for coronaviruses. In Leicester, Nicholson studied acute upper respiratory tract viral illness in 11 homes for the elderly (74). Two or three peaks of acute respiratory illness in the homes were identified, with the first (during weeks 39–48) coinciding with peak activity of HRV infection. Although lower respiratory illness complicated only 1 of 11 HRV infections, one patient progressively deteriorated and died from pneumonia. Coronavirus OC43 cocirculated with RSV and influenza during a second peak of activity. Reinfection with the same or related strain of coronavirus is common and outbreaks typically occur during the winter and early spring when influenza is generally prevalent. Human coronaviruses are noted for their pronounced coryza, but in this study population the illness was clinically indistinguishable from RSV and influenza, and lower respiratory tract complications occurred in one-quarter.

The Wisconsin Veterans Home studies did not include serological studies for coronaviruses, but as in Leicester they used cultures for HRVs (32). Culture is particularly insensitive for HRVs (four to five times as many HRV infections can be identified by PCR) and thus estimates of the burden of HRV without PCR must be interpreted with caution. In Wisconsin, HRV infections occurred sporadically throughout influenza seasons, but an outbreak involving 67 residents occurred in August, 1993. Throat and nasopharyngeal virus cultures yielded HRV from 33 of the 67 and no other respiratory virus was implicated. Overall 100% had upper respiratory symptoms, 34% gastrointestinal symptoms, 71% had systemic symptoms, 66% had lower respiratory symptoms (a rate virtually identical to that for community-dwelling elderly (31)), and 52% had new abnormalities on lung auscultation. The residents with chronic obstructive pulmonary disease had more severe illnesses: 2 of 17 required transfer to hospital and 1 died of respiratory failure. Throughout the 7 year study only 1 of 61 residents with HRV infections died (32). A study conducted in a 591-bed nursing home in Rochester (USA) identified HRV to be the second most frequent virus isolate after RSV (70). In contrast to RSV, HRV illness was rather mild, and all 14 patients recovered without sequelae. Lennox briefly describes an analysis of cases of ILI in eight continuing-care wards for the elderly on two hospital sites during the winter months of 1986–1987 (87). HRVs were the most common isolates, but no details of their outcome are provided. Loeb makes no reference to HRV as a cause of any of the outbreaks in five nursing homes in Toronto (75).

In contrast to HRV and coronavirus infections, there are abundant data on the burden of influenza in residential care. Many reports describe influenza outbreaks, often with high attack rates despite high uptake of influenza vaccine. Since outbreaks with what are described as high attack rates and/or high morbidity/mortality are more likely to be reported in the literature than ones with low attack rates, the available data must be treated with caution. Zadeh conducted a questionnaire survey of 1017 randomly selected nursing homes in nine states in the United States (88). The response rate was 78%. Overall 116 (15%) nursing homes reported having a suspected or laboratory-confirmed influenza A outbreak in at least one influenza season between 1995 and 1998.

Possibly a better indication of the burden of influenza is provided by prospective, double blind, placebo-controlled trials of antivirals; prospective nonrandomized studies of vaccine efficacy that include nonvaccinated controls; and prospective observational (surveillance) studies. Two studies of rimantadine and the neuraminidase inhibitor oseltamivir in heavily immunized residential facilities suggest attack rates for symptomatic virologically confirmed influenza of ~4.5% (89,90). Deguchi studied 22,462 subjects in 301 public nursing homes during an influenza A (H3N2) epidemic in Japan (91). Overall 694 cases of influenzal illness were confirmed as influenza, for an attack rate of 5.9% by virus culture or serology among 11,723 unvaccinated controls. Prospective observational studies indicate annual incidence rates for symptomatic influenza of between 0.4 and 7.7% (32,33,74,80,92). As noted above, influenza often cocirculates in residential care with other respiratory viruses and is difficult to differentiate clinically. While many patients with influenza are febrile, fever was not prominent during an outbreak of influenza B involving 66 virologically confirmed cases in vaccinated residents in Wisconsin; 39% of the cases had low-grade fever at presentation and one-third were never febrile (93).

The availability of effective antivirals against influenza A and B requires that influenza can be reliably diagnosed. Analysis of so-called outbreaks in homes that have been shown by laboratory tests to be associated with influenza in the facility indicate that approximately half of those with acute respiratory infections or influenza-like illness do indeed have influenza (80,94–102).

There have been numerous reports of high influenza attack rates in residential care facilities, and mortality rates of greater than 4% are common (86,96). Nguyen Van Tamme and Nicholson examined certified influenza deaths in Leicestershire during the 1989–1990 epidemic (103). The estimated mortality for the fit elderly was ~7 per 100,000 population. Among nonresidential subjects the rate for certified influenza deaths was 11.6 and 23.1 per 100,000 for those with lung and heart disease, respectively. The major impact of influenza was in residential care facilities, where the rates were 343, 499, and 2703 per 100,000, respectively, for people with one, two, and three or more medical conditions. In further studies conducted in people with influenza as a certified cause of death in five health regions in England, and in patients admitted to Leicestershire hospitals with P & I related conditions, Ahmed found that more than half of those who died lived in residential care (odds ratio [OR] 2.08, 95%CI 1.48–2.9), as did over 15% of the P & I admissions in Leicester (OR 2.96, CI 1.35–6.53) (104,105). Since only about 5% of the elderly population in England live in residential care, it is evident that this group is at the greatest risk of serious morbidity and mortality. Homes that experience influenza outbreaks tend to be larger (>100 beds) and less well vaccinated (<80% of residents immunized) than other establishments (96,102).

Employees represent one of the most important routes of influenza virus entry (and presumably other viruses) into nursing homes. During 1993–1994, a comparatively mild epidemic season in Scotland, serological evidence of influenza infection was found in 23% of 970 healthcare workers at four acute care hospitals in Glasgow (34). More than half (59%) of these could not recall having influenza or taking sick (52%) leave for a respiratory infection. Moreover, two other studies have shown that ≥70% of healthcare workers with laboratory evidence of influenza or influenza-like illness have continued to work (106,107). It is therefore not surprising that healthcare workers have been implicated as the source of influenza infections in nursing home influenza outbreaks (108), or that vaccination of staff benefits residents (109).

B. Asthmatics

Research into the effects of respiratory viral infections, particularly HRVs, in chronic lung disease has been hampered by difficulties in laboratory diagnosis. HRVs, the major causative agents of the common cold, are fastidious for certain growth conditions and cells, and the large number of serotypes—at least 102—precludes serological examination for epidemiological studies. Rates of HRV identification that rely on culture have accordingly remained low, especially in adults. ARI are commonly implicated as the precipitating factor for episodes of exacerbation and bronchoconstriction in asthmatic patients. Two comparable prospective studies in asthmatic patients identified viruses in 55% of symptomatic respiratory tract infections in children less than 11 years of age, but in only 26% of such infections in subjects aged 3–60 years (110,111).

The role of respiratory viruses in causing asthma exacerbations in adults is less clear than in children with older studies showing RTI associated with asthma exacerbations in only 10–21% (112,113). However, the percentage of laboratory-confirmed viral infections that resulted in exacerbations of asthma was similar in adults with asthma (60%) to those reported for children (48–53%) (111). Beasley, in a longitudinal outpatient study, showed an incidence of viral RTI of 36% in acute severe adult asthma exacerbations and 10% in mild asthma exacerbations (114). The weak association between asthma and upper respiratory tract infections in these older studies could be due to difficulties in isolating human HRVs and coronaviruses.

During influenza outbreaks, hospital admission rates for respiratory illnesses including asthma increase. Asthma excess mortality was increased during influenza A outbreaks of 1957–1966 and deaths attributed to asthma increased by 19–46% during peak influenza A activity (115,116). Uncomplicated influenza infection and RSV in healthy young adults can result in peripheral airway dysfunction, increased airway hyperreactivity, and abnormalities in gas exchange. These changes may persist for weeks after clinical recovery from the infection (117–120).

Prospective Community Studies

Nicholson and colleagues were the first to apply coronavirus serology and a reverse transcription–polymerase chain reaction (RT-PCR) for picornaviruses to the study of respiratory viruses in asthma (121). Previously these investigators had shown that the RT-PCR increased the diagnostic rate for HRVs two- to fivefold (122). Virus isolation was also attempted and the relatively insensitive complement fixation test was used on paired acute and convalescent sera for antibodies to adenovirus, influenza A and B, RSV, parainfluenza virus types 1–3, *Mycoplasma pneumoniae*, and *Chlamydia psittaci*. Colds were reported in 80% (223 of 280) of episodes with symptoms of wheeze, chest tightness, or breathlessness, and 89% (223 of 250) of colds were associated with asthma symptoms. Forty-four percent of episodes with mean decreases in flow rate of ≥50l/min were associated with laboratory-confirmed infections. Of 119 virus infections, 66% (78) subsequently had statistically significant drops in peak flow. A virus pathogen was identified in 43% of 49 episodes that were sufficiently severe to be treated with oral prednisolone and in 31 (44%) of 70 patients who consulted their physician. Infections with HRVs, coronaviruses OC43 and 229E, influenza B, RSV, parainfluenza virus, and *Chlamydia* were all associated with objective evidence of an exacerbation of asthma. Because of the limitations of the serological tests applied, these investigators speculated that more sensitive tests would find these and other nonbacterial pathogens to have a much greater role than their results indicate (121).

Further studies using newer diagnostic techniques to evaluate the frequency of viral infections in adults with acute exacerbations of asthma have been performed in the United States and Japan. Atmar recruited 29 asthmatic adults from the pulmonary clinic of an urban county hospital and followed them in a longitudinal cohort study for signs and symptoms of asthma and acute respiratory virus infection (123). An exacerbation of asthma was defined by an increase in wheezing and/or dyspnea. Respiratory secretions and paired serum samples were collected from subjects with acute wheezing episodes and evaluated using virus culture, serological testing, and RT-PCR for HRV, influenza A, and coronavirus OC43. As in the Leicester study, 44% of 87 asthma exacerbations were associated with an acute respiratory virus infection. Forty-six (60%) of the 77 picornavirus infections and 22 (71%) of the 31 coronavirus infections were identified only using RT-PCR (121). Kuga similarly applied RT-PCR to study the role of picornaviruses (including HRVs and enteroviruses). Overall 40 of 65 (61.5%) asthmatics with symptomatic colds had an asthma exacerbation, and picornavirus RNA was recovered from 16 of 52 (30.8%) patients experiencing exacerbation (124).

A longitudinal cohort study of 76 cohabiting couples (one healthy and one asthmatic) by Corne and colleagues found that during the HRV peak season of autumn–early winter, 32 of 378 (8.5%) and 38 of 375 (10.1%) samples from healthy and asthmatic sufferers, respectively, were positive for HRV (125). The groups did not differ in frequency, duration, or severity of symptoms of upper respiratory illness. However, HRV infection in asthmatic subjects was associated with more frequent lower respiratory tract infections (p = 0.051) that were of longer duration than in healthy individuals (median 2.5 days; range 0–35 vs. median 0 days; range 0–22; p < 0.005).

"Emergency Department" and Hospital Admission Studies

Abramson, in a case-control study of 38 patients >10 years admitted to the hospital with acute asthma and 90 controls admitted for road trauma or endoscopy, identified positive viral cultures or viral immunofluorescence in 8 asthmatic patients and 2 controls (126). The asthmatic group had 6.2 times more chance of having an acute viral respiratory infection than controls.

Teichtahl carried out a prospective study over a 12 month period to assess the incidence of respiratory tract infection [RTI] in adults with acute asthma exacerbation requiring admission to a general hospital in metropolitan Melbourne, Australia (127). A control group was studied from elective surgical inpatients. Thirty-seven percent of adult patients with acute asthma admitted to the Department of Respiratory Medicine over a 12-month period had evidence of recent RTI. Influenza A (n = 13) and HRV (n = 9) were the most common infectious agents. Other agents identified were RSV, influenza B, adenovirus, and *Mycoplasma*. The authors considered that the incidence of 37% RTI occurring in adult patients with acute exacerbation of asthma requiring hospitalization was underestimated because a number of the patients failed to return for their convalescent serum sample, thus some viral infections may have been missed.

As a second component of their investigations, Atmar studied 122 asthmatic adults who presented to the hospital emergency department with acute symptoms of asthma (123). Overall 148 asthma exacerbations were evaluated; 55% were associated with an acute respiratory virus infection and a virus infection was identified in 21 (50%) of 42 of the subjects who were hospitalized. El-Sahly conducted a prospective cohort study to determine the prevalence of HRV and coronavirus infections in patients of all ages hospitalized in Houston, Texas, for acute respiratory illnesses (128). A total of 61 HRV and coronavirus infections were identified from 1198 respiratory illnesses. Of these illnesses, 408 (34.1%) had paired sera available for testing for coronavirus infection. Underlying cardiopulmonary diseases were present in 93% of patients aged between 5 and 35 years, and in 73% aged >35 years. For the 15 patients between the ages of 5 and 35 years, the primary reason for admission was for the treatment of asthma (n = 14); 1 patient had pneumonia. For the 26 aged greater than 35 years, admissions were precipitated by exacerbations of chronic obstructive airways disease, pneumonia, heart failure, and congestive cardiac failure. The use of RT-PCR assays for HRV and coronavirus has increased the frequency with which these virus infections were identified, but it was not performed in this study. Moreover, since serological testing was only performed on a subset, the burden of infections detected in this study must be regarded as an underestimate.

In marked contrast to the above studies of asthma and hospital admissions with HRV and coronavirus infections, a study of 33 patients in Cleveland, who presented to the emergency room with 35 exacerbations of asthma, failed to identify any viral pathogens by culture or rapid antigen testing despite 56% of patients having symptoms suggestive of viral illness. The investigators suggested as a possible explanation the lack of sensitivity of the available diagnostic tests and culture techniques (129).

Rossi evaluated the involvement of viral and *Mycoplasma* infections in exacerbations of asthma in 112 adult patients admitted to Oulu University Central Hospital; a virus or *Mycoplasma* was implicated in 29% of cases (130).

There is overwhelming evidence that asthma exacerbations in adults are frequently triggered by an acute respiratory virus infection. All respiratory viruses, *Chlamydia pneumoniae*, and *Mycoplasma pneumoniae* evidently exacerbate asthma, but because of the large number of different HRVs these pathogens are the most important overall. The role of influenza infection in this group supports the view that in adults with significant long-term asthma, annual influenza vaccination is advisable.

C. Chronic Cardiopulmonary Conditions

Exacerbations of chronic obstructive pulmonary disease (COPD) have been repeatedly linked to respiratory virus infections. Exacerbations are generally considered to be viral, bacterial, and mixed viral–bacterial infections of the respiratory tract. As noted above, research into the effects of respiratory viral infections, particularly HRVs and coronaviruses, in chronic lung disease has been hampered by difficulties in laboratory diagnosis, so the association between exacerbations of chronic obstructive airways disease and upper respiratory tract infections is probably an underestimate.

One of the earliest studies of the association between respiratory viral disease and chronic bronchitis was conducted by Carilli in 1964 who studied 30 subjects with chronic bronchitis and 10 controls (131). HRV infections were not diagnosed in this study, but virus infections including 8 RSV, 4 influenza A, 2 parainfluenza type 3, and 10 other infections caused by adenovirus, *Chlamydia psittaci, Coxiella burnetii,* and *Mycoplasma pneumoniae* were identified in 24 (52%) of 46 exacerbations. Shortly thereafter HRV infections were found to be associated with exacerbations of chronic bronchitis (132) and an association between coronaviruses and exacerbations of chronic bronchitis was established in the 1970s (133).

The extent to which acute respiratory viral infections cause exacerbations of COPD appears comparable to that for exacerbations of asthma, with studies revealing an association with up to two-thirds of exacerbations (68,131–139). A thorough analysis by Lieberman revealed the presence of one or more pathogens in 73% of 249 hospitalizations for acute exacerbations of COPD (140). In 117 (48.8%) hospitalizations at least one of seven viral pathogens was identified. In 72 (30.0%) cases at least one of *Legionella* spp, *Mycoplasma pneumoniae,* or *Coxiella burnetii* was identified. More than one pathogen was identified in one-third of the cases. The investigators concluded that in most cases of hospitalization for an exacerbation, the pathogen is usually a virus or an atypical bacteria, and is a classic bacteria in only a minority of cases. Essentially all viruses known to cause respiratory illness (with the possible exception of adenovirus) have been shown to be capable of causing exacerbations.

Several studies have shown more severe viral illness and increased illness rates or susceptibility (32,68,136,138,141) in patients with chronic lung disease than in those without. Patients with COPD experience 2.2–2.4 acute respiratory illnesses per person per year compared with 1.4 illnesses in age-matched controls. For those with moderate–severe airways disease, the number of illnesses per person per year increases to 3.0 (68,141). The reason(s) why patients with chronic bronchitis suffer from an increased illness rate and a greater number of seroconversions than healthy controls is unclear, but it is possible that the long-standing lower respiratory tract disease disrupts normal defense mechanisms.

Respiratory tract infections are associated with both acute and chronic deterioration in pulmonary function in healthy individuals and those with chronic bronchitis and cystic fibrosis (119,141–146). Although acute respiratory virus infections are generally perceived as mild, for those with underlying chronic medical conditions they cause a substantial number of visits to physicians and represent a leading cause of hospitalization (116,139,147). Glezen found that the risk for hospital admission was 19.7:10,000 for those with underlying chronic medical illnesses compared to 9.3:10,000 in controls (116,248). The greatest risk for hospital admissions occurred in those over 65 years with chronic pulmonary conditions (87.5:10,000) and 27.5:10,000 for those aged 45–64 years. The hospitalization rate of 311.6:10,000 for those from low-income groups was significantly higher than that for middle-income families: 44.7:10,000. Influenza, parainfluenza, and RSV accounted for 75% of all virus infections identified.

In a study by Walsh, 134 community-dwelling elderly adults in Rochester with chronic cardiopulmonary disease were monitored over two consecutive winters, 1996–1997 and 1997–1998 for the presence of respiratory viruses (136). The incidence of documented viral infection was significantly higher in those with congestive heart failure than with chronic airways disease (31 vs. 16 infections per 100 person-winters, p = 0.02). Of positive samples, there were 13 of 39 (33%, incidence of 7.0 per 100 person-winters) influenza A, 8 of 39 (21%, incidence of 4.3 per 100 person-winters) RSV, 9 of 39 (23%, incidence of 4.9 per 100 person-winters) coronavirus, and 7 of 39 (18%, incidence of 3.8 per 100 person-winters) HRVs identified. These incidences were found to be statistically similar; however, 9 of 21 with influenza A or RSV were hospitalized compared to 0 of 17 with other viruses, suggesting the greatest clinical impact from influenza A and RSV infection.

Between 9 and 43% of exacerbations of chronic bronchitis are associated with HRV infection (68,131,136,141,148–150). The number of inflammatory cells in the bronchial mucosa increases after experimental infection of the upper respiratory tract (151), but it is unclear whether HRV invades the lower airways to cause exacerbations of asthma or chronic bronchitis or pneumonia through direct enhancement of local inflammatory responses (152). HRV was recovered more often from sputum of children during attacks of wheezy bronchitis than from the nose and throat, suggesting that virus replication occurs in the lower respiratory tract (153). HRV has also been recovered from the lower respiratory tract of infected individuals (154–156), but pneumonia is evidently rare in adults, occurring almost always in the immunocompromised (157). HRV infection in patients with COPD causes small statistically insignificant declines in spirometric results (143). HRV infection is generally more severe among those with underlying lung disease. Wald showed that persons with lung disease are more likely than those without lung disease to report dyspnea (42%), and they have a longer duration of illness (144).

Utilizing diagnostic PCR for HRV and serological means for coronavirus, El-Sahley in Texas evaluated 1198 respiratory illnesses in 1068 hospitalized patients, including 546 adults >35 years of age (128). There were 13 (2.3%) cases each of HRV and coronavirus infection. Nineteen of 26 cases had underlying asthma, congestive heart failure, or chronic airways disease. Eight patients were admitted with pneumonia and one required ventilation support. A study by Falsey of 316 elderly persons hospitalized with cardiopulmonary illnesses found 61 (19%) and 22 (7%) cases of influenza A and RSV, respectively (158). Of the 249 remaining cases, 100 were evaluated for HRV and coronaviruses by PCR. Twelve (12%) of these were positive. All had significant underlying disease and although all recovered, the mean length of stay was 8 days; four had pneumonia and one required ventilation. These data clearly associate HRV and coronavirus with severe respiratory illness, particularly in the frail elderly with underlying chronic cardiopulmonary diseases.

Overall, the prevalence of specific viruses in a number of studies of patients with chronic medical conditions has ranged from 11 to 33% influenza A, 6 to 8% influenza B, 0.8 to 21% RSV, 9 to 30% HRV, 6 to 23% coronavirus, 5 to 29% parainfluenza, and 0 to 1% for adenovirus. No significant differences in the distribution of specific viruses between subjects with mild or moderate/severe COPD have been noted during these various studies (68,136,141,148–150).

Although infrequently identified as an acute cause precipitating an exacerbation of airways disease, DNA viruses such as adenovirus, target airway epithelial cells, and portions of their genome can persist in these cells in a latent form after infection has cleared. The presence of this latent viral protein amplifies cigarette-smoke-induced inflammation and is associated with development of emphysema. The presence of detectable latent DNA virus infection is associated with steroid unresponsiveness of allergen-induced inflammatory lung disease and therefore may contribute to the pathogenesis of COPD (159).

D. The Immunocompromised

Respiratory virus infections have become an increasingly recognized problem in immunocompromised adults. The prevalence and severity of illness vary with degrees of immunosuppression, affecting most severely bone marrow transplant recipients and those with myelosuppression. Although respiratory viral infections in the immunocompromised typically occur during outbreaks in the community, PIV infections, in particular, have been reported throughout the year (160). Adenovirus infection may result from reactivation rather than newly acquired community or nosocomial infection.

Prior to 1988, only sporadic case reports of RSV in immunosuppressed patients had been published (161,162). The first series of RSV infections in 11 immunocompromised adults aged 21–50 years was reported by Englund in Minnesota in 1988 (163). Underlying conditions included six bone marrow transplants, three renal transplants, one pancreas transplant, and one T-cell lymphoma. All had lower respiratory tract involvement, 8 of 11 had progressive disease associated with bilateral changes on chest radiography, and four died.

Bone Marrow Transplant Recipients

Couch reported the results of 3 years' surveillance from 1992 to 1995 of respiratory viruses in patients with leukemia or following bone marrow transplantation (BMT) at the MD Anderson Cancer Center in Houston (164). Of 668 nasal and throat swabs cultures, 56 (31%) yielded RSV, 52 (28%) picornaviruses, 33 (18%) influenza, 15 (15%) parainfluenza, and 14 (8%) adenoviruses. RSV and influenza were confined to winter and spring, but HRVs, adenoviruses, and PIV-3 tended to occur throughout the year. Pneumonia and death complicated 58–78% and 22–44% of infections, respectively, with possibly greater morbidity for RSV than other viruses.

Whimbey cultured community respiratory viruses from 67 of 217 (31%) adult BMT recipients over two winters, 1992–1994 (165,166). RSV was isolated most frequently, accounting for 49%. Subsequently the incidence of RSV declined, attributed by the authors to improved infection control, but almost half the picornavirus, influenza, parainfluenza, and adenovirus infections were nosocomial. During the winter months, the incidence of pneumonia and deaths was fourfold higher than associated with respiratory cytomegalovirus (CMV) infection. During 1993–1995, 60 (18%) of 335 hospitalized adults with leukemia had positive cultures, with infections due to influenza (32%), RSV (30%), picornaviruses (17%), parainfluenza (10%), and adenoviruses (3%). As in BMT patients, temporal occurrence of each virus reflected community activity; RSV and influenza occurred only in the winter months.

Of 61 patients with culture-confirmed PIV during 1991–1994 from the MD Anderson Cancer Center, 53% occurred in the spring or summer. During peak PIV activity, 32 of 96 (33%) adult BMT recipients presenting with ARI had positive PIV cultures. The overall mortality was 39% and 66% in BMT and leukemia patients, respectively (166). Some 8221 hospital laboratory reports of PIV infections from England and Wales between 1975 and 1997 to PHLS were analyzed by Laurichesse (167). PIV-3 accounted for 71% of reports compared to 17%, 7.5%, and 1.1% for PIV-1, PIV-2, and PIV-4, respectively. Only 186 (2.4%) PIV reports were from persons >45 years of age. Many of these involved immunosuppressed patients including those with malignancy, transplant recipients, and AIDS. Pneumonia was the most common diagnosis in the immunocompromised subjects; 64% of these reports were associated with PIV-3.

Bowden at the Fred Hutchinson Cancer Research Center in Seattle cultured and performed direct antibody fluorescence on nasopharyngeal samples from all post-BMT patients with respiratory symptoms and bronchoalveolar lavage from those with radiographic abnormalities (160). Between 1990 and 1996, the most frequently observed infection was RSV, which occurred in 44 (35%) samples followed by PIV (30%) with types 1 and 3 occurring equally; HRVs and influenza A accounted for 25% and 11%, respectively. RSV and PIV had the highest rates of progression from upper to lower tracts; virtually all HRVs were isolated from the upper respiratory tract.

Respiratory viruses are also recognized as important pathogens following bone marrow transplantation in Europe (168). Ljungman identified 39 respiratory virus infections among 545 BMT recipients at the Huddinge Centre in Sweden, but did not culture for HRVs. Pneumonia caused by RSV and adenoviruses was associated with the highest mortality rates of 60% and 75%, respectively. A substantial proportion of the RSV infections occurred late following transplantation after the period of most intense chemotherapy. The same study group performed a prospective study at 37 centers to determine the frequency and outcome of infections following 819 allogeneic and 1154 autologous stem cell transplantations (169). The mortality from RSV and influenza was 30% and 23%, respectively.

Although most HRV infections in immunocompromised subjects are associated with upper respiratory tract illness, they are increasingly recognised as causing lower tract complications. In one study of BMT recipients, HRV infections accounted for 12 (18%) illnesses with a proven viral cause; 7 of these (58%) had pneumonia and 3 (25%) died from progressive viral pneumonia (165). A 5 year retrospective study of hematology patients including BMT recipients identified 23 HRV infections. All had upper respiratory tract symptoms but 8 (35%) developed respiratory failure and histological changes consistent with viral pneumonia at postmortem (170).

At the University of Virginia Health Center, only 17 of 431 adults with one or more respiratory viruses identified in bronchoalveolar lavage (BAL) fluid were positive for HRVs (157). Of these patients, 70% had dual pathogens identified. All had immunosuppressive disease, including six solid organ transplants, three malignancies, and two with AIDS. All had radiographic evidence of pneumonia, 60% required ventilation, and 25% died. Histological findings in bronchial biopsies ranged from fibropurulent inflammation to diffuse alveolitis.

PCR is more sensitive than viral culture or antigen or serological testing for the detection of respiratory viruses in patients with hematological malignancies. Van Elden retrospectively analyzed the value of PCR to detect PIV 1-3, RSV, HRV, influenza viruses A and B, enteroviruses, and coronaviruses in BAL samples from 43 patients with hematological cancer (171). Culture or antigen testing revealed four RSV, three rhinovirus, and two influenza infections in 8 of 43 (19%) patients. PCR identified additional HRV, enterovirus, PIV, RSV, and coronavirus infections and increased the overall identification rate from 19% to 35% (p < 0.005).

Adenovirus infections are frequently encountered, although the relative contribution of primary or latent reactivation is unclear. A large series of 118 adult and 83 pediatric BMT recipients in Wisconsin found that the overall incidence of adenovirus infection was 21% (172), exceeding earlier rates estimated at 4–8% (164,166,173,174). Adenoviruses were cultured from 14% of the adult recipients, with most cases occurring more than 90 days posttransplantation. In BMT recipients, adenovirus serotypes 1, 2, 5, 11, and 31 tend to predominate. Lung, liver, and gastrointestinal disease represent the most usual manifestations, dissemination occurs frequently, and the case fatality rate may approach 60% (175,176).

Solid Organ Transplants

Immunosuppressive therapy, exposure of the graft to the environment, reduced lymphatic and ciliary clearance, and absent cough reflexes all contribute to the increased risk of lung transplant recipients to respiratory virus infections. Case reports indicate that RSV, parainfluenza, influenza, and adenoviruses may cause serious and fatal disease (177–181). During 1992–1998, 182 lung transplants were performed at Duke University hospital. Matar et al. identified 21 respiratory viral infections including nine PIV, eight RSV, five adenovirus, and two influenza infections (180). PIV and RSV were associated with mild respiratory illness, typically without radiographic changes, and full recovery. Adenovirus was symptomatic in all cases, resulting in progressive fulminant pulmonary disease and 80% mortality. A patient with dual infection with influenza and parainfluenza developed fatal respiratory failure.

Opportunistic respiratory virus infections have been found in adult cardiac, liver, and renal transplant recipients. Ljungman reported 12 cases of influenza in renal transplant recipients; 1 had severe illness and 11 cases were clinically uncomplicated (182). A prospective study of 51 consecutive liver transplant recipients submitting weekly clinical swabs following transplant for 3 months found 2 of 323 (0.62%) RSV positive by culture/PCR, but no other respiratory viruses were identified (183).

Transmission

Outbreaks on BMT units with at least RSV, PIV-3, and influenza have been attributed to nosocomial spread. In excess of 50% immunocompromised patients may acquire infection by this means (163,165,184–189). At times of virus activity in the general community, infections may be introduced by visitors and hospital staff (190). In immunocompromised hosts, the respiratory viral infection may be protracted with prolonged viral shedding and virus transmission may continue after the virus has disappeared from the community. The shedding of respiratory virus may be intermittent and not necessarily associated with respiratory illness, thereby delaying diagnosis and initiation of control measures (164,185). Nosocomial transmission of PIV-3 and RSV is generally caused by direct contact with the virus itself, usually hand-to-hand contact, and physical transfer of viable organisms to a susceptible host from an infected person (190,191). Transmission from contaminated fomites is also an important route. Droplet transmission can occur as a result of virus-containing large-particle droplets or small-particle aerosols generated during sneezing or speaking. Large-droplet transmission, as with adenovirus, generally requires close contact between source and recipient because these particles do not remain suspended in the air or travel in excess of 1 m (191).

Given the frequency, morbidity, and mortality of nosocomial infection, an aggressive multifaceted infection control strategy is required. Community virological surveillance will initially identify the period of risk when local virus activity increases. Educational updates to staff working on high-risk units are important to ensure compliance with infection control programs. Important central control measures include isolation or cohort nursing of infected patients and rigorous hand washing. The Centers for Disease Control (CDC, Atlanta) also advise the use of contact precautions, in addition to standard nursing procedures. Recommendations include wearing of gloves, gowns, and eye protection where possible (191). Family and visitor restrictions, particularly children, either during outbreaks or the entire winter season have been advocated. Individual institutions usually assess the relative benefit and practicality of each measure (192).

IV. Clinical Spectrum of Infection

Respiratory virus infections may be subclinical or cause symptoms ranging from mild self-limiting upper respiratory illness to severe, systemic illness with appreciable morbidity, complications, and occasional mortality. Respiratory virus infections cause overlapping syndromes that correspond to the site of infection. Upper respiratory tract infection is characterized by the presence of low-grade fever with coryza, nasal congestion, and discharge. Additional features include otitis media, middle ear effusion, and acute sinusitis. Laryngopharyngitis presents with sore throat and hoarseness. Tracheobronchitis with middle and lower respiratory airway inflammation gives symptoms including cough, dyspnea, and sputum production, but radiographically clear lung fields. Lower respiratory tract complications include exacerbations of COPD, asthma, viral pneumonitis, and secondary bacterial pneumonia. Respiratory viruses are rarely identified outside the respiratory tract.

Influenza has been traditionally associated with the most severe illnesses and the highest frequency of complications, but as diagnostic techniques have improved other viruses have been shown to cause clinically indistinguishable disease, with an overall burden approaching or even exceeding that of influenza. Influenza A is characteristically abrupt in onset after an incubation period of several days. An overview of symptoms recorded by 579 adults with H1N1, H2N2, and H3N2 subtypes of influenza A is summarized in Figure 2. Some 70–84% of patients experience early systemic features at onset including myalgia, fever, chills, headache, and general malaise. Fever is a prominent sign in the infection, peaking at the time of systemic features and lasting for 1–5 days. Systemic features are generally accompanied by an unproductive cough, nasal discharge, stuffiness, and, to a lesser extent, sore throat. Ocular symptoms such as conjunctivitis, lacrimation, grittiness, and photophobia occur in up to 20% of affected individuals. Gastrointestinal upset including diarrhea and abdominal pain occurs less frequently (in around 6% of infected indi-

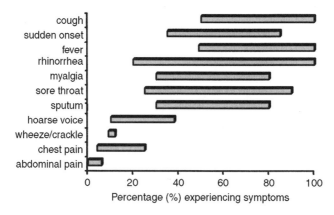

Figure 2 Overall clinical characteristics of virologically confirmed influenza infection in adults. (Data from Refs. 14, 26, 29, 31, 38, 80, 144, 193–196.)

viduals). Mild attacks of influenza are associated with a 20–40% impairment of reaction times for a number of tasks (197). Monto and colleagues pooled clinical data from 3744 subjects enrolled into zanamivir treatment studies; to be enrolled, patients had to have a predefined influenza-like illness (196). Subjects with influenza were more likely to have cough (93% vs. 80%), fever (68% vs. 40%), or nasal congestion (91% vs. 81%) than those without influenza. After multivariate analysis, cough and fever had a positive predictive value (PPV) of 79% (p < 0.001). A study in Quebec enrolled 100 subjects with influenza-like illness, of whom 79% had confirmed influenza. Fever and cough were independently associated with a positive diagnosis, and the PPV for the combination was 89% (195). In contrast, in settings outside clinical trials, a physician-based surveillance study of ARI in France during periods of high and low influenza activity found a PPV for influenza of ~40% for respiratory symptoms with cough and fever (39). In a study in community-dwelling elderly, the complex of myalgia, fever, sweats, and respiratory symptoms had a PPV of 33% during the time of influenza activity, but fell to 9% during the nonepidemic period (31).

Observations in young adults indicate that RSV infection is usually mild with symptoms confined to the upper respiratory tract (198–200). Hall prospectively evaluated 2960 New York healthy working adults aged 18–60 years for respiratory virus infections, 211 (7%) and 59 (2%) had RSV and influenza infections, respectively (201). Nasal congestion, productive cough, otalgia, and sinus pain were significantly associated with RSV infection; fever and headache were associated with influenza. RSV illness was of significantly longer duration than influenza (9.5 vs. 6.8 days). In keeping with this finding, an outbreak of RSV among healthy hospital staff found persisting fatigue, exertional dyspnea and exaggerated airways reactivity on pulmonary function tests for up to 8 weeks following infection (120). In Dowell's study of RSV-associated community acquired pneumonia, clinical features clearly separating RSV-infected patients were the presence of wheeze and rhonchi on examination (p = 0.009 and 0.002, respectively, after controlling for variables including underlying disease); RSV subjects reported more cough, but less fever than influenza cases (p < 0.05 each (57).

Limited comparative descriptions of adenovirus illness in military populations have failed to identify specific features, although there is a trend to greater frequency of high fever >38.1°C (91–100%) and conjunctivitis (up to 56%) than with other pathogens (61,202). There are few comparative studies on clinical findings of community-dwelling elderly adults with acute respiratory infections. Nicholson prospectively followed 533 subjects, aged 60–90 years; there were 497 ARIs of which 211 (43%) were positive for pathogens (31). Although there were no pathognomonic features for pathogens (coronavirus, influenza, rhinovirus, RSV, and unknown) that were compared, RSV was associated with a greater frequency of sneezing and lower respiratory involvement, and systemic features including sweating, myalgia and rigors, and impact on daily activities, were more prominent in those with influenza. In community-dwelling elderly with cardiopulmonary disease, comparison of presenting symptoms of influenza, rhinovirus and RSV infections likewise revealed similar illness, with influenza associated with more systemic features and fever.

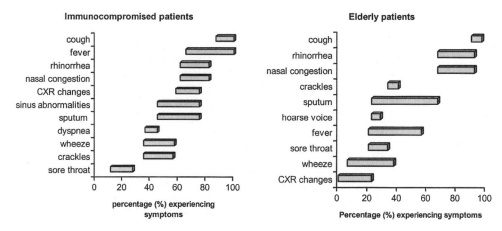

Figure 3 Clinical manifestations of RSV infections in immunocompromised (from Refs. 163, 184, 190, 203) and elderly subjects (from Refs. 31, 57, 70, 71, 80, 144, 198, 199, 204–206).

Rhinovirus tended to cause milder illness with more upper respiratory features such as rhinorrhea and sore throat (136).

Studies in nursing homes have afforded the opportunity to compare clinical characteristics associated with particular viral infections. The clinical syndromes are broadly equivalent with no clear identifying features (32,70,74,75,80). Clinical manifestations of RSV infection are greatest in the frail elderly, those with underlying chronic medical conditions, and immunosuppression (Fig. 3). Approximately 67–92% of elderly sufferers have nasal congestion or rhinorrhea and up to one-third have laryngopharyngitis. Cough is predominant in 90–97% of elderly patients. Lower respiratory tract involvement is frequent with wheezing and crackles on auscultation in 33–40% patients in the community and radiographic abnormalities in around 20% of elderly patients in the hospital (71,74,205,207).

The primary symptomatic illness of rhinovirus or coronavirus infection is the so-called common cold syndrome; around one-third of infections are subclinical (20,208,209). In a self-reported illness study; 41%, 17%, and 15% of rhinovirus-positive healthy adults reported the first symptoms to be sore throat, stuffy nose, and sneezing respectively; 31%, 22%, 19%, and 10% considered runny nose, stuffy nose, sore throat, and malaise, respectively, to be the most troublesome symptoms (210). There is potential for lower respiratory tract involvement in young adults: 10% of experimentally induced rhinovirus infection was associated with sputum, dyspnea, and chest pain (155). Cough is more common and persistent in smokers who develop symptomatic rhinovirus infection (220,221). Among the frail elderly attending day care, Falsey found no difference in clinical features of HRV or coronavirus infections (69); many had evidence of lower respiratory tract involvement including sputum (58%), crackles (48%), and dyspnea (36%). Among elderly patients hospitalized with acute respiratory illness, Falsey found no difference between those infected with rhinovirus or coronavirus and influenza except for the presence

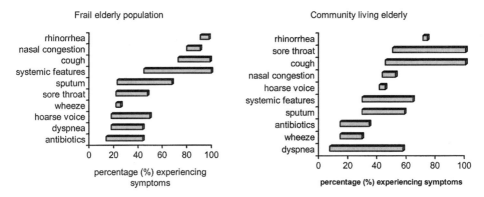

Figure 4 Clinical characteristics of rhinovirus- or coronavirus-associated acute respiratory tract infections in community-dwelling and frail elderly populations. (Refs. 31,69,70,136.)

of higher temperature with influenza (158). In the hospitalized elderly, there is a tendency to more severe lower respiratory tract symptoms and, in some cases, respiratory failure requiring ventilator support (128,158). Figure 4 illustrates the characteristics of rhinovirus infection in elderly populations.

A prospective study, described earlier in this chapter, by Marx enrolled 7927 adult patients admitted with acute respiratory tract illness to 15 regional hospitals between 1991 and 1992 (58). A total of 18 of 721 (2.5%) and 24 of 705 (3.1%) patients had serological evidence of PIV-1 and PIV-3 infection. The mean age of the patients was 69 years. Excluding patients with dual infections, clinical characteristics of 22 PIV-3 infected subjects were compared to those infected with other respiratory viruses. The spectrum of illness was very similar to other respiratory viruses (RSV, influenza, adenovirus, rhinovirus). Wheezing was more commonly reported among PIV-3-infected subjects (86% vs. 73%), but the presence of auscultatory rhonchi was significantly increased among the PIV-3 subjects. In Falsey's prospective study, six PIV (three each of types 1 and 2) were isolated. Although the numbers were small, PIV-2 illnesses were all mild with main complaints of sore throat and hoarseness compared to PIV-1 and RSV (70).

A.   Features in Immunosuppression

Distinctive clinical features of respiratory viral infections in immunocompromised patients are the relatively high frequency of nosocomial transmission rates, prolonged duration of viral shedding, and higher frequency of complicating pneumonia and death.

RSV infection is possibly responsible for the greatest morbidity, particularly in BMT recipients in whom pneumonia and mortality rates may approach 80% (163,165,166,185,190,212,213). RSV disease is associated with a high fever, cough, and lower respiratory symptoms (Fig. 3). The risk of pneumonia and outcome is related to degree of immunosuppression of the host, type of virus, presence of concurrent infections, and the posttransplant time in adult BMT recipients. The frequency of pneumonia and associated mortality falls from 70% to 24% as time from graft rises from the first week to beyond 2 months (166). High rates of progression to pneumonia and death are likewise associated with influenza in immunocompromised adults (Table 6). Neutropenia and recent chemotherapy increase the complication rate (214,215).

Influenza viruses, parainfluenza, and adenovirus have been associated with acute rejection of organ transplants, usually arising from the temporary withdrawal of immunosuppressive therapy or as a consequence of direct infection (213,215–220). Adenovirus infection in some organ transplant recipients has been associated with hemorrhagic cystitis (renal transplants) and hepatic necrosis (liver transplants), resulting in rejection rather than increased pulmonary manifestations (221,222).

B. HIV

Although influenza vaccination is recommended for those with HIV, few data indicate a generalized increase in incidence or severity of influenza or other respiratory viruses (with the possible exception of adenoviruses) in this population (223). A prospective bronchoscopic study of community-based lower respiratory tract disease from 47 consecutive HIV-infected patients presenting during a period of community RSV and influenza activity failed to detect influenza, RSV, adenovirus, PIV, or enterovirus in any BAL specimen (224). There have been several case reports of influenza in HIV-infected adults, but overall presentation appears similar to that in the general population (223,224). A cluster of seven cases of influenza in HIV-infected adults found viral pneumonitis and secondary bacterial infection to be less severe than described during pandemic influenza (225). An increase in pneumonia-related deaths among 25–44-year-olds was observed in US cities with the highest HIV/AIDS incidence during peak influenza activity 1981–1987, although causes of pneumonia were not noted (226). RSV illness in an HIV-infected male was associated with a prolonged lower tract infection and viral shedding for 17 days (227). By screening 431 BAL specimens with PCR from hospitalized subjects with lower respiratory tract illness, Malcolm identified 17 adult rhinovirus infections, of which two were in AIDS patients, indicating a potential role for rhinoviruses in this population (157). Adenovirus in HIV-infected adults is most frequently associated with severe gastroenteritis or colitis, although terminal respiratory failure has been reported with serotype 29 (175,228).

V. Complications

A. Respiratory

Acute Otitis Media

Although primarily complications of children, abnormalities of middle ear pressures (MEP) and otitis media have been identified in adults following respiratory virus infection. Following experimental influenza H1N1, increased MEP and eustachian

Table 6 RSV-Associated Pneumonia in Hospitalized Adults

Author (Ref.)	Country	Year	Age (years)	Diagnostic test	Number in study	Number of illness due to RSV (% positive)
Fransen (205)	Sweden	1963–66	>60	serology	216	16 (7.4)
Hers (248)	Holland	1967–68	>18	serology	207	10 (4.3)
Vikerfors (20)	Sweden	1971–80	>18	serology, Ag[a]	2400	57 (2.4)
Kimball (249)	U.S.	1980–81	>18	serology, culture	100	2 (2)
Zaroukian (250)	U.S.	1987–88	>18	serology, culture, Ag	55	3 (5.4)
Melbye (251)	Norway	1988–89	>18	serology	36	5 (13.9)
Falsey (71)	U.S.	1989–92	>65	serology, Ag, culture	483	69 (14.3)
Dowell (57)	U.S.	1990–92	All	serology	1195	53 (4.4)
			18–59		616	18 (2.9)
			>60		39	966 (4)
Ruiz (252)	Spain	1996–97	>18	serology	204	5 (2.4)
Lerida (253)	Spain	1995–97	All	serology	250	17 (6.8)
			18–64			7
			>65			10

[a] Antigen detection on respiratory samples.

tube dysfunction occur in 70–80% adults; up to 20% had otoscopic features consistent with otitis media (229,230). RSV, HRV, and other respiratory viruses are associated with the development of earache during symptomatic infection (57,70,211,231). Increased MEP occurs in up to 60% of those infected (232,233).

Acute Sinusitis

Nose blowing during rhinovirus infection has been demonstrated to propel nasal fluid from the middle meatus into the sinuses and probably contributes to the pathogenesis of sinusitis (234). It is difficult to differentiate between primary viral rhinosinusitis and secondary bacterial infection. However, radiographic studies of subjects with common cold syndrome found that 33–85% of adults have detectable abnormalities of the sinus cavities, showing that colds are a viral rhinosinusitis (235,236).

Pneumonia

The incidence and case fatality rate of respiratory virus-associated pneumonia vary considerably and depend on the age, immune status, and presence of pre-existing chronic medical conditions of the host and the properties of the virus. There are two major recognized patterns of pneumonia: primary viral and secondary bacterial pneumonia. During the second wave of the Spanish influenza pandemic of 1918, the incidence of pneumonia approached 18%, with morbidity and mortality concentrated in those aged 24–40 years (237,238). More recent studies in general practice have identified rates of 2–2.9% (239–241), a figure comparable to rates identified in recent trials of neuraminidase inhibitors. However, this may be an underestimate since when chest radiographs were used to assess patients, the incidence of pneumonia increased to around 5% (242). Significantly higher incidences of pneumonia (21–38%) have been reported during influenza outbreaks among soldiers (243) and in nursing homes (80). Primary influenzal pneumonia is considered to be clinically and radiologically indistinguishable from those with bacterial infection (244,245). Interstitial fibrosis may complicate primary influenza pneumonia (246,247).

Reports of RSV-associated pneumonia are summarized in Table 6. In the United States, the annual cost of RSV pneumonia, excluding any exacerbations of underlying cardiopulmonary disease, is estimated to be $150–680 million (254). In RSV outbreaks in long-term residential homes, attack rates and frequency of complications are of variable severity and incidence. Outbreaks in such facilities may result in attack rates of 12–89%, with high rates of pneumonia (range, 13–55%) and mortality (range, 3–53%) (76–79,82,255). Overall pneumonia and death rates from outbreak and prospective studies are summarized on Table 7.

Secondary Bacterial Pneumonia

This may occur either with or following primary viral pneumonitis. Overall, studies since the Asian influenza pandemic have revealed that up to 75% of patients with severe influenzal pneumonia had secondary bacterial infection (71). A review of staphyloccocal pneumonia found that 32 (52%) of 61 patients had evidence of in-

Table 7 Incidence of Pneumonia and Death in RSV Infections Affecting Those Living in Long-Term-Care Facilities

Type of study	Number of positive RSV cases	Pneumonia Pneumonia/ RSV cases (%)	Deaths Deaths/ RSV cases (%)
Prospective studies in nursing homes	204	15/186 (8%)	6/195 (3%)
Outbreak studies in nursing homes	230	42/109 (39%)	36/230 (16%)
Total	434	57/295 (19%)	42/425 (10%)

Sources: Refs. 69, 70, 74, 76–80, 82, 83, 86, 92, 144, 255–257.

fluenza infection (258). *Staphylococcus aureus*, *Streptococcus pneumoniae*, *Haemophilus influenzae*, *Pseudomonas aeruginosa*, and haemolytic streptococci groups have been cultured from blood or sputum following influenza or rhinovirus infections, particularly in hospitalized elderly patients (71,127,128,158). An outbreak of parainfluenza 1 virus in a nursing home was implicated in the pathogenesis and development of *Streptococcus pneumoniae* pneumonia, and bacteremia was identified in 20% of the cases (259).

B. Nonpulmonary Complications

Cardiovascular

Excess mortality from ischemic heart disease has been identified in association with influenza (260–262). Electrocardiograph (ECG) abnormalities have been found in over half of hospital patients and 43% of community patients with influenza (263,264). Abnormalities including T-wave inversion, sinus bradycardia or tachycardia, extrasystolic beats, and dysrhythmias such as atrial fibrillation are generally unaccompanied by cardiac symptoms. These are usually transient, but have been identified as persisting for several months after infection. Echocardiographic changes compatible with myocarditis and rises in levels of cardiac enzymes occur in 14% and 7% of influenza patients with ECG abnormalities, respectively.

A study into the effectiveness of influenza immunization in the elderly suggested a 28.6% reduction in hospitalizations due to congestive cardiac failure in vaccine recipients (265).

Chronic cardiac disease is also an important risk factor for RSV infection. In one study of 134 chronic cardiopulmonary patients, RSV infections were twice as common in those with congestive cardiac failure as in those with chronic airways disease (136).

Neurological

Neurological complications of influenza infections in adults include viral encephalitis, postinfective immune-mediated encephalomyelitis, and Guillain-Barré syndrome. These occur in <0.1% of influenza infections and after a median duration of 5 days (range, 0–21) following infection (266). Myalgia is a recognized feature of early influenza infection in adults; diffuse myositis is a rare complication. Influenza virus has been isolated from skeletal muscle with accompanying microscopic features suggestive of virus-induced inflammation (267). There is an association with influenza A and subsequent meningococcal infection (268).

Significant decreases in functional abilities follow influenza infection (71,269,270). Up to three-quarters of community-dwelling elderly people with influenza are unable to cope with activities of daily living and are confined to bed (31). During RSV illness, one-third of elderly sufferers are confined to bed and almost half are unable to cope with daily activities (31). In those with influenza B, simple measures of performance such as reaction times are reduced compared to controls to a degree comparable with alcohol consumption (197,271).

Diabetes Mellitus

Patients with diabetes are more likely to develop complications and pneumonia following influenza than the general population (53,272). Excess mortality among patients with diabetes increased by 5–15% during epidemics in the period 1957–1966 in the United States and by about 30% during epidemics in England and Wales in 1989–1990 (260,273,274). Fourfold increases in deaths from influenza and pneumonia were found in those patients with cardiac disease and diabetes compared to those only with cardiac disease (275). Furthermore, influenza vaccination was estimated to reduce the number of respiratory admissions in diabetic patients by 79% during the epidemics in 1989–1990 and 1993 (276).

Pregnancy

Influenza illness may be severe in pregnancy and pregnant women appear to be at increased risk of hospitalization, complications, and death during epidemics. The Asian influenza pandemic in 1957-1958 was associated with doubling of the expected mortality for pregnant women in the United Kingdom and Netherlands (277,278). An American study similarly found a three- to fourfold increase in pneumonia associated with influenza in pregnancy (279). Analysis of maternal deaths in the United Kingdom suggested a fourfold increase during the 1989–1990 epidemic and attributed to it about 90 excess deaths during pregnancy (280).

VI. Immunity

For influenza, the risk of reinfection and illness is related to serum hemagglutination-inhibition antibody titers (281). Infection with influenza A (H1N1) during its re-emergence in 1977 rarely produced symptoms in those who had lived through the previous H1N1 period ending in 1957. Although most positive H1N1 cultures were in those with symptomatic illnesses born after 1956, there were significant infection rates for those born before 1956 as detected by seroconversion. However, the peak of hospitalizations of older people was associated with the peak of H1N1 activity, suggesting that reinfection does occur and immunity is incomplete (13,282,283). Both influenza B/Singapore and influenza A/Bangkok (H3N2) caused severe epidemics with considerable excess mortality in 1979–1980 and 1980–1981, respectively (55,284,285). However, some immunity must have persisted since there was no excess mortality detected during the re-emergence of influenza B/Singapore in 1981–1982 and a much reduced mortality during the return of influenza A/Bangkok (H3N2) in 1982–1983 (286,287).

Protective immunity to RSV infection is complex and the relative importance of humoral and cellular components is debated. All adults have detectable RSV antibody titers and the elderly are capable of eliciting anti-RSV IgA and IgG antibody responses (256,288–290). High levels of circulating neutralizing antibody to RSV appear correlated with protection in the elderly and support the view that boosting by immunization may be of potential benefit in reducing infection (290). Cell-mediated responses appear important in recovery and viral clearance and defective T-cell responses to RSV have been noted in older subjects (291).

Reinfection with rhinovirus and coronaviruses occurs throughout adult life because of multiple serotypes and the development of partial immunity (30,185,292,293). Over the duration of the 1965–69 Seattle surveillance family studies, there was a gradual rise in the proportion of higher-numbered rhinovirus serotypes isolated in patients, suggesting progressive antigenic shift and evasion of pre-existing immunity (20,21). The most frequent rhinovirus serotypes causing illness were different in the New York, Seattle, and Tecumseh studies, suggesting local differences in serotype prevalence. Rhinovirus serotypes numbers 6, 8, 19, 28, and 81 cause illness in >75% of those infected contrasting with serotype 36, which produces symptomatic illness in <30% of those infected (21). Although titers of antibody to coronavirus rise with age, the level of pre-existing antibody level does not appear to influence occurrence of reinfection: reinfection with the same strain is common after a period of months since previous infection, suggesting only short-term immunity (30,208).

VII. Control

A. Vaccines

The existence of large numbers of diverse viral serotypes makes vaccine preparation difficult. Frequent mutations, as with influenza, may require regular updates of vaccine antigens. Locally delivered live vaccines may offer immunological advantages: they deliver a larger dose of antigen to bronchial lymphoid tissue than parenteral vaccine and induce a broader immunological response. This includes higher or equal serum antibody, neutralizing antibody, and local mucosal secretory IgA responses reducing the amount and frequency of viral shedding (294–296). Potential vaccine may need to be adapted to target groups since optimally attenuated live vaccines designed for infants may be over-attenuated for adults.

Three types of inactivated influenza vaccine are available: whole virus, split product, and purified surface antigen vaccines. Early whole-virus inactivated vaccines were associated with adverse effects, particularly in children, and are little used. Most influenza vaccines are supplied as so-called split vaccines, produced from disrupted highly purified virus, or as surface antigen vaccines containing purified hemagglutinin and neuraminidase. Protective efficacy of 70–95% in young healthy subjects can be achieved when there is a good match between vaccine and circulating strains (297). Vaccination of the elderly is associated with a 19–63% reduction in hospitalization for pneumonia and influenza, 17–39% reduction in hospitalization for all respiratory conditions, and 27–75% reduction in all causes of mortality (298). However, influenza outbreaks have occurred in well-immunized nursing homes. A US study found that 58% of hospitalized patients >65 years who were culture-positive for influenza had been recently immunized (299). Attempts are being made to augment protection through the use of adjuvants, virosomal delivery, and live vaccines. One approach is the use of live, cold-adapted (*ca*) vaccines generated by genetic reassortment between a wild-type and a *ca* donor that has been extensively passaged at 25°C and 33°C (i.e., is unable to replicate at core body temperature). Coadministration of intranasal live vaccine and parenteral conventional vaccine has proved effective in elderly subjects (300). Various adjuvants have been used in an attempt to enhance immunogenicity. MF-59, an oil-in-water emulsion, has a marked effect on the antibody responses of immunologically naive subjects. A study of two doses (7.5–30 µg), three weeks apart, of subunit H5N3 vaccine and MF-59 adjuvanted vaccine found that the numbers in patients who attained HI titers of ≥1:40 or neutralizing antibody titers ≥1:20 were significantly higher on day 42 after the adjuvanted vaccine (301). Virosomes created by inserting influenza HA into a liposome bilayer can serve as delivery systems. Two small randomized trials comparing the immunogenicity of virosomal influenza vaccine with that of whole and subunit vaccines in the elderly found improved antibody responses following virosomal formulation (302,303). Mucosal delivery of influenza vaccine may improve compliance. Nontoxic enterotoxins as adjuvants are being developed and clinical trials are in progress.

Several RSV vaccine candidates incorporating epitopes from the F and G glycoproteins currently under clinical investigation include purified subunit proteins, subunit peptide fragments, and chimeric proteins. Purified RSV fusion F protein-(PFP-2) derived vaccine has been demonstrated to be safe and to induce stimulation of neutralization antibody to RSV in seropositive children and those with cystic fibrosis (304,305). A purified subunit PFP-2 vaccine has been well tolerated in elderly trials in which 53–87% vaccinees produced a fourfold or greater rise in serum IgG and 47–61% produced neutralizing antibody titers to RSV (306). Adjuvanted subunit vaccines composed of purified F, G, and M RSV A proteins formulated with either aluminium phosphate or polydicarboxylatophenoxyphosphazene (PCPP) have been evaluated in two randomized placebo-controlled trials of eighty 18–45-year-old healthy adults. Both vaccines are well tolerated and elicit fourfold rises in neutralizing antibody to RSV A and B in >75% of recipients postvaccination (307).

Two live attenuated PIV-3 vaccines have been developed. A cold-passaged, cold-adapted, temperature-sensitive mutant of PIV-3 has been found to be well tolerated in seronegative children with good immunogenic seroconversion rates (81%). However, in seropositive children, who may reflect the adult population more closely, only 11% developed significant rises in hemagglutinin titers and 22% acquired nasal IgA antibodies (308). Recombinant bovine PIV-3 is being evaluated as a vector for the delivery of other viral antigens including RSV proteins.

The development of highly effective live oral type 4 and 7 adenovirus vaccines, extensively used in military recruitment centers, virtually eliminated adenovirus outbreaks. However, due to commercial reasons, production of vaccine was halted in 1996 and resulted in re-emergence of adenovirus as a major cause of illness in this group (309).

B. Antiviral Therapy

Amantadine and rimantadine are tricyclic primary amines that inhibit influenza viral uncoating and are active against influenza A subtypes, but at therapeutic doses have no effect on influenza B. They are effective in treatment of influenza A if commenced within 24 h of onset of the illness. They can be used as chemoprophylaxis during the influenza season and reduce infection rates by 50–90%. However, rapid emergence of drug-resistant strains may render prophylaxis and treatment in outbreaks ineffective (310–313). The neuraminidase has been targeted for antiviral therapy because of its role in viral replication and transmission. Competitive inhibitors have been developed and are discussed in another chapter of this book. They are active against a broad range of human, avian, and amantadine-resistant influenza strains and are effective for treatment and prophylaxis of influenza (314–317), although there is limited data on their use in high-risk populations. Emergence of clinical resistance appears rare, although a zanamivir-resistant influenza B virus was recovered from a BMT recipient following 2 weeks of treatment (318).

Passive immunization against RSV can be achieved with polyclonal or monoclonal antibodies. Intravenous immunoglobulin produced from donors with high titers of RSV has shown protective efficacy and has been licensed in the United States. Palivizumab is a humanized monoclonal IgG_1 directed against the F protein that blocks virus-induced cell fusion and has neutralizing activity against RSV A and B. Palivizumab is of proven efficacy in prevention of severe RSV disease in children (319). Ribavirin is a guanosine analog with anti-RSV activity, which can be administered orally, intravenously, or by inhalation, although only the inhaled route is licensed for treatment. In immunocompromised patients following BMT, prompt combination therapy of aerosolized ribavirin and intravenous immunoglobulin appears to reduce progression of RSV infection to pneumonia and death, although studies are small, nonrandomized and are based on observed reductions in outcomes compared to expected mortality (320). Patients with ventilatory-dependent RSV pneumonia have a 100% mortality even following therapy and consequently it is not recommended.

Therapies currently available for the common cold ease symptoms. Antihistamines reduce rhinorrhea and weight of nasal secretions but have little effect on other symptoms. Intranasal ipratropium bromide reduces nasal drainage and sneezing but duration of relief is limited (321,322). α-Adrenergic decongestants are effective in natural and experimental colds by shrinking the mucosal swelling of the nasal turbinates, although rebound rhinitis occurs following prolonged use (323). Nonsteroidal anti-inflammatory drugs may actually increase viral shedding, nasal symptoms, and decrease neutralizing antibody responses in rhinovirus-infected volunteers (324). Pleconaril is a novel capsid binder with broad antipicornaviral activity (inhibits 93% rhinovirus serotypes) by blocking virus attachment and uncoating. Two placebo-controlled trials of pleconaril treatment found it to be well tolerated, with the most common adverse effects of diarrhea, nausea, abdominal pain, and headache being only slightly more common than in the placebo group. Early pleconaril therapy in picornavirus-positive subjects was associated with a significant reduction of illness duration of 1.5 days (8.5 vs. 10 days; p = 0.029) and total symptoms score (325,326). In phase II trials, 2096 adults presenting within 24 h were recruited and 62–69% were positive for picornaviruses. The time to alleviation of illness was 1 day shorter in the treated group (6.3 vs. 7.3 days; p < 0.001) (327). Another antipicornaviral agent is ruprintrivir, a 3C protease inhibitor with broad antirhinovirus activity. Intranasal ruprintrivir was tested in 868 patients presenting within 36 h of coldlike symptoms. There were no significant differences in the course of the illness, although only 27% of participants were picornavirus positive (328). Overall, these agents have produced only modest clinical improvements and further studies of such agents in higher-risk populations are needed.

References

1. Stockton J, Ellis J, Saville M, Clewley JP, Zambon MC. Multiplex PCR for typing and subtyping influenza and respiratory syncytial virus. J Clin Microbiol 1998; 36: 2990–2995.
2. Carmen WF, Wallace LA, Walker J, McIntyre S, Noone A, Christie P, Millar J, Douglas JD. Rapid virological surveillance of community influenza infection in general practice. Br Med J 2000; 321:736–739.
3. Zambon MC, Stockton JD, Clewley JC, Fleming DM. Contribution of influenza and respiratory syncytial virus to community cases of influenza-like illness: an observational study. Lancet 2001; 358:1410–1417.
4. Van Hoogen BG, De Jong JC, Groen J, Kuiken T, De Groot R, Fourchier RAM, Osterhaus ADME. A newly discovered human pneumovirus isolated from young children with respiratory tract disease. Nature Medicine 2001; 7:719–724.
5. Reid A, Fanning TG, Hultin JV, Taubenberger JK. Origin and evolution of the 1918 Spanish influenza virus haemagglutinin gene. Proc Natl Acad Sci 1999; 96:1651–1655.
6. Nokes D, Enquselassie F, Nigatu W, Vyse A, Cohen B, Brown D, Cutts F. Has oral fluid the potential to replace serum for the evaluation of population immunity levels. Bull WHO 2001; 79:588–595.
7. Monto AS, Ullman BS. Acute respiratory illness in an American community: the Tecumseh study. JAMA 1974; 227:164–169.
8. Fox JP, Hall CE. 1980. Viruses in Families, Surveillance of Families as a Key to Epidemiology of Virus Infections. Littleton, MA: PSG Publishing Company.
9. Fox JP, Hall CE, Cooney MK, Foy HM. Influenzavirus infections in Seattle families

1975–1979. I. Study designs, methods and the occurrence of infection by time and age. Am J Epidemiol 1982; 116:212–227.

10. Frank AL, Taber LH, Glezen WP. Reinfection with influenza A (H3N2) virus in young children and their families. J Infect Dis 1979; 140:829–836.

11. Jennings LC, MacDiarmid RD, Miles JA. A study of acute respiratory disease in the community of Port Chalmers. Illness within a group of selected families and the relative incidence of respiratory pathogens in the whole community. J Hyg (Lond) 1978; 31:49–66.

12. Mann PG, Pereira M, Smith J, Hart RJ, Williams W. A five year study of influenza in families. Joint Public Health Laboratory/Royal College of General Practitioners Working Group. J Hyg (Lond) 1981; 87:191–200.

13. Monto AS, Sullivan KM. Acute respiratory illness in the community. Frequency of illness and the agents involved. Epidemiol Infect 1993; 110:145–160.

14. Monto AS, Kioumehr F. The Tecumseh study of respiratory illness. IX Occurrence of influenza in the community 1966–1971. Am J Epidemiol 1975; 102:553–563.

15. Longini IM, Halloran ME, Nizam A. Estimation of the efficacy of live attenuated influenza vaccine from a multicentre two year vaccine trial: implications for influenza epidemics control. Vaccine 2000; 17:1902–1909.

16. Taber LH, Paredes A, Glezen WP. Infection with influenza A/Victoria virus in Houston families. J Hyg Camb 1981; 86:307–313.

17. Buescher EL. Respiratory disease and adenovirus. Med Clin North Am 1967; 51:759.

18. Glezen WP, Payne AA, Synder DN. Mortality and influenza. J Infect Dis 1982; 146:313–322.

19. Glezen, WP, Couch RB, Taber LH, Paredes A, Allison JE, Frank AL. Epidemiological observations of influenza B infections in Houston, Texas 1976–1977. Am J Epidemiol 1980; 111:13–22.

20. Fox JP, Cooney MK, Hall CE, Foy HM. Rhinoviruses in Seattle families 1975–1979. Am J Epidemiol 1985; 122:830–846.

21. Fox JP, Cooney MK, Hall CE. The Seattle Virus watch. V. Epidemiologic observations of rhinovirus infections 1965–1969 in families with young children. Am J Epidemiol 1975; 101:122–145.

22. Hendley OM, Gwaltney J, Jordan WS. Rhinovirus in an industrialised population. IV. Infections within families of employees during two fall peaks of respiratory illness. Am J Epidemiol 1996; 89:184–196.

23. Gardner G, Frank AL, Taber LH. Effects of social and family factors on viral respiratory infection and illness in the first year of life. J Epidemiol Community Health 1984; 38:42–48.

24. Goings SA, Kulle T, Bascom R, Sauder L, Green D, Hebel J, Clements M. Effect of nitrogen dioxide exposure on susceptibility to influenza A infection in adults. Am Rev Respir Dis 1989; 139:1075–1081.

25. Leigh M, Carson J, Denny FW. Pathogenesis of respiratory infections due to influenza virus: implications for developing countries. Rev Infect Dis 1991; 13(S6)S501–S508.

26. Lina B, Valette M, Foray S, Luciani J, Stagnara J, See DM, Aymard M. Surveillance of community acquired viral infections due to respiratory viruses in Rhone-Alps during winter 1994 to 1995. J Clin Microbiol 1996; 34(12):3007–3011.

27. Monto AS, Bryan ER, Ohmit S. Rhinovirus infections in Tecumseh, Michigan: frequency of illness and number of serotypes. J Infect Dis 1987; 156:43–49.

28. Glezen WP, Keitel WA, Taber LH, Piedra PA, Clover RD, Couch RB. Age distribution

of patients with medically attended illnesses caused by sequential variants of influenza A/H1N1 comparison to age specific infection rates, 1978–1989. Am J Epidemiol 1991; 133:296–304.

29. Monto AS, Koopman JS, Longini IM. Tecumseh study of illness XIII. Influenza infection and disease 1976–1981. Am J Epidemiol 1985; 121:811–822.

30. Hamre D, Beem M. Virologic studies of acute respiratory disease in young adults. V. Coronaviruses 229E infections during six years of surveillance. Am J Epidemiol 1972; 96:94–106.

31. Nicholson KG, Kent J, Hammersley V. Acute viral infections of upper respiratory tract in elderly people living in the community: comparative, prospective, population based study of disease burden. Br Med J 1997; 315:1060–1064.

32. Drinka PJ, Gravenstein S, Krause P, Langer EH, Barthels L, Dissing M, Shult P, Schilling M. Noninfluenza respiratory viruses may overlap and obscure influenza activity. J Am Geriatr Soc 1999; 47:1087–1093.

33. Fox JP, Cooney MK, Hall CE. Influenza virus infections in Seattle families 1975–1979 II. Pattern of infection in invaded households and relation of age and prior antibody to occurrence of infection and related illness. Am J Epidemiol 1982; 116:228–243.

34. Elder AG, O'Donnell B, McCruden EA, Symington IS, Carmen W. Incidence and recall of influenza in a cohort of Glasgow healthcare workers during the 1993–94 epidemic: results of serum testing and questionnaire. Br Med J 1996; 313:1241–1242.

35. Glezen WP, Cough RB. Interpandemic influenza in the Houston area 1974–76. N Engl J Med 1978; 298:587–592.

36. Marine WM, McGowan JE, Thomas JE. Influenza detection: a prospective comparison of surveillance methods and analysis of isolates. Am J Epidemiol 1976; 104:248–255.

37. Frank AL, Taber LH, Glezen WP. Influenza B virus infections in the community and the family. Am J Epidemiol 1983; 118:313–325.

38. Wright PF, Thompson J, Karzon DT. Differing virulence of H1N1 and H3N2 influenza strains. Am J Epidemiol 1980; 112:814–819.

39. Carrat F, Tachet A, Rouzioux C, Housset B, Valleron AJ. Evaluation of clinical case definitions of influenza: investigation of patients during the 1995–96 epidemic in France. Clin Infect Dis 1999; 28:283–290.

40. Frank AL, Taber LH, Wells J. Comparison of infection rates and severity of illness for influenza A H1N1 and H3N2. J Infect Dis 1985; 151:73–80.

41. Simonsen L, Fukuda K, Shonberger L, Cox N. The impact of influenza epidemics on hospitalisations. J Infect Dis 2000; 181:831–837.

42. Simonsen L, Clarke M, Stroup D, Wiliamson GD, Arden N, Cox NJ. A method for timely assessment of influenza-associated mortality in the United States. Epidemiol 1997; 8:390–395.

43. Fleming DM, Zambon MC, Bartelds AIM. Population estimates of persons presenting to general practitioners with influenza-like illness, 1987–96: a study of the demography of influenza-like illness in general practice networks in England and Wales, and The Netherlands. Epidemiol Infect 2000; 124:245–253.

44. Monto AS, Cavallaro JJ. The Tecumseh study of respiratory illness. II. Patterns of occurrence of infection with respiratory pathogens, 1965–1969. Am J Epidemiol 1971; 94(3):280–289.

45. Monto AS, Bryan ER, Ohmit S. Rhinovirus infections in Tecumseh, Michigan: frequency of illness and number of serotypes. J Infect Dis 1987; 156:43–49.

46. Fleming DM. Weekly returns service of the Royal College of General Practitioners. Community Dis Public Health 1999; 2: 96–100.
47. Birmingham Research Unit of RCGP. Influenza (Collective research in General Practice). J R Coll Gen Pract 1977; 27:544-551.
48. Fleming DM, Cross KW. Respiratory syncytial virus or influenza. Lancet 1993; 342: 1507–1510.
49. Fleming DM, Cross KW, Crombie DL, et al. Respiratory illness and mortality in England and Wales. Eur J Epidemiol 1993; 9:571–576.
50. Nicholson KG. Impact of influenza and respiratory syncytial virus on mortality in England and Wales for January 1975 to December 1990. Epidemiol Infect 1996; 116: 51–63.
51. Fleming DM. The contribution of influenza to combined acute respiratory infections, hospital admissions and deaths in winter. Community Dis Public Health 2000; 3:32–38.
52. Nguyen Van Tamme JS, Brockway CR, Pearson JG, Hayward AC, Fleming DM. Excess hospital admissions for pneumonia and influenza associated with influenza epidemics in persons > 65 years in three English health districts. Options for Control of Influenza IV. Crete, September 2000.
53. Meier C, Jefferson T, Napalkov P, Wegmuller Y. A population based study on the incidence and risk factors for influenza and clinical complications in the UK. Options for the control of influenza IV. Crete, September 2000.
54. Szucs TD. Influenza: the role of burden-of-illness research. Pharmacoeconomics 1999; 16 (suppl) 1:27–32.
55. Glezen WP, Decker M, Joseph SW, Mercready RG. Acute respiratory disease associated with influenza epidemics in Houston, 1981–1983. J Infect Dis 1987; 155:1119–1126.
56. Johnson KM, Bloom KH, Mufson MA. Natural reinfection of adults by respiratory syncytial virus: possible relation to mild upper respiratory diseases. N Engl J Med 1962; 267:68–72.
57. Dowell SF, Anderson LJ, Gary HEJ, Erdman DD, Plouffe JF, File TMJ. Respiratory syncytial virus is an important cause of community acquired lower respiratory tract infection among hospitalised patients. J Infect Dis 1996; 174:456–462.
58. Marx A, Gary HE, Marston B, Erdman D, Breiman RF, Torok TJ, Plouffe JF, File TM, Anderson L. Parainfluenza virus infection among adults hospitalised for lower respiratory tract infection. Clin Infect Dis 1999; 29:134–140.
59. Boivin G, Osterhaus ADME, Gaudreau A, Jackson HC, Groen J, Ward P. Role of picornaviruses in flu-like illnesses of adults enrolled in an oseltamivir treatment study who had no evidence of influenza virus infection. J Clin Microbiol 2002; 40:330–334.
60. Hilleman M, Werner J, Adair C, Dreisbach A. Outbreak of acute respiratory illness caused by RI-67 and influenza viruses. Fort Leonard Wood. Am J Hyg 1955; 61:163–173.
61. Mogabagab WJ. M pneumoniae and adenovirus illnesses in military and university personnel, 1959–66. Am Rev Respir Dis 1968; 97:645–652.
62. Grayston J, Woolridge RL, Loosli C, Gundelfinger BF, Johnston PB, Pierce WE. Adenovirus infections in naval recruits. J Infect Dis 1959; 105:61–65.
63. Woolridge RL, Grayston J, Whiteside J, Loosli C, Friedman M, Pierce WE. Studies on acute respiratory illness in naval recruits with emphasis on adenoviruses (APC-RI). J Infect Dis 1956; 98:182–185.
64. Gray GC, Callahan JD, Hawksworth AW, Fisher CA, Gaydos J. Respiratory disease

among US military personnel: countering emerging threats. Emerg Infect Dis 1999; 5:379–387.

65. Ryan M. Adenoviral respiratory infections in young adults in US military training. In: Ison M, ed. Current Research on Respiratory Viral Infections. Fourth International Symposium. Antiviral Res 2002; 55:227–228.

66. Gray CG, Goswami P, Malasig M, Hawksworth AW, Trump D, Ryan M, Schnurr D. Adults adenovirus infections: loss of orphaned vaccines precipitates military respiratory diseases epidemics. Clin Infect Dis 2000; 31:633–670.

67. Ryan M, Gray C, Malasig M. Two fatal cases of adenovirus-related illness in previously healthy adults—Illinois 2000. MMWR 2001; 50:553–555.

68. Greenberg SB, Allen M, Wilson J, Atmar RL. Respiratory viral infections in adults with and without chronic obstructive pulmonary diseases. Am J Respir Crit Care Med 2000; 162:167–173.

69. Falsey AR, McCann RM, Hall WJ, Criddle MM, Formica MA, Wycoff D, Kolassa JE. The common cold in frail older persons: impact of rhinovirus and coronavirus in a senior day care centre. J Am Geriatr Soc 1997; 45:706–711.

70. Falsey AR, Treanor JJ, Betts RF, Walsh EE. Viral respiratory infections in the institutionalised elderly: clinical and epidemiology findings. J Am Geriatr Soc 1992; 40: 115–119.

71. Falsey AR, Cunningham CK, Barker WH, Kouides RW, Yuen JB, Menegus M, Weiner LB, Bonville CA, Betts RF. Respiratory syncytial virus and influenza A infections in the hospitalised elderly. J Infect Dis 1995; 172:389–394.

72. Peret T, Boivin G, Li Y, Couillard M, Humphrey C, Osterhaus ADME, Erdman D, Anderson L. Characterisation of human metapneumovirus isolated from patients in North America. J Infect Dis 2002; 185:1660–1663.

73. Stockton JD, Stephenson I, Zambon MC, Fleming DM. Human metapneumovirus as a cause of community acquired respiratory illness in 2000–01. Emerg Infect Dis 2002; 8:897–901.

74. Nicholson KG, Baker DJ, Farquahar A, Hurd D, Kent J, Smith SH. Acute upper respiratory tract illness and influenza immunisation in homes for the elderly. Epidemiol Infect 1990; 105:609–618.

75. Loeb M, McGreer A, Mcarthur M. Surveillance for outbreaks of respiratory tract infections in nursing homes. CMAJ 2000 18;192:1133–1137.

76. Garvie DG, Gray J. Outbreak of respiratory syncytial virus infection in the elderly. Br Med J 1980; 281:1253–1254.

77. PHLS CDSC. Respiratory syncytial virus in the elderly 1976-82. Br Med J 1983: 27: 1618–1619.

78. Hart RJ. An outbreak of respiratory syncytial virus infection in an old people's home. J Infect 1984; 8:259–261.

79. CDC. Respiratory syncytial virus—Missouri. MMWR 1978; 26:351.

80. Mathur U, Bentley DW, Hall CB. Concurrent respiratory syncytial virus and influenza A infections in the institutionalised elderly and chronically ill. Ann Intern Med 1980; 3:49.

81. Morales F, Calder M, Ingles JM, Murdock P, Williamson J. A study of respiratory infections in the elderly to assess the role of respiratory syncytial virus. J Infect 1983; 7:236–247.

82. Sorvillo FJ, Huie SF, Strassburg MA, Butsumyo A, Shandera WX. An outbreak of RSV pneumonia in a nursing home for the elderly. J Infect Dis 1984; 9:252–256

83. Osterweil D, Norman D. An outbreak of an influenza like illness in a nursing home. J Am Geriatr Soc 1990; 38:659–662.

84. Drinka PJ, Gravenstein S, Langer E, Krause P, Shult P. Mortality following isolation of various respiratory viruses in nursing home residents. Infect Control Hosp Epidemiol 1990; 20:812–815.

85. Glasgow K, Tamblyn SE, Blair G. A respiratory outbreak due to parainfluenza 3 in a home for the aged—Ontario. Can Commun Dis Rep 1995; 21:57–61.

86. Gross P, Rodenstein M, LaMontague JR, Kaslow RA, Saah A, Wallenstein S. Epidemiology of acute respiratory illness during an influenza outbreak in a nursing home. Arch Intern Med 1988; 148:559–661.

87. Lennox IM, MacPhee GJ, McAlpine CH, Cameron SO, Leask BG, Somerville R. Use of influenza vaccine in longstay geriatric units. Age Aging 1990: 19:169–172.

88. Zadeh MM, Buxton Bridges C, Thompson WW, Arden N, Fukuda K. Influenza outbreak detection and control measures in nursing homes in the United States. J Am Geriatr Soc 2000; 48:1310–1315

89. Monto AS, Omhit SE, Hornbuckle K, Pearce CL. Safety and efficacy of long-term use of rimantidine for prophylaxis of influenza A in nursing homes. Antimicrob Agents Chemother 1995; 39:2224–2228.

90. Peters P, Gravenstein S, Norwood P, de Bock V, Van Couter A, Gibbens M, von Planta T, Ward P. Safety and efficacy of longterm use of rimantadine for prophylaxis of influenza in a frail vaccinated older population. J Am Geriatr Soc 2001; 49:1025–1031.

91. Deguchi Y, Nishimura K. Efficacy of influenza vaccine in elderly persons in welfare nursing homes: reduction in risk of mortality and morbidity during an influenza A epidemic. J Geront A Biol Sci Med Sci 2001; 56:M391–394.

92. Arroyo JC, Jordan W, Milligan L. Upper respiratory tract infection and serum antibody responses in nursing home patients. Am J Infect Control 1988; 16;152–158.

93. Drinka PJ, Gravenstein S, Krause P, Schilling M, Miller BA, Shult P. Outbreaks of influenza A and B in a highly immunized nursing home population. J Fam Pract 1997 Dec; 45(6):509–514.

94. Kohn M, Farley TA, Sundin D, Tapia R, McFarland LM, Arden N. Three summertime outbreaks of influenza type A. J Infect Dis 1995; 172:246–249.

95. Mast EE, Harmon M, Gravenstein S, Wu SP, Arden N, Circo R, Tyszka G, Kendal AP, Davis J. Emergence and possible transmission of amantadine-resistant viruses during nursing home outbreaks of influenza A H3N2. Am J Epidemiol 1991; 134:988–997.

96. Patriarca P, Weber J, Parker RA, Orenestein WA, Hall W, Kendal AP, Schonberger LB. Risk factors for outbreaks of influenza in nursing homes. A case control study. Am J Epidemiol 1986; 124:114–119.

97. Horman J, Stetler H, Isreal E, Sorley D, Schiper M, Joseph M. An outbreak of influenza A in nursing homes. Am J Public Health 1986; 76:501–504.

98. Strassburg M, Greenalnd S, Sorvillo F, Lieb L, Habel LA. Influenza in the elderly: report of an outbreak and a review of vaccine effectiveness reports. Vaccine 1986; 4:38–44.

99. Goodman R, Orenstein W, Munro T, Smith SC, Sike RK. Impact of influenza A in a nursing home. JAMA 1982; 247:1451–1453.

100. Hall WN, Goodman R, Noble GR, Kendal AP, Steece RS. An outbreak of influenza B in an elderly population. J Infect Dis 1981; 144:297–302.

101. Read C, Mohsen A, Nguyen-van-Tamme J, McKendrick M, Kudesia G. Outbreak of

influenza A in nursing homes in Sheffield during the 1997–98 season: implications for diagnosis and control. J Public Health Med 2000; 22:116–120.

102. Arden N, Monto A, Ohmit SE. Vaccine use and the risk of outbreaks in a sample of nursing homes during an influenza epidemic. Am J Public Health 1995; 85:399–401.

103. Nguyen Van Tamme JS, Nicholson KG. Influenza deaths in Leicestershire during the 1989/90 epidemic. Implications for prevention. Epidemiol Infect 1992; 108:537–545.

104. Ahmed AH, Nicholson KG, Nguyen-van-Tamme JS. Reduction in mortality associated with influenza vaccine during 1989–90 epidemic. Lancet 1995; 346:591–595.

105. Ahmed A, Nicholson KG, Nguyen-van-Tamme J, Pearson J. Effectiveness of influenza vaccine in reducing hospital admissions during the 1989–90 epidemic. Epidemiol Infect 1997; 118:27–33.

106. Wilde JA, McMillan JA, Serwint J, Butta J, O'Riordan MA, Steinhoff MC. Effectiveness of influenza vaccine in health care professionals—a randomised trial. JAMA 1999; 281:908–913.

107. Weingarten S, Riedinger M, Bolton LB, Miles P, Ault M. Barriers to influenza vaccine acceptance. A survey of physicians and nurses. Am J Infect Control 1989; 17:202–207.

108. Coles F, Balzano G, Morse DL. An outbreak of influenza H3N2 in a well immunised nursing home population. J Am Geriatr Soc 1992; 40:589–592.

109. Oshitani H, Saito R, Seki N, Tanabe N, Yamazaki O, Hayashi S, Suzuki H. Influenza vaccination levels and influenza-like illness in long-term care facilities for elderly people in Niigata, Japan during influenza A epidemic. Infect Control Hosp Epidemiol 2000; 21:728–733.

110. Minor TE, Dick EC, Baker JW, Ouellette JJ, Cohen M, Reed CE. Rhinovirus and influenza type A infections as precipitants of asthma. Am Rev Respir Dis 1976; 113: 149–153.

111. Minor T, Baker J, Dick EC, DeMeo A, Ouellette J, Cohen M, Reed C. Greater frequency of viral respiratory infections in asthmatic children as compared with their nonasthmatic siblings. J Paediatr 1974; 85:472–477.

112. Hudgel DW, Langston L, Selner JC, McIntosh K. Viral and bacterial infections in adults with chronic asthma Am Rev Respir Dis 1979; 120:393–397.

113. Huhti E, Mokka T, Nikoskelainen J, Halonen P. Association of viral and mycoplasma infections with exacerbations of asthma. Ann Allergy 1974; 33:145–149.

114. Beasley R, Coleman ED, Hermon Y, Holst PE, O'Donnell TVO, Tobias M. Viral respiratory tract infection and exacerbation of asthma in adults. Thorax 1988; 43:679–683.

115. Houseworth J, Langmuir AD. Excess mortality from epidemic influenza 1957–66. Am J Epidemiol 1974; 100:40–43.

116. Glezen P, Decker M, Perrotta D. Survey of underlying conditions of persons hospitalised with acute respiratory disease during the influenza epidemics in Houston 1978–81. Am Rev Respir Dis 1987; 136:550–555.

117. Little JW, Hall WJ, Douglas RJ, Mudholkar GS, Speers DM, Patel K. Airway hyperreactivity and peripheral airway dysfunction in influenza A infection. Am Rev Respir Dis 1978; 118:295–303.

118. Utell MJ, Aquilina AT, Hall WJ, Speers DM, Douglas RG, Gibb FR, Morrow PE, Hyde RW. Development of airway reactivity to nitrates in subjects with influenza A. Am Rev Respir Dis 1980; 121:233–241.

119. Hall WJ, Douglas RJ, Hyde RW, Roth RK, Cross AS, Speers DM. Pulmonary function

mechanics after uncomplicated influenza A infection. Am Rev Respir Dis 1976; 113: 141–147.

120. Hall WJ, Hall CB. Respiratory syncytial virus infections in adults: virologic and serial pulmonary function studies. Ann Intern Med 1990; 56:203–205.

121. Nicholson KG, Kent J, Ireland DC. Respiratory viruses and exacerbations of asthma in adults. Br Med J 1993; 307:982–986.

122. Ireland DC, Kent J, Nicholson KG. Improved detection of rhinovirus in throat swabs by semi nested RT-PCR. J Med Virol 1993; 40:96–102.

123. Atmar RL, Guy E, Guntupalli KK, Zimmerman JL, Bandi V, Baxter B, Greenberg SB. Respiratory tract infections in inner-city asthmatics. Arch Intern Med 1998; 158: 2453–2459.

124. Kuga H, Hoshiyama Y, Kokubu F, Imai T, Tokunga H, Matsukura S, Kawaguchi M, Adachi M, Kawaguchi T. The correlation between exacerbation of bronchial asthma and picornavirus infection in throat gargles by PCR. Arerugi Jpn J Allergol 2000; 49(4):358–364.

125. Corne JM, Marshall C, Smith S, Schrieber J, Sanderson G, Holgate ST, Johnston SL. Frequency, severity and duration of rhinovirus infections in asthmatic and nonasthmatic individuals: a longitudinal cohort. Lancet 2002; 359:831–835.

126. Abramson M, Pearson L, Kutin J, Czarny D, Dziukas L, Bowes G. Allergies, upper respiratory tract infections and asthma. J Asthma 1994; 31:367–374.

127. Teichtahl H, Buckmaster N, Pertnikovs E. The incidence of respiratory tract infection in adults requiring hospitalisation for asthma. Chest 1997; 112:591–596.

128. El-Sahly HM, Atmar RL, Glezen WP, Greenburg SB. Spectrum of clinical illness in hospitalised patients with common cold infections. Clin Infect Dis 2000; 31:96–100.

129. Sokhandan M, McFadden ER, Huang YT, Mazanec MB. The contribution of respiratory viruses to severe exacerbations of asthma in adults. Chest 1995; 107:1570–1575.

130. Rossi OV, Kinnula V, Tuokko H, Huhti E. Respiratory viral and mycoplasma infection in patients with acute asthma. Monaldi Arch Chest Dis 1994; 49:107–111.

131. Carilli A, Gohd R, Gordon W. A virologic study of chronic bronchitis. N Engl J Med 1964; 170:123–127.

132. Stenhouse AC. Rhinovirus infection in acute exacerbations of chronic bronchitis: a controlled prospective study. Br Med J 1967; 3:461–463.

133. Gump DW, Philips CA, Forsyth B, McIntosh K, Lamborn KR, Stouch WH. Role of infection in chronic bronchitis. Am Rev Respir Dis 1976; 113:465–474.

134. Buscho RO, Saxtan D, Shultz PS. Infections with viruses and mycoplasma infections during exacerbations of chronic bronchitis. J Infect Dis 1978; 137:377–383.

135. Smith CB, Golden M, Klauber MR, Kanner R, Renzetti A. Interactions between viruses and bacteria in patients with chronic bronchitis. J Infect Dis 1976; 134:552–561.

136. Walsh EE, Falsey AR, Hennessey PA. Respiratory syncytial and other virus infections in persons with chronic cardiopulmonary disease. Am J Respir Crit Care Med 1999; 160:791–795.

137. Ross CA, McMicheal S, Eadie M, Lees A, Murray E, Pinkerton I. Infective agents and chronic bronchitis. Thorax 1966; 21:461–464.

138. Monto AS, Higgins MW, Ross HW. Tecumseh study of respiratory illnesses. VIII. Acute infection in chronic respiratory diseases and comparison groups. Am Rev Respir Dis 1975; 111:27–36.

139. Lamy ME, Pouthier-Simon F, Debacker-Willame E. Respiratory viral infections in hospital patients with chronic bronchitis. Chest 1973; 63:336–341.

140. Lieberman D, Ben-Yaakov M, Lazarovich Z, Hoffman S, Ohana B, Friedman M, Dvoskin B, Leinonen M, Boldur I. Infectious aetiologies in acute exacerbation COPD. Diagn Microbiol Infect Dis 2001; 40(3):95–102.

141. Smith CB, Golden M, Kanner R, Renzetti A. Association of viral and mycoplasma infections in acute respiratory illness in patients with chronic obstructive airways diseases. Am Rev Respir Dis 1980; 121:225–232.

142. Sterk PJ. Viral induced airway hyperresponsiveness in man. Eur Respir J 1993; 6: 894–902.

143. Blair HT, Greenberg SB, Stevens PM, Bilunos PA, Couch RB. Effects of rhinovirus infection on pulmonary function of healthy human volunteers. Am Rev Respir Dis 1976; 114:95–102.

144. Hall WJ, Hall CB. Clinical significance of pulmonary function tests. Alterations in pulmonary function following respiratory viral infection. Chest 1979; 76:458–465.

145. Collinson, J, Nicholson KG, Cancio E, Ashman J, Ireland DC, Hammersley V, Kent J, O'Callaghan C. Effects of upper respiratory tract infections in patients with cystic fibrosis. Thorax 1996; 51:1115–1122.

146. Wiselka MJ, Kent J, Cookson JC, Nicholson KG. Impact of respiratory virus infection in patients with chronic chest diseases. Epidemiol Infect 1993; 111:337–346.

147. Simonsen L, Conn LA, Pinner RW, Teutsch S. Trends in infectious disease hospitalisations in the United States 1980–1984. Arch Intern Med 1998; 158:1923–1928.

148. Glezen WP, Greenberg SB, Atmar RL, Piedra PA, Couch RB. Impact of respiratory virus infections on persons with chronic underlying conditions. JAMA 2000; 283: 499–505.

149. Monto AS, Ross HW. Tecumseh study of respiratory illness. X. Relation of acute infections to smoking, lung function and chronic symptoms. Am J Epidemiol 1978; 107; 57–64.

150. Monto AS, Higgins MW, Ross HW. Tecumseh study of respiratory illness. VIII. Acute infection in chronic respiratory disease and comparison groups. Am Rev Respir Dis 1975; 111:27–35.

151. Fraenkel DJ, Bardin PG, Sanderson G, Lange F, Johnston SL, Holgate JT. Lower airways inflammation during rhinovirus colds in normal and in asthmatic subjects. Am J Respir Crit Care Med 1995; 151:879–886.

152. Kaiser L, Hayden FG. Rhinovirus pneumonia—a clinical entity? Clin Infect Dis 1999; 29:533–553.

153. Horn MEC, Reed SE, Taylor P. Role of viruses and bacteria in acute wheezy bronchitis in childhood: a study of sputum. Arch Dis Child 1979; 54:587–592.

154. Halperin SA, Eggleston PA, Hendley JO. Pathogenesis of lower respiratory tract symptoms in experimental rhinovirus infection. Am Rev Respir Dis 1983; 128:806–810.

155. Gern JE, Galagan DM, Jarjour NN. Detection of rhinovirus RNA in lower airways cells during experimentally induced infection. Am J Crit Care Med 1997; 155:1159–1161.

156. Las Heras J, Swanson VL. Sudden death of an infant with rhinovirus infection complicating bronchial asthma: case report. Paediatr Pathol 1983; 1:319–323.

157. Malcolm E, Arruda E, Hayden F, Kaiser K. Clinical features of patients with acute respiratory illness and rhinovirus in their bronchoalveolar lavages. J Clin Virol 2001; 21:9–16.

158. Falsey AR, Walsh EE, Hayden F. Rhinovirus and coronavirus infection associated hospitalisations among older adults. J Infect Dis 2002; 185:1338–1341.

159. Hogg JC. Role of latent viral infections in chronic obstructive pulmonary diseases and asthma. Am J Respir Crit Care Med 2001; 164:S71–80.

160. Bowden RA. Respiratory virus infections after marrow transplant; the Fred Hutchison cancer research centre experience. Am J Med 1997; 102(3A):27–30.

161. Soloman L, Rafety AT, Mallick NP, Johson RW, Longson M. Respiratory syncytial virus infection following renal transplantations. J Infect 1981; 3:280–282.

162. Spelman DW, Stanley PA. Respiratory syncytial virus pneumonitis in adults. Med J Aust 1983; 1:430–431.

163. Englund JA, Sullivan CJ, Jordan C, Dehner LP, Vercellotti GM, Balfour HH. Respiratory syncytial virus infection in immunocompromised adults. Ann Intern Med 1988; 109:203–208.

164. Couch RB, Englund JA, Whimbey E. Respiratory viral infections in immunocompetent and immunocompromised persons. Am J Med 1997; 102:2–9.

165. Whimbey E, Champlin RE, Couch RB, Englund J, Goodrich J, Raad I, Przepiorka D, Lewis V, Mirza M, Yousuf Y, Tarrand J, Bodey G. Community respiratory virus infections among hospitalised adult bone marrow transplant recipients. Clin Infect Dis 1996; 22:778–782.

166. Whimbey E, Englund JA, Couch RB. Community respiratory virus infections in immunocompromised patients with cancer. Am J Med 1997; 102(3A):10–18.

167. Laurichesse H, Dedman D, Watson J, Zambon MC. Epidemiological features of parainfluenza virus infections: laboratory surveillance in England and Wales 1975–97. Eur J Epidemiol 1999; 15:475–483.

168. Ljungman P. Respiratory virus infections in bone marrow transplant recipients: the European perspective. Am J Med 1997; 102:44–47.

169. Ljungman P, Ward K, Crooks BN, Parker A, Martino R, Shaw P, Brinch L, Brune M, et al. Respiratory virus infections after stem cell transplantation: a prospective study from the Infectious Disease Working party of the European Group for Blood and Marrow Transplantation. Bone Marrow Transplant 2001; 5:479-484.

170. Ghosh S, Champlin RE, Couch RB, Englund J, Raad I, Malik S, Luna M, Whimbey E. Rhinovirus infections in myelosuppressed adult blood and marrow transplant recipients. Clin Infect Dis 1999; 29:528–532.

171. van Elden J, van Kraaij MG, Nijhuis M, Hendriksen KA, Dekker AW, Rozenberg-Arska M, van Loon AM. Polymerase chain reaction is more sensitive than viral culture and antigen testing for the detection of respiratory viruses in adults with hematological cancer and pneumonia. Clin Infect Dis 2002; 34(2):177–183.

172. Flomberg P, Babbit J, Dorbyski W. Increasing incidence of adenovirus disease in bone marrow transplant recipients. J Infect Dis 1994; 169:775–781.

173. Shields AF, Hackman RC, Fife K. Adenovirus infections in patients undergoing bone marrow transplantation. N Engl J Med 1985; 312:529–533.

174. Ambinder R, Burns W, Forman M. Haemorrhagic cystitis associated with adenovirus infection in bone marrow transplantation. Arch Intern Med 1986; 146: 1400–1401.

175. Hierholzer JC. Adenoviruses in imunocompromised host. Clin Microbiol Rev 1992; 262–274.

176. Rude V, Ross S, Trenschel R, Lagemann E, Basu O, Renzing K, Schafer U, Roggendorf M, Holler E. Adenovirus infection after allogenic stem cell transplantation (SCT): report on 130 patients from a single SCT unit involved in a prospective multi centre surveillance study. Bone Marrow Transplant 2001; 28:51–57.

177. Wendt CH, Fox JMK, Hertz MI. Paramyxovirus infection in lung transplant recipients. J Heart Lung Transplant 1995; 14:479–485.

178. Doud JR, Hinkmap T, Garrity ER. Respiratory syncytial virus pneumonia in a lung transplant recipient. J Heart Lung Transplant 1992; 11:77–79.

179. Aschan J, Ringden O, Ljungman P, Influenza B in transplant patients. Scand J Infect Dis 1989; 21:349–350.

180. Matar L, McAdams H, Palmer S, Howell D, Henshaw N, Davis DD, Tapson V. Respiratory viral infections in lung transplant recipients: radiological findings with clinical correlation. Radiology 1999; 213;735–742.

181. Simsir A, Greenebaum E, Nuova G, Schulmann L. Late fatal adenovirus pneumonitis in a lung transplant recipient. Transplantation 1998; 65:592–594.

182. Ljungman P, Andersson J, Aschan JS. Influenza A in immunocompromised patients. Clin Infect Dis 1993; 17;244–247.

183. Singhal S, Muir DA, Ratcliffe DA, Shirley JA, Cane PA, Hastings JG, Pillay D, Mutimer DJ. Respiratory viruses in adult liver transplant recipients. Transplantation 1999; 68:981–984.

184. Whimbey E, Couch RB, Englund JA. Respiratory syncytial virus pneumonia in hospitalised adult patients with leukaemia. Clin Infect Dis 1995; 21:376–379.

185. Jones BL, Clark S, Curran ET, McNamee S, Horne G, Thaaker B, Hood J. Control of an outbreak of respiratory syncytial virus infection in immunocompromised adults. J Hosp Infect 2000; 44:53–57.

186. Whimbey E, Elting LS, Couch RB. Influenza A virus infection among hospitalised adults adult bone marrow transplant recipients. Bone Marrow Transplant 1994; 13:437–440.

187. Elting LS, Whimbey E, Lo W. Epidemiology of influenza A virus infection in patients with acute or chronic leukaemia. Supportive Care Cancer 1995; 3:198–202.

188. Alford RH, Kasel JA, Gerone PJ, Knight V. Human influenza resulting from aerosol inhalation. Proc Soc Exp Biol Med 1966; 122:800–824.

189. Ladisla B, Englund JA, Couch RB. RSV disease among hospitalised adults immunocompromised patients with leukaemia. Infectious Diseases Society of America, 34th meeting 1996; 45 (abstract 10).

190. Tablan OC, Anderson LJ, Arden NH. Guideline for prevention of nosocomial pneumonia. Part 1. Issues on prevention of nosocomial pneumonia—1994. Am J Infect Control 1994; 22:247–292.

191. Garner JS. Guidelines for isolation precautions in hospitals. Infect Control Hosp Epidemiol 1996; 17:53–80.

192. Hall CB. Nosocomial respiratory syncytial virus infections: the cold war has not ended. Clin Infect Dis 2000; 31:590–596.

193. Weingarten S, Friedlander M, Rascon D, Ault M, Morgan M, Meyer RD. Influenza surveillance in an acute hospital. Arch Intern Med 1988; 148:113–116.

194. Ksiazek TG, Olson JG, Irving GS, Settle CS, White R, Petrusso R. An influenza outbreak due to A/USSR/77 like (H1N1) virus aboard a US Navy ship. Am J Epidemiol 1980; 112:487–494.

195. Boivin G, Hardy I, Tellier G, Maziade J. Predicting influenza infections during epidemics with a clinical case definition. Clin Infect Dis 2000; 31:1166–1169.

196. Monto AS, Gravenstein S, Elliot M, Colopy M, Schweinle J. Clinical signs and symptoms predicting influenza infection. Arch Intern Med 2000; 160:3243–3247.

197. Smith AP, Thomas M, Brockman P, Kent J, Nicholson KG. Effect of influenza B virus infection on human performance. Br Med J 1993; 306:760–761.

198. Mills J, Van Kirk J, Wright PF, Chanock RM. Experimental respiratory Syncytial virus infection of adults. J Immunol 1971; 107:123–130.

199. Kravetz H, Knight V, Chanock RM, Morris AJ, Johnson K, Rifkind D. Respiratory Syncytial Virus: III. Production of illness and clinical observations in adult volunteers. JAMA 1961; 176:657–663.

200. Hall C, Geiman J, Biggar RJ. Respiratory virus infections within families. N Engl J Med 1976; 294:414–419.

201. Hall CB, Long C, Schnabel KC. Respiratory syncytial virus infections in previously healthy working adults. Clin Infect Dis 2001; 33:792–796.

202. Sanchez JL, Binn L, Innis BL, Reynolds R, Lee T, Mitchell-Raymundo F, Craig S, Marquez JP, Shepherd G, Polyak CS, Connoly J, Kohlhase K. Epidemic of adenovirus-induced respiratory illness among US military recruits: epidemiological and immuno-logical risk factors in healthy young adults. J Med Virol 2001; 65:710-718.

203. Hertz MI, Englund JA, Snover P, Bitterman PB, McGlave P. Respiratory syncytial virus induced acute lung injury in adult patients with bone marrow transplants: clinical approach and review of literature. Medicine 68:269–281.

204. Falsey AR, McCann RM, Hall MJ, Tanner MA, Criddle MM. Acute respiratory tract infection in day centers for older person. J Am Geriatr Soc 1995; 43:30–36.

205. Fransen H, Heigel Z, Wolontis S, Forsgren M, Svedmyr A. Infections with viruses in patients hospitalised with acute respiratory illness in Stockholm 1963–1967. Scand J Infect Dis 1969; 1:127–136.

206. Vikerfors T, Grandien M, Olan P. Respiratory syncytial virus infections in adults. Am Rev Resp Dis 1987; 136:561–564.

207. McConnochie KM, Hall CB, Walsh EE. Variation in severity of respiratory syncytial virus with subtype. J Paediatr 1990; 117:52–58.

208. Schmidt OW, Allan ID, Cooney MK, Foy HM, Fox JP. Rises in titres of antibody to human coronaviruses OC43 and 229E in Seattle families during 1975–1979. Am J Epidemiol 1986; 123:862–879.

209. Gwaltney JM, Hendley JO, Simon G, Jordan WS. Rhinovirus infections in an industrial population. II. Characteristic of illness and antibody response. JAMA 1967; 202:158–164.

210. Arruda E, Pitkaranta A, Witek TJ, Doyle CA, Hayden FG. Frequency and natural history of rhinovirus infections in adults in the autumn. J Clin Microbiol 1997; 2864–2868.

211. Nicholson KG, Kent J, Hammersley V, Cancio E. Risk factors for lower respiratory complications of rhinovirus infections in elderly people living in the community: prospective cohort study. Br Med J 1993; 313:1119–1123.

212. Fouillard L, Mouthon L, Isnard LF, Strachowiak M, Aoudjhane M, Lucet JC. Severe respiratory syncytial virus pneumonia after autologous bone marrow transplantation: a report of three cases and review. Bone Marrow Transplant 1992; 9:97–100.

213. Wendt CH. Community respiratory viruses in organ transplant recipients. Am J Med 1997; 102(3A):31–38.

214. Apalsch AM, Green M, Ledsma J, Nour B, Wald ER. Parainfluenza and influenza virus infections in paediatric organ transplant recipients. Clin Infect Dis 1995; 20:394–399.

215. Yousuf HM, Englund JA, Couch RB. Influenza among hospitalised adults with leukaemia. Clin Infect Dis 1997; 24:1095–1099.

216. Mauch TJ, Bratton S, Myers T. Influenza B virus infection in paediatric solid organ transplant recipients. Paediatrics 1994; 994:225–229.

217. DeFabritus AM, Riggio RR, David DS. Parainfluenza type 3 in a transplant unit. JAMA 1979; 241:384–386.

218. Gabriel R, Selwyn S, Brown D. Virus infections and acute renal transplant rejection. Nephron 1976; 16:282–286.
219. Feldman S, Webster RG, Sugg M. Influenza A in children and young adults with cancer. Cancer 1977; 39:350–353.
220. Keane WR, Helderma JH, Luby J, Gailiunas P, Hull AR, Kokko JP. Epidemic renal transplant rejection associated with influenza A Victoria. Proc Clin Dialysis Transplant Forum 1978; 8:232–236.
221. Yagisawa T, Takahashi K, Yamaguchi Y. Adenovirus induced nephropathy in kidney transplant recipients. Transplant Proc 1989; 21:2097–2099.
222. Carnes B, Rahier J, Burtomboy G. Acute adenovirus hepatitis in liver transplant recipients. J Paediatr 1992; 120:33–37.
223. King JC. Community respiratory viruses in individuals with human immunodeficiency virus infection. Am J Med 1997; 102:19–24.
224. Miller RF, Loveday C, Holton J, Sharvell Y, Pate G, Brink GS. Community based respiratory viral infections in HIV positive patients with lower respiratory tract diseases. Genitourin Med 1996; 72:9–11.
225. Radwan HM, Cheeseman S, Kwe Lai K, Ellison RT. Influenza in HIV infected patients during the 1997–98 influenza season. Clin Infect Dis 2000; 31:604–606.
226. Increase in pneumonia mortality among young adults and the HIV epidemic—New York, US. MMWR 1988; 37:593–595.
227. Murphy D, Rose RC. Respiratory syncytial virus pneumonia in HIV infected man. JAMA 1989; 261:1147.
228. Valainis GT, Carlisle J, Daroca P, Gohd R, Enelow T. Respiratory failure complicated by adenovirus serotype 29 in a patient with AIDS. J Infect Dis 1989; 160:349–351.
229. Petersdorf RG, Fusco JJ, Harter DH, Albrink WS. Pulmonary infections complicating Asian influenza. Arch Intern Med 1959; 103:262–272.
230. Doyle WJ, Skoner DP, Hayden FG. Nasal and otologic effects of experimental influenza A virus infection. Ann Otol Rhinol Laryngol 1994; 103:59–69.
231. Gwaltney JM, Hendley JO, Simon G, Jordan WS. Rhinoviruses in an industrial population. I. The occurrence of illness. N Engl J Med 1966; 275:1261–1268.
232. Chonmaitree T. How do respiratory viruses cause otitis media. Dec 1999 Program and abstracts of the Second International Symposium on Influenza and Respiratory viruses, Grand Cayman, British West Indies.
233. Buchman CA, Doyle WJ, Pilcher O, Gentile DA, Skoner DP. Nasal and otologic effects of experimental respiratory syncytial virus infection in adults. Am J Otolaryngol 2002; 23:70–75.
234. Gwaltney J, Hendley JO, Philips CD, Bass CR, Mygind N, Winther B. Nose blowing propels nasal fluid into the paranasal sinuses. Clin Infect Dis 2000; 30:387–391.
235. Gwaltney M, Philips CD, Miller RD. Computed tomographic study of the common cold. N Engl J Med 1994; 330:25–30.
236. Turner RW, Cail WS, Hendley JO. Physiologic abnormalities in paranasal sinuses during experimental rhinovirus infection. J Allergy Clin Immunol 1992; 90:474–478.
237. Cole CEC. Preliminary report on the influenza epidemic at Bramshott in September-October 1918. Br Med J 1918; 2:566–568.
238. Abrahams A, Hallows N, French N. A further investigation into the influenza-pneumococcal and influenza-streptococcal septicaemia. Lancet 1919; 1–11.
239. Bendkowski B. Asian influenza in allergic patients. Br Med J 1958; 2;1314–1315.
240. Fry J. Clinical and epidemiological features in a general practice. Br Med J 1958; I: 259–261.

241. Guthrie J, Forsyth DM, Montgomery H. Asiatic influenza in the middle east: an outbreak in a small community. Lancet 1957; 2:590–592.
242. Gilroy J. Asian influenza. Br Med J 1957; 2:997–998.
243. Gaydos JC, Hodder RA, Top FH. Swine influenza A at Fort Dix New Jersey. Case finding and clinical study of cases. J Infect Dis 1976; 136:S356–S362
244. Louria DB, Bulmenfeld HL, Ellis JT, Kilbourne ED, Rogers DE. Studies on influenza in the pandemic of 1957–58. II. Pulmonary complications of influenza. J Clin Invest 1958; 38:213–265.
245. Martin CM, Kunin CM, Gottieb LS, Barnes MW, Liu C, Finland M. Asian influenza A in Boston 1957–58. Observations in 32 influenza associated fatal cases. Arch Intern Med 1959; 103:515–518.
246. Pinsker KL, Schneyer B, Becker N, Kamholz SL. Usual interstitial pneumonia following Texas A2 infection. Chest 1981; 80:123–126.
247. Luksza AR, Jones DK. Influenza B virus infection complicated by pneumonia, acute renal failure and disseminated intravascular coagulation. J Infect 1984; 9:174–176.
248. Hers J, Masurel N, Gans JC. Acute respiratory disease associated with pulmonary involvement in military servicement in the Netherlands. Am Rev Respir Dis 1969; 100:499–506.
249. Kimball AM, Foy HM, Cooney MK, Allan M, Matlock M, Plorde JJ. Isolation of respiratory syncytial virus from the sputum of patients hospitalised with pneumonia. J Infect Dis 1983; 147:181–184.
250. Zaroukian MH, Leader I. Community acquired pneumonia and infection with respiratory syncytial virus. Ann Intern Med 1988; 109:515–516.
251. Melbye HB, Berdal BP, Straumme H, Russell L, Vorland L, Thacker WL. Pneumonia—clinical or radiological diagnosis. Scand J Infect Dis 1992; 24:647–655.
252. Ruiz M, Ewig S, Marcos MA, Martinez J, Arancibia F, Mensa J. Etiology of community acquired pneumonia: impact on age, comorbidity and severity. Am J Respir Crit Care 1999; 160:397–405.
253. Lerida A, Marron A, Casanova A, Roson B, Carratala J, Gudiol F. Respiratory syncytial virus infection in adult patients hospitalised with community acquired pneumonia. Enferm Infecc Microbiol Clin 2000; 18:177–181.
254. Han LL, Alexander JP, Anderson LJ. Respiratory syncytial virus pneumonia among the elderly: an assessment of disease burden. J Infect Dis 1999; 179:25–33.
255. Mandal SK, Joglekar VM, Khan AS. An outbreak of respiratory syncytial virus infection in a continuing care geriatric ward. Age Aging 1985; 14:184–186.
256. Falsey AR, Walsh EE, Betts RF. Serologic evidence of respiratory syncytial virus infection in nursing home patients. J Infect Dis 1990; 162:568–569.
257. Orr PH, Peeling RW, Fast M, Bruna J, Duckworth H, Harding G. Serological study of responses to selected pathogens causing respiratory tract infection in the elderly. Clin Infect Dis 1996; 23:1240–1245.
258. Woodhead MA, Radvan J, Macfarlane JT. Adult community acquired staphylococcal pneumonia in the antibiotic era: a review of 61 cases. Q J Med 1987; 64:783–790.
259. Fiore AE, Iverson C, Messmer T, Erdman D, Lett SM, Talkington DF, Anderson LJ, Fields B, Carlone GM. Outbreak of pneumonia in a long-term facility: antecedent human parainfluenza virus 1 infection may predispose to bacterial pneumonia. J Am Geriatr Soc 1998; 46:1112–1117.
260. Housworth J, Langmuir AD. Excess mortality from epidemic influenza 1957–1966. Am J Epidemiol 1974; 100:40–48.

261. Glezen WP. Serious morbidity and mortality associated with influenza epidemics. Epidemiol Rev 1982; 4:25–44.

262. Bainton D, Jones GR, Hole D. Influenza and ischaemic heart disease—a possible trigger for acute myocardial infarction? Int J Epidemiol 1978; 7:231–239.

263. Karjalainen J, Nieminen MS, Heikkila J. Influenza Al myocarditis in conscripts. Acta Med Scand 1980; 207:27–30.

264. Verel D, Warrack AJN, Potter CW, Ward C, Rickards DF. Observations on the A2 England influenza epidemic. Am Heart J 1976; 92:290–296.

265. Nichol KL, Margolis KL, Woremna J, von Sternberg T. Effectiveness of influenza vaccine in the elderly. Gerontology 1996; 42:274–279.

266. Nicholson KG. Human influenza. In: Nicholson KG, Webster RJ, Hay AJ, eds. Textbook of Influenza. Oxford: Blackwell Publication, 1998:219–264.

267. Lindsay MI, Hermman EC, Morrow GW, Brown AL. Hong Kong influenza: clinical, microbiology and pathologic features in 127 cases. JAMA 1970; 214:1825–1832.

268. Cartwright KA, Jones DM, Smith AJ, Stuart JM, Kaczmarski EB, Palmer SR. Influenza A and meningococcal disease. Lancet 1991; 338;554–557.

269. Gladman JRF, Barer D, Venkatesan P. The outcome of pneumonia in elderly: a hospital review. Clin Rehab 1991; 5:201–205.

270. Barker WH, Borisute H, Cox C. A study of the functional impact of influenza on the functional status of frail older people. Arch Intern Med 1998; 158:645–651.

271. Smith AP, Tyrrell DAJ, Al-Nakib W. Effects and after effects of the common cold and influenza on human performance. Neuropsychobiology 1989; 21:90–93.

272. Moss SE, Klein R, Klein BEK. Cause specific mortality in a population based study of diabetes. Am J Pub Health 1991; 81:1158–1162.

273. Curwen M. Dunnell K, Ashley J. Hidden influenza deaths 1989–90. Popul Trends 1990; 61:31–33.

274. Clifford RE, Smith JWG, Tillett HE, et al. Excess mortality associated with influenza in England and Wales. Int J Epidemiol 1977; 6:115–128.

275. Barker WH, Mullooly JP. Pneumonia and influenza deaths during influenza epidemics. Implications for prevention. Arch Intern Med 1982; 142:85–89.

276. Nicholson KG, Stone AJ, Botha JL, Raymond NT. Effectiveness of influenza vaccine reducing hospital admissions in people with diabetes. In: Brown LE, Hampson AW, Webster RG, eds. Options for the Control of Influenza III. Amsterdam: Elsevier, 113–118.

277. Public Health Laboratory Service. Deaths from Asian influenza 1957. Br Med J 1958; 1:915–919.

278. Polak MF. Influenzaasterfte in de herfst van 1957. Ned Tijdschr Geneeskd 1959; 103:1098–1099.

279. Petersdorf RG, Fusco JJ, Harter DH, Albrink WS. Pulmonary infections complicating Asian influenza. Arch Intern Med 1959; 103:262–272.

280. Ashley J, Smith T, Dunnell K. Deaths in Great Britain associated with the influenza epidemic 1989–90. Popul Trends 1991; 65:16–20.

281. Fox JP, Hall CE, Cooney MK, Foy HM. Influenza virus infections in Seattle families 1975–1979. I Study designs, methods and the occurrence of infection by time and age. Am J Epidemiol 1982; 116:212–227.

282. Kendal AP, Joseph JM, Kobayashi G. Laboratory based surveillance of influenza virus in the United States during the winter of 1977–78. I Periods of prevalence of H1N1 and H3N2 influenza A strains, their relative rates of isolation in different age groups and detection of antigenic variants. Am J Epidemiol 1979; 110:449–461.

283. Glezen WP, Keitel WA, Taber LH, Piedra PA, Clover RD, Couch RB. Age distribution of patients with medically attended illnesses caused by sequential variants of influenza A/H1N1 comparison to age specific infection rates, 1978–1989. Am J Epidemiol 1991; 133:296–304.

284. Nolan TF, Goodman RA, Hinman AR, Noble GR, Kendal AP, Thacker SB. Morbidity and mortality associated with influenza B in the United States 1979–1980. J Infect Dis 1980; 142:360–362.

285. Centers of Disease Control. Influenza surveillance July 1979-June 1981. Publication number CDC-84–8295, Washington DC: US Department of Health and Human Services: 16–19.

286. Influenza surveillance summary 1981–1982. MMWR CDC Surveill Summ 1982: 31: 375–379.

287. Influenza surveillance summary—United States 1982–1983. MMWR CDC Surveill Summ 1983; 32:373–377.

288. Agius G, Dindinaud G, Biggar RJ, et al. An epidemic of respiratory syncytial virus in elderly people: clinical and serological findings. J Med Virol 1990; 30:117–127.

289. Falsey AR, Walsh EE. Humoral immunity to respiratory syncytial virus infection in the elderly. J Med Viol 1992; 36;39–43.

290. Falsey AR, Walsh EE. Relationship of serum antibody to risk of respiratory syncytial virus infection in elderly adults. J Infect Dis 1998; 177:463–466.

291. Looney RJ, Falsey AR, Walsh EE, Campbell D. Effect of aging on cytokine production in response to respiratory syncytial virus infection. J Infect Dis 2002; 185:682–685.

292. Callow KA, Parry HF, Seargant M, Tyrrell DAJ. The time course of the immune response to experimental coronavirus infection in man. Epidemiol Infect 1990; 105: 435–446.

293. Reed S. The behaviour of recent isolates of human respiratory coronavirus in vitro and in volunteers: evidence of heterogeneity among 229E-related strains. J Med Virol 1984; 13:179–192.

294. Clements ML, Betts RF, Murphy BR. Advantage of live attenuated cold adapted influenza A virus over inactivated vaccine for A/Washington/80. Lancet 1984; 1:705–709.

295. Treanor JJ, Kotloff K, Betts RF, et al. Evaluation of live cold adapted and inactivated influenza vaccines in prevention of virus infection and illness following challenge with wild-type influenza A (H1N1), A (H3N2) and B viruses. Vaccine 1999; 18:899–906.

296. Belshe RB, Gruber WL, Mendelson PM, et al. Correlates of immune protection induced by live attenuated cold adapted trivalent intranasal influenza virus vaccine. J Infect Dis 2000; 181:1133–1137.

297. Meiklejohn G. Viral respiratory disease at Lowry Air Force base in Denver 1952–82. J Infect Dis 1983; 148:775–784.

298. Nicol KL. Efficacy/clinical effectiveness of inactivated influenza virus vaccines in adults. In: Nicholson KG, Webster RG, Hay AJ, eds. Textbook of Influenza. Oxford: Blackwell, 1998:358–372.

299. Betts RF, O'Brien D, Menegus M. A comparison of the protective benefit of influenza vaccine in reducing hospitalisation of patients infected with influenza A or B. Clin Infect Dis 1993; 17:573.

300. Treanor JJ, Mattison HR, Dumyati G. Protective efficacy of combined live intranasal and inactivated influenza A virus vaccines in the elderly. Ann Intern Med 1992; 117: 625–633.

301. Nicholson KG, Colegate AC, Podda A, Stephenson I, Ypma E, Wood JM, Zambon MC. Safety and antigenicity of non-adjuvanted and MF59-adjuvanted influenza A/Duck/Singapore/97 (H5N3) vaccine: a randomised trial of two potential vaccines against H5N1 influenza. Lancet 2001; 357:1937–1942.

302. Conne P, Gauthey L, Vernet P. Immunogenicity of trivalent subunit versus virosome-formulated influenza vaccines in geriatric patients. Vaccine 1997; 15:1675–1679.

303. Gluck R, Mischler R, Finkel B. Immunogenicity of new virosome influenza vaccine in elderly people. Lancet 1994; 344:160–163.

304. Piedra PA, Grace S, Jewell A. Purified fusion protein vaccine protects against lower respiratory tract illness during respiratory syncytial virus season in children with cystic fibrosis. Pediatr Infect Dis J 1996; 15:23–31.

305. Belshe RB, Anderson EL, Walsh EE. Immunogenicity of purified F glycoprotein of respiratory syncytial virus: clinical and immune responses to subsequent natural virus: clinical and immune responses to subsequent natural infection in children. J Infect Dis 1993; 168:1024–1029.

306. Falsey AR, Walsh EE. Safety and immunogenicity of a respiratory syncytial virus subunit vaccine (PFP-2) in the ambulatory elderly. Vaccine 1996; 14:1214–1218.

307. Sales V. Safety and immunogenicity of a RSV A vaccine in adults—two phase I clinical studies. In Current research on respiratory viral infections: Fourth International Symposium. Antiviral Res 2002; 55:227–278.

308. Karron RA, Wright PF, Newman FK. A live attenuated human parainfluenza type 3 virus vaccine is attenuated and immunogenic in healthy children and infants. J Infect Dis 1995; 172:1445–1450.

309. Katz JM. A tale of two vaccines. Clin Infect Dis 2000; 31:671–672.

310. Dolin R, Reichman RC, Madore HP, et al. A controlled trial of amantadine and rimantadine in prophylaxis of influenza A infection. N Engl J Med 1982; 307:580–584.

311. Togo Y, Hornich RB, Dawkins AT. Double blind studies designed to assess prophylactic efficacy of amantadine hydrochloride against A2/Rockville/1/65 strain. JAMA 1968; 203:1095–1099.

312. Clover RD, Crawford SA, Abell TD, et al. Effectiveness of rimantadine prophylaxis of children within families. Am J Dis Child 1986: 140:706–709.

313. Hayden FG, Belshe RB, Clover RD, et al Emergence and apparent transmission of rimantadine-resistant influenza A in families. N Engl J Med 1989; 321:1696–1702.

314. MIST Study Group. Randomised trial of efficacy and safety of inhaled zanamivir in treatment of influenza A and B virus infection. Lancet 1998; 352:1877–1884.

315. Monto AS, Robinson DP, Hollocher ML, et al. Zanamivir in prevention of influenza among healthy adults—a randomised controlled trial. JAMA 1999; 282(1):31–38.

316. Nicholson KG, Aoki FY, Osterhaus ADME, et al. Efficacy and safety of oseltamivir in treatment of acute influenza: a randomised controlled trial. Lancet 2000; 355:1845–1850.

317. Hayden FG, Atmar RL, Schilling M, et al. Use of selective oral neuraminidase inhibitor oseltamivir to prevent influenza. N Engl J Med 1999; 341(18): 1336–1345.

318. Gubareva LV, Matrosovich MN, Brenner MK, Bethell RC, Webster RG. Evidence for zanamivir resistance in an immunocompromised child infected with influenza B virus. J Infect Dis 1998; 178:1257–1262.

319. Impact RSV study group. Palivizumab a humanised respiratory syncytial virus monoclonal antibody reduces hospitalisation from respiratory syncytial virus infection in high risk infants. Paediatrics 1998; 102:531–537.

320. Ghosh S, Champlin R, Englund J, Giralt S, Rolston K, Raad I, Jacobsen K, Neumann J, Ippoliti C, Mallik S, Whimbey E. RSV upper respiratory tract illness in adult blood and marrow transplant recipients: combination therapy with aerosolised ribavirin and intravenous immunoglobulin. Bone Marrrow Transplant 2000; 25:751–755.

321. Howard JC, Kantner TR, Lilienfiled LS, Princiotto JV, Krum RE, Crutcher JE. Effectiveness of antihistamines in the management of the common cold. JAMA 1979; 242: 2414–2417.

322. Gwaltney JM, Park J, Paul RA, Edelman DA, O'Connor RR, Turner RB. Randomised controlled trial of clemastine for treatment of experimental rhinovirus colds. Clin Infect Dis 1996; 22:656–662.

323. Hayden FG, Diamond L, Wood PB, Korts DC, Wecker MT. Effectiveness and safety of intranasal ipratropium bromide in common colds: a randomised double blind placebo-controlled trial. Ann Intern Med 1996; 125:89–97.

324. Graham NMH, Burrell CJ, Douglas RM, Debelle P, Davies L. Adverse effects of aspirin, acetaminophen and ibuprofen on immune function, viral shedding and clinical status in rhinovirus infected volunteers. J Infect Dis 1990; 162:1277–1282.

325. Hayden FG, Hassman H, Coats T, Mendez R, Bock T. In 39th Interscience Conference on Antimicrobial Agents and Chemotherapeutics. San Francisco, 1999, LB-3.

326. Hayden FG, Kim K, Coats T, Blatter M, Drehobl M. In 41st Interscience Conference on Antimicrobial Agents and Chemotherapeutics. Toronto, Ontario, 2000, 1161.

327. Hayden FG, Kim K, Hudson S. In 41st Interscience Conference on Antimicrobial Agents and Chemotherapeutics. Chicago, 2001, H659.

328. Patrick A. Antipicornal virus agents. In Current research on respiratory viral infections: Fourth International Symposium. Antiviral Res 2002; 55:227–278.

20

The Common Cold and Its Relationship to Rhinitis, Sinusitis, Otitis Media, and Asthma

NIELS MYGIND

Vejle Hospital
Vejle, Denmark

JACK M. GWALTNEY, Jr., BIRGIT WINTHER, and J. OWEN HENDLEY

University of Virginia
Charlottesville, Virginia, U.S.A.

I. Introduction

In this chapter, we will focus on the common cold, an upper airway tract infection mainly caused by rhinovirus (RV), the clinical manifestations of this infection, and its complications in the airways: acute sinusitis, acute otitis media, and exacerbations of asthma. Acute sinusitis is prevalent in both children and adults, and acute otitis media is the most frequent bacterial disease in childhood. In patients with asthma, a common cold can have serious consequences and result in considerable morbidity and in increased mortality.

We will start this chapter with a description of the pathophysiology of the common cold/RV infection, its transmission, and its treatment, as knowledge of these issues is of importance for a full understanding of the relationship between a common cold and its complications.

II. The Common Cold

A. Definition

A common cold is a viral disease, which causes symptoms mainly involving the upper airways. The common cold is the leading cause of acute morbidity and medical visits in the world. The "common" part of the term comes from the commonality of the illness. The "cold" comes from the belief that catching a cold is associated with getting chilled, but this is without scientific support (1). More important than the disease itself are the complications that often result from a common cold.

B. Virology

It has been described in textbooks and review articles that RV is responsible for 50–60% of acute viral upper respiratory tract illnesses, and coronavirus for about 10–20%, while respiratory syncytial virus (RSV), influenza virus, parainfluenza virus, and adenovirus account for a minor proportion of common colds (1). Viruses can now be identified by very sensitive molecular biology techniques (polymerase chain reaction [PCR] for DNA virus, and reverse transcription polymerase chain reaction [RT-PCR] for RNA virus) (2). Using the RT-PCR technique, a recent study has shown RV to be more important than earlier believed and has identified this virus in 80% of adults with cold symptoms during the autumn (3).

RV is one of the best-described viruses on the molecular level (1). It is a nonenveloped 30 nm RNA picornavirus. The surface of the virus has deep canyons, containing the ligand for the RV receptor on the epithelial cells, which in 90% of the cases is intercellular adhesion molecule-1 (ICAM-1) (4).

RV has more than 100 immunotypes. Infection with each type provides immunity, but vaccination is not realistic due to the considerable antigen diversity (1).

C. Transmission

Introduction of RV into the eye or the nose is a highly efficient way of initiating an experimental infection (5). By contrast, inoculation of RV into the mouth or exposure to infected volunteers, for example, by prolonged kissing, is an inefficient method of initiating infection (5).

Children are the major reservoir for RV. Young children experience 8–12 colds a year, while adults have 2–3 colds (6). In addition, children easily get a runny nose since they have the same number of nasal glands as adults (7) but a smaller mucosal area and therefore a lower mucociliary transport capacity. Consequently, virus transmission occurs readily in families with young children (5,8), especially when they attend a kindergarten.

During colds, nasal secretions containing RV contaminate the fingers and the environment of the infected person. Although a non-enveloped virus is more sensitive to dessication than an enveloped virus, RV retains infectivity for up to 3 days, for example, on a plastic surface (5).

Attempts to transmit RV infection by experimental exposure have shown that a 15 s hand-to-hand contact between a virus-infected and an antibody-negative person, followed by touching the eye or the nostril, is a very efficient way to transmit RV (9).

The hand contact self-inoculation model, proposed by Gwaltney and Hendley (9), has been used to test virucidal hand treatment (10), environmental disinfectants (11), and virucidal handkerchiefs (12). The findings in these studies support the finger-to-eye and finger-to-nose inoculation routes of RV transmission, and they indicate that stopping virus transmission may be one way to reduce the number of cold-induced complications.

The portal of entry for RV can be either the eye or the nose, where the virus can be placed by a finger during eye rubbing and nose picking, respectively. The relative importance of these two sites of entry, in different age groups, is unknown. RV and other respiratory viruses can be detected in secretions from the paranasal sinuses, the middle ear, and the lower airways, but still an open question is to what degree the mucous membranes of these tissues are infected by RV and, if so, whether it is by direct inhalation or by spread of infectious secretions from the nose (13). Spread of virus from the nose to the paranasal sinuses, the middle ear, and the lower airways has to occur against the direction of the movement of mucociliary transport.

D. Rhinovirus Entry to the Body

Entry Through the Nose

When RV is placed in the nostril, it comes in direct contact with skin or with squamous epithelium in the mucous membrane. It does not seem possible for a finger to reach the ciliated epithelium, which can transport the virus to the adenoid area, where infection appears to be initiated. One can speculate, however, that virus particles, placed in the nostril, are carried to the ciliated epithelium by the sniffing of nasal secretions, running to the nostrils. Cold air induces glandular hypersecretion by a cholinergic reflex (14). It can be hypothesized that this is why it is commonly believed that exposure to cold air predisposes to the development of a viral infection, or why a cold is called a cold. When radioactive material is placed in the nostril by a finger, it can be shown by a gammacamera in the nasal cavity after exposure to cold air (B. Winther, N. Mygind, unpublished data).

Entry Through the Eye

When RV is placed in the eye, it will pass through the nasolacrimal duct to the nasal cavity. In a study of the spread of RV in the nose, we inoculated virus in the conjunctiva on one side. Virus could then be detected in brush biopsy samples from the nasopharyngeal mucosa earlier, more frequently, and longer (for up to 3 weeks) than in samples from the nasal cavities (15). The more frequent detection of virus in the nasopharynx than in the nose may be simply because the nasopharynx is the end point of the mucociliary clearance from the nasal passages. On the other hand, RV replication has been demonstrated by in situ hybridization in surface cells, probably M cells, in the lymphoepithelium of the adenoids (16). This indicates that the adenoid may hold a key position regarding initial RV infection. The nose acts as a filter for inhaled particles, and the mucociliary system is designed in such a way that all deposited particles are conveyed to the adenoids, which acts as the primary immune organ of the upper airways.

E. ICAM-1 Is the Major Receptor for Rhinovirus

It is of considerable interest that the receptor for 90% of the RV types is ICAM-1 (17). In addition, ICAM-1 has a central role in recruitment of inflammatory cells

(18). Conjunctival cells and columnar epithelial cells in the nose do not constitutively express ICAM-1, but they do so when they are antigen stimulated, for example, by allergen exposure of IgE-sensitized individuals (19,20). Also an RV-infection will upregulate ICAM-1 in airway epithelial cells, dependent upon upregulation of NF-κB proteins (18).

ICAM-1 is present in basal epithelial cells in the airways, but it is uncertain whether the virus can reach and infect these cells. It can be hypothesized that ICAM-1 receptors in the nasopharynx hold a key position in the initial contact between virus and host cells, as surface cells (possibly M cells) with constitutively high ICAM-1 expression have been demonstrated on the surface of the normal adenoid (21).

F. Rhinovirus Infection of Cells

RV replication occurs in the nasopharynx and in the ciliated and the nonciliated columnar epithelial cells of the nasal passages. The newly formed viruses are shed into respiratory secretions (22,23). One infected cell can produce up to 100,000 virus particles by 8 h after infection (24). In spite of this, the number of infected epithelial cells seems to be low. Turner and colleagues (23), utilizing immunohistochemical staining of sloughed epithelial cells from patients with experimental RV-induced colds, found that less that 2% of the cells were positive for RV antigen. By in situ hybridization, Bardin and co-workers (25) found RV replication in a few cells in nasal biopsies from only half of the patients with RV-induced colds. Arruda and co-workers (16,22) examined multiple nasal scrape biopsies from volunteers with colds and demonstrated RV replication in only a few cells, providing further evidence for virus infection in a limited number of epithelial cells. In two studies, Winther and co-workers (15,26) took several brush biopsies and found virus growth only in a part of the biopsies, showing that the RV infection of the nasal lining is not universal but spotty.

G. Viral Cytopathological Effect

The effect of cold viruses on nasal epithelial cells has been studied in vitro by Winther and co-workers (27). Experimental infection with RV and with coronavirus does not result in visual damage of the epithelial cells. The cilia continue to beat on the nasal tissue fragments (27) and the nasal epithelial cell monolayer remains confluent. Thus, RV has no or only a small cytopathological effect on ciliated cells.

In contrast, infection of nasal cultures with influenza and adenovirus results in a complete destruction of the epithelial cells within a few days (27,28). Infection with RSV has an intermediate effect (29).

This difference in cytopathological effect may explain, in part, why RV and coronavirus usually cause a common cold (i.e., a trivial disease with upper airway symptoms), while influenza virus causes a more severe disease with fever and symptoms from both upper and lower airways.

H. Conclusions

The common cold is a viral disease with symptoms predominantly from the upper airways. It is mainly transmitted by hand–(object)–hand contact and self-inoculation of eyes or nose. The most frequently occurring viruses, RV and coronavirus, do not cause any marked cytopathological effect on epithelial cells.

III. Relationship Between Common Cold and Rhinitis

A. Inflammation and Pathophysiology

The first study of nasal histological findings in naturally occurring colds dates from 1930. In this work, substantial separation and sloughing of the nasal epithelium were reported (30). Largely based on this study, it was assumed for more than 50 years that the cold viruses damage the nasal epithelial lining, directly causing the cold symptoms, and also impairing mucociliary clearance, which results in a secondary bacterial infection with neutrophilia and purulent secretions.

It was not until 1984 that a subsequent study of common cold was published using light and scanning electron microscopy (31). This study showed a largely intact and continuous epithelial surface. There was accumulation of neutrophils in spite of the absence of a concomitant bacterial infection (32). Based on these observations, we hypothesized that the virus infection of the epithelial cells does not cause symptoms due to damage of epithelial cells with impairment of the mucociliary transport, causing a bacterial infection and neutrophilia, but indirectly by a series of inflammatory cytokines and mediators, released predominantly from epithelial cells. This hypothesis has been supported by the in vitro studies, mentioned above, which show that RV does not cause any gross damage of epithelial cells (27).

Ciliated Epithelial Cells

Nasal biopsies from patients with naturally acquired colds (31,33) have shown an intact and continuous epithelium by light and by scanning electron microscopy. Considering the dynamics of airway epithelium, showing closure of cell defects within hours after trauma (34), these findings do not exclude an increased turnover rate and shedding of epithelial cells during a RV cold. In fact, in a study of naturally acquired colds, Pedersen and co-workers (35) found a reduced number of ciliated cells in nasal scrape biopsies during and for some weeks after the cold. It is possible that this study was undertaken during a period with an epidemic of influenza, parainfluenza, or adenovirus infection. It needs confirmation with the use of modern diagnostic tests for establishing the virus etiology, because the results differ from the in vitro studies, showing no or very little cytopathological effect of RV and coronavirus on ciliated cells. Some early studies of nasal smears from patients with naturally acquired colds of undetermined cause have shown shed ciliated cells with signs of damage (ciliocytophthoria) (36).

The apparent contradiction between the findings of viable epithelial cells in in vitro studies of RV infection and the reduced mucociliary clearance in in vivo studies of naturally acquired colds may be explained by a transmission electron microscopic study by Afzelius (37). Among hundreds of nasal biopsies he found a single biopsy with infection of the columnar cells with a virus (coronavirus?). The infected cells looked viable without destruction, but the cilia were retracted from the surface into the cytoplasm.

Neutrophils

Infiltration of neutrophils in the nasal mucosa seems to be an early and transient event. In our first study of naturally acquired colds, the number of neutrophils was clearly increased in the surface epithelium and in the lamina propria by day 2 of the disease (31).

In experimental RV infection one study showed a slightly increased number of neutrophils in nasal biopsies on day 1 and day 2 of infection (38), while another study (39) failed to show any change in the number of neutrophils on day 4 of the illness.

Within 24 h of RV inoculation, Naclerio and co-workers (40) found an increase of neutrophils in nasal washes obtained every 4 h around the clock, and the number had already begun to decrease by day 3. An increased number of neutrophils was found by Levandowsky and co-workers (41) in nasal washes from patients with experimental RV colds on day 4 after virus inoculation.

It is important to include sham-inoculation in these types of studies because a biopsy procedure in itself can induce neutrophilia, probably by perturbation of epithelial cells and subsequent release of IL-8 (38).

Experimental RV infection is associated with an increase in neutrophils not only in the nose but also in the blood (42,43).

Mast Cells and Eosinophils

Studies have shown no changes in the number of mast cells and eosinophils in the nasal epithelium and lamina propria during a cold (31,39). This suggests that these cells are not involved in the pathogenesis of a common cold. However, it cannot be excluded that an RV cold enhances allergen-induced degranulation of basophils and mast cells. An in vitro study has shown that interferon, released by peripheral blood cells incubated with virus, promotes basophil histamine release (44). In addition, antihistamines have a therapeutic effect on common cold symptoms (see later).

Lymphocytes

The lymphocytes in lamina propria of the nasal mucous membrane have been examined by immunohistochemistry in two studies of RV colds (39,45). No changes in the total number of cells or in lymphocyte subsets (CD3$^+$, CD4$^+$, CD8$^+$, CD22$^+$) were detected.

The published data on the number of circulating lymphocytes in experimental RV infection are conflicting. In three studies (41–43), the number of T cells was reduced early during the infection. Winther and co-workers (45), on the other hand, did not find any change in CD3$^+$, CD4$^+$, CD8$^+$, CD22$^+$ (B cells), and CD57$^+$ (natural killer cells). However, Skoner and co-workers (46) found an increased number of both total lymphocytes and of the CD4$^+$ and CD8$^+$ subsets.

A recent study by Vianna and co-workers (47) showed a decreased peripheral blood T-cell response to phytohemagglutinin and reduced cytokine formation during a common cold. One can speculate that this reduced T-cell activity may be part of the explanation why common colds induce complications in tissues not infected by virus, such as reactivation of labial herpes (cold sore).

Proinflammatory Cytokines

RV infection of the nasal epithelial cells triggers the synthesis and release of cytokines and mediators, causing a cascade of inflammatory reactions assumed to be responsible for the cold symptoms (47).

The cytokines, some of which function as neutrophil chemoattractants and activators, are of particular interest since the number of neutrophils in nasal lavage fluid correlates with symptoms in experimental RV colds (40). In this respect, IL-8 is of the greatest importance, since it is a strong chemoattractant for neutrophils and it also activates these cells.

In vitro studies of cell cultures have shown that an RV infection induces IL-8 production in both epithelial cells (49,50) and in fibroblasts (51). In vivo studies of naturally acquired colds (52,53) and of experimental RV colds (54) have shown an increased level of IL-8 in nasal lavage fluid.

Infection with RSV induces significant IL-8 production in epithelial cells both in the nose (53) and in the bronchi (54).

Viral infections stimulate the release of other cytokines (IL-1β, IL-6, tumor necrosis factor-α, interferon-γ) into nasal secretions (52,53,55–61) but their role in the pathogenesis of common cold is not clear. Interferon-γ probably plays an important role in terminating the virus infection, which occurs before the formation of specific antibodies. IL-6 may be important in stimulating T lymphocytes (62). It has been shown that IL-6 and IL-8 are generated following virus-induced activation of the transcription factor NF-κB (58).

Studies are needed to characterize the cytokine profile of RV-induced infection compared to other types of inflammation of the nasal mucosa. One study of nasal lavage fluid has shown a different cytokine profile in experimental colds (interferon-γ and IL-1β) and in allergic rhinitis (GM-CSF and IL-1β) (63).

Inflammatory Mediators

Kinins

Kinin levels are increased in nasal lavage fluid from patients with experimental (40) and with natural RV colds (64). The concentration of kinins peaks at the same time as the symptoms.

Intranasal challenge with bradykinin in normal subjects produces nasal irritation, rhinorrhea, nasal obstruction and a sore throat (65). Since these symptoms imitate cold symptoms, it provides suggestive evidence that kinins might contribute to the symptoms of viral colds. However, a possible causal role for kinins in the development of cold symptoms cannot be established until it is possible to block their action by specific antagonists.

Histamine

There is no histological evidence of mast cell degranulation during a common cold (31), and the level of histamine in nasal lavage fluid is not increased during an experimental RV infection (66–68).

The usefulness of H_1 antihistamines for the treatment of common cold has been the subject of controversy (69). There are now three double-blind, placebo-controlled, and randomized studies with adequate statistical power that show a beneficial effect of first-generation sedating antihistamines on cold symptoms (70–72). However, second-generation nonsedating antihistamines appear not to be clinically effective and, therefore, it is possible that the treatment with first-generation antihistamines is effective because, due to the sedative effect and a CNS blockage of reflexes, it reduces sneezing and watery rhinorrhea.

Leukotrienes

Sulfidoleukotrienes sprayed into the nose do not cause irritation and sneezing but they induce vascular changes (73) and also act as secretagogues (74). It is possible that drugs inhibiting the synthesis of leukotrienes and drugs blocking the leukotriene receptor may have a beneficial effect on nasal blockage and mucus hypersecretion in colds. This hypothesis can now be tested because leukotriene receptor antagonists are commercially available.

Prostaglandins

Intranasal challenge with prostaglandin D_2 and with prostaglandin $F_{2\alpha}$ results in sneezing and coughing (75). The role played by prostaglandins in the common cold can be judged by the clinical effect of nonsteroidal anti-inflammatory drugs (NSAIDs). These drugs seem to have some beneficial effect on coughing (76) and on sneezing, but not on blockage and rhinorrhea (77).

Nasal Hyperresponsiveness

Although several reports have shown that a common cold can increase the nonspecific bronchial responsiveness in asthma, the possibility that a viral infection of the nose also induces nasal hyperresponsiveness has not received much attention.

Grønborg and colleagues (78) performed nasal challenges with histamine and methacholine during and after a naturally acquired cold. Both the sneezing and the secretory response to histamine were significantly increased, but only during the first 3 days of the disease, while the secretory response to methacholine was increased for 9 days. In a study of experimental RV infection, Doyle and co-workers (79) found an increased nasal responsiveness to histamine challenge for sneezing and rhinorrhea but not for blockage. The mean number of histamine-induced sneezes increased from 4.5 to 10.5 in nonallergic volunteers, but the increase in allergic rhinitis patients (studied outside the pollen season) was from 10.0 to 19.5.

Mucosal Permeability

It is well established that the nasal inflammation in a common cold is associated with increased passage of molecules (e.g., albumin) from the tissue to the airway lumen. In addition, Greiff and co-workers (80), who measured histamine-induced mucosal exudation of plasma before and during a coronavirus infection, found that the concentration of plasma components in nasal lavage fluid was significantly increased during the infection, indicating the existence of an exudative hyperresponsiveness. These authors also studied the permeability of the mucous membrane from the lumen to the tissue (81). In contrast to common belief, the permeability, measured as the ability to absorb $_{51}$Cr-EDTA, was not increased during the viral infection. Thus, virus-induced inflammation promotes epithelial permeability from the tissue to the airway lumen but not from the lumen to the tissue.

B. Symptoms and Signs

The first symptom of a common cold is often throat irritation without pain on swallowing, indicating that the irritation is located in the nasopharynx. The throat irritation diminishes in a few days even though the adenoidal region remains infected for up to 3 weeks (15).

Nasal irritation, sneezing, and watery rhinorrhea, running from the nostrils, are the next symptoms followed by nasal blockage and a sensation of stuffiness (Table 1). After some days the watery rhinorrhea is replaced by blown nasal mucoid secretions that may become purulent. In uncomplicated colds, the symptoms subside within 5–10 days.

C. Diagnosis

Although people usually know when they have caught a cold, it is not always easy for the doctor to make the diagnosis with certainty. Exposure to cold air and inhaled irritants can cause symptoms similar to cold symptoms. The diagnosis is particularly difficult in patients with perennial rhinitis. In clinical trials, it is necessary to use well-defined criteria in order to make the diagnosis with a sufficient degree of certainty.

D. Treatment

Therapy of a common cold has three purposes, to reduce symptoms, to prevent complications, and to decrease viral shedding and spread of the infection.

Decongestants

α-Adrenoceptor agonists significantly reduce the severity of nasal blockage (82–84), showing that this symptom is due to vasodilatation and not edema formation.

Table 1   Effect of RV Infection on Various Tissues

Nose
   Infection of epithelial cells
   Rhinitis symptoms
Nasopharynx
   Infection of epithelial cells (M cells)
   Initial mild pharyngitis symptoms
Paranasal sinuses
   Infection of epithelial cells
   Sinus pathology seen on imaging
   Mild sinusitis symptoms that recover without treatment
   Predisposes to acute bacterial sinusitis
Middle ear
   Infection of epithelial cells
   Reduced middle ear pressure
   Predisposes to acute bacterial otitis media
Lower airways
   Infection of epithelial cells
   Predisposes to exacerbation of asthma
   Predisposes to exacerbation of chronic obstructive pulmonary disease

Intranasal application has a definitely better therapeutic index than oral administration, but a nasal spray should only be used for 1–2 weeks due to the risk of rhinitis medicamentosa.

Anticholinergics

Intranasal ipratropium bromide is effective in stopping watery nasal discharge in the initial phase of a cold by blocking the cholinergic innervation of the submucosal glands (85). This is clear evidence that the rhinorrhea in common cold is a glandular product and not plasma exudation. Ipratropium bromide has no effect on viscous and mucopurulent secretions (85). Because watery nasal secretions are the main source of infective viruses, it is theoretically possible that ipratropium treatment may reduce virus transmission to other persons.

Antihistamines and NSAIDs

These agents are described above.

Corticosteroids

A series of cytokines are upregulated in the common cold, and the important IL-8 is generated following virus-induced activation of NF-κB in epithelial cells (58). Corticosteroids interact with this transcription factor and can, in theory, be expected to have an anti-inflammatory effect and to be useful for symptomatic treatment of the common cold. However, in practice, corticosteroids are not or are only marginally effective in treating cold symptoms. In one study, intranasal corticosteroid treatment, begun prior to RV inoculation, showed trends towards fewer symptoms during the first 2 days, but this was followed by a normal progression of manifestations of the common cold (86). In another study, a high doze of intranasal corticosteroid had no clinically recognizable effects on the symptoms of a naturally acquired cold, but it produced prolonged shedding of viable RV (87). Oral prednisone (60 mg daily) did not improve cold symptoms in volunteers with experimentally induced RV colds but it did increase viral shedding (88). One can speculate that the marked reduction in the number of epithelial Langerhans cells, which is induced by intranasal corticosteroid treatment (89), may result in impaired antigen presentation to lymphocytes, and in reduced and delayed antibody formation.

It is difficult to explain why corticosteroids have no or little symptomatic effect in the common cold (a cytokine-driven neutrophil-dominated inflammatory disease), while these drugs have a marked effect in allergic rhinitis (a cytokine-driven eosinophil-dominated inflammatory disease), considering that NF-κB is a pathway for drug activity in both diseases.

Interferon-α

Interferon-α has antiviral activity against RV. Prophylactic intranasal administration, beginning when one family member develops cold symptoms, reduces the risk of acquiring a cold by 60% among other family members (90). When used in the initial phase of a cold, intranasal interferon-α decreases RV shedding but has little effect on alleviating the symptoms (91). The reason for the limited symptomatic response to interferon-α, in spite of the antiviral effect, may be because the viral infection already had triggered the inflammatory cascade responsible for the cold symptoms.

Combined Therapy

Probably the most effective treatment of common cold consists of a combination of antiviral and antimediator drugs, as proposed by Gwaltney (92). In a study of volunteers with experimentally induced RV infection combined treatment with intranasal interferon-α, intranasal ipratropium bromide and oral naproxen significantly reduced the viral titer and the overall cold symptoms (92).

Antiviral drugs are not yet commercially available to treat the common cold. A combination of a long-acting first-generation antihistamine (chlorpheniramine 12 mg) and an NSAID (ibuprofen 400 mg), started at the first symptoms of a cold and continued every 12 h for several days, is an effective treatment.

E. Conclusions

The mediators of the clinical symptoms and signs of a common cold are largely unknown. An important pathogenic mechanism is a neutrophil-dominated inflammation, characterized by upregulation and release of IL-8 and other cytokines, causing local neutrophilia. At present, there is only symptomatic therapy for the common cold.

IV. Relationship Between Common Cold and Conjunctivitis

It is well known clinically that an adenovirus infection can cause conjunctivitis, and there are hundreds of publications on this association (93,94). Also some enterovirus types cause conjunctivitis.

With regard to the other respiratory viruses, the published data are less clear. We have not been able to find a single publication showing an association between an infection with RV or coronavirus and conjunctivitis.

When RV is placed in the eye, it will pass through the nasolacrimal duct to the nasal cavity. This occurs apparently without a clinical infection of the epithelial cells in the conjunctiva. This is difficult to understand because the receptor for RV, ICAM-1, can be upregulated in conjunctival cells (95) in the same way as in the nasal mucosa.

V. Relationship Between Common Cold and Sinusitis

A. Definition

Sinusitis, defined as inflammation of one or more sinuses, has been characterized as acute when lasting 3–4 weeks and chronic when lasting longer (96). This review will consider acute sinusitis. Most cases of acute sinusitis are considered to result from bacterial disease secondary to a preceding viral upper respiratory tract infection.

B. Acute Viral Sinusitis

The common cold has traditionally been considered to be a viral rhinitis. Recent imaging data, however, have shown that it is, in fact, a viral rhinosinusitis. This has been convincingly shown by Gwaltney and co-workers. In one study, using magnetic resonance imaging, it was found that 33% of adult volunteers experimentally infected with RV had sinus abnormality (97). In another study, computed tomographic (CT) scan imaging was performed in patients with naturally acquired colds (98). There were extensive abnormalities in the paranasal sinuses in 87% of the patients in the 3–5 days after onset of nasal symptoms. The abnormalities resolved spontaneously without antibiotics within 3 weeks.

Puhakka et al. (99) studied 197 young adults with a common cold. Repeated x-ray examinations showed radiological sinus abnormalities in 39% of the patients. A viral cause was demonstrated in 82% of the patients with radiographic sinusitis. Patients with and without radiological sinusitis could not be differentiated based on symptoms, serum C reactive protein concentration, or total white cell blood count. All patients made a clinical recovery within 3 weeks without antibiotic treatment. The authors conclude that viral sinusitis frequently occurs in the early days of a common cold, but it is a self-limited illness. It is emphasized that the sinuses should not be imaged in patients with a common cold if the signs and symptoms of illness gradually become less severe and no specific signs of bacterial sinusitis occur.

Shopfner and co-workers (100) found sinus abnormalities on radiographs in 75% of children with a common cold. Using the more sensitive CT scan, Winther et al. (101) showed that sinus abnormalities are present in most children with RV colds.

Pitkäranta et al. (102) studied 20 adults with acute naturally acquired sinusitis and detected RV by RT-PCR in 50%, including maxillary aspirates from 40% and nasal swabs from 45%.

These studies show that RV infections frequently cause disease of the paranasal sinuses, although the pathogenesis of this viral rhinosinusitis is incompletely defined, and it is uncertain how often active viral replication occurs in the sinus mucosa.

C. Acute Bacterial Sinusitis

The common bacterial flora of acute bacterial sinusitis are well established, *Streptococcus pneumoniae*, *Haemophilus influenzae*, and *Moxaxella catarrhalis* being most frequently involved (103).

Most cases of acute bacterial sinusitis result from a preceding viral upper airway infection. It has been estimated that 0.5–2.5% of common-cold cases lead to secondary bacterial infection (104). Bacterial sinusitis is typically seen after a common cold with purulent secretions persisting beyond 7–10 days, or showing a biphasic pattern.

D. Inflammation and Pathophysiology

The surface epithelium in the sinuses is similar to that of the nose, and one can expect that the inflammatory changes in the sinuses are similar to those described in the nasal mucosa during a common cold. But this issue has not been addressed in controlled studies.

There is an anatomical difference between the two sites: the nose has a high capacity for producing watery secretions from a large number of seromucous glands, while mucus produced in the sinuses is mainly derived from goblet cells, since there are very few glands in the sinus mucosa (7). Consequently, secretions from the sinuses are more mucoid and viscous than the watery nasal secretions.

It is commonly believed that swelling of the nasal mucous membranes may obstruct drainage from and ventilation of the paranasal sinuses, causing mucus to collect in the sinuses and sinus pressure to decrease. However, another mechanism may also be at work. In the cold study of Gwaltney and co-workers (98), the CT abnormalities, which consisted of opacities in the ostiomeatal complex and paranasal sinuses, could be due to accumulation of mucus, to mucosal congestion/edema, or to both. The presence of air bubbles in the opacities indicated an accumulation of mucus. It is difficult to explain the occurrence of air bubbles without assuming a simultaneous introduction of fluid and air from the nasal cavity during nose blowings. This issue was therefore analyzed in a study of normal volunteers (105). Sinus CT scans were performed after instillation of radiopaque contrast medium into the nose and nasopharynx followed by nose blowing. A nose blow could increase nasal pressure to 65 mmHg and propel up to 1 ml viscous fluid from the nose into the maxillary sinus. If such a mechanism is at work for introducing secretions into the sinus cavities, viruses and bacteria may be introduced by the same mechanism.

E. Symptoms and Signs

Symptoms of acute sinusitis include nasal congestion, purulent nasal secretions, postnasal drainage, tenderness over the sinus cavities, and nocturnal cough (96). While viscous postnasal drainage is a sign of sinusitis, watery rhinorrhea is a sign of rhinitis.

F. Diagnosis

The diagnosis of acute sinusitis is based primarily on the clinical history. Endoscopy is a quick and safe way to visualize the condition of the nasal mucosa and the presence of secretions and may aid the diagnosis. Generally, imaging is not necessary in making the diagnosis of acute sinusitis and should be avoided during a common cold. Maxillary aspiration for culture is definitive but is indicated only when precise microbial identification is essential.

Berg and Carenfeldt (106) studied 55 adults patients referred to a university ear, nose, and throat (ENT) department for acute sinusitis. They found that unilateral pain and purulent secretion could predict the existence of maxillary empyema with an 85% overall reliability.

Recently, Niehaus et al. (107) examined lactoferrin in nasal secretions and found it elevated in 4% of patients with uncomplicated colds and in 79% of patients with clinical sinusitis. The authors conclude that nasal lactoferrin helps to differentiate sinusitis from colds. This may be the biochemical equivalent to purulent secretion.

Clinically, it is difficult to differentiate between rhinitis and sinusitis, and it is even more difficult to differentiate a viral sinusitis from a bacterial sinusitis. Complaints of sinus pressure, postnasal drainage, and discolored nasal discharge lasting for more than 7–10 days, or showing a biphasic pattern, is associated with the diagnosis of bacterial sinusitis (108). Especially unilateral pain and purulent secretion are reliable signs. It is now realized that imaging techniques are not helpful unless they show the presence of empyema.

G. Treatment

The aim of treatment is to relieve symptoms, re-establishing ventilation and drainage of the sinuses and eradicating the infection.

Antibiotics

If untreated, acute bacterial sinusitis may become chronic or lead to severe complications. Therefore, antibiotics are generally considered necessary for its medical management (109). Recent findings, however, have made the benefit of antibiotics questionable (110). Imaging studies have clearly shown that a viral sinusitis resolves without antibiotic treatment.

Decongestants

Both topical and oral vasoconstrictors are often used in the therapy of acute sinusitis because they reduce nasal blockage and it is thought that they may widen ostial patency and improve sinus ventilation and drainage. However, controlled studies to show this are lacking, which is astonishing considering the very frequent use of this therapy.

Corticosteroids

There is a single study of intranasal corticosteroid treatment of acute sinusitis. Meltzer et al. (111) gave amoxicillin with and without momethasone furoate nasal spray to 407 adults with recurrent sinusitis experiencing a new episode of acute sinusitis. There was a significant effect of the intranasal corticosteroid on sinusitis symptoms.

A few recent studies have suggested that the addition of intranasal corticosteroid to antibiotic therapy is beneficial in the treatment of chronic sinusitis (112,113). However, the effect has been clinically marginal, and it is dubious whether intranasal medication can reach the osteomeatal complex.

Other Treatments

It can be hypothesized that early treatment during a cold with ipratropium bromide or perhaps a first-generation antihistamine, reducing the amount of nasal fluid, may reduce sinus involvement during colds (105), and, more importantly, may reduce virus transmission to other persons.

H. Conclusions

A viral infection usually precedes an acute bacterial sinusitis. Virus, predominantly rhinovirus, can by sensitive methods (PCR and RT-PCR) be identified in a large proportion of affected paranasal sinuses. It is now well established that the viral infection itself can cause abnormal pressure and sinus pathology, and that a viral sinusitis resolves spontaneously without antibiotic treatment. However, it is not known by which mechanisms the viral infection can predispose to an acute bacterial sinusitis.

VI. Relationship Between Common Cold and Otitis Media

A. Definition

Otitis media is classified as acute otitis media (AOM), chronic otitis media, and otitis media with effusion. This review covers AOM. AOM is defined as an inflammatory disease of the middle ear mucosa, which traditionally is considered to be a bacterial infection preceded by a viral respiratory tract infection. AOM is the most frequent bacterial infection in early childhood and the most common disease in children who seek medical care. In addition, more prescriptions are written for antimicrobial agents for AOM than for any other disease (114).

B. Viral Otitis Media

Viruses Reduce Middle Ear Pressure

Experimental RV infection of adult volunteers has shown development of eustachian tube dysfunction and reduced middle ear pressure in 40–50% of the infected volunteers (115,116). Inoculation with influenza A virus likewise induces the development of abnormal middle ear pressure in 80% of volunteers (116,117). However, no subject developed evidence of middle ear effusion or otitis symptoms.

Elkhatieb et al. (118) measured middle ear pressure in adults with natural RV colds. They found major abnormalities in 50–60%, which resolved by day 14 without treatment. Only 1 of 91 patients developed clinically apparent otitis media. The authors conclude that natural RV colds in adults are frequently associated with transient abnormalities in middle ear pressure.

Occurrence of Virus in Acute Otitis Media

Pitkäranta et al. (119) sampled middle ear fluids and nasopharyngeal aspirates from children with AOM. The samples were examined for bacteria and for viruses by RT-PCR. Bacterial pathogens were detected in 62%. Virus RNA was detected in 75% of the nasopharyngeal samples and in 48% of the middle ear samples. Among the virus-infected children, RV were found in 64%, RSV in 57%, and coronavirus in 36%. Viral DNA was detected in similar percentages of bacteria-positive and bacteria-negative samples. The authors conclude that these findings highlight the importance of virus, particularly RV and RSV, in predisposing to and causing AOM in young children.

Heikkinen et al. (120) studied 456 children with AOM. Specimens of nasopharyngeal washing and middle-ear fluid were obtained for viral culture. A specific viral cause of respiratory symptoms was identified in 41%. RSV was found in nasal washing/middle ear fluid in 14%/11%, parainfluenza virus in 6%/3%, enterovirus in 6%/1%, influenza virus in 5%/2%, and adenovirus in 5%/0.2%. In a subsequent letter to the editor, it was pointed out by Pitkäranta and Hayden (121) that in this study sensitive methods were not used to identify RV and coronavirus.

Chonmaitree et al. (122) used a commercially available RT-PCR to detect seven common respiratory viruses (RSV-A, RSV-B, parainfluenza virus 1, 2 and 3, influenza virus A and B) in 65 middle ear specimens from 40 children with AOM. The authors found positive virus DNA in 18 children (parainfluenza virus in 9, RSV in 6, and influenza virus in 3). Testing for RV and coronavirus was not included.

The above studies clearly show that a viral respiratory disease is present in the large majority of patients with AOM. RV and RSV are the most frequently found viruses. Coronavirus, parainfluenza virus, and influenza virus are found less frequently (123).

C. Bacterial Otitis Media

Bacteria can be detected in middle ear fluid in about 75% of patients with AOM, while no bacterial pathogen can be isolated in the remaining 25% of the patients (120). In the study by Heikkinen et al. (120), the bacteria identified were *Streptococcus pneumoniae* in 25%, *Haemophilus influenzae* in 23%, *Moxaxella catarrhalis* in 15%, and a mixture in 10%.

D. Inflammation and Pathophysiology

It is commonly believed that swelling of the nasal mucous membrane may obstruct drainage from and ventilation of the eustachian tube, causing mucus to collect in the middle ear and pressure to decrease.

It can be hypothesized that viruses are responsible for some of the pathological changes in the middle ear, by an effect on eustachian tube function and/or by an infection of the middle ear mucosa. Studies have clearly shown the occurrence of viruses in middle ear fluid during a large proportion of AOM cases. It is still unclear, however, whether the detection of virus in the middle ear fluid merely reflects passive passage from the nasopharynx, or how often virus replicates in the middle ear mucosa, causing an active infection. The similarity between the epithelial linings of the nose and that of part of the middle ear favors the latter possibility. So too does the finding that respiratory viruses have the ability to induce the production of several mediators and cytokines in the middle ear mucosa (124).

An artificial virus infection can cause an abnormal middle ear pressure (116,125), but clinical otitis media rarely develops. In community-acquired AOM, a virus is the only identifiable pathogen in about 10% of cases (126), and it is likely that most of the 25% bacteria-negative cases are merely virus-induced when sensitive tests are used for all respiratory viruses. In these cases, the viral disease is probably the only cause of the clinical middle ear disease.

E. Symptoms and Signs

McCormick et al. (127) studied 80 children with AOM for bacterial pathogens and viruses in the middle ear fluid and their relationship to symptoms and otoscopic findings. Bacteria were detected in 50% of the ears, bacteria and virus in 12%, and virus alone in 7%. In this study, RV was detected in only one ear and coronavirus in none. A bacterial cause was associated with bulging of the ear drum (p = 0.001), which had a predictive value of a bacterial infection with a positive value of 74% and a negative value of 45%. There was no correlation among microbiology and symptoms, body temperature, and middle ear fluid volume, color, or viscosity. This study indicates that mild cases of AOM without a bulging eardrum are likely to be of viral origin. However, it is difficult or impossible even for experienced clinicians to differentiate AOM caused by bacterial infection alone from AOM caused by viral infection alone (126).

F. Treatment

Antibiotics

Because AOM has traditionally been considered exclusively a bacterial disease, antibiotic treatment has been recommended for decades without support from controlled clinical trials. The first placebo-controlled study by Mygind et al. (128) of the effect of penicillin treatment of AOM in children, published in 1981, showed merely a marginal effect on pain score on day 2 and day 3 of the disease and no effect on the resolution of the middle ear disease, visualized by otoscopy and tympanometry. These findings are in accord with the demonstration of a viral otitis media as the only cause of otitis in a part of the patients and with the policy of more restrained use of antibiotics in the routine treatment of AOM (129).

Decongestants

Although decongestants alone or in combination with antihistamines have been used extensively in the treatment of AOM, based on the rationale that vasoconstriction and improved nasal patency improve eustachian tube function and middle ear pathology, the first placebo-controlled study of treatment with an oral vasoconstrictor failed to show any effect on the symptoms or the course of AOM in children (130).

This finding has been confirmed in three placebo-controlled studies of added use of an oral vasoconstrictor and an antihistamine (131–133) and in one study of an intranasal vasoconstrictor (134). A single study showed a mild effect of combined use of an oral vasoconstrictor and an antihistamine on nasal congestion and the course of middle ear effusion (135). Together, the published studies do not support the use of vasoconstrictors and antihistamines in AOM (136).

Corticosteroids

It is believed that virus-induced host inflammatory response in the nasopharynx plays a key role in the pathogenesis of AOM. In theory, suppression of this inflammatory process might prevent the development of AOM as a complication of a common cold. Ruohola et al. (137) tested this hypothesis by treating 210 children with a common cold with either intranasal fluticasone propionate or placebo, starting within 48 h after the first cold symptoms. The results clearly showed that intranasal corticosteroid treatment does not prevent the development of AOM. On the contrary, children infected with RV developed AOM in 46% in the fluticasone propionate group and in 15% in the placebo group ($p = 0.005$).

In children with chronic middle ear effusion a single placebo-controlled study has shown that intranasal beclomethasone dipropionate improved middle ear pressure ($p = 0.004$) and gave a quicker resolution of middle ear effusions at 4 and 8 weeks ($p = 0.05$) (138).

Intranasal Interferon-β

In a study of adults with an experimental RV infection, treatment with interferon-β nose drops reduced the number of abnormal middle ear pressures from 38% to 18% (139), indicating that antiviral therapy may alter the course of middle-ear dysfunction associated with experimental RV colds.

G. Otitis Media with Effusion

Otitis media with effusion often follows an AOM which, as a rule, is initiated by a viral respiratory tract infection. In a study of 100 children with otitis media with effusion virus was detected in middle ear fluid in 30 of the children (RV in 19, RSV in 8, and coronavirus in 3) (140). It is concluded that virus is present in a larger percentage of these children than previously suspected. A single study has indicated that intranasal corticosteroid treatment may be useful in the treatment of otitis media with effusion (138).

H. Conclusions

A viral infection usually precedes a bacterial AOM. Virus, predominantly RV, can be identified by sensitive methods (PCR and RT-PCR) in a large proportion of affected middle ears. It is now well established that the viral infection itself can cause abnormal middle ear pressure, and that a viral otitis media resolves spontaneously without antibiotic treatment. However, it is not known by which mechanisms the viral infection can predispose to an AOM.

VII. Relationship Between Common Cold and Asthma Exacerbations

A. Magnitude of the Problem

Clinical experience has indicated that a viral airway infection precedes the majority of acute episodes of wheezing in infants and children, and that it also is an important cause of exacerbations of asthma in adults (141).

The study of the association between viral airway infections and wheezy episodes/exacerbations of asthma has been hampered by the lack of sensitive diagnostic tests for virus infection (142). More recently, the very sensitive PCR and RT-PCR techniques have been used in clinical studies.

Johnston and co-workers (143) studied 108, children aged 9–11 years with asthma. In more than 80% of the episodes with wheezing and reduced peak flow, polymerase chain reaction PCR on respiratory secretions was positive for virus, and this was RV in two-thirds of the cases. Thus, this study showed that at least 80% of reported exacerbations of asthma in schoolchildren are associated with an upper airway infection, mainly caused by RV.

Nicholson and co-workers (144) studied the role of a common cold in exacerbations of asthma in 138 adults in a longitudinal study. The patients reported clinical colds in 80% of episodes with asthma symptoms. A virus was identified in 57% of subjects with symptomatic colds, and in these cases RV was found in 64% and coronavirus in 30%. Thus, at least half of the asthma exacerbations are associated with a virus infection, predominantly with RV.

Atmar et al. (145) studied 122 adult patients admitted to the hospital with acute exacerbations of asthma. The exacerbation was associated with a viral infection in 55% RT-PCR. RV, coronavirus, and influenza virus were the most frequently identified causes.

In conclusion, recent studies using the highly sensitive PCR technique have indicated that a viral airway infection, mainly with RV, is an important precipitator of asthma episodes both in children and in adults, and that this connection is even more important than believed earlier.

B. Lower Airways in Naturally Acquired Colds

While studies have convincingly shown that colds can increase asthma severity, there is little information on the direct effect of a naturally acquired virus infection on the pathology of the lower airways.

Trigg and co-workers (146) studied whether naturally acquired colds increase lower airway inflammation in nonasthmatic subjects. Twenty subjects (12 normal persons, 8 atopics and 4 of these rhinitics) had bronchoscopy before and during a cold. A viral infection was diagnosed in eight of the subjects (six normal and two atopics). In bronchial biopsies, during the colds, eosinophils and $CD8^+$ T cells increased significantly and neutrophils increased in bronchial washings.

The authors conclude that lower airway inflammation is present in subjects with a cold, and that many subjects with symptoms traditionally thought to indicate upper airway infection have evidence of lower airway inflammation. However, the atopic subjects in this study had more activated eosinophils and fewer positive virological tests than the nonatopic controls, which raises a question about the validity of the study. Symptoms of a virus cold and of allergic rhinitis are similar, and allergic subjects may have reported symptoms of allergic inflammation as a cold.

In a study of children with virus-induced asthma exacerbations, Teran et al. (147) found an increased level of eosinophil chemoattractants (regulated on activation, normal T-cell expressed and secreted [RANTES], migration inhibition factor [MIF-1]) and of the eosinophil major basic protein (MBP) in nasal secretions. In another study of 70 wheezing children admitted to the emergency room, Rakes et al. (148) found an RSV infection in 82% of infants (<2 year) and an RV infection in 71% of children (>2 year). There were strong odds for wheezing in infected children who also had a positive radioallergosorbent test (RAST), nasal eosinophilia, or elevated nasal eosinophil cationic protein (ECP).

Induced sputum can be used as a clinically accessible method to measure the inflammatory response in the lower airways to a viral respiratory tract infection (149).

C. Lower Airways in Experimental Rhinovirus Infection

A number of studies have investigated experimental RV infection, lower airway inflammation, and bronchial responsiveness. In these studies virus inoculation has been performed using standard methods. The inoculum is dripped or sprayed into the nasal cavity, which makes bronchial deposition of the virus unlikely. RV 16 (150–152) and RV 39 (153) have been used.

Enhanced Bronchial Inflammation

Bronchoscopy studies during an experimental RV infection have shown an increase in mucosal $CD3^+$, $CD4^+$, and $CD8^+$ cells (43), in epithelial eosinophils (43), and in the concentration of ECP in induced sputum (152). The epithelial eosinophil numbers were elevated for a prolonged period in asthmatic volunteers (43), and there seems to be a positive correlation between the concentration of sputum ECP and the change in bronchial responsiveness (PC_{20} histamine) (154). While these results indicate that a viral infection can activate eosinophils in vivo, RV has little effect on eosinophil activation in vitro (155). The concentration of IL-6 and IL-8 in induced sputum is also increased during an experimental RV infection (152).

Based on these studies it has been hypothesized that an immunological response, involving T cells and eosinophils, may be responsible for the virus-induced increase in airway responsiveness in asthmatics (43), described below.

It is difficult to explain why RV, which primarily infects the upper airways and causes rhinitis symptoms, induces a T-cell/eosinophil inflammation in the bronchi but not in the nose.

Increased Bronchial Response to Histamine and Methacholine

Asthma symptoms are closely associated with bronchial hyperresponsiveness, making measurement of PC_{20} or PD_{20} to inhaled histamine or methacholine a useful parameter for studying the link between common cold and asthma.

Normal Subjects

Gern et al. (151) and Skoner et al. (153) did not find any change in nonspecific bronchial responsiveness during an experimental RV infection of normal volunteers.

Allergic Rhinitis

Lemanske and colleagues (150) studied 10 ragweed allergic subjects outside the pollen season. An RV infection resulted in a significantly increased bronchial responsiveness to histamine. Gern and co-workers (151) got a similar result in 18 subjects with a positive skin test to ragweed, cat, or housedust mite but without rhinitis symptoms. In contrast, Skoner et al. (153), in a study of 46 subjects with seasonal allergic rhinitis studied outside the pollen season, were unable to find any significant change in bronchial responsiveness during an RV infection. Thus, the results are conflicting, probably due to differences in the selection of patient populations (mild or severe rhinitis).

Allergic Asthma

Although Halperin and co-workers (156) found increased responsiveness to histamine in only 4 of 22 asthma subjects after experimental RV infection, three other studies of asthma patients have all shown a significant reduction in PC_{20} or PD_{20} to inhaled histamine or methacholine (42,43,152). The increase in bronchial responsiveness in these studies has been modest, which may be due to the selection of patients. For safety reasons, only patients with mild asthma have been studied. Grünberg et al. (152) found an increased bronchial responsiveness after RV inoculation in atopic asthmatics in conjunction with augmented airway inflammation, as reflected by an increase in ECP, IL-6, and IL-8 in sputum. The results suggest that the RV-enhanced airway hyperresponsiveness is associated with eosinophil inflammation.

Asthma patients who increase their bronchial sensitivity to nonspecific stimuli also do so to a specific challenge with allergen, especially demonstrated by an increased late-phase responsiveness (150).

Increased Bronchial Response to Antigen

Busse and colleagues (157–159) performed segmental bronchial provocation with allergen during bronchoscopy in volunteers with and without an experimental RV infection. During the viral infection there was an increased symptom response to the allergen challenge (both early and late response), an increased level of histamine and protein, and an increased number of eosinophils in bronchoalveolar lavage fluid. The authors conclude that these data show an increase in inflammatory response during the RV infection, which indicates that RV upregulates the inflammatory response to allergen, and this may be due to an increased generation of cytokines. The findings imply that viral infection and allergy have a synergistic effect on lower-airway inflammation.

Variable Airway Obstruction

It was shown by Grünberg et al. (160) that an experimental RV infection in asthmatics augments variable airway obstruction, which is a sign of active asthma. This observation favors a causative role for RV colds in asthma exacerbations, and is in keeping with RV-induced worsening of airway inflammation and hyperresponsiveness.

D. Mechanisms by Which Viruses Precipitate Asthma

A number of mechanisms have been proposed to explain how a common cold can induce asthma, but so far no explanation is satisfactory. In principle, a common cold can induce asthma exacerbations in two different ways: directly by a virus infection of the lower airways; and indirectly by an infection, limited to the upper airway, that by immunological and neurogenic mechanisms induces lower airway inflammation, hyperresponsiveness, and asthma symptoms.

E. Does Rhinovirus Infect the Lower Airways?

This is an important question for our understanding of the link between the common cold and asthma. Earlier, most evidence on the ability of RV and coronavirus to infect the lower airways was equivocal on the question (1). It has been difficult to determine whether virus growth occurs in the bronchi because of the problem of obtaining lower airway specimens that are not contaminated with nasopharyngeal secretions during sampling (156).

Several lines of evidence now point to the fact that RV may indeed replicate in the lower airways. Gern and co-workers (161) used RT-PCR to identify RV in bronchoalveolar lavage cells from volunteers inoculated intranasally with RV. The RT-PCR was positive in eight of eight inoculated volunteers, and negative in the controls. Although these results suggest that RV can infect the lower airways, it is necessary to remember that RT-PCR is an extremely sensitive test and that contamination from the upper airways cannot be completely excluded.

Stronger evidence that RV do replicate in the lower airways has now been provided by in situ hybridization studies showing presence of RV in bronchial biopsies from experimentally infected human volunteers (162).

Because RV have an optimum replication temperature at 33°C, this has been taken as an argument against replication in the lower airways. However, it has now been shown that RV can replicate in bronchial epithelial cell lines in vitro at 37°C (24).

F. Direct Effect of Lower Airway Infection on Asthma

Hypotheses have been advanced placing the bronchial epithelial cell in a central position. However, there are some problems with most of these hypotheses, described below. First, it is not known with certainty how often bronchial epithelial cells are infected by virus. Second, considering the minor cytopathological effect of RV and coronavirus on the epithelial lining in the nose and on epithelial cells in vitro, it seems unlikely that there are any marked structural and functional changes in the bronchial epithelium.

Cytokines

Epithelial cells are able to secrete a broad array of cytokines, as discussed earlier. In vitro studies indicate that RV induces secretion of IL-1, IL-6, IL-8, IL-11, RANTES, and granulocyte–macrophage colony-stimulating factor (GM-CSF) from epithelial cells (161). IL-11 is secreted in large amounts and may have a direct effect on bronchial hyperresponsiveness (163). Respiratory viruses have the ability to induce the release of cytokines also from other cell types. Balfour-Lynn and co-workers (164) reported that tumor necrosis factor-α, a proinflammatory cytokine produced primarily by mononuclear phagocytes, is detectable in nasopharyngeal secretions in three-quarters of infants with wheezing illness.

Mediators

Epithelial cells produce biochemical mediators, such as products of 15-lipoxygenase activity (15-HETEs and leukotriene B_4), that can directly contract bronchial smooth muscles (165).

Bronchodilator Factor

It has been reported that the airway epithelium is a source of a regulator protein (endogenous bronchodilator factor) with a protective role that maintains bronchial patency. Also it has been speculated that epithelial damage may reduce the synthesis of this protein, resulting in bronchoconstriction (166).

Neurogenic Inflammation

Based on rodent studies, it has been hypothesized that epithelial damage, by loss of neutral endopeptidase and reduced breakdown of neuropeptides, such as substance P, results in the development of neurogenic inflammation. However, neurogenic inflammation has not been described in humans.

Vagal Reflex

It seems reasonable to assume that perturbation of the surface epithelium may induce airway hyperresponsiveness by exposing sensory nerve endings to irritants and inflammatory mediators. This enhanced stimulation of afferent fibers may cause increased vagal activity and bronchoconstriction.

In addition, the M_2 muscarinic receptors on the vagal nerve endings, which normally inhibit acetylcholine release, are dysfunctional during a viral infection (167).

Antigen Absorption

It has long been believed that epithelial stripping aids penetration of antigens into the mucous membrane, but Greiff and co-workers (80) have now clearly shown that mucosal absorption of macromolecules is not increased during an infection with coronavirus.

Effect on Airway Smooth Muscle Responsiveness

Hakonarson et al. (168) inoculated human airway smooth muscle tissue with RV and found that it induced increased muscle constrictor responsiveness to acetylcholine and attenuated the dose–response relaxation of smooth muscles to beta$_2$-adrenoceptor stimulation. These RV-induced changes were largely prevented by pretreating the tissue with a monoclonal antibody to ICAM-1. The findings provide new evidence that RV directly induces asthma by changed smooth muscle responsiveness and that this effect is triggered by binding of RV to the ICAM-1 receptor.

G. Indirect Effect of Upper Airway Infection on Asthma

In theory, an indirect effect from an RV infection, limited to the upper airways, can be mediated by the following mechanisms: impaired nasal physiology; a nasobronchial reflex; aspiration of infectious secretions; and absorption of cytokines and mediators, causing recruitment and activation of immune cells, which may have an effect not only in the nose but also in the lower airways, as well as in other parts of the body. We find the last possibility most likely. A systemic effect of an RV cold on host defense factors is supported by the observation that a common cold not only induces an exacerbation of asthma but also can reactivate a herpes infection on the lip.

H. Does Allergy Predispose to Common Cold?

Increased Frequency

The Th1-cytokine interferon-γ induces a marked and persistent downregulation of ICAM-1 expression on RV-infected epithelial cells. The Th2-cytokine IL-13 and allergen exposure induce a marked upregulation of ICAM-1 (19,20,169). One can therefore speculate that antigen-stimulated persons are particularly suceptible to RV infections. However, it is an important counterargument that almost all normal sero-negative volunteers can be infected by experimental inoculation of RV (1). As in the nose, ICAM-1 is not constitutively expressed by surface epithelial cells in the bronchi, but it is upregulated in symptomatic asthma (170). In theory, this could make asthmatic bronchial airways more sensitive than normal airways to direct infection with RV. However, there are no data in support of this hypothesis, and it is not common clinical experience that allergic patients have more colds than normal persons. Because it can be difficult to differentiate between an attack of allergic rhinitis and a viral infection, modern and sensitive diagnostic virus tests (RT-PCR) are necessary in studies of the frequency of RV infections in atopic and in nonatopic individuals.

Increased Severity

One can also speculate that allergic rhinitis, associated with upregulation of ICAM-1 and with the presence of inflammatory cells in the surface epithelium, leads to more cold symptoms during a virus infection, because it is amplified by concurrent inflammation.

Some support for this hypothesis comes from a study by Bardin and co-workers (25), who inoculated 11 volunteers (5 atopic and 6 asthmatic patients) with RV. The authors conclude that the results "suggest heightened suceptibility to the detrimental effects of a cold in the atopic/asthmatic patients." However, Doyle and co-workers (79) found that experimentally induced RV colds are clinically similar in normal and in allergic subjects.

Hinriksdottir (171) studied 64 patients with allergic rhinitis and 23 nonallergic individuals who recorded symptoms of upper airway infections for 1 year. There was no difference between the two groups in the number of upper airway infections or the duration of the disease.

Together, these studies indicate that allergic rhinitis cannot be considered to increase the frequency or the severity of upper respiratory infections.

I. Prevention and Treatment of Common Cold-Induced Asthma

Reduced Transmission

When mothers who had been exposed to a child with a common cold at home regularly dipped their fingers in 2% aqueous iodine, the number of new colds was reduced by 67% (5). Another study of the hand-contact route of cold transmission was performed under natural conditions in asthmatic children (172). One group of children was trained to avoid self-inoculatory (finger/nose) behavior and were then compared with untrained controls. Following the training period, the groups were evaluated for several months during which time the trained group had significantly less self-inoculatory behavior, fewer viral respiratory infections, and fewer attacks of asthma.

Washing hands after an infectious contact can be recommended, as well as avoiding finger-to-eye and finger-to-nose contact. As an alternative right-handed asthmatics could touch their eyes and nose only with the left hand, adapting the practice of using a clean hand for this purpose and a dirty hand for contact with the surroundings.

The high frequency of respiratory tract viral infections suggests that strategies for the prevention of viral infections should be targeted to the asthmatic population. It is possible that an asthmatic mother with a small child, in the future may be able to reduce the number of asthma exacerbations by use of an antiviral hand lotion, or an intranasal interferon-α spray when the child gets cold symptoms. Finally, kindergartens are not suitable places for patients with severe asthma, either children or adults.

Corticosteroids

It is general practice, recommended in international consensus reports (173), to treat severe exacerbations of asthma with corticosteroids in a high dosage. A rationale for this is a reduced sensitivity of T cells to corticosteroid treatment during a common cold (47). An in vitro study has shown that corticosteroid treatment of epithelial cells prevents the RV-induced increased expression of ICAM-1 (174), while another study has failed to show this effect (175).

Most but not all placebo-controlled trials have shown a beneficial effect of corticosteroids in treating acute severe asthma (176). Although airway infections, including common colds, are known to be important causes of asthma exacerbations, there does not seem to be any placebo-controlled study on the use of corticosteroids in this specific situation. A Medline search of published articles gave the following number of publications: asthma 61,043; asthma and corticosteroid 4,377; asthma and common cold (or RV) 123; asthma and common cold (or RV) and corticosteroid 5.

In an open study of preschool children who experienced repeated asthma attacks related to upper airway infections, Brunette and co-workers (177) found that a short burst of oral prednisone (1 mg/kg), given as soon as the first symptoms of an infection appeared, resulted in a significant decrease in the number of wheezing days and visits to the emergency room.

More recently, Doull and co-workers (178) performed a double-blind study of the prophylactic effect of inhaled beclomethasone dipropionate (400 µg/day) on wheezing episodes associated with viral infection in 104 children aged 7–9 years. Although there was a significant increase in forced expiratory volume in 1 s (FEV_1) and in methacholine PD_{20}, the authors conclude that the treatment offered no clinically significant benefit on the wheezing episodes.

Because of the limited effect of corticosteroids during virus-induced asthma exacerbations, new therapeutic interventions need to be developed based on the increasing pathophysiological knowledge about the role of viruses in asthma. Recent in vitro data have shown an RV-induced downregulation of glucocorticoid receptors on peripheral lymphocytes (Pontus Stierna, personal communication), which may explain the relative resistance to this treatment in viral-induced asthma exacerbations.

J. Conclusions

Studies of the link between a common cold and asthma are few and our knowledge is remarkably insufficient, considering the important clinical significance of this issue. We have shown that RV and coronavirus, in contrast to influenza virus, parainfluenza virus, and adenovirus, cause little damage to epithelial cells in the airways. It remains to be established whether an RV infection causes wheezing by a direct infection of the lower airways or by alternative mechanisms through which an upper airway infection can cause changes in lower airway function. It is hypothesized that virus-induced generation of cytokines, mainly by epithelial cells, amplifies the T-cell-driven eosinophil inflammation in asthma. But it is unclear how the virus-induced inflammation, characterized by a Th1-type cytokine response, enhances inflammation in asthma, characterized by a Th2-type cytokine response. Considering the hypothesis that the common cold is a virus-induced and cytokine-driven disease, it is remarkable that corticosteroids have no or little effect on the nasal symptoms of a common cold. Clinical experience shows that corticosteroids have a beneficial effect on common cold-induced asthma exacerbations, but placebo-controlled studies have not clearly shown this to be the case. Intervention studies are needed to show whether attempts at stopping virus transmission to asthma patients can reduce the number of colds and asthma exacerbations.

References

1. Gwaltney JM Jr, Ruckert RR. Rhinovirus. In: Richman DD, Whitley RJ, Hayden FG, eds. Clinical Virology. New York: Churchill Livingstone, 1997:1025–1047.
2. Johnston SL, Sanderson G, Pattemore PK, et al. Use of polymerase chain reaction for diagnosis of picornavirus infection in subjects with and without respiratory symptoms. J Clin Microbiol 1993; 31:111–117.
3. Arruda E, Pitkäranta A, Witek TJ Jr, Doyle CA, Hayden FG. Frequency and natural history of rhinovirus infections in adults during autumn. J Clin Microbiol 1997; 35: 2864–2868.

4. Rossman MG, Palmenberg AC. Conservation of the putative receptor attachment site in picornaviruses. Virol 1988; 164:373–382.
5. Hendley JO, Gwaltney JM Jr. Mechanisms of transmission of rhinovirus infection. Epidemiol Rev 1988; 10:242–258.
6. Dingle JH, Badger GF, Jordan WS Jr. Illness in the Home. A Study of 25,000 Illnesses in a Group of Cleveland Families. Cleveland: The Press of Western Reserve University, 1964.
7. Tos M. Distribution of mucus producing elements in the respiratory tract. Differences between upper and lower airways. Eur J Respir Dis 1983; 64(suppl 128):269–279.
8. Hendley JO, Gwaltney JM Jr, Jordan WS Jr. Rhinovirus infections in an industrial population. IV. Infections within families of employees during two fall peaks of respiratory illness. Am J Epidem 1969; 89:184–196.
9. Gwaltney JM Jr, Moskalski PB, Hendley JO. Hand-to-hand transmission of colds. Ann Intern Med 1978; 88:463.
10. Gwaltney JM Jr, Moskalski PB, Hendley JO. Interruption of experimental rhinovirus transmission. J Infect Dis 1980; 142:811.
11. Gwaltney JM Jr, Hendley JO. Transmission of experimental rhinovirus infection by contaminated surfaces. Am J Epidemiol 1982; 116:828.
12. Hayden FG, Hendley JO, Gwaltney JM Jr. The effect of placebo and virucidal paper handkerchiefs on viral contamination of the hand and transmission of experimental rhinoviral infection. J Infect Dis 1985; 152:403.
13. Gern JE, Galagan DM, Jarjour NN, Dick EC, Busse WW. Detection of rhinovirus RNA in lower airway cells during experimentally induced infection. Am J Respir Crit Care Med 1997; 155:1159–1161.
14. Østberg B, Winther B, Mygind N. Cold air-induced rhinorrhea and high-dose ipratropium. Arch Otorhinolaryngol 1987; 113:160–162
15. Winther B, Gwaltney JM Jr, Mygind N, Turner RB, Hendley JO. Sites of rhinovirus recovery after point-inoculation of the upper airways. JAMA 1986; 256:1763–1767.
16. Arruda E, Mifflin TE, Gwaltney JM, Winther B, Hayden FG. Localization of rhinovirus replication in vitro with in situ hybridization. J Med Virol 1991; 34:38–44.
17. Greve JM, Davis G, Mayer AM. The major human rhinovirus receptor is ICAM-1. Cell 1989; 56:839.
18. Papi A, Johnston S. Rhinovirus infection induces expression of its own receptor, intercellular adhesion molecule-1 (ICAM-1) via increased NF-kappaB-mediated transcription. J Biol Chem 1999; 274:9707–9720.
19. Ciprandi G, Pronzato C, Ricca V, Bagnasco M, Canonica GW. Evidence of intracellular adhesion molecule-1 expression on nasal epithelial cells in acute rhinoconjunctivitis caused by pollen exposure. J Allergy Clin Immunol 1994; 99:738–746.
20. Bianco A, Whiteman SC, Sethi SK, Allen JT, Knight RA, Spiteri MA. Expression of intercellular adhesion molecule-1 (ICAM-1) in nasal epithelial cells of atopic subjects: a mechanism for increased rhinovirus infection? Clin Exp Allergy 2000; 121:339–345.
21. Winther B, Greve JM, Gwaltney JM Jr, Innes DJ, Eastman RJ, McClelland A, Hendley JO. Surface expression of ICAM-1 on epithelial cells in the human adenoid. J Infect Dis 1997; 176:523–525.
22. Arruda E, Boyle TR, Winther B, Pevear DC, Gwaltney JM Jr, Hayden FG. Localization of human rhinovirus replication in the upper respiratory tract by in situ hybridization. J Infect Dis 1995; 171:1329–1333.
23. Turner RB, Hendley JO, Gwaltney JM Jr. Shedding of infected ciliated epithelial cells in rhinovirus colds. J Infect Dis 1982; 145:849.

24. Bates PJ, Johnston SL. Common colds and respiratory viruses. In: Busse WW, Holgate ST, eds. Asthma and Rhinitis. Oxford: Blackwell Science, 2000:1481–1492.

25. Bardin PG, Johnston SL, Sanderson G, Robinson BS, Pickett MA, Fraenkel DJ, Holgate ST. Detection of rhinovirus infection of the nasal mucosa by oligonucleotide in situ hybridization. Am J Respir Cell Mol Biol 1994; 10:207–213.

26. Turner RB, Winther B, Hendley JO, Mygind N, Gwaltney JM Jr. Sites of virus recovery and antigen detection in epithelial cells during experimental rhinovirus infection. Acta Otolaryngol (Stockh) 1984; suppl 413:9–14.

27. Winther B, Gwaltney JM Jr, Hendley JO. Respiratory virus infection of monolayer cultures of human nasal epithelial cells. Am Rev Respir Dis 1990; 141:839–845.

28. Hoorn B, Tyrrell DA. Effects of some viruses on ciliated cells. Am Rev Respir Dis 1966; 93:156–161.

29. Becker S, Soukup J, Yankaskas JR. Respiratory syncytial virus infection of human primary nasal and bronchial epithelial cell cultures and bronchoalveolar macrophages. Am J Respir Cell Mol Biol 1992; 6:369–374.

30. Hilding A. The common cold. Arch Otolaryngol 1930; 12:133–150.

31. Winther B, Brofeldt S, Christensen B, Mygind N. Light and scanning electron microscopy of nasal biopsy material from patients with naturally acquired common colds. Acta Otolaryngol (Stockh) 1984; 97:309–318.

32. Winther B, Brofeldt S, Grønborg H, Mygind N, Pedersen M, Vejlsgaard R. Study of bacteria in the nasal cavity and nasopharynx during naturally acquired common colds. Acta Otolaryngol (Stockh) 1984; 98:315–320.

33. Carson JL, Collier AM, Hu SS. Acquired ciliary defects in nasal epithelium of children with acute viral upper respiratory infections. N Engl J Med 1985; 312:463–468.

34. Persson PGA. Asthma the important questions: epithelial cells, barrier functions and shedding-restitution mechanisms. Am J Respir Crit Care Med 1998; 153:100–106.

35. Pedersen M, Sakakura Y, Winther B, Brofeldt S, Mygind N. Nasal mucociliary transport, number of ciliated cells, and beating pattern in naturally acquired common colds. Eur Respir J 1983; 64(suppl 128):355–364.

36. Bryan WTK, Bryan MP, Smith CA. Human ciliated epithelial cells in nasal secretions. Ann Otol Rhinol Laryngol 1964; 73:474.

37. Afzelius B. Ultrastructure of human nasal epithelium during an episode of coronavirus infection. Virch Arch 1994; 424:295–300.

38. Winther B, Farr B, Turner RB, Hendley JO, Gwaltney JM Jr, Mygind N. Histopathologic examination and enumeration of polymorphonuclear leukocytes in the nasal mucosa during experimental rhinovirus colds. Acta Otolaryngol (Stockh) 1984; (Suppl 413):19–24.

39. Fraenkel DJ, Bardin PG, Sanderson G, Lampe F, Johnston SL, Holgate ST. Immunohistochemical analysis of nasal biopsies during rhinovirus experimental colds. Am J Respir Crit Care Med 1994; 150:1130–1136.

40. Naclerio RM, Proud D, Lichtenstein LM, Kagey-Sobotka A, Hendley JO, Sorrentino J, Gwaltney JM Jr. Kinins are generated during experimental rhinovirus colds. J Infect Dis 1988; 157:133–142.

41. Levandowski RA, Ou DW, Jackson GG. Acute-phase decrease of T-lymphocyte subsets in rhinovirus infection. J Infect Dis 1986; 153:743–748.

42. Cheung D, Dick EC, Timmers MC, de Klerk EPA, Spaan WJM, Sterk PJ. Rhinovirus inhalation causes long-lasting excessive airway narrowing in response to methacholine in asthmatic subjects in vivo. Am J Respir Crit Care Med 1995; 152:1490–1496.

43. Fraenkel DJ, Bardin PG, Sanderson G, Lampe F, Johnston SL, Holgate ST. Lower

airways inflammation during rhinovirus colds in normal and asthmatic subjects. Am J Respir Crit Care Med 1995; 151:879–886.

44. Folkert G, Busse WW, Nijkamp FP, Sorkness R, Gern JE. Virus-induced airway hyper-responsiveness and asthma. Am Rev Respir Crit Care Med 1998; 157:1708–1720.

45. Winther B, Innes DF, Bratsch J, Hayden FG. Lymphocyte subsets in the nasal mucosa and peripheral blood during experimental rhinovirus infection. Am J Rhinol 1992; 6: 149–156.

46. Skoner DP, Whiteside TL, Wilson JW, Doyle WJ, Herberman RB, Fireman P. Effect of rhinovirus 39 infection on cellular immune parameters in allergic and nonallergic subjects. J Allergy Clin Immunol 1993; 92:732–743.

47. Vianna EO, Westcott J, Martin RJ. The effects of upper respiratory infection on T-cell proliferation and steroid sensitivity in asthmatics. J Allergy Clin Immunul 1998; 102:592–597.

48. Winther B. The effect on the nasal mucosa of respiratory viruses (common cold). Dan Med Bull 1994; 41:193–204.

49. Subauste MC, Jacoby DB, Richards SM, Proud D. Infection of a human respiratory epithelial cell line with rhinovirus. Induction of cytokine release and modulation of susceptibility to infection by cytokine exposure. J Clin Invest 1995; 96:549–557.

50. Zhu Z, Tang W, Gwaltney JM Jr, Elias JA. Rhinovirus stimulation of interleukin-8 in vivo and in vitro: role of NF-κB. Am J Physiol 1997; 273:L814–824.

51. Turner RB. Rhinovirus infection of human embryonic lung fibroblast induces the production of a chemoattractant for polymorphonuclear leukocytes. J Infect Dis 1988; 157:346–350.

52. Röseler S, Holtappels G, Wagenmann M, Bachert C. Elevated levels of interleukins IL-1beta, IL-6 and IL-8 in naturally acquired viral rhinitis. Eur Arch Otorhinolaryngol 1995; 252 (Suppl 1):S61–S63.

53. Noah TL, Henderson FW, Wortman IA, Devlin RB, Handy J, Koren HS, Becker S. Nasal cytokine production in viral acute upper respiratory infection of childhood. J Infect Dis 1995; 171:584–592.

54. Turner RB, Weingand KW, Yeh CH, Leedy DW. Association between interleukin-8 concentration in nasal secretions and severity of symptoms of experimental rhinovirus colds. Clin Infect Dis 1998; 26:840–846.

55. Choi AMK, Jacoby DB. Influenza virus A infection induces interleukin-8 gene expression in human airway epithelial cells. FEBS Letts 1992; 309:327–329.

56. Kenney JS, Baker C, Welch MR, Altman LC. Synthesis of interleukin-1 alpha, interleukin-6, and interleukin-8 by cultured human nasal epithelial cells. J Allergy Clin Immunol 1994; 93:1060–1067.

57. Proud D, Gwaltney JM Jr, Hendley JO, Dinarello CA, Gillis S, Schleimer RP. Increased levels of interleukin-1 are detected in nasal secretions of volunteers during experimental rhinovirus colds. J Infect Dis 1994; 169:1007–1013.

58. Zhu Z, Tang W, Ray A, Wu Y, Einarsson O, Landry M, Gwaltney JM Jr, Elias JA. Rhinovirus stimulation of interleukin-6 in vivo and in vitro: Evidence for NFκB-dependent transcriptional activation. J Clin Invest 1996; 97:421–430.

59. Cheung D, Hiemstra PS, Dick EC, de Klerk EPA, Sterk PJ. Effects of experimental rhinovirus infection on IL-8 in nasal washings in asthmatic subjects in vivo. Eur Respir J 1994; 7:481s.

60. Teran L, Johnston S, Shute J, Church M, Holgate S. Increased levels of interleukin-8 in nasal aspirates of children with viral associated asthma. J Allergy Clin Immunol 1994; 93:272.

61. Lau L, Corne J, Scott S, Davies R, Friend E, Howarth P. Nasal cytology in the common cold. Am J Respir Crit Care Med 1996; 153:A697.

62. Muraguchi A, Hirano T, Tang B, Matsuda T, Horii Y, Nakajima K, Kishimoto K. The essential role of B cell stimulatory factor 2 (BSF-2/IL-6) for the terminal differentiation of B cells. J Exp Med 1988; 167:332–344.

63. Linden M, Greiff L, Andersson M, Svensson C, Åkerlund A, Bende M, Andresson E, Persson CGA. Nasal cytokines in common cold and allergic rhinitis. Clin Exp Allergy 1995; 25:166–172.

64. Proud D, Naclerio RM, Gwaltney JM Jr, Hendley JO. Kinins are generated in nasal secretions during natural rhinovirus colds. J Infect Dis 1990; 161:120–123.

65. Proud D, Reynolds CJ, Lacapra S, Kagey-Sobotka A, Lichtenstein LM, Naclerio RM. Nasal provocation with bradykinin induces symptoms of rhinitis and a sore throat. Am Rev Respir Dis 1988; 137:613–616.

66. Eggleston PA, Hendley JO, Gwaltney JM Jr, Eggleston AW, Leavell BS Jr. Histamine in nasal secretions. In Arch Allergy Appl Immunol 1978; 57:193–200.

67. Naclerio RM, Proud D, Kagey-Sobotka A, Lichtenstein LM, Hendley JO, Gwaltney JM Jr. Is histamine responsible for the symptoms of rhinovirus colds? A look at the inflammatory mediators following infection. Pediatr Infect Dis J 1988; 7:218–222.

68. Igarashi Y, Skoner DP, Fireman P, Kaliner MA. Analysis of nasal secretions during experimental rhinovirus upper respiratory infections. J Allergy Clin Immunol 1993; 92:722–731.

69. Smith MB, Feldman W. Over-the-counter cold medications. A critical review of clinical trial between 1950 and 1991. JAMA 1993; 269:2258–2263.

70. Eccles R, van Cauwenberge P, Tetzloff W, Borum P. A clinical study to evaluate the efficacy of the antihistamine doxylamine succinate in the relief of runny nose and sneezing associated with upper respiratory tract infection. J Pharm Pharmacol 1995; 47:990–993.

71. Gwaltney JM Jr, Park J, Paul RA, Edelman DA, O'Connor RR, Turner RB. Randomized controlled trial of clemastine fumarate for treatment of experimental rhinovirus colds. Clin Infect Dis 1996; 22:656–662.

72. Gwaltney JM Jr, Druce HM. Efficacy of brompheniramine maleate treatment for rhinovirus colds. Clin Infect Dis 1997; 25:1188–1194.

73. Bisgaard H, Olsson P, Bende M. Effect of leukotriene D4 on nasal mucosal blood flow, nasal airway resistance and nasal secretion in humans. Clin Allergy 1986; 16:289–298.

74. Lundgren JD, Shelhammer JH. Pathogenesis of airway mucus hypersecretion. J Allergy Clin Immunol 1990; 85:399–417.

75. Doyle WJ, Boehm S, Skoner DP. Physiologic response to intranasal dose-response challenge with histamine, methacholine, bradykinin, and prostaglandin in adult volunteers with and without nasal allergy. J Allergy Clin Immunol 1990; 86:924–935.

76. Sperber SJ, Hendley JO, Hayden FG, Riker DK, Sorrentino JV, Gwaltney GM Jr. Effects of naproxen on experimental rhinovirus colds. Ann Intern Med 1992; 117:37.

77. Winther B, Mygind N. Placebo-controlled trial of the effect of ibuprofen on the symptoms of naturally acquired common cold. Am J Rhinol 2001; 15:239–242.

78. Grønborg H, Borum P, Winther B, Mygind N. Nasal methacholine and histamine reactivity during a common cold. Eur J Respir Dis 1983; 64(suppl 128):406–408.

79. Doyle WJ, Skoner DP, Seroky JT, Fireman P, Gwaltney JM. Effect of experimental rhinovirus 39 infection on the nasal response to histamine and cold air challenges in allergic and nonallergic subjects. J Allergy Clin Immunol 1994; 93:534–542.

80. Greiff L, Andersson M, Åkerlund A, Wollmer P, Svensson C, Alkner U, Persson CGA. Microvascular exudative hyperresponsiveness in human coronavirus-induced common cold. Thorax 1994; 49:121–127.

81. Persson CGA, Andersson M, Greiff L, Svensson C, Erjefält JS, Sundler F, Wollmer P, Erjefält I, Gustafsson B. Airway permeability. Clin Exp Allergy 1995; 25:807–814.

82. Grønborg H, Winther B, Brofeldt S, Mygind N. Effects of oral norephedrine on common cold symptoms. Rhinology 1983; 21:3–12.

83. Åkerlund A, Klint T, Olén L, Rundcrantz H. Nasal decongestant effect of oxymethazoline in the common cold: An objective dose–response study in 106 patients. J Laryngol Otol 1989; 103:743–746.

84. Sperber SJ, Sorrentino JV, Riker DK, Hayden FG. Evaluation of an alpha agonist alone and in combination with a nonsteroidal antiinflammatory agent in the treatment of experimental rhinovirus colds. Bull NY Acad Med 1989; 65:145–160.

85. Borum P, Olsen L, Winther B, Mygind N. Ipratropium nasal spray: A new treatment for rhinorrhea in the common cold. Am Rev Respir Dis 1981; 123:418–420.

86. Farr BM, Gwaltney JM Jr, Hendley JO, Hayden FG, Naclerio RM, McBride T, Doyle WJ, Sorrentino JV, Riker DK, Proud D. A randomized controlled trial of glucocorticoid prophylaxis against experimental rhinovirus infection. J Infect Dis 1990; 162:1173–1177.

87. Puhakka T, Makela MJ, Malmström K, Uhari M, Savolainen J, Terho EO, Pulkkinen M, Ruuskanen O. The common cold: effect of intranasal fluticasone propionate treatment. J Allergy Clin Immunol 1998; 101:726–731.

88. Gustafson LM, Proud D, Hendley JO, Hayden FG, Gwaltney JM Jr. Oral prednisone therapy in experimental rhinovirus infections. J Allergy Clin Immunol 1996; 97:1009–1014.

89. Holm AF, Fokkens WJ, Godthelp T, Mulder PGH, Vroom TH, Rijnges E. Effect of 3 months nasal steroid therapy on T cells and Langerhans cells in patients suffering from allergic rhinitis. Allergy 1995; 50:204–209.

90. Hayden FG, Albrecht JK, Kaiser DL, Gwaltney JM Jr. Prevention of natural colds by contact prophylaxis with intranasal alpha2-interferon. N Engl J Med 1986; 314:71.

91. Hayden FG, Gwaltney JM Jr. Intranasal interferon-alpha$_2$ treatment of experimental rhinoviral colds. J Infect Dis 1984; 150:174–180.

92. Gwaltney JM Jr. Combined antiviral and antimediator treatment of rhinovirus colds. J Infect Dis 1992; 166:776–782.

93. Hallsworth PG, McDonald PJ. Rapid diagnosis of viral infections with fluorescent antisera. Pathology 1985; 17:629–632.

94. Elnifro EM, Cooper RJ, Klapper PE, Yeo AC, Tullo AB. Multiplex polymerase chain reaction for diagnosis of viral and chlamydial keratoconjunctivitis. Invest Ophthalmol Vis Sci 2000; 41:1818–1822.

95. Canonica GW, Ciprandi G, Pesce GP, Buscaglia S, Paolieri F, Bagnasco W. ICAM-1 on epithelial cells in allergic subjects: a hallmark of allergic inflammation. Int Arch Allergy Immunol 1995; 107:99–102.

96. Spector SL, Bernstein IL, Li JT, Berger WE, Kaliner MA, Schuller DE, et al. Sinusitis practice parameters. Complete guidelines and references. J Allergy Clin Immunol 1998; 102:S117–144.

97. Turner RW, Cail WS, Hendley JO, Gwaltney JM Jr, et al. Physiologic abnormalities in the paranasal sinuses during experimental rhinovirus colds. J Allergy Clin Immunology 1992; 90:474–478.

98. Gwaltney JM Jr, Phillips CD, Miller RD, Riker DK. Computed tomographic study of the common cold. N Engl J Med 1994; 330:25–30.

99. Puhakka T, Mäkelä J, Alanen A, Kallio T, Korsoff L, Arstila P, et al. Sinusitis in the common cold. J Allergy Clin Immunol 1998; 102:403–408.

100. Shopfner CE, Rossi JO. Roentgen evaluation of paranasal sinuses in children. Am J Roentgenol Radium Ther Nucl Med 1973; 118;176–186.

101. Winther B, Schwartz R, Pitkäranta, et al. Computerized thomography (CT) imaging of paranasal sinuses and microbiology in children with acute purulent rhinorrhea. Proceedings of the 7th International Congress of Pediatric Otorhinolaryngology 1998, Helsinki, Finland.

102. Pitkäranta A, Arruda F, Malmberg H, Hayden FG. Detection of rhinovirus in sinus brushings of patients with acute community-acquired sinusitis by reverse transcription-PCR. J Clin Microbiol 1997; 35:1791–1793.

103. van Cauwenberge P, Ingels K. Effects of viral and bacterial infection on nasal and sinus mucosa. Acta Otolaryngol 1996; 116:316–321.

104. Kalliner MA, Osguthorpe JD, Fireman P, Anon J, Georgitis J, Davis ML, et al. Sinusitis: bench to bedside. Current findings, future directions. J Allergy Clin Immunol 1997; 99:S829–847.

105. Gwaltney JM Jr, Hendley JO, Phillips CD, Bass CR, Mygind N, Winther B. Nose blowing propels nasal fluids into the paranasal sinuses. Clin Infect Dis 2000; 30:387–391.

106. Berg O, Carenfeldt C. Analysis of symptoms and clinical signs in maxillary sinus empyema. Acta Otolaryngol (Stockh) 1988; 105:343–349.

107. Niehaus MD, Gwaltney JM Jr, Hendley JO, Newman MJ, Heymann PW, Rakes GP, Platts-Mills TA, Guerrant RL. Lactoferrin and eosinophil cationic protein in nasal secretions from patients with experimental rhinovirus colds, natural colds, and presumed acute community-acquired bacterial sinusitis. J Clin Microbiol 2000; 38:3100–3102.

108. Hueston WJ, Eberlein C, Johnston D, Mainous AG. Criteria used by clinicians to differentiate sinusitis from viral upper respiratory tract infections. J Fam Pract 1998; 46:487–492.

109. Gwaltney JM Jr, Scheld WM, Sande MA, Sydnor A. The microbial etiology and antimicrobial therapy of adults with acute community-acquired sinusitis: a fifteen-year experience at the University of Virginia and review of other selected studies. J Allergy Clin Immunol 1992; 90:457–461.

110. van Buchem FL, Knottnerus JA, Schrijnemaekers VJ, Peeters MF. Primary-care based randomised placebo-controlled trial of antibiotic treatment in acute maxillary sinusitis. Lancet 1997; 349:683.

111. Meltzer EO, Charous BL, Busse WW, Zinreich SJ, Lorber RR, Danzig M. Added relief in the treatment of acute recurrent sinusitis with adjunctive momethasone furoate nasal spray. J Allergy Clin Immunol 2000; 106:630–637.

112. Meltzer EO, Orgel HA, Backhaus JW, et al. Intranasal flunisolide spray as an adjunct to oral antibiotic therapy for sinusitis. J Allergy Clin Immunol 1993; 92:812–823.

113. Berlan IB, Erkan E, Bakir M, Berrak S, Basran MM. Intranasal budesonide spray as an adjunct to oral antibiotic therapy for acute sinusitis in children. Ann Allergy Asthma Immunol 1997; 78:598–601.

114. Bluestone CD. Treatment of otitis media with effusion. Scand J Infect Dis Suppl 1983; 39:26–33.

115. Buchman CA, Doyle WJ, Skoner D, Fireman P, Gwaltney JM. Otologic manifestations of experimental rhinovirus infection. Laryngoscope 1994; 104:1295–1299.

116. Doyle WJ, Alper CM, Buchman CA, Moody SA, Skoner DP, Cohen S. Illness and otological changes during upper respiratory virus infection. Laryngoscope 1999; 109:324–328.

117. Doyle WJ, Skoner DP, Hayden F, Buchman CA, Seroky JT, Fireman P. Nasal and otologic effects of experimental influenza A virus infection. Ann Otol Rhinol Laryngol 1994; 103:59–69.

118. Elkhatieb A, Hipskind G, Woerner D, Hayden FG. Middle ear abnormalities during natural rhinovirus colds in adults. J Infect Dis 1993; 168:618–621.

119. Pitkäranta A, Virolainen A, Jero J, Arruda E, Hayden FG. Detection of rhinovirus, respiratory syncytial virus, and coronavirus infections in acute otitis media by reverse transcriptase polymerase chain reaction. Pediatrics 1998; 102:291–295.

120. Heikkinen T, Thint M, Chonmaitree T. Prevalence of various respiratory virusus in the middle ear during acute otitis media. N Engl J Med 1999; 340:260–264.

121. Pitkäranta A, Hayden FG. Respiratory viruses in acute otitis media. Letter to the editor. N Engl J Med 1999; 340:2001–2002.

122. Chonmaitree T, Hendickson KJ. Detection of respiratory viruses in the middle ear fluids of children with acute otitis media by multiplex reverse transcription: polymerase chain reaction assay. Pediatr Infect Dis J 2000; 19:258–260.

123. Arola M, Ruuskanen O, Ziegler T, et al. Clinical role of respiratory virus infection in acute otitis media. Pediatrics 1990; 86:848–855.

124. Chonmaitree T, Heikkinen T. Role of viruses in middle-ear disease. Ann NY Acad Sci 1997; 830:143–157.

125. Buchman CA, Doyle WJ, Skoner D, Fireman P, Gwaltney JM. Otologic manifestations of experimental rhinovirus infection. Laryngoscope 1994; 104:1295–1299.

126. Ramilo O. Role of respiratory viruses in acute otitis media: implications for management. Pediatr Infect Dis J 1999; 18:1125–1129.

127. McCormick DP, Lim-Melia E, Saeed K, Baldwin CD, Chonmaitree T. Otitis media: can clinical findings predict bacterial or viral etiology? Pediatr Infect Dis J 2000; 19: 256–258.

128. Mygind N, Meistrup-Larsen K-I, Thomsen J, Thomsen JF, Josefsson K, Sørensen H. Penicillin in acute otitis media. A double-blind, placebo-controlled trial. Clin Otolaryngol 1981; 6:5–13.

129. Glaszion PP, Hayem M, Del Mar CB. Antibiotics for acute otitis media in children. Cochrane Database Syst Rev 2000; (2):CD000219.

130. Meistrup-Larsen, Mygind N, Thomsen J, Sørensen H, Vesterhauge S. Oral norephedrine in the treatment of acute otitis media. Results of a double-blind placebo-controlled trial. Acta Otolaryngol (Stockh) 1978; 86:248–250.

131. Schnore SK, Sangster JF, Gerace TM, Bass MJ. Are antihistamine-decongestants of value in the treatment of acute otitis media in children? J Fam Pract 1986; 22:39–43.

132. Chilton LA, Skipper BE. Antihistamines and alpha-adrenergic agents in treatment of otitis media. South Med J 1979; 72:953–955.

133. Bhambhani K, Foulds DM, Swany KN, Eldis FE, Fischel JE. Acute otitis media in children: are decongestants or antihistamines necessary? Ann Emerg Med 1983; 12:13–16.

134. Hayden F, Randall JE, Randall JC, Hendley JO. Topical phenylephrine for the treatment of middle ear effusion. Arch Otolaryngol 1984; 110:512–514.

135. Moran DM, Mutchie KD, Higbee MD, Paul LD. The use of an antihistamine-decongestant in conjunction with an anti-infective drug in the treatment of acute otitis media. J Pediatr 1982; 101:132–136.

136. Karma P, Palva T, Kouvalainen K, Karja J, Makela PH, Prinssi VP, Ruuskanen O, Launiala K. Finnish approach to the treatment of acute otitis media. Report of the Finnish Consensus Conference. Ann Oto Rhinol Laryngol Suppl 1987; 129:1–19.

137. Ruohola A, Heikkinen T, Waris M, Puhakka T, Ruuskanen O. Intranasal fluticasone

propionate does not prevent acute otitis media during viral upper respiratory tract infection in children. J Allergy Clin Immunol 2000; 106:467–471.

138. Tracy JM, Demain JG, Hoffman KM, Goetz DW. Intranasal beclomethasone as an adjunct to treatment of chronic middle ear effusion. Ann Allergy Asthma Immunol 1998; 80:198–206.

139. Sperber SJ, Doyle WJ, McBride TP, Sorrentino JV, Riker DK, Hayden FG. Otologic effects of interferon beta serine in experimental rhinovirus colds. Arch Otolaryngol Head Neck Surg 1992; 118:933–936.

140. Pitkäranta A, Jero J, Arruda E, Virolainen A, Hayden FG. Polymerase chain reaction-based detection of rhinovirus, respiratory syncytial virus, and coronavirus in otitis media with effusion. J Pediatr 1998; 133:390–394.

141. Pattemore PK, Johnston SL, Bardin PG. Viruses as precipitants of asthma symptoms. I. Epidemiology. Clin Exp Allergy 1992; 22:325–336.

142. Minor TE, Dick EC, Baker JW, Ouellette JJ, Cohen M, Reed CE. Rhinovirus and influenza type A infections as precipitants of asthma. Am Rev Respir Dis 1976; 113: 149–153.

143. Johnston S, Pattemore PK, Sanderson G, et al. Community study of role of viral infections in exacerbations of asthma in 9–11 year old children. Br Med J 1995; 310:1225–1229.

144. Nicholson KG, Kent J, Ireland DC. Respiratory viruses and exacerbations of asthma in adults. Br Med J 1993; 307:982–986.

145. Atmar RL, Guy E, Guntupalli HH, Zimmerman JL, Bandi VD. Respiratory tract viral infections in inner-city asthmatic adults. Arch Intern Med 1998; 158:2453–2459.

146. Trigg CJ, Nicholson KG, Wang JH, Ireland DC, Jordan S, Duddle JM, Hamilton S, Davies RJ. Bronchial inflammation and the common cold: a comparison of atopic and non-atopic individuals. Clin Exp Allergy 1996; 26:665.

147. Teran LM, Seminario MC, Shute JK, et al. RANTES, MIP-1 and the eosinophil product MBP are released into upper respiratory secretions during virus-induced asthma exacerbations in children. J Infect Dis 1999; 179:677–681.

148. Rakes GP, Arruda E, Ingram JM, Hoover GE, Zambrano JC, Hayden FG, Platts-Mills TAE, Heyman PW. Rhinovirus and respiratory syncytial virus in wheezing children requiring emergency care. Am J Respir Dis Crit Care Med 1999; 159:785–790.

149. Pizzichini MM, Pizzichini E, Efthimiadis A, Chauhan AJ, Johnston SL, Hussack P, Mahony J, Dolovich J, Hargreave FE. Asthma and natural colds. Inflammatory indices in induced sputum: a feasibility study. Am J Respir Crit Care Med 1998; 158:1178–1184.

150. Lemanske RF, Dick EC, Swenson CA, Vrtis RF, Busse WW. Rhinovirus upper respiratory infection increases airway hyperreactivity and late asthmatic reactions. J Clin Invest 1989; 83:1–10.

151. Gern JE, Calhoun W, Swenson C, Shen G, Busse WW. Rhinovirus infection preferentially increases lower airway responsiveness in allergic subjects. Am J Respir Crit Care 1997; 155:1872–1876.

152. Grünberg K, Timmers MC, Smits HH, et al. Effect of experimental rhinovirus 16 on airway hyperresponsiveness to histamine and interleukin-8 in nasal lavage in asthmatic subjects in vivo. Clin Exp Allergy 1997; 27:36–45.

153. Skoner DP, Doyle WJ, Seroky J, Van Deusen MA, Fireman P. Lower airway responses to rhinovirus 39 in healthy allergic and nonallergic subjects. Eur Respir J 1996; 9: 1402–1406.

154. Grünberg K, Smits HH, Timmers MC, et al. Experimental rhinovirus 16 infection.

Effects on cell differentials and soluble markers in sputum in asthmatic subjects. Am J Respir Crit Care Med 1997; 156:609–616.

155. Handzel ZT, Busse WW, Sedgwick JB, Vritris R, Lee WM, Kelley EAB, Gern JE. Eosinophils bind rhinovirus and activate virus-specific T cells. J Immunol 1998; 160: 1279–1284.

156. Halperin SA, Eggleston PA, Hendley JO, Gwaltney JM Jr, et al. Pathogenesis of lower respiratory tract symptoms in experimental rhinovirus infection. Am Rev Respir Dis 1983; 128:806.

157. Busse WW, Calhoun WJ, Dick EC. Effect of an experimental rhinovirus 16 infection on airway mediator response to antigen. Int Arch Allergy Immunol 1992; 99:422–424.

158. Calhoun WJ, Dick EC, Schwartz LB, Busse WW. A common cold, rhinovirus 16, potentiates airway inflammation after segmental antigen bronchoprovocation in allergic subjects. J Clin Invest 1994; 94:2200–2208.

159. Calhoun WJ, Swenson CA, Dick EC, Schwartz LB, Lemanske RF, Busse WW. Experimental rhinovirus 16 infections potentiates histamine release after antigen bronchoprovocation in allergic subjects. Am Rev Respir Dis 1991; 144:1267–1273.

160. Grünberg K, Timmers MC, de Klerk EP, Dick EC, Sterk PJ. Experimental rhinovirus 16 infection causes variable airway obstruction in subjects with atopic asthma. Am J Respir Crit Care Med 1999; 160:1375–1380.

161. Gern JE, Lemanske Jr RF, Busse WW. The role of rhinoviruses in virus-induced asthma. In: Marone G, Austen KF, Holgate ST, Kay AB, Lichtenstein LM, eds. Asthma and Allergic Diseases. San Diego: Academic Press, 1998:293–307.

162. Papadopoulos NG, Bates PJ, Bardin PG, et al. Rhinoviruses infect the lower airways. J Infect Dis 2000; 181:1875–1888.

163. Einarsson O, Geba GP, Zhu Z, Landry M, Elias JA Interleukin-11: stimulation in vivo and in vitro by respiratory virusus and induction of airways hyperresponsiveness. J Clin Invest 1996; 97:915–924.

164. Balfour-Lynn L, Valman H, Wellings R, et al. Tumour necrosis factor-α and leukotriene E4 production in wheezy infants. Clin Exp Allergy 1994; 24:121–126.

165. Shannon V, Chanez P, Bousquet J, et al. Histochemical evidence for induction of arachidonate 15-lipoxygenase in airways disease. Am Rev Respir Dis 1993; 147:1024–1028.

166. Butler GB, Adler KB, Evans JN. Modulation of rabbit airway smooth muscle responsiveness by respiratory epithelium. Am Rev Respir Dis 1987; 135:1099–2007.

167. Jacoby DB, Fryer AD. Interaction of viral infections with muscarinic receptors. Clin Exp Allergy 1999; 29(suppl 2):59–64.

168. Hakonarson H, Maskeri N, Carter C, Hodinka RL, Cambell D, Grünstein MM. Mechanisms of rhinovirus-induced changes in airway smooth muscle responsiveness. J Clin Invest 1998; 102:1732–1741.

169. Bianco A, Spiteri MA. A biological model to explain the association between human rhinovirus respiratory infections and bronchial asthma. Monaldi Arch Chest Dis 1998; 53:83–87.

170. Campell AM, Vignola AM, Chanez P. HLA-DR and ICAM-1 expression on bronchial epithelial cells in asthma and chronic bronchitis. Am Rev Respir Dis 1993; 148:689–694.

171. Hinriksdottir I, Melen I. Allergic rhinitis and upper respiratory tract infections. Acta Otolaryngol (Stockh) 1994; suppl 515:30–32.

172. Corley DL. Prevention of postinfectious asthma in children by reducing self-inoculatory behavior. J Pediatr Psychol 1987; 12:519–531.

173. McFadden Jr ER. Dosages of corticosteroids in asthma. Am Rev Respir Dis 1993; 147:1306–1310.
174. Papi A, Papadopoulos NG, Degitz K, Holgate ST, Johnston SL. Corticosteroids inhibit rhinovirus-induced intercellular adhesion molecule-1 up-regulation and promotor activation on respiratory epithelial cells. J Allergy Clin Immunol 2000; 105:318–326.
175. Grünberg K, Sharon RF, Hiltermann TJ, Brahim JJ, Dick EC, Sterk PJ, Van Krieken JH. Experimental rhinovirus 16 infection increases intercellular adhesion molecule-1 expression in bronchial epithelium of asthmatics regardless of inhaled steroid treatment. Clin Exp Allergy 2000; 30:1015–1023. 2000; 105:318–326.
176. Engel T, Heinig JH. Glucocorticoid therapy in acute severe asthma—a critical review. Eur Respir J 1991; 4:881–889.
177. Brunette MG, Lands L, Thibodeau LP. Childhood asthma: prevention of attacks with short-term corticosteroid treatment of upper airway respiratory tract infection. Pediatrics 1988; 81:624–629.
178. Doull IJM, Lampe FC, Smith S, Schreiber J, Freezer NJ, Holgate ST. Effect of inhaled corticosteroids on episodes of wheezing associated with viral infection in school age children: randomized double blind placebo controlled trial. Br Med J 1997; 315:858–862.

21

Role of Virus Infections in Early Life and the Development of Asthma
Epidemiology

ERIKA VON MUTIUS

University Children's Hospital
Munich, Germany

I. Introduction

Respiratory illnesses are a very common cause of consultation in pediatric practice and of hospital admissions in children under the age of 6 years. Infections of the respiratory tract, largely observed as common colds, are the most frequent cause of illness in humans in general. Children in particular go through a series of these viral infections within their first years of life. Respiratory syncytial virus (RSV), human rhinovirus, coronavirus, parainfluenza virus type 1–3, adenovirus, and influenza virus type A and B have all been associated with infections of the respiratory tract in children (1–4). In general, any respiratory virus can cause any picture of acute respiratory infection, but certain viruses tend to associate with a particular group of diseases (5).

A number of studies have shown that childhood wheeze is often associated with viral respiratory tract infections (5–7). Subjects on their first visit to a clinic because of wheezing often present rhinorrhea, nasal congestion, mild fever, cough, and other features of viral upper respiratory tract infection. A significant proportion of these children will be affected by recurrent episodes of wheeze and some will become atopic and develop airway hyperresponsiveness and asthma subsequent to the initial viral illness. The factors that determine the prognosis and further progression or remission of the disease relate to both intrinsic and extrinsic characteristics.

567

Intrinsic host factors will determine a subject's capability to limit the clinical response to a viral infection to no symptoms or only local signs of infection such as rhinorrhea and sneezing, or to extend the response to the lower respiratory tract and other organ systems. Johnston and colleagues have recently elegantly shown that although rhinovirus could be detected with equal frequency in nasal washes of asthmatic and nonasthmatic subjects, it was the asthmatics who were at much higher risk of developing lower respiratory tract symptoms than the exposed nonasthmatic control subjects (8). In addition to these intrinsic factors which are determined by host characteristics, extrinsic factors are likely to contribute to the disease process by interacting with the host. Extrinsic factors may be attributable to different virus species eliciting diverse immune responses or to environmental conditions that may either alter a host's susceptibility or enhance harmful characteristics of certain viruses.

The first section of this chapter will discuss the different phenotypes of wheezing illness in infancy and childhood. The second part is concerned with the incidence and type of viral infections detected in wheezing lower respiratory tract illnesses in various age groups in children. The potential harmful or protective role of such infections for the incidence of wheeze, asthma, and atopy will be discussed.

II.   Wheezing Illnesses in Infancy and the Childhood Years

The lack of a universally accepted definition of asthma that can be used to study the epidemiology of this childhood disease reflects a continued uncertainty about causal factors and underlying mechanisms. The definition of asthma as an obstructive lung disease with hyperreactivity of the airways to a variety of stimuli and a high degree of reversibility of the obstructive process either spontaneously or as a result of treatment has been used extensively in clinical practice. However, in epidemiological studies relying mostly on questionnaire information this type of information is often unavailable. Furthermore, in population-based studies different objective features of the so-called asthma syndrome such as atopy and airway hyper-responsiveness are not exclusively found among asthmatic subjects but also occur as separate traits in nonasthmatic individuals. Moreover, in prospective studies different patterns of wheezing illnesses have been identified in various age groups of children, pointing to the developmental nature of this disease. There is in fact growing evidence that childhood wheezing illnesses are not one homogeneous disease, as will be discussed in the following sections.

III.   Transient Wheezing of Infancy

In children up to 2–3 years of age wheeze is a very common respiratory symptom. For example, in the random population sample enrolled into the prospective Tucson Children's Respiratory Study, 19.3% of infants up to the age of 2 years were wheezing (9). In a European population-based survey this proportion amounted to 7.5%

(10). More boys than girls are affected as shown in many surveys (10–12). Furthermore, hospital admissions due to wheezing illnesses are particularly high in this young age group (13).

Wheezing in infancy is associated with a number of characteristics that are different from factors related to wheezing in older children. Several host and environmental risk factors have been identified, the effects of which are most likely attributable to reduced lung function prior to the occurrence of any wheeze. Using the rapid thoracic compression technique Martinez and colleagues reported that in the neonatal period percentage of expiratory time necessary to reach peak tidal expiratory flow (T_{me}/T_E), an indirect measure of airway conductance, was predictive of subsequent wheeze during the first 3 years of life (14). Wheezy infants also showed limited flows during tidal expiration in the first year of life, as demonstrated by a reduced size-corrected V_{max} functional residual capacity (FRC) (14).

Two other prospective studies have provided further supportive evidence that early-life lung function abnormalities are present prior to the first wheezing episodes in infancy (15–17). In the British study infants underwent pulmonary function testing at age 1–3 months prior to any respiratory illness (16). These children were then followed up to the age of 1 year. Mean specific airway conductance was significantly reduced among infants who subsequently wheezed (16). The odds ratio for wheeze was 2.1 (95% confidence interval [CI]: 1.1–3.8) for every unit decline in specific airway conductance. In this study impaired premorbid lung function was also associated with an earlier age at onset of wheezing symptoms. Significant determinants of reduced lung function were a parental history of asthma and maternal smoking.

In the Australian study infants underwent lung function testing at the age of 1, 6, and 12 months of age and were followed up to the age of 2 years (15). As in the British and American studies, the authors also found flow limitations (i.e., decreases in V'_{max}, FRC) among infants subsequently developing wheeze over the first and second year of life. It was interesting that differences in lung function existed between infants wheezing only in the first year of life as compared to infants commencing to wheeze after the first birthday or continuing to wheeze up to age 2 years. The abnormal lung function observed in the infants who wheezed only in the first year of life improved within 12 months, whereas persistent small airway dysfunction was a feature of those who wheezed during the second year of life. These findings suggest that in fact pulmonary function is a strong determinant of the appearance of wheezing symptoms in infancy.

From the cohort studies available it has become evident that a substantial proportion of infants outgrow their symptoms around the age of 1–3 years (9,10,15,18,19). In the large prospective study in Tucson (AZ, USA), many children wheezing at age 1–2 years lost their symptoms around their third birthday (9). Likewise, in a smaller European cohort most of the 21 children who wheezed before their second birthday never wheezed again and did not show airway hyperresponsiveness at age 11 years (18). Follow-up of this population into adult years showed that subjects younger than 2 years with wheeze were no more likely to become adults with asthma than those without wheeze (19).

A. Role of Viral Infections for Infant Wheeze

Most wheezing in infancy is related to viral infections. Several epidemiological surveys have shown that children exposed to infections early in life in daycare settings or through older siblings are at risk of developing wheezing (12,20–25). In a large population-based survey enrolling all newborns of the main birth clinics in Oslo, Norway, parental questionnaires were used to assess daycare attendance, number of siblings and infectious diseases at ages 6, 12, 18, and 24 months and relate these exposures prospectively to episodes of airway obstruction at 2 years of age (23). Having older siblings (aOR=1.8, 95%CI: 1.3–2.6) and attendance at day care at age 1 year [adjusted odds ratio (aOR=1.6, 95%CI: 1.1–2.4)] were positively associated with episodes of airway obstruction at age 2 years, as was a history of lower respiratory tract infections (bronchiolitis, bronchitis, pneumonia) (aOR=11.6, 95%CI: 8.3–16.2), otitis media (aOR=1.4, 95%CI: 1.0–1.9), and croup (aOR=2.3, 95%CI: 1.3–3.9) during the first year of life.

Likewise in a large population-based cohort of children followed to 2 years of age in the United States, children in daycare were at twice the risk of developing lower respiratory tract illnesses of children looked after at home (20). The rate ratio for wheezing associated respiratory illness was 2.3 (95% CI: 1.8–3.0) comparing infants in daycare to nonexposed children. Virus infections are furthermore the chief cause of hospitalization for respiratory tract illnesses in young children (26).

Up to 70% of wheezing episodes in the first year of life have been found to be associated with evidence of viral respiratory infections (27). These epidemiological observations have been confirmed by two subsequent emergency visit studies detecting viruses in nasal washes of infants under the age of 2 years (28,29). The authors demonstrated that in wheezing patients 70–82% of the cultures were positive for virus compared to 20% of a nonwheezing control group. The predominant pathogen in the washes of these symptomatic infants was respiratory syncytial virus (RSV) as recognized by a positive antigen test in 68% of the samples. Rhinoviruses were detected by reverse transcriptase–polymerase chain reaction (RT-PCR) in equal proportion (41%) among wheezing and control infants in the latter study (29).

Two major hypotheses are conceivable to explain the relation between viral infections and subsequent respiratory abnormalities (30). One could argue that viral infections early in life damage the growing lung or alter host immune regulation and are thus the causal insult to the airways. The second hypothesis holds that respiratory infections are more severe in susceptible infants and children with certain underlying predispositions. In this case, the symptomatic viral infection is merely an indicator of an otherwise silent condition, whereas viral infections were causal risk factors if the first hypothesis holds true. In infants with premorbid reduced lung function the most likely explanation is that the mucosal swelling induced by viral infections contributes to substantial narrowing of airways resulting in clinically manifest wheeze. The host factors become less important over toddler years as lung tissues and airways grow. These children subsequently seem to outgrow their wheeze and are asymptomatic even in the presence of viral infections later in life.

IV. Wheeze in Preschool Children Aged 3 to 6 Years

There are few epidemiological studies available that have investigated preschool-aged children for respiratory symptoms. Part of the limitations to perform such studies is the difficult approach to a random sample of the general population in this age group, which can only be attained by census records, since in most countries not all preschoolers are enrolled in activities such as kindergarten or vaccination programs. Moreover, only few longitudinal studies have investigated children at these ages. Therefore, most of the information available is derived from clinical studies and a few longitudinal surveys.

It has been shown in prospective and retrospective cohort studies that wheezing at the age of 3–6 years is determined by other factors than transient infant wheezing (9,10). The association between wheeze and markers of atopy such as infant eczema (10) and skin test reactivity at age 6 years (9) was much stronger among toddlers than infants. Likewise, in the Tucson Cohort the relation between wheeze and a family history of atopy was stronger among toddlers than infants (9).

Both determinants were more weakly associated with wheeze among children with late-onset symptoms than in children with recurrent and persisting wheeze from infancy into school age. These findings suggest that in toddler years two wheezing phenotypes may occur: one being closely associated with the development of atopy among predisposed subjects, the other possibly related to other factors, particularly viral infections. Toddler wheezing may thus represent a transition period in the continuum from infant years in which viral infections are the predominant trigger of wheezing symptoms to school age when atopy is the main predictor of wheeze.

A. Role of Virus Infections in Preschool Wheeze

As discussed earlier viral infections, particularly with RSV, are a major determinant of wheeze in infancy. Several researchers have followed children with proven RSV bronchiolitis to study their outcome after several years. There is evidence to suggest that infants with RSV bronchiolitis are at increased risk for additional episodes of wheeze in preschool years. Most authors, however, documented that wheezing tends to diminish over time and no significant increase in wheezing compared to controls is seen by school age or adolescence (31–34). For example, in the study by Pullen and co-workers (32), who followed 130 infants admitted to hospital at a mean age of 14 weeks with proven RSV bronchiolitis and compared them to matched controls, 6.2% of the RSV group were wheezing at the age of 10 years compared to 4.5% of the control group. A slightly increased prevalence of repeated mild episodes of wheeze was found during the first 4 years of age (38 vs. 15%), but no increased rate of atopic sensitization was seen in the cases compared to the controls. A recent meta-analysis of 10 controlled studies of children hospitalized for RSV bronchiolitis came to the same conclusion that wheezing is common after RSV bronchiolitis, but that no significant difference between the RSV bronchiolitis and the control group was observed regarding recurrent wheezing by 5 years of follow-up (34)

Sigurs and colleagues from Sweden came to conflicting conclusions. These investigators followed 47 infants hospitalized for RSV bronchiolitis in infancy and a matched control group of 93 children up to the age of 7.5 years (35). The prevalence of current wheeze at age 7.5 years amounted to 38% among former RSV hospitalized children compared to 2% of control subjects. Skin test reactivity also differed markedly between groups: whereas 20% of the cases reacted to a panel of aeroallergens, only 2% of the controls were skin test positive. Although the investigators selected the controls very carefully, the low prevalence of both wheeze and skin test reactivity in this group is astonishing. The prevalence of wheeze among random samples of 6–7-year-old children in Sweden was estimated at 11–15% in the ISAAC survey in 1994/95 (36). Therefore, residual selection bias may have affected these results.

Potential bias in the studies referred to above may furthermore have occurred through selection of hospitalized patients who are likely to be sicker than other infected symptomatic children. Studies in a general population sample, including the whole spectrum of RSV illness, may therefore be more informative. In the large longitudinal cohort in Tucson, 472 children with lower respiratory tract illness underwent testing for the infecting organism (37). RSV infection was documented in 43.9% of the subjects and significantly increased the risk for wheezing during preschool years. No effect on atopic sensitization was found.

Not only RSV infections were detected among children with lower respiratory illnesses in the Tucson Children's Respiratory Study. Parainfluenza and other infectious agents (adenovirus, influenza, *Chlamydia*, cytomegalovirus, rhinovirus, and mixed infection) were also found in 14.4% and 27.3% of subjects, respectively (37). Likewise, in these children an increased risk of repeated wheezing episodes, but not atopy in preschool years, was reported. These findings support the notion that in preschool children the distinction between wheezy bronchitis as an illness triggered by viral infections only and asthma as a wheezing illness triggered by viral infections as well as other factors such as allergens, exercise, or odors may be useful.

V. Persistent Wheeze from Infancy to School Age

In a substantial proportion of infants wheezing episodes starting early in life persist into school-age years. In the Tucson cohort a group of children showed recurrent episodes of wheeze from birth up to the age of 6 years. These infants had normal lung function and cord-serum IgE levels at birth, but developed significantly higher IgE levels at 9 months of age and skin test reactivity to a panel of aeroallergens at the age of 6 years. This condition was furthermore associated with a maternal history of asthma and the occurrence of eczema during the first year of life in the child (9). For this group, pulmonary function was within normal limits in the first year of life. More boys than girls were affected.

Many studies have consistently shown that the production of specific IgE antibodies to environmental allergens is strongly associated with childhood asthma. In cross-sectional and clinical studies atopic sensitization was related to an increased prevalence of asthma, bronchial hyperresponsiveness (BHR), and a greater severity of respiratory symptoms than with the absence of atopy (38–40). In a cross-sectional survey from Australia early sensitization (developing before the age of 6–8 years) was found to be a stronger predictor for asthma than sensitization, being only detectable thereafter (41). In the prospective German Cohort study the onset of atopic sensitization was investigated earlier: from age 1 to 7 years (42). The onset of atopic sensitization in children with current asthma at the age of 7 years occurred significantly earlier than in atopic children without development of asthma. Approximately 39% of asthmatic children had detectable IgE antibodies to either foods or inhalants at age 1 year compared to only 21% of nonasthmatic individuals (p = 0.015). Thus, factors enhancing the production of specific IgE antibodies or the lack of protective mechanisms to induce tolerance towards environmental allergens early in life may also increase the risk for asthma.

In several cross-sectional studies an inverse relation between school age asthma and the overall burden of respiratory infections has been reported. In Papua New Guinea Anderson observed that respiratory infections were more common among children in the Highlands, where the asthma rate was exceedingly low, than in the coastal regions of the country where asthma occurred more frequently (43). In the Fiji Islands, Flynn studied two groups of children: the indigenous Fijians, who showed a high hospital admission rate for pneumonia; and the Fiji Indians, whose asthma admission rate was three times higher than in the Fijians (44,45). Consistent with the hospitalization rates, Indian children had a threefold higher prevalence of asthma and airway hyperresponsiveness than Fijians, whereas respiratory infections were more than twice as common in Fijian than Indian children. In the East European countries a higher prevalence of bronchitis and respiratory infections was found, whereas asthma and BHR were significantly lower than in Sweden and West Germany (46–48). Recently published findings showing markedly lower prevalences of asthma and wheeze in the Finnish part of Karelia compared to the Russian part of Karelia corroborate the East–West European differences (49).

As described earlier, attendance at daycare early in life is associated with a significant risk of infectious illnesses, including lower respiratory tract illnesses such as croup, bronchitis, pneumonia, and wheezing illnesses. A report from the longitudinal follow-up of the Tucson cohort has recently opened the perspective from infant and toddler years into school age and adolescence. These investigators showed that children in day care very early in life, (i.e., in the first 6 months of life) were at increased risk of wheezing in the first years of life as discussed in previous sections of this chapter (24). The relation, however, reversed around the 6th birthday at which time attendance at daycare early in life proved to be protective against the occurrence of wheezing illnesses. This beneficial effect increased up to the age of 13 years, when the risk of wheezing among former daycare attendees was less than one-third that of other children raised at home.

An Italian retrospective cohort study confirmed these findings (10). Whereas having siblings and attending a daycare center were both risk factors for transient early wheeze up to the age of 2 years (aOR=1.41, 95% CI: 1.21–1.64 and aOR=1.70, 95% CI: 1.48–1.96, respectively), both exposures were protective for wheezing occurring after the age of 2 years (aOR=0.83, 95% CI: 0.70–0.97 and aOR=0.72, 95% CI: 0.59–0.88, respectively).

Recent analyses of the German longitudinal MAS Study are in line with these findings and suggest that repeated episodes of rhinitis in the first year of life and viral infections of the herpes type in the first 3 years of life are associated with a significant decrease in the risk of subsequent wheezing up to the age of 7 years (50). The risk estimates at school age of both prospective surveys are very comparable, indicating that exposed children are at approximately half the risk of nonexposed children.

In cross-sectional surveys of young men, a positive serological response to hepatitis A has been inversely related to allergic asthma (51). The timing of exposure to the virus has not been assessed; therefore, it remains open whether early life exposure or also later exposure to hepatitis A can protect from the development of asthma. As an alternative, a positive serological response to hepatitis A is merely an indicator of a nonhygienic lifestyle, in which case other microbial (bacterial as well as viral) exposures may account for the inverse association between hepatitis A and allergic asthma.

Most of these studies have shown a concomitant decrease in the prevalence or incidence of atopy among exposed compared to nonexposed subjects, suggesting that the characteristics of the atopic wheezing phenotype can beneficially be influenced by viral exposures. The mechanisms that underlie these inverse relations remain to be elucidated. Whether certain viruses and particularly repeated viral exposures induce a Th1-like immune response that can counteract allergic responses needs further investigation. The results of the German MAS Cohort Study positively linking very early onset of sensitization to asthma (42) and inversely relating very early exposure to repeated rhinitis episodes to asthma (50) may support this notion. As an alternative, other features of atopic wheeze may be affected by viral infections, thereby conferring the protection.

VI. Summary

Wheezing with upper respiratory tract infections is a very common childhood condition. A multitude of viral agents have been associated with these episodes, although the methods to detect viral infections have been cumbersome until recent advances introducing PCR techniques. These new methods may in the future allow us to understand better the role of viruses in triggering and eliciting wheezing episodes in children predisposed either by anatomical abnormalities of airway size and lung parenchyma or by reactive airway disease. Future studies will also have to address differences in wheezing phenotypes over childhood years, because effect modification is likely to occur. While in infants and some toddlers virus infections are positively linked to wheeze and lower respiratory tract illnesses, atopic asthma at school age has mostly been inversely related to repeated viral episodes. The mechanisms by which virus infections trigger symptoms among infants with transient wheeze will differ from those conferring protection from atopy and asthma. Carefully designed longitudinal studies may in the future contribute to a better understanding of the complex interactions between a host's susceptibility and the invading virus's characteristics.

References

1. Horn M, Brain E, Gregg I, Inglis J, Yealland S, Taylor P. Respiratory viral infection and wheezy bronchitis in childhood. Thorax 1979; 34:23–28.
2. Carlsen K, Orstavik I, Leegaard J, Hoeg H. Respiratory virus infections and aeroallergens in acute bronchial asthma. Arch Dis Child 1984; 59:310–315.
3. Pattemore P, Johnston S, Bardin P. Viruses as precipitants of asthma symptoms. I. Epidemiology Clin Exp Allergy 1992; 22:325–36.
4. Kabesch M, von Mutius E. Risk factors for wheezing with upper respiratory tract infections in children. In: Asthma and Respiratory Infections. New York: Marcel Dekker, 2000.
5. Busse W. Viral infections in humans. Am J Respir Crit Care Med 1995; 151:1675–1677.
6. Minor T, Dick E, Baker J, Ouellette J, Cohen M, Reed C. Rhinovirus and influenza type A infections as precipitants of asthma. Am Rev Respir Dis 1976; 113:149–153.
7. Johnston S, Pattemore P, Sanderson G, Smith S, Lampe F, Josephs L, Symington P, O'Toole S, Myint S, Tyrrell D, et al. Community study of role of viral infections in exacerbations of asthma in 9–11 year old children. Br Med J 1995; 310:1225–1229.
8. Corne J, Marshall C, Smith S, Schreiber J, Sanderson G, Holgate S, Johnston S. Frequency, severity, and duration of rhinovirus infections in asthmatic and non-asthmatic individuals: a longitudinal cohort study. Lancet 2002; 359:831–834.
9. Martinez F, Wright A, Taussig L, Holberg C, Halonen M, Morgan W, Personnel G. Asthma and wheezing in the first six years of life. N Engl J Med 1995; 332:133–138.
10. Rusconi F, Galassi C, Corbo G, Forastiere F, Biggeri A, Ciccone G, Renzoni E. Risk factors for early, persistent, and late-onset wheezing in young children. SIDRIA Collaborative Group. Am J Respir Crit Care Med 1999; 160:1617–1622.
11. Tariq S, Matthews S, Hakim E, Stevens M, Arshad S, Hide D. The prevalence of and risk factors for atopy in early childhood: a whole population birth cohort study. J Allergy Clin Immunol 1998; 101:587–593.
12. Celedon J, Litonjua A, Weiss S, Gold D. Day care attendance in the first year of life and illnesses of the upper and lower respiratory tract in children with a familial history of atopy. Pediatrics 1999; 104:495–500.
13. Wickman M, Farahmand B, Persson P, Pershagen G. Hospitalization for lower respiratory disease during 20 yrs among under 5 yr old children in Stockholm County: a population based survey. Eur Respir J 1998; 11:366–370.
14. Martinez F, Morgan W, Wright A, Holberg C, Taussig L. Diminished lung function as a predisposing factor for wheezing respiratory illness in infants. N Engl J Med 1988; 319:1112–1117.
15. Young S, Arnott J, O'Keeffe P, Le Souef P, Landau L. The association between early life lung function and wheezing during the first 2 yrs of life. Eur Respir J 2000; 15:151–157.
16. Dezateux C, Stocks J, Dundas I, Fletcher M. Impaired airway function and wheezing in infancy. The influence of maternal smoking and a genetic predisposition to asthma. Am J Respir Crit Care Med 1999; 159:403–410.

17. Clarke J, Reese A, Silverman M. Bronchial responsiveness and lung function in infants with lower respiratory tract illness over the first 6 months of life. Arch Dis Child 1992; 67:1454–1458.

18. Sporik R, Holgate S, Cogswell J. Natural history of asthma in childhood—a birth cohort study. Arch Dis Child 1991; 66:1050–1053.

19. Rhodes H, Thomas P, Sporik R, Holgate S, Cogswell J. A birth cohort study of subjects at risk of atopy: twenty-two-year follow-up of wheeze and atopic status. Am J Respir Crit Care Med 2002; 165:176–180.

20. Marbury M, Maldonado G, Waller L. Lower respiratory illness, recurrent wheezing, and day care attendance. Am J Respir Crit Care Med 1997; 155:156–161.

21. Koopman L, Smit H, Heijnen M, Wijga A, van Strien R, Kerkhof M, Gerritsen J, Brunekreef B, de Jongste J, Neijens H. Respiratory infections in infants: interaction of parental allergy, child care, and siblings— The PIAMA study. Pediatrics 2001; 108:943–948.

22. Nafstad P, Hagen J, Oie L, Magnus P, Jaakkola J. Day care centers and respiratory health. Pediatrics 1999; 103:753–758.

23. Nafstad P, Magnus P, Jaakkola J. Early respiratory infections and childhood asthma. Pediatrics 2000; 106(3):E38.

24. Ball T, Castro-Rodriguez J, Griffith K, Holberg C, Martinez F, Wright A. Siblings, daycare attendance, and the risk of asthma and wheezing during childhood. N Engl J Med 2000; 343:538–543.

25. McKeever T, Lewis S, Smith C, Collins J, Heatlie H, Frischer M, Hubbard R. Siblings, multiple births, and the incidence of allergic disease: a birth cohort study using the West Midlands general practice research database. Thorax 2001; 56:758–762.

26. Glezen W, Greenberg S, Armar R, Piedra P, Couch R. Impact of respiratory virus infections on persons with chronic underlying conditions. JAMA 2000; 283:499–505.

27. Wright A, Holberg C, Martinez F, Morgan W, Taussig L, GHMA. Breast feeding and lower respiratory tract illness in the first year of life. Br Med J 1989; 299:946–949.

28. Duff A, Pomeranz E, Gelber L, Price W, Farris H, Hayden F, Platts-Mills T, Heymann P. Risk factors for acute wheezing in infants and children: viruses, passive smoke, and IgE antibodies to inhalant allergens. Pediatrics 1993; 92:535–540.

29. Rakes G, Arruda E, Ingram J, Hoover G, Zambrano J, Hayden F, Platts-Mills T, Heymann P. Rhinovirus and respiratory syncytial virus in wheezing children requiring emergency care. IgE and eosinophil analyses. Am J Respir Crit Care Med 1999; 159:785–790.

30. Long C, McBride J, Hall C. Sequelae of respiratory syncytial virus infections. A role for intervention studies. Am J Respir Crit Care Med 1995; 151:1678–1681.

31. Hall C, Hall W, Gala C, Magill F, Leddy J. Long term prospective study in children after respiratory syncytial virus infection. J Pediatr 1984; 105:358–364.

32. Pullen C, Hey E. Wheezing, asthma and pulmonary dysfunction 10 years after infection with respiratory syncytial virus in infancy. Br Med 1982; 284:1665–1669.

33. Wennergren G, Kristjansson S. Relationship between respiratory syncytial virus bronchiolitis and future obstructive airway diseases. Eur Respir J 2001; 18:1044–1058.

34. Kneyber M, Steyerberg E, de Groot R, Moll H. Long-term effects of respiratory syncytial virus (RSV) bronchiolitis in infants and young children: a quantitative review. Acta Paediatr 2000; 89:654–660.

35. Sigurs N, Biarnason R, Sigurbergsson F, Kjellman B. Respiratory syncytial virus bronchiolitis in infancy is an important risk factor for asthma and allergy at age 7. Am J Respir Crit Care Med 2000; 161:1501–1507.

36. Isaac SC. Worlwide variations in the prevalence of asthma symptoms: the International

Study of Asthma and Allergies in Childhood (ISAAC). Eur Respir J 1998; 12:315–335.

37. Stein R, Sherrill D, Morgan W, Holberg C, Halonen M, Taussig L, Wright A, Martinez F. Respiratory syncytial virus in early life and risk of wheeze and allergy by age 13 years. Lancet 1999; 354:541–545.

38. Clough J, Williams J, Holgate S. Effect of atopy on the natural history of symptoms, peak expiratory flow, and bronchial responsiveness in 7- and 8- year-old children with cough and wheeze. Am Rev Respir Dis 1991; 143:755–760.

39. Kelly W, Hudson I, Phelan P, Pain M, Olinsky A. Atopy in subjects with asthma followed to the age of 28 years. J Allergy Clin Immunol 1990; 85:548–557.

40. Van Asperen P, Kemp A, Mukhi A. Atopy in infancy predicts the severity of bronchial hyperresponsiveness in later childhood. J Allergy Clin Immunol 1990; 85:790–795.

41. Peat J, Salome C, Woolcock A. Longitudinal changes in atopy during a 4-year period: Relation to bronchial hyperresponsiveness and respiratory symptoms in a population sample of Australian schoolchildren. J Allergy Clin Immunol 1990; 85:65–74.

42. Illi S, von Mutius E, Lau S, Nickel R, Niggemann B, Sommerfeld C, Wahn U, a. t. M. S. Group. The pattern of atopic sensitization is associated with the development of asthma in childhood. J Allergy Clin Immunol 2001; 108:709–714.

43. Anderson H. The epidemiological and allergic features of asthma in the New Guinea Highlands. Clin Allergy 1974; 4:171–183.

44. Flynn M. Respiratory symptoms, bronchial responsiveness, and atopy in Fijan and Indian children. Am J Respir Crit Care Med 1994; 150:415–420.

45. Flynn M. Respiratory symptoms of rural Fijian and Indian children in Fiji. Thorax 1994; 49:1201–1204.

46. von Mutius E, Martinez FD, Fritzsch C, Nicolai T, Roell G, Thiemann HH. Prevalence of asthma and atopy in two areas of West and East Germany. Am J Respir Crit Care Med 1994; 149(2 Pt 1):358–364.

47. Braback L, Breborowicz A, Dreborg S, Knutsson A, Pieklik H, Bjorksten B. Atopic sensitization and respiratory symptoms among Polish and Swedish school children. Clin Exp Allergy 1994; 24(9):826–835.

48. Nowak D, Heinrich J, Jorres R, Wassmer G, Berger J, Beck E, Boczor S, Claussen M, Wichmann HE, Magnussen H. Prevalence of respiratory symptoms, bronchial hyperresponsiveness and atopy among adults: west and east Germany. Eur Respir J 1996; 9(12):2541–2552.

49. Vartiainen E, Petäys T, Haahtela T, Jousilahti P, Pekkanen J. Allergic diseases, skin prick test responses, and IgE levels in North Karelia, Finland, and the Republic of Karelia, Russia. J Allergy Clin Immunol 2002; 109:643–648.

50. Illi S, vonMutius E, Lau S, Bergmann R, Niggemann B, Sommerfeld C, Wahn U, a. t. M. S. Group. Early childhood infectious diseases and the development of asthma up to school age: a birth cohort study. Br Med J 2001; 322:390–395.

51. Matricardi P, Rosmini F, Riondino S, Fortini M, Ferrigno L, Rapicetta M, Bonini S. Exposure to foodborne and orofecal microbes versus airborne viruses in relation to atopy and allergic asthma: epidemiological study. Br Med J 2000; 320:412–417.

22

Does Respiratory Syncytial Virus Cause Asthma?

ROBERT C. WELLIVER

Children's Hospital
State University of New York at Buffalo
Buffalo, New York, U.S.A.

I. Introduction

Respiratory syncytial virus (RSV) infection in infancy frequently causes bronchiolitis, an illness characterized by airway obstruction and wheezing. Whether this illness is related to the eventual development of childhood asthma, another illness with prominent airway obstruction and wheezing, has been the subject of debate for decades.

In support of an association is the high frequency with which infantile bronchiolitis is followed by both recurrent episodes of wheezing and by evidence of dysfunction of the small airways, which may persist into school age. Some prospective studies have suggested that RSV infection may be a more important determinant of the development of childhood asthma and atopy than even the allergic characteristic of the parents. Also experimental RSV infection in mice that were previously sensitized to an allergen provokes airway eosinophilia and enhances airway hyperreactivity, each of which is characteristic of asthma.

In contrast, the development of wheezing following bronchiolitis might reasonably be related to some congenital trait that predisposes to airway obstruction both at the time of RSV infection in infancy as well as at the time of exposure to other stimuli during childhood. These hereditary factors might include smaller airway diameter, increased airway reactivity, aberrant immunological responses, or other features.

Table 1   Questions Regarding Bronchiolitis and Childhood Asthma

Does RSV bronchiolitis result in recurrent wheezing?
Bronchiolitis is associated with recurrent wheezing through school ages, but not into
  adolescence.
Does RSV bronchiolitis result in persistent airway dysfunction?
The development of multiple wheezing LRI in childhood is associated with small-airway
  dysfunction in later childhood. However, a single episode of bronchiolitis is not
  associated with abnormal long-term lung function.
Does RSV bronchiolitis cause airway hyperreactivity?
Bronchiolitis is associated with airway hyperreactivity in childhood, but factors such as
  atopy and exposure to cigarette smoke may be more important determinants.
Does RSV bronchiolitis induce a persistent TH2 bias?
Feature of TH2 responses are observed after bronchiolitis. However, bronchiolitis itself is
  not associated with induction of TH2 cytokine responses.
Does RSV bronchiolitis enhance sensitization to allergens?
A brief period of enhanced sensitization may occur in animals shortly after RSV infection,
  but is not related to enhanced TH2 responses. Similar data are lacking in humans.

This review will summarize the current information in support of and disputing
the idea that RSV bronchiolitis in infancy is a cause of childhood asthma. The report
will focus on five questions regarding the connection of bronchiolitis to asthma
(Table 1). These questions concern the development of recurrent wheezing following
bronchiolitis, the development of long-term airway dysfunction or airway hyperreactivity following bronchiolitis, the induction of T-helper lymphocyte type 2 (TH2)
immune responses by RSV infection, and the possibility that RSV infection may
sensitize the host to allergens.

II.   Is Bronchiolitis in Infancy Associated with Recurrent Wheezing?

A.   Evidence Favoring a Causative Role for Bronchiolitis in Recurrent Wheezing

Early studies of infants with RSV bronchiolitis readily demonstrated that these infants were prone to the development of recurrent episodes of wheezing. Zweiman
and colleagues, studying infants with bronchiolitis 3–4 years later, found that 50 %
of infants still experienced episodic wheezing (1). Rooney and Williams followed
62 infants with bronchiolitis up to 7 years of age, and found that 56% had at least
one subsequent episode of wheezing, while that 43% wheezed on three or more
occasions (2). Sims and colleagues followed 35 infants with bronchiolitis and an
equal number of controls without bronchiolitis through the age of 8 years (3). Eighteen (51%) of the index cases and only one (6%) of the controls experienced wheezing at any time in this interval (p $<$ 0.0005). The authors noted that 10 of the 18
(56%) index cases with recurrent wheezing had remained free of wheezing in the

2 years preceding the study; therefore only 8 (23%) of the original 35 infants were still wheezing at age 8 years. McConnochie and Roghmann similarly followed 59 infants with bronchiolitis and 177 controls to the ages of 6–9 years (4). In contrast to the previous studies, all subjects followed by McConnochie and Roghmann had experienced only mild bronchiolitis that did not require hospitalization. At the time of follow-up 44% of former bronchiolitis patients and 13.6% of controls (p < 0.0001) were experiencing wheezing. Therefore subjects with mild bronchiolitis managed as outpatients had the same rate of recurrent wheezing as those infants whose initial illness was severe enough to require hospitalization.

In all of these studies, these recurrent wheezing spells began shortly after the initial bronchiolitis episode, and were almost never so severe that hospitalization was required for management. Zweiman and colleagues (1) found that eosinophilia in nasal secretions was observed more frequently in children with recurrent wheezing after bronchiolitis than in those who had no further wheezing. Rooney and Williams (2) found that subsequent wheezing was more frequent in infants who had immediate family members with asthma. In contrast, Sims et al. (5) and McConnochie and Roghmann (4) found no relationship between a personal or family history of atopy and the development of recurrent wheezing. Thus it was clear from these initial investigations that recurrences of wheezing were common following infantile bronchiolitis, although the role of atopy in determining whether or not repeated wheezing occurs was less certain. Most importantly, these studies do not identify whether recurrent wheezing is a direct result of RSV infection itself, or an expression of some underlying tendency which results in wheezing both at the time of RSV infection in infancy and in later childhood.

Perhaps the most convincing evidence that bronchiolitis is associated, in a manner independent of atopy, with recurrent wheezing comes from the studies of Sigurs and colleagues (6). This investigative team identified 47 children who were hospitalized for bronchiolitis in infancy, and a comparison group of 93 children who did not require hospitalization for bronchiolitis. All children were followed through the age of 7 years. At this age, comparisons were made between groups regarding the number of subjects in whom a diagnosis of asthma had been made, the number of children with positive skin tests to allergens, and the presence of immunoglobulin (IgE) antibodies to allergens.

At the time of follow-up, asthma (defined as three or more episodes of wheezing occurring at any age) was diagnosed in 23% of the children with bronchiolitis, and only 2% of the controls. Multivariate analysis of the data revealed that RSV bronchiolitis was the only factor predictive of a diagnosis of asthma, and was a stronger predictor of any recurrent wheezing than a history of asthma in the parents. These findings imply that RSV bronchiolitis itself is an independent risk factor for the development of asthma.

B. Evidence Against a Causal Association of Bronchiolitis and Recurrent Wheezing

A major problem in interpreting the nature of the association of bronchiolitis and asthma is that not all wheezing that follows bronchiolitis persists and becomes childhood asthma. Early investigations of the natural history of bronchiolitis demonstrated that the incidence of wheezing-associated respiratory illness fell continuously with increasing age throughout childhood (3,7).

This is illustrated in greater detail by the prospective studies of large numbers of infants in the Tucson area by Martinez and colleagues (8). Following a population of 1246 newborns through the age of 6 years (Table 2), this team found that 425 children (52%) never experienced wheezing. An additional 164 (20%) enrollees had so-called transient wheezing, defined as one or more wheezing episodes occurring before the age of 3 years but none thereafter. Another 124 (15%) subjects had no wheezing during the first 3 years of life, but began wheezing thereafter (late-onset wheezing), and 113 participants had wheezing beginning in infancy that persisted thorough 6 years of age (persistent wheezing).

In comparison to the group of children without wheezing, the group with transient wheezing had diminished airway function both before the age of 1 year, and again at the age of 6 years. These transient wheezers were more likely to have mothers who smoked during pregnancy, but did not have evidence of atopy at age 6 years. In contrast, children with persistent wheezing had normal lung function in the first year of life, but were more likely to have mothers with asthma, as well as personal evidence of atopy. Their lung function had become reduced by the time of the 6 year evaluation. Finally, the late-onset wheezing group had normal lung function throughout, but also had evidence of personal atopy.

These findings, which have been recently confirmed (9), suggested that wheezing following bronchiolitis has different causes. In the case of transient wheezing, RSV infection might promote airway obstruction by acting on airways that are already narrowed as a result of intrauterine exposure to components of tobacco smoke. However, the long-term prognosis for wheezing (although perhaps not for normal airway function) in these children appears to be reasonably benign. In contrast, the combination of RSV infection occurring in an atopic infant may be associated with persistent wheezing and limited airway function as well. This hypothesis is supported by the results of two studies (10,11) indicating that the presence of eosinophilia in peripheral blood at the time of RSV bronchiolitis identifies those infants who will still have wheezing at school age.

Table 2 Maximal Airflow FRC at Age 1 and 6 Years Analyzed by Wheezing History

Age at time of testing (yr)	No wheezing	Transient wheezing	Late-onset wheezing	Persistent wheezing
<1	123	71[a]	107	104
6	1262	1097[b]	1174	1069[b]

[a]p < 0.05 vs. any other group.
[b]p < 0.05 vs. group with no wheezing.
Source: Data adapted from. Ref. 8.

The significance of these studies is that RSV bronchiolitis itself does not appear to be the critical factor in determining the presence of wheezing at 6 years of age. The risk of recurrent wheezing is the same in infants with milder initial episodes of bronchiolitis as it is in infants with more severe forms of bronchiolitis not requiring hospitalization. Therefore, the severity of the initial RSV infection does not appear to influence the rate of subsequent asthma. Rather the atopic status of the infant appears to determine the prognosis for childhood wheezing following bronchiolitis, although not necessarily the self-limited recurrent wheezing that ceases before 3 years of age.

Furthermore, the results of two studies suggest that even if RSV bronchiolitis in infancy confers an increased risk of wheezing in school age, by adolescence the risk is reduced almost to that of the general population (that is, those without a history of bronchiolitis) (12,13). In each of these studies, the relative risk conferred by infantile bronchiolitis for asthma at age 13 was approximately 1.5, and not statistically different from control populations. A slightly increased risk for wheezing at age 13 could not be excluded entirely. In general, lower respiratory illness in childhood has not been associated with chronic lung disease in adult life, if the contributions of asthma and smoke exposure are considered simultaneously (14,15).

Most studies of the relationship of bronchiolitis to recurrent wheezing and asthma have not determined the effects of one vs. several bouts of wheezing in infancy on the development of asthma. In a study of 770 children in the East Boston area, a single episode of bronchiolitis in infancy was not associated with the presence of asthma at age 5–9 years (16). This was confirmed by McConnochie and Roghmann (17), who found that children who had only one episode of wheezing before the age of 2 years were not at an increased risk for wheezing in childhood. Thus a single episode of bronchiolitis, in the absence of other factors, does not appear to increase the risk of childhood asthma.

In addition, it might be expected that the earlier an episode of bronchiolitis occurred, the more lung dysfunction might be induced. However, Tager and colleagues found no association with age at the time of bronchiolitis and the frequency of subsequent lower respiratory illnesses (18).

In summary, RSV bronchiolitis in infancy is associated with an increased risk of wheezing persisting through school age, but probably not into adolescence. A single episode of bronchiolitis may not confer this increased risk. The development of asthma during school age appears to be more directly related to heredity for asthma and personal evidence of atopy.

III. Does Bronchiolitis Result in Long-Term Airway Damage or Hyperreactivity?

A. Evidence Favoring a Causative Role for Bronchiolitis in Persistent Lung Dysfunction and Bronchial Hyperreactivity

Lung function has been determined in infants during the acute phase of bronchiolitis. Studying hospitalized, but not intubated, infants, Dezateux and colleagues (19) found expiratory obstruction (reduced ratio of time to maximum expiratory flow to total expiratory time) but normal resistance, compliance and airflow at functional residual capacity. In contrast, Hammer and colleagues (20) studying infants with endotracheal tubes in place, found increased resistance, reduced compliance, reduced airflow in small airways, and evidence of air trapping. These two studies therefore agree in finding that RSV bronchiolitis is associated with small airway obstruction during the acute phase of illness.

Shortly after the discovery of an association between bronchiolitis and recurrent wheezing, investigators at several institutions became interested in whether bronchiolitis was also associated with long-term reductions in lung function. Pullan and Hey (21) found that infants with a previous history of bronchiolitis (severe enough to require hospitalization) had normal airflow in large airways, but reduced airflow in the terminal airways 10 years after the initial bronchiolitis episode. Small studies (also in infants initially hospitalized for bronchiolitis) by Sims et al. (3) and Hall and colleagues (22) confirmed these findings. The degree of airflow reduction in the small airways was comparatively minor, with most studies reporting values for maximum expiratory flow (MEF_{25-75}) of approximately 50% of that predicted for the age of the child. This is a milder reduction than that typically seen in children with asthma, in whom airflows in the small airways are often 25–30% of predicted values.

More recently, long-term pulmonary function has been assessed in children with histories of lower respiratory illness before the age of 2 years. In all of these children, the initial episode did not require hospitalization. Henderson and colleagues (23) found that, at age 9, boys (but not girls) with histories of multiple wheezing lower respiratory infections (LRI) before 2 years of age had approximately 20% reductions in forced expiratory volume in 1 s (FEV_1) and airflows in small airways in comparison to control children. Voter and colleagues (24) and Gold et al. (25) reported similar findings, with greater abnormalities again observed in boys. McConnochie (26) found that airflows in small airways were 64% of predicted values in similar patients. These studies demonstrate that boys with multiple wheezing episodes in early life have reduced small airway function at school age, and imply that RSV infection at an early stage of airway development may cause this persistent dysfunction. It should be noted that these changes are much more mild in degree than those observed in children with atopic asthma.

In addition to airflow limitations, persistent hypoxia (22,27) was noted more commonly in infants with histories of bronchiolitis than in those without such a history.

B. Evidence Against an Association of Bronchiolitis with Long-Term Airway Dysfunction and BHR

In many of the studies of spirometry in school children with a history of bronchiolitis, a history of a single episode of bronchiolitis in infancy without subsequent recurrent episodes of LRI was not associated with long-term airway dysfunction. Thus Henderson and colleagues (23) found that children with zero or one episode of wheezing LRI in the first 2 years of life had normal lung function (forced vital capacity [FVC], FEV_1, MEF_{25-75}, $V_{max}50$, and FEV_1/FVC) when tested at the age of

Table 3 Lung Function at Age 6 Years Analyzed by Number of Wheezing LRI Before 2 Years of Age

Wheezing LRI before age 2 years	Boys		Girls	
	FEV_1	MEF_{25-75}	FEV_1	MEF_{25-75}
0	0.95	1.05	0.95	1.07
1	0.95	1.07	0.84	0.93
2+	0.86[a]	0.81[a]	0.92	1.02

[a]$p < 0.05$ vs. any group.
Source: Data from Ref. 23.

6 years (Table 3). Only those children with two or more episodes of wheezing LRI before the age of 2 years had reduced lung function subsequently. Voter and colleagues (24) found that a single episode of RSV LRI before the age of 2 years did not influence the results of spirometry performed on 57 boys between the ages of 11 and 22 years. Both Strope and colleagues, in a study of 89 boys and 70 girls evaluated between the ages of 6 and 18 years (28), and Gold and colleagues in a study of 801 children followed to the age of 13 years (25), found that a single episode of wheezing before the age of 2 years was not associated with long-term lung dysfunction. These results would seem to indicate rather clearly that a single episode of RSV bronchiolitis is not associated with long-term lung dysfunction.

It also might be assumed that more severe episodes of bronchiolitis might be more likely to damage the airway of infants, and therefore result in long-term lung dysfunction. However, the existing data seem to indicate that the degree of lung dysfunction in childhood is unrelated to the severity of the initial RSV episode. Hall and colleagues (22) studied children whose initial RSV infection was severe enough to require hospitalization, and found that indices of small airway function were between 67 and 80% of that predicted for normal children of the same age. Pullan and Hey (21) also studied children who had been hospitalized for bronchiolitis as infants, and found that small airway function was approximately 80% of that predicted for age. Henderson and colleagues (23), Voter et al. (24), and McConnochie and Roghmann (17) all studied infants with histories of milder bronchiolitis managed without hospitalization. In all three of these latter studies, small airway function was also reduced by 10–20% in comparison to that of normal control children. Therefore the small-airway dysfunction that follows bronchiolitis is not apparently related to the severity of the initial RSV infection. This in turn suggests that some other factor besides the RSV infection itself is responsible for long-term airway dysfunction following bronchiolitis.

Several studies have been directed at determining whether lung dysfunction following bronchiolitis is related to the atopic status of the host. Welliver and Duffy (29) found that large airway function at 7–9 years after bronchiolitis was related to the number of positive skin tests to allergens, while small-airway dysfunction was related to maternal smoking. Henderson and colleagues (23) found reduced lung function in males with previous histories of LRI in infancy. Among those subjects with multiple wheezing LRI in infancy, lung function appeared to be determined by the presence of atopy. In contrast, lung function in those with zero to one episode of wheezing LRI was unrelated to atopy.

The findings of Martinez and colleagues (8) are also of interest. Among non-atopic children, wheezing in infancy was associated with reduced airflow on a hereditary basis (that is, present before the episode of bronchiolitis occurred). A mild degree of limited airflow was still present in childhood. In contrast, atopic children with infantile wheezing had normal airflow in infancy, but began to lose function in later childhood. Therefore mild airflow reductions after bronchiolitis were related to hereditary differences in the airway, while more serious reductions in airflow in childhood were related to atopy. In neither case could long-term reductions in airflow be related to bronchiolitis itself. The results of all these studies suggest that atopy, not bronchiolitis, is the principal determinant of postbronchiolitic lung dysfunction.

Welliver and Duffy (29) determined the degree of oxygen saturation at the age of 7–9 years in infants who had been hospitalized for bronchiolitis in infancy. All subjects had normal oxygen saturation determinations. This study used transcutaneous pulse oximetry, which is less invasive and more accurate than the methods used in earlier studies (22,27) to determine oxygenation following bronchiolitis. It seems unlikely that uncomplicated viral bronchiolitis in infancy results in chronic hypoxia.

IV.   Does RSV Infection Induce Bronchial Hyperreactivity?

A.   Evidence Favoring a Causative Role for Bronchiolitis in BHR

In adults, natural RSV infection results in a brief period of increased airway responsiveness to nonspecific bronchoconstricting agents (30). Similar studies of bronchial reactivity have not been performed in infants during the acute phase of bronchiolitis because of the potential risk involved. However, two follow-up studies have demonstrated greater airway reactivity in children with a past history of bronchiolitis than in a control group without such a history (3,31). The degree of airway hyperreactivity observed in subjects previously hospitalized with bronchiolitis was greater than that of control subjects, but less than that commonly observed in children with asthma (31).

Tepper and colleagues (32) also evaluated BHR several months after an episode of bronchiolitis in infancy. They found that the normal decrease in airway reactivity (which occurs with increasing age in childhood) was impeded among infants with bronchiolitis. The degree of increase in BHR was rather minimal, and did not correlate with recurrent wheezing following bronchiolitis.

McConnochie and Roghmann (26) also evaluated BHR in a cohort of 25 children at the age of 8–12 years who had mild, outpatient bronchiolitis in infancy. The airway reactivity in these subjects with outpatient bronchiolitis was not different from control children who had never experienced bronchiolitis. Infants with milder forms of bronchiolitis may not develop persistent airway hyperreactivity, while reactivity may be mildly increased in those subjects who had more severe forms of illness originally.

B. Evidence Against a Causative Role for Bronchiolitis in BHR

All infants have increased airway reactivity to nonspecific challenges in comparison to older children and adults (33,34). The degree of airway reactivity appears to decrease with age, but may then increase again following an episode of wheezing illness (24). Thus it is not necessarily true that BHR measured several years after an episode of bronchiolitis can be attributed to the bronchiolitis episode itself. Indeed airway reactivity following wheezing LRI has been associated with personal evidence of atopy (23) and with passive exposure to cigarette smoke (29), in addition to recent wheezing illnesses (24). In the study by Tepper and colleagues (32) the BHR observed immediately following bronchiolitis did not account for recurrent wheezing. Two other small studies did not find an association of BHR in young children with the development of more frequent wheezing episodes (35,36), although a significant association could not be excluded.

In summary, bronchial reactivity may be increased following bronchiolitis, but may have been in existence before the episode of bronchiolitis occurred, may be related to factors other than bronchiolitis (such as atopy and exposure to cigarette smoke), and has not been demonstrated to be of clinical significance as far as the development of childhood asthma is concerned. However, McConnochie and Roghmann (26) found no difference in BHR between control infants and those who had mild outpatient bronchiolitis in infancy, while other studies have found greater reactivity among children formerly hospitalized with bronchiolitis. It is therefore possible that greater degrees of bronchial reactivity may contribute to the expression of more severe forms of illness at the time of the initial episode of bronchiolitis.

V. Does RSV Infection Induce T-Helper Type 2 Responses?

A. Evidence Suggesting That RSV Induces TH2-Like Responses

A current theory of asthma pathogenesis is that an over-production of cytokines released by T-helper type 2 (TH2) lymphocytes is responsible for many of the pathological features of this illness (37). More specifically, the release of interleukins 4 and 5 (among others) may account for both the increase in IgE production as well as the migration of eosinophils into the respiratory tract.

Several features of a TH2 response have been described in infants with bronchiolitis, including the development of RSV-specific IgE antibody responses (38-43), the release of histamine (39,44) and cysteinyl leukotrienes (45,46), and the degranulation of eosinophils (47-49). Renzi and associates (50) studied infants 5 months after an episode of bronchiolitis, and found persistently elevated expression of CD23 (the IgE receptor) and evidence of continued lymphocyte activation. Rabatic and colleagues (42) also found increased expression of CD23 in infants with bronchiolitis, particularly those who exhibited RSV-specific IgE responses. Roman and co-workers (51) found a reduced number of suppressor lymphocytes in infants with RSV bronchiolitis.

These findings might suggest that RSV infection results in the unmasking of an allergic diathesis, consisting of unregulated lymphocyte activity, eosinophilia, and increased IgE production, possibly to a variety of allergens. In this regard, it has also been suggested that the development of asthma might result from a failure of the host to be exposed in early life to an adequate number of infections that promote TH1 cytokine responses (52). These infants would then be unable to prevent the development of TH2 cytokine responses upon exposure to allergens, and therefore to prevent the development of atopy (52).

B. Evidence Against the Induction of a TH2 Response by RSV

One limitation of these studies of TH2 responses to RSV infection is that they cannot determine whether the immunological biases identified were induced by RSV infection, or if they were already present beforehand, representing the inherent immunological status of the host. In this regard, several studies have demonstrated that infants of asthmatic or atopic parents have elevated IgE antibody titers in cord blood specimens, greater expression of CD23 antigen on B-lymphocytes, and reduce interferon-γ (IFN-γ) synthesis by peripheral blood mononuclear cells (53,54). This suggests that the TH2-like responses observed during convalescence from RSV infection may predate, rather than be induced by, the infection. Also against the induction of TH2 response as a result of RSV infection are data indicating that severe RSV infection is characterized by a relative increase in production of the TH1 cytokine IFN-γ rather than TH2 cytokines. In opposition to a role for TH2 cytokines in virus-induced wheezing, one study found higher concentrations of IFN-γ in nasopharyngeal secretions of infants and children with bronchiolitis or recurrent wheezing due to RSV, while IL-4 was the predominant cytokine in those with upper respiratory infection (URI) alone and in healthy control infants (46). IFN-γ was also found to be present in greater quantities than IL-4 in samples of serum obtained during acute RSV bronchiolitis in a separate study by Renzi and associates (50).

Studies of cytokine responses in peripheral blood lymphocytes at the time of RSV infection have led to conflicting results. Renzi and colleagues (55) and colleagues found increased production of IFN-γ by lymphocytes from infants with bronchiolitis who would not subsequently develop asthma. No differences in IL-4 production were noted between groups. Aberle and colleagues (43) found greater IFN-γ production in cells from infants with moderate bronchiolitis than in cells from healthy infants, whereas IFN-γ production was equal in infants with severe bronchiolitis and in controls. Bendelja and colleagues found more IL-4 production by lymphocytes from subjects with URI alone due to RSV, and greater IFN-γ production by those with bronchiolitis or pneumonia (56). Brandenburg and associates (57) found no difference in cellular production of IL-4 or IFN-γ among infants with mild or more severe bronchiolitis.

It seems possible to conclude that current evidence does not support the hypothesis that RSV infection induces a persistent TH2 response. Therefore the development of asthma following bronchiolitis probably cannot be accounted for on this basis.

VI. Does RSV Infection Sensitize the Host to the Effects of Allergens?

In humans, sensitization of infants to environmental allergens takes place over several years (58). Thus human infants are exposed to allergens such as house dust mite with no ill effects for several years, only later developing allergic manifestations.

There is suggestive evidence from animal studies that RSV infection occurring during the interval in which animals are being sensitized to an allergen may enhance the effects of exposure to the allergen. Various species of animals develop airway hyperreactivity to methacholine after a prolonged period of exposure to ovalbumin. The degree of airway reactivity is increased if the animals are infected with RSV during the sensitization procedure (59-6l). The allergen-induced airway reactivity is associated with airway eosinophilia, and the enhancement of airway reactivity by RSV infection is associated with a further increase in the number of airway eosinophils.

If similar events occurred in humans, this would offer a possible explanation for the link between RSV bronchiolitis and asthma. No evidence in support of this has been generated in humans to date. Even in animals, the effects of viral infection seem to be temporary, lasting for only 1–2 weeks after experimental infection.

VII. Conclusion: What Is the Nature of the Link Between RSV Bronchiolitis and Childhood Asthma?

There is no convincing evidence (and some counterevidence) that a single RSV infection in infancy is a direct cause of recurrent wheezing, persistent airway dysfunction, prolonged airway hyperreactivity, or the development of atopy. Yet there is clearly an association between infantile bronchiolitis and childhood wheezing. We suspect that the nature of the association consists of similarities in the nature of the inflammatory response to virus infections and allergen exposures.

In a fashion similar to asthma, viral infections result in the appearance of CD4-positive lymphocytes (62), eosinophils or eosinophil degranulation products (47-49), histamine (39,44,63), and cysteinyl leukotrienes (45,46) in the airway. It is not surprising that susceptible individuals (perhaps those with hyperreactive airways) would develop airway obstruction at the time of both viral infections and allergen exposures if the nature of the inflammatory response to each inciting agent were similar.

The mechanism by which the same terminal inflammatory response is induced may differ between asthma and virus-induced wheezing. In asthma, TH2 cytokines appear to initiate the allergic response. Recent evidence suggests that the concentration of chemokines such as macrophage inflammatory protein 1-alpha and eotaxin is increased in secretions of infants with severe (hypoxic) forms of RSV bronchiolitis

(64). These chemokines are chemotactic for lymphocytes and eosinophils, and can cause degranulation of mast cells, basophils, and eosinophils (65,66). The release of these chemokines during bronchiolitis may therefore provide an alternative method (not involving TH2 cytokines) for inciting the same type of inflammatory response as is observed in asthma.

Our conclusion, therefore, is that RSV bronchiolitis does not bear a causal relationship to the development of asthma. We suggest that the apparent cause–effect relationship of bronchiolitis and asthma is actually due to the induction of similar terminal inflammatory responses at the time of viral infections in infancy and during allergen exposures in childhood, resulting in airway obstruction in susceptible hosts on both occasions. The false appearance of a causal relationship is due to similar pathological responses to different stimuli resulting in the same disease manifestations.

References

1. Zweiman B, Schoenwetter WF, Hildreth EA. The relationship between bronchiolitis and allergic asthma. J Allergy 1966; 37:48.
2. Rooney JC, Williams HE. The relationship between proved viral bronchiolitis and subsequent wheezing. J Pediatr 1971; 79:744–747.
3. Sims DG, Downham MAPS, Gardner PS, Webb JKG, Weightman D. Study of 8-year-old children with a history of respiratory syncytial virus bronchiolitis in infancy. Br Med J 1978;1:11–14.
4. McConnochie KM, Roghmann KJ. Bronchiolitis as a possible cause of wheezing in childhood: new evidence. Pediatrics 1984; 74:1–10.
5. Sims DG, Gardner PS, Weightman, D, Turner MW, Soothill JF. Atopy does not predispose to RSV bronchiolitis or postbronchiolitis wheezing. Br Med J 1981; 282:2086–2088.
6. Sigurs N, Bjarnason R, Sigurbergsson F, Kjellman B. Respiratory syncytial virus bronchiolitis in infancy is an important risk factor for asthma and allergy at age 7. Am J Respir Crit Care Med 2000;161:1501–1507.
7. Henderson FW, Clyde WA, Jr, Collier AM, Denny FW, Senior RJ, Sheaffer CI, Conley WG, III, Christian RM. The etiologic and epidemiologic spectrum of bronchiolitis in pediatric practice. J Pediatr 1979; 95:183–190.
8. Martinez FD, Wright AL, Taussig LM, Holberg CJ, Halonen M, Morgan WJ, The Group Health Medical Associates. N Eng J Med 1995; 332:133–138.
9. Rusconi F, Galassi C, Corbo GM, Forastiere F, Biggeri A, Ciccone G, Renzoni E, SIDRIA Collaborative Group. Risk Factors for early, persistent, and late-onset wheezing in young children. Am J Respir Crit Care Med 1999; 160:1617–1622.
10. Martinez FD, Stern DA, Wright AL, Taussig LM, Halonen M. Differential immune responses to acute lower respiratory illness in early life and subsequent development of persistent wheezing and asthma. J Allergy Clin Immunol 1998; 102:915–920.
11. Ehlenfield DR, Cameron K, Welliver RC. Eosinophilia at the time of respiratory syncytial virus bronchiolitis predicts childhood reactive airway disease. Pediatrics 2000; 105: 79–83.
12. McConnochie KM, Roghmann KJ. Wheezing at 8 and 13 years: changing importance of bronchiolitis and passive smoking. Pediatr Pulmonol 1989; 6:138–146.

13. Stein RT, Sherrill D, Morgan WJ, Holberg CJ, Halonen M, Taussig LM, Wright AL, Martinez FD. Respiratory syncytial virus in early life and risk of wheeze and allergy by age 13 years. Lancet 1999; 354:541–545.

14. Strachan DP, Anderson HR, Bland JM, Peckham C. Asthma as a link between chest illness in childhood and chronic cough and phlegm in young adults. Br Med J 1988; 196:890–893.

15. Mann SL, Wadsworth MEJ, Colley JRT. Accumulation of factors influencing respiratory illness in members of a national birth cohort and their offspring. J Epidemiol Community Health 1992; 46:286–292.

16. Sherman CB, Tosteson TD, Tager IB, Speizer FE, Weiss ST. Early childhood predictors of asthma. Am J Epidemiol 1990; 132:83–95.

17. McConnochie KM, Roghmann KJ. Predicting clinically significant lower respiratory tract illness in childhood following mild bronchiolitis. Am J Dis Child 1985; 139:625–631.

18. Tager IB, Hanrahan JP, Tosteson TD, Castile RG, Brown RW, Weiss ST, Speizer FE. Lung function, pre- and post-natal smoke exposure, and wheezing in the first year of life. Am Rev Respir Dis 1993; 147:811–187.

19. Dezateux C, Fletcher ME, Dundas I, Stocks J. Infant respiratory function after RSV-proven bronchiolitis. Am J Respir Crit Care Med 1997; 155:1349–1355.

20. Hammer J, Numa A, Jewth CJL. Albuterol responsiveness in infants with respiratory failure caused by respiratory syncytial virus infection. J Pediatr 1995; 127:485–490.

21. Pullan CR, Hey EN. Wheezing, asthma and pulmonary dysfunction 10 years after infection with respiratory syncytial virus in infancy. Br Med J 1982; 284:1665–1669.

22. Hall CB, Hall WJ, Gala CL, MaGill FB, Leddy JP. Long-term prospective study in children after respiratory syncytial virus infection. J Pediatr 1984; 105:358–364.

23. Henderson FW, Stewart PW, Burchinal MR, Voter KZ, Strope GL, Ivins SS, Morris R, Wang O-L, Henry MM. Respiratory allergy and the relationship between early childhood lower respiratory illness and subsequent lung function. Am Rev Respir Dis 1992; 145:283–290.

24. Voter KZ, Henry MM, Stewart PW, Henderson FW. Lower respiratory illness in early childhood and lung function and bronchial reactivity in adolescent males. Am Rev Respir Dis 1988; 137:302–307.

25. Gold DR, Tager IB, Weiss ST, Tosteson TD, Speizer FE. Acute lower respiratory illness in childhood as a predictor of lung function and chronic respiratory symptoms. Am Rev Respir Dis 1989; 140:877–884.

26. McConnochie KM, Mark JD, McBride JT, Hall WJ, Brooks JG, Klein SJ, Miller RL, McInerny TK, Nazarian LF, MacWhinney JB. Normal pulmonary function measurements and airway reactivity in childhood after mild bronchiolitis. J Pediatr 1985; 107:54–58.

27. Kattan M, Keens TG, Lapierre J-G, Levison H, Bryan AC, Reilly BJ. Pulmonary function abnormalities in symptom-free children after bronchiolitis. Pediatrics 1977; 59:683–688.

28. Strope GL, Stewart PW, Henderson FW, Ivins SS, Stedman HC, Henry MM. Lung function in school-age children who had mild lower respiratory illnesses in early childhood. Am Rev Respir Dis 1991; 144:655–662.

29. Welliver RC, Duffy L. The relationship of RSV-specific immunoglobulin E antibody response in infancy, recurrent wheezing, and pulmonary function at age 7–8 years. Pediatr Pulmonol 1993; 15:19–27.

30. Hall WJ, Hall CB, Speers DM. Respiratory syncytial virus infection in adults: clinical, virologic, and serial pulmonary function studies. Ann Intern Med 1978; 88:203–205.

31. Gurwitz D, Mindorff C, Levison H. Increased incidence of bronchial reactivity in children with a history of bronchiolitis. J Pediatr 1981; 98:551–555.

32. Tepper RS, Rosenberg D, Eigen H. Airway responsiveness in infants following bronchiolitis. Pediatr Pulmonol 1992;13:6–10.

33. Young S, LeSouef PN, Geelhoed GC, Stick SM, Chir B, Turner KJ, Landau LI. The influence of a family history of asthma and parental smoking on airway responsiveness in early infancy. N Engl J Med 1991; 324:1168–1173.

34. Clarke JR, Reese A, Silverman M. Bronchial responsiveness and lung function in infants with lower respiratory tract illness over the first six months of life. Arch Dis Child 1992; 67:1454–1458.

35. Wilson NM, Phagoo SB, Silverman M. Atopy, bronchial responsiveness, and symptoms in wheezy 3 year olds. Arch Dis Child 1992; 67:491–495.

36. Stick SM, Arnott J, Turner DJ, Young S, Landau LI, Lesouef PN. Bronchial responsiveness and lung function in recurrently wheezy infants. Am Rev Respir Dis 1991; 144:1012–1015.

37. Robinson DS, Hamid Q, Ying S, Tsicopoulos A, Barkans J, Bentley AM, Corrigan C, Durham SR, Kay AB. Predominant TH2-like bronchoalveolar T-lymphocyte population in atopic asthma. N Engl J Med 1992; 326:298–204.

38. Welliver RC, Kaul TN, Ogra PL. The appearance of cell-bound IgE in respiratory-tract epithelium after respiratory-syncytial virus infection. N Engl J Med 1980; 303:1198–1202.

39. Welliver RC, Wong DT, Sun M, Middleton E Jr, Vaughan RS, Ogra PL. The development of respiratory syncytial virus-specific IgE and the release of histamine in nasopharyngeal secretions after infection. N Engl J Med 1981; 305:841–846.

40. Bui RHD, Molinaro GA, Kettering JD, Heiner DC, Imagawa DT, St Geme JW Jr. Virus-specific IgE and IgG4 antibodies in serum of children infected with respiratory syncytial virus. J Pediatr 1987; 110:87–90.

41. Russi JC, Delfraro A, Borthagaray MD, Velazqu4es B, Garcia-Barreno B, Hortal M. Evaluation of immunoglobulin E-specific antibodies and viral antigens in nasopharyngeal secretions of children with respiratory syncytial virus infections. J Clin Microbiol 1993; 31:819–823.

42. Rabatic S, Gagro A, Lokar-Kolbas R, Krusulovic-Hresic V, Vrtar Z, Popow-Kraupp T, Drazenovic V, Mlinaric-Galinovic G. Increase in CD23[+] B cells in infants with bronchiolitis is accompanied by appearance of IgE and IgG4 antibodies specific for respiratory syncytial virus. J Infect Dis 1997; 175:32–37.

43. Aberle JH, Aberle SW, Dworzak MN, Mandl CW, Rebhandl W, Vollnhofer G, Kundi M, Popow-Kraupp T. Reduced interferon-γ expression in peripheral blood mononuclear cells of infants with severe respiratory syncytial virus disease. Am J Respir Crit Care Med 19991; 160:1263–1268.

44. Skoner DP, Fireman P, Caliguiri L, Davis H. Plasma elevations of histamine and a prostaglandin metabolite in acute bronchiolitis. Am Rev Respir Dis 1990; 142:359–364.

45. Volovitz B, Welliver RC, DeCastro G, Krystofik DA, Ogra PL. The release of leukotrienes in the respiratory tract during infection with respiratory syncytial virus: role in obstructive airway disease. Pediatr Res 1988; 24:504–507.

46. van Schaik SM, Tristram DA, Nagpal IS, Hintz KM, Welliver RC III, Welliver RC.

Increased production of IFN-γ and cysteinyl leukotrienes in virus-induced wheezing. J Allergy Clin Immunol 1999; 103:630–636.

47. Garofalo R, Kimpen JLL, Welliver RC, Ogra PL. Eosinophil degranulation in the respiratory tract during naturally acquired respiratory syncytial virus infection. J Pediatr 1992; 120:28–32.

48. Garofalo R, Dorris A, Ahlstedt S, Welliver RC. Peripheral blood counts and eosinophil cationic protein content of respiratory secretions in bronchiolitis: relationship to severity of disease. Pediatr Allergy Immunol 1994; 5:111–117.

49. Colocho Zelaya EA, Orvell C, Strannegard O. Eosinophil cationic protein in nasopharyngeal secretions and serum of infants infected with respiratory syncytial virus. Pediatr Allergy Immunol 1994; 5:100–106.

50. Renzi P, Turgeon JP, Yang JP, Drblik SP, Marcotte JE, Pedneault L, et al. Cellular immunity is activated and a TH-2 response is associated with early wheezing in infants after bronchiolitis. J Pediatr 1977; 130:584–93.

51. Roman M, Calhoun WJ, Hinton KL, Avendano LF, Simon V, Escobar AM, Gaggero A, Diaz PV. Respiratory syncytial virus infection in infants is associated with predominant Th-2–like response. Am J Respir Crit Care Med 1997; 156:190–195.

52. Prescott SL, Macaubas C, Smallacombe T, Holt BJ, Sly PD, Holt PG. Development of allergen-specific T-cell memory in atopic and normal children. Lancet 1999; 353:196–200.

53. Rinas U, Horneff G, Wahn V. Interferon-γ production by cord-blood mononuclear cells is reduced in newborns with a family history of atopic disease and is independent from cord blood IgE-levels. Pediatr Allergy Immunol 1993; 4:60–64.

54. Koning H, Baert MRM, Oranje AP, Savelkoul HFJ, Neijens HJ. Development of immune functions related to allergic mechanisms in young children. Pediatr Res 1996; 40:363–375.

55. Renzi PM, Turgeon JP, Marcotte JE, Drblik SP, Berube D, Gagnon MF, Spier S. Reduced interferon- production in infants with bronchiolitis and asthma. Am J Respir Crit Care Med 1999; 159:1417–1422.

56. Bendelja K, Gagro A, Bace A, Lokar-Kolbas R, Krsulovic-Hresic V, Drazenovic V, Mlinaric-Galinovic G, Rabatic S. Predominant type-2 response in infants with respiratory syncytial virus (RSV) infection demonstrated by cytokine flow cytometry. Clin Exp Immunol 2000; 121:332–338.

57. Brandenberg AH, Kleinjan A, van het Land B, Moll HA, Timmerman HH, de Swart RL, Neijens HJ, Fokkens W, Osterhaus ADME. Type 1-like immune response is found in children with respiratory syncytial virus infection regardless of clinical severity. J Med Virol 2000; 62:267–277.

58. Sporik R, Holgate ST, Platts-Mills TAE, Cogswell JJ. Exposure to house-dust mite allergen (Der p I) and the development of asthma in childhood: a prospective study. N Engl J Med 1990; 323:502–507.

59. Robinson PJ, Hegele RG, Schellenberg RR. Allergic sensitization increases airway reactivity in guinea pigs with respiratory syncytial virus bronchiolitis. J Allergy Clin Immunol 1997; 100:492–498.

60. Schwarze J, Hamelmann E, Bradley KL, Takeda K, Gelfand EW. Respiratory syncytial virus infection results in airway hyperresponsiveness and enhanced airway sensitization to allergen. J Clin Invest 1997; 100:226–233.

61. Peebles RS Jr, Sheller JR, Johnson JE, Mitchell DB, Graham BS. Respiratory syncytial virus infection prolongs methacholine-induced airway hyperresponsiveness in ovalbumin-sensitized mice. J Med Virol 1999; 57:186–192.

62. Everard ML, Swarbrick A, Wrightham M, McIntyre J, Dunkley C, James PD, Sewell HF, Milner AD. Analysis of cells obtained by bronchial lavage of infants with respiratory syncytial virus infection. Arch Dis Child 1994; 71:428–432.

63. Counil FP, Lebel B, Segondy M, Peterson C, Voisin M, Bousquet J, Arnoux B. Cells and mediators from pharyngeal secretions in infants with acute wheezing episodes. Eur Respir J 1997; 10:2592–2595.

64. Garofalo R, Olszewska-Pazdrak B, Ogra PL, Welliver RC. Beta-chemokines in nasal secretions of infants with respiratory syncytial virus-induced upper respiratory illness and bronchiolitis. Pediatr Allergy Asthma Immunol 2001; 15:43–50.

65. Rot A, Krieger M, Brunner T, Bischoff SC, Schall TJ, Dahinden CA. RANTES and macrophage inflammatory protein-1α induce the migration and activation of normal human eosinophil granulocytes. J Exp Med 1992; 176:1489–1495.

66. Alam R, Forsythe PA, Stafford S, Lett-Brown MA, Grant JA. Macrophage inflammatory protein-1α activates basophils and mast cells. J Exp Med 1992; 176:781–786.

23

Microbiology and Epidemiology of *Mycoplasma pneumoniae* and *Chlamydia pneumoniae* in Normal and Asthmatic Subjects

PEKKA SAIKKU

University of Oulu
Oulu, Finland

I. Introduction

Bacterial agents causing so-called atypical pneumonias are usually considered to include *Mycoplasma pneumoniae*, *Chlamydia* (*Chlamydophila*) spp., and *Legionella* spp. In recent years, the two most common agents in human respiratory infections, *M. pneumoniae* and *C. pneumoniae*, have also been associated with asthma. They are both capable of causing frequent reinfections. Both pathogens are extremely common and no one seems to avoid contact with them. The outcome of infection is mainly dependent on the host response. Persistent infections are typical for chlamydiae, and the possibility of chronic mycoplasmal infections has recently also received attention. In these chronic infections, the activated immune defence mechanisms are evidently mainly responsible for the damage seen.

M. pneumoniae has been known since 1944 (1). Because it passed bacteriological filters, it was originally believed to be a virus. In 1962, it was shown to grow on cell-free medium and its mycoplasmal nature was confirmed (1). *C. pneumoniae* is a relatively recently discovered bacterium. Although the first isolation was done as early as 1965, the first studies on its association with respiratory infections were only published in 1985 (2) and 1986 (3). Both *M. pneumoniae* and *C. pneumoniae* have been studied by a few expert laboratories only. The problems in growing these agents, both of which require specialized techniques, and the difficulties in the diag-

Table 1 General Properties of *Mycoplasma pneumoniae* and *Chlamydia pneumoniae*

	M. Pneumoniae	C. Pneumoniae
Genome	860 000 kb	1 200 000 kb
Related bacteria	Gram-positive	Gram-negative
Cell wall	Devoid of peptidoglycan trilamellar membrane exogenous cholesterol "Tip" structure of P1 protein 46 putative lipoprotein genes	Devoid of peptidoglycan gram-negative cell wall cystine-rich proteins Type III secretion sysytem 21 putative outer membrane genes, LPS present
Replication	Slow, binary fission No amino acid synthesis	Slow, reticulate body binary fission using peptidoglycan, elementary body nonreplicative
Mode of parasitism	Cell surface, found intracellulary	Obligatory intracellular parasitism, use of ADP/ATP translocase for acquiring ATP
Acute infection	Common in childhood and early adulthood	Common in childhood, severe pneumonias in elderly
Persistent infection	Described	Common

nostics of *C. pneumoniae* have been some reasons for this neglect. The recent advent of molecular microbiology has profoundly altered our knowledge of these agents, and their properties and pathogenetic mechanisms will, in the future, be more easily accessible for further studies (4,5) (Table 1).

II. *M. pneumoniae*

A. Natural History

Mycoplasma pneumoniae is one of the 13 species found in humans of the 102 currently recognized species of genus *Mycoplasma* in the order Mycoplasmatales in the Class Mollicutes. Mycoplasmas are widespread parasites in nature. Mycoplasmas are small bacteria, 120–150 nm in diameter, without a rigid peptidoglycan wall and thus resistant to beta-lactam antibiotics. Instead, they have a triple-layered cell membrane containing sterols, are deformable (*mollis*, soft; *cutis*, skin) and can thus pass bacteriological filters. They are not visible in Gram's staining. They are able to grow in cell-free media and are the smallest self-replicating organisms with small genomes (580–1350 kb). The genome sequences of three mycoplasmas have been published (6-8). The *M. pneumoniae* genome is 816 kb, codes about 700 proteins, but is devoid of genes responsible for amino acid synthesis, which explains its total dependency on exogenous amino acids. In cultivation, they grow in rich media containing serum, peptone, and yeast extract. *M. pneumoniae* is also dependent on the fatty acids and cholesterol of its host. Cholesterol is used as the buffer of membrane fluidity. Mycoplasmal membranes have, for a long time, been used as models of biological membranes. The small defective genome without gene duplications is reflected in their relatively slow growth rate. The lack of DNA repair enzymes is, moreover, associated with an increased mutation rate (7). *M. pneumoniae* is close to the minimal cell concept of the simplest self-replicating organism (8).

M. pneumoniae colonizes mucous membranes in the ororespiratory tract. The minute mycoplasmas have the impressive ability to maintain a surface architecture that is both antigenically and functionally versatile. The elongated mycoplasma has a tip containing P1 protein as a main adhesin, with which it attaches to cell surfaces. P1 is organized into two gene families, and it shows a strong immune response during infection (9). The adhered *M. pneumoniae* inhibits cilial motility. Cytoadherence and fusion with the cellular membrane have been speculated as a mode to acquire a membrane similar to the host cell for mimicry and intracellular invasion. Mycoplasmal enzymes may lead to clastogenic effects in the cell (10). While *M. pneumoniae* has been demonstrated intracellularly and shown to be alive for at least 7 days, it is not known if it can replicate intracellularly. The intracellular location promotes the establishment of latent or chronic infection states and circumvents mycoplasmacidal immune mechanisms and selective drug therapies (11). Mycoplasmal infection leads to a powerful induction of different cytokines. The induction of IL-10, a downregulating cytokine, is also noteworthy. The clinical picture is suggestive of damage to the host's immune and inflammatory responses rather than a direct toxic effect of the mycoplasmal cell components. Various autoantibodies, especially ones against neural tissue (12), are commonly produced in *M. pneumoniae* infections, and the roles of these antibodies have mainly been studied in view of neurological complications.

B. Epidemiology and Diagnosis

M. pneumoniae usually causes a mild respiratory disease. Most cases will not require a medical visit, and confirmed diagnosis is often not accomplished in daily practice. Thus, the available data reveal only a minor part of actual instances of disease. *M. pneumoniae* infections occur in temperate climates throughout the year, but the absolute number of infections is higher in the winter season. Since other respiratory tract pathogens also cause disease in wintertime, the proportion of *M. pneumoniae* infections is highest in the summer. Protective immunity may be acquired in daycare centers. Epidemics occur at intervals of 4–5 years. More severe infections occur predominantly in school-aged children, with another peak in young adults. Only 5–10% of infected persons develop pneumonia, depending on the age and presence of underlying diseases. Antibody titers in older people are significantly lower than in younger people (Fig. 1), and recent studies suggest that in the older age group and in young children serological diagnosis may be inadequate (13,14). The incubation period of *M. pneumoniae* is approximately 3 weeks. Spread in communities is slow, but microepidemics may arise.

Since the culturing of *M. pneumoniae* is difficult, serological testing has been

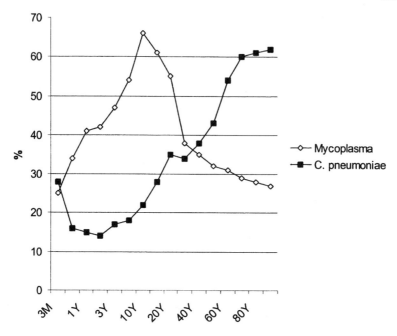

Figure 1 Prevalence of complement fixing antibodies in relation to age against *Mycoplasma pneumoniae* in 58,500 patients with suspected viral illness and microimmunofluorescence antibodies against *Chlamydia pneumoniae* in 5203 patients, respectively. (From Ukkonen et al., 1984; Saikku, 1994). M=months, Y=years.

traditionally utilized as a diagnostic tool. In several laboratories, a viral antigen panel for complement fixation (CF) test has also included the CF antigen for *M. pneumoniae*, which is a purified lipid antigen. Cross-reactivity with a human brain tissue antigen (12) has been reported, and low titered seroconversions remain doubtful. Enzyme-linked immunosorbent assays (ELISA) have the advantage of being able to differentiate between immunoglobulin classes, and IgM titrations can avoid the need for a second sample to show significant seroconversion. A rapid immunofluorescence test for IgM antibodies has a low positive predictive value (15). ELISA tests can be made more specific by using isolated P1 protein or parts of it as antigens. Immunoblotting has been used to verify the specificity of antibodies to *M. pneumoniae* (16).

Direct detection by a species-specific nucleic acid (NA) probe (17) and by enzyme immunoassay (ELA) for antigen (18) are or were available commercially. Polymerase chain reaction (PCR) methods have been used for *M. pneumoniae* for over 10 years (19), but they seem to be quite slow in replacing the older methods. In-house NA amplification methods may be vulnerable, which explains the notably variable results obtained. However, they are more sensitive than antigen detection and culture and should be available commercially. The first commercial kits have already appeared on the market, and their application may alter our notion of *M.*

pneumoniae-associated diseases. One should remember that after acute mycoplasmal infection the agent is often carried for months in respiratory tract and is demonstrable during epidemics also in asymptomatic contacts (17)

III. *C. pneumoniae*

A. Natural History

Chlamydiae are small gram-negative eubacteria that have, in their evolution, developed several adaptations to their parasitism. The classification of chlamydiae is under modification, and close relatives of human *C. pneumoniae* have been found in horse (20), koala (21), and frogs (22). Their relevance for human disease (21) and, moreover, the ability of human *C. pneumoniae* to multiply in environmental amebae (23) found swarming in walls of what are called sick buildings are totally open questions. Hypothetically the spore forms of these amebae could transmit *Chlamydia* in these houses.

The recent sequencing of chlamydial genomes (5) has altered our earlier notions of these organisms. Chlamydiae have a sporelike form, called elementary body (EB), which is the infective particle. It is devoid of peptidoglycan and the rigidity of the cell wall is due to S–S bridges of cysteine-rich proteins. A rough-type lipopolysaccharide of gram-negative bacteria is in the wall. It is outside cell inert, but *C. pneumoniae* EBs are adsorbed to a susceptible cell with glycosaminoglycan receptors (24). The bridging heparin is derived from host cells. The mannose receptor does not seem to be as important as in the adsorption of other chlamydiae (25), and the final triggers of engulfment of the EB are not known. Inside the cell, the *C. pneumoniae* endosome is able to avoid lysosomal fusion, travels along microtubules, and associates with the exocytic Golgi compartment and sphingomyelin-containing vesicles (26). In the formation of the chlamydial vacuole, the EB transforms into a reticulate body (RB), which start to parasitize the cell, grows and divides by binary fission. *C. pneumoniae* inhibits host cell apoptosis via IL-10 (27) and NF–κB (28), induces cytokines (29) and uses the type III secretion system (30) to control the host cell. In the end of a slow cycle taking about 70 h the RBs start to condense to EBs. An eukaryote-related histone takes part in packing the chromosome and excess lipopolysaccharide (LPS) is left over. In the end chlamydia activates proteinases (31,32) and apoptosis of the cell, leading to its destruction and liberation of free EBs. The elusive persistent form of *Chlamydia* has been described for *C. pneumoniae* also in lungs (33,34). The persistent form may differ profoundly from the actively dividing form (35,36) and is very resistant to antibiotics (37). It is hoped that genomic studies can find its weak points in the future (38). Pathogenetic studies on *C. pneumoniae* have concentrated on the pathogenesis of vascular diseases (39), and relatively few studies on the pathology of chronic pulmonary diseases have been published (34,40). However, the inflammatory responses of mononuclear cells and macrophages are similar (41,42). Chronic obstructive pulmonary disease is associated with coronary heart disease (43) and abdominal aortic aneurysms (44), both of which diseases are also associated with chronic *C. pneumoniae* infection. Ciliostasis is naturally seen in the lungs only (45). There are several animal models for acute lung infection (46–50). Large inoculum or repeated inoculations lead to a chronic lung infection (51), in which the agent cannot be isolated but its presence can be demonstrated by PCR (52), and it can be activated by immunosuppressive cortisone treatment (53,54). However, these chronic infection models in animals have been utilized mostly in studies on atherosclerosis (55). Chronic *C. pneumoniae* lung infections have remained inadequately studied.

B. Epidemiology and Diagnosis

The asymptomatic carrier rate has been reported to be low, and it has been characterized by a study in Japan. In this study on medical students and hospital staff, the asymptomatic carrier rate detected by PCR varied from 0 % to 3.2% in the different years, and the carriers did not show serological criteria for acute infection (56). Up to 70% of infections have been estimated to be asymptomatic (57). However, asymptomatic infections by *C. pneumoniae* need not be harmless. In *C. trachomatis* infection in women, asymptomatic infections may lead to severe sequelae. In the first *C. pneumoniae* epidemic described, 17% of the patients felt themselves asymptomatic. However, they also had radiographic pneumonic infiltrates indicating that the agent had invaded into their lungs (2). The precise role of *C. pneumoniae* in upper respiratory tract infections is not well characterized, but the part it plays in acute bronchitis and pneumonias is now well established on all continents (58-60). In elderly patients, *C. pneumoniae* pneumonia may be fatal (61). Since *C. pneumoniae*, tends to cause persistent infections, there often remains a question in acute episodes in adults: reinfection or reactivation of chronic infection? Since the behavior of *C. pneumoniae* is uniform in serological tests, only molecular biology methods can be expected to give an answer to the question of whether the strain is an old reactivated one or a new one. There are already some published studies on this issue (62). Indirect evidence can be obtained in connection with epidemics, which have been described in schools (2,63,64), in military garrisons (65,66), and nursing homes (61). In Scandinavia, countrywide epidemics have been described (67,68).

The current diagnostic guidelines have recently been reviewed by the Centers for Disease Control (CDC) (69). Improved, standardized, commercially available diagnostic kits are lacking. The uncertainties created by sloppy reading of the microimmunofluorescence (MIF) test mastered only by experts (70), and the differences seen in findings by in-house immunocytochemistry and especially PCR tests (71) have highlighted the difficulties in diagnosis. The MIF serology has remained the so-called gold standard in the diagnosis of acute infections caused by *C. pneumoniae*. Only fourfold seroconversions detected in an experienced laboratory are reliable markers of acute infections. The high titer ($\geq$512) for the indication of an acute infection (58) was originally estimated with a low-powered transillumination fluorescence microscope. It has repeatedly been found, in other laboratories, to be only suggestive of acute infection and often a better marker of chronic infection. The new enzyme immunoassay (EIA) methods on the market nowadays seem to be equally as or even more sensitive than MIF in acute infections, though there are some reservations on the specificity of these tests. The application of these test kits to the study of chronic infections has, however, generally been a disappointment (72). It has been suggested earlier that short-lived IgA antibodies typical of the Th2 type response could be better markers in chronic conditions, and several recent studies favor this concept (73,74). A pitfall is the variable quality of the anti-IgA conjugates available. At this moment, we do not have a simple test that allows us to tell from a single serum sample whether this very patient has an active *C. pneumoniae* disease possibly requiring treatment with antichlamydial drugs. Local antibodies have remained poorly studied (75,76). According to several seroepidemiological studies in cardiology, a combination of serological markers with those of inflammation [C-reactive protein (CRP)] and/or autoimmunity to heat shock protein 60 (Hsp60) seem to be better markers of risk. This may also be true in chronic pulmonary diseases, and IgA antibodies against chlamydial Hsp60 seem to be a marker of the severity of asthma (77).

The nucleic acid amplification (NAA) methods for *C. pneumoniae* have been repeatedly shown to be quite variable in their results (71). There are several reasons for this. The agent is possibly present patchily and in small amounts, inhibitors may be present, the extraction methods are not optimal, and primers and probes vary between laboratories. No commercially available kit system is currently on the market. However, NA amplification methods are the most sensitive diagnostic test and, in the future, they may shed light especially on chronic *C. pneumoniae* infections. NAA methods are suitable for testing bronchoalveolar lavage (BAL) samples and induced sputa (Table 2).

IV. Treatment

The lack of structural peptidoglycan renders beta-lactam antibiotics ineffective, and treatment with macrolides and tetracyclines is recommended (78,79). *C. pneumoniae* apparently uses peptidoglycan in replication, and in an animal model, amoxicillin-clavulanic acid was as effective in the acute phase as other antibiotics (80). However, beta-lactams only prevent the agent from dividing, and it starts to develop when the antibiotic is removed, promoting the development of chronic infections. This is reflected in relapses and recurrences of the disease after beta-lactam treatment of *C. pneumoniae* infection (59). Prolonged courses (up to 3 weeks) have been recommended in the treatment of *C. pneumoniae* pneumonias. New fluoroquinolones and ketolides are also effective. The treatment of chronic infections is problematic. In animal experiments, combination therapy with rifampicin and macrolide improved the eradication of *C. pneumoniae* (81). In cardiovascular diseases, treatments for *C. pneumoniae* for up to 1 year have been tried (82). Cortisone in animal experiments is known to activate chronic *C. pneumoniae* infection and to produce infectious progeny (53,54). This effect has not been studied in detail. There is a possibility, that when *C. pneumoniae* activates in persistently infected cell, it kills its host cell and is released. Fortunately the number of persistently infected cells is quite low in chronic *C. pneumoniae* infections. Moreover, the released EBs are now attacked

Table 2 Diagnostic Methods Used for *Mycoplasma pneumoniae* and *Chlamydia pneumoniae*

	M. pneumoniae	C. pneumoniae
Culture	+	+
Serology		
complement fixation	+++	+
EIA	+++	++
IF	++	+++
latex agglutination	+	−
Antigen detection		
LPS	−	+
IF	−	+
EIA	+	++
Nucleic acid detection		
direct hybridization	+++	−
NAA	+++	+++

⁻Not reported.
⁺Possible.
⁺⁺Usable.
⁺⁺⁺Recommended.

by antibodies typical for chronic infections and could be neutralized. It has even been speculated that one should try combined cortisone–antibiotic treatment in order to activate the persistent form to multiply. Then it would be vulnerable to the usual antibiotic treatment.

V. Association of Atypical Pathogens with Asthma

These pathogens discussed in detail in other chapters. For decades, *M. pneumoniae* has been associated with asthma, and interest in it has been revived recently, since asthma is nowadays classified as an inflammatory disease. *M. pneumoniae* is able to cause reinfections, and it has earlier been sought mainly in asthma exacerbations (83,84). The earlier reports were cautious and mainly based on follow-up studies showing persistent damage to the airways and on IgE antibody findings (85). In *M. pneumoniae* pneumonia, a tendency to a Th2 type immune response with a tendency to IgE production has been reported (86). Only after Kraft et al. reported the common presence of *M. pneumoniae* in the airways of adults with chronic asthma did the possible chronic presence of the agent as an allergen attract renewed interest (87). The NAA detection methods made this advent possible, since both cultures and serological tests remained negative in asthma. Moreover, PCR-positive asthmatics showed a kind of edema not seen in PCR-negative individuals, and this could be effected by clarithromycin treatment (88). Cytokine induction in chronic mycoplasmal infection has been speculated to be due to monocytic cells recruited into a chronically inflamed area (89). Asthma patients with positive PCR, whether for *M. pneumoniae* or *C. pneumoniae*, had an accumulation of mast cells in their lungs when compared to PCR negative patients (90). Recently, a mouse model was reported in which *M. pneumoniae* caused a chronic infection that led in 530 days to infection-associated reactive airway disease (91). In mice, *M. pneumoniae* persisted in a cultivable state. The final form in which noncultivable *M. pneumoniae* possibly persists in asthmatic lungs is not known.

Persistent infection means continuous presence of foreign proteins and other bacterial components deep in the lungs. Chlamydiae are well known for their capability to cause persistent infections. There is evidence based on local antibodies (75,76), PCR(92), immunohistochemistry (34), and electron microscopy (33) that *C. pneumoniae* can be found in lung tissue and its amount is increased in diseased conditions. The presence of *C. pneumoniae* DNA in white blood cells of apparently healthy people has been reported repeatedly. Although the amount of circulating nucleic acid is increased in atherosclerotic conditions, there is a clearer correlation with smoking and seasonality, since the amount of circulating DNA increases in the winter months (93). This fits well with the concept that the majority of the NA found in white blood cells is possibly derived from lungs, where *C. pneumoniae* can be shown to be present in alveolar macrophages. Smoking is known to impair the action of immunological defense mechanisms, and this could provoke the multiplication of the pathogen (94). Since *C. pneumoniae* epidemics are known to occur years apart, to be prolonged and not to be seasonal, there is a possibility that the respiratory viruses occurring during the wintertime or the stress caused by cold air alone can activate persistent *C. pneumoniae* infection. The outcome would depend mainly on the individual carrying the pathogen. If the person is immunologically susceptible to respond with asthmatic symptoms to an allergen in the lungs, activation of the pathogen could at least worsen the asthma attack. Archives of histological samples should be studied for the presence of *M. pneumoniae* and *C. pneumoniae*. These agents are not detected in light microscopy and are difficult to find in electron microscopy, but immunohistochemistry and in situ hybridization could give the sought-after answers.

VI. Conclusions

It is difficult to prove the presence of chronic infection caused by atypical agents in the lungs. *M. pneumoniae* does not seem to induce an antibody response, is not cultivable, and can be demonstrated only by NA amplification methods. *C. pneumoniae* is able to multiply in macrophages and is repeatedly found in the circulation. This can explain the differences in antibody patterns found between these two agents in relation to age. The presence of IgG antibodies is not, however, diagnostic, since the prevalence may also be extremely high in asymptomatic patients. IgA antibodies may be better indicators in that sense (95). Apart from possibly reflecting a process on mucosal membranes, their presence in the circulation may also be a sign that immunological defense has been directed to a Th2 type response, which is inefficient in defense against intracellular pathogens. Local IgA antibodies could be even better markers and they should be sought in asthma and chronic obstructive pulmonary disease (COPD). The availability of sputum is a limiting factor, and the presence of secretory IgA in saliva has so far remained unstudied. The advent of NAA-based techniques may solve many problems. A demand for them would lead to both commercially available kits and to a decrease in their costs. There are suggestions that early proper treatment can improve the prognosis (96), and this necessitates the availability of rapid and sensitive diagnostic means. The first large intervention trial with antibiotics effective against atypical pathogens in patients with established asthma did not conclusively answer the question of whether antimicrobial treatment could modify the course of asthma (97), as has been anecdotally reported (98). Large, controlled trials are indicated (99).

References

1. Chanock RM, Hayflick L, Barile MF. Growth on artifical medium of an agent associated with atypical pneumoniae and its identification as a PPLO. Proc Natl Acad Sci 1962; 48:41–49.
2. Saikku P, Wang SP, Kleemola M, Brander E, Rusanen E, Grayston JT. An epidemic of mild pneumonia due to an unusual strain of *Chlamydia psittaci*. J Infect Dis 1985; 151:832–839.
3. Grayston JT, Kuo CC, Wang SP, Altman J. A new *Chlamydia psittaci* strain, TWAR, isolated in acute respiratory tract infections. N Engl J Med 1986; 315:161–168.
4. Razin S, Yogev D, Naot Y. Molecular biology and pathogenicity of mycoplasmas. Microbiol Mol Biol Rev 1998; 62:1094–1156.
5. Rockey DD, Lenart J, Stephens RS. Genome sequencing and our understanding of chlamydiae. Infect Immun 2000; 68:5473–5479.
6. Chambaud I, Heilig R, Ferris S, Barbe V, Samson D, Galisson F, Moszer I, Dybvig K, Wroblewski H, Viari A, Rocha EP, Blanchard A. The complete genome sequence of the murine respiratory pathogen *Mycoplasma pulmonis*. Nucleic Acids Res 2001; 29:2145–2153.
7. Himmelreich R, Hilbert H, Plagens H, Pirkl E, Li BC, Herrmann R. Complete sequence analysis of the genome of the bacterium *Mycoplasma pneumoniae*. Nucleic Acids Res 1996; 24:4420–4449.
8. Fraser CM, Gocayne JD, White O, Adams MD, Clayton RA, Fleischmann RD, Bult CJ, Kerlavage AR, Sutton G, Kelley JM, et al. The minimal gene complement of *Mycoplasma genitalium*. Science 1995; 270:397–403.
9. Krause DC. Mycoplasma pneumoniae cytadherence: unravelling the tie that binds. Mol Microbiol 1996; 20:247–253.
10. Stewart SD, Watson HL, Cassell GH. Investigation of clastogenic potential of *Ureaplasma urealyticum* on human leukocytes. IOM Lett 1994; 3:662–663.
11. Baseman JB, Tully JG. Mycoplasmas: sophisticated, reemerging, and burdened by their notoriety. Emerg Infect Dis 1997; 3:21–32.
12. Biberfeld G. *Mycoplasma pneumoniae* infections and antibodies to brain. Lancet 1969; 2:1202.
13. Dorigo-Zetsma JW, Wilbrink B, van der Nat H, Bartelds AI, Heijnen ML, Dankert J.

Results of molecular detection of *Mycoplasma pneumoniae* among patients with acute respiratory infection and in their household contacts reveals children as human reservoirs. J Infect Dis 2001; 183:675–678.

14. Layani-Milon MP, Gras I, Valette M, Luciani J, Stagnara J, Aymard M, Lina B. Incidence of upper respiratory tract *Mycoplasma pneumoniae* infections among outpatients in Rhone-Alpes, France, during five successive winter periods. J Clin Microbiol 1999; 37:1721–1726.

15. Dorigo-Zetsma JW, Zaat SA, Wertheim-van Dillen PM, Spanjaard L, Rijntjes J, van Waveren G, Jensen JS, Angulo AF, Dankert J. Comparison of PCR, culture, and serological tests for diagnosis of *Mycoplasma pneumoniae* respiratory tract infection in children. J Clin Microbiol 1999; 37:14–17.

16. Jacobs E, Bennewitz A, Bredt W. Reaction pattern of human anti-*Mycoplasma pneumoniae* antibodies in enzyme-linked immunosorbent assays and immunoblotting. J Clin Microbiol 1986; 23:517–522.

17. Kleemola SR, Karjalainen JE, Raty RK. Rapid diagnosis of *Mycoplasma pneumoniae* infection: clinical evaluation of a commercial probe test. J Infect Dis 1990; 162:70–75.

18. Kok TW, Varkanis G, Marmion BP, Martin J, Esterman A. Laboratory diagnosis of *Mycoplasma pneumoniae* infection. 1. Direct detection of antigen in respiratory exudates by enzyme immunoassay. Epidemiol Infect 1988; 101:669–684.

19. Bernet C, Garret M, de Barbeyrac B, Bebear C, Bonnet J. Detection of *Mycoplasma pneumoniae* by using the polymerase chain reaction. J Clin Microbiol 1989; 27:2492–2496.

20. Storey C, Lusher M, Yates P, Richmond S. Evidence for *Chlamydia pneumoniae* of non-human origin. J Gen Microbiol 1993; 139:2621–2626.

21. Coles KA, Timms P, Smith DW. Koala biovar of *Chlamydia pneumoniae* infects human and koala monocytes and induces increased uptake of lipids in vitro. Infect Immun 2001; 69:7894–7897.

22. Berger L, Volp K, Mathews S, Speare R, Timms P. *Chlamydia pneumoniae* in a free-ranging giant barred frog (*Mixophyes iteratus*) from Australia. J Clin Microbiol 1999; 37:2378–2380.

23. Essig A, Heinemann M, Simnacher U, Marre R. Infection of *Acanthamoeba castellanii* by *Chlamydia pneumoniae*. Appl Environ Microbiol 1997; 63:1396–1399.

24. Wuppermann FN, Hegemann JH, Jantos CA. Heparan sulfate-like glycosaminoglycan is a cellular receptor for *Chlamydia pneumoniae*. J Infect Dis 2001; 184:181–187.

25. Kuo CC, Puolakkainen M, Lin TM, Witte M, Campbell LA. Mannose-receptor positive and negative mouse macrophages differ in their susceptibility to infection by *Chlamydia* species. Microb Pathog 2002; 32:43–48.

26. Al-Younes HM, Rudel T, Meyer TF. Characterization and intracellular trafficking pattern of vacuoles containing *Chlamydia pneumoniae* in human epithelial cells. Cell Microbiol 1999; 1:237–247.

27. Geng Y, Shane RB, Berencsi K, Gonzol E, Zaki MH, Margolis DJ, Trinchieri G, Rook AH. *Chlamydia pneumoniae* inhibits apoptosis in human peripheral blood mononuclear cells through induction of IL-10. J Immunol 2000; 164:5522–5529.

28. Wahl C, Oswald F, Simnacher U, Weiss S, Marre R, Essig A. Survival of *Chlamydia pneumoniae*-infected Mono Mac 6 cells is dependent on NF-kappaB binding activity. Infect Immun 2001; 69:7039–7045.

29. Kaukoranta-Tolvanen SS, Teppo AM, Laitinen K, Saikku P, Linnavuori K, Leinonen M. Growth of *Chlamydia pneumoniae* in cultured human peripheral blood mononuclear cells and induction of a cytokine response. Microb Pathog 1996; 21:215–221.

30. Subtil A, Parsot C, Dautry-Varsat A. Secretion of predicted Inc proteins of *Chlamydia pneumoniae* by a heterologous type III machinery. Mol Microbiol 2001; 39:792–800.

31. Vehmaan-Kreula P, Puolakkainen M, Sarvas M, Welgus HG, Kovanen PT. *Chlamydia pneumoniae* proteins induce secretion of the 92-kDa gelatinase by human monocyte-derived macrophages. Arterioscler Thromb Vasc Biol 2001; 21:E1–E8.

32. Fan P, Dong F, Huang Y, Zhong G. *Chlamydia pneumoniae* secretion of a protease-like activity factor for degrading host cell transcription factors required for major histocompatibility complex antigen expression. Infect Immun 2002; 70:345–349.

33. Theegarten D, Mogilevski G, Anhenn O, Stamatis G, Jaeschock R, Morgenrot K. The role of chlamydia in the pathogenesis of pulmonary emphysema. Electron microscopy and immunofluorescence reveal corresponding findings as in atherosclerosis. Virchows Arch 2000; 437:190–193.

34. Wu L, Skinner SJ, Lambie N, Vuletic JC, Blasi F, Black PN. Immunohistochemical staining for *Chlamydia pneumoniae* is increased in lung tissue from subjects with chronic obstructive pulmonary disease. Am J Respir Crit Care Med 2000; 162:1148–1151.

35. Byrne GI, Ouellette SP, Wang Z, Rao JP, Lu L, Beatty WL, Hudson AP. *Chlamydia pneumoniae* expresses genes required for DNA replication but not cytokinesis during persistent infection of HEp-2 cells. Infect Immun 2001; 69:5423–5429.

36. Kutlin A, Flegg C, Stenzel D, Reznik T, Roblin PM, Matthews S, Timms P, Hammerschlag M. Ultrastructural study of *Chlamydia pneumoniae* in a continuous-infection model. J Clin Microbiol 2001; 39:3721–3723.

37. Gieffers J, Fullgraf H, Jahn J, Klinger M, Dallhof K, Katus HA, Solbach W, Maass M. *Chlamydia pneumoniae* infection in circulating human monocytes is refractory to antibiotic treatment. Circulation 2001; 103:351–356.

38. Molestina RE, Klein JB, Miller RD, Pierce WH, Ramirez JA, Summersgill JT. Proteomic analysis of differentially expressed *Chlamydia pneumoniae* genes during persistent infection of HEp-2 cells. Infect Immun 2002; 70(6):2976–2981.

39. Leinonen M, Saikku P. Evidence for infectious agents in cardiovascular diseases and atherosclerosis. Lancet Infec Dis 2002; 2:11–17.

40. Pizzichini MM, Pizzichini E, Efthimiadis A, Clelland L, Mahony JB, Dolovich J, Hargreave FE. Markers of inflammation in induced sputum in acute bronchitis caused by *Chlamydia pneumoniae*. Thorax 1997; 52:929–931.

41. Mahony JB, Coombes BK. *Chlamydia pneumoniae* and atherosclerosis: does the evidence support a causal or contributory role? FEMS Microbiol Lett 2001; 197:1–9.

42. Shor A. The pathology of *Chlamydia pneumoniae* lesions in humans and animal models. Trends Microbiol 2000; 8:541–542.

43. Jousilahti P, Vartiainen E, Tuomilehto J, Puska P. Symptoms of chronic bronchitis and the risk of coronary disease. Lancet 1996; 348:567–572.

44. Lindholt JS, Heickendorff L, Antonsen S, Fasting H, Henneberg EW. Natural history of abdominal aortic aneurysm with and without coexisting chronic obstructive pulmonary disease. J Vasc Surg 1998; 28:226–233.

45. Shemer-Avni Y, Lieberman D. *Chlamydia pneumoniae*-induced ciliostasis in ciliated bronchial epithelial cells. J Infect Dis 1995; 171:1274–1278.

46. Kaukoranta-Tolvanen S-SE, Laurila AL, Saikku P, Leinonen M, Liesirova L, Laitinen K. Experimental infection of *Chlamydia pneumoniae* in mice. Microb Pathog l993; 15: 293–302.

47. Yang ZP, Kuo CC, Grayston JT. A mouse model of *Chlamydia pneumoniae* strain TWAR pneumonitis. Infect Immun 1993; 61:2037–2040.

48. Yang ZP, Cummings PK, Patton DL, Kuo CC. Ultrastructural lung pathology of experimental *Chlamydia pneumoniae* pneumonitis in mice. J Infect Dis 1994; 170:464–467.

49. Penttila JM, Anttila M, Puolakkainen M, Laurila A, Varkila K, Sarvas M, Makela PH, Rautonen N. Local immune responses to *Chlamydia pneumoniae* in the lungs of BALB/c mice during primary infection and reinfection. Infect Immun 1998; 66:5113–5118.

50. Geng Y, Berencsi K, Gyulai Z, Valyi-Nagy T, Gonczol E, Trinchieri G. Roles of interleukin-12 and gamma interferon in murine *Chlamydia pneumoniae* infection. Infect Immun 2000; 68:2245–2253.

51. Kaukoranta-Tolvanen S-SE, Laurila AL, Saikku P, Leinonen M, Laitinen K. Experimental *Chlamydia pneumoniae* infection in mice: effect of reinfection and passive immunization. Microb Pathog 1995; 18:279–288.

52. Moazed TC, Kuo C, Grayston JT, Campbell LA. Murine models of *Chlamydia pneumoniae* infection and atherosclerosis. J Infect Dis 1997; 175:883–890.

53. Malinverni R, Kuo CC, Campbell LA, Grayston JT. Reactivation of *Chlamydia pneumoniae* lung infection in mice by cortisone. J Infect Dis 1995; 172:593–594.

54. Laitinen K, Laurila AL, Leinonen M, Saikku P. Reactivation of *Chlamydia pneumoniae* infection in mice by cortisone treatment. Infect Immun 1996; 64:1488–1490.

55. Campbell LA, Blessing E, Rosenfeld M, Lin T, Kuo C. Mouse models of *C. pneumoniae* infection and atherosclerosis. J Infect Dis 2000; 181 Suppl 3:S508-S513.

56. Miyashita N, Niki Y, Nakajima M, et al. Prevalence of asymptomatic infection with *Chlamydia pneumoniae* in subjectively healthy adults. Chest 2001; 119:1416–1419.

57. Hahn DL, Azenabor AA, Beatty WL, Byrne GI. *Chlamydia pneumoniae* as a respiratory pathogen. Front Biosci 2002; 7:e66–e76.

58. Grayston JT, Campbell LA, Kuo C-C, Mordhorst CH, Saikku P, Thom DH, Wang S-P. A new respiratory tract pathogen: *Chlamydia pneumoniae*, strain TWAR. J Infect Dis 1990; 161:618–625.

59. Kauppinen M, Saikku P. Pneumonia due to *Chlamydia pneumoniae*: prevalence, clinical features, diagnosis and treatment. Clin Infect Dis 1995; 21:S244-S252.

60. Macfarlane J, Holmes W, Gard P, Macfarlane R, Rose D, Weston V, Leinonen M, Saikku P, Myint S. Prospective study of the incidence, aetiology and outcome of adult lower respiratory tract illness in the community. Thorax 2001; 56:109–114.

61. Troy CJ, Peeling RW, Ellis AG, Hockin JC, Bennett DA, Murphy MR, Spika JS. *Chlamydia pneumoniae* as a new source of infectious outbreaks in nursing homes. JAMA. 1997; 277:1214–1218.

62. Miyashita N, Fukano H, Hara H, Yoshida K, Niki Y, Matsushima T. Recurrent pneumonia due to persistent *Chlamydia pneumoniae* infection. Intern Med 2002; 41:30–33.

63. Pether JV, Wang SP, Grayston JT. *Chlamydia pneumoniae*, strain TWAR, as the cause of an outbreak in a boys' school previously called psittacosis. Epidemiol Infect 1989; 103:395–400.

64. Hagiwara K, Ouchi K, Tashiro N, Azuma M, Kobayashi K. An epidemic of a pertussis-like illness caused by *Chlamydia pneumoniae*. Pediatr Infect Dis J 1999; 18:271–275.

65. Ekman M-R, Grayston JT, Visakorpi R, Kleemola M, Kuo C-c, Saikku P. An epidemic of infections due to *Chlamydia pneumoniae* in military conscripts. Clin Infect Dis 1993; 17:420–425.

66. Gray GC, Schultz RG, Gackstetter GD, McKeehan JA, Alridge KV, Hudspeth MK, Malasig MD, Fuller JM, McBride WZ. Prospective study of respiratory infections at the U.S. Naval Academy. Mil Med 2001; 166:759–763

67. Grayston JT, Mordhorst C, Bruu AL, Vene S, Wang SP. Countrywide epidemics of

Chlamydia pneumoniae, strain TWAR, in Scandinavia, 1981–1983. J Infect Dis 1989; 159:1111–1114.

68. Bruu AL, Haukenes G, Aasen S, Grayston JT, Wang SP, Klausen OG, Myrmel H, Hasseltvedt V. *Chlamydia pneumoniae* infections in Norway 1981–87 earlier diagnosed as ornithosis. Scand J Infect Dis 1991; 23:299–304.

69. Dowell SF, Peeling RW, Boman J, Carlone GM, Fields BS, Guarner J, Hammerschlag MR, Jackson LA, Kuo CC, Maass M, Messmer TO, Talkington DF, Tondella ML, Zaki SR. Standardizing *Chlamydia pneumoniae* assays: recommendations from the Centers for Disease Control and Prevention (USA) and the Laboratory Centre for Disease Control (Canada). Clin Infect Dis 2001; 33:492–503.

70. Peeling RW, Wang SP, Grayston JT, Blasi F, Boman J, Clad A, Freidank H, Gaydos CA, Gnarpe J, Hagiwara T, Jones RB, Orfila J, Persson K, Puolakkainen M, Saikku P, Schachter J. *Chlamydia pneumoniae* serology: interlaboratory variation in microimmunofluorescence assay results. J Infect Dis 2000; 181 Suppl 3:S426–S429.

71. Apfalter P, Blasi F, Boman J, Gaydos CA, Kundi M, Maass M, Makristathis A, Meijer A, Nadrchal R, Persson K, Rotter ML, Tong CY, Stanek G, Hirschl AM. Multicenter comparison trial of DNA extraction methods and PCR assays for detection of *Chlamydia pneumoniae* in endarterectomy specimens. J Clin Microbiol 2001; 39:519–524.

72. Wald NJ, Law MR, Morris JK, Zhou X, Wong Y, Ward ME. *Chlamydia pneumoniae* infection and mortality from ischaemic heart disease: large prospective study. Br Med J 2000; 321:204–207

73. Danesh J, Whincup P, Lewington S, Walker M, Lennon L, Thomson A, Wong YK, Zhou X, Ward M. *Chlamydia pneumoniae* IgA titres and coronary heart disease. Prospective study and meta-analysis. Eur Heart J 2002; 23:371–375

74. Hahn DL, Anttila T, Saikku P. Association of *Chlamydia pneumoniae* IgA antibodies with recently symptomatic asthma. Epidemiol Infect 1996; 117(3):513–517

75. von Hertzen L, Leinonen M, Surcel HM, Karjalainen J, Saikku P. Measurement of sputum antibodies in the diagnosis of acute and chronic respiratory infections associated with *Chlamydia pneumoniae*. Clin Diagn Lab Immunol 1995; 2:454–457.

76. Cunningham AF, Johnston SL, Julious SA, Lampe FC, Ward ME. Chronic *Chlamydia pneumoniae* infection and asthma exacerbations in children. Eur Respir J. 1998; 11: 345–349.

77. Huittinen T, Hahn D, Anttila T, Wahlstrom E, Saikku P, Leinonen M. Host immune response to *Chlamydia pneumoniae* heat shock protein 60 is associated with asthma. Eur Respir J 2001; 17:1078–1082.

78. Ferwerda A, Moll HA, de Groot R. Respiratory tract infections by *Mycoplasma pneumoniae* in children: a review of diagnostic and therapeutic measures. Eur J Pediatr 2001; 160(8):483–491.

79. Hammerschlag MR. Antimicrobial susceptibility and therapy of infections caused by *Chlamydia pneumoniae*. Antimicrob Agents Chemother 1994; 38:1873–1878.

80. Masson ND, Toseland CD, Beale AS. Relevance of *Chlamydia pneumoniae* murine pneumonitis model to evaluation of antimicrobial agents. Antimicrob Agents Chemother 1995; 39:1959–1964.

81. Bin XX, Wolf K, Schaffner T, Malinverni R. Effect of azithromycin plus rifampin versus amoxicillin alone on eradication and inflammation in the chronic course of *Chlamydia pneumoniae* pneumonitis in mice. Antimicrob Agents Chemother 2000; 44: 1761–1764

82. Grayston JT. Secondary prevention antibiotic treatment trials for coronary artery disease. Circulation 2000; 102:1742–1743.

83. Berkovich S, Millian SJ, Snyder RD. The association of viral and mycoplasma infections with recurrence of wheezing in the asthmatic child. Ann Allergy 1970; 28:43–49.

84. Freymuth F, Vabret A, Brouard J, Toutain F, Verdon R, Petitjean J, Gouarin S, Duhamel JF, Guillois B. Detection of viral, *Chlamydia pneumoniae* and *Mycoplasma pneumoniae* infections in exacerbations of asthma in children. J Clin Virol 1999; 13:131–139.

85. Tipirneni P, Moore BS, Hyde JS, Schauf V. IgE antibodies to *Mycoplasma pneumoniae* in asthma and other atopic diseases. Ann Allergy 1980; 45:1–7.

86. Koh YY, Park Y, Lee HJ, Kim CK. Levels of interleukin-2, interferon-gamma, and interleukin-4 in bronchoalveolar lavage fluid from patients with *Mycoplasma pneumoniae*: implication of tendency toward increased immunoglobulin E production. Pediatrics 2001; 107:E39.

87. Kraft M, Cassell GH, Henson JE, Watson H, Williamson J, Marmion BP, Gaydos CA, Martin RJ. Detection of *Mycoplasma pneumoniae* in the airways of adults with chronic asthma. Am J Respir Crit Care Med 1998; 158:998–1001.

88. Chu HW, Kraft M, Rex MD, Martin RJ. Evaluation of blood vessels and edema in the airways of asthma patients: regulation with clarithromycin treatment. Chest 2001; 120: 416–422.

89. Kazachkov MY, Hu PC, Carson JL, Murphy PC, Henderson FW, Noah TL. Release of cytokines by human nasal epithelial cells and peripheral blood mononuclear cells infected with *Mycoplasma pneumoniae*. Exp Biol Med (Maywood) 2002; 227:330–335.

90. Martin RJ, Kraft M, Chu HW, Berns EA, Cassell GH. A link between chronic asthma and chronic infection. J Allergy Clin Immunol 2001; 107:595–601.

91. Hardy RD, Jafri HS, Olsen K, Hatfield J, Iglehart J, Rogers BB, Patel P, Cassell G, McCracken GH, Ramilo O. *Mycoplasma pneumoniae* induces chronic respiratory infection, airway hyperreactivity, and pulmonary inflammation: a murine model of infection-associated chronic reactive airway disease. Infect Immun 2002; 70:649–654.

92. Schmidt SM, Muller CE, Bruns R, Wiersbitzky SK. Bronchial *Chlamydia pneumoniae* infection, markers of allergic inflammation and lung function in children. Pediatr Allergy Immunol 2001; 12:257–265.

93. Smieja M, Mahony JB, Goldsmith CH, Chong S, Petrich A, Chernesky M. Replicate PCR testing and probit analysis for detection and quantitation of *Chlamydia pneumoniae* in clinical specimens. J Clin Microbiol 2001; 39:1796–1801.

94. Hertzen von L, Surcel H-M, Kaprio J, Koskenvuo M, Bloigu A, Leinonen M, Saikku P. Immune responses to *Chlamydia pneumoniae* in twins in relation to gender and smoking. J Med Microbiol 1998; 47:441–446.

95. Hahn DL, Peeling RW, Dillon E, McDonald R, Saikku P. Serologic markers for *Chlamydia pneumoniae* in asthma. Ann Allergy Asthma Immunol 2000; 84:227–233.

96. Principi N, Esposito S, Blasi F, Allegra L. Role of *Mycoplasma pneumoniae* and *Chlamydia pneumoniae* in children with community-acquired lower respiratory tract infections. Clin Infect Dis 2001; 32:1281–1289.

97. Johnston SL. Is *Chlamydia pneumoniae* important in asthma? The first controlled trial of therapy leaves the question unanswered. Am J Respir Crit Care Med 2001; 164:513–514.

98. Hahn DL. Treatment of *Chlamydia pneumoniae* infection in adult asthma: a before-after trial. J Fam Pract 1995; 41:345–351.

99. Richeldi L, Ferrara G, Fabbri LM, Gibson PG. Macrolides for chronic asthma (Cochrane Review). Cochrane Database Syst Rev 2002; (1):CD002997.

24

Chlamydia/Mycoplasma
Do They Precipitate Acute Asthma Attacks?

LUIGI ALLEGRA, FRANCESCO BLASI, ROBERTO COSENTINI, and PAOLO TARSIA

Policlinico Hospital
University of Milan
Milan, Italy

The association between respiratory infections and asthma exacerbations was first observed in the early 1970s. In particular, the role of viral upper respiratory tract infections has been evaluated both in pediatric and adult populations. More recently, evidence of *Mycoplasma* and *Chlamydia pneumoniae* involvement in asthma attacks has been reported. We will review the role of these so-called atypical pathogens in the pathogenesis of acute asthma exacerbations in both children and adults.

I. Findings in Children

During the last few decades, wheezing has become one of the most frequent causes of consultation in pediatric practice (1,2). A number of epidemiological and clinical studies have highlighted that most episodes of wheezing occurring in early life are associated with viral infections, the most frequently encountered agents being respiratory syncytial virus, adenovirus, parainfluenza viruses 1, 2, and 3, influenza viruses type A and B, and rhinovirus (3,4). The possibility that viruses may interact with the immune and respiratory systems in early life to initiate the complex pathogenetic mechanism leading to asthma has been the matter of considerable study and debate (5). It is generally recognized that viral respiratory infections often exacerbate established asthma, and there is speculation that they may be associated with initiation and maintenance of asthma.

Nonviral respiratory pathogens such as *Mycoplasma pneumoniae* and *Chlamydia pneumoniae* have also been associated with possible initiation and promotion of asthma (6-9). Both *M. pneumoniae* and *C. pneumoniae* are the causative agents in a number of respiratory diseases, including upper respiratory tract illnesses such as rhinitis, pharyngitis, or otitis, as well as bronchitis and atypical pneumonia (10). These pathogens are plausible candidates as causative agents in asthma because of their tropism for the human respiratory tract and their demonstrated ability to produce chronic respiratory tract infection and inflammation. Further evidence for the role of these pathogens in asthma comes from the observation of improvement in asthma symptoms after antimicrobial therapy active against *M. pneumoniae* and *C. pneumoniae* (11,12).

Most of the published information linking *M. pneumoniae* or *C. pneumoniae* infection to asthma is derived from studies of adult patients (6,7,11,12). Few data are available regarding childhood (8,9).

In a large prospective study involving 75 children hospitalized for a severe attack of asthma, Freymuth et al. evaluated the incidence of viruses, *Mycoplasma pneumoniae*, and *C. pneumoniae* applying immunofluorescence assays, isolation, and molecular biology techniques on nasal aspirates (13). More than two-thirds of exacerbations were positive for an infectious agent, mainly viruses. *C. pneumoniae* was found in 4.5% of nasal aspirates with positive identification.

Cunningham et al. (9), in a large prospective study on school-aged children with asthma, showed that chronic *C. pneumoniae* infection was common in this population and the immune response to *C. pneumoniae* was positively associated with the frequency of asthma exacerbations. The authors suggest that the immune response to chronic *C. pneumoniae* infection may interact with allergic inflammation to increase asthma symptoms. Furthermore, a number of episodes by each child during the 13 months of the study were positively associated with the levels of secretory IgA towards *C. pneumoniae*.

More recently, our group analyzed 71 children aged 2–14 years presenting to the pediatric emergency department with an acute episode of wheezing (defined by cough and/or dyspnea with expiratory rales and wheezes) associated with fever and signs or symptoms of upper respiratory tract infection (14). During the same time interval, 80 healthy subjects of similar gender and ages without any history of respiratory tract infection in the 3 months before enrollment, seen at our institution for minor surgical problems, were evaluated as control group. On admission and after 4–6 weeks, sera for determination of antibodies to *M. pneumoniae* and *C. pneumoniae* and nasopharyngeal aspirates for *M. pneumoniae* and *C. pneumoniae* DNA detection were obtained from all the participants in the study. Acute *M. pneumoniae* infection was demonstrated in 16 of 71 (22.5%) children with wheezing: it was serologically determined in all the 16 infected patients (IgM-specific antibody $\geq$ 1:100 in 12 children and IgG titer $\geq$ 1:400 in 4), and confirmed by polymerase chain reaction (PCR) in one subject (who presented with an IgG titer $\geq$ 1:400). In none of the patients was *M. pneumoniae* DNA detected without any evidence of seroconversion. Among controls, 6 of 80 (7.5%) children showed evidence of acute *M. pneumoniae* infection without any respiratory symptom (children with wheezing vs. controls: p = 0.01, using χ^2 test): all the 6 subjects presented serological evidence of acute infection (IgM specific antibody $\geq$ 1:100 in 2 children and IgG titer $\geq$ 1:400 in 4); in none of the controls was *M. pneumoniae* DNA detected.

Acute *C. pneumoniae* infection was shown in 11 of 71 (15.5%) patients with wheezing: it was serologically determined in 9 of the 11 infected children (IgG specific antibody $\geq$ 1:512 in 1 child and a fourfold rise in IgG titer in 8 patients), and confirmed by PCR in 4 of 9 (in the child with IgG specific antibody $\geq$ 1:512 and in 3 of those with a fourfold rise in IgG titer); in 2 more patients, *C. pneumoniae* DNA was detected without any evidence of seroconversion. Among controls, 2 of 80 (2.5%) children showed evidence of acute *C. pneumoniae* infection without any respiratory symptom (children with wheezing vs. controls: p = 0.01, using χ^2 test): both the subjects showed *C. pneumoniae* DNA without seroconversion.

Among the infected children, three patients with wheezing and none of the controls had *M. pneumoniae* and *C. pneumoniae* coinfection.

Considering studies that have shown the highest incidence of atypical bacteria infections in children older than 5 years (15,16), we performed a subanalysis comparing subjects with wheezing and controls aged 2–4 years and those older than 5 years. Table 1 summarizes the incidence of acute *M. pneumoniae* or *C. pneumoniae* infection in the study population in different age groups. Despite the higher incidence of infection due to either pathogen in children with wheezing than in controls in both the age groups, the difference was significant only in subjects aged more than 5 years.

Fifteen of the 16 (93.7%) wheezing patients with acute *M. pneumoniae* infection had a history of recurrent wheezing, defined as acute episodes of wheezing-related symptoms (i.e., cough, dyspnea, and wheezes) compared to only 16 of the 55 (29.1%) without (p < 0.0001, using χ^2 test); results were similar in the case of acute *C. pneumoniae* infection: 8 of 11 (72.7%) vs. 23 of 60 (38.3%) (p = 0.04, using χ^2 test).

Table 1 Incidence of Acute *M. pneumoniae* or *C. pneumoniae* Infection in Children with Acute Wheezing Episodes and in Control Children in Different Age Groups

Infection/age group	Children with wheezing (%)	Controls (%)	p value
M. pneumoniae			
2–4 years	4/40 (10.0)	2/34 (5.9)	0.68[a]
$\geq$ 5 years	12/31 (38.7)	4/46 (8.7)	0.0003[b]
C. pneumoniae			
2–4 years	4/40 (10.0)	2/34 (5.9)	0.68[a]
$\geq$5 years	7/31 (22.6)	0/46	0.001[b]

[a]Fisher's exact test.
[b]χ^2 test.

Table 2 Incidence of Recurrent Episodes in Children Presenting with Acute Wheezing Episodes in Different Age Groups

Age group	*M. pneumoniae* and/or *C. pneumoniae* infected (%)	*M. pneumoniae* and/or *C. pneumoniae* not infected (%)	p value
2–4 years	8/8 (100.0)	9/32 (28.1)	0.003[a]
≥5 years	12/16 (75.0)	2/15 (13.3)	0.002[b]

[a]Fisher's exact test.
[b]χ^2 test.

Table 2 describes the incidence of recurrent episodes in the children with wheezing in different age groups. In both age groups, history of recurrent wheezing was significantly more frequent in the patients infected by one of the two pathogens than in those without either infection.

No significant difference in the prevalence of atopy was found between the wheezing subjects with and without infections due to these pathogens. In the group of 16 patients with wheezing and acute *M. pneumoniae* infection, 6 (37.5%) appeared to be atopic, whereas among the 55 with wheezing but no *M. pneumoniae* infection 16 (29.1%) were atopic (p=0.54, using Fisher exact test). Among the 11 patients with wheezing and acute *C. pneumoniae* infection, 4 (36.7%) were atopic, whereas in the 60 with no *C. pneumoniae* infection 18 (30.0%) subjects showed evidence of atopy (p = 0.72, using Fisher's exact test).

The finding of a relationship between wheezing episodes and acute *M. pneumoniae* or *C. pneumoniae* infection is intriguing and suggests the potential role for these pathogens in the exacerbation of childhood asthma. It is likely that *M. pneumoniae* and *C. pneumoniae* can trigger what is termed the wheezing process in subjects who are predisposed either by their genetic background or by events that have primed their immune systems and lungs. In agreement with previous reports, our results also show that in children with wheezing the incidence of acute *M. pneumoniae* and *C. pneumoniae* infections increases with age and occurs mainly after 5 years of age.

II. Findings in Adults

Seggev et al. (17) evaluated the possible role of infection with *Mycoplasma pneumoniae* in exacerbations of bronchial asthma in adults in 95 patients hospitalized due to acute asthma. The authors found that approximately 20% of the patients had evidence of a recent *M. pneumoniae* infection and concluded that this infection may be significant in exacerbations of asthma. A more recent study suggested that in addition to causing exacerbations, *M. pneumoniae* may be associated with the initial onset of bronchial asthma (18).

Data suggesting the association between *C. pneumoniae* infection and asthma in adult patients was first put forward by Hahn et al. in the early 1990s (7). The result of this study showed a dose–response relationship between specific antibody titer level and prevalence of wheeze; moreover, 4 of 19 patients with acute *C. pneumoniae* infection subsequently developed asthma, and four others had exacerbation of previously diagnosed asthma. Our group later studied 74 adult asthma patients and found *C. pneumoniae* seroconversion in association with asthma exacerbation in 8% of patients (19). These results were further confirmed by Miyashita et al., who found evidence of acute *C. pneumoniae* infection in 15 of 168 (8.9%) adult patients with acute asthma exacerbations (20). In this controlled study the incidence of acute infection was significantly higher in asthmatics than in controls (p = 0.048), but the main findings of the study were the higher prevalence and geometric mean titers for both IgG and IgA antibodies in asthmatic patients. These data confirm the role of *C. pneumoniae* in asthma exacerbations and suggest the possibility of persistent chronic infection in these patients. *C. pneumoniae* chronic infection may play a role in the natural history of the disease by contributing to chronic inflammatory derangement of the airways. This hypothesis was highlighted by Hahn et al., who found that in some patients *C. pneumoniae* acute infection is associated with new onset of asthma (21). During a 9 year study period, they found ten patients with de novo wheezing and acute infection. Four of them did not develop asthma during the observation period, whereas five developed chronic asthma and one chronic bronchitis. The authors conclude that acute *C. pneumoniae* respiratory tract infection in previously nonasthmatic subjects can result in chronic asthma.

The association between *C. pneumoniae* infection and asthma has been addressed in a further large study involving 430 subjects who attended the hospital with symptoms suggestive for asthma, rhinitis, and allergy (22). The population was organized in three groups: recent asthmatics (224 subjects), long-standing asthmatics (108 subjects), and nonasthmatics (98 subjects). Logistic regression analysis controlling for age, gender, and smoking showed that asthma was significantly associated with elevated IgG antibody levels to *C. pneumoniae*. More interesting was that when atopics and nonatopics were analyzed separately, an even stronger relationship with long-standing asthma was obtained in the nonatopic group odds ratio ([OR] 6.0, 95% confidence interval [CI] 2.1–17.1). The relationship between atopic asthma, irrespective of asthma past history, and IgG titers was not significant, indicating that asthma per se is not a predisposing factor to *C. pneumoniae* infection. These data indicate the involvement of the micro-organism in the development of nonatopic asthma. The possible role of *C. pneumoniae* chronic infection on asthma severity in adults has been hypothesized by Black et al. (23). The authors describe 619 asthmatic subjects screened in a large multinational study on the effect of antibiotic treatment of asthmatic subjects seropositive for *C. pneumoniae*. In the screened population IgG and IgA antibodies to *C. pneumoniae* were associated with asthma severity markers. A positive association was found between antibodies to *C. pneumoniae* and the use of high-dosage inhaled steroids, higher daytime symptom scores, and an inverse association with forced expiratory volume in 1s (FEV_1) as percentage of predicted. These findings once again raise the possibility that chronic *C. pneumoniae* infection may lead to an increase in asthma severity. Hahn et al., in a case series study, reported that prolonged antibiotic treatment (6–12 weeks) with a macrolide may induce a significant improvement in asthma control in patients with severe steroid-dependent asthma and serological evidence of *C. pneumoniae* infection (24).

We recently studied 35 consecutive patients with severe (peak expiratory flow [PEF] $\leq$ 50% of predicted, respiratory rate $\geq$ 25 breaths/min, heart rate > 110 beats/min) (group 1 = 15 patients) or nonsevere (group 2 = 20 patients) acute asthma exacerbation. All patients underwent the following tests on admission and at follow-up: spirometry, microimmunofluorescence *C. pneumoniae* antibody determination, serum *Mycoplasma pneumoniae* antibody titers; nested PCR for *C. pneumoniae* DNA detection on pharyngeal swab specimens (admission only).

The *C. pneumonaie* seroprevalence (IgG $\geq$ 1:64) was similar in group 1 and group 2, whereas acute infection was significantly more common in the former (9 of 15 vs 2 of 20, p = 0.02). We found *C. pneumonia* DNA in six of nine group 1 patients and in one of two group 2 patients with acute infection serological pattern. No evidence of acute *Mycoplasma pneumoniae* infection was found in the patients with acute asthma. We also evaluated *C. pneumoniae* seroprevalence in 120 adult patients with stable asthma and in 163 healthy blood donors by microimmunofluorescence determination of *C. pneumoniae* antibodies, and a nested PCR for *C. pneumoniae* DNA detection on pharyngeal swab specimens. *C. pneumoniae* IgG seroprevalence was significantly higher in stable asthma subjects than in blood donors: 34.2% and 22%, respectively (p = 0.034). *C. pneumoniae* DNA was detected in five seropositive asthmatic patients but PCR was negative in both seronegative asthma patients and control subjects (p = 0.005).

Follow-up lung function testing showed a similar improvement in respiratory function in both patients subgroups. Therefore, group 1 and group 2 asthma patients presumably differed functionally only in the intensity of the acute exacerbation and not in terms of baseline severity of the disease. This is further suggested by the fact that inhaled steroid use prior to admission was similar in both study groups. We suggest that, in our study population, the diversity in exacerbation intensity may have been associated with the presence of *C. pneumoniae* infection. In summary, taking into account the limited population size in the study, *C. pneumoniae* infection appears to be associated with severe asthma exacerbations. Should this be confirmed by further studies, appropriate anti-*C. pneumoniae* antibiotic treatment may have to be considered in patients with severe asthma exacerbations.

All the reported studies indicate the need for new investigations aimed at assessing whether antibiotic treatment reaching bacterial eradication may lead to an improvement in asthma control. It must however be considered that eradication of intracellular pathogens such as *C. pneumoniae* may be difficult to obtain.

References

1. Milgrom H, Wood II RP, Ingram D. Respiratory conditions that mimic asthma. Immunol Allergy Clin North Am 1998; 18:113–132.
2. Martinez FD, Helms PJ. Types of asthma and wheezing. Eur Respir J 1998; 12 (Suppl 27): 3S–8S.

3. Duff AL, Pomeranz ES, Gelber LE, Price GW, Farris H, Hayden FG, Platts-Mills TA, Heymann PW. Risk factors for acute wheezing in infants and children: viruses, passive smoke, and IgE antibodies to inhalant allergens. Pediatrics 1993; 92: 535–540.
4. Newson R, Strachan D, Archibald E, Emberlin J, Hardaker P, Collier C. Acute asthma epidemics, weather and pollen in England, 1987–1994. Eur Respir J 1998; 11:694–701.
5. Martinez FD. Viral infections and the development of asthma. Am J Respir Crit Care Med 1995; 151:1644–1648.
6. Kraft M, Cassell GH, Henson JE, Watson H, Williamson J, Maarmion BP, Gaydos CA, Martin RJ. Detection of *Mycoplasma pneumoniae* in the airways of adults with chronic asthma. Am J Respir Crit Care Med 1998; 158:998–1001.
7. Hahn DL, Dodge RW, Goulgjatnikov R. Association of *Chlamydia pneumoniae* (Strain TWAR) infection with wheezing, asthmatic bronchitis, and adult-onset asthma. JAMA 1991; 266:225–230.
8. Emre U, Roblin PM, Gelling M, Dumornay W, Rao M, Hammerschlag M, Schachter J. The association of *Chlamydia pneumoniae* infection and reactive airway disease in children. Arch Pediatr Adolesc Med 1994; 148:727–732.
9. Cunningham AF, Johnston SL, Julious SA, Lampe FC, Ward ME. Chronic *Chlamydia pneumoniae* infection and asthma exacerbations in children. Eur Resp J 1998; 11:345–349.
10. File TM, Tan JS, Plouffe JF. The role of atypical pathogens: *Mycoplasma pneumoniae*, *Chlamydia pneumoniae*, and *Legionella pneumophila* in respiratory infection. Infect Dis Clin North Am 1998; 12:569–592.
11. Hahn DL. Treatment of *Chlamydia pneumoniae* infection in adult asthma: a before–after trial. J Fam Prac 1995; 41:345–351.
12. Black PN, Bagg B, Brodie SM, Robinson E, Cooper B. A double-blind, crossover study of roxithromycin in the treatment of asthma. Eur Respir J 1998; 12 (Suppl 28):190S.
13. Freymuth F, Vabret A, Brouard J, Toutain F, Verdon R, Petitjean J, et al. Detection of viral, *Chlamydia pneumoniae* and *Mycoplasma pneumoniae* infections in exacerbations of asthma in children. J Clin Virol 1999; 13:131–139.
14. Esposito S, Blasi F, Arosio C, Fioravanti L, Fagetti L, Droghetti R, Tarsia P, Allegra L, Principi N. Importance of acute *Mycoplasma pneumoniae* and *Chlamydia pneumonia* infections in children with wheezing. Eur Respir J 2000; 16:1142–1146.
15. Block S, Hedrick J, Hammerschlag MR, Cassell GH, Craft JC. *Mycoplasma pneumoniae* and *Chlamydia pneumoniae* in pediatric community-acquired pneumonia: comparative efficacy and safety of clarithromycin vs. erythromycin ethylsuccinate. Pediatr Infect Dis J 1995; 14:471–477.
16. Normann E, Gnarpe J, Gnarpe H, Wettergren B. *Chlamydia pneumoniae* in children with acute respiratory tract infections. Acta Paediatr 1998; 87:23–27.
17. Seggev JS, Lis I, Siman-Tov R, Gutman R, Abu-Samara H, Schey G, Naot Y. *Mycoplasma pneumoniae* is a frequent cause of exacerbation of bronchial asthma in adults. Ann Allergy 1986; 57: 263–265.
18. Yano T, Ichikawa Y, Komatu S, Arai S, Oizumi K. Association of *Mycoplasma pneumoniae* antigen with initial onset of bronchial asthma. Am J Respir Crit Care Med 1994; 149:1348–1353.
19. Allegra L, Blasi F, Centanni S, Cosentini R, Denti F, Raccanelli R, Tarsia P, Valenti V. Acute exacerbations of asthma in adults: role of *Chlamydia pneumoniae* infection. Eur Respir J 1994; 7:2165–2168.
20. Miyashita N, Kubota Y, Nakajima M, Niki Y, Kawana H, Matshima T. *Chlamydia*

pneumoniae and exacerbations of asthma in adults. Ann Allergy Asthma Immunol 1998; 80:405–409.

21. Hahn DL, McDonald R. Can acute *Chlamydia pneumoniae* respiratory tract infection initiate chronic asthma?. Ann Allergy Asthma Immunol 1998; 81:339–344.

22. Von Hertzen L, Toyryla M, Gimishanov A, Bloigu A, Leinonen M, Saikku P, et al. Asthma, atopy and *Chlamydia pneumoniae* antibodies in adults. Clin Exp Allergy 1999; 29:522–528.

23. Black PN, Scicchitano R, Jenkins CR, Blasi F, Allegra L, Wlodarczyk J, Cooper BC. Serological evidence of infection with *Chlamydia pneumoniae* is related to the severity of asthma. Eur Respir J 2000; 15:254–259.

24. Hahn DL, Bukstein D, Luskin A, Zeit H. Evidence for *Chlamydia pneumoniae* infection in steroid-dependent asthma. Ann Allergy Asthma Immunol 1998; 80:45–49.

25

Chlamydia/Mycoplasma
Do They Chronically Infect and Contribute to Asthma Severity?

E. RAND SUTHERLAND and RICHARD J. MARTIN

National Jewish Medical and Research Center
Denver, Colorado, U.S.A.

I. Introduction

The question that forms the title of this chapter has not yet been answered. However, respiratory tract infection with the atypical bacteria *Mycoplasma pneumoniae* and *Chlamydia pneumoniae* has recently emerged as an important clinical issue in patients with chronic asthma. The exact contribution of chronic atypical bacterial infection to asthma pathogenesis and phenotype remains to be determined, but a growing body of both clinical and basic scientific data implicates atypical pathogens as potentially important factors in asthma.

The challenges faced in elucidating the relationship between atypical bacterial infection and asthma are numerous. Animals models of chronic atypical bacterial infection are still in the process of being developed. Although analogies to airway damage from viral respiratory tract infections may be appropriate when forming hypotheses about atypical bacteria and asthma, further development and study of animal models are required to elucidate the role of atypical bacteria in asthma. An additional challenge is that many of the methods of detecting atypical bacteria in humans are either insensitive or nonspecific, particularly in the setting of the low organism burdens seen with chronic infection. This leads to difficulties in identifying these pathogens in population-level studies of stable asthmatics. Reliable detection often requires invasive diagnostic procedures such as bronchoscopy with airway biopsy. Furthermore, since asthma is a final common clinical pathway that may be influenced by a host of intrinsic and acquired insults, determining the importance of infectious agents relative to other risk factors in the pathogenesis of this syndrome of airway inflammation, airway responsiveness, and reversible airflow limitation continues to pose a challenge.

This chapter will review the current evidence on the importance of chronic *Mycoplasma* and *Chlamydia* infection in the pathogenesis and clinical phenotype of asthma. We will review the biology of *M. pneumoniae* and *C. pneumoniae* and present the current state of research into the association between these organisms and asthma, based on both basic scientific and epidemiological evidence for this association. Analogies to viral pathogens and their putative role in asthma pathogenesis will be made, and mechanisms that may explain the relationship between atypical bacteria and asthma severity will be described. We will conclude by briefly addressing the potential role of anti-infective agents in the treatment of asthma.

II. Biology of *Mycoplasma pneumoniae*

Mycoplasma pneumoniae was the first *Mycoplasma* species for which a role as an agent of human disease was demonstrated. Reports in the late 1930s (1) and early 1940s (2) noted that some cases of acute pneumonitis in young adults were atypical in both their clinical course and lack of response to penicillin and sulfonamide antibiotics. In 1944 Eaton and colleagues demonstrated the infectious nature of an agent of atypical pneumonia (3), which was later observed by Marmion and Goodburn to be similar to *Mycoplasma mycoides*, the agent that causes contagious bovine pleuropneumonia (4). In 1961, Koch's postulates were satisfied after laboratory-isolated *M. pneumoniae* were used to infect human volunteers, resulting in atypical pneumonia (5). *Mycoplasma pneumoniae* is now known as an important cause of pneumonia, tracheobronchitis, and pharyngitis (6). It has also been associated with a variety of extrapulmonary manifestations, including articular, hepatopancreatic, exanthematic, cardiovascular, and central nervous system syndromes (7).

Mycoplasmas have a filamentous shape with specialized polar tip organelles that facilitate attachment to host target cells by means of adhesion proteins called adhesins (8). These adhesins mediate mycoplasmal colonization of mucous membranes and share significant sequence homology with mammalian structural proteins, which may trigger an anti-self response to structural proteins such as myosin, keratin, and fibrinogen (9) and form the basis for bacterially mediated autoimmune disease. Cell adherence is the initial step in *Mycoplasma* infection, which is followed by the potential for induction of a wide range of immunomodulatory events, including lymphocyte activation and cytokine production (10).

Mycoplasmas are fastidious organisms that are highly dependent on the surrounding host or culture microenvironment for growth. Mycoplasmas appear to be capable of fusing with host cells due to characteristics of their cholesterol-containing cell membranes, and their intracellular location allows them to survive long courses of appropriate antibiotic treatment (10). Intact mycoplasma have been demonstrated in the cytoplasm and perinuclear regions of human cells both in vitro and in vivo (11).

The absence of an acute antibody response to *M. pneumoniae* has been reported (12,13). In adults and children with community-acquired pneumonia, up to 60% of subjects will demonstrate evidence of infection by polymerase chain reaction analysis (PCR) or culture while remaining seronegative (14). In 1999 Doriga-Zetsma and colleagues reported the results of a study in which they prospectively compared the utility of PCR, culture, and serology for the diagnosis of *Mycoplasma pneumoniae* respiratory tract infection in children (15). In the setting of active respiratory tract infection, and using a gold standard for active *M. pneumoniae* infection of positive culture and/or positive complement fixation, they demonstrated a sensitivity of PCR of 78%, with specificity and positive predictive values of 100%. Immunoglobulin M immunofluorescence antibody (IgM IFA) testing demonstrated a sensitivity equal to that of PCR, but it had a specificity of 92% and a positive predictive value of only 57%. The authors concluded that the IgM IFA should not be utilized as a single assay to make the diagnosis of acute *Mycoplasma* infection, and that the sensitivity of PCR is increased when used in concert with complement fixation assays (15).

The test characteristics described above have been determined in the setting of acute infection, where the organism load is presumably higher than that seen in states of chronic *Mycoplasma* colonization. The diagnosis of active *M. pneumoniae* infection becomes more challenging in states in which chronic carriage, with lower total organism burdens, is the case. As noted previously, *M. pneumoniae* is present in the airways of approximately 55% of subjects with chronic, stable asthma (12). Detection of *M. pneumoniae* in these subjects was by PCR; the organism could not be cultured from lower respiratory specimens of any subjects. Culture of *M. pneumoniae* from the airways of chronic asthmatics has been an ineffective means of detecting the pathogen, and it was the least sensitive of the methods used to detect *Mycoplasma* in the cohort of Kraft and colleagues (12). This is likely due to a combination of factors, including the organism's extreme fastidiousness and dependence on an intracellular environment for growth, as well as the low level of organisms present in the airways of subjects without acute infection. Although culture methods are now well-standardized, the low burden of organisms in the setting of chronic infection further complicates the diagnosis of this infection by culture alone. It should be noted that lidocaine, commonly used to anesthetize the airways of subjects undergoing bronchoscopy with lavage and biopsy to obtain lower respiratory tract specimens, does not inhibit the growth of *M. pneumoniae* in vitro. It is unlikely to contribute to the difficulties encountered in culturing *M. pneumoniae* from the airways of asthmatics (16).

III. Biology of *Chlamydia pneumoniae*

The first clinical isolate of *Chlamydia pneumoniae* to cause respiratory disease, AR-39, was isolated in 1983. It and other chlamydiae grow only intracellularly, again leading to challenges with culture and diagnosis. *Chlamydia pneumoniae* was first though to be a strain of *Chlamydia psittaci*, but subsequent investigation revealed it to be a separate species. There is <10% sequence homology between *C. pneumoniae* and other chlamydiae, and its morphology differs from that of other chlamydiae as well. The elementary body of *C. pneumoniae* is pear-shaped and contains a periplasmic space, unlike other chlamydiae. There is only one serovar of *C. pneumoniae* (17).

Chlamydiae are obligate intracellular pathogens that survive in the host cell within the confines of a membrane-bound inclusion. Host cell invasion is affected by the elementary body of *C. pneumoniae*, which then differentiates to a more metabolically active reticulate body. This reticulate body then replicates by binary fission and ultimately returns to the elementary body form, which is then released from infected host cells to continue the cycle of infection and replication (18). Respiratory epithelium appears to be the primary target of *C. pneumoniae* infection, but other host cells including smooth muscle cells, vascular endothelium, and mononuclear cells can be infected by the organism in vitro (19).

Diagnostic techniques for *C. pneumoniae* vary somewhat from those utilized for *M. pneumoniae*. In the setting of acute respiratory tract infection, Gaydos and colleagues (20) evaluated PCR–enzyme immunoassay (PCR-EIA) and serology in 56 subjects with respiratory symptoms and 80 control subjects. Using a gold standard for diagnosis of either positive broth culture or positive direct fluorescent antibody (DFA), they reported a sensitivity of 74.2% and a specificity of 96.2% for PCR-EIA. Serology testing with microimmunofluorescence, using the criteria of Grayston and colleagues (IgM 1:16 or IgG 1:512) (21) did not perform as well. Of asymptomatic subjects 75% had some level of antibody response to *C. pneumoniae*, and 18.8% of asymptomatic subjects had antibody levels considered to be diagnostic of acute infection with *C. pneumoniae*. The authors concluded that PCR-EIA was more reliable than serology for the diagnosis of acute *C. pneumoniae* infection (20). More recently, Verkooyen and colleagues, based on the results of their prospective study of 156 subjects with community-acquired pneumonia, reported that recombinant lipopolysaccharide enzyme-linked immunosorbent assay may be the test of choice for diagnosis of acute *C. pneumoniae* infection, and that microimmunofluorescence was the test of choice for the diagnosis of *C. pneumoniae* infection in the community (22).

Less information is available about the utility of these tests in individuals who are chronically infected. In the study of chronic stable asthmatics by Kraft and colleagues, a high prevalence (33%) of serological response to *C. pneumoniae* was seen. The prevalence of positive PCR and culture was lower or zero, respectively, perhaps due to a lower organism load than is seen in acute infection (12). Similar findings were reported in 1993 by Kern and colleagues (23).

A number of potential explanations for these findings exist. In the general population, overall seropositivity for *C. pneumoniae* increases over each decade of life, with a peak prevalence of 50–60% seropositivity (17). This serves to reduce the sensitivity and specificity of serological criteria for the diagnosis of acute infection in adults. The criteria that have been proposed for the serological diagnosis of *C. pneumoniae* infection (particularly those using a single immunoglobulin titer) are arbitrary and may in fact lead to the overdiagnosis of acute *C. pneumoniae* infection in population-based studies, as described above. The serological assays utilized for *C. pneumoniae* have also been complicated by cross-activity of antibodies to bacterial lipopolysaccharide antigens of a variety of different *Chlamydia* species (23), making accurate identification of *C. pneumoniae* more difficult. In a recent study, Routes and colleagues reported a lack of correlation between *C. pneumoniae* antibody titers and adult-onset asthma, providing further indication that serology alone is an inadequate means of strengthening the evidence for a relationship between. *C. pneumoniae* and asthma (24). Further studies are required to determine the most reliable means of detecting chronic infection with *C. pneumoniae* in subjects with asthma.

IV. Is Respiratory Tract Infection an Important Factor in Asthma Pathogenesis?

The exact role of respiratory tract infections in asthma pathogenesis is controversial, but basic scientific, epidemiological, and clinical research all support the conclusion that there is an association between early childhood respiratory infection and asthma. Two distinct observations have been made at the clinical level. First, early childhood respiratory tract infections, especially those occurring before 6 months of age, are associated with wheezing during active infection (25). Second, patients with recurrent wheezing and diminished lung function often have a history of respiratory tract infections in early life (26). These observations have led to the conclusion that childhood respiratory tract infections may predispose to subsequent asthma.

In contrast, a number of investigators have also reported that the frequency of allergic diseases is inversely related to the number of early-life respiratory tract infections, and that these infections may actually protect against the subsequent development of asthma (27). These investigators postulate that bacterial and viral infections occurring during the first 6 months of life provide important signals to the developing immune system. They change the immunological phenotype to a predominantly T-helper 1 (TH1) or a more balanced TH1/TH2 phenotype in response to intracellular bacteria and viruses, resulting in reduced IgE synthesis and a less prominent so-called allergic response (28,29). In 1995, Martinez and colleagues reported that a history of recurrent nonwheezing respiratory tract infections was associated with decreased levels of serum IgE and skin test reactivity (30).

Similar conclusions were drawn recently by Ball and colleagues from their questionnaire study of asthma incidence and wheezing prevalence in children participating in the Tucson Children's Respiratory Study (31). They found that the presence of one or more older siblings at home (which presumably increases the exposure of the youngest child to infectious agents) appeared to protect against the development of asthma (based on a parent-reported doctor's diagnosis of asthma or a reported exacerbation within the previous year. There was an adjusted relative risk of 0.8 per each older sibling (95% confidence interval [CI] = 0.7–1.0, p = 0.04). Attendance at daycare within the first 6 months of life was also associated with a reduction in the risk of subsequent asthma, with an adjusted relative risk of 0.4, 95% CI = 0.2–1.0, p = 0.04. Serum IgE levels were reported as being lower in children with two or more older siblings or daycare exposure, with a relative risk of high IgE (serum levels above the 95th percentile) of 0.8 (relative risk 0.8, 95% CI = 0.6–1.0, p = 0.03).

The authors concluded that their results confirmed the observation that early-life infectious exposure protects against the later development of asthma. However, the authors also reported the conflicting observation that children with increased exposure to others at home or daycare were more likely to demonstrate frequent (parent-reported) wheezing at age 2 years than children with little or no exposure (adjusted relative risk 1.4, 95% CI = 1.1–1.8, p = 0.01), although this wheezing was less likely to persist in these children from ages 6 through 13 years (31). The observations of these and other authors bring forth the potentially important interaction between infection and allergy and the possibility of this interaction somehow affecting the clinical expression of asthma and wheezing. The interaction between infection and allergic sensitization may be crucial in the development of the asthma phenotype, although much work remains to be done to clarify this relationship further.

In attempts to delineate the relative importance of infection and allergic sensitization, a significant body of research has focused on the role of viral pathogens in inducing both acute and chronic airway inflammation and airway responsiveness. The importance of *Mycoplasma pneumoniae* and *Chlamydia pneumoniae* in asthma, however, is a question researchers have only begun to address. The mechanisms by which atypical bacteria induce or worsen asthma may ultimately be shown to differ from those by which viruses have their effect. However, one approach to generating hypotheses about the relationship between atypical bacteria and asthma is to review current theories about the relationship between viral respiratory tract infection and asthma.

V. Animal Models of Viral Respiratory Tract Infection–Induced Airway Damage

Acute respiratory tract infection with agents such as rhinovirus, coronavirus, influenza, and respiratory syncytial virus (RSV) causes significant damage to respiratory tract epithelium (32), resulting in epithelial necrosis and local airway inflammatory responses during acute infection that result in airway obstruction and airflow limitation. Epithelial necrosis can lead to sloughing of cellular debris into the airway. Virus-mediated damage to ciliated epithelial cells decreases the effectiveness of the mucociliary elevator, allowing mucus, inflammatory cells, and plasma exudate to accumulate within the airway lumen. Both bronchial epithelial and vascular endothelial permeability are increased as a result of the inflammatory response, allowing exudation of plasma and proteinaceous fluid into the airway. Epithelial damage exposes normally protected afferent neurons within the airway wall to environmental stimuli, resulting in the release of neuropeptides such as neurokinins and substance

P. These then mediate vascular smooth muscle contraction and further exacerbate capillary endothelial permeability. Damage to airway epithelium has also been shown to result in altered expression of adhesion molecules such as the intracellular adhesion molecule 1 (ICAM-1) (33) and increased production of chemoattractant cytokines (34). This combination of epithelial damage and resultant airway obstruction leads to the clinical manifestations of asthma, including airways responsiveness, wheezing, and dyspnea (32) (Fig. 1).

Viral respiratory tract infection not only to leads to the airway changes described above (32) but also allows sensitization to inhaled allergens (35) and facilitates subsequent allergic airway inflammation (36). In 1984, Sakamoto and colleagues (35) demonstrated that sensitization to inhaled antigen could be induced during the acute phase of viral respiratory tract infection. Following experimental respiratory tract infection with influenza A, C3H mice were exposed to inhaled ovalbumin and ovalbumin-specific immunoglobulin E (IgE) production was measured. Ovalbumin-specific IgE production was seen in those mice exposed to inhaled ovalbumin following viral infection, and specific IgE production could not be demonstrated in the absence of preceding viral infection. The authors concluded that viral

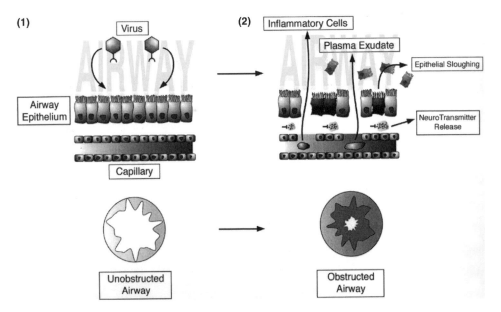

Figure 1 Viral respiratory tract infection causes airway obstruction. In panel 1, virus infects airway epithelium. Viral infection leads to necrosis and sloughing of epithelial cells into the airway lumen, as well as increased capillary endothelial permeability resulting in exudation of plasma and inflammatory cells into the airway lumen and submucosa (panel 2). Neurotransmitter release mediates smooth muscle contraction. These mechanisms of airway obstruction may also be relevant to respiratory infection with atypical bacteria. Bottom images in each panel show airway cross-sections.

damage of the respiratory tract epithelial lining was necessary for allergic sensitization to occur, and that airway epithelial damage was likely a critical factor in the etiology of certain atopic disorders (35) (Fig. 2).

Suzuki and coinvestigators infected BALB/c mice with two different strains of influenza A (H_1N_1 and H_3N_2) and then sensitized the animals to inhaled ovalbumin. They subsequently measured ovalbumin-specific IgE production and airway responsiveness (37). They demonstrated that inhalation of ovalbumin in the setting of influenza A infection led to a 10-fold increase in ovalbumin-specific IgE production over baseline ($p < 0.01$) in those mice infected with influenza A strain H_1N_1 and a sixfold increase in ovalbumin-specific IgE production over baseline ($p < 0.01$) in those mice infected with influenza A strain H_3N_2. This phenomenon was not seen in mice exposed to ovalbumin in the absence of prior influenza A infection. The combination of influenza A infection and ovalbumin sensitization also led to airways responsiveness as measured by changes in specific airway resistance in response to methacholine challenge ($p < 0.01$), a phenomenon not seen with either viral infection or ovalbumin sensitization alone. These data further strengthened the hypotheses that viral infection altered immune response to inhaled allergen and predisposed to airway responsiveness (37).

In an extensive study of the relationship between viral respiratory tract infection, allergen sensitization and airway responsiveness, Schwarze and coinvestigators infected BALB/c mice with human respiratory syncytial virus (RSV)(strain A) and measured a number of variables including airway reactivity, the cellular response to infection, and mononuclear cell cytokine production (36). They showed that the airways of infected mice became reactive, with a 5.33 ± 2.41-fold increase in reactivity to methacholine in those mice infected with RSV compared with a 2.75 ± 1.42-fold increase in reactivity to methacholine in sham-infected animals ($p < 0.05$). The authors also demonstrated that there was influx of both eosinophils and neutrophils into the lungs in response to RSV infection. Eosinophils increased 1.87-fold in lung isolates of infected animals compared with controls ($p < 0.05$), and neutrophils increased 2.57-fold ($p < 0.05$) compared with controls. The level of the eosinophilic response was reported to correlate closely with increased airway responsiveness, with a correlation coefficient of 0.89 for days 11–20 following infection ($p < 0.001$) and a correlation coefficient of 0.96 for days 21–30 following infection ($p < 0.001$) (36).

Acute RSV infection also caused a transient increase in the production of interferon gamma (IFN-γ) by mononuclear cells in peribronchial lymph nodes (PBLN), with levels 7860 ± 1901.7 pg/mL in infected animals vs. 4269.6 ± 2654.8 pg/mL in controls ($p = 0.04$). There was also a transient decrease in the production of interleukin (IL)-4 (10.7 ± 1.55 pg/mL in infected vs. 71.0 ± 24.7 pg/mL in controls, $p = 0.02$) and IL-5 (686.0 ± 322.8 pg/mL in infected vs. 1996.3 ± 536.7 pg/mL in controls, $p = 0.03$), resulting in a predominantly TH1-type cytokine response. This deviation to a TH1 response was short-lived, however, and by day 12 postinfection, cytokine levels had returned to normal. The authors went on, however, to demonstrate that sensitization to inhaled ovalbumin after RSV infection alters the immune response of mononuclear cells towards a TH2-type cytokine response.

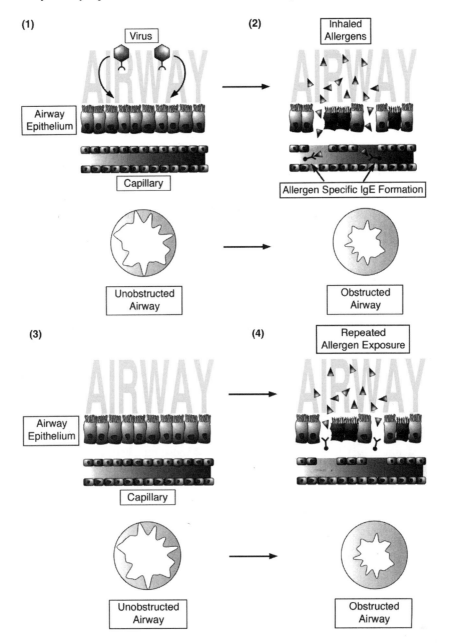

Figure 2 Viral infection amplifies sensitization to inhaled allergens. In panel 1, virus infects airway epithelium. This results in airway epithelial and capillary endothelial damage, facilitating inhaled allergen-specific IgE formation (panel 2). Following infection, airways return to normal (panel 3). Repeated exposure to inhaled allergen evokes allergic airways inflammation and subsequent airway obstruction (panel 4). Similar mechanisms of allergic sensitization in atypical bacterial infection have not yet been proven. Bottom images in each panel show airway cross-sections.

Ovalbumin sensitization after RSV infection resulted in a significantly decreased production of IFN-γ compared to ovalbumin sensitization alone (20.63 ± 12.7 pg/mL vs. 63.3 ± 15.49 pg/mL, p=0.02). The production of IL-4 was significantly increased from 1.08 ± 0.13 pg/mL to 5.33 ± 1.08 pg/mL (p = 0.02). No significant differences in IL-5 production were detected (36).

The authors of this study were able to demonstrate conclusively that acute RSV infection resulted in a significant increase in airway responsiveness, and that the kinetics of this increase in airway responsiveness was closely associated with the development of an eosinophilic and neutrophilic inflammatory response in the airways. In the setting of acute RSV infection the cytokine response was shown to be transiently of the TH1 type, with a return to normal levels by day 12 postinfection. Eosinophilic inflammation is typically seen in the setting of a TH2-type cytokine response and not in the context of a TH1-type response, as was demonstrated in this study. The eosinophilic response to RSV infection may have been mediated by virus-induced epithelial changes with altered expression of adhesion molecules and chemokines (36).

VI. Are Models of Virus-Induced Airway Damage Relevant to the Study of Atypical Bacterial Airway Infection?

If atypical bacteria induce alterations in airway epithelium or inflammatory response similar to those seen following viral respiratory tract infection, mechanisms of chronic airway damage and allergic sensitization may be relevant to models of atypical bacterial infection and asthma pathogenesis. Although animal models of *Mycoplasma* and *Chlamydia* infection will be discussed in further detail later in this chapter, *Mycoplasma* infection does cause significant damage to airway epithelium with inflammatory cell infiltration, mucosal thickening, and ultimately extensive airway remodeling (38). Changes in cytokine similar to those seen with viral infection have also been demonstrated. In their murine model of *M. pneumoniae* respiratory infection (described in further detail later in this chapter), Martin and colleagues (39) reported that *M. pneumoniae* infection also suppressed production of IFN-γ and that this suppression was correlated with increased airways responsiveness.

Few studies of airway epithelial changes following *Mycoplasma* infection have been published. In 1990, Söderberg and colleagues (40) published a study in which they obtained bronchial mucosal biopsies from 12 subjects who had recently sustained respiratory tract infection with influenza A (n=7), parainfluenza (n = 1), or *M. pneumoniae* (n = 4). All subjects had recovered from infection at the time of biopsy, and the only remaining symptom was that of cough, seen in only five subjects. Airway responsiveness testing was normal in all but two subjects. Morphometric analysis was performed on biopsy specimens, and the features of airway epithelial damage resulting from each infection were compared both with each other, and with endobronchial biopsies of healthy subjects. The authors were unable to demonstrate significant differences in the degree of epithelial damage or basement membrane thickness between subjects who had recently had respiratory tract infection and healthy volunteers (40).

This study may appear at first viewing to indicate that airway epithelial disruption is minimal in the setting of both viral and mycoplasma airway infection in humans. However, these subjects had all recovered from acute infection, and a significant amount of epithelial healing may have already occurred by the time of biopsy. Furthermore, since no differences were found between viral and mycoplasma infection, it remains unclear from this study whether there are significant differences in mechanisms of airway epithelial damage or allergic sensitization in viral vs. *Mycoplasma* infection. This study was unable to resolve whether the effects of *Mycoplasma* infection on airway epithelium are uniform, or whether individuals with more severe clinical infections are more likely to have severe airway epithelial damage and subsequent airway responsiveness or asthma.

The inflammatory profile of the airways in subjects with *M. pneumoniae* infection has been described recently by Martin and colleagues (41). The authors performed bronchoalveolar lavage and endobronchial biopsies on 55 asthmatic and 11 control subjects and evaluated subjects for the presence of *M. pneumoniae* by PCR, culture, and serology. There were no differences in the BAL inflammatory cell characteristics between subjects who demonstrated evidence of M. pneumoniae DNA by PCR and those who did not. In endobronchial biopsy specimens there was a significantly higher number of mast cells, as documented by AA1 immunohistochemical staining for mast cell tryptase, in the airways of *M. pneumoniae* PCR-positive subjects (29.1 cells/mm^2 [18.3–63.4 interquartile range [IQR] vs. 9.8 cells/mm^2 (0–41.3 IQR), p = 0.04). The was also a trend toward a significant increase in CD3-positive T-lymphocytes in subjects who were PCR positive for *M. pneumoniae* when compared with those without evidence of *M. pneumoniae* DNA in the airways (20.9 cells/mm^2 [0–54.6 IQR] vs. 0 cells/mm^2 [0–46.2 IQR], p = 0.09). IgE levels were slightly, but not significantly, elevated in PCR-positive subjects compared with PCR-negative subjects. The authors concluded that the increased number of tissue mast cells found in the airways of subjects with PCR evidence of continuing *M. pneumoniae* infection may suggest an interaction between infection and allergic sensitization (41).

VII. What Is the Clinical and Epidemiological Evidence for an Association Between Respiratory Infection and Asthma?

Respiratory infections are associated with discrete episodes of wheezing and may also predispose to the development of chronic asthma. In previously healthy, nonatopic adults, upper respiratory tract infection with common viral pathogens results in airways responsiveness during histamine challenge testing (42). In adults with established asthma, clinical and spirometric worsening of airflow limitation is seen commonly during acute viral respiratory tract infection (43). Similar findings have been demonstrated in adults with acute *Mycoplasma* infection (44).

Viral infections sustained in childhood are associated with subsequent development of airway responsiveness and asthma. In 1982, Pullan and Hey reported longitudinal follow-up on a series of children with RSV infections in infancy who were evaluated for 10 years after initial presentation. Forty-two percent of subjects with prior RSV infection had had further episodes of wheezing 10 years later, compared with 19% of control subjects (p < 0.001). There was a threefold increase in airways responsiveness by histamine challenge testing in subjects with prior RSV infection compared with controls (45). In 1995 Sigurs and co-workers confirmed this observation, reporting a prospective series in which a significantly greater percentage of children (23% vs. 1%, p < 0.001) with prior RSV infection sustained later episodes of asthma than did controls (46).

VIII. Association Between *Mycoplasma pneumoniae* and Asthma

Mycoplasma pneumoniae is a common cause of so-called atypical pneumonia and tracheobronchitis (10). It attaches to ciliated airway epithelial cells by means of a terminal organelle, infecting the cell and causing epithelial damage and ciliary stasis (47). Over the last three decades, a number of reports have demonstrated an association between airway reactivity and *M. pneumoniae* infection. *M. pneumoniae* has been implicated as a cause of wheezing in asthmatic (48) and nonasthmatic (49) children, has been associated with impaired pulmonary function up to 3 years after acute infection (50), and has been detected repeatedly in the lower airways of adults with chronic asthma (12). It now appears that *M. pneumoniae* can be detected in up to 25% of all community-acquired pneumonias across all age groups (51), whereas historically this was thought to be primarily an infection of the young. In the past this prevalence figure was also much lower, because identification techniques were not as sensitive as those in use today (e.g., PCR). Although *M. pneumoniae* is clearly an important cause of pneumonia, no conclusive causative link has yet been established between *M. pneumoniae* and chronic asthma.

In 1963, Wenner et al. concluded that *Mycoplasma pneumoniae* infection was associated with the onset of wheezing in children without a previous history of asthma (49). *M. pneumoniae* can also exacerbate airflow limitation in asthmatics. In a series of children with pre-existing asthma, *M. pneumoniae* infection was seen in 7 of 40 (18%) episodes of acute exacerbation (48). In addition to causing a decrement in pulmonary function during acute infection, *M. pneumoniae* may result in long-term impairment of pulmonary function in both asthmatics and nonasthmatics. In a series of 108 children with lower respiratory tract infection caused by *M. pneumoniae* (detected by increased complement fixation titers), 40% of subjects presented with wheezing as an initial clinical finding, and at both 3 months and 3 years of age there were significant decrements in forced vital capacity (FVC) (93.1% vs. 100.8% of predicted, p < 0.01) and forced expiratory volume in 1 s (FEV_1) (94.5% vs. 100.6% of predicted, p < 0.02) in nonasthmatic subjects with previous *Mycoplasma* pneumonia compared to controls (50). However, a separate series of 50 children evaluated 1.5–9.5 years after clinical and radiographic recovery from *M. pneumoniae* pneumonia did not demonstrate persistent reductions in FVC or FEV_1 (52).

M. pneumoniae infection has been reported to precede directly the onset of asthma. In 1994, Yano and colleagues reported a previously healthy patient in whom *Mycoplasma pneumoniae* infection was associated with the subsequent development of asthma (53). Following serologically documented *Mycoplasma* pneumonia, this patient developed reversible airflow limitation, *M. pneumoniae*-specific IgE, and bronchial hyperresponsiveness to inhaled mycoplasmal antigens after his acute infection (53). The authors did not rule out concurrent viral infection, however, so allergic sensitization to *Mycoplasma* antigens in the setting of an acute viral respiratory tract infection cannot be completely excluded.

Asthmatics have been shown to have significantly higher levels of IgE antibodies specific to *M. pneumoniae* than control populations (54). An increased prevalence of *M. pneumoniae* in both the upper and lower airways of asthmatics has also been demonstrated by means of culture. When Gil and colleagues cultured the upper airway of 77 asthmatics, they were able to isolate *M. pneumoniae* in a significantly greater number of asthmatics than controls (24.7% vs. 5.7%, p < 0.01) (55).

In 1998, Kraft et al. (12) published the first systematic evaluation of *Mycoplasma* infection in the upper and lower airways of adults with chronic, stable asthma. The investigators evaluated 18 asthmatics and 11 normal controls for the presence of *M. pneumoniae* and *C. pneumoniae*, assaying serology and performing culture and PCR for these organisms on specimens obtained from the naso- and oropharynx, bronchoalveolar lavage, and endobronchial biopsy of the lower airway. *M. pneumoniae* was detected by PCR in 55.6% of asthmatic subjects compared with 9% of controls (p = 0.02) (12). Cultures, serologies, and enzyme-linked immunoassays for *M. pneumoniae* were negative in all subjects, and common respiratory viruses were excluded by enzyme immunoassay in all subjects. On the basis of these data, the authors concluded that a majority of adults with chronic, stable asthma are chronically infected with *M. pneumoniae* with a significantly greater frequency than nonasthmatic subjects. At this time, more study is needed to evaluate whether *Mycoplasma* infection is a pathogenic factor in asthma or merely a epiphenomenon somehow related to the enhanced airway inflammation seen in patients with chronic asthma.

The investigation of Kraft and colleagues (12) was driven by several difficult cases of asthma encountered in the outpatient setting. The first patient was a 22-year-old woman with a diagnosis of childhood-onset asthma. She had been corticosteroid-dependent for 13 years, requiring between 24 and 80 mg of oral methylprednisolone daily. She also required high-dosage inhaled corticosteroids, long-acting beta-2 agonists, theophylline, cromolyn sodium, ipratropium bromide, and as-needed albuterol. Diagnoses other than asthma were excluded, and she ultimately underwent bronchoscopy and endobronchial biopsy, which revealed intraluminal *M. pneumoniae*. She was treated with clarithromycin, 500 mg orally per day, and a gradual improvement in her lung function was seen with antibiotic treatment. When antibiotics were discontinued her lung function worsened, however, so continuous therapy with macrolide antibiotics was initiated. The patient is now approaching 9 years of continuous antibiotic treatment and has noted a tremendous improvement in her asthma. She has been able to discontinue oral corticosteroids and currently requires only moderate dosages of inhaled corticosteroids and long-acting beta-2 agonists. Furthermore, she has now become corticosteroid-sensitive, requiring only short (3–5 days) courses of oral corticosteroids for the treatment of asthma exacerbations.

The second patient was a 31-year-old fitness instructor who had adult-onset corticosteroid-dependent asthma. Alternative diagnoses were again excluded. Bronchoscopy with biopsy did not demonstrate *M. pneumoniae*, although at that time we were not aware of the potential association of *C. pneumoniae* and asthma and therefore did not test for it. An empirical trial of macrolide antibiotic therapy was initiated, and the patient improved dramatically. Corticosteroids were tapered, and after 2 years antibiotic therapy was discontinued. The patient has done well after discontinuation of antibiotic therapy.

The third patient was a retired oral surgeon with debilitating asthma and fixed airway obstruction. He required approximately 10 days of oral corticosteroids per month, but after the addition of clarithromycin he no longer required oral corticosteroids. He was able to discontinue clarithromycin after 6 months and has continued to note a significant improvement in his asthma.

The final illustrative case is that of a 55-year-old woman with severe persistent asthma requiring multiple medications and unresponsive to systemic or inhaled corticosteroids. After the initiation of macrolide antibiotic therapy her lung function improved steadily over the course of a year, with morning peak flows improving from 270 L/min to 450 L/min over that time period. She has been maintained on clarithromycin with continued improvement of her asthma.

Although these cases are anecdotal, they provide clinical context for the observations made by clinical and epidemiological investigators. They also raise interesting questions about the possibility of chronic latent infection influencing steroid responsiveness. Furthermore, it appears that the short courses of antibiotics normally used for the treatment of acute atypical bacterial infection may not be appropriate in the setting of chronic infection, given that these patients required, at a minimum, 6 months of treatment to sustain improvements in airflow.

IX. Association Between *Chlamydia pneumoniae* and Asthma

Like *M. pneumoniae*, *Chlamydia pneumoniae* infection has also been associated with subsequent wheezing illness. *C. pneumoniae* is a common cause of bronchitis and atypical pneumonia, and may result in chronic infections as well (56)(Table 1).

C. pneumoniae also causes exacerbations of pre-existing asthma. In a cohort of 70 adults presenting with asthma exacerbation, 10% were shown by serology to be acutely infected with *C. pneumoniae* (57). In a community-based cohort of patients with lower respiratory tract illness, 47% of patients with acute *C. pneumoniae* infection were found to have subjective evidence of bronchospasm during the course of the infection. There was a strong positive correlation between the level of *C. pneumoniae* titers and wheezing at the time of enrollment. There was also an association of *C. pneumoniae* antibody titers and subsequent development of asthmatic

Table 1   *Chlamydia pneumoniae-*
Associated Conditions

Established	Possible
Bronchitis	Asthma
Otitis	Atherosclerosis
Pharyngitis	Endocarditis
Pneumonia	Myocarditis
Sinusitis	Erythema nodosum
	Sarcoidosis

bronchitis after the acute illness, which was seen in 32% of cases (odds ratio = 7.2, 95% CI = 2.2–23.4) (58).

In 1998, Hahn and McDonald reported a series of 163 primary care outpatients with acute wheezing illnesses or chronic asthma and showed that 12% had evidence of *C. pneumoniae* infection by culture and/or serology. Of these patients, 50% had not been diagnosed previously with airflow obstruction, and 30% were subsequently given the diagnosis of asthma (59). In the study by Kraft et al. cited above, culture and PCR for *C. pneumoniae* were negative in all asthmatic and control subjects. In their cohort, nine asthmatics (50%) and one control (9%) were positive for *C. pneumoniae* by serology (p = 0.05). Recent work in our laboratory has shown that approximately 13% of patients with chronic asthma demonstrate evidence of *C. pneumoniae* DNA within the airways by PCR. Individuals with PCR evidence of *C. pneumoniae* in lower-airway specimens demonstrate greater degrees of airflow limitation and airway inflammation than do subjects who manifest only serological evidence of infection (60).

X. Additional Epidemiological Data from Large Cohort Studies

In 1999, von Mutius and colleagues published a cohort study in which they utilized core questions from the ISAAC phase II survey to evaluate the relationship between childhood fever and antibiotic treatment and asthma prevalence. They showed that surrogate markers of infection, such as repeated episodes of fever and antibiotic treatment in early life, were strongly associated with asthma and recurrent wheezing episodes. There was an odds ratio of up to 7.95 (95% confidence interval [CI] 6.02–10.50, p value not reported) in children who had received ≥ six antibiotic courses in the first 3 years of life (61). Subjects were not stratified by the pathogen causing the febrile illness, however, and the site of infection and type of antibiotic used were not reported. It is therefore difficult to attribute this increased in asthma prevalence to respiratory tract infection alone. However, since respiratory tract infections account for a significant fraction of antibiotic prescriptions in childhood, since 20–25% of community-acquired pneumonias (across all age groups) are caused by *Mycoplasma pneumoniae* (51), and since *Chlamydia pneumoniae* has been isolated from 15–20%

of adults and children with community-acquired pneumonia (17), *Mycoplasma* and *Chlamydia* infections may be implicated in a large number of the febrile episodes resulting in antibiotic prescription.

A 1999 cohort study by Castro-Rodriguez and colleagues demonstrated a significant association between lower respiratory tract infection (LRI) and decreased pulmonary function in later childhood (26). A birth cohort of 888 subjects were followed for the development of LRI. Over the course of the first 3 years of life, 7.4% of the cohort developed LRI that met radiographic criteria for pneumonia, and 44.7% developed LRI that did not meet criteria for pneumonia. In each group, respiratory syncytial virus was the most common pathogen, seen in 36.4% of patients with LRI and pneumonia and 35.6% of patients with LRI and no pneumonia. The exact prevalence of atypical bacterial infection in the cohort was not reported, and 43.6% and 37.6% of infectious causes went unidentified in the pneumonia and LRI without pneumonia groups, respectively.

Subjects were subsequently surveyed via questionnaire for a physician's diagnosis of asthma at ages 6 and 11 years. Children who had LRI, both with and without evidence of pneumonia in the first 3 years of life, demonstrated an increased prevalence of asthma, with 13.6% of all subjects carrying an asthma diagnosis at age 6 years (OR = 3.3, 95% CI = 1.4–7.8, p < 0.01) and 25.9% of all subjects carrying an asthma diagnosis at age 11 years (OR = 2.8, 95% CI = 1.4–5.6, p < 0.01). Subjects with LRI (with or without pneumonia) also demonstrated lower values of FEV_1 than control subjects (26). Based on data from this study, and given the prevalence of *Mycoplasma* and chlamydial infection in pediatric community-acquired pneumonia, atypical bacterial infection may be contributing to the increased risk of asthma following early childhood pneumonia. This conclusion is limited by the fact that a high prevalence of atypical bacterial infection was not reported in this cohort. However, difficulties with detection of atypical bacterial pathogens may lead to underdetection of these agents, complicating efforts at determining the prevalence of atypical bacterial infection in cohort studies such as this one.

Most epidemiological studies have been limited in their ability to determine the strength of the association between *Mycoplasma* and *Chlamydia* infection and asthma because of limitations in the ability to characterize the microbiological exposure status of subjects well enough to determine the relative prevalence of viral, typical, and atypical bacterial pathogens in subjects with lower respiratory tract infections or pneumonia. We are currently investigating the association between atypical bacterial pneumonia caused by *M. pneumoniae* and *C. pneumoniae* and subsequent asthma at the population level. We have identified a small cohort (n = 260) of pediatric subjects who were enrolled in a prior drug treatment trial (13) of community-acquired pneumonia. All members of this cohort had both clinical and radiographic evidence of community-acquired pneumonia at the time of enrollment. All were tested for active *Mycoplasma* and *Chlamydia* infection with culture and PCR of respiratory tract secretions, as well as serology. Utilizing a questionnaire-based retrospective follow-up study design, we are in the process of determining the prevalence of doctor-diagnosed asthma in subjects with and without *M. pneumoniae* and *C. pneumoniae* as the cause of their pneumonia. Although our research is underway, preliminary results from a questionnaire-based study of subjects who demonstrated evidence of active atypical bacterial pneumonia by positive sputum culture or PCR indicates that the prevalence of asthma in these subjects 7–8 years postinfection is similar to that of subjects with viral pneumonia (62). If these results are borne out by more extensive follow-up of this cohort, they may provide evidence for an association between atypical bacterial infection and asthma that is at least as strong as the association between viral infection and asthma.

XI. Animal Models of *Mycoplasma pneumoniae* Infection

Animal models are critical to expanding our knowledge of the association between atypical bacterial infection and asthma. *Mycoplasma* species have been used to study respiratory tract infection in laboratory animals, including mice, leading to insights into mechanisms by which atypical bacteria lead to airway inflammation and responsiveness. *Mycoplasma pulmonis*, a natural pathogen in mice, has been used in a murine model of *Mycoplasma* respiratory tract infection. These models have demonstrated that *Mycoplasma* infection can lead to chronic airway inflammation typified by lymphocytic airway infiltration, mucosal thickening, airway vessel angiogenesis, and extensive remodeling of the airways (38). *M. pulmonis* also causes neurogenic airway inflammation with substance P-mediated leakage of plasma exudate into the airways (38). *M. pulmonis*, however, is not a human respiratory tract pathogen. Recent efforts in our laboratory and by other investigators have been directed at establishing a murine model of *M. pneumoniae* infection with the goal of using this model to investigate both the mechanisms by which this infection may become chronic and to understand the mechanisms of airways inflammation and responsiveness seen following *M. pneumoniae* infection.

Although *M. pneumoniae* is not a natural mouse pathogen, Wubbel and colleagues demonstrated that intranasal introduction of *M. pneumoniae* into BALB/c mice results in acute respiratory tract infection. This was based on positive broth culture data from BAL specimens performed up to 15 days following infection (63). Murine infection with *M. pneumoniae* also results in an active immunological response. Some 62% of animals demonstrated enzyme–linked immunosorbent assay (ELISA) evidence of *M. pneumoniae*-specific IgM production, and 97% of animals demonstrated positive immunoblots for *M. pneumoniae*. Many animals also demonstrated histological evidence of airway epithelial disruption following *M. pneumoniae* infection (63). The investigators concluded that *M. pneumoniae* in mice provided a model by which histological and immunological responses to *Mycoplasma* infection could be studied.

Pietsch and colleagues studied the inflammatory response of BALB/c mice during acute primary and secondary infection with *M. pneumoniae*. Following infection, the investigators evaluated in vivo cytokine gene expression in the spleens and lungs of these animals (64). During the acute phase of infection, the authors found elevated expression of tumor necrosis factor-alpha (TNF-α), interleukin-1 (IL-1), IL-6, and interferon-gamma (IFN-γ). IL-2 and IL-2 receptor gene expression was seen only during reinfection. Expression of cytokines also varied over the course of infection; IL-2 mRNA levels fell over the first 24 h of infection and were not detectable after 24 h and IL-10 mRNA levels rose over this same period. Furthermore, during reinfection with *M. pneumoniae* mRNA levels of IL-6 and TNF-α were 10-fold higher than those seen during acute infection. IFN-γ mRNA levels were 50-fold higher following reinfection than with acute infection (64). These data support the assertion that infection with *M. pneumoniae* can lead to the production of proinflammatory cytokines, many of which have also been implicated in the pathogenesis of asthma. These results indicate that although *M. pneumoniae* is not a natural murine pathogen, it produces inflammatory responses similar to those seen in human asthma and provides an adequate model with which to study the effects of *Mycoplasma* infection on the airways.

Recent efforts in our laboratory (39) have been directed at determining the alterations in airways responsiveness and inflammatory responses over a 3-week time interval in a mouse model of *M. pneumoniae* respiratory infection. BALB/c mice were infected with *M. pneumoniae* and airway responsiveness testing to increasing dosages of methacholine was performed at 3, 7, 14, and 21 days postinfection. After methacholine challenge, BAL was performed and fluid was analyzed for cell count and differential as well as mycoplasma culture and PCR for *M. pneumoniae*. After lavage, lungs were excised and histological analysis for severity of inflammation was performed. A portion of the lung was utilized for reverse transcription-polymerase chain reaction for IFN-γ.

Mice infected with *M. pneumoniae* demonstrated significant increases in airways responsiveness at days 3, 7, and 14 postinfection when compared with sham-infected controls. There were no differences in airways responsiveness at day 21. The cellular inflammatory response varied with time, with a predominantly neutrophilic response to infection seen at days 3 and 7, followed by an increase in macrophages and lymphocytes in infected tissue at days 14 and 21. The lung tissue at day 3 demonstrated intense neutrophilic and mononuclear peribronchiolar, bronchial, and perivascular infiltrates, as well as bronchial luminal exudate. At subsequent days, a decrease in inflammatory response was seen, with infiltration noted primarily at the bronchioles and adjacent blood vessels. At all time points eosinophils were only rarely seen. Furthermore, there was a highly significant correlation ($r = 0.78$, $p < 0.0001$) between lung tissue inflammation score and airways responsiveness to methacholine (39).

The expression of IFN-γ mRNA in the lung tissue was significantly depressed in the infected groups on days 3 and 7 compared to control animals ($p < 0.03$). In infected animals, the degree of IFN-γ mRNA expression was significantly higher on day 21 than on days 3, 7, or 14 ($p < 0.002$). There was a significant negative correlation ($r = -0.5$, $p = 0.022$) between IFN-γ and airways responsiveness to methacholine (39).

This murine model of *M. pneumoniae* infection demonstrated that inflammation was most prominent through day 14 following infection. Infection with *M. pneumoniae* significantly increased airways responsiveness for up to 14 days, and the degree of tissue inflammation was closely correlated with the degree of airways responsiveness. Finally, the suppression of IFN-γ in the week following infection may provide a regulatory mechanism for determining airway responsiveness, with the increase in IFN-γ expression after day 14 playing a pivotal role in regulating the decrease in airway responsiveness seen later in the course of infection (39).

XII. Animal Models of *Chlamydia pneumoniae* Infection

Although no animal reservoir has been implicated in the transmission of *Chlamydia pneumoniae* (65), animal models of *C. pneumoniae* have been successfully established in mice, rabbits, and monkeys. Kuo and colleagues have demonstrated homogenous infection in mice following nasal inoculation with *C. pneumoniae*, with interstitial pneumonitis on the third day after inoculation, parenchymal pneumonia on the fifth day following inoculation, and a strong antibody response that peaked 3–4 weeks following intranasal inoculation (66). In this model, histological analysis demonstrated primarily perivascular and peribronchial lymphocytic infiltration. These pathological changes were observed for several weeks after the acute infection (66). These investigators have also demonstrated that *C. pneumoniae* DNA can be detected in lungs by PCR and in situ DNA hybridization, even after the organism can no longer be cultured from the lungs (67). *Chlamydia pneumonia* also appears to establish chronic latent infection in mice; if immunosuppressive medications such as corticosteroids are administered after recovery from primary infection, *C. pneumoniae* can once again be cultured from lung tissue within 14 days following immunosuppression (68).

XIII. Can *Mycoplasma pneumoniae* Cause Chronic Airway Infection?

In an investigation designed to describe the natural evolution of untreated *M. pneumoniae* infection in the mouse, Hardy and colleagues established a murine model of chronic *M. pneumoniae* infection (69). At 28 days postinfection, they were able to demonstrate positive BAL culture or PCR in 100% of mice. At 84 days 70% of animals remained positive on BAL culture or PCR for *M. pneumoniae*. Histopathological scoring of tissue inflammation was most severe in the acute phase of infection, with the level of tissue inflammation decreasing to control levels at day 84. After the acute phase the infection seems to be contained largely in the airways, with BAL cultures positive but minced lung cultures negative following acute infection. All mice demonstrated *M. pneumoniae* IgG at 35 days postinfection and beyond (69). Development of a murine model of chronic airway infection with *M. pneumoniae* is critical to understanding the immunopathogenesis of the infection and will continue to provide insights into the mechanisms by which *M. pneumoniae* establishes chronic infection and contributes to the asthma phenotype.

XIV. Role of Antimicrobial Therapy in Modifying the Clinical Expression of Asthma

Current treatment guidelines do not recommend antibiotics as a component of asthma therapy, either in the chronic, stable state or during exacerbations (70,71). In 1975, Berman and colleagues (72) published the results of a cohort study of 26 subjects with asthma exacerbations presumed to be secondary to infection. They performed transtracheal aspiration to obtain specimens for culture of aerobic, anaerobic, and atypical bacteria, as well as mycobacteria, fungi, and viruses. In asthmatic subjects, 55.6% of specimens yielded microbial growth, and in normal controls 66.7% of specimens yielded microbial growth. Approximately 50% of specimens in each group yielded polymicrobial culture results, and in all cases bacterial growth was sparse. Multiple different bacteria were cultured, with alpha-hemolytic *Streptococcus* being the most common organism (present in 6 of 27 asthmatic subjects and 4 of 12 control subjects). In no subjects was *Mycoplasma* or respiratory viruses cultured (72). Although the culture methods used in this now more than 20-year-old study are likely less sensitive than those in use today, this study suggests that bacterial infection of the upper airway is not a significant factor in most acute asthma exacerbations.

In 1982, Graham and co-workers published a randomized, placebo-controlled trial of amoxicillin (500 mg orally three times daily) in 60 adult subjects with acute asthma exacerbations (73). Patients were continued on corticosteroid and bronchodilator therapy throughout the course of the trial, and the authors were unable to demonstrate any significant improvement in spirometric indices (peak expiratory flow rate, FEV_1 and FVC), symptom scores, or length of stay in patients treated with amoxicillin vs. conventional therapy. At the time of discharge from the hospital, FEV_1 values were actually significantly greater in the placebo group than the antibiotic group (65.6% of predicted vs. 52.3% of predicted, p = 0.039). The authors concluded that the routine use of antibiotics in acute asthma exacerbations was unwarranted (73).

There is some evidence, however, that indices of airway inflammation in asthma may improve when patients who have atypical bacterial infection as a cofactor in their asthma are treated with macrolide antibiotics (74). Kraft et al. treated 15 asthmatics who had countinuing lower airway infection with *Mycoplasma pneumoniae* or *Chlamydia pneumoniae* (diagnosed by PCR performed on lower airway biopsy) with clarithromycin (500 mg orally twice daily)for 6 weeks. At the end of the treatment course there was a significant reduction in the expression of proinflammatory cytokine TNF-α and IL-5 by airway epithelial cells in these patients (74). We are continuing to study the clinical utility of the addition of antibiotic therapy to standard asthma therapy in our laboratory.

XV. Conclusion

Infection is an important acquired factor in the pathogenesis and clinical expression of asthma, and there is mounting evidence that atypical bacterial pathogens are important contributors to asthma pathogenesis and severity. It is clear that respiratory tract infections can induce airway epithelial damage that results in airway obstruction and signs and symptoms of asthma. Viral infection also facilitates sensitization to inhaled allergens that may predispose to atopic asthma later in life. Antibiotics are not recommended for the treatment of either stable or acutely exacerbated asthma, but the role of macrolide antibiotics in the treatment of some asthmatics will likely expand as we further understand the role of atypical bacterial pathogens in the clinical expression of asthma.

There is little doubt that future research will serve to further elucidate this relationship. Ever-improving methods of detecting and culturing *Mycoplasma* and *Chlamydia* will improve our efforts to determine the prevalence of both acute and chronic infection in patients with asthma. They will also make easier research into the link between respiratory tract infections and asthma. Research currently underway into the importance of atypical bacterial pathogens in asthma will answer coucial questions about whether these infections are important in asthma pathogenesis or whether their prevalence is simply increased in asthmatics due to chronic airway inflammation or other, yet unidentified, predisposing factors. Should airway infection with atypical bacterial pathogens be shown to be a significant primary factor in asthma pathogenesis or critical in determining asthma severity, significant changes will occur in therapeutic recommendations for the treatment of this disease. This may provide a potentially important role for antibiotics in the prophylaxis and management of this disease.

References

1. Reimann HA. An acute infection of the respiratory tract with atypical pneumonia. JAMA 1938; 111:2377–2384.
2. Gallagher RJ. Acute pneumonitis: a report of 87 cases among adolescents. Yale J Biol Med 1941; 13:663–678.
3. Eaton MD, Meiklejohn G, van Herick W. Studies on the etiology of primary atypical pneumonia. A filterable agent transmissable to cotton rats, hamsters and chicken embryos. J Exp Med 1944; 79:649–668.
4. Marmion BP, Goodburn GM. Effect of an inorganic gold salt on Eaton's primary atypical pneumonia agent and other observations. Nature 1961; 189:247–248.
5. Chanock RM, Rifkind D, Kravetz HM, Knight V, Johnson KM. Respiratory disease in volunteers infected with the Eaton agent; a preliminary report. Proc Natl Acad Sci USA 1961; 48:41–49.
6. Baseman JB, Reddy SP, Dallo SF. Interplay between mycoplasma surface proteins, airway cells, and the protean manifestations of mycoplasma-mediated human infections. Am J Respir Crit Care Med 1996; 154:S137–44.
7. Murray HW, Masur H, Senterfit LB, Roberts RB. The protean manifestations of *Mycoplasma pneumoniae* infection in adults. Am J Med 1975; 58:229–242.
8. Baseman JB. The cytadhesins of *Mycoplasma pneumoniae* and *M. genitalium*. In: Rottem S, Kahane I, eds. Subcellular Biochemistry. New York: Plenum Press, 1993:243–259.

9. Tully JG, Rose DL, Baseman JB, Dallo SF, Lazzell AL, Davis CP. *Mycoplasma pneumoniae* and *Mycoplasma genitalium* mixture in synovial fluid isolate. J Clin Microbiol 1995; 33:1851–1855.

10. Baseman JB, Tully JG. Mycoplasmas: Sophisticated, reemerging, and burdened by their notoriety. Emerg Infect Dis 1997; 3:21–32.

11. Baseman JB, Lange M, Criscimagna NL, Giron JA, Thomas CA. Interplay between mycoplasmas and host target cells. Microb Pathog 1995; 19:105–116.

12. Kraft M, Cassell GH, Henson JE, et al. Detection of *Mycoplasma pneumoniae* in the airways of adults with chronic asthma. Am J Respir Crit Care Med 1998; 158:998–1001.

13. Block S, Hedrick J, Hammerschlag MR, Cassell GH, Craft JC. *Mycoplasma pneumoniae* and *Chlamydia pneumoniae* in pediatric community-acquired pneumonia: comparative efficacy and safety of clarithromycin versus erythromycin ethylsuccinate. Pediatr Infect Dis J 1995; 14:471–447.

14. Marmion BP, Williamson J, Worswick PA, Kok TW, Harris RJ. Experience with newer techniques for the laboratory detection of *Mycoplasma pneumoniae* infection: Adelaide, 1978–1991. Clin Infect Dis 1993; 17:S90–S99.

15. Dorigo-Zetsma JW, Zaat SAJ, Wertheim-van Dillen PME, et al. Comparison of PCR, culture and serological tests for diagnosis of *Mycoplasma pneumoniae* respiratory tract infection in children. J Clin Microbiol 1999; 37:14–17.

16. Cassell GH, Waites KB, Crouse DT. Mycoplasmal Infections. In: Remington JS, Klein JO, eds. Infectious Diseases of the Fetus and Newborn Infant. Philadelphia: WB Saunders, 1994:619–655.

17. Grayston JT. Infections caused by *Chlamydia pneumoniae* strain TWAR. Clin Infect Dis 1992; 15:757–761.

18. LaVerda D, Kalayoglu MV, Byrne GI. Chlamydial heat shock proteins and disease pathology: New paradigms for old problems? Infect Dis Obstet Gynecol 1999; 7:64–71.

19. Redecke V, Dalhoff K, Bohnet S, Braun J, Maass M. Interaction of *Chlamydia pneumoniae* and human alveolar macrophages: Infection and inflammatory response. Am J Respir Cell Mol Biol 1998; 19:721–727.

20. Gaydos CA, Roablin PM, Hammerschlag MR, et al. Diagnostic utility of PCR-enzyme immunoassay, culture and serology for detection of *Chlamydia pneumoniae* in symptomatic and asymptomatic patients. J Clin Microbiol 1994; 32:903–905.

21. Grayston JT, Campbell LA, Kuo CC, et al. A new respiratory tract pathogen: *Chlamydia pneumoniae*, strain TWAR. J Infect Dis 1990; 161:618–625.

22. Verkooyen RP, Willemse D, Hiep-van Casteren SC, et al. Evaluation of PCR, culture, and serology for diagnosis of Chlamydia pneumoniae respiratory infections. J Clin Microbiol 1998; 36:2301–2307.

23. Kern DG, Neill MA, Schachter J. A seroepidemiologic study of *Chlamydia pneumoniae* in Rhode Island: evidence of serologic cross-reactivity. Chest 1993; 104:208–213.

24. Routes JM, Nelson HS, Noda JA, Simon FT. Lack of correlation between *Chlamydia pneumoniae* antibody titers and adult onset asthma. J Allergy Clin Immunol 2000; 105:392.

25. Wright AL, Taussig LM, Ray CG, Harrison HR, Holberg CJ. The Tucson Children's Respiratory Study, II: Lower respiratory tract illnesses in the first year of life. Am J Epidemiol 1989; 129:1232–1246.

26. Castro-Rodriguez JA, Holberg CJ, Wright AL, et al. Association of radiologically ascertained pneumonia before age 3 yr with asthmalike symptoms and pulmonary function during childhood: a prospective study. Am J Respir Crit Care Med 1999; 159:1891–1897.

27. Shaheen SO, Aaby P, Hall AJ, et al. Measles and atopy in Guinea-Bissau. Lancet 1996; 347:1792–1796.

28. Holt PG. Environmental factors and primary T-cell sensitisation to inhalant allergens in infancy: reappraisal of the role of infections and air pollution. Pediatr Allergy Immunol 1995; 6:1–10.

29. Romagnani S. Human TH1 and TH2 subsets: regulation of differentiation and role in protection and immunopathology. Int Arch Allergy Immunol 1992; 98:279–285.

30. Martinez FD, Wright AL, Taussig LM, Holberg CJ, Halonen M, Morgan WJ. Asthma and wheezing in the first six years of life. The Group Health Medical Associates. N Engl J Med 1995; 332:133–138.

31. Ball TM, Castro-Rodriguez JA, Griffith KA, Holberg CJ, Martinez FD, Wright AL. Siblings, day-care attendance, and the risk of asthma and wheezing during childhood. N Engl J Med 2000; 343:538–543.

32. Hegele RG, Hayashi S, Hogg JC, Pare PD. Mechanisms of airway narrowing and hyper-responsiveness in viral respiratory tract infections. Am J Respir Crit Care Med 1995; 151:1659–1664.

33. Arnold R, Werchau H, Koenig W. Expression of adhesion molecules (ICAM-1, LFA-3) on human epithelial cells (A549) after respiratory syncytial virus infection. Int Arch Allergy Immunol 1995; 107:392–393.

34. Noah TL, Becker S. Respiratory syncytial virus-induced cytokine production by a human bronchial epithelial cell line. Am J Physiol 1993; 265:L472–L478.

35. Sakamoto M, Ida S, Takishima T. Effect of influenza virus infection on allergic sensitization to aerosolized infection in mice. J Immunol 1984; 132:2614–2617.

36. Schwarze J, Hamelmann E, Bradley KL, Takeda K, Gelfand EW. Respiratory syncytial virus infection results in airway hyperresponsiveness and enhanced airway sensitization to allergen. J Clin Invest 1997; 100:226–233.

37. Suzuki S, Suzuki Y, Yamamoto N, Matsumoto Y, Shirai A, Okubo T. Influenza A virus infection increases IgE production and airway responsiveness in aerosolized antigen-exposed mice. J Allergy Clin Immunol 1998; 102:732–740.

38. Bowden JJ, Schoeb TR, Lindsey JR, McDonald DM. Dexamethasone and oxytetracycline reverse the potentiation of neurogenic inflammation in airways of rats with *Mycoplasma pulmonis* infection. Am J Respir Crit Care Med 1994; 150:1391–1401.

39. Martin RJ, Chu HW, Honour JM, Harbeck RJ. Airway inflammation and bronchial hyperresponsiveness following *Mycoplasma pneumoniae* infection in a murine model. Am J Respir Crit Care Med 2000; 161:A606.

40. Söderberg M, Hellstrom S, Lundgren R, Bergh A. Bronchial epithelium in humans recently recovering from respiratory infections caused by influenza or mycoplasma. Eur Respir J 1990; 3:1023–1028.

41. Martin RJ, Kraft M, Chu HW, Berns EA, Cassell GH. A link between chronic asthma and chronic infection. J Allergy Clin Immunol 2001; 107:595–601.

42. Empey DW, Laitinen LA, Jacobs L, Gold WM, Nadel JA. Mechanisms of bronchial hyperreactivity in normal subjects after upper respiratory tract infection. Am Rev Respir Dis 1976; 113:131–139.

43. Nicholson KG, Kent J, Ireland DC. Respiratory viruses and exacerbations of asthma in adults. Br Med J 1993; 307:982–986.

44. Rossi OV, Kinnula VL, Tuokko H, Huhti E. Respiratory viral and mycoplasma infections in patients hospitalized for acute asthma. Monaldi Arch Chest Dis 1994; 49:107–111.

45. Pullan CR, Hey EN. Wheezing, asthma, and pulmonary dysfunction 10 years after infection with respiratory syncytial virus in infancy. Br Med J 1982; 284:1665–1669.

46. Sigurs N, Bjarnason R, Sigurbergsson F, Kjellman B, Bjorksten B. Asthma and immunoglobulin E antibodies after respiratory syncytial virus bronchiolitis: a prospective cohort study with matched controls. Pediatrics 1995; 95:500–505.

47. Andersen P. Pathogenesis of lower respiratory tract infections due to chlamydia, mycoplasma, legionella and viruses. Thorax 1998; 53:302–307.

48. Berkovich S, Millian SJ, Snyder RD. The association of viral and mycoplasma infections with recurrence of wheezing in the asthmatic child. Ann Allergy 1970; 28:43–49.

49. Wenner H. The etiology of respiratory illnesses occurring in infancy and childhood. Pediatrics 1963; 31:4.

50. Sabato AR, Martin AJ, Marmion BP, Kok TW, Cooper DM. *Mycoplasma pneumoniae*: acute illness, antibiotics, and subsequent pulmonary function. Arch Dis Child 1984; 59: 1034–1037.

51. Cassell GH. Infectious causes of chronic inflammatory diseases and cancer. Emerg Infect Dis 1998; 4:475–487.

52. Mok JY, Waugh PR, Simpson H. *Mycoplasma pneumonia* infection. A follow-up study of 50 children with respiratory illness. Arch Dis Child 1979; 54:506–511.

53. Yano T, Ichikawa Y, Komatu S, Arai S, Oizumi K. Association of *Mycoplasma pneumoniae* antigen with initial onset of bronchial asthma. Am J Respir Crit Care Med 1994; 149:1348-1353.

54. Tipirneni P, Moore BS, Hyde JS, Schauf V. IgE antibodies to *Mycoplasma pneumoniae* in asthma and other atopic diseases. Ann Allergy 1980; 45:1–7.

55. Gil JC, Cedillo RL, Mayagoitia BG, Paz MD. Isolation of *Mycoplasma pneumoniae* from asthmatic patients. Ann Allergy 1993; 70:23–25.

56. Grayston JT, Kuo CC, Wang SP, Altman J. A new *Chlamydia psittaci* strain, TWAR, isolated in acute respiratory tract infections. N Engl J Med 1986; 315:161–168.

57. Allegra L, Blasi F, Centanni S, et al. Acute exacerbations of asthma in adults: role of *Chlamydia pneumoniae* infection. Eur Respir J 1994; 7:2165–2168.

58. Hahn DL, Dodge RW, Golubjatnikov R. Association of *Chlamydia pneumoniae* (strain TWAR) infection with wheezing, asthmatic bronchitis, and adult-onset asthma. JAMA 1991; 266:225–230.

59. Hahn DL, McDonald R. Can acute *Chlamydia pneumoniae* respiratory tract infection initiate chronic asthma? Ann Allergy Asthma Immunol 1998; 81:339–344.

60. Langmack EL, Kraft M, Gaydos CA, Martin RJ. Significance of PCR positivity for *Chlamydia pneumoniae* in the lower airways of stable asthmatics. Am J Respir Crit Care Med 2000; 161:A898.

61. von Mutius E, Illi S, Hirsch T, Leupold W, Weiland SK. Frequency of infections and risk of asthma, atopy, and airway hyperresponsiveness in children. Eur Resp J 1999; 14:4–11.

62. Sutherland ER, Brandorff JM, Cassell GH, Weiss ST, Martin RJ. Asthma prevalence following atypical bacterial versus viral pneumonia of childhood. American Thoracic Society International Conference. San Francisco, California, 2001.

63. Wubbel L, Jafri HS, Olsen K, et al. *Mycoplasma pneumoniae* pneumonia in a mouse model. J Infect Dis 1998; 178:1526–1529.

64. Pietsch K, Ehlers S, Jacobs E. Cytokine gene expression in the lungs of BALB/c mice during primary and secondary intranasal infection with *Mycoplasma pneumoniae*. Microbiology 1994; 140:2043–2048.

65. Kuo CC, Jackson LA, Campbell LA, Grayston JT. *Chlamydia pneumoniae* (TWAR). Clin Microbiol Rev 1995; 8:451–461.

66. Kishimoto T. Studies on *Chlamydia pneumoniae*, strain TWAR, infection. I. Experimental infection of *C. pneumoniae* in mice and serum antibodies against TWAR by MFA. Kansenshogaku Zasshi 1990; 64:124–131.

67. Kaukoranta-Tolvanen SE, Laurila AL, Saikku P, Leinonen M, Laitinen K. Experimental *Chlamydia pneumoniae* infection in mice: effect of reinfection and passive immunization. Microb Pathog 1995; 18:279–288.

68. Malinverni R, Kuo CC, Campbell LA, Grayston JT. Reactivation of *Chlamydia pneumoniae* lung infection in mice by cortisone. J Infect Dis 1995; 172:593–594.

69. Hardy RD, Jafril H, Wordemann M, et al. *Mycoplasma pneumoniae*: chronic infection in the mouse pneumonia model. 39th ICAAC, American Society of Microbiology. San Francisco, California, 1999.

70. Lipworth BJ. Treatment of acute asthma. Lancet 1997; 350:18–23.

71. Guidelines for the diagnosis and management of asthma. National Heart, Lung and Blood Institute, 1997.

72. Berman SZ, Mathison DA, Stevenson DD, Tan EM, Vaughan JH. Transtracheal aspiration studies in asthmatic patients in relapse with "infective" asthma and in subjects without respiratory disease. J Allergy Clin Immunol 1975; 56:206–214.

73. Graham VAL, Knowles GK, Milton AF, Davies RJ. Routine antibiotics in hospital management of acute asthma. Lancet 1982; 1:418–420.

74. Kraft M, Hamid Q, Cassell GH, et al. Mycoplasma and chlamydia cause increased airway inflammation that is responsive to clarithromycin. Am J Respir Crit Care Med 1999; 159:A516.

26

Chlamydia/Mycoplasma
Do They Cause New-Onset Asthma in Adults?

DAVID L. HAHN

University of Wisconsin Medical School
Madison, Wisconsin, U.S.A.

I. Introduction

The origins of adult-onset asthma are obscure. Five to six decades ago, some clinicians believed that asthma was primarily related to infection and that allergy, while important, played a secondary role (1,2). A decade ago, expert opinion held that asthma was a noninfectious allergic disease whose root cause was inflammation (3). Since then a growing body of evidence, reviewed in this book, has emerged to suggest again a significant role for viral and atypical infections in the pathogenesis of asthma.

Regarding the atypical organism *Chlamydia pneumoniae* (*Cpn*), Chapter 23 reviews the evidence that acute *Cpn* infection is associated with asthma exacerbations and Chapter 24 presents evidence relevant to a potential role for chronic *Cpn* infection as an asthma promoter. The focus of this chapter is on a third question about atypical infections and asthma: can these infections cause (initiate) new-onset asthma in adulthood?

II. Definitions of New-Onset Asthma

What is meant by new-onset asthma in adults? In the context of infection as a possible cause for asthma, it must be stated at the outset that many are exposed (infected) but only some get asthma. This is particularly germane for *Cpn*, to which the majority of people worldwide are exposed one or more times during life (4). Thus, host reponse must be assumed to play a major role in this complex multifactorial syndrome. In defining new-onset asthma, therefore, pre-existing characteristics such as asymptomatic bronchial hyperreactivity, atopy, or other covariates may be contributing factors but are insufficient to define new-onset asthma. A reasonable working definition of new-onset asthma ideally includes the history of a first attack of characteristic symptoms (e.g., wheeze, shortness of breath, chest tightness, or cough) accompanied by objective evidence of reversible airway obstruction either spontaneously or after treatment. A weakness of this definition in the clinical setting is the retrospective nature of the history, with the possibility of unremembered or unrecognized previous symptomatic episodes. This weakness also applies to any prospective epidemiological study that does not begin at birth. This limitation notwithstanding, careful history-taking from reliable informants reporting new-onset asthma can produce consistent correlations with microbiological findings (5).

For purposes of this discussion, it is worthwhile to differentiate between new-onset asthma in adulthood (adult-onset asthma; AOA) and childhood-onset asthma that persists into adulthood (COA). AOA and COA have characteristically distinct clinical and epidemiological features, although there appear to be major overlaps between these syndromes for asthma appearing during the middle years (roughly ages 20–40). Compared to COA, AOA is associated with fewer markers of atopy (6), more likely to affect women (7), more clinically severe (8,9), less likely to remit (10,11), and associated with more fixed obstruction (12–14). It is unclear, however, whether COA and AOA are different diseases with different underlying causes or different clinical presentations of the same underlying cause. Nor do we know what factors determine whether a child with asthma will go into remission, reactivate asthma later, or persist with symptoms into adulthood.

AOA is a clinical entity that, unlike classic COA, does not fit cleanly into the rubric of asthma as a noninfectious atopic disease. From the perspective of the primary care clinician, patients with AOA often deny previous respiratory problems, do not have a history of clinical allergy, and are skin test negative. Furthermore, patients developing AOA often recall that their asthma symptoms started after an acute respiratory illness such as acute bronchitis, pneumonia, or an influenza-like illness (15). This description applies most clearly to AOA beginning after age 40. Clinical observations (16,17) and prospective epidemiological studies (18-20) also support an association between bronchitis/pneumonia and subsequent adult asthma. While these observations have often been interpreted to suggest that the preceding illnesses were actually misdiagnosed asthma symptoms or merely viral exacerbations of previously unrecognized asthma, a third possibility is that acute infectious illnesses might actually play a role in asthma initiation. Of additional interest are the facts that epidemiological associations of respiratory illness and subsequent asthma also pertain to children (21) and adolescents (22) and that the association of atopy with asthma in both children and adults is not as great as previously believed (23).

III. Illness Burden Due to Various Forms of Asthma

The economic burden (direct and indirect costs) of asthma illness in adults is equivalent to the economic burden in children (24,25). What proportion of the economic burden of adult asthma is borne by those with AOA, compared to those with COA persisting into adulthood, is an open question. In adults with active asthma, AOA may account for a greater proportion of active disease than COA (26). It is likely that the morbidity and economic burden due to AOA are disproportionately greater than that of persistent COA since, as mentioned earlier, AOA tends to be more severe and more associated with fixed obstruction (i.e., chronic obstructive pulmonary disease; COPD), the consequences of which (disability and premature death) have not been accounted for in current economic analyses of asthma (24,25,27). An example of the long-term consequences of severe AOA is given in the following clinical case report.

IV. Asthma or COPD?

A. Asthma

On July 15, 1981, a previously healthy 55-year-old nonsmoking man was seen for complaints of nasal congestion, sore throat, and cough lasting 2 weeks. He was diagnosed with acute bronchitis and treated with antihistamines, decongestants, and a 1-week course of erythromycin. Respiratory symptoms improved temporarily and then relapsed to include wheezing, shortness of breath, and nocturnal awakening with respiratory trouble. On September 21 his pulmonary function was normal (forced expiratory volume in 1 s [FEV_1] 87% predicted) with no significant bronchodilator response. On October 19 he presented with a severe exacerbation of asthma symptoms and had decreased pulmonary function (FEV_1 25%) that responded to a burst of oral prednisone (postprednisone FEV_1 119% predicted). He later continued to experience severe exacerbations of asthma requiring steroid pulses and was hospitalized in late 1981. This description of a patient I encountered is characteristic of the so-called infectious asthma syndrome (15) and also typifies the often rapid deterioration in lung function noted in AOA in older adults (28).

B. COPD

On December 18, 1997, I again encountered this patient, now 71 and retired. He was being treated with theophylline 300 mg three times daily, inhaled albuterol 2 puffs four times daily, terbutaline sulfate 5 mg orally three times daily, and prednisone 10 mg alternating with 5 mg orally each day. His FEV_1 while taking steroids was 50% predicted and his FEV_1/forced vital capacity (FVC) ratio was 48%. His medications controlled, but did not eliminate, persistent cough, wheezing, shortness of breath, and chronic sputum production. He appeared emaciated, older than his stated age, and was unable to engage in vigorous physical activity. He suffered from multiple lumbar compression fractures due to osteoporosis. He met diagnostic criteria for chronic bronchitis. His *Chlamydia pneumoniae* IgG titer was 1:64, without an IgM response. On May 24 1998, he died unexpectedly in cardiac arrest with documented ventricular fibrillation, presumably from an acute myocardial infarction. Postmortem examination was not performed.

This case illustrates the shortcomings of cross-sectional diagnostic thinking that does not acknowledge the natural history of disease. Morbidity attributable to AOA should include long-term complications including loss of lung function, decreased quality of life, complications of anti-inflammatory therapy, and decreased life expectancy. This patient's story also highlights known epidemiological associations among asthma, chronic bronchitis, and heart disease (29-32) that remain unexplained.

V. Asthma Temporal Trends

A key factor motivating publication of this book is the observed increase in asthma in westernized countries. Indeed, a consensus has emerged that asthma prevalence in both children and adults has increased worldwide in recent decades (33). This increase cannot be satisfactorily explained by changes in traditional asthma risk factors (34). Since one purpose of this book is to stimulate research into interactions between infectious agents and increasing asthma, it is worthwhile noting an association between the increasing population burden of *Cpn* infection and increases in asthma, in both adults and children of both genders (Fig. 1). While these ecological data (from different study groups in the same place and times) cannot prove causality, the data presented in Figure 1 do support the suggestion that research into the current asthma epidemic should include a search for infectious agents as a cause.

Figure 1 Temporal trends in *Chlamydia* antibodies and asthma in Finland over two decades. (A) *Chlamydia* complement fixation titers in sera sent for virus serological screening 1971–1987 (5000–14,000 patients annually, total number of sera studied: 162,401). These data almost certainly represent *Cpn* infection, as *Chlamydia trachomatis* and *C. psittaci* infections are rare in Finland and another epidemic of CF titer in Denmark was *Cpn*. [Mordhorst CH, Wang SP, Grayston JT. Epidemic "ornithosis" and TWAR infection, Denmark, 1976-85. In Oriel D and Ridgeway G (eds). Chlamydial Infections: Proceedings of the Sixth International Symposium on Human Chlamydial Infections. Cambridge, Cambridge University Press, 1986, pp 325-328]. (From Puolakkainen M, Ukkonen P, Saikku P. The seroepidemiology of Chlamydiae in Finland over the period 1971 to 1987. Epidemiol Infect 1989; 102: 287–295.) (B) The self-reported prevalence of chronic asthma in the Finnish population, by age and gender, in 1976 and 1987. The samples were representative of the Finnish noninstitutionalized population and the number of interviewed adults was 16,413 in 1976 and 13,138 in 1987. (Adapted from Klaukka T, Peura S, Martikainen J. Why has the utilization of anti-asthmatics increased in Finland? J Clin Epidemiol 1991; 44:859-863.)

(A) CHLAMYDIA COMPLEMENT FIXATION TITERS (%)

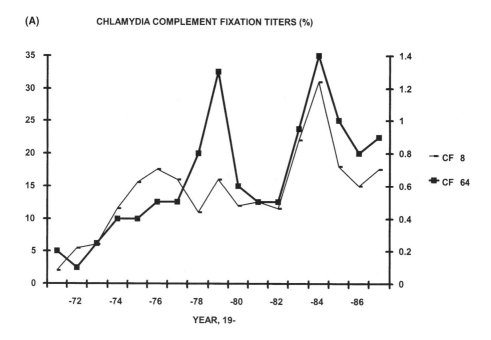

(B) CHRONIC ASTHMA (%)

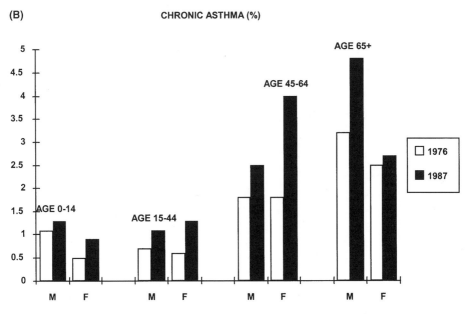

VI. *Chlamydia/Mycoplasma* and Asthma Initiation in Adults

The amount of available information on whether *Cpn/Mpn* can intiate asthma is much smaller than the body of evidence for chronic atypical infection in asthma (35). Factors contributing to the paucity of available data include the facts that initial episodes are relatively rare compared to prevalent disease episodes, patients do not always seek medical attention for them, and if an initial encounter does occur, it is usually in a primary care setting where research does not often occur. Initiating events may be obscured or undetectable years later when chronic asthma presents to academic medical centers, where most asthma research is currently performed. Thus, current published evidence for an infectious initiation for AOA is limited to case reports and case series from primary care settings (Table 1).

Table 1 Evidence That *Chlamydia/Mycoplasma* Can Cause New-Onset Asthma in Adults

Reference	Type of study	Findings
Mpn		
(36)	Case series	*Mpn* infection in eight adults admitted with wheezing, four had no prior hx of asthma. No long-term follow-up.
(37)	Case report	Association of *Mpn* antigen with initial onset of bronchial asthma and with *Mpn*-specific IgE antibodies
Mpn/Cpn		
(38)	Case report	A case having initial onset of bronchial asthma, probably induced by prolonged *Mpn* infection, accompanied by concurrent highly suspicious chlamydial infection (in Japanese)
Cpn		
(39)	Case report	Serological proven acute *Cpn* infection initiated severe chronic asthmatic bronchitis in an adult
(40)	Case series	Nine patients wheezed during serologically acute *Cpn* infection: of these, four had newly diagnosed asthma after illness
(41)	Case report	38-year old previously nonasthmatic physician developed prolonged asthmatic bronchitis following culture and serologically proven acute primary *Cpn* infection; positive culture persisted despite prolonged doxycycline treatment
(42)	Case report	An adult with persistent symptoms of new-onset reactive airways disease following a culture and serologically proven acute primary *Cpn* infection
(5)	Case series	10 adults with new-onset wheezing had serological proven acute primary (8) or secondary (2) infection: of these, 5 developed chronic asthma and 1 chronic bronchitis along with serological profiles compatible with chronic infection.

A. Case Reports and Case Series

Mycoplasma pneumoniae

While ample evidence exists for acute *Mpn* infection exacerbating established asthma (43,44) only a few reports suggest that *Mpn* can initiate asthma in adults (36-38). Buckmaster et al. (36), described eight adults with wheezing and *Mpn* infection, four of whom had no prior history of asthma, but no long-term follow-up was available. Yano et al. 1994 (37) presented a meticulously detailed case report of a previously nonasthmatic 37-year-old man with community-acquired pneumonia and hemolytic anemia who had serologically diagnosed acute *Mpn* infection. One month after macrolide treatment and resolution of pneumonia, the patient developed asthma symptoms and reversible airways obstruction. Two months later, and then again 1 year after initial onset of asthma, bronchial hyperresponsiveness to methacholine was demonstrated. IgE antibody against *Mpn* was detected 1 and 7 months after illness onset and a skin prick test to *Mpn* was positive 2 years after onset. Further evidence for direct involvement of *Mpn* in the patient's asthma symptoms was demonstration of bronchial hyperreactivity to inhaled *Mpn* antigen but lack of response to inhaled *Mycoplasma salivarium* antigen. Lastly, IgE antibodies to *Mpn* were demonstrated in an additional 7 of 13 patients with pneumonia (not asthma) compared to none of 10 controls, suggesting that IgE antibody can be generated also in *Mpn*-infected nonasthmatic patients. The authors also made the interesting observation that, in total, six of the eight patients with detectable *Mpn*-specific IgE had persistent cough lasting 3 months, although only the one case patient had symptoms or signs of asthma. This case report could not answer the question of whether the case patient's atopic state (ability to produce IgE) preceded or followed the acute *Mpn* infection. This report also suggests that prescence of *Mpn*-specific IgE was not always sufficient to cause asthma, since other infected patients with *Mpn*-specific IgE did not develop asthma after pneumonia.

In another report, the same authors (38) described a case of new-onset asthma that appeared to be associated with *Mpn* and chlamydial coinfection. This observation has potential significance since coinfections with *Cpn* and other respiratory pathogens are common (45) and it has been speculated that *Cpn* may serve as a cofactor to enhance pathogenicity of these other agents (46).

Chlamydia pneumoniae

Evidence that *Cpn* can intiate asthma is more common than for *Mpn* but it is unclear whether this is due to a true difference in incidence or to the fact that *Cpn* has been more often studied. Several case reports (39,41,42) have documented new-onset reactive airways disease, sometimes called asthmatic bronchitis, in patients with serological, culture, and/or polymerase chain reaction (PCR) test-proven acute infection. As part of a prospective study into the role of *Cpn* and *Mpn* in community-acquired respiratory illnesses (bronchitis and pneumonia), Hahn et al. (40) described nine patients with serologically proven acute *Cpn* infection who wheezed: four of these patients were newly diagnosed with chronic asthma after the reported infection episode. No comparable associations were found for acute *Mpn* infection, however. The diagnostic accuracy of these findings was obscured, however, by the fact that pulmonary function testing was not routinely performed as part of the study. Furthermore, serological criteria for acute infection used in the study included both a fourfold titer rise (universally accepted as valid) and a single high titer of 1:512 or greater (not universally accepted as valid, since it might indicate previous exposure or ongoing chronic infection). In a follow-up analysis of the significance of the two different titer categories in asthma, Hahn et al. (5) reported that incident wheezing and prevalent asthma, confirmed by pulmonary function testing, demonstrated different serological patterns of so-called acute *Cpn* antibodies in adults. Of 20 adults meeting serological criteria for acute infection (both titer categories) 10 adults had a first ever (incident) wheezing episode and 10 others had chronic (prevalent) asthma. Notable was that none of the chronic asthmatics had evidence of a fourfold titer rise whereas all 10 of the first ever wheezers had a fourfold rise in titer, of whom 8 also had detectable IgM antibody indicating an acute primary infection. The other two had no detectable IgM, indicating an acute secondary (re)infection. Another significant finding was the prospective observation that 6 of these 10 patients with incident wheezing subsequently developed chronic asthma (n = 5) or chronic bronchitis (n = 1) along with a serological profile that resembled that of the 10 patients who already had chronic asthma. This report provides the strongest available evidence that acute *Cpn* infection can lead to new-onset chronic asthma in adults. The likelihood of a causal association between the acute infection and development of chronic asthma is further strengthened by the additional observation that prolonged courses of antichlamydial antibiotics administered to those who developed new-onset asthma resulted in disappearance of asthma symptoms and return of normal pulmonary function (47).

B. Epidemiological Data

The available epidemiological evidence suggests that the population-based proportion of asthma cases attributable to atopy is usually less than 50% (23). The (more limited) seroepidemiological data for *Cpn* in asthma suggest that half of adult asthma cases could be attributable to this infection (48).

What proportion of AOA is attributable to *Cpn* or *Mpn* infection is unknown and can only be answered conclusively by large prospective studies. In the absence of such studies it is worthwhile examining some indirect evidence. Melbye et al. (49) performed a prospective microbiological and clinical study in over 500 adult general practice patients without known asthma or COPD to determine the occurrence of airflow limitation and the frequency of significant reversibility during acute upper and lower respiratory illnesses. They measured spirometry (before and after bronchodilator) during illness and at follow-up after the acute phase (4–5 weeks later). They compared results of pulmonary function testing with microbiological testing for five respiratory viruses (influenza A and B, RSV, parainfluenza 3, and adenovirus), *Mpn*, and *Cpn*. Patient Groups with detectable viral or *Mpn* infections showed improvement in pulmonary function at follow-up. Only patients with evidence for *Cpn* infection had worse pulmonary function at follow-up than during acute illness, suggesting a unique ability for *Cpn* to produce long-lasting obstruction after acute infection. Furthermore, *Cpn*-infected patients had the lowest rate of clinical recovery at follow-up (71% for *Cpn,* 84% for viral infection, and 92% for *Mpn*).

Additional unpublished epidemiological evidence relating to the topic of this chapter is presented here for the first time. In a retrospective study, I have investigated relationships between asthma duration and the quantities of IgG and IgA antibodies against *Cpn* in seroreactive adults with asthma to determine any associations that might support or reject the hypothesis that asthma began after acute *Cpn* infection that had occurred sometime in the past.

Methods

Adult outpatients (104) (mean age 42 years) with acute asthmatic bronchitis (AAB, 24 patients) or chronic asthma (CA, 80 patients) were selected from a community-based primary care clinic. AAB was defined as acute bronchitis with wheezing in a patient without a previous diagnosis of asthma. CA was diagnosed based on persistent asthma symptoms and results of pulmonary function testing. The date of first reported wheezing symptoms was used to calculate asthma duration. *Cpn*-specific IgG and IgA antibodies were measured using the microimmunofluorescence (MIF) test (50). IgG was adsorbed prior to IgA testing (51).

Patients who were seroreactive against *Cpn*-specific IgA (titer of 1:16 or greater in the MIF test) were categorized by asthma duration (<1 year, 1 to <3 years, 3 to <10 years, and 10+ years). Geometric mean antibody titers (GMT) were calculated separately for these patient groups. The correlation between asthma duration and antibody titer level (after ordinal transformation) was calculated, and analysis of covariance (ANOCOVA) was used to control for potential confounders such as age of asthma onset and smoking. P values less than 0.05 are reported as significant.

Results

Fifty-five patients (53%) with reactive airways disease were IgA seropositive. All 55 patients who were IgA seropositive were also IgG seropositive (1:16 or greater). There was no significant correlation between asthma duration and IgA titer levels. However, these was a significant inverse correlation of asthma duration and IgG titer levels ($r = -0.34$, $p < 0.001$) that persisted after controlling for IgA titer magnitude, age of asthma onset, and smoking by ANOCOVA. The relationship between asthma duration and IgG titer was not strictly linear, however (see Fig. 2). Patients with asthma duration between 1 and 3 years had the highest IgG GMT titer level, and patients with asthma more than 10 years had the lowest titers. As previously noted, IgA titer levels were similar for all categories of asthma duration, even for patients with asthma for more than 10 years. These data suggest that asthma duration is, along with age, gender, and smoking, an additional confounder of the association between *Cpn* IgG antibodies and asthma. This confounding is a possible

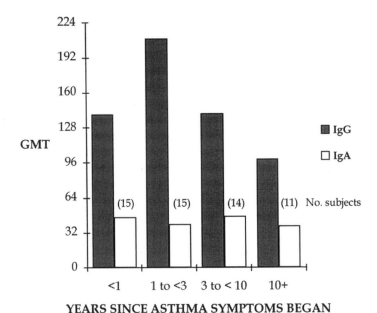

Figure 2 *Chlamydia pneumoniae* antibodies (GMT, y axis) and asthma duration (x axis) in 55 adult patients with asthma encountered in a family practice outpatient setting. All subjects were IgG and IgA seroreactive (titers ≥ 1:16) against *Cpn*. Figures in parentheses are the number of asthma patients in each group.

explanation for the observation that when both IgA and IgG antibodies against Cpn are measured in case–control studies of asthma, significant associations are more often reported for IgA than for IgG (35,52).

Had these data been obtained prospectively on the same cohort over time, it would be proper to conclude that IgG titers initially increased over the first to third year after symptom onset, then declined significantly over the remainder of the 10 year period, whereas IgA titers remained constant. Since IgA titers have a relatively short half-life (7 days) and reflect mucosal antigen stimulation, it would also have been reasonable to conclude that persistent detection of Cpn-specific IgA was evidence for persistent infection. It would also be reasonable to suggest that the initial rise and subsequent fall in IgG titer provided evidence that acute infection might have occurred around the time that asthma symptoms first began. These interpretations cannot be made, however, since the data were actually collected retrospectively on different patient groups. The data are, however, suggestive and illustrate the importance of performing prospective microbiological and clinical studies.

A recent prospective study (the Caerphilly Prospective Heart Disease Study) followed a cohort of 2512 middle-aged Welshmen for almost 14 years, but did not collect information on chronic respiratory symptoms or diagnoses (53). Nevertheless, *Cpn* IgG and IgA antibodies were measured on stored sera obtained at entry from a subgroup of subjects, and titers were analyzed in relation to self-reported use of a broad range of medications that might have been prescribed for respiratory symptoms (beta-adrenergic or antimuscarinic bronchodilators, theophyllines, inhaled steroids, cromoglycate, or oxygen). Death certificate information on deaths from respiratory illnesses and lung function decline between entry and the 5 year visit (no further lung function testing was available) were also analyzed. Positive quantitative associations were found between *Cpn*-specific IgA titer magnitude and medication use at baseline ("prevalent") and new medication use during follow-up ("incident") but neither trend attained statistical significance. Using IgA seronegative (<1:8) patients as the reference group, the odds ratio (95% confidence interval) associating IgA titers ≥ 1:16 with "incident" cases was 1.7 (0.83–3.48). No comparable trends were noted for IgG antibodies nor were any antibody associations found for respiratory deaths or lung function decline. Given the nonspecific nature of medication use as a proxy for asthma or COPD, the short (5 year) interval over which lung function decline was measured and the small number of respiratory deaths, these results are hard to interpret. They do not conclusively exclude a role for *Cpn* infection as a cause for "incident" respiratory disease in adults, and they do illustrate the need for further prospective studies.

VII. Future Prospects

A. Prospective Studies

Two types of prospective studies could help to answer the question of whether *Cpn/ Mpn* can cause new-onset asthma in adults. The first type of study is the classic population-based prospective study, resembling the Tucson Epidemiologic Study that has provided insight into the natural history (28,54) and immunopathology (6) of asthma. A prospective study should include (in addition to detailed clinical information, pulmonary function testing, and measures of atopy) microbiological testing for *Cpn* and *Mpn* including serial serology and PCR on respiratory secretions and on peripheral blood mononuclear cells (PBMCs) (55). Since the incidence of AOA is about 1:1000 per year (56), this study will need to follow 10,000 adults over a decade to accrue approximately 100 cases of new-onset adult asthma. This study would therefore be expensive.

An alternative strategy that might yield comparable information at a reduced cost would be to enroll-high risk patients via a large geographically dispersed practice-based research network (PBRN). This strategy might decrease the required sample size and, possibly, the follow-up interval needed to accrue 100 new cases of AOA. Although PBRN populations are not random samples of the general population, the study sample can nevertheless be representative of a random sample of the adult primary care population, as long as the sample is large (57,58). Since AOA often begins after an acute respiratory illness that persists (15), it is reasonable to suggest that one recruitment strategy would be to enroll as high risk those patients encountered with acute bronchitis or pneumonia who deny a prior history of asthma symptoms. The risk of being diagnosed with asthma within 3–4 years after acute bronchitis was 3.7% per year in a primary care study (16) and 4–6% in a prospective cohort study (20). Risk of asthma diagnosed after pneumonia, at least in children and teenagers, may be even greater (59). An advantage of this strategy is the ability to study relationships between these acute lower respiratory tract illnesses and other chronic sequelae such as chronic bronchitis and chronic sinusitis. A disadvantage is the possibility that clinical interventions might confound the results. This problem can also occur in classic epidemiological studies that, unlike PBRN studies, do not have comparable access to treatment details.

This type of PBRN study might not have been feasible (at least in North America) one or two decades ago. Currently, however, a growing number of North American PBRNs have a track record of performing quality research on a variety of primary care topics, including asthma (60). European centers have a successful track record of collaboration between general practitioners and specialists in the study of respiratory illnesses (61) and asthma (62). Prospective studies on infectious causes for asthma in adults would be an ideal framework for international collaboration between PBRNs.

Previously published prospective epidemiological studies that have investigated a role for *Cpn* in asthma onset or in airflow limitation have been limited by lack of any clinical respiratory diagnoses (53) or by dependence on a history of a physician diagnosis of asthma without any supporting pulmonary function evidence (63). A properly conducted PBRN study can include detailed clinical information (16,40) along with objective evidence for reversible airway obstructions (5,17,49,64,65) to support a diagnosis of asthma, thus increasing both internal and external validity.

B. Animal Studies

Another approach to the question of whether *Cpn* infection initiates asthma is to explore the effects of *Cpn* infection in existing animal models of asthma. This approach requires choosing an animal model in which both asthma and infection can be established. For example, Hsiue et al. (66) recently isolated *Cpn* from lung homogenate and from alveolar macrophages obtained by bronchoalveolar lavage after intranasal inoculation of *Cpn* in guinea pigs. Further studies of infection and bronchial hyperresponsiveness are planned. Mouse and rabbit models have been commonly used to study *Cpn* lung infection (67,68). Animal models for asthma are also available. To my knowledge, however, there are as yet no published studies on the effects of *Cpn* acute primary, secondary, or chronic infections on bronchial hyperreactivity or airway obstruction in animal models.

VIII. In Vitro and In Vivo Observations Relating to Pathogenesis

A growing body of in vitro experimental evidence demonstrates that *Cpn* infection of relevant human cell lines is capable of inducing inflammatory mediators that are

Table 2 *Chlamydia pneumoniae*: Potential Mechanisms in Asthma Pathogenesis

Observations(s)	Potential role in asthma
Cpn induces pulmonary epithelial ciliary stasis (69)	Mucociliary clearance is impaired in adult asthma (70)
Cpn-specific IgE antibodies are associated with culture-positive childhood asthma (71)	IgE incites acute bronchospasm and may lead to chronic inflammation
Cpn-specific IgE antibody is associated with adult-onset asthma (65)	IgE, but not skin test positivity, is associated with adult-onset asthma: the "missing antigen"? (6)
Cpn infects human monocytes and induces TNFa, IL1-b and IL-6 in vitro (72)	Pulmonary inflammation is the hallmark of asthma
Cpn infects human alveolar macrophages in vivo and in vitro and induces reactive oxygen species, TNF α, IL-1β, and IL-8 in vitro (73)	Inflammation and free radical production; upregulation of IgE reponses by dysregulation of alveolar macrophage function? (74)
Cpn infects human smooth muscle cells in vivo (75)	Demonstrated in vascular smooth muscle; effect on bronchial smooth muscle hyperreactivity?
Cpn infects human bronchial smooth muscle cells in vitro, to produce IL-6 and basic fibroblast growth factor (76)	Inflammation and airway remodeling
Cpn heat shock protein 60 (hsp60) antibodies are associated with adult asthma (65,77,78)	Chlamydial hsp60 has been implicated in other chronic inflammatory chlamydial diseases (pelvic inflammatory disease, tubal infertility, trachoma)
Cpn contains a chlamydial lipopolysaccharide (LPS) related to gram negative endotoxin	Bacterial LPS augments IgE response to allergen in an animal model (79) and induces bronchial hyperresponsiveness in humans correlated with release of IL-6 and IL-8 from alveolar macrophages and monocytes in vitro (80)

thought to play a key role in asthma pathogenesis (Table 2). Less is known about the ability of *Mpn* in this regard, but the lack of evidence is related more to the difficulty in studying this slow growing organism than to an established body of negative evidence. Regarding asthma initiation specifically, several mechanisms could be important. As well as generating an inflammatory response, acute *Cpn* infection can damage bronchial epithelium and impair mucociliary clearance by producing ciliary stasis (69). It has been hypothesized that bronchial epithelial disruption could produce hyperreactivity and enhance penetration of allergens after viral infection (81), a hypothesis that applies also to acute atypical infections. As described elsewhere in this book, a growing body of evidence suggests significant interactions between viral infections and the atopic immune response (82). Preliminary studies suggest that a similar interaction may be operative for *Cpn* lung infection (65,71,79). Of potential importance are observations that *Cpn* infection of human bronchial smooth muscle cells can induce basic fibroblast growth factor (76) and that heat shock protein 60 is associated with asthma (65,77,78). Both observations may be relevant to production of airway remodeling and accelerated decline of lung function in asthma. Thus, current in vitro evidence is consistent with a role for *Cpn* not only in asthma initiation but also over the long course.

IX. Conclusions

Prospective clinical observations drawn mainly from primary care settings show that acute *Cpn* (and to a lesser extent *Mpn*) infections are associated with de novo wheezing that, in some patients, becomes persistent and leads to a diagnosis of asthma with all the typical clinical and spirometric characteristics to support that diagnosis. Of considerable additional interest are a limited number of examples of induction of complete remissions (at least for a year or two) in some of these patients following prolonged courses of antibiotics with activity against atypical infections. Some of these reports have even documented microbial eradication associated with asthma remission. Thus, the available evidence strongly supports a role for acute atypical infections in asthma initiation, at least in a small subset of patients, and this possibility is supported by a limited number of in vitro pathogenesis studies, outlined above.

A role for initiation cannot be considered proven, however, because none of the clinical observations summarized above can rule out the possibility of low-grade so-called asymptomatic asthma that was exacerbated but not initiated by atypical infection. Thus, long-term prospective studies of nonasthmatic subjects are necessary to determine the quantitative role of *Cpn/Mpn* infection as a cause of new-onset asthma in adults.

References

1. Bivings L. Asthmatic bronchitis following chronic upper respiratory infection. JAMA 1940; 115:1434–1436.
2. Chobot R, Uvitsky IH, Dundy H. The relationship of the etiologic factors in asthma in infants and children. J Allergy 1951; 22:106–110.
3. Expert Panel Report. National Asthma Education Program: guidelines for the diagnosis and management of asthma. Office of Prevention, Education, and Control. National Heart. Lung, and Blood Institute. Bethesda, MD: National Institutes of Health. Publication No. 91-3042, 1991.
4. Wang S-P, Grayston JT. Population prevalence antibody to Chlamydia pneumoniae, strain TWAR. In: Bowie WR, Caldwell HD, Jones RP, et al. eds. Chlamydial Infections. Cambridge: Cambridge University Press, 1990:402–405.
5. Hahn DL, McDonald R. Can acute *Chlamydia pneumoniae* infection initiate chronic asthma? Ann Allergy Asthma Immunol 1998; 81:339–344.
6. Burrows B, Martinez F, Halonen M, et al. Association of asthma with serum IgE levels and skin-test reactivity to allergens. N Engl J Med 1989; 320:271–277.
7. de Marco R, Locatelli F, Sunyer J, et al. Differences in incidence of reported asthma related to age in men and women. Am J Respir Crit Care Med 2000; 162:68–74.

8. Toogood JH, Jennings B, Baskerville J, et al. Personal observations on the use of inhaled corticosteroid drugs for chronic asthma. Eur J Respir Dis 1984; 65:321–338.

9. Cline MG, Lebowitz MD, Burrows B. Determinants of the percent predicted FEV1 in asthma. Am J Respir Dis 1993; 147 (part 2 of 2 parts):A380.

10. Bronnimann S, Burrows B. A prospective study of the natural history of asthma. Remission and relapse rates. Chest 1986; 90:480–484.

11. Rönmark E, Jönsson E, Lunbbäck B. Remission of asthma in the middle aged and elderly: report from the Obstructive Lung Disease in Northern Sweden study. Thorax 1999; 54:611–613.

12. Burrows B. Epidemiologic evidence for different types of chronic airflow obstruction. Am J Resp Dis 1991; 143:1452–1455.

13. Rijcken B, Schouten JP, Rosner B, et al. Is it useful to distinguish between asthma and chronic obstructive pulmonary disease in respiratory epidemiology? Am J Respir Dis 1991; 143:1456–1457.

14. Frazier EA, Vollmer WM, Wilson SR, et al. Characteristics of older asthmatics with moderate-severe disease. Am J Respir Crit Care Med 1997; 155 (part 2 of 2 parts): A286.

15. Hahn DL. Infectious asthma: a reemerging clinical entity? J Fam Pract 1995; 41:153-157.

16. Williamson HA, Schultz P. An association between acute bronchitis and asthma. J Fam Pract 1987; 24:35–38.

17. Williamson HA. Pulmonary function tests in acute bronchitis: evidence for reversible airway obstruction. J Fam Pract 1987; 25:251–256.

18. Burrows B, Knudson RJ, Leibowitz M. The relationship of childhood respiratory illness to adult obstructive airway disease. Am Rev Respir Dis 1977; 115:751–760.

19. Sherman CB, Tosteson TD, Tager IB, et al. Early childhood predictors of asthma. Am J Epidemiol 1990; 132:83–95.

20. Jónsson JS, Gíslason T, Gíslason D, et al. Acute bronchitis and clinical outcome three years later: prospective cohort study. Br Med J 1998; 317:1433.

21. Infante-Rivard C. Childhood asthma and indoor environmental factors. Am J Epidemiol 1993; 137:834–844.

22. Dodge RR, Burrows B, Lebowitz MD, et al. Antecedent features of children in whom asthma develops during the second decade of life. J Allergy Clin Immunol 1993; 92: 744–749.

23. Pearce N, Pekkanen J, Beasley R. How much asthma is really attributable to atopy? Thorax 1999; 54:268–272.

24. Weiss KB, Gergen PJ, Hodgson T. An economic evaluation of asthma in the United States. N Engl J Med 1992; 326:862–866.

25. Stempel DA, Hedblom EC, Durcanin-Robbins JF, et al. Use of a pharmacy and medical claims database to document cost centers for 1993 annual asthma expenditures. Arch Fam Med 1996; 5:36–40.

26. Bodner C, Ross S, Douglas G, et al. The prevalence of adult onset wheeze: longitudinal study. Br Med J 1997; 314:792–793.

27. Smith DH, Malone DC, Lawson KA, et al. A national estimate of the economic cost of asthma. Am J Resp Crit Care Med 1997; 156:787–793.

28. Burrows B, Lebowitz MD, Barbee RA, et al. Findings before diagnosis of asthma among the elderly in a longitudinal study of a general population sample. J Allergy Clin Immunol 1991; 88:870–877.

29. Torén K, Lindholm NB. Increased mortality due to ischemic heart diseases among pa-

tients with steroid-dependent asthma. Am Rev Respir Dis 1992; 145 (part 2 of 2 parts): A297.

30. Enright PL, Ward BJ, Tracy RP, et al. Asthma and its association with cardiovascular disease in the elderly. J Asthma 1996; 33:45–53.

31. Jousilahti P, Vartiainen E, Tuomilehto J, et al. Symptoms of chronic bronchitis and the risk of coronary disease. Lancet 1996; 348:567–572.

32. Tockman MS, Pearson JD, Fleg JL, et al. Rapid decline in FEV_1: a new risk factor for coronary heart disease mortality. Am J Respir Crit Care Med 1995; 151:390–398.

33. Cookson JB. Prevalence rates of asthma in developing countries and their comparison with those of Europe and North America. Chest 1987; 91:97S–103S.

34. Strachan DP. Time trends in asthma and allergy: ten questions, fewer answers. Clin Exp Allergy 1995; 25:791–794.

35. Hahn DL. *Chlamydia pneumoniae*, asthma and COPD: what is the evidence? Ann Allergy Asthma Immunol 1999; 83:271–292.

36. Buckmaster N, McLaughlin P, Tai E, et al. Exacerbation or initiation of asthma by Mycoplasma pneumoniae infection. Am Rev Respir Dis 1993; 147 (part 2 of 2 parts): A380.

37. Yano T, Ichikawa Y, Komatsu S, et al. Association of *Mycoplasma pneumoniae* antigen with initial onset of bronchial asthma. Am J Respir Crit Care Med 1994; 149:1348–1353.

38. Yano T, Ichikawa Y, Komatsu S, et al. A case having initial onset of bronchial asthma, probably induced by prolonged mycoplasmal infection, accompanied with concurrent highly suspicious chlamydial infection {Japanese}. Kansenshogaku Zasshi 1990; 64: 1566–1571.

39. Frydén A, Kihlström E, Maller R, et al. A clinical and epidemiological study of "ornithosis" caused by *Chlamydia psittaci* and *Chlamydia pneumoniae* (strain TWAR). Scand J Infect Dis 1989; 21:681–691.

40. Hahn DL, Dodge R, Golubjatnikov R. Association of *Chlamydia pneumoniae* (strain TWAR) infection with wheezing, asthmatic bronchitis and adult-onset asthma. JAMA 1991; 266:225–230.

41. Hammerschlag MR, Chirgwin K, Roblin PM, et al. Persistent infection with *Chlamydia pneumoniae* following acute respiratory illness. Clin Infect Dis 1992; 14:178–182.

42. Thom DH, Grayston JT, Campbell LA, et al. Respiratory infection with *Chlamydia pneumoniae* in middle-aged and older adult outpatients. Eur J Clin Microbiol Infect Dis 1994; 13:785–792.

43. Gil JC, Cedillo RL, Mayagoitia BG, et al. Isolation of *Mycoplasma pneumoniae* from asthmatic patients. Ann Allergy 1993; 70:23–25.

44. Seggev JS, Lis I, Siman-Tov R, et al. *Mycoplasma pneumoniae* is a frequent cause of exacerbation of bronchial asthma in adults. Ann Allergy 1986; 57:263–265.

45. Kauppinen M, Herva E, Kujala P, et al. The etiology of community-acquired pneumonia among hospitalized patients during a *Chlamydia pneumoniae* epidemic in Finland. J Infect Dis 1995; 172:1330–1335.

46. Kauppinen M, Saikku P, Kujala P, et al. Clinical picture of community-acquired *Chlamydia pneumoniae* pneumonia requiring hospital treatment: a comparison between chlamydial and pneumococcal pneumonia. Thorax 1996; 51:185–189.

47. Hahn DL. Treatment of *Chlamydia pneumoniae* infection in adult asthma: a before–after trial. J Fam Pract 1995; 41:345–351.

48. Hahn DL. Intracellular pathogens and their role in asthma: *Chlamydia pneumoniae* in adult patients. Eur Respir Rev 1996; 6:224–230.

49. Melbye H, Kongerud J, Vorland L. Reversible airflow limitation in adults with repiratory infection. Eur Respir J 1994; 7:1239–1245.
50. Wang SP, Grayston JT. Microimmunofluorescence serological studies with the TWAR organism. In: Oriel D, Ridgeway G, eds. Chlamydial Infections: Proceedings of the Sixth International Symposium on Human Chlamydial Infections. Cambridge: Cambridge University Press: 1986, 329–332.
51. Jauhiainen T, Tuomi T, Leinonen M, et al. Interference of immunoglobulin G (IgG) antibodies in IgA antibody determinations for *Chlamydia pneumoniae* by microimmunofluorescence test. J Clin Microbiol 1994; 32:839–840.
52. Petitjean J, Vincent F, Le Moël G, et al. *Chlamydia pneumoniae* and acute exacerbation of chronic obstructive pulmonary disease or asthma in adults. In: Saikku P, ed. Proceedings: Fourth Meeting of the European Society for Chlamydia Research, Helsinki, Finland, 2000. Bologna, Italy: Esculapio, 2000:285.
53. Strachan DP, Carrington D, Mendall M, et al. *Chlamydia pneumoniae* serology, lung function decline, and treatment for respiratory disease. Am J Respir Crit Care Med 2000; 161:493–497.
54. Burrows B. The natural history of asthma. J Allergy Clin Immunol 1987; 80:375S–377S.
55. Blasi F, Arioso C, Cavallaro G, et al. *Chlamydia pneumoniae* DNA detection in peripheral blood mononuclear cells is predictive of bronchial infection. In: Saikku P, ed. Proceedings: Fourth Meeting of the European Society for Chlamydia Research, Helsinki, Finland, 2000. Bologna, Italy: Esculapio, 2000:243.
56. Dodge RR, Burrows B. The prevalence and incidence of asthma and asthma-like symptoms in a general population sample. Am J Respir Dis 1980; 122:567–575.
57. Green LA, Miller RS, Reed FM, et al. How representative of typical practice are practice-based research networks? A report form the Ambulatory Sentinel Practice Network (ASPN). Arch Fam Med 1993; 2:939–949.
58. Hahn DL, Beasley JW. Diagnosed and possible undiagnosed asthma: a Wisconsin Research Network (WReN) study. J Fam Pract 1994; 38:373–379.
59. Clark CE, Coote JM, Silver DAT, et al. Asthma after childhood pneumonia: six year follow up study. Br Med J 2000; 320:1514–1516.
60. Green LA, Hames Sr. CG, Nutting PA. Potential of practice-based research networks: experience from ASPN. J Fam Pract 1994; 38:400–406.
61. van Weel C, van den Bosch WJHM, M vdHHJ, et al. Development of respiratory illness in childhood–a longitudinal study in general practice. J R Coll Gen Prac 1987; 37:404–408.
62. van Schayck CP, Dompeling E, Van Herwaarden CLA, et al. Interacting effects of atopy and bronchial hyperresponsiveness on the annual decline in lung function and the exacerbation rate in asthma. Am Rev Respir Dis 1991; 144:1297–1301.
63. Mills GD, Lindeman JA, Fawcett JP, et al. *Chlamydia pneumoniae* serological status is not associated with asthma in children or young adults. Int J Epidemiol 2000; 29:280–284.
64. Melbye H, Aasebø U, Straume B. Symptomatic effect of inhaled fenoterol in acute bronchitis: a placebo-controlled double-blind study. Fam Pract 1991; 8:216–222.
65. Hahn DL, Peeling RW, Dillon E, et al. Serologic markers for *Chlamydia pneumoniae* in asthma. Ann Allergy Asthma Immunol 2000; 84:227–233.
66. Hsiue TR, Lin TM, Chen CW, et al. *Chlamydia pneumoniae* respiratory infection in guinea pigs. Eur Respir J 2000; 16, Suppl 31:20s (abstract P312).
67. Moazed TC, Kuo C-C, Grayston JT, et al. A pathogenic role of mononuclear phagocytes

in *Chlamydia pneumoniae* infection in a mouse model. In Abstracts of the 96th General Meeting of the American Society for Microbiology, New Orlean, Louisiana, May 19-23, 1996, abstract D-15, page 244.

68. Laitinen K, Laurila A, Pyhälä L, et al. *Chlamydia pneumoniae* infection induces inflammatory changes in the aortas of rabbits. Infect and Immun 1997; 65:4832–4835.

69. Shemer-Avni Y, Lieberman D. *Chlamydia pneumoniae*-induced ciliostasis in ciliated bronchial epithelial cells. J Infect Dis 1995; 171:1274–1278.

70. O'Riordan TG, Zwang J, Smaldone GC. Mucociliary clearance in adult asthma. Am Rev Respir Dis 1992; 146:598–603.

71. Emre U, Sokolovskaya N, Roblin P, et al. Detection of *Chlamydia pneumoniae*-IgE in children with reactive airway disease. J Infect Dis 1995; 172:265–267.

72. Kaukoranta-Tolvanen S-S, Teppo AM, Leinonen M, et al. *Chlamydia pneumoniae* induces the production of TNFα, IL-1b, and IL-6 by human monocytes. Proc Eur Soc Chlamydia Res 1992; 2:85.

73. Redecke V, Dalhoff K; Bohnet S, et al. Interaction of *Chlamydia pneumoniae* and human alveolar macrophages: infection and inflammatory response. Am J Respir Cell Mol Biol 1998; 19:721–727.

74. Thepen T, McMenamin C, Girn B, et al. Regulation of IgE production in pre-sensitized animals: in vivo elimination of alveolar macrophages preferentially increases IgE responses to inhaled allergen. Clin Exp Allergy 1992; 22:1107–1114.

75. Kuo C-C, Gown AM, Benditt EP, et al. Detection of *Chlamydia pneumoniae* in aortic lesions of atherosclerosis by immunocytochemical stain. Arterioscler Thromb 1993; 13: 1501–1504.

76. Rödel J, Woytas M, Groh A, et al. Production of basic fibroblast growth factor and interleukin 6 by human smooth muscle cells following infection with *Chlamydia pneumoniae*. Infect Immun 2000; 68:3635–3641.

77. Huittinen T, Harju T, Paldanius M, et al. *Chlamydia pneumoniae* HSP60 antibodies in adults with stable asthma. In: Saikku P, ed. Proceedings: Fourth Meeting of the European Society for Chlamydia Research, Helsinki, Finland, 2000. Bologna, Italy: Esculapio, 2000:185.

78. Roblin PM, Witkin SS, Weiss SM, et al. Immune response to *Chlamydia pneumoniae* in patients with asthma: role of heat shock proteins (HSPs). In: Saikku P, ed. Proceedings: Fourth Meeting of the European Society for Chlamydia Research, Helsinki, Finland, 2000. Bologna, Italy: Esculapio, 2000:209.

79. Slater JE, Paupore EJ, Elwell MR, et al. Lipopolysaccharide augments IgG and IgE responses of mice to the latex allergen Hev b 5. J Allergy Clin Immunol 1998; 102: 977–983.

80. Kline JN, Cowden JD, Hunninghake GW, et al. Expression of sensitive or hyporesponsive phenotypes in individuals challenged with inhaled lipopolysaccharide correlates with differential response of alveolar macrophages and monocytes in vitro. Eur Respir J 1998; 12:46s (abstract P370).

81. Busse WW. Respiratory infections and bronchial hyperreactivity. J Allergy Clin Immunol 1988; 81:770–775.

82. Busse WW. The relationship between viral infections and onset of allergic diseases and asthma. Clin Exp Allergy 1989; 19:1–9.

27

Therapeutic Trials for *Chlamydia pneumoniae* in Asthma

PETER N. BLACK

University of Auckland
Auckland, New Zealand

I. Introduction

In recent years a number of observational studies have suggested an association between infection with *Chlamydia pneumoniae* and the development of asthma (1,2) while other studies have found an association between infection with *C. pneumoniae* and the severity of asthma (3–5). These observations beg the question of whether treatment with antibiotics that are active against *C. pneumoniae* will lead to an improvement in the severity of asthma in individuals with evidence of infection with *C. pneumoniae*. In vitro activity against *C. pneumoniae* has been demonstrated with macrolides, tetracyclines, and quinolones (6,7), although most clinical studies of treatment for *C. pneumoniae* in patients with asthma have used macrolide antibiotics including roxithromycin, clarithromycin, erythromycin, and azithromycin. Interest in a role for macrolide antibiotics in the treatment of asthma, however, predates the recognition of *Chlamydia pneumoniae* as a respiratory pathogen.

II. Macrolide Antibiotics and Asthma

In 1959 Kaplan and Goldie reported a case series of patients treated with troleandomycin (TAO)(8). They observed that TAO, a macrolide antibiotic, was useful in the treatment of what was termed infectious asthma. They noted that it led to a reduction in the requirement for medication including corticosteroids. The first controlled trial of TAO as a treatment for asthma was conducted by Itkin and Menzel (9). This was a randomized, controlled, cross-over study with 12 subjects and they were able to demonstrate significant improvements in lung function. They suggested that TAO might act by inhibiting the metabolism of corticosteroids. Spector et al. conducted a larger study with 74 steroid-dependent asthmatics and confirmed that treatment with TAO allowed a reduction in the dosage of methylprednisolone (10). Szefler et al. demonstrated that TAO did indeed inhibit the metabolism of methylprednisolone, with an increase in the half-life of methylprednisolone from 2.46 to 4.63 h (11).

Although the benefits of TAO are due primarily to the inhibition of the metabolism of corticosteroids, there has been a debate about whether this agent has other actions that are useful in the treatment of asthma. There have been a number of uncontrolled studies suggesting that TAO has effects above and beyond the inhibition of metabolism of corticosteroids. When Zeiger et al. commenced 16 steroid-dependent patients on TAO there was a more than fourfold reduction in the dosage of methylprednisolone (12). This is a greater reduction than one would expect in a medicine that doubles the half-life of methylprednisolone. In another uncontrolled study Flotte and Loughlin reduced the dosage of methylprednisolone from 15.3 to 1.4 mg per day in nine children treated with TAO (13).

Erythromycin has also been studied as a treatment for asthma. In an open, uncontrolled study Miyatake et al. treated 23 patients with 200 mg erythromycin three times daily for 10 weeks (14). The use of erythromycin was associated with an improvement in bronchial responsiveness with an increase in the PC_{20} for histamine from 0.13 to 0.35 mg/L. In a similar study Shimuzu et al. found a threefold decrease in bronchial hyperresponsiveness in children treated for 8 weeks with roxithromycin, another macrolide antibiotic. None of the subjects were being treated with oral corticosteroids and theophylline levels did not change during the study (15). This study also has the limitation of being an open, uncontrolled study, as is another that reported a decrease in bronchial hyperresponsiveness with roxithromycin (16).

With open, uncontrolled studies, however, not all of the improvement may be due to the effect of the study medicine. In addition to the placebo effect, participation in a study may improve compliance with other treatments. Nelson and his colleagues addressed this by conducting a double-blind, randomized, placebo-controlled study of TAO in subjects with steroid-dependent asthma (17). Seventy five subjects were randomized to treatment. Fifty seven subjects remained in the study at the end of 1 year and at this time the mean dosage of methylprednisolone was 6.3 mg/day in the subjects on TAO compared with 10.4 mg/day in the subjects receiving placebo. In addition steroid side effects were greater in the TAO group. In this study all of the apparent steroid-sparing effects of TAO can be explained by its effects on the metabolism of methylprednisolone. In another double-blind, placebo controlled trial of TAO undertaken in 18 children, the reduction in the dosage of methylprednisolone was likewise no greater than one would anticipate from the effect of TAO on steroid metabolism (18). More recently we have undertaken a randomized, placebo-controlled, crossover study of roxithromycin in subjects with uncontrolled asthma. These subjects were not receiving treatment with oral corticosteroids (19). Subjects were eligible to take part in the study if they were receiving treatment with ≥ 400 µg inhaled beclomethasone dipropionate or budesonide, had daily symptoms and a forced expiratory volume in 1 s (FEV_1) < 80% of predicted. There were 19 subjects with a mean age of 51.8 ± 2.8 years and a mean FEV_1 of $60.3 \pm 3.6\%$ predicted. The study involved two 4 week treatment periods separated by a 4 week washout period. Subjects received treatment with 150 mg roxithromycin twice daily in the first treatment period and the alternative treatment in the second treatment period. During the last 2 weeks of each treatment period the mean morning peak expiratory flow rate (PEFR) was 323 L/min with roxithromycin and 336 L/min with placebo ($p = 0.06$). Other end points also favored placebo. These findings do not favor the idea that roxithromycin is useful for the treatment of unselected patients with asthma. None of these studies addresses the question of whether macrolide antibiotics are effective for the treatment of patients with asthma and evidence of infection with *C. pneumoniae*.

III. Treatment of Infection with *C. pneumoniae* in Asthma

The observation that infection with *C. pneumoniae* may influence the severity of asthma has kindled interest in the idea that antibiotics that are active against *C. pneumoniae* may be useful in treating patients who have evidence of persistent infection with *C pneumoniae*. The first study looking at the effect of antibiotics in patients with asthma and infection with *C. pneumoniae* was conducted by Hahn (20). He enrolled 46 patients with adult-onset asthma who were seropositive for *C. pneumoniae*. The subjects had a mean duration of asthma of 5.5 years. This was an open, uncontrolled study in which subjects were treated with doxycycline, erythromycin, or azithromycin for 3–9 weeks. Eighteen subjects had a marked improvement in their symptoms and another seven had a complete remission. The second study by Emre and colleagues involved the treatment of children presenting to the Emergency Department with wheezing (21). A total of 118 children between 5 and 16 years of age presented to the Emergency Department during the course of the study. One hundred ten children had been previously diagnosed as having asthma. *C. pneumoniae* was grown from nasopharyngeal swabs in 13 children. Seven of the children who were culture positive did not *have* circulating antibodies to *C. pneumoniae*. Twelve of the children who were culture-positive were treated with either erythromycin or clarithromycin for 10 days to 3 weeks and all became culture-negative. Nine of these children had a substantial improvement in their symptoms. This did not just reflect the resolution of their acute exacerbation, since many were substantially better than they had been prior to the exacerbation. Both of these studies have the limitation that they are open, uncontrolled studies. Nonetheless the improvements seen in these studies provide a strong argument for conducting further studies in this area.

IV. CARM Study

The largest study of antibiotic treatment for patients with asthma and evidence
of infection with *C. pneumoniae* is the CARM study (*Chlamydia pneumoniae,
Asthma, Roxithromycin, Multinational Study*) (22). Subjects (n = 232) were randomized to treatment in the study that was conducted in Australia, New Zealand,
Italy, and Argentina. Subjects were eligible for the study if they fit the following
criteria:

1. A diagnosis of asthma
2. $FEV_1 > 50\%$ of predicted.
3. An increase in $FEV_1 \geq 15\%$ following inhaled salbutamol or diurnal variation in peak expiratory flow (PEF) of $\geq 15\%$ on 7 of 14 days during
   the run-in period.
4. IgG antibodies to *C. pneumoniae* $\geq$ 1:64 and/or IgA antibodies $\geq$ 1:16
5. Remained symptomatic during the run-in period.

Subjects were not eligible if they had been receiving treatment with any macrolide, quinolone, or tetracycline in the 4 weeks before study entry or for more than
3 weeks in the preceding 4 months. They were also excluded if they had a smoking
history of $\geq$ 20 pack years, bronchiectasis, any other serious systemic diseases,
hypersensitivity to macrolides, or any significant change in asthma medication in
the previous month including a course of oral corticosteroids. In addition they were
not eligible if they had a respiratory tract infection (with increased cough and increased volume and/or purulence of sputum) during the run-in or if they had abnormal liver function tests or a serum creatinine > 200 μmol/L. The baseline characteristics of the subjects are shown in Tables 1 and 2.

Subjects were randomized to receive treatment with roxithromycin 150 mg
twice daily or matching placebo for 6 weeks. Following the end of treatment the
subjects were followed up for a further 6 months. The subjects recorded their PEF,
symptom score, and use of rescue medicine twice a day for the duration of the study.

Table 1 CARM Study Baseline Characteristics of Patients

	Placebo	Roxithromycin
No. of Subjects	114	105
Mean age (SD)	42(11.9)	40(11.6)
M/F	57/57	47/58
Percentage receiving inhaled steroids	84.2%	77.1%
IgG antibodies to *C. pneumoniae*	109.2	96.2
Geometric mean titer (95% CI)	(88.8–134.2)	(80.7–115.1)
IgA antibodies to *C. pneumoniae*	12.5	11.4
Geometric mean titer (95% CI)	(10.6–14.6)	(9.8–13.2)

Table 2 CARM Study Baseline Clinical Characteristics

	Placebo	Roxithromycin
Mean FEV$_1$, L (SD)	2.53 (0.76)	2.62 (0.9)
Mean FEV$_1$, % predicted (SD)	75.3% (17.4)	79.0% (19.3)
Mean PEFR		
Morning L/min (SD)	358.1 (112)	364.0 (104)
Evening L/min (SD)	373.5 (115)	378 (101)
Mean symptom score		
Daytime (SD)	1.7 (0.8)	1.7 (0.9)
Nighttime (SD)	0.8 (0.6)	0.8 (0.5)
Rescue medication		
Mean no. puffs daytime (SD)	3.5 (2.9)	3.0 (2.7)
Mean no. puffs nighttime (SD)	1.6 (1.5)	1.2 (1.4)

An analysis of baseline characteristics showed that the subjects from Australia and New Zealand subjects had more severe asthma than those from Italy and Argentina. As a result, an analysis was performed for the Australasian subjects as well as the whole intention-to-treat population.

From baseline to the end of the 6 week treatment period there was an increase in the mean morning PEF of 14 L/min in the roxithromycin group compared with 8 L/min in the placebo group. Although the morning PEF continued to improve in both groups over the next 6 months, the difference between the two groups decreased. At 6 months after the end of treatment the improvement over baseline was 21 L/min in the roxithromycin group and 18 L/min in the placebo group. The differences between the two groups were not significant at any time point. A greater effect of roxithromycin on the morning PEF was seen in the Australasian subjects. In the Australasian population the change in the morning PEF from baseline to the end of the 6 week treatment period was 18 L/min with roxithromycin and 2 L/min for the placebo group (p = 0.04). Six months after the end of treatment, the morning PEF had increased by 15 L/min from baseline with roxithromycin compared with 9 L/ min in the baseline group and this difference was not significant.

With the evening PEF the greatest difference between the two treatment groups was again seen at the end of treatment. In the whole study population the increase in the mean evening PEF was 15 L/min with roxithromycin and 3 L/min with placebo (Fig. 1). At 6 months after the end of treatment the values were 18 L/min and 20 L/min, respectively. The effect of roxithromycin on evening PEF was significant at the end of 6 weeks treatment, but not at subsequent endpoints. In the Australasian population the effect of roxithromycin at the end of 6 weeks treatment was even clearer with an increase in evening PEF of 19 L/min compared with a change of 1 L/min with placebo (p = 0.01). Again, as with the whole study population, the difference between the two groups diminished following the end of treatment and was not significant at subsequent time points. Changes in the symptom

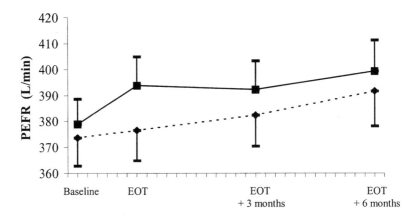

Figure 1 Evening peak expiratory flow rate (mean ± s.e.m.) for roxithromycin (■) and placebo (◆) at baseline, end of treatment (EOT), 3 months after the end of treatment, and 6 months after the end of treatment. Evening peak expiratory flow rate was significant with roxithromycin at end of treatment (p=0.02) but not at other time points.

scores also favored roxithromycin, although the differences were not statistically significant.

There were no significant differences in the number of adverse events reported for placebo (184 events) and roxithromycin (216 events). The most common adverse events were exacerbation of asthma, headache, rhinitis, infection, and flu syndrome and these were equally distributed between the two groups. Adverse events that were reported as possibly related to study medicine included diarrhea (10 reports with placebo and 6 with roxithromycin), nausea (5 reports with placebo and 13 with roxithromycin), and changes in liver function test (1 patient receiving placebo and 6 patients receiving roxithromycin). In only two of these subjects did a change in transaminases or bilirubin result in a value outside the normal range. Neither subject was symptomatic and in both cases the values had returned to normal following the end of treatment.

This study showed that treatment with roxithromycin led to a small but significant improvement in PEF but the effect was not sustained after the end of treatment. Although the effect seen with roxithromycin was not large, it is comparable in magnitude to the benefit seen when a leukotriene antagonist is added to treatment with an inhaled corticosteroid (23,24) or when the dosage of inhaled steroid is doubled in patients whose asthma is not adequately controlled (25). The absence of sustained benefit following the 6 week course of roxithromycin does not suggest that this approach is likely to find a place in the routine treatment of asthma. It is conceivable that long-term treatment with roxithromycin (or other macrolide antibiotics) may lead to continued benefit, but this has to be weighed against well-founded concerns about the development of antibiotic resistance (26).

V. Mechanism of Action of Roxithromycin

The findings of this study do raise the question of why roxithromycin led to an improvement in asthma control. If roxithromycin was acting to eradicate *C. pneumoniae*, one would expect to see sustained benefit after the end of treatment. It may, however, be unduly optimistic to expect 6 weeks of treatment with roxithromycin to eradicate *C. pneumoniae*. Hammerschlag et al. described a number of individuals who remained culture-positive for *C. pneumoniae* despite having several courses of antibiotics of 10–21 days' duration (27). In vitro antibiotics can inhibit the growth of *C. pneumoniae* in endothelial and vascular smooth cells (28). It appears to be more difficult to clear *C. pneumoniae* from monocytes. Gieffers et al. infected monocytes with *C. pneumoniae* and then cultured the monocytes with azithromycin or rifampicin (29). Culture in the presence of antibiotics did not prevent the *C. pneumoniae* from remaining viable within the monocytes, although an aberrant morphology was seen. The same workers identified two patients whose circulating monocytes were polymerase chain reaction-PCR-positive for *C. pneumoniae*. Despite treatment with 500 mg/day azithromycin for 3 days (on two occasions), it was still possible to culture *C. pneumoniae* from the monocytes from these patients. This raises the concern that even if antibiotics cleared infection from epithelial cells, reinfection could occur from circulating monocytes. Kraft et al. also highlighted the problems of trying to treat chronic infection with *C. pneumoniae*. They identified three subjects whose bronchial biopsies were PCR positive for *C. pneumoniae*(30). Following treatment for 6 weeks with clarithromycin, they became PCR-negative. Several months later, however, two of the subjects again had biopsies that were PCR-positive.

Infection of cultured epithelial cells by *C. pneumoniae* leads to increased production of proinflammatory cytokine such as granulocyte–macrophage colony-stimulating factor (GM-CSF) and interleukin (IL) 16(31). It is not difficult to envisage how chronic infection with *C. pneumoniae* could promote airways inflammation in asthma. In the CARM study the improvement that occurred may have been due to short-term suppression of infection with *C. pneumoniae*. This in turn could lead to a reduction in airways inflammation. Failure to eradicate *C. pneumoniae* would mean that the benefit would not be sustained. This is, however, not the only possible explanation for the findings of the CARM study. The benefit seen with roxithromycin could be due to the anti-inflammatory actions of roxithromycin independent of any effect on *C. pneumoniae*. Anti-inflammatory effects have been reported in vitro with roxithromycin and other macrolide antibiotics (32). Roxithromycin inhibits the neutrophil oxidant burst (33,34) and reduces the formation of cytokines including IL-6, IL-8, and GM-CSF (35) from airway epithelial cells and of IL-5 from splenocytes (36). In animal models roxithromycin inhibits the formation of edema in the rat paw in response to carageenin (37) or poly-L-arginine (38). Macrolides may have other actions relevant to asthma. Erythromycin inhibits the secretion of mucus from human airways in vitro (39). In another study erythromycin (3×10^{-5} M) led to a decrease in the response to electrical field stimulation of 93% (40).

Other macrolides, including roxithromycin and clarithromycin, are reported to have similar effects (41).

The failure of previous randomized, controlled trials to show any benefit with macrolide antibiotics in unselected patients with asthma (above and beyond any effects on corticosteroid metabolism) (17,19) argues against the importance of the anti-inflammatory actions of macrolides. These were, however, small studies and the possibility that the actions of roxithromycin are not due to its antimicrobial actions cannot be dismissed.

VI. Other Recent Studies

In a preliminary report, Kraft et al. described a randomized, controlled trial of 39 subjects with asthma who were treated for 6 weeks with clarithromycin or placebo. Bronchial biopsies and bronchoalveolar lavage were performed prior to treatment (41). Twenty of the 39 subjects had evidence on PCR of biopsy or lavage fluid of infection with *Mycoplasma pneumoniae*. In addition seven of the subjects were PCR-positive for *C. pneumoniae*. Subjects who were PCR-positive for *C. pneumoniae* or *Mycoplasma pneumoniae* had a significant improvement in FEV_1 from 2.52 $\pm$ 0.19 L to 2.78 $\pm$ 0.22 L (p = 0.03). The subjects who were PCR-negative also improved but to a lesser extent (2.49 $\pm$ 0.32 L to 2.62 $\pm$ 0.24 L, p = 0.24). *M. pneumoniae* is an intracellular pathogen and, like *C. pneumoniae*, it can give rise to chronic infection. Consideration needs to be given to the possibility that chronic infection with *M. pneumoniae* may also influence the severity of asthma.

VII. Design of Future Studies

In any future study of treatment for chronic infection with *C. pneumoniae*, a key question will be how to identify the subjects who should be included in the study. In the CARM study subjects were eligible for inclusion if they had high titers of antibodies to *C. pneumoniae*. There are problems with this approach. Some individuals can be culture-positive even though they do not have detectable antibodies for *C. pneumoniae* (21). It is also possible that individuals may clear infection with *C. pneumoniae* while remaining seropositve (although it has yet to be proven that this happens). In future studies it may be better to select on the basis of a positive PCR for *C. pneumoniae* rather than the presence of antibodies to *C. pneumoniae*. Certainly a positive PCR is not uncommon in patients with airway disease. Cunningham et al. found that nasopharyngeal aspirates were PCR positive for *C. pneumoniae* in 20% of children with asthma and positivity rates are likely to be even higher in adults. Von Hertzen et al. reported that almost half of patients with severe chronic obstructive pulmonary disease (COPD) were PCR-positive for *C. pneumoniae* in their sputum (42). In ideal circumstances, it would be preferable if *C. pneumoniae* was cultured from sputum or nasopharyngeal swabs before subjects were included in studies, but most laboratories have not been successful in culturing *C. pneumoniae* from biological samples. The use of PCR may be a more convenient approach.

If patients are selected for studies on the basis of PCR positivity in sputum, it also begs the question of whether changes in the sputum PCR should be an end point for studies of antibiotic treatment for *C. pneumoniae*. It is not clear, however, whether it is possible to eradicate infection with *C. pneumoniae*. Studies described above suggest that treatment with a single antibiotic for a few weeks is unlikely to eradicate infection with *C. pneumoniae* permanently. Future studies should consider treatment for longer periods and treatment with more than one antibiotic. Newer antibiotics such as telithromycin, which is bactericidal for *C. pneumoniae* rather than bacteriostatic, may have advantages and need to be studied. If it is not possible to eradicate C pneumoniae it may still be appropriate to try to reduce the bacterial load. The development of a quantitative PCR for *C. pneumoniae* should facilitate this approach (43).

One approach to identifying a role for *C. pneumoniae* in asthma is to determine if treatment with antichlamydial antibiotics can eradicate infection with *C. pneumoniae* and if this leads to sustained improvement in asthma control after the antibiotic has been discontinued. If this were to happen, it would argue that the antibiotics were not simply having an anti-inflammatory effect. An alternative approach would be to study derivatives of the macrolide antibiotics that have anti-inflammatory actions without having an antibacterial effect. This approach has already been successfully used with chemically modified tetracyclines that inhibit matrix metalloproteases without having antibacterial actions (44).

VIII. Conclusions

There is an association between infection with *C. pneumoniae* and the severity of asthma. This has raised the question of whether antibiotic treatment directed against *C. pneumoniae* would lead to an improvement in asthma control. In a randomized, controlled trial, 6 weeks of treatment with roxithromycin in patients with high titers of antibodies to *C. pneumoniae* led to modest improvements in asthma control, but the benefit was not sustained beyond the end of treatment. It is still not clear whether the lack of sustained benefit was due to failure to eradicate *C. pneumoniae* or whether the improvements seen were due to the anti-inflammatory effect of roxithromycin. Further studies are needed to elucidate the role of antichlamydial therapy in the treatment of asthma.

References

1. Hahn DL, Dodge R, Golubjatnikov R. Association of Chlamydia pneumoniae (strain TWAR) infection with wheezing, asthmatic bronchitis and adult onset asthma. JAMA 1991; 266: 225–230.
2. Hahn DL, Antilla T, Saikku P. Association of Chlamydia pneumoniae IgA antibodies with recently symptomatic asthma. Epidemiol Infect 1996; 117: 513–517.
3. Cunningham AF, Johnston SL, Julious SA, Lampe FC, Ward ME. Chronic *Chlamydia pneumoniae* and asthma exacerbations in children. Eur Respir J 1998; 11: 345–349.

4. Cook PJ, Davies P, Tunnicliffe W, Ayres JG, Honeybourne D, Wise R. Chlamydia pneumoniae and asthma. Thorax 1998; 53: 254–259.
5. Black PN, Jenkins CR, Schiccitano R, Allegra L, Blasi F, Wlodarzyck J, Cooper BC. Serological evidence of infection with *Chlamydia pneumoniae* is related to the severity of asthma. Eur Respir J 2000; 15:256–259.
6. Hammerschlag MR, Qumei KK, Roblin PM. In vitro activities of azithromycin, clarithromycin, L-ofloxacin and other antibiotics against *Chlamydia pneumoniae*. Antimicrob Agents Chemother 1992; 36: 1573–1574.
7. Roblin PM, hammeschlag MR. In vitro activity of a new ketolide antibiotic HMR 3647 against *Chlamydia pneumoniae*. Antimicrob Agents Chemother 1998; 48: 1515–1516.
8. Kaplan MA, Goldin M. The use of triacetyloleandomycin in chronic infectious asthma. In: Welch H, Marti-Ibauez F, eds. Antibiotic Annual 1958–1959. New York: Interscience Publishers, 1959: 273–276.
9. Itkin IH, Menzel ML. The use of macrolide antiiotic substances in the treatment of asthma. J Allergy 1970; 45: 146–162.
10. Spector SL, Katz FH, Farr RS. Troleandomycin: effectiveness in steroid dependent asthma and bronchitis. J Allergy Clin Immunol 1974; 54: 367.
11. Szefler SJ, Rose JQ, Ellis EF, Spector SL, Green AW, Jusko WJ. The effect of troleandomycin on methylprednisolone elimination. J Allergy Clin Immunol 1980; 66: 447–451.
12. Zeiger RS, Schatz M, Sperling W, Simon RA, Stevenson DD. Efficacy of troleandomycin in out-patients with severe corticosteroid-dependent asthma. J Allergy Clin Immunol 1980; 66: 438–446.
13. Flotte TR, Loughlin GM. Benefits and complications of troleandomycin in young children with steroid dependent asthma. Pediatr Pulmonol. 1991; 10; 178–182.
14. Miyatake H, Taki F, Taniguchi H, Sizuki R, Takagi K, satake T. Erthromycin reduces the severity of bronchial hyperresponsiveness in asthma. Chest 1991; 99: 670–673.
15. Shimuzu T, Kato M, Mochizuki H, Tokuyama K, Morikawa A, Kuroume T. Roxithromycin reduces the degree of bronchial hyperresponsiveness in children with asthma. Chest 1994; 106; 458–461.
16. Kamoi H, Kurihara N, Fujiwara H, Hirata K, Takeda T. The macrolide antibacterial roxithromycin reduces bronchial hyperresponsivenes in children with asthma. J Asthma 1995; 32: 191–197.
17. Nelson HS, Hamilos DL, Corsello PR, Levesque NV, Buchmeier AD, Bucher BL. A double-blind study of troleandomycin and methylprednisolone in asthmatic subjects who require daily corticosteroids. Am Rev Respir Dis 1993; 147: 398–404.
18. Kamada AK, Hill MR, Ikle DN, Manon Bremner A, Szefler SJ. Efficacy and safety of low dose troleandomycin therapy in children with severe steroid-requiring asthma. J Allergy Clin Immunol 1993; 91: 873–882.
19. Black PN, Bagg B, Brodie SM, Robinson E, Cooper B. A double-blind crossover study of roxithromycin in the treatment of asthma (abstract) Eur Respir J 1998; 12 (Suppl 28): 190s.
20. Hahn DL. Treatment of *Chlamydia pneumoniae* infection in adult asthma: a before–after trial. J Fam Pract 1995; 41: 345–351.
21. Emre U, Roblin PM, Gelling M, Dumornay W, Rao M, Hammerschlag MR, Schacter J. The association of Chlamydia pneumoniae infection and reactive airway disease in children. Arch Pediatr Adolesc Med 1994; 148: 727–732.
22. Black PN, Blasi F, Jenkins CR, Scicchitano R, Allegra L, Mills GD, Rubinfeld AR, Ruffin AR, Mullins PR, Dangain J, Bem-David D, Cooper BC. Trial of roxithromycin

in subjects with asthma and serological evidence of infection with Chlamydia pneumoniae. Am J Respir Crit Care Med 2001; 164: 536–541.

23. Laviolette M, Malmstrom K, Chervinsky P, Pujet JC, Zhange J, Reiss TF. Monetlukast added to inhaled beclomethasone in the treatment of asthma. Am J Respir Crit Care Med 1999; 160: 1862–1868.

24. Christian Virchow J, Prasse A, Naya I, Summerton L, Harris A. Zafirkulast improves asthma control in patients receiving high dose inhaled corticosteroids. Am J Respir Crit Care Med 2000; 162: 578–585.

25. Fabbri L, Burge PS, Croonenborgh L, Warlies F, Wecke B, Ciaccia A, Parker C. Comparison of fluticasone propionate with beclomethasone dipropionate in moderate to severe asthma treated for one year. Thorax 1993; 48:817–823.

26. Seppala H, Klaukka T, Vuopio-Varkila J, Muotiala A, Helenius H, Lager K, Huovinen P. The effect of changes in ther consumption of macrolide antibiotics on erythromycin resistance in group A streptococci in Finland. N Engl J Med 1997; 337: 491–492.

27. Hammerschlag MR, Chirgwin K, Roblin PM et al. Persistent infection with *Chlamydia pneumoniae* following acute respiratory illness. Clin Infect Dis 1992; 14: 178–182.

28. Gieffers J, Solbach W, Maass M. Activity of antibiotics in eliminating Chlamydia pneumoniae cardiovascular strains from cell types involved in the pathogenesis of arteriosclerosis. Clin Microbial Infect 1999; 5(suppl 3): 381 (abstr).

29. Gieffers J, Füllgraf, Jahn J, Klinger M, Dalhoff K, Katus HA, Solbach W, Maass M. *Chlamydia pneumoniae* infection in circulating human monocytes is refractory to antibiotic treatment. Circulation 2001; 103: 351–356.

30. Langmark EL, Kraft M, Gaydos CA, Martin RJ. Significance of PCR positivity for Chlamydia pneumoniae in the lower airways of stable asthmatics. Am J Respir Crit Care Med 2000 161: A898 (abstr).

31. Biscione G, Hussain IR, Papi A, Johnston SL. Pathophysiology of *Chlamydia pneumoniae*. Proceedings, 4th International Conference on Macrolides, Streptogrammins & Ketolides, 1998 (abstr).

32. Black PN. Antinflammatory effects of macrolide antibiotics. Eur Respir J 1997; 10: 971–972.

33. Lambro MT, El Benna J, Babin-Chevaye C. Comparison of the in vitro effects of several macrolides on the oxidative burst of human neutrophils. J Antimicrob Chemother 1989; 24: 561–572.

34. Anderson R. Erythromycin and roxithromycin potentiate human neutrophil locomotion in vitro by inhibition of leukoattractant activated superoxide generation and autooxidation. J Infect Dis 1989; 5: 966–972.

35. Kawasaki S, Takizawa H, Takayuki O, et al. Roxithromycin inhibits cytokine production by and neutrophil attachment to human neutrophil attachment to human bronchial epithelial cells in vitro. Antimicrob Agents Chemother 1988; 42: 1499–1502.

36. Konno S, Adachi M, Asano K, Okamoto K, Takahashi T. Antiallergic activity of roxithromycin: inhibition of interleukin-5 production from mouse T-lymphocytes. Life Sci 1993; 52: 25–30.

37. Scaglione F, Rossoni G. Comparative anti-inflammatory effects of roxithromycin, azithromycin and clarithromycin. J Antimicrob Chemother 1998; 41 (Suppl B): 47–50.

38. Agen C, Danesi R, Blandizzi C, et al. Macrolide antibiotics as anti-inflammatory agents: roxithromycin in an unexpected role. Agents Actions 1993; 147: 153–159.

39. Goswami SK, Kivity S, Marom Z. Erthromycin inhibits respiratory glyconjugate secretion from human airways in vitro. Am Rev Respir Dis 1990; 141: 72–78.

40. Tamaoki J, Tagaya E, Sakai A, Konno K. Effects of macrolide antibiotics on neurally

mediated contraction of human isolated bronchus. J Allergy Clin Immunol 1995; 95: 853–859.

41. Kraft M, Cassell GH, Duffy LB, Metze T, Pak J, Gaydos CA, Martin RJ. Mycoplasma and Chlamydia are present in the airways of chronic, stable asthmatics. Am J Respir Crit Care Med 1999; 159: A517 (abstr).

42. Von Hertzen L, Alakarppa H, Koskinen R, Liippo K, Surcel HM, Leinonen M, Saikku P. Chlamydia pneumoniae infection in patients with chronic obstructive pulmonary disease. Epidemiol Infect 1997; 118: 155–164.

43. Berger M, Schroder B, Daeschlein G, Schneider W, Busjahn A, Buchwalow I, Luft FC, Haller H. Chlamydia pneumoniae DNA in non-coronary atherosclerotic plaques and circulating leukocytes. J Lab Clin Med 2000; 136: 194–200.

44. Golub LM, Ranamurthy NS, Llavaneras A, Ryan ME, Lee HM, Liu Y, Bain S, Sorsa T. A chemically modified nonantimicrobial tetracycline (CMT-8) inhibits gingival matrix metalloproteinases, periodontal breakdown and extra-oral bone loss in ovariectomized rats. Ann NY Acad Sci 1999; 878: 290–310.

28

Treatment of the Common Cold
Prospects and Implications for the Treatment of Asthma Exacerbations

DEAN D. CREER

Royal London Hospital
London, England

COLIN M. GELDER

University of Wales College of Medicine
Cardiff, Wales

SEBASTIAN L. JOHNSTON

National Heart and Lung Institute
Imperial College London
London, England

I. Introduction

Upper respiratory viral infections are now known to be the major precipitants of exacerbations of asthma in all age groups (1,2). However, with the exception of the neuraminidase inhibitors and the adamantanes for influenza, no treatment for common cold viruses that is clinically effective has yet made it to the market place. The mechanisms of virus-induced asthma are beginning to be understood and involve a number of inflammatory pathways. Both antiviral and anti-inflammatory therapies potentially offer hope for intervention after the onset of symptoms, but a combination of both therapies may offer the best hope. Prophylaxis, either in the form of vaccination or of prophylactic therapy, offers the best hope of a major impact in disease prevention. Advances in molecular biology, virology, and immunology are identifying mechanisms and generating new avenues for developing treatment of common cold viruses for populations at risk, particularly those with asthma.

The chief obstacle to successful intervention is the enormous number of organisms associated with the acute respiratory viral infections (around 300 different viruses or atypical bacteria; see Table 1). Other problems that demand attention are the identification of appropriate target groups for therapy, and determining optimal timing of therapy for prophylactic and interventional therapy (early onset of treat-

Table 1   Agents Causing the Common Cold

Agent[a]	Number of serotypes	Incidence (% of infections)	Comments
Viruses			
Rhinoviruses	100+	60	Year round with autumn and spring peaks
Coronaviruses	2	15	Year round, winter peaks
Influenza viruses	3	$1-10^b$	Annual epidemic
Parainfluenza viruses	4	$1-10^b$	Parainfluenza 1 & 2 winter peaks, parainfluenza 3 summer peak
Respiratory syncytial virus	2	$1-10^b$	Discrete yearly winter epidemic
Adenoviruses	47	$1-10^b$	Sporadic
Enteroviruses	40+	$1-10^b$	Sporadic
Atypical bacteria			
Mycoplasma pneumoniae	1	$1-10^b$	5-yearly epidemic cycle
Chlamydia pneumoniae	1	$1-10^b$	New organism, true incidence uncertain

[a] Each agent has been reviewed in detail in Myint S, Taylor-Robinson D, eds. Viral and Other Infections of the Human Respiratory Tract. London: Chapman Hall, 1996.
[b] Variable incidence depending on age, immunity, and seasonality.

ment is essential if any benefit is to ensue). An accurate and timely viral diagnosis is required for appropriate targeting of specific antiviral therapies. Other obstacles include the rapid mutation rates of viruses leading to the emergence of resistant strains (3,4), difficulties with drug delivery, expense, and efficacy of candidate drugs. These problems have in the past persuaded many pharmaceutical companies to abandon research programs. However, there is now renewed interest because of the increasing appreciation of the morbidity and mortality associated with these infections both in asthma and other chronic cardiorespiratory diseases, particularly chronic obstructive pulmonary disease (COPD).

This chapter will briefly review the epidemiology and morbidity associated with common cold virus infections, the mechanisms involved in virus-induced asthma exacerbations, and will discuss recent advances made in the development of both specific antiviral therapies and the alternative approaches of attempting to downregulate the inflammatory responses to these viral infections.

II.   Epidemiology and Complications

The common cold is probably the most frequent illness afflicting mankind. Upper respiratory tract infections are the most common of the respiratory tract infections in community-based studies (5). Respiratory tract infections are the number one cause of consultations with primary care medical practitioners (6,7). The majority of these are upper respiratory tract infections such as the common cold (8). Respiratory tract infections are estimated to cost $10–15 billion in the United States annually (9,10) and are associated with significant industrial and school absenteeism (10), accounting for an estimated 150 million lost workdays annually (9). Based on current estimates, adults are thought to have an average of two to five per annum (11), school-aged children 8–12 (12), with infants suffering even more frequently (10). Numerous factors influence the epidemiology of viral upper respiratory tract infections including individual and community immunity, seasonal variation, smoking, psychological stress, socioeconomic factors such as nutrition, population density, and family structure. It is well known that preschool and school-aged children are the most frequent introducers of new viruses into families. In addition to the common cold, upper respiratory viral infections are associated with more severe lower respiratory symptoms and reductions in lung function in asthmatic compared to normal subjects (13). Virus infections have been associated with as many as 85% of exacerbations of asthma in children (12) and 40–60% of exacerbations in adults (14). Other common complications include otitis media (15) and sinusitis (16), and lower respiratory tract infections such as bronchitis, pneumonia (17) and exacerbations of COPD (18). Detailed epidemiological studies have not so far been carried out to enable accurate quantification of the risk for individual agents except influenza, for which the excess deaths associated with epidemics and pandemics are well described (19).

III. Mechanisms of Virus-Induced Inflammation

The symptoms of the common cold principally involve rhinorrhea, resulting from vascular leakage and later mucus secretion (20); nasal blockage, chiefly a result of mucosal edema consequent upon vascular engorgement and inflammatory cell infiltration; general malaise and fever, thought to result from systemic proinflammatory cytokine release; and cough resulting from neural pathway activation combined with increased mucus production. Sore throat, probably resulting in part from local inflammatory mediator release, is also a common symptom.

A. Inflammatory Mediators

Several studies have looked for inflammatory mediators in upper respiratory tract infections: kinins (21), histamine (in atopic subjects) (20), and leukotriene C_4 (22) have been detected in nasal secretions. More recently several cytokines including interleukin (IL)-1, -6, -10, -11, -16, granulocyte colony-stimulating factor (G-CSF), tumor necrosis factor α (TFN-α), interferon-α (IFN-α) as well as the chemokines IL-8, RANTES, and macrophage inflammatory protein 1α (MIP1α) have all been found in the nasal secretions of subjects with common colds (23–29).

B. Inflammatory Cell Infiltration

Neutrophil infiltration and peripheral blood leukopenia have long been recognized in upper respiratory tract infections. Grunberg has demonstrated increased neutrophil numbers and IL-8 secretion as well as an association with induction of bronchial hyperresponsiveness in asthmatic subjects undergoing experimental rhinovirus infection (30). Teran studied children with naturally occurring asthma exacerbations and noted increased nasal aspirate IL-8 production, increased myeloperoxidase levels (a marker of neutrophil activation), and a correlation between IL-8 levels and severity of upper respiratory symptoms (31). These studies together implicate neutrophil activation in the pathogenesis of virus-associated asthma and suggest that blocking IL-8 production or activity could be a productive therapeutic approach.

Levandowski demonstrated elevated numbers of lymphocytes in nasal secretions using flow cytometry (32). However studies in nasal biopsies have failed to demonstrate a mucosal lymphocytosis during common colds (33). This may be because of technical problems such as the timing of the biopsies, or because inflammatory cell infiltrates are not important in producing nasal congestion directly. In contrast, in the lower airway, $CD3^+$, $CD4^+$, and $CD8^+$lymphocyte infiltration has been demonstrated in the bronchial mucosa of normal and asthmatic subjects undergoing experimental rhinovirus infection (34). The mechanisms regulating this lymphocyte infiltration have not yet been clarified. However, it is likely that, following virus infection of respiratory epithelial cells; local induction of lymphocyte chemotactic and activating factors such as IL-16 and RANTES leading to a chemotactic gradient attracting lymphocytes to the airway plays an important role (27). Eosinophils and eosinophil products, such as eosinophil cationic protein and major basic protein, have also been implicated in virus-associated wheezing episodes (35,36). A bronchial mucosal eosinophilia has been demonstrated during experimental colds in both normal and asthmatic subjects (34). Calhoun also demonstrated an impressive eosinophilia in response to allergen challenge in the context of rhinovirus experimental infections (37). Again the chemotactic factors regulating the eosinophil infiltrate in this context have not been clarified, but a number of candidates exist, including G-CSF, RANTES, and eotaxin (27,29). These data suggest that, in addition to antiviral therapy, factors regulating inflammatory cell infiltration in to the airway during virus-induced asthma may be attractive targets for therapeutic intervention.

C. Upper Versus Lower Airways: Drug Delivery

The optimal route of drug delivery for treatment of the common cold has not been established in the absence of adequate treatment. For many years it has been thought that treatment should only need to be effective at the level of the upper respiratory tract and could therefore be effectively delivered by nasal spray. However, the high frequency of lower respiratory tract complications of common colds, such as cough, acute bronchitis, and exacerbations of asthma and COPD, suggests that common cold viruses usually infect the lower as well as the upper respiratory tract. A number of studies have confirmed this to be the case for rhinoviruses (29,38,39), although no similar studies have been carried out for other common cold viruses, particularly coronaviruses. This information strongly suggests that for both antiviral and nonspecific treatment drugs would ideally need to be delivered to the lower airways as well as the upper. The oral route should achieve both and is therefore the preferred mode of delivery as long as absorption, tissue penetration, drug interactions, and side effects/toxicity permit it. Indeed the options are frequently directed more by the pharmokokinetics of the drug than by choice, as is the case with the anti-influenza drugs zanamivir, which is not absorbed orally; and oseltamivir, which is. This has provided an interesting opportunity to study the efficacy of intranasal combined with orally inhaled zanamivir compared with that of orally delivered oseltamivir. As will be discussed later in this chapter, orally inhaled zanamivir was just as effective as intranasal combined with orally inhaled and efficacy was comparable to the orally delivered oseltamivir. This suggests that, at least for influenza, lower-airway delivery alone is sufficient. Similar studies will be required with new antiviral therapies for other respiratory viruses as they emerge.

The site of drug delivery could be particularly relevant for anti-inflammatory treatments if the local effects of treatment could be potentially beneficial in reducing the symptoms of the common cold. Conversely, the effects of anti-inflammatory treatments may be less desirable if they reduce host immunity. While the value to the host of the inflammatory response associated with respiratory tract infections remains poorly understood, this issue will remain unresolved.

D. Acute Therapy Versus Prophylaxis

The demand for acute therapy of the common cold remains extremely high as evidenced by the high rates of physician consultation, prescription of antibiotics, and widespread use of over the counter preparations as well as so-called alternative and health medicines. There are also a number of reasons why prophylaxis remains a key target for drug development. The prevention of disease offers the greatest potential benefit in prevention of morbidity and mortality associated with respiratory viral infections. This is particularly true for at-risk populations including asthmatics, those with chronic heart and lung disease, the elderly, and those living in crowded conditions where the spread of viruses is facilitated. Prophylactic treatment of household or work contacts could have an enormous effect in terms of reducing the morbidity in the community, with massive cost savings for the state and industry. A major problem of specific antiviral therapy is the difficulty in identifying the causative pathogen early enough to provide effective prophylaxis. While empirical decisions can be made based on the local epidemiology for a given virus, this has a limited specificity, at best approaching 70% in clinical trials of influenza (40). The specificity of a clinical diagnosis would be significantly less for other common cold viruses, particularly in average day-to-day medical practice. Should cost-effective, rapid, near-patient diagnostic tests be developed this would potentially be a key area for their use. The following therapies have been demonstrated to be effective in preventing virus infection when given prophylactically: interferon, neuraminidase inhibitors and the adamantanes. Although these agents are highly effective, the side effects of interferons have prohibited their use, as discussed below. The neuraminidase inhibitors are effective for the prophylaxis of influenza caused by influenza A and B but require an early diagnosis for an illness that is indistinguishable from that caused by the remainder of pathogens responsible for the common colds. This limitation is even more relevant to the adamantanes, which are effective only against influenza A, albeit the more common of the two and more likely to cause more severe illness.

IV. Therapeutic Options

A major obstacle to the more widespread use of antiviral therapies has been their specificity. Specific antiviral therapies ideally need to be used in the context of rapid viral diagnosis. For the majority of agents, especially the most common (rhinoviruses and coronaviruses) presently available methods are inadequate. The development of the polymerase chain reaction (PCR) for viral diagnosis may change this, and make early diagnosis and appropriate specific treatment possible in the future (12). This is especially important, as even in influenza type A epidemics and respiratory syncytial (RS) virus bronchiolitis, the contribution of rhinovirus infections is being increasingly recognized (41,42). The knowledge that rhinoviruses are responsible for around 60% of colds has made them a particularly attractive target for therapy. Many compounds have been studied that inhibit rhinoviral infection by preventing virus uncoating or virus entry into the cell, or that inhibit various stages in virus replication once the virus has gained entry to the cell. Most of the early compounds were abandoned because of a combination of factors. The most important of these are limitations in drug potency and delivery, drug toxicity (viruses are dependent on host cell machinery to replicate; compounds that are toxic to viruses can also often be toxic to humans), and the emergence of resistant viruses (3). Many therapies for the common cold have been tried, although none so far has been very successful.

A. Over-the-Counter Remedies

Vitamin C

Perhaps the most controversial treatment of the common cold has been vitamin C, which has been extensively investigated. A recent review claims that consuming vitamin C can reduce the duration of illness by an average of 1 day (43). A systematic review of 30 clinical trials found that even prolonged courses of high-dosage vitamin C had "no consistent beneficial effect on the incidence of the common cold." This review did confirm that both preventative and therapeutic trials of vitamin C appear to reduce the cold symptom days by 8–9%, representing a reduction of half a day per cold (44).

Zinc

Zinc gluconate has also been shown to reduce symptom duration by 2 days. The mechanism is unknown, although it is possible that it has an antiviral effect (45).

In a systematic review of seven randomized controlled studies performed between 1984 and 1997 investigating the role of zinc as treatment for the common cold, the authors found the evidence to be inconclusive with conflicting data and methodological differences between the different studies (46). Treatment with zinc was found not to reduce the duration of the common cold in this meta-analysis that included studies showing benefit and those without. One possible explanation for the contradictory results that has been suggested is that some studies have used inadequate dosages or incorrect formulations. More recent studies investigating the effect of zinc on common colds addressed this issue. A small randomized, double-blind, placebo-controlled study involved 50 patients taking either placebo or 12.8 mg zinc acetate (every 2–3 h while awake) within 24 h of developing common cold symptoms and taken thereafter for the duration of symptoms. It found a statistically significant reduction in the overall duration of symptoms (4.5 vs. 8.1 days, $p < 0.01$). There was also a $>50\%$ reduction in cough (3.1 [95% confidence interval] (CI), 2.1–4.1] vs. 6.3 [CI, 4.9–7.7] days), a significant reduction in nasal discharge, and decreased severity of overall symptoms ($p < 0.002$) in favor of zinc (47). Although this treatment was required to be taken very frequently, it did demonstrate impressive results. The role of zinc requires further study, particularly in the light of evidence from the same investigators indicating that zinc deficiency may be related to impaired antiviral immunity (48).

Echinacea

Echinacea, a plant extract and popular herbal remedy, has been reported to be beneficial for the treatment of common cold symptoms due to immunomodulatory effects (49). The results of published data are conflicting, with studies using both different Echinacea preparations and study designs (50;51). Echinacea was found to be ineffective in the prevention or therapy of human rhinovirus infection in a study of experimental HRV23 infection, in which volunteers (n = 92) were treated with either placebo or Echinacea 300 mg three times per day for 2 weeks prior to virus challenge and for 5 days subsequently (51). More recently a systematic review of Echinacea reviewed 16 trials. The majority of studies found positive results in favor of Echinacea in the prevention and treatment of upper respiratory tract infections (52). This at best weak recommendation suggests a limited role for Echinacea. However, firm conclusions cannot be drawn in view of the great variability in dosages and preparations studied so far.

Nasal Decongestants

Numerous nasal decongestants (sympathomimetic amines and imidazoline derivatives) are marketed for the relief of nasal blockage, which is a common symptom of the common cold. These drugs act by constricting nasal mucosa vessels, relieving the congestion due to sinusoidal vasodilatation. A recent meta-analysis of four randomized placebo-controlled trials of oral and topical nasal decongestants (all of which were performed in adults with common cold), showed a significant reduction in subjective symptoms and nasal airways resistance after a single dose of active treatment. Repeated doses, however, were found to be no better than placebo at relieving nasal congestion. The overall conclusion was that there was no evidence to support use over several days, nor could treatment be recommended in young children due to a lack of studies in patients in this age group (53).

Antihistamines

Although early studies failed to show any elevation of histamine levels in common colds (54), more recent studies have found an increase (55), particularly among atopic subjects (20). Furthermore it has been suggested that the effect of antihistamines may be related to anticholinergic activity in earlier-generation compounds that have an atropine-like action on nasal mucosa (56). Randomized, placebo-controlled experimental human rhinovirus (HRV) infection studies in healthy volunteers studies have demonstrated a reduction in rhinorrhea, sneezing, and nasal secretion weight only with first-generation compounds. Chlorpheniramine was found to reduce sneezing and nasal mucus weights compared to placebo but had no effect on the objective measures of nasal congestion in one experimental HRV infection randomized controlled trial (57). An earlier experimental infection randomized controlled trial investigating oral chlorpheniramine found no effect on nasal symptoms and mucus production (58). Clemastine fumarate (1.34 mg twice daily) reduced sneeze severity score, sneeze counts, rhinorrhea, and nasal secretion weights but was associated with a high incidence of side effects (dry mouth 6%, dry nose 19%, dry throat 17%) (59). Brompheniramine maleate (12 mg twice daily) significantly reduced total symptom scores on days 1 and 2 and cough on day 1 but with more adverse effects particularly somnolence (60). Overall, antihistamine treatment in common colds has shown relatively little benefit, with significant side effects (56,58,61), a conclusion that was supported in a critical review of studies published since 1975 (62). Since these studies, more potent nonsedating antihistamines have been introduced. These have the potential benefit of reduced side effects and they reduce epithelial cell intracellular adhesion molecule1 (ICAM-1) expression in vitro (63). These compounds appear ineffective in common cold studies (64). Given the role of ICAM-1 in inflammation and as the cellular receptor for major group rhinoviruses, it would be interesting to reassess these compounds, particularly in virus-induced wheezing episodes.

B. Nonspecific Remedies

Anticholinergics

Anticholinergic nasal sprays have been shown to reduce rhinorrhea and sneezing in naturally occurring common colds (65,66). Atropine methonitrate administered intranasally in two separate small studies using different dosages (125 µg three times daily and 250 µg four times daily) in randomized placebo-controlled experimental HRV39 infection studies found that the higher dosage was associated with a reduction in nasal mucus production and nasal dryness (67). A slightly larger (n = 63) randomized placebo-controlled HRV39 experimental infection study using intranasal ipratropium bromide administered three times per day was associated with lower nasal mucus weights and rhinorrhea scores compared to placebo, although these did not reach statistical significance. Overall total nasal symptom scores were similar in the two groups (68). These data suggest that anticholinergics at best have potential for partial symptomatic relief of the common cold. They could also be suited for use in combination products.

Hyperthermic Treatment

An interesting treatment that has been tested is the inhalation of humidified hot air at 43°C, which has been shown to reduce the severity of symptoms in natural and experimental common colds (69). The effect of hyperthermic treatment has subsequently been disputed after further studies were unable to demonstrate an improvement in symptoms (70,71) or on viral shedding (72). The mechanism of the hyperthermic anti-HRV effect is unknown. However, the profound inhibitory effect of hyperthermia on HRV replication in HeLa cells has been associated with the production of hsp70, a heat shock protein postulated to be involved in cytoprotective intracellular defense mechanisms during HRV infection (73). The role of pyrexia and heat shock proteins are potential targets for common cold treatment strategies. They also have theoretical potential in virus infections in allergic individuals, since hyperthermia has also been shown to have beneficial effects in allergic rhinitis and asthma (74,75).

C. Antibiotics

The role of antibiotics in the treatment of the common cold should be obvious: as a predominantly viral and self-limiting illness, treatment with antibiotics is both counterintuitive and unnecessary. However, there is evidence that macrolide antibiotics have an anti-inflammatory effect inhibiting both cytokine production (IL-6) (76) and the production of ICAM-1 (77). The macrolide antibiotic bafilomycin A_1 is a vacuolar ATPase inhibitor that blocks HRV and influenza virus infection in vitro. Vacuolar ATPases are ATP-driven proton pumps that acidify eukaryotic cell intracellular compartments. This process is necessary for numerous essential cell functions and for entry of many viruses into their host cells. The mechanism of the anti-HRV activity was confirmed by demonstrating reduced HRV14 titers in infected human tracheal epithelial cells with inhibition of virus-induced cytokine, NFκB and ICAM-1 due to bafilomycin A_1 (78). An antiviral effect for another macrolide antibiotic has been reported in vitro (79) with the inhibition of rhinovirus (RV14) infection of human tracheal epithelial cell cultures by erythromycin.

An antiviral effect was not been found in vivo in a double-blind placebo-controlled study of healthy volunteers with experimental HRV16 infection: no significant difference was found in cold symptoms or the degree of neutrophilic nasal inflammation when treated with clarithromycin (80). Furthermore, a recent Cochrane review of seven trials with over 2000 adults and children does not support the use of antibiotics for the treatment of the common cold. Overall the studies do not demonstrate an improvement or higher rates of cure in the antibiotic limbs of these placebo-controlled studies. Only two studies evaluated the effect of antibiotics on purulent nasal discharge, with conflicting results. There was also a significant increase in side effects in those receiving antibiotics (OR 2.72, CI 1.02–7.27) (81).

The in vitro data suggest that macrolide antibiotics do have an antiviral effect, and the mechanisms by which this occurs require further investigation. It remains to be established whether this would have any clinical benefit and whether the benefit may be specific to groups at risk such as asthmatics. Until further controlled studies clarify these issues the prescription of antibiotics for upper respiratory tract infections is not recommended.

D. Anti-Inflammatory Agents

Anti-Inflammatory Versus Antiviral

The majority of treatments for the common cold are symptomatic. These treatments are often directed toward reducing the inflammatory response mounted against the virus responsible. A major advantage is that the treatment is not specific to the pathogen and can be taken even when viral titers are falling when antiviral therapies would have no benefit, but when anti-inflammatory treatment may still have symptomatic benefit. The potential disadvantage is that the inflammatory response may also have beneficial effects, which on being suppressed could increase viral replication. This theory is supported by data on steroids on which treatment has been shown to be associated with higher viral titers (82). Anti-inflammatories have no role in reducing spread to contacts and are less likely than antivirals to be successful for prophylaxis, except perhaps in those with underlying inflammatory diseases such as asthma and COPD.

An important benefit of antiviral treatment is that the source of infection is addressed directly, thereby reducing both the inflammatory response and the infectivity of the illness. Additional potential advantages are that the same agent can be used for both therapy and prophylaxis. Again, a major obstacle is the problem of identifying the causative pathogen early enough in the natural history of the illness. A further theoretical problem with both antiviral and anti-inflammatory treatment is that it could result in loss of the protective immune response resulting in increased susceptibility to serotypes of an organism they would otherwise have been immune to. To date, data from trials with the neuraminidase inhibitors (83) and with pleconaril (84) suggest that this is not a problem with antiviral therapy where there was no loss in protective immune responses with equally high seroconversion rates in both treatment and placebo arms.

Corticosteroids

Corticosteroids are known to have widespread anti-inflammatory effects, including the reduction of inflammatory cell infiltration and cytokine production. The effectiveness of corticosteroids in therapy of the common cold has been assessed in randomized controlled trials. In one study, although they reduced inflammation and symptoms during the first 2 days of treatment, there appeared to be a rebound effect when treatment was stopped, and no overall benefit was demonstrated (85). In a second recent study comparing oral prednisolone and placebo in experimental rhinovirus infections, steroids were reported to reduce sneezing and mucus weights on day 1, but there was no overall difference in symptoms. Furthermore, steroids were associated with increased viral titers (82). The use of high-dosage oral steroids for the common cold is therefore clearly not justified, in view of their lack of efficacy and their known side effects.

Topical use of steroids has also been investigated. Intranasal corticosteroid (Fluticasone propionate 200 μg mcg QDS) had no marked positive effects on symptoms in naturally occurring common colds in adults compared to placebo in a randomized controlled trial. Active treatment was associated with reduced cough and nasal congestion on some days as well as persistent viral shedding (86), thus demonstrating the same patterns with oral steroid treatment.

Steroids may have a more effective and logical place in the treatment of virus-associated wheezing illness. There have been several recent studies of inhaled steroids in virus-associated wheeze in children of varying ages. High-dosage inhaled steroids started immediately on the onset of upper respiratory or lower respiratory symptoms have shown partial benefit (87,88), but other studies with lower-dosage prophylactic therapy have shown no benefit (89).

Nonsteroidal Anti-Inflammatories

Prostanoid inflammatory mediators have been detected in common colds and mimic many of the symptoms of common colds when administered topically. A recent study has also implicated this class of inflammatory mediators in the pathogenesis of the common cold by finding increased levels of the synthetic enzyme cyclooxygenase-2 (COX-2) regulating prostanoid synthetic pathways in experimental rhinovirus infections in normal subjects (90). A simple treatment such as the antiprostaglandin, nonsteroidal anti-inflammatories (NSAIDS) would therefore seem a logical choice for the treatment and amelioration of symptoms. Naproxen, a cyclo-oxygenase inhibitor, was investigated in a randomized double-blind placebo-controlled experimental HRV study (n = 79) in which treatment was taken for 5 days following viral challenge. There was no difference in the viral titers or antibody response in the two arms. However, symptoms (headache, malaise, myalgia, and cough) were significantly reduced in the naproxen treated group with a 29% reduction in the 5 day total symptom score (91). Whether a similar magnitude of symptomatic benefit would be seen in patients who take treatment only when symptoms develop rather than early after exposure to virus would seem unlikely. As such it is possible the benefit reported in this study may be greater than would be observed in the clinical situation. However, these data suggest that NSAIDS may have a role to play for the partial relief of symptoms, most likely as a component in mixed preparations. NSAIDS may theoretically increase synthesis of leukotrienes, which are also implicated in the pathogenesis of common colds and virus-induced wheezing. Studies with the new generation COX-2 specific compounds would therefore be of great interest in both contexts.

Antileukotrienes

Leukotrienes have been implicated in virus-induced wheezing illness (92) but not until recently in the common cold alone (90). However, the study referred to above also showed increased expression of 5-lipoxygenase, the major enzyme regulating leukotriene synthesis in normal subjects undergoing rhinovirus infections (90). Clinical trials with leukotriene antagonists in virus-induced wheezing illness are now underway. Similar studies in the common cold would also be of great interest.

Bradykinin Antagonists

Elevated levels of kinins have been found in association with natural and experimental colds (21,93). However, only one small trial ($n = 22$) of a bradykinin antagonist (intranansal NPC 567) has been carried out in experimental rhinovirus colds. This study reported negative results, with the further suggestion that the drug exacerbated the symptoms (94). Further studies with more potent bradykinin antagonists are awaited.

Cromolyns

Cromolyns are antiallergic and anti-inflammatory drugs with effects on mast cells, eosinophils, epithelial cells, and sensory nerves. There are two in use clinically at present, and their mechanism of action is thought to involve inhibition of chloride channels (95). Intranasal nedocromil sodium reduces symptoms and improves psychomotor performance in experimental colds (96). A recent study of intranasal and inhaled sodium cromoglycate in adults with symptoms of a common cold for less than 24 h showed that patients treated with cromoglycate for 7 days produced swifter resolution of symptoms and reduced the severity of symptoms in the last 3 days of treatment. The treatment was very well tolerated with no significant side effects (97). These studies are encouraging in demonstrating an effect after symptoms had begun. The mechanisms involved in the protective effect of cromolyns in common colds are currently unknown.

MAP Kinase Inhibitors

The mitogen-activated protein (MAP) kinases are signal transduction mediators involved in the regulation of cytokine synthesis, cell apoptosis, and proliferation. p38 kinase, a serine–threonine MAP kinase is inhibited by pyridinyl imidazoles such as SB239063 and SB203580 (MAP kinase inhibitors). The role of p38 kinase in virus-induced cytokine induction and regulation was recently reported in vitro, in which infection of bronchial epithelial cell cultures by HRV39 was associated with a time- and dose-dependent increase in p38 kinase phosphorylation. Treatment of infected cells with MAP kinase inhibitors resulted in inhibition of cytokine production (IL-6, IL-8, G-CSF, GM-CSF, GRO$\propto$ and ENA-78). However, there was no inhibition of viral replication seen (98). These early data provide further insight into the regulation of virus induced cytokine induction in the pathogenesis of the common cold and may provide targets for drug development.

Combination Therapy

Gwaltney proposed that a combined antiviral, anticholinergic, and anti-inflammatory effect would be required for effective suppression of common cold symptoms, since these agents appear poorly effective on their own (99). He studied intranasal IFN-α combined with intranasal ipratropium (an anticholinergic) and oral naproxen (an NSAID) begun 24 h after experimental rhinovirus infection. An antiviral effect was demonstrated. Virus shedding was significantly reduced and the mean virus titer was also reduced. The number of clinical colds, the mean symptom score, mucus secretion, cough, and general malaise were all significantly reduced in treated subjects and the medications were well tolerated. The symptom that was least effectively treated in this study was sneezing, as antihistamines are effective at treating sneezing in allergic rhinitis, their addition to the cocktail tested above may render it more effective.

This has also been recently tested. A randomized, controlled, clinical trial was conducted with a combination of intranasal IFN-α2b (6 $\times 10^6$ U every 12 h) plus oral chlorpheniramine (12 mg extended release) and ibuprofen (400 mg) every 12 h for 4.5 days ($n = 59$ subjects) compared with intranasal placebo and oral chlorpheniramine and ibuprofen ($n = 61$ subjects) or intranasal and oral placebos ($n = 30$ subjects). Treatment was started 24 h after intranasal rhinovirus challenge in healthy men and women (aged 18–51 years). During the 4.5 days of treatment with IFN-α2b, chlorpheniramine, and ibuprofen, the daily mean total symptom score was reduced by 33–73%, compared with placebo. Treatment reduced the severity of rhinorrhea, sneezing, nasal obstruction, sore throat, cough, and headache and reduced nasal mucus production, nasal tissue use, and virus concentrations in nasal secretions. IFN-α2b added to the effectiveness of chlorpheniramine and ibuprofen and was well tolerated (100). These studies suggest that the use of combined therapies should be investigated in naturally occurring common colds.

E. Licensed Antiviral Therapies

The only specific virus antagonists currently licensed for use are those active against influenza A and B (zanamivir and oseltamivir), influenza type A (amantidine and rimantidine), and RS virus (ribavarin).

Adamantanes

Amantidine and rimantidine are the two licensed adamantanes. Amantidine was discovered in 1964 and is an acyclic amine. Rimantidine is a methylated derivative that does not cross the blood–brain barrier, and therefore does not induce the jitteriness sometimes associated with amantidine. Both compounds are thought to act after virus–cell attachment, but before uncoating, probably by interfering with ion flux mediated via the M2 protein (101). Amantidine and rimantidine are effective only against influenza type A, and are recommended for prophylactic and therapeutic use only in the presence of clear virological and epidemiological evidence of influenza A infection in the community. They should be used prophylactically for 6–8 weeks by at-risk populations such as the elderly, those with chronic ill health (including asthma or chronic bronchitis), those within community groups and health care workers in frequent contact with influenza (whether vaccinated or not). In these situations they prevent 23% of clinical cases and 63% of cases of serologically confirmed influenza A (102). Therapy for patients with a clinical diagnosis of influenza should be initiated in the first 24–48 h of symptoms and given for 10 days. These agents reduce the duration of symptoms by 1–2 days overall if commenced early, a finding confirmed in a recent meta-analysis (102). These drugs should not replace vaccination, as they are inactive against influenza type B.

The adamantanes have had limited clinical use because of a combination of factors. Although influenza A is considered more important clinically, because its infections are considered more severe as well as occurring more frequently than influenza B (103), the isolated anti-influenza A action requires that attending physicians be up to date with local seroprevalence rates of influenza infection. There are also a number of side effects, particularly gastrointestinal and central nervous system symptoms. These side effects stop with discontinuation of treatment and are limited by using lower dosages. The rapid emergence of resistance has been associated with treatment failure and is another reason for low prescription rates.

Neuraminidase Inhibitors

Uncomplicated influenza is characterized by the abrupt onset of constitutional and respiratory signs and symptoms (fever, malaise, myalgia, headache, nonproductive cough, sore throat, and rhinorrhea)(104). Outbreaks of influenza occur nearly every year during the winter months in temporal climates. During typical outbreaks 10–20% of the population develop serological evidence of infection (105). Among at-risk groups such as the elderly and those with chronic respiratory disease the risk for hospitalization may approach 1:300 and the risk of death in those hospitalized 1:15 (105). Influenza is a well-described trigger for asthma attacks in all age groups (12,14,106,107). During the 1957 Asian influenza pandemic excess deaths were identified in young asthmatics (108,109). Influenza A and B viruses are highly infectious and spread by respiratory secretions. The virus replicates throughout the respiratory tract causing widespread damage to the respiratory epithelium even in apparently mild cases. Viral replication peaks early (within 48 h of infection) in normal individuals and the systemic symptoms of influenza are due to the host immune response.

Influenza viruses enter cells by the interaction of its surface coat protein hemagglutinin with sialic acid on the surface of the host cell. This leads to viral entry into the cell inside a small vesicle. Once inside a host cell vesicle, the influenza viruses M2 protein acts as an ion channel and alters the surrounding vesicles pH. The hemagglutinin undergoes a pH change-induced change in structure, which allows virus–host cell fusion. Viral RNA then enters the host cell leading to the production of new viral genes, messenger RNA, and proteins. Influenza exits via the luminal surface of the respiratory epithelial cell, and as it leaves it is enveloped in host cell membrane. Because the host cell membranes have sialic acid molecules embedded in them, the emerging viruses form inactive bunches. Neuraminidase, the second influenza surface coat protein, functions as a glycohydrolase enzyme and cleaves the sialic acid molecules from the new (host-cell-derived) viral surface membrane allowing viral escape (110). Neuraminidase also inactivates sialic acid present in respiratory mucus, thus increasing influenza virus infectivity (111).

Neuraminidase inhibitors block the actions described above, and thus decrease the capacity of influenza viruses to infect respiratory cells. Attempts have been made for at least 20 years to block the function of influenza neuraminidase. A major step forward in drug design occurred following the resolution of the three-dimensional structure of neuraminidase (112) and the identification and characterization of its active site (113). This work revealed that the active site in the molecule contained 11 key amino acids that are unchanged among all known naturally occurring influenza viruses (114,115). This finding suggested that any drug that could inhibit this site would have a broad action against influenza A and B viruses. Using a computer modeling program, chemists designed 4-guanidino-NeuAc2en (zanamivir) specifically to inactivate this site (116). Zanamivir binds to influenza neuraminidase with high specificity (116) and is at least $100\times$ more potent than amantadine in vitro when tested against a panel of H1N1, H2N2, H3N2 influenza A, and influenza B viruses (117). Zanamivir is poorly absorbed orally and is therefore administered by inhalation. It is thought to function topically. Following inhalation 7–21 % of the administered drug reaches the bronchi and lungs, 70–87% is deposited in the oropharynx (118). Approximately 4–17% of the total administered dose is systemically absorbed (119). Systemically absorbed zanamivir has a half life of 2.5–5.1 h and is excreted unchanged in the urine (119). Zanamivir is believed to have few drug interactions and dosage reduction is not required in patients with renal or hepatic failure or in the elderly (118–121). Even though only approximately 13% of the drug reaches the lower respiratory tract, the resulting concentration of zanamivir in the lung is $1000\times$ in excess of the in vitro IC_{50} (118).

In contrast to zanamivir, the second neuraminidase inhibitor oseltamivir is administered orally. As oseltamivir carboxylate, the active compound has low oral bioavailability (122). It is administered as an ethyl ester prodrug oseltamivir that undergoes rapid metabolism to the active parent drug in the liver following absorption (118). Oseltamivir also inhibits the action of neuraminidase by binding to its active site. Binding affinity is enhanced by the presence of a lipophilic side chain that binds to a hydrophobic pocket in the active site of neuraminidase (123). Oseltamivir is also highly selective for influenza neuraminidase (124). Following oral administration peak plasma concentrations occur within 2.5–6 h. Among patients with impaired renal function, serum concentrations of oseltamivir increase with declining renal function (125).

F. Treatment with Neuraminidase Inhibitors

Zanamivir

The clinical efficacy of zanamivir has been reported in several placebo-controlled randomized controlled trials. These trials were all conducted in patients with influenza-like symptoms for less than 48 h (less than 36 h in the MIST study). Monto and co-workers compared zanamivir 10 mg inhaled and 6.4 mg by nasal drops in twice- and four-times daily regimens with placebo (126). In the intention to treat group (ITT, n = 834) zanamivir decreased the duration of clinically significant symptoms by a median of 1 day compared to placebo (equivalent to a 14% reduction, p < 0.02). There was no significant difference between two and four times a day regimens, and in all later studies the drug was admnistered twice daily. In patients receiving zanamivir twice a day who were febrile at enrollment (>37.8 °C, n = 155) a 1.5 day difference was reported compared to placebo (21% reduction, p < 0.05).

Hayden and colleagues compared inhaled zanamivir 10 mg twice daily, inhaled zanamivir plus nasal zanamivir 6.4 mg twice daily and placebo (127). They found no significant difference between inhaled zanamivir alone and combined inhaled and nasal administration, and in all future studies the drug was only administered by oral inhalation. In this study in the ITT group (*n* = 132) inhaled zanamivir alone reduced the duration of clinically significant symptoms by a mean of 0.7 days compared to placebo (11.5% reduction, p < 0.05). In patients febrile at enrollment (*n* = 46) a 1.5 day difference was reported (22% reduction, p = 0.01). In patients treated within 30 h (*n* = 43), zanamivir reduced symptoms by 1.9 days compared to placebo (27% reduction, p = 0.001).

In the MIST study, a phase III trial, 10 mg twice daily inhaled zanamivir was compared with placebo (128). On an ITT analysis (*n* = 228) zanamivir reduced the duration of clinically significant symptoms by a median of 1.5 days (equivalent to a 23% reduction, p = 0.01). In patients febrile at enrollment (*n* = 128), zanamivir reduced symptoms by 2 days (31% reduction, p < 0.001). Zanamivir shortened the time to return to normal activities by 2 days (p < 0.001). The MIST study included 76 high-risk patients (57 had a respiratory disorders [mostly mild asthma], 14 were >65 years, 11 had an endocrine or metabolic disorder, 8 had a cardiovascular disorder other than hypertension, and 2 were immunocompromised). High-risk patients treated with zanamivir had fewer complications than placebo (placebo 18/39, zanamivir 5/37, difference 32%, p = 0.004). High-risk patients treated with zanamivir used fewer antibiotics than placebo (placebo 15/39, zanamivir 5/37, difference 25% p = 0.025).

Makela and colleagues also compared 10 mg twice daily inhaled zanamivir to placebo (129). The trial included 455 subjects, 55% of whom were febrile at enrollment. In the ITT population zanamivir reduced the duration of clinically significant symptoms by a median of 2.5 days (p < 0.001) over placebo.

A pooled analysis of all material from phase II and III studies (130) showed that the time for alleviation of clinically significant symptoms was reduced from 6 days in the placebo group (*n* = 1102) to 5 days in the treatment group (*n* = 1133) (p < 0.001). Overall there was a 1 day benefit in patients not considered severely ill (*n* = 555 zanamivir and *n* = 543 placebo, p < 0.001) and a 3 day benefit in those considered severely ill at enrollment (*n* = 252 zanamivir and n = 222 placebo, p < 0.001). A 3 day benefit was seen in those >50 years old (p = 0.003), compared to a 1 day benefit in those less than 50 (p < 0.001).

Hedrick and co-workers have investigated the efficacy of zanamivir in children aged 5–12 years (131). In this study zanamivir reduced the median time to symptom alleviation by 1.25 days compared to placebo in patients with confirmed influenza (p < 0.001), and by 1 day in ITT group (p = 0.002).

In the trials discussed above a total of 1,334 patients received zanamivir. Adverse events in all three trials were comparable to placebo and where symptoms were reported they were very similar to the classic symptoms of influenza. Recently it has been reported that elderly subjects have difficulty using the diskhaler used to administer zanamivir, which may limit the use of the drug in the elderly (132). A meta-analysis of zanamivir in high-risk patients (133) (69% with respiratory disease) revealed a treatment benefit of 2.5 days compared to placebo (p = 0.015) and a reduction in the use of antibiotics for complications of 43% (p = 0.045). Adverse events were similar between the two groups.

A pooled analysis of the effectiveness of zanamivir in patients with asthma and COPD was carried out by Murphy and colleagues (134). They identified 525 subjects with asthma and/or COPD aged >12 years. In these subjects zanamivir reduced the median symptom duration time by 1.5 days (p = 0.009) and reduced the overall influenza assessment score compared to placebo (p = 0.004). A similar frequency and pattern of adverse events were observed in the active treatment and placebo groups, and no adverse effect was seen on pulmonary function. Patients treated with zanamivir had a significant increase in mean morning peak expiratory flow rate (PEFR) (mean adjusted for baseline 346.1 vs. 333 L/min, p = 0.011) and mean evening PEFR (mean adjusted for baseline 357.0 vs. 343.9 L/min, p = 0.007) compared with the placebo during the treatment period (days 1–5).

The issue of the safety of zanamivir in patients with respiratory disease has been raised. There have been a few case reports of severe bronchospasm following treatment with zanamivir, including a case of severe respiratory distress in a 63-year-old man with oxygen-dependent COPD (135). It is of course extremely difficult to separate the effects of influenza virus infection itself (which is known to cause airway narrowing) from any putative effects of a drug used in the context of acute influenza infection. Using postmarketing surveillance data, the manufacturers of zanamivir estimate the risk of bronchospasm following administration of zanamivir via the diskhaler is to be less than 1 : 10,000 in normal subjects and 1 : 1,000–1 : 10,000 in asthmatic subjects. The latter figure is lower than the reported incidence of bronchospasm following administration of other commonly used inhaled therapies (e.g., 1% asthma associated with Seretide [Seretide product monograph, Allen & Hanbury's Stockley Park West, Uxbridge, UK]. These safety concerns have been recently reviewed by a panel of experts. They concluded that use of zanamivir in patients with asthma or COPD with influenza was associated with reduced respiratory adverse events and that the drug should continue to be used in those high risk groups that need it most: patients with asthma and COPD (136). UK guidelines issued by the Department of Health (www.doh.gov.uk//zanimivirguidance/index.htm) in conjunction with the National Institute for Clinical Excellence (NICE, November 2000) (www.nice.org.uk) likewise recommend zanamivir for at-risk adults who are able to take the medication within 48 h of symptom onset. The at-risk population is defined as: those over 65, those with chronic respiratory disease requiring medication, those with significant cardiovascular disease, the immunocompromised, and diabetics.

To date no influenza strains resistant to zanamivir have been detected in clinical trials despite intensive monitoring. There is one report of a zanamivir-resistant strain being found after prolonged treatment in an immunosuppressed child (137).

Oseltamivir

The efficacy of oseltamivir has been investigated in two double-blind randomized controlled trials (138) investigating 629 nonimmunized adults aged 18–65 years with a febrile illness of less than 36 h duration, a temperature of at least 38°C plus at least one respiratory and one constitutional symptom. They compared oral oseltamivir 7 mg twice daily and 150 mg twice daily with placebo. They showed a reduction in duration of illness by 30% with oseltamivir 75 mg twice daily (median 71.5 h, p < 0.001) and with 150 mg twice daily (median 69.9 h, p = 0.006) compared with placebo (median 103.3 h). They likewise showed a reduction in the severity of symptoms by 38% in patients receiving the 75 mg twice daily dose (p < 0.001). Complications requiring treatment were 7% in the combined oseltamivir groups and 15% in the placebo group (p = 0.03). However, upper gastrointestinal (GI) effects (nausea or nausea with vomiting) were 7.4 % for placebo and 17% for the 75 mg group and 19% for 150 mg groups (p = 0.002 and p < 0.001), respectively. Nicholson et al. (139) investigated 726 healthy nonimmunized adults with a febrile illness of up to 36 h duration. Duration of illness was shortened by treatment in influenza-positive patients : a 29 h (25%) reduction in the 75 mg b group (median duration 87.4 h, p = 0.02) and 35 h (30%) in the 150 mg group (median duration 81.8 h, p = 0.01) compared to placebo (median duration 116.5 h). Nausea and vomiting were again more common in the treatment groups (nausea: placebo 4% vs. 12% in both oseltamivir groups and vomiting: placebo 3% vs. 10%).

Whitley and colleagues investigated the efficacy of oral oseltamivir in children 1–12 years with fever (≥38°C) and a history of cough or coryza of <48 h duration in a randomized double-blind, placebo-controlled study (83). Subjects received oseltamivir 2 mg/kg or placebo twice daily for 5 days. Among infected children the median duration of illness was reduced by 36 h (26%) in oseltamivir compared with placebo recipients (101 h; 95% CI, 89–118 vs. 137 h; 95% CI, 125–150; p < 0.0001). Oseltamivir treatment also reduced cough, coryza, and duration of fever. New diagnoses of otitis media were reduced by 44% (12% vs. 21%). The incidence of physician-prescribed antibiotics was significantly lower in influenza-infected oseltamivir (68 of 217, 31%) than placebo (97 of 235, 41%, p = 0.03) recipients. Oseltamivir therapy was generally well tolerated, although associated with an excess frequency of emesis (5.8%). Discontinuation because of adverse events was low in both groups (1.8% with oseltamivir vs. 1.1% with placebo). Oseltamivir treatment did not affect the influenza-specific antibody response.

In challenge studies of human subjects infected with influenza virus, 3% of the posttreatment isolates showed emergence of influenza variants with decreased neuraminidase susceptibility to oseltamivir. Genetic analysis of these isolates showed that reduced susceptibility to oseltamivir is due to mutations in neuraminidase. In clinical studies of naturally acquired influenza 1.3% of posttreatment isolates showed emergence of variants with decreased susceptibility to oseltamivir (Roche product information 2001: http://www.rocheusa.com/products/tamiflu/pi _only.htm).

Summary of Clinical Trial Data

Both oseltamivir and zanamivir must be administered early in infection. There is little evidence for efficacy if the drugs are administered 48 h after symptoms develop in normal individuals. This reflects the fact that viral replication peaks within 48 h of infection in adults with an intact immune system. In the immunocompromised prolonged viral shedding is well recognized. One author (CG) has used zanamivir successfully 4 weeks after the onset of symptoms in a renal transplant patient with documented influenza B infection. In the clinical trials described above both drugs were more effective in febrile patients.

G. Prevention with Neuraminidase Inhibitors

Zanamivir

Two randomized controlled trials have investigated the role of zanamivir in the prevention of influenza. Monto and co-workers investigated 1107 healthy adults and randomized them to receive inhaled zanamivir 10 mg once per day for 4 weeks or placebo (126). Zanamivir was 67% efficacious in preventing laboratory-confirmed influenza ($p < 0.001$) and 87% efficacious in preventing laboratory-confirmed influenza with fever ($p = 0.03$). Adverse events did not differ between the two groups.

Hayden and colleagues enrolled families before the influenza season (140). If one family member developed influenza-like illness, the others were randomized to receive either zanamivir 10 mg for 10 days or placebo. The index case was treated with zanamivir 10 mg twice daily or placebo. The proportion of families with at least one initial healthy household contact in whom influenza developed was smaller in the zanamivir treatment group (4% vs. 19%, $p < 0.001$). This represents a 79% reduction in the proportion of families affected. Index cases receiving treatment had a 2.5 days shorter median duration of symptoms than the placebo group (5 vs. 7.5 days, $p = 0.01$). The study drug was well tolerated and there was no evidence of the emergence of resistant viruses.

Oseltamivir

Hayden and colleagues randomly assigned 1559 healthy nonimmunized adults aged 18–65 to receive either oral oseltamivir (75 mg od or twice daily) or placebo for 6 weeks during the peak period of local influenza virus activity (141). The risk of influenza among subjects assigned to either once or twice a day oseltamivir (1.2% and 1.3% respectively) was lower than among subjects who received placebo (4.8%, $p < 0.001$, and $p = 0.001$ for comparison with once and twice daily treatment). The protective efficacy overall was 74% and 87% for laboratory-confirmed influenza. Oseltamivir was well tolerated but associated with a greater frequency of nausea (12.1% and 14.6%, respectively, for once and twice a day treatment) than was placebo (7.1%). Vomiting occurred at rates of 2.5% and 2.7% vs. 0.8% in placebo group. However, the discontinuation rate was similar among all three groups (3.1–4%).

Welliver and co-workers (142) investigated the efficacy of oseltamivir in the prevention of influenza in household contacts of 377 index cases, of whom 43% had laboratory confirmed influenza. Household contacts (n = 955) aged >12 years of whom 415 were contacts of influenza-positive patients, were randomized to receive oral oseltamivir 75 mg od or placebo. In the contacts of influenza-positive cases the efficacy of oseltamivir was 89% for individuals (p < 0.001) and 84% for households (p < 0.001). In contacts of all index cases efficacy was 89% in preventing clinical influenza (p < 0.001). Gastrointestinal symptoms were similar in active treatment and placebo groups (9.3% vs. 7.2%).

What Can Be Achieved in Asthmatic Subjects?

Influenza is an important cause of asthma exacerbations during winter outbreaks (12,14,106,107). During pandemics death rates increase in asthmatics (108,109). This has led the UK Advisory Committee on Immunisation Practices (ACIP) (143) to recommend that all asthmatics should be vaccinated each winter against influenza. However, not all asthmatics are vaccinated (144), in part because some refuse vaccination because they perceive that the vaccine causes asthma exacerbations. Indeed bronchoprovocation tests show increased reactivity after vaccination (145,146) and anecdotal reports suggest an association between vaccination and exacerbation (147,148). A randomized placebo-controlled crossover trial on the effects of inactivated influenza vaccine on pulmonary function in asthma demonstrated that deterioration in lung function may rarely occur as a result of influenza vaccination. However, the risk was small and outweighed by the benefits of vaccination (149).

Vaccines are only 70–90% effective in young adults and 50% effective in the elderly (150). There is very good evidence for efficacy of neuraminidase inhibitors in the normal population (discussed in detail above). Since the drug works on the virus and not the host, there is little reason to believe the action will be less than in nonasthmatics. Moreover, what evidence there is from randomized controlled studies with zanamivir points to increased benefit of active treatment in patients with respiratory disease (although this included patients with COPD) (128,134). Bronchospasm associated with zanamivir appears to be a rare event and the incidence compares favorably with other inhaled therapies (e.g., 1% asthma associated with Seretide [Seretide product monograph, Allen & Hanbury's, Stockley Park West, Uxbridge, UK]).

Oseltamivir has recently been studied in influenza-like illness in asthmatic children aged 6–12 years. This randomized, double-blind, placebo-controlled study enrolled children with asthma requiring regular medical follow-up or hospital care who presented with influenza symptoms (fever ≥37.8°C with cough or coryza) of less than 48h duration. Children received either oseltamivir 2mg/kg or placebo twice daily for 5 days. Spirometry was measured at study entry and at the end of study treatment. Peak flow measurements were recorded daily in the morning for 28 days. Analysis was performed on children with laboratory-confirmed influenza to investigate whether anti-influenza treatment could influence the outcome of influenza-induced asthma exacerbations in asthmatic children. The improvement in forced expiratory volume in 1 s (FEV_1) between entry and end of study treatment was significantly greater in oseltamivir recipients than among placebo recipients (median improvement from entry of 10.8% vs. 4.7%, respectively, p = 0.0148). There were also reduced asthma exacerbations in the oseltamivir-treated patients (p = 0.031). Improvements were greater among those treated within 24h of onset of symptoms (S. L. Johnston, unpublished data).

Zanamivir and oseltamivir are both very useful treatments for both the prevention and active treatment of influenza. There is plentiful evidence that influenza viruses cause asthma exacerbations and increased deaths among asthmatics. There is also evidence that both drugs improve respiratory outcomes in patients with asthma and acute influenza infections. A good case can therefore be made for supplying asthmatics with these drugs to be used prophylactically if family members or other close contacts develop influenza-like illness or therapeutically if the patient develops influenza-like illness at a time when influenza is known to be circulating in the community.

Ribavarin

Ribavarin is a nucleoside analog active against RS virus and hepatitis C virus in vivo, but also against influenza and herpes viruses in vitro. The mechanism of action is unknown, but there is evidence that it interferes with protein translation from mRNA, possibly by interfering with the 5′ cap. Ribavarin is relatively toxic, and its use is therefore restricted to an aerosol in infants and children within the first 3 days of RS virus bronchiolitis. The cost, lack of antirhinoviral activity, and concerns regarding toxicity are factors that make ribavarin an unsuitable candidate in treatment of the common cold.

H. Unlicensed Antivirals

Interferons

Nasal IFN-α has perhaps been the most successful treatment used, having been first tested over 20 years ago. It is undoubtedly effective when given shortly before or after exposure to the virus, and also when given prophylactically to contacts in family outbreaks (151,152). In a recent systematic review Jefferson and Tyrrell identified 81 interferon studies that were included in a meta-analysis (153). Nasal interferon was highly efficacious in preventing experimental colds caused by rhinovirus, coronavirus, influenza, parainfluenza, and coxsackie viruses with a protective efficacy of 46% (95% CI: 37–54%) and slightly less so for naturally occurring colds in all age groups with a protective efficacy of 24% (95% CI: 21–27%). However, it has not gained favor with pharmaceutical companies or clinicians, owing to a number of drawbacks including the expense of production, frequency of dosage, and side effects.

The side effect profile of nasal interferon appears worse when treating naturally occurring colds to experimental colds as reported in the above meta-analysis. It found that nasal stuffiness (OR 3.07, 2.09–4.51), increased sneezing, and nasal irritation (OR 2.58, 1.88 to 3.52) occurred with a statistically significantly greater frequency in the interferon-treated groups. Interferon therapy therefore causes some of the symptoms it is meant to treat. Of more concern is the significantly greater frequency of blood-stained nasal mucus (OR 4.52, 3.78–5.41) and nasal erosions (OR 2.58, 1.71–3.91) caused by interferon (153).

IFN Inducers

The IFN inducers stimulate endogenous production of IFN by white blood cells and can be administered orally and intranasally. In a recent systematic review Jefferson and Tyrrell identified 10 randomized controlled trials investigating the effects of IFN inducers (153) and found no prophylactic benefit for the IFN inducers studied (Poly-I.Poly-C, propanediamine, intranasal BRL 5907) in the prevention of experimental colds. What evidence there was for the reduction in illness severity in experimental infection was considered impossible to interpret due to the small size of the studies. The preventive effect of the antiplatelet medication dipyridamole was investigated in three simultaneous community-based double-blind placebo-controlled randomized controlled trials in kindergarteners ($n = 264$), older schoolchildren ($n = 405$), and adults ($n = 432$) with acute respiratory tract infections with dosages ranging from 25 to 100 mg/day for 8 days according to age (154). These studies found that dipyridamole prevented naturally occurring colds with a preventive efficacy of 49% (95% CI: 30–62%) compared to placebo (153). According to the analyses performed in the meta-analysis, dipyridamole had the most protective effect in naturally occurring colds of all the antivirals studied.

Pleconaril

Pleconaril is an orally active capsid-binding compound that inhibits capsid function of picornaviruses by binding to a hydrophobic pocket of VP1 a major viral capsid protein. Pleconaril exerts an antiviral effect by blocking the virus's ability to attach to the cellular receptor and by blocking viral uncoating (155). This ultimately blocks the ability of the virus to insert its genetic material into the infected cell, thereby interrupting the virus replication cycle. Pleconaril has been found to have a broad-spectrum antipicornaviral activity (84) and is effective against a wide range of human rhinovirus isolates (156).

In an experimental coxsackie virus A21 respiratory infection, a randomized, controlled, double-blind study of 33 adults showed significant reductions in viral shedding, nasal mucus production, and symptom scores in the pleconaril arm compared to the placebo arm (84). In this study the infection rate, as determined by seroconversion, was not reduced by treatment commenced 14 h prior to inoculation.

However, in a meta-analysis including the data from this study, the protective efficacy of pleconaril against experimental colds was 71% (95% CI: 15–90%) (153).

The efficacy and tolerability of oral pleconaril in treating acute viral respiratory illness (VRI) have recently been evaluated in two double-blind, placebo-controlled trials. Otherwise healthy subjects, 14 years of age or older, who presented within 36 h of VRI symptom onset were randomized to receive pleconaril or placebo for 7 days. Among the subset of subjects with proven picornaviral infection in both studies (42% of total enrolled), pleconaril 400 mg three times daily ($n = 323$) reduced the time to alleviation of illness (no rhinorrhea and other symptoms mild or absent for ≥48 h) compared with placebo ($n = 264$) (median: 10.0 days for placebo and 8.5 days for pleconaril; p = 0.029). In addition, pleconaril reduced the time to a ≥50% reduction from baseline in total symptom severity score (median: 4.5 days for placebo and 3.5 days for pleconaril, p = 0.038). Significant reductions in the number of tissues used for nose-blowing (20% reduction) and in nights of disturbed sleep (16% reduction) were also observed. Pleconaril was generally well tolerated but was associated with a greater incidence of nausea (3% for placebo vs. 7% for pleconaril, p = 0.003). Pleconaril 400 mg administered three times daily reduced the duration and severity of picornaviral VRI in adolescents and adults (157).

Although these data are encouraging, there are some concerns regarding drug safety (158), particularly in the context of a self-limiting illness such as the common cold, as well as the degree of clinical benefit compared with cost. It is likely that pleconaril will have its most significant beneficial role in the treatment or prevention of virus-induced asthma, which is caused by picornaviruses in the majority of cases, especially in children. Studies of this agent in this context would clearly be of great interest.

Blocking Virus–Receptor Binding

Following the identification of several cell surface proteins that act as virus receptors and are involved in virus entry into the cell, efforts have been targeted at blocking virus–receptor binding. One particular focus of attention has been rhinovirus and its binding to ICAM-1, which is the receptor for 90% of rhinoviruses. Blocking this interaction would treat about 50% of common colds (reviewed in 159). Trials with monoclonal antibodies and soluble ICAM-1 have been encouraging in vitro (160) and in animal studies.

Soluble ICAM-1

Soluble ICAM-1 has been found to have a broad spectrum of antirhinovirus activity against both field isolates and laboratory strains (161). Turner et al. recently reported on four randomized, double-blind, placebo-controlled trials of intranasal sICAM-1 (tremacamra) in experimental HRV39 infection in healthy human volunteers (162). Treatments were administered 7 h preinoculation and postinoculation with HRV39 for 7 days. There was no significant difference in infection rates between those receiving sICAM-1 and those receiving placebo, although the rate of clinical colds was significantly higher in the placebo arm (67% vs. 44%, p < 0.001), as were the total symptom scores and nasal mucus weights (p < 0.001). A note of caution, however, is the possible emergence of resistant strains. It had been thought that any mutations producing resistance would result in nonviability, because receptor binding is an essential step to virus replication. However, there is a report of in vitro selection of strains of rhinovirus resistant to neutralization by soluble receptor (163).

A comparison of the antirhinoviral activity of sICAM-1 and a chimeric ICAM-1/immunoglobulin A molecule found the chimeric molecule not only inhibited most HRVs studied with greater potency than sICAM-1 but also was able to inhibit the sICAM-1-resistant strain of HRV (164). Problems with sICAM-1 are that it is expensive to produce and may therefore not be cost-effective particularly as it has to be given six times a day. In addition, the need for frequent dosing is likely to reduce compliance.

ICAM-1 Monoclonal Antibody

The potential for an antirhinovirus effect has been investigated with a rhinovirus receptor murine monoclonal antibody (RRMA) in double-blind, placebo-controlled experimental HRV39 studies of healthy volunteers. Intranasal RRMA administered prophylactically did not prevent infection. Only a higher dosage (1 mg vs. 135 µg) was found to delay viral shedding and cold symptoms by 1–2 days in addition to significant reductions in viral titers, nasal symptoms, and mucus weights with no toxicity seen (165). Further clinical trials have not been published.

HRV Protease Inhibitors

Infection by HRV results in the translation of the viral genome into a large (220 kDa) polyprotein that is cleaved by viral proteases (2A and 3C) to produce viral proteins essential for viral replication. These viral proteases have been identified as antiviral chemotherapy targets and to date a number of 3C protease inhibitors have been studied including peptide aldehydes, isatins, and homopthalimides. Ag7088 is a novel irreversible inhibitor of 3C protease with antipicornavirus effects in vitro. Ag7088 has been shown to reduce significantly the levels of infectious virus and inhibit the production of IL-6 and IL-8 in a human bronchial epithelial cell line (BEAS-2B) infected with HRV14 (166). A broad antipicornaviral activity of Ag7088 has been demonstrated in vitro where it inhibited all 48 HRV serotypes and picornaviruses (coxsackie A21 and B3, enterovirus 70, and echovirus 11) studied in cell culture (167). In addition the anti-HRV effect was equal to or significantly better than both pirodavir and pleconaril with a broader anti-HRV and antipicornavirus activity. These data are supported by Kaiser et al., who reported significantly better cytopathic effect (CPE) inhibition of numbered HRV serotypes and clinical HRV isolates for Ag7088 than pleconaril (156).

Pharmacokinetic and safety data have been reported for ruprintrivir (Ag7088) in healthy human volunteers with no significant adverse events reported in single and multiple dosing regimens (168). Multiple dosing of six times per day was shown to provide adequate nasal levels of the drug, although less frequent dosing regimens may also be possible. Clinical studies are currently awaited.

Pirodavir

Pirodavir, an aerosol (formerly R77975), is a synthetic phenoxy-pyridazinamine antiviral with broad-spectrum antipicornaviral activity in vitro, although limited in part to specific rhinovirus serotypes (169). The results of a randomized, double-blind placebo-controlled study of naturally occurring rhinovirus common colds in adults investigating the efficacy of pirodavir aerosol (administered six times per day) was disappointing with no significant clinical effects. This was despite significantly lower frequencies of viral shedding in the actively treated arm on days 3 and 5 (p < 0.002) (170). The mean duration of illness was 7 days in both groups, with no difference in symptom scores or in the resolution of respiratory symptoms. Additional factors were that the pirodavir arm has higher rates of nasal dryness, bloody mucus, and unpleasant taste.

I. Vaccines

Vaccine development has long been thought the most effective way of controlling virus-induced disease. However, apart from the case of influenza, vaccine development programs for respiratory viruses have had little success. Killed whole or split virus influenza vaccine is effective but requires intensive vigilance and annual revaccination because of the antigenic drift of this virus.

RS virus has been a priority for vaccine production. A major setback occurred when formalin-inactivated vaccines were found to be associated with increased morbidity and mortality on subsequent natural exposure to the virus. Considerable research has been undertaken to determine why such adverse effects resulted from this vaccine (reviewed recently in 171). Present thoughts suggest that different RS virus proteins are capable of inducing different cellular immune responses and that the formalin inactivation resulted in immunopathological immune responses rather than protective ones (172-174). Clinical studies with F subunit vaccines are now underway, and it is hoped that a safe and effective vaccine may not be too long in being developed. There are also initial trials with parainfluenza type 3 vaccines; recent progress with both vaccine types has been reviewed extensively elsewhere (175). The other respiratory viruses have commanded relatively little attention. Rhinoviruses in particular have been very difficult targets for vaccine design, since there are well over 100 different serotypes, each of which is specific in its induction of neutralizing antibody. Recent work, however, has suggested that T-cell responses are relatively conserved across serotypes; this may be a fruitful area for future research (176).

V. Future Avenues for Treatment Development

Molecular biological tools have enormously increased our knowledge of respiratory virology and immunology, and have suggested several avenues that may profitably be explored in the search for new treatments.

Novel methods of inhibiting viral replication are continuously being investigated. The recognition of low-density lipoprotein receptors as receptors for cell entry of minor group human rhinoviruses has identified one such alternative. There is recent in vitro evidence of inhibition of human rhinovirus infection by very-low-density lipoprotein receptor fragments in cell culture (177). Whether blocking this minor group receptor pathway has realistic therapeutic potential and will eventually have a clinical impact as a treatment option will remain unknown until further developmental studies are carried out.

The inflammatory mediators and cytokines involved in the response to viral infection could also be potential sites for inhibition of virus-induced inflammation. The development of specific inhibitors of candidate molecules (such as anti-IL-8 therapies) will permit evaluation of the inhibitors as therapeutic options. They will also shed further light on the importance of the candidates themselves and thus further advance our mechanistic understanding. If inhibitors of virus-induced inflammatory pathways are shown to be therapeutically effective, this could be of huge clinical potential; they would almost certainly be applicable to a generic viral respiratory tract infection.

VI. Targeting At-Risk Populations

The cure for common colds is still a long way off. However, as and when effective treatments become available, a productive approach is likely to be one that targets populations most at risk. The elderly, the young, and those with significant respiratory disease, such as asthma or COPD, are most likely to benefit from treatment. They are also groups most likely to be motivated to take treatments correctly, thereby giving the greatest chance of success. As is currently the case for influenza vaccination, a strategy that should be encouraged is to concentrate treatment or prophylaxis regimens at the times of year when the risk is greatest: the annual epidemics of influenza and RSV, and for rhinoviruses most particularly the second to fourth weeks after children have returned to school (178).

VII. Conclusion

Success in terms of prevention or treatment for common colds has so far evaded research and development, with the exception of influenza vaccines. The major barriers to development of effective treatments are the multiplicity of agents involved; difficulties with drug delivery, potency, and toxicity; the fact that viral replication peaks on the first day or two of symptoms; and the emergence of resistant strains. Newer molecular methods and a better understanding of viral immunology are leading to encouraging developments in vaccine research and to the synthesis of more potent antagonists.

References

1. Johnston SL, Sanderson G, Pattemore PK, Smith S, Bardin PG, Bruce CB, Lambden PR, Tyrrell D A, Holgate S.T. Use of polymerase chain reaction for diagnosis of picor-

navirus infection in subjects with and without respiratory symptoms. J Clin Microbiol 1993; 31(1), 111–117.

2. Woodhead M. Management of lower respiratory tract infections in out-patients. Monaldi Arch Chest Dis 1997; 52(5), 486–491.

3. Dearden C, al-Nakib W, Andries K, Woestenborghs R, Tyrrell DA. Drug resistant rhinoviruses from the nose of experimentally treated volunteers. Arch Virology 1989; 109:71–81.

4. Hayden FG, Belshe RB, Clover RD, Hay AJ, Oakes MG, Soo W. Emergence and apparent transmission of rimantadine-resistant influenza A virus in families. N Engl J Med 1989; 321(25):1696–1702.

5. Monto AS, Napier JA, Metzner HL. The Tecumseh Study of Respiratory Illness: I. Plan of study and observations on syndromes of acute respiratory illness. Am J Physiol 1971; 94(3):269–279.

6. Davey P, Rutherford D, Graham B, Lynch B, Malek JM. Repeat consultations after antibiotic prescribing for respiratory infection: A study in one general practice. Br J Gen Pract 1994; 44:509–513.

7. McCormick A, Fleming D, Charlton J. Morbidity Statistics from General Practice, 4th national study, 1991–1992. London: HMSO, 1995.

8. Howie JGR. Respiratory illness and antibiotic use in general practice. J R Coll Gen Pract 1971; 21:657–663.

9. Garibaldi RA. Epidemiology of community-acquired respiratory tract infections in adults. Am J Med 1985; 78:32–37.

10. Graham NMH. The epidemiology of acute respiratory infections in children and adults: a global perspective. Epidemiol Rev 1990; 12:149–178.

11. Myint S, Taylor-Robinson D. Viral and other infections of the human respiratory tract. ed. London: Chapman and Hall, 1996.

12. Johnston SL, Pattemore PK, Sanderson G, Smith S, Lampe F, Josephs L, et al. Community study of role of viral infections in exacerbations of asthma in 9–11 year old children. BMJ 1995; 310:1225–1229.

13. Corne JM, Marshall C, Smith S, Schreiber J, Sanderson G, Holgate ST, et al. Frequency, severity, and duration of rhinovirus infections in asthmatic and non-asthmatic individuals: a longitudinal cohort study. Lancet 2002; 359:831–834.

14. Nicholson KG, Kent J, Ireland DC. Respiratory viruses and exacerbations of asthma in adults. BMJ 1993; 307:982–986.

15. Arola M, Ziegler T, Puhakka H, Lehtonen OP, Ruuskanen O. Rhinovirus in otitis media with effusion. Ann Otol Rhinol Laryngol 1990; 99(6 Pt1):451–453.

16. Gwaltney JMJ, Phillips CD, Miller RD, Riker DK. Computed tomographic study of the common cold. N Engl J Med 1994; 330(1):25–30.

17. Monto A S, Cavallaro J J. The Tecumseh study of respiratory illness. II. Patterns of occurrence of infection with respiratory pathogens, 1965–1969. Am J Epidemiol 1994(3):280–289.

18. Seemungal TAR, Harper-Owen R, Bhowmik A, Moric I, Sanderson G, Message S, et al. Respiratory viruses, symptoms and inflammatory markers in acute exacerbations and stable chronic obstructive pulmonary disease. Am J Respir Crit Care Med 2001; 164(9):1618–1623.

19. Stockton J, Ellis JS, Saville M, Clewley JP, Zambon MC. Multiplex PCR for typing and subtyping influenza and respiratory syncytial viruses. J Clin Microbiol 1998; 36(10):2990–2995.

20. Igarashi Y, Skoner DP, Doyle WJ, White MV, Fireman P, Kaliner MA. Analysis of

nasal secretions during experimental rhinovirus upper respiratory infections. J Allergy Clin Immunol 1993; 92(5):722–731.

21. Naclerio RM, Proud D, Lichtenstein LM, Kagey-Sobotka A, Hendley JO, Sorrentino J, et al. Kinins are generated during experimental rhinovirus colds. J Infect Dis 1988; 157(1):133–142.

22. Volovitz B, Welliver RC, De Castro G, Krystofik DA, Ogra PL. The release of leukotrienes in the respiratory tract during infection with respiratory syncytial virus: role in obstructive airway disease. Pediatr Res 1988; 24(4):504–507.

23. Lau L C K, Corne J M, Scott S J, Davies R, Friend E, Howarth P H. Nasal cytokines in common cold. Am J Respir Critical Care Med 1996; 153(4): A697.

24. Teran LM, Johnston SL, Holgate ST. Immunoreactive RANTES and MIP-1 are increased in the nasal aspirates of children with virus-associated asthma. Am J Respir Crit Care Med 1995; 151(4):A385.

25. Einarsson O, Geba GP, Panuska JR, Zhu Z, Landry M, Elias JA. Asthma-associated viruses specifically induce lung stromal cells to produce interleukin-11, a mediator of airways hyperreactivity. Chest 1995; 107(3 Suppl):132S–133S.

26. Taylor CE, Webb MS, Milner AD, Milner PD, Morgan LA, Scott R, et al. Interferon alfa, infectious virus, and virus antigen secretion in respiratory syncytial virus infections of graded severity. Arch Dis Child 1989; 64(12):1656–1660.

27. Papadopoulos NG, Papi A, Meyer J, Stanciu LA, Salvi S, Holgate ST, Johnston SL. Rhinovirus infection up-regulates eotaxin and eotaxin-2 expression in bronchial epithelial cells. Clin Exp Allergy 2001; 31(7):1060–1066.

28. Corne JM, Lau L, Scott SJ, Davies R, Johnston SL, Howarth PH. The relationship between atopic status and IL-10 nasal lavage levels in the acute and persistent inflammatory response to upper respiratory tract infection. Am J Respir Crit Care Med 2001; 163(5):1101–1107.

29. Scroth MK, Grimm E, Frindt P, Galagan DM, Konno SI, Love R, et al. Rhinovirus replication causes RANTES production in primary bronchial epithelial cells Am J Respir Cell Mol Biol 1999; 20:1220–1228.

30. Grunberg K, Timmers MC, Smits HH, de Klerk EP, Dick EC, Spaan WJ, et al. Effect of experimental rhinovirus 16 colds on airway hyperresponsiveness to histamine and interleukin-8 in nasal lavage in asthmatic subjects in vivo. Clin Exp Allergy 1997; 27: 36–45.

31. Teran LM, Johnston SL, Schroder JM, Church M K, Holgate ST. Role of nasal interleukin-8 in neutrophil recruitment and activation in children with virus-induced asthma. Am J Respir Crit Care Med 1997; 155(4), 1362–1366.

32. Levandowski RA, Weaver CW, Jackson GG. Nasal-secretion leukocyte populations determined by flow cytometry during acute rhinovirus infection. J Med Virol 1988; 25(4):423–432.

33. Fraenkel DJ, Bardin PG, Sanderson G, Lampe F, Johnston SL, Holgate ST. Immunohistochemical analysis of nasal biopsies during rhinovirus experimental colds. Am J Respir Crit Care Med 1994; 150(4):1130–1136.

34. Fraenkel D J, Bardin P G, Sanderson G, Lampe F, Johnston S L, Holgate S T. Lower airways inflammation during rhinovirus colds in normal and in asthmatic subjects. Am J Respir Crit Care Med 1995; 151(3 Pt 1), 879–886.

35. Heymann PW, Rakes GP, Hogan AD, Ingram JM, Hoover GE, Platts-Mills TA. Assessment of eosinophils, viruses and IgE antibody in wheezing infants and children. Int Arch Allergy Immunol 1995; 107(1–3):380–382.

36. Teran LM, Seminario MC, Shute JK, Papi A, Compton SJ, Low JL, Gleich GJ, John-

ston SL. RANTES, macrophage-inhibitory protein 1alpha, and the eosinophil product major basic protein are released into upper respiratory secretions during virus-induced asthma exacerbations in children. J Infect Dis 1999; 179(3), 677–681.

37. Calhoun WJ, Dick EC, Schwartz LB, Busse WW. A common cold virus, rhinovirus 16, potentiates airway inflammation after segmental antigen bronchoprovocation in allergic subjects. J Clin Invest 1994; 94(6):2200–2208.

38. Papadopoulos NG, Bates PJ, Bardin PG, Papi A, Leir SH, Fraenkel DJ, Meyer J, Lackie PM, Sanderson G, Holgate ST, Johnston SL. Rhinoviruses infect the lower airways. J Infect Dis 2000; 181(6):1875–1884.

39. Gern JE, Galagan DM, Jarjour NN, Dick EC, Busse WW. Detection of rhinovirus RNA in lower airway cells during experimentally induced infection. Am J Respir Crit Care Med 1997; 155(3):1159–1161.

40. Monto AS, Gravenstein S, Elliott M, Colopy M, Schweinle J. Clinical signs and symptoms predicting influenza infection. Arch Intern Med 2000; 160(21):3243–3247.

41. Papadopoulos NG, Moustaki M, Tsolia M, Bossios A, Astra E, Prezerakou A et al. Association of rhinovirus infection with increased disease severity in acute bronchiolitis. Am J Respir Crit Care Med 2002; 165(9): 1285–1289.

42. Boivin G, Osterhaus AD, Gaudreau A, Jackson HC, Groen J, Ward P. Role of picornaviruses in flu-like illnesses of adults enrolled in an oseltamivir treatment study who had no evidence of influenza virus infection. J Clin Microbiol 2002; 40(2):330–334.

43. Hemila H, Herman ZS. Vitamin C and the common cold: a retrospective analysis of Calmers' review. J Am Coll Nutr 1995; 14(2):116–123.

44. Douglas RM, Chalker EB, Treacy B. Vitamin C for preventing and treating the common cold (Cochrane Review). In: The Cochrane Library Issue 1. Oxford: Update Software, 2002.

45. Godfrey JC, Conant Sloane B, Smith DS, Turco JH, Mercer N, Godfrey NJ. Zinc gluconate and the common cold: a controlled clinical study. J Int Med Res 1992; 20(3): 234–246.

46. Marshall, I. Zinc for the common cold (Cochrane Review). In: The Cochrane Library Issue 1. Oxford: Update Software, 2002.

47. Prasad AS, Fitzgerald JT, Bao B, Beck FW, Chandrasekar PH. Duration of symptoms and plasma cytokine levels in patients with the common cold treated with zinc acetate. A randomized, double-blind, placebo-controlled trial. Ann Intern Med 2000; 133(4): 245–252.

48. Prasad AS. Effects of zinc deficiency on Th1 and Th2 cytokine shifts. J Infect Dis 2000; 182(Suppl 1):S62–68.

49. Burger RA, Torres AR, Warren RP, Caldwell VD, Hughes BG. Echinacea-induced cytokine production by human macrophages. Int J Immunopharmacol 1997; 106:138–143.

50. Hoheisel O, Sandberg M, Bertram S, Bulitta M, Schafer M. Echinagard treatment shortens the course of the common cold: a double-blind, placebo-controlled clinical trial. Eur J Clin Res 1997; 9:261–278.

51. Turner RB, Riker DK, Gangemi JD. Ineffectiveness of Echinacea for prevention of experimental rhinovirus colds. Antimicrob Agents Chemother 2000; 44(6):1708–1709.

52. Melchart D, Linde K, Fischer P, Kaesmayr J. Echinacea for preventing and treating the common cold (Cochrane Review). In: The Cochrane Library Issue 1. Oxford: Update Software, 2002.

53. Taverner D, Bickford L, Draper M. Nasal decongestants for the common cold. (Cochrane Review). In: The Cochrane Library Issue 1. Oxford: Update Software, 2002.

54. Welliver RC. The role of antihistamines in upper respiratory tract infections. J Allergy Clin Immunol 1990; 86:633–637.
55. Smith TF, Remigio LK. Histamine in nasal secretions and serum may be elevated during viral respiratory tract infections. Int Arch Allergy Appl Immunol 1982; 67(4): 380–383.
56. Gaffey MJ, Kaiser DL, Hayden FG. Ineffectiveness of oral terfenadine in natural colds: evidence against histamine as a mediator of common cold symptoms. Pediatr Infect Dis J 1988; 7:223–228.
57. Doyle WJ, McBride TP, Skoner DP. A double-blind, placebo-controlled clinical trial of the effect of chlorpheniramine on the response of the nasal airway, middle ear and eustachian tube to provocative rhinovirus challenge. Pediatr Infect Dis J 1988; 7:215–242.
58. Gaffey MJ, Gwaltney JM, Sastre A, Dressler WE, Sorrentino JV, Hayden FG. Intranasally and orally administered antihistamine treatment of experimental rhinovirus colds. Am Rev Respir Dis 1987; 136(3):556–560.
59. Gwaltney JMJ, Park J, Paul RA, Edelman DA, O'Connor RR, Turner RB. Randomised controlled trial of clemastine fumerate for treatment of experimental rhinovirus colds. Clin Infect Dis 1996; 22(4):656–662.
60. Gwaltney JMJ, Druce HM. Efficacy of brompheniramine maleate for the treatment of rhinovirus colds. Clin Infect Dis 1997; 25(5):1188–1194.
61. Berkowitz RB, Tinkelman DG. Evaluation of oral terfenadine for treatment of the common cold. Ann Allergy 1991; 67:593–597.
62. Luks D. Antihistamines and the common cold. A review and critique of the literature. J Gen Intern Med 1996; 11(4):240–244.
63. Vignola AM, Crampette L, Mondain M, Sauvere G, Czarlewski W, Bousquet J, et al. Inhibitory activity of loratadine and descarboethoxyloratadine on expression of ICAM-1 and HLA-DR by nasal epithelial cells. Allergy 1995; 50(3):200–203.
64. Muether PS, Gwaltney JM Jr. Variant effect of first- and second-generation antihistamines as clues to their mechanism of action on the sneeze reflex in the common cold Clin Infect Dis 2001; 33(9):1483–1488.
65. Duckhorn R, Grossman J, Posner M, Zinny M, Tinkleman D. A double-blind, placebo-controlled study of the safety and efficacy of ipratropium bromide nasal spray versus placebo in patients with the common cold. J Allergy Clin Immunol 1992; 90:1076–1082.
66. Hayden FG, Diamond L, Wood PB, Korts DC, Wecker MT. Effectiveness and safety of intranasal ipratropium bromide in common colds: a randomised, double-blind, placebo controlled trial. Ann Intern Med 1996; 125, 89–97.
67. Gaffey MJ, Gwaltney JMJ, Dressler WE, Sorrentino JV, Hayden FG. Intranasally administered atropine methonitrate treatment of experimental rhinovirus colds. Am Rev Respir Dis 1987; 135(1):241–244.
68. Gaffey MJ, Hayden FG, Boyd JC, Gwaltney JMJ. Ipratropium bromide treatment of experimental rhinovirus infection. Antimicrob Agents Chemother 1988; 32(11):1644–1647.
69. Tyrrell DAJ, Barrow I, Arthur J. Local hyperthermia benefits natural and experimental common colds. BMJ 1989; 298:1280–1283.
70. Macknin ML, Mathew LS, Menendrop S. Effect of inhaling heated vapour on symptoms of the common cold. JAMA 1990; 264:989–991.
71. Forstall GJ, Macknin ML, Yen-Lieberman BR, Menendrop S. Effect of inhaling heated vapour on symptoms of the common cold. JAMA 1994; 271:1109–1111.

72. Hendley JO, Abbott RD, Beasley PP, Gwaltney JM. Effect of inhalation of hot humidified air on experimental rhinovirus infection. JAMA 1994; 271:1112–1113.

73. Conti C, de Marco A, Mastromarino P, Tomao P, Santoro MG. Antiviral effect of hyperthermic treatment in rhinovirus infection. Antimicrob Agents Chemother 1999; 43(4):822–829.

74. Johnston SL, Perry D, O'Toole S, Summers QA, Holgate ST. Attenuation of exercise induced asthma by local hyperthermia. Thorax 1992; 47(8):592–597.

75. Johnston S L, Price J N, Lau L C, Walls A F, Walters C, Feather I H, Holgate S T, Howarth P H, The effect of local hyperthermia on allergen-induced nasal congestion and mediator release. J Allergy Clin Immunol 1993; 92(6), 850–856.

76. Takizawa H, Desaki M, Ohtoshi T, Kikutani T, Okazaki H, Sato M, et al. Erythromycin suppresses interleukin 6 expression by human bronchial epithelial cells: a potential mechanism of its anti-inflammatory action. Biochem Biophys Res Commun 1995; 210: 781–786.

77. Khair OA, Devalia JL, Abdelaziz MM, Sapsford RJ, Davies RJ. Effect of erythromycin on Haemophilus influenzae endotoxin-induced release of IL-6, IL-8 and sICAM-1 by cultured human bronchial epithelial cells. Eur Respir J 1995; 8:1451–1457.

78. Suzuki T, Yamaya M, Sekizawa K, Hosoda M, Yamada N, Ishizuka S, et al. Bafilomycin A1 inhibits rhinovirus infection in human airway epithelium: effects on endosome and ICAM-1. Am J Physiol Lung Cell Mol Physiol 2001; 280:L1115–L1127.

79. Suzuki T, Yamaya M, Sekizawa K, Hosoda M, Yamada N, Ishizuka S, et al. Erythromycin inhibits rhinovirus infection in cultured human tracheal epithelial cells. Am J Respir Crit Care Med 2002; 165:1113–1118.

80. Abisheganaden JA, Avila PC, Kishiyama JL, Liu J, Yagi S, Schnurr D, et al. Effect of clarithromycin on experimental rhinovirus-16 colds: a randomised, double-blind, controlled trial. Am J Med 2000; 108(6):453–459.

81. Arroll, B. and Kenealy, T. Antibiotics for the common cold (Cochrane Review). In: The Cochrane Library, Issue 2. Oxford: Update Software, 2001.

82. Gustafson M, Proud D, Hendley JO, Hayden FG, Gwaltney JMJ. Oral prednisolone therapy in experimental rhinovirus infections. J Allergy Clin Immunol 1996; 97:1009–1014.

83. Whitley RJ, Hayden FG, Reisinger KS, Young N, Dutkowski R, Ipe D, et al. Oral oseltamivir treatment of influenza in children. Pediatr Infect Dis J 2001; 20(2):127–133.

84. Schiff GM, Sherwood JR. Clinical activity of pleconaril in an experimentally induced coxsackievirus A21 respiratory infection. J Infect Dis 2000; 181:20–26.

85. Farr BM, Gwaltney JM, Hendley JO, Hayden FG, Nacleri RM, McBride TP, et al. A randomised controlled trial of glucocorticoid prophylaxis against experimental rhinovirus infection. J Infect Dis 1990; 162:1173–1177.

86. Puhakka T, Makela MJ, Malmstrom K, Uhari M, Saolainen J, Terho EO, et al. The common cold: effects of intranasal fluticasone propionate treatment. J Allergy Clin Immunol 1998; 101:726–731.

87. Wilson NM, Silverman M. Treatment of episodic asthma in preschool children using intermittant high dose inhaled steroids. Arch Dis Child 1990; 65:407–410.

88. Connett G, Lenney W. Prevention of viral induced asthma attacks using inhaled budesonide. Arch Dis Child 1993; 68:85–87.

89. Wilson N, Sloper K, Silverman M. Effect of continuous treatment with topical corticosteroid on episodic viral wheeze in preschool children. Arch Dis Child 1995; 72:317–320.

90. Seymour ML, Gilby N, Bardin PG, Fraenkel DJ, Sanderson G, Penrose JF, et al. Rhino-

virus infection increases 5-lipoxygenase and cyclooxygenase-2 in bronchial biopsy specimens from nonatopic subjects. J Infect Dis 2002; 185(4):540–544.

91.   Sperber SJ, Hendley JO, Hayden FG, Riker DK, Sorrentino JV, Gwaltney JMJ. Effects of naproxen on experimental rhinovirus colds. Ann Intern Med 1992; 117(1): 37–41.

92.   van Schaik SM, Tristram DA, Nagpal IS, Hintz KM, Welliver RC2, Welliver RC. Increased production of IFN-gamma and cysteinyl leukotrienes in virus-induced wheezing. J Allergy Clin Immunol 1999; 103(4):630–636.

93.   Proud D, Naclerio RM, Gwaltney JM, Hendley JO. Kinins are generated in nasal secretions during natural rhinovirus colds. J Infect Dis 1990; 161(1):120–123.

94.   Higgins PG, Barrow GI, Tyrrell DAJ. A study of the efficacy of the bradykinin antagonist NPC 567 in rhinovirus infection in human volunteers. Antiviral Res 1990; 14: 339–344

95.   Norris AA, Alton EW. Chloride transport and the action of sodium cromoglycate and nedocromil sodium in asthma. Clin Exp Allergy 1996; 26(3):250–253

96.   Barrow GI, Higgins PG, Al-Nakib W, Smith AP, Wenham PBM, Tyrrell AJ. The effect of intranasal nedocromil sodium on viral upper respiratory tract infections in human volunteers. Clin Exp Allergy 1990; 20:45–51.

97.   Aberg N, Aberg B, Alestig K. The effect of inhaled and intranasal sodium chromoglycate on symptoms of upper respiratory tract infections. Clin Exp Allergy 1996; 26: 1045–1050.

98.   Griego SD, Weston CB, Adams JL, Tal-Singer R, Dillon SB. Role of p38 mitogen-activated protein kinase in rhinovirus-induced cytokine production by bronchial epithelial cells. J Immunol 2000; 165:5211–5220.

99.   Gwaltney JMJ. Combined antiviral and antimediator treatment of rhinovirus colds. J Infect Dis 1992; 166:656–662.

100. Gwaltney JMJ, Winther B, Patrie JT, Hendley JO. Combined antiviral-antimediator treatment for the common cold. J Infect Dis 2002; 186(2):147–154.

101. Pinto LH, Holsinger LJ, Lamb RA. Influenza virus M2 protein has ion channel activity. Cell 1992; 69:517–528.

102. Jefferson T, Demicheli V, Deeks J, Rivetti D. Amantadine and rimantadine for preventing and treating influenza. (Cochrane Review). In: The Cochrane Library Issue. Oxford: Update Software, 2002.

103. Anonymous. Recent increases in influenza and other respiratory infections. Communicable disease report. CDR Weekly 1999; 9(3):17.

104. Cox NJ, Subbarao K. Influenza. Lancet 1999; 354(9186):1277–1282.

105. Couch RB. Advances in influenza virus vaccine research. Ann NY Acad Sci 1993; 685:803–812.

106. Minor TE, Dick EC, Baker JW, Ouellette JJ, Cohen M, Reed CE. Rhinovirus and influenza type A infections as precipitants of asthma. Am Rev Respir Dis 1976; 113(2): 149–153.

107. Minor TE, Dick EC, DeMeo AN, Ouellette JJ, Cohen M, Reed CE. Viruses as precipitants of asthmatic attacks in children. JAMA 1974; 227(3):292–298.

108. Housworth J, Langmuir AD. Excess mortality from epidemic influenza, 1957–1966. Am J Epidemiol 1974; 100(1):40–48.

109. Quarles van Ufford WJ, Savelberg PJ. Asiatic influenza in allergic patients with bronchial asthma. Int Arch Allergy Appl Immunol 1959; 15:189–192.

110. Palese P, Tobita K, Ueda M, Compans RW. Characterization of temperature sensitive influenza virus mutants defective in neuraminidase. Virology 1974; 61(2):397–410.

111. Klenk HD, Rott R. The molecular biology of influenza virus pathogenicity. Adv Virus Res 1988; 34:247–281.

112. Varghese JN, Laver WG, Colman PM. Structure of the influenza virus glycoprotein antigen neuraminidase at 2.9 A resolution. Nature 1983; 303(5912):35–40.

113. Colman PM, Varghese JN, Laver WG. Structure of the catalytic and antigenic sites in influenza virus neuraminidase. Nature 1983; 303(5912):41–44.

114. Colman PM, Hoyne PA, Lawrence MC. Sequence and structure alignment of paramyxovirus hemagglutinin- neuraminidase with influenza virus neuraminidase. J Virol 1993; 67(6):2972–2980.

115. Govorkova EA, Leneva IA, Goloubeva OG, Bush K, Webster RG. Comparison of efficacies of RWJ-270201, zanamivir, and oseltamivir against H5N1, H9N2, and other avian influenza viruses. Antimicrob Agents Chemother 2001; 45(10):2723–2732.

116. von Itzstein M, Wu WY, Kok GB, Pegg MS, Dyason JC, Jin B, et al. Rational design of potent sialidase-based inhibitors of influenza virus replication. Nature 1993; 363: 418–423.

117. Woods JM, Bethell RC, Coates JA, Healy N, Hiscox SA, Pearson BA et al. 4-Guanidino-2,4-dideoxy-2,3-dehydro-N-acetylneuraminic acid is a highly effective inhibitor both of the sialidase (neuraminidase) and of growth of a wide range of influenza A and B viruses in vitro. Antimicrob Agents Chemother 1993; 37(7):1473–1479.

118. Cass LM, Brown J, Pickford M, Fayinka S, Newman SP, Johansson CJ, et al. Pharmacoscintigraphic evaluation of lung deposition of inhaled zanamivir in healthy volunteers. Clin Pharmacokinet 1999; 36(Suppl 1):21–31.

119. Cass LM, Efthymiopoulos C, Bye A. Pharmacokinetics of zanamivir after intravenous, oral, inhaled or intranasal administration to healthy volunteers. Clin Pharmacokinet 1999; 36(Suppl 1):1–11.

120. Bergstrom M, Cass LM, Valind S, Westerberg G, Lundberg EL, Gray S, et al. Deposition and disposition of [11C]zanamivir following administration as an intranasal spray. Evaluation with positron emission tomography. Clin Pharmacokinet 1999; 36(Suppl 1):33–39.

121. Daniels MJ, Barnett JM, Pearson BA. The low potential for drug interactions with Zanamivir. Clin Pharmacokinet 1999; 36 (Suppl) 1:41–51.

122. Li W, Escarpe PA, Eisenberg EJ, Cundy KC, Sweet C, Jakeman KJ, et al. Identification of GS 4104 as an orally bioavailable prodrug of the influenza virus neuraminidase inhibitor GS 4071. Antimicrob Agents Chemother 1998; 42(3):647–653.

123. Kim CU, Lew W, Williams MA, Wu H, Zhang L, Chen X, et al. Structure-activity relationship studies of novel carbocyclic influenza neuraminidase inhibitors. J Med Chem 1998; 41(14):2451–2460.

124. Mendel DB, Tai CY, Escarpe PA, Li W, Sidwell RW, Huffman JH, et al. Oral administration of a prodrug of the influenza virus neuraminidase inhibitor GS 4071 protects mice and ferrets against influenza infection. Antimicrob Agents Chemother 1998; 42(3):640–646.

125. Bardsley-Elliot A, Noble S. Oseltamivir. Drugs 1999; 58(5):851–860.

126. Monto AS, Robinson DP, Herlocher ML, Hinson JM Jr, Elliott MJ, Crisp A. Zanamivir in the prevention of influenza among healthy adults: a randomized controlled trial. JAMA 1999; 282(1):31–35.

127. Hayden FG, Osterhaus AD, Treanor JJ, Fleming DM, Aoki FY, Nicholson KG, et al. Efficacy and safety of the neuraminidase inhibitor zanamivir in the treatment of influenzavirus infections. GG167 Influenza Study Group. N Engl J Med 1997; 337(13): 874–880.

128. Randomised trial of efficacy and safety of inhaled zanamivir in treatment of influenza A and B virus infections. The MIST (Management of Influenza in the Southern Hemisphere Trialists) Study Group. Lancet 1998; 352:1877–1881.

129. Makela MJ, Pauksens K, Rostila T, Fleming DM, Man CY, Keene ON, et al. Clinical efficacy and safety of the orally inhaled neuraminidase inhibitor zanamivir in the treatment of influenza: a randomized, double- blind, placebo-controlled European study. J Infect 2000; 40(1):42–48.

130. Monto AS, Webster A, Keene O. Randomized, placebo-controlled studies of inhaled zanamivir in the treatment of influenza A and B: pooled efficacy analysis. J Antimicrob Chemother 1999; 44 (Suppl B):23–29.

131. Hedrick JA, Barzilai A, Behre U, Henderson FW, Hammond J, Reilly L, et al. Zanamivir for treatment of symptomatic influenza A and B infection in children five to twelve years of age: a randomized controlled trial. Pediatr Infect Dis J 2000; 19(5):410–417.

132. Diggory P, Fernandez C, Humphrey A, Jones V, Murphy M. Comparison of elderly people's technique in using two dry powder inhalers to deliver zanamivir: randomised controlled trial. BMJ 2001; 322:577–579.

133. Lalezari J, Campion K, Keene O, Silagy C. Zanamivir for the treatment of influenza A and B infection in high-risk patients: a pooled analysis of randomized controlled trials. Arch Intern Med 2001; 161(2):212–217.

134. Murphy KR, Eivindson A, Pauksens K, Stein WJ, Tellier G, Watts R, et al. Efficacy and safety of inhaled zanamivir for the treatment of influenza in patients with asthma or chronic obstructive pulmonary disease. Clin Drug invest 2000; 20(5):337–349.

135. Williamson JC, Pegram PS. Respiratory distress associated with zanamivir. N Engl J Med 2000; 342(9):661–662.

136. Gravenstein S, Johnston SL, Loeschel E, Webster A. Zanamivir: a review of clinical safety in individuals at high risk of developing influenza-related complications. Drug Safety 2001; 24(15):1113–1125.

137. Gubareva LV, Matrosovich MN, Brenner MK, Bethell RC, Webster RG. Evidence for zanamivir resistance in an immunocompromised child infected with influenza B virus. J Infect Dis 1998; 178(5):1257–1262.

138. Treanor JJ, Hayden FG, Vrooman PS, Barbarash R, Bettis R, Riff D, et al. Efficacy and safety of the oral neuraminidase inhibitor oseltamivir in treating acute influenza: a randomized controlled trial. US Oral Neuraminidase Study Group. JAMA 2000; 283(8):1016–1024.

139. Nicholson KG, Aoki FY, Osterhaus AD, Trottier S, Carewicz O, Mercier CH, et al. Efficacy and safety of oseltamivir in treatment of acute influenza: a randomised controlled trial. Neuraminidase Inhibitor Flu Treatment Investigator Group. Lancet 2000; 355:1845–1850.

140. Hayden FG, Gubareva LV, Monto AS, Klein TC, Elliot MJ, Hammond JM, et al. Inhaled zanamivir for the prevention of influenza in families. Zanamivir Family Study Group. N Engl J Med 2000; 343(18):1282–1289.

141. Hayden FG, Atmar RL, Schilling M, Johnson C, Poretz D, Paar D, et al. Use of the selective oral neuraminidase inhibitor oseltamivir to prevent influenza. N Engl J Med 1999; 341(18):1336–1343.

142. Welliver R, Monto AS, Carewicz O, Schatteman E, Hassman M, Hedrick J, et al. Effectiveness of oseltamivir in preventing influenza in household contacts: a randomized controlled trial. JAMA 2001; 285(6):748–754.

143. Prevention and control of influenza: recommendations of the Advisory Commitee on Immunization Practices (ACIP). MMWR Morbid Mortal Wkly Rep 2000; 49(RR-3):1–38.

144. Nguyen-Van-Tam JS, Nicholson KG. Influenza immunization; vaccine offer, request and uptake in high-risk patients during the 1991/2 season. Epidemiol Infect 1993; 111(2):347–355.

145. Ouellette JJ, Reed CE. Increased response of asthmatic subjects to methacholine after influenza vaccine. J Allergy 1965; 36(6):558–563.

146. Anand SC, Itkin IH, Kind LS. Effect of influenza vaccine on methacholine (mecholyl) sensitivity in patients with asthma of knowm and unknown origin. J Allergy 1968; 42:187–192.

147. Hassan WU, Henderson AF, Keaney NP. Influenza vaccination in asthma. Lancet 1992; 339:194.

148. Daggett P. Influenza and asthma. Lancet 1992; 339:367.

149. Nicholson KG, Nguyen-Van-Tam JS, Ahmed AH, Wiselka MJ, Leese J, Ayres J, et al. Randomised placebo-controlled crossover trial on effect of inactivated influenza vaccine on pulmonary function in asthma. Lancet 1998; 351:326–331.

150. Nicholson KG. Efficacy/clinical effectiveness of inactivated influenza vaccines in adults. In: Nicholson KG, Webster RG, Hay AJ, eds. Textbook of Influenza. Oxford: Blackwell Science, 1998:358–372.

151. Sperber SJ, Hayden FG. Chemotherapy of rhinovirus colds. Antimicrob Agents Chemother 1988; 32(4):409–419.

152. Douglas RM, Moore BW, Miles HB, Davies LM, Graham NM, Ryan P et al. Prophylactic efficacy of intranasal alpha 2-interferon against rhinovirus infections in the family setting. N Engl J Med 1986; 314(2):65–70.

153. Jefferson TO, Tyrrell D. Antivirals for the Common Cold (Cochrane Review). In: The Cochrane Library, Issue 1. Oxford: Update software, 2002.

154. Kuzmov K, Galabov AS, Radeva Kh, Kozhukharova M, Milanov K. [Epidemiological trial of the prophylactic effectiveness of the interferon inducer dipyridimole with respect to influenza and acute respiratory diseases]. [Russian]. Zh Mikrobiol Epidemiol Immunobiol 1985; 6:26–30.

155. McKinlay MA, Pevear DC, Rossmann MG. Treatment of the picornavirus common cold by inhibitors of viral uncoating and attachment. Annu Rev Microbiol 1992(46): 635–654.

156. Kaiser L, Crump CE, Hayden FG. In vitro activity of pleconaril and AG7088 against selected serotypes and clinical isolates of human rhinoviruses. Antiviral Res 2000; 47(3):215–220.

157. Hayden FG, Coats T, Kim K, Hassman HA, Blatter MM, Zhang B, et al. Oral pleconaril treatment of picornavirus-associated viral respiratory illness in adults: efficacy and tolerability in phase II clinical trials. Antiviral Ther 2002; 7(1):53–65.

158. Senior K. FDA panel rejects common cold treatment. Lancet 2002; 2(5):264.

159. Johnston SL, Bardin PG, Pattemore PK. Viruses as precipitants of asthma symptoms. III. Rhinoviruses: molecular biology and prospects for future intervention. Clin Exp Allergy 1993; 23(4):237–246.

160. Arruda E, Crump CE, Marlin SD, Merluzzi VJ, Hayden FG. In vitro studies of the antirhinovirus activity of soluble intercellular adhesion molecule-1. Antimicrob Agents Chemother 1992; 36(6):1186–1191.

161. Ohlin A, Hoover-Litty H, Sanderson G, Paessens A, Johnston SL, Holgate ST, Huguenel E, Greve JM. Spectrum of activity of soluble intercellular adhesion molecule-1 against rhinovirus reference strains and field isolates. Antimicrob Agents Chemother 1994; 38(6), 1413–1415.

162. Turner RB, Wecker MT, Pohl G, Witek TJ, McNally E, St. George R, et al. Efficacy

of tremacamra, a soluble intercellular adhesion molecule 1, for experimental rhinovirus infection. JAMA 1999; 281:1797–804.

163. Arruda E, Crump CE, Hayden FG. In vitro selection of human rhinovirus relatively resistant to soluble intercellular adhesion molecule-1. Antimicrob Agents Chemother 1994; 38(1):66–70.

164. Crump CE, Arruda E, Hayden FG. Comparative antirhinoviral activities of soluble intercellular adhesion molecule-1 (sICAM-1) and chimeric ICAM-1/immunoglobulin A molecule. Antimicrob Agents Chemother 1994; 38(6):1425–1427.

165. Hayden FG, Gwaltney Jr JM, Colonno RJ. Modification of experimental rhinovirus colds by receptor blockade. Antiviral Res 1988; 9:233–247.

166. Zalman LS, Brothers MA, Dragovich PS, Zhou R, Prins TJ, Worland STPAK. Inhibition of human rhinovirus-induced cytokine production by AG7088, a human rhinovirus 3C protease inhibitor. Antimicrob Agents Chemother 2000; 44:1236–1241.

167. Patick AK, Binford SL, Brothers MA, Jackson RL, Ford CE, Diem MD, et al. In vitro antiviral activity of AG7088, a potent inhibitor of human rhinovirus 3C protease. Antimicrob Agents Chemother 1999; 43:2444–2450.

168. Hsyu P-H, Pithavala YK, Gersten M, Penning CA, Kerr BM. Pharmacokinetics and safety of an antirhinoviral agent, Ruprintrivir, in healthy volunteers. Antimicrob Agents Chemother 2002; 46(2):392–397.

169. Andries K, Dewindt B, Snoeks J, Willebrords R, van Eemeren K, Stokbroekx R, et al. In vitro activity of pirodavir (R77975), a substituted phenoxy-pyridazinamine with broad-spectrum antipicornaviral activity. Antimicrob Agents Chemother 1992; 36(1):100–107.

170. Hayden FG, Hipskind GJ, Woerner DH, Eisen GF, Janssens M, Janssen PA, et al. Intranasal pirodavir (R77.975) treatment of rhinovirus colds. Antimicrob Agents Chemother 1995; 39(2):290–294.

171. Graham BS. Immunological determinants of disease caused by respiratory syncytial virus. Trends Microbiol 1996; 4(8):290–293.

172. Openshaw PJ. Immunity and immunopathology to respiratory syncytial virus. The mouse model. Am J Respir Crit Care Med 1995; 152(4 Pt 2):S59–62.

173. Graham BS. Pathogenesis of respiratory syncytial virus vaccine-augmented pathology. Am J Respir Crit Care Med 1995; 152(4 Pt 2):S63–66.

174. Alwan WH, Kozlowska WJ, Openshaw PJ. Distinct types of lung disease caused by functional subsets of antiviral T cells. J Exp Med 1994; 179(1):81–89.

175. Murphy BR, Hall SL, Kulkarni AB, Crowe JEJ, Collins PL, Connors M, et al. An update on approaches to the development of respiratory syncytial virus (RSV) and parainfluenza virus type 3 (PIV3) vaccines. Virus Res 1994; 32(1):13–36.

176. Hastings GZ, Rowlands DJ, Francis MJ. Proliferative responses of T cells primed against human rhinovirus to other rhinovirus serotypes. J Gen Virol 1991; 72(12):2947–2952.

177. Marlovits TC, Abrahamsberg C, Blaas D. Very-low-density lipoprotein receptor fragment shed from HeLa cells inhibits human rhinovirus. J Virol 1998; 72(12):10246–10250.

178. Johnston SL, Pattemore PK, Sanderson G, Smith S, Campbell MJ, Josephs LK, Cunningham A, Robinson BS, Myint SH, Ward ME, Tyrrell DA, Holgate ST. The relationship between upper respiratory infections and hospital admissions for asthma: a time-trend analysis. Am J Respir Crit Care Med 1996; 154(3 Pt 1):654–660.

29

Therapy for Virus-Induced Asthma Exacerbations
Current Status and Future Prospects

IOLO J. M. DOULL

University Hospital of Wales
Cardiff, Wales

I. Background

Our understanding of what constitutes asthma appears to have turned full circle in recent years, with a rediscovery of previously discarded conditions and diagnoses. With a greater understanding of the epidemiology, pathophysiology, and natural history of asthma has come a reassessment of its heterogeneous nature, and a recognition that many individuals wheeze only in association with viral infections. This is particularly relevant in pediatrics, where there is increasing evidence for a differentiation between classic asthma and viral-associated wheezing episodes. With this understanding has come a reappraisal of asthma therapies, and the realization that therapies that increase indices of pulmonary function may not necessarily be beneficial for virus-induced asthma attacks. Osler's aphorism that "all that wheezes is not asthma" seems even more relevant today.

II. Differences Between Asthma and Virus-Associated Wheeze

To appreciate the difficulty in interpreting the treatment options for episode of virus-induced asthma, it is helpful to understand the changes in the understanding of childhood asthma that have taken place in the last 40 years, with the see-sawing between lumping and splitting of wheezing phenotypes. Historically there had always been a dichotomy between asthma in adults and older children, and bronchitis in younger children. Starr's *Diseases of Children* published in 1894 contains separate chapters on bronchitis and asthma. In 1968 Jolly stated that "acute spasmodic bronchitis . . . . has nothing to do with asthma and it's prognosis is quite different."

However from the late 1960s onward there was a reappraisal of the differentiation between infant bronchitis and asthma. Two studies were pivotal in lumping the two conditions. In 1969 Williams and McNicol (89) reported their comparison of Melbourne school children diagnosed as asthmatic, children diagnosed as wheezy bronchitic, and normal children. The children diagnosed as having wheezy bronchitis showed greater similarity to the children diagnosed with asthma than to the normal children. Longitudinal follow-up revealed that bronchitic children frequently exhibited an asthmatic pattern, and vice versa. The authors concluded that both groups arose from the same population, and that differences between groups reflected severity and not pathogenesis.

In 1983 Speight et al. (73) highlighted the underdiagnosis and undertreatment of asthma in school-aged children, noting that many children diagnosed as having wheezy bronchitis, responded to antiasthma prophylaxis. They described the relationship of treatment and morbidity in a cross-sectional study of 2700 children in the north of England. Half of the children with more than four episodes of wheeze per year had missed more than 50 days of school in the previous year because of wheeze. When these children were commenced on continuous prophylactic anti-asthma therapy, school absenteeism fell 10-fold. As a result there was a perception that "all that wheezes is probably asthma," and all that wheezes should be treated as asthma. This lumping of the wheezing phenotypes blurred our understanding of the treatment of virus-induced asthma attacks.

The 1990s have seen the resplitting of wheezing phenotypes, particularly in children (52), between classic asthma and viral-associated wheeze (VAW) often referred to as respiratory viral-induced wheeze, wheezy bronchitis, or virus-induced asthma). Although the case for considering VAW and asthma as separate entities has been clearly proposed by Silverman (70), there are at present no universally accepted diagnostic criteria. The classic asthma of childhood is characterized by the chronicity of clinical features, with atopy being a major risk factor. There may be persistent symptoms, even if relatively mild. There may be persistent abnormalities in pulmonary function, either in day-to-day or diurnal variation, or diminished pulmonary function following exercise or allergen exposure. Although respiratory viral infections may exacerbate symptoms and worsen pulmonary function, some symptoms and pulmonary function anomalies remain even in the absence of respiratory viral infections.

In contrast, the pattern of VAW would appear to be short episodes of acute respiratory symptoms, characterized by upper respiratory symptoms leading to lower respiratory symptoms and a decrease in pulmonary function, interspersed between longer periods with no respiratory symptoms (16). During such asymptomatic periods pulmonary function (including diurnal and day-to-day variation in peak expiratory flow measurement) is frequently within normal limits (16,23,41). However, the differences between VAW and asthma are not clear cut or mutually exclusive.

The pattern of viral-associated wheezing continues through childhood (16, 23,41) and into adulthood (33). In a follow-up study over 25 years conducted in Aberdeen, children who had wheeze only, in the presence of infection had a better prognosis than children labeled as having asthma (33). They were more likely to report wheeze (OR 3.8) and phlegm (OR 4.4) than subjects with no respiratory symptoms in childhood. However, they had normal pulmonary function, normal bronchial responsiveness to methacholine, and the reported symptoms did not interfere with normal activities. It is therefore likely that although children with VAW may have less severe symptoms in adulthood and that their pulmonary function may be normal, they do nevertheless have persisting symptoms.

It has long been acknowledged by both asthmatic patients, and their doctors, that viral upper respiratory tract infections (URTI) are critical to the initiation of asthmatic attacks. There is strong epidemiological and pathophysiological evidence to link respiratory virus infections to exacerbations in childhood wheezing and asthma (see previously). Asthma in adults is an inflammatory disorder, even in mild cases (21), and there is increasing evidence that the disease processes is similar in childhood asthma (62). Ethical considerations have precluded biopsy studies in children, but induced sputum and bronchoalveolar lavage studies demonstrate epithelial shedding and an inflammatory infiltrate of eosinophils, mast cells, and neutrophils. Furthermore, the degree of inflammation (particularly eosinophil inflammation) appears inversely correlated with pulmonary function, bronchial hyper-responsiveness (BHR)and asthma symptoms. There are fewer data in children with viral-associated wheeze, but a suggestion is that they have decreased numbers of bronchoalveolar lavage mast cells and eosinophils compared to atopic asthma (74).

III. Therapies for Virus-Associated Wheezing Syndrome

There are a number of clear published guidelines on the treatment of asthma (9,35), with emphasis on prophylactic anti-inflammatory therapy. In contrast, the treatment of VAW remains contentious. A consequence of the previous lumping of asthma phenotypes is a relative paucity of studies assessing therapeutic options for treating virus-induced asthma exacerbations. Studies assessing therapeutic options in preschool wheezing have limited objective outcome measures, due to the technical difficulties in performing reliable indices of pulmonary function in children of this age. As a result studies in preschool children are reliant on parent-reported symptoms and physician assessment of benefit, although in reality these are probably downstream measures of virus-induced asthma exacerbations. In contrast, measures of pulmonary function in older children and adults are simple and reproducible, and studies in older subjects have used changes in pulmonary function as primary outcome measures. Only recently have studies in older children and adult asthmatics begun to assess the effects of various therapies on asthma exacerbations. Consequently this review is based on two basic assumptions:

1. The response to therapy for a respiratory virus-induced asthma attack is the same regardless of whether the underlying process is asthma or virus-

associated wheeze. There is a large body of evidence testifying to the benefits of therapy of chronic symptoms in classic asthma, but few studies have specifically addressed the effect of therapies on episodes of viral-induced wheezing in either classic asthma or viral-associated wheeze. Although the clinical manifestations and time course of a respiratory viral infection in a classic asthma and a virus-associated wheeze appear similar, it is unclear at present whether the underlying pathophysiology, or the end result, are the same. It is uncertain whether a therapy effective for respiratory viral infection in a classic asthmatic is also effective for viral-associated wheeze, and vice versa. The difficulties with this assumption are discussed later.

2. Acute exacerbations of asthma are primarily due to respiratory viral infections. Longitudinal epidemiological studies suggest that respiratory virus infections account for up to 80% of acute exacerbations of cough or wheezing in children (41) and 50% of adults with asthma (58). Virtually no therapeutic studies have performed simultaneous viral identification, but it is assumed that the majority of acute exacerbations are precipitated by respiratory viral infections.

One unique clinical scenario of virus-associated wheezing is of respiratory syncytial virus (RSV) infection in the first year of life. To date there is no evidence that anything other than supportive treatment is effective in RSV-induced wheezing. Specifically there is no benefit from either short-acting bronchodilators, beta$_2$ agonists or ipratropium bromide (38), nebulized or systemic corticosteroids (55).

A. β$_2$-Agonists

Both systemic and inhaled β$_2$-agonists decrease symptoms and improve pulmonary function in acute asthma in children and adults. Because the majority of such episodes are likely to be virally mediated, it is likely that β$_2$-agonists ameliorate the acute effects of virus-induced asthma exacerbations. However, their effect is relatively short-lived, and their regular use in persistent asthma may increase the frequency of acute exacerbations. In a 1 year study of 64 adult asthmatics (54 of whom were also receiving regular inhaled corticosteroids), regular fenoterol 400 µg four times a day was associated with a significantly shorter period to first asthma exacerbation of 33 vs. 66 days compared to those taking fenoterol as required (p = 0.04) (83). Compared to regular inhaled corticosteroids, a regular long-acting beta$_2$ agonist (LABA) used alone (without concurrent inhaled corticosteroids) in a group of 35 asthmatic children resulted in a significantly greater frequency of asthma exacerbation (need for oral corticosteroids) (17 vs. 2 exacerbations, p < 0.001) (86). The role of LABAs when used in conjunction with inhaled corticosteroids in preventing viral induced wheezing is discussed below.

B. Anticholinergics

Anticholinergics are effective during acute wheezing exacerbations in adult (88) and childhood asthma (1), decreasing symptoms and improving indices of pulmonary function. Their action appears greatest when used in conjunction with inhaled β_2-agonists in more severe asthma (63). The effect of ipratropium bromide is relatively short-lived, and there is no evidence to support its regular use in preventing virus-induced asthma exacerbations.

C. Methylxanthines

The methylxanthines aminophylline and theophylline have bronchodilator effects in acute asthma (64,92). Theophylline has mild anti-inflammatory effects, and improves indices of pulmonary function in asthmatics with persistent symptoms receiving regular inhaled corticosteroids (26). Although they may have a role in acute asthma exacerbations, and in persistent asthma, there is to date no evidence to support their use in virus-induced asthma exacerbations.

D. Cromolyns

Disodium cromoglycate (DSCG) has been used as maintenance therapy for persistent asthma since 1967, and more recently as prophylaxis against exercise-induced bronchoconstriction. Initial studies were in adults with chronic asthma who were frequently dependent on oral corticosteroids, but with time usage moved into the school-aged and then preschool age groups. A major difficulty with disodium cromoglycate is its relatively short half-life, requiring a four times daily dosing regimen. Consequently nedocromil sodium was viewed as an advance, given its twice or thrice daily dosing regimen and more potent anti-inflammatory effects than disodium cromoglycate.

The long-held belief in disodium cromoglycate's role as maintenance therapy in persistent asthma has been seriously questioned by a recent systematic review of 24 randomized placebo-controlled trials of sodium cromoglycate in childhood asthma (81). Older studies were more in favor of benefit for DSCG than recent studies, which the authors interpreted as a publication bias and concluded that the superiority of DSCG over placebo in the maintenance treatment of children with asthma was not proven. However, the older studies were nearly all in school-aged children, while the recent studies were mostly in preschool children. The authors were challenged to recalculate the size of effect separately for trials involving school-aged and preschool children (69). The reanalysis suggested that DSCG might be more effective in school-aged children than preschool children. What are we to make of these statistical meditations? A reasonable interpretation would be that DSCG might have a small and extremely limited effect in chronic asthma, but that it has no effect at all in the preschool population with a predominately viral-associated wheezing phenotype. It is noticeable that the few trials of DSCG in infants labeled as having wheezy bronchitis or recurrent wheezing show no benefit at all (4,17,31,37).

The benefits of regular nebulized nedocromil sodium in children with VAW are likewise limited (46). A randomized, double-blind placebo-controlled comparative study of thrice daily nebulized 0.5% nedocromil sodium versus placebo in 93 children aged 6–12 years with moderate asthma showed modest benefits in favor of nedocromil for improving asthmatic symptoms, but had little effect on episodes of virus-induced asthma exacerbations. All children had asthma diagnosed on the basis of symptoms, with both a 15% improvement in forced expiratory volume in 1 second (FEV$_1$) following an inhaled bronchodilator and a 20% fall in FEV$_1$ after methacholine challenge. In addition, the children were required to have a history of two respiratory virus infections in the preceding 12 months, but none in the preceding 6 weeks. The study was targeted at the respiratory viral season, and ran from September/October, 1989, to March/April, 1990. On each day the children recorded a daytime asthma, sleep asthma, and cough diary, from which a summary score from 0–6 was constructed. They also recorded the best of three peak expiratory flow measurements each morning and evening. Symptomatic respiratory infections (SRI) were defined as a symptom complex of two or more symptoms of stuffy nose, runny nose, sneezing, throat discomfort, headaches, fever, malaise. Based on the diary scores, the children had mild asthma with mean baseline asthma summary scores of 1.25 out of a maximum of 6.

There were small and statistically significant benefits in daytime asthma scores, sleep asthma scores, and cough symptom scores in favor of nedocromil during the first 4 weeks after commencing therapy, although these benefits did not persist for the rest of the study. There were no consistent effects on either morning or evening peak expiratory flow rate (PEFR), spirometry, or methacholine responsiveness. Over the 24 weeks of the study the subjects experienced a total of 59 SRIs. The mean asthma symptom score peaked at day 3 of the onset of the SRI, and declined to baseline by day 10. The peak mean symptom score on day 3 was slightly higher in the nedocromil-treated group, and so the decline in symptom score from day 3 to day 5 was significantly greater in the nedocromil-treated group. There were no other significant differences in either severity or duration of symptom episodes or PEFR episodes of the SRI between the two groups. Although nasopharyngeal swabs were obtained for viral culture, no virological results are supplied.

Interpretation of this important study is hampered by the absence of predefined outcome variables, and the large number of possible outcome variables that were analyzed. It is likely that the small differences reported are the result of type I error rather than true effect. It is regrettable that the findings for virus identification during SRIs are not supplied. Consistent features are of a marginal improvement in parent-reported symptom scores and symptom-free days, but there is little evidence for efficacy in viral-induced asthma exacerbations.

The most extensive assessment of the use of nedocromil in childhood asthma was reported by the Childhood Asthma Management Program (15). Over a 4–6 year period, over 1000 children with persistent asthma (defined as symptoms and need for bronchodilator twice weekly with bronchial responsiveness to methacholine less than 12.5 mg/mL) were randomized to receive budesonide 200 µg nedocromil 8 mg, or placebo twice daily. Compared with placebo, regular inhaled nedocromil resulted in decreased need for courses of oral prednisolone (102 vs. 122:100 person years, $p < 0.01$) and decreased urgent care visits for asthma (16 vs. 22:100 person years, $p < 0.02$) but had no effect on hospitalization due to asthma (4.3 vs. 4.4: 100 person years, $p = 0.99$). However, the protective effect of nedocromil was not as beneficial as regular inhaled corticosteroids (see below).

What might be the reason for the discrepancy in findings between the studies reported by König and CAMP, since as both studied similar populations? It may simply reflect the differences in size and duration of the two studies. It does, however, seem likely that regular nedocromil sodium has a small effect on virus-induced asthma exacerbations in persistent asthmatic children, but insufficient to affect the rate of hospitalization for such children.

E. Corticosteroids

Rationale for Use

Corticosteroids are the mainstay of the treatment of asthma in adults and in children (9,35). Systemic corticosteroids, usually delivered via the oral route, are extremely effective at decreasing symptoms, improving pulmonary function, decreasing bronchial hyperresponsiveness, and decreasing airway inflammation. Inhaled corticosteroids offer advantages comparable to systemic corticosteroids in maintaining therapeutic efficacy while decreasing the possibility of significant side effects. Like systemic corticosteroids, inhaled corticosteroids decrease symptoms, improve pulmonary function, decrease bronchial hyperresponsiveness, and decrease airway inflammation (2).

Respiratory virus infections result in an inflammatory response in the upper and lower airways (29). Corticosteroids are potent anti-inflammatory agents, and thus it is logical that their use should be extended from control of asthma to preventing or treating virus-induced asthma exacerbations. Although there is now a considerable body of evidence that regular inhaled corticosteroids decrease the frequency of virus-induced asthma exacerbations in adults (49,60), school-aged children (15), and preschool children (5,57), the evidence for their effect on such exacerbations in subjects with isolated VAW is not as clear-cut (23,9).

F. Intermittent Systemic Corticosteroids

There is clear and consistent evidence of benefit for both systemic (50,66,67) and inhaled corticosteroids (25) in decreasing symptoms and the need for additional therapies in established asthma exacerbations. A possible explanation for these findings is the observation that corticosteroids ameliorate experimental virus infections when given prophylactically to healthy adult volunteers (27). In a randomized placebo-controlled trial corticosteroids were administered to 44 healthy adult volunteers prior to an innoculum of either rhinovirus type 39 or rhinovirus HH, dependent on antibody status. For corticosteroid prophylaxis, nasal beclomethasone was administered for 4 days prior and 5 days following viral inoculation, and systemic corticosteroids (prednisone 30 mg daily) were administered for 1 day prior and 2 days following the viral inoculation. Viral infection rate was similar in the corticosteroid and placebo-treated groups (82% vs. 86% viral shedding). Significantly fewer corticosteroid-treated volunteers felt they had a cold compared to those receiving placebo (53% vs. 83%, p = 0.046). Although there was a trend towards decreased nasal mucus and kinin production in the first 2 days, there were few significant objective benefits. The relevance of these benefits in healthy controls compared to asthmatics is unclear, but it would suggest that benefits in asthmatics are potentially greater.

A pivotal retrospective clinical study was reported by Brunette and colleagues (10). In an open manner they assessed the effects of oral prednisone 1 mg/kg/day in preventing viral-associated wheezing in preschool children. The subjects were aged 2–6 years (mean 38 months), had all experienced at least four severe wheezing attacks per year over a 2-year period, two or more of which had required hospitalization. Children whose wheezing attacks were not usually precipitated by URTIs were excluded. Over a 4-year period 32 suitable children were identified, of whom the parents of 16 agreed to allow their children to receive prednisone at the onset of any URTI symptoms. The control group consisted of 16 children whose parents were unhappy with the use of systemic corticosteroids. During the first year of the study all children had received theophylline and orciprenaline at the onset of symptoms. During the second year the prednisone group received oral prednisone 1 mg/kg/day from the onset of any URTI symptoms until the child was asymptomatic. For the control group, outcome measures during both years were remarkably similar. However, the prednisone-treated children had significantly fewer days wheezing (65 vs. 23, $p < 0.001$), fewer wheezing attacks (6.8 vs. 15.4, $p < 0.002$), fewer emergency room visits (3.6 vs. 9.3, $p < 0.001$), and fewer hospitalizations (0.7 vs. 7.6, $p < 0.001$) during the second year. Although the study was retrospective and relied on historical control data, it clearly demonstrates that high-dosage systemic corticosteroids administered at the onset of an URTI have the ability to modify and ameliorate the severity of the lower airway symptoms: specifically, to decrease the severity and duration of wheezing attacks.

Although the numbers of wheezing attacks were decreased by approximately 50%, the numbers of emergency room visits were decreased by 66% and the number of hospitalizations decreased by 90%. The benefits of systemic corticosteroids have to be weighed against their side effects (22).

G. Inhaled Corticosteroids: Continuous

Adult Studies

When inhaled corticosteroids were first introduced there were concerns that their use might depress the normal immune response to viral infections. Thus small surveillance studies such as that reported by Tarlo and colleagues (80) of respiratory infections in adult asthmatics were designed to determine if there was an increased frequency of URTI. Over a 1-year period a similar number of symptomatic colds was reported in those receiving regular inhaled or oral corticosteroids as in those receiving no maintenance therapy. It is difficult to draw meaningful conclusions from studies such as this since it was not interventional, was very small, and, with the viral isolation methods available at the time, a viral cause was identified in only 3 of the 21 colds.

Since then inhaled corticosteroids have become the mainstay of the management of persistent asthma. Although originally introduced in oral-corticosteroid-dependent adult asthmatics, their use has extended to milder cases with the recognition that even mild asthmatics have significant airway inflammation. In adult asthmatics, inhaled corticosteroids reduce symptoms, decrease use of rescue medication, and increase pulmonary function measurements (11,36). This is accompanied by a decrease in airway inflammation and bronchial hyperresponsiveness (40,47).

However, their beneficial effects on asthma exacerbation rates has really come to the fore with more recent studies such as the OPTIMA study (60). This demonstrated that for subjects with persistent asthma symptoms not previously receiving corticosteroids, budesonide decreased the risk of first asthma exacerbation by 60% (RR = 0.40, 95% confidence interval [CI] = 0.27–0.59) compared to patients receiving placebo. Over the year of the study the exacerbation rate decreased from 0.77 for placebo to 0.29 per year for budesonide (RR = 0.38, 95% CI = 0.25–0.57). Similar results have been reported by Malstrom (49), who documented an approximately 60% decrease in asthma exacerbations (defined as requiring oral corticosteroids or an unscheduled medical contact) with beclomethasone 400μg per day via metered dose inhaler and spacer compared to placebo in nearly 900 adult patients with asthma and an FEV_1 of between 50% and 85% predicted (see below). It is likely that there is a dose–response curve for inhaled corticosteroids for preventing asthma exacerbations. In both the FACET (61) study and that reported by Foresi (28) the use of budesonide 400 μg twice daily compared to 100 μg twice daily decreased the proportion of subjects experiencing an asthma exacerbation by approximately 50% (see below). There appear to be no therapeutic studies on isolated RVIW in adults.

Studies in School-Aged Children

The use of continuous inhaled corticosteriods (ICS) is of proven benefit in older children with a classic asthmatic phenotype (42,43,85), with benefits in control of symptoms, improved pulmonary function, and decreased bronchial hyperresponsiveness (15). The trial reported by the childhood asthma management program is particularly convincing, demonstrating as it does that regular inhaled corticosteroids significantly decrease virus-associated asthma exacerbations in children with persistent asthma (15). Over a 4–6 year period, over 1000 children with persistent asthma (defined as symptoms and need for bronchodilator twice weekly with bronchial responsiveness to methacholine less than 12.5 mg/mL) were randomized to receive budesonide 200 μg nedocromil 8 mg, or placebo twice daily. Compared with placebo, regular inhaled budesonide resulted in a decreased need for courses of oral prednisolone (70 vs. 122:100 person years, p < 0.001), a decrease in urgent care visits for asthma (12 vs. 22:100 person years, p < 0.001), and a decreased rate of hospitalization due to asthma (2.5 vs. 4.4:100 person years, p = 0.04). The beneficial effects on need for oral prednisolone and urgent care visits appear greater than for nedocromil, and unlike nedocromil their use results in significantly fewer hospitalizations.

Only one study in older children has attempted to assess the effects of regular inhaled corticosteriods on isolated VAW, which utilized symptom diaries and changes in PEFR to define such episodes (23). In a randomized double-blind, placebo-controlled study, the effect of inhaled beclomethasone dipropionate (BDP) 400 µg/day was determined on episodes of respiratory symptoms and PEFR in a group of school children with VAW (23). The treatment period was designed to cover the period of maximum respiratory virus-induced wheezing episodes, from returning to school after the summer through until the Easter of the following year.

The children were recruited on the basis of reported symptoms, not doctor-diagnosed asthma. A simple respiratory questionnaire was sent to the parents of 5727 children aged 7–9 years in the Southampton (UK) area, resulting in 4830 replies (84.3% response). Children were selected on the basis of either five or more wheezing episodes, or an episode of wheezing lasting for 3 or more days in the preceding year. All children were reported by their parents to develop respiratory symptoms in association with upper respiratory tract infections. One hundred sixty children fulfilled the enrolment criteria, of whom 104 agreed to participate and were randomized to receive either BDP 200 µg or placebo twice daily as dry powder via a Diskhaler.

During the study the children completed a daily symptom diary on upper and lower respiratory symptoms, scored as 0, none; 1, mild; 2, moderate; 3, severe. The sum of upper respiratory symptoms (blocked nose, runny nose, sore throat, hoarse voice, fever, watery eyes) was calculated (maximum score 18), as was the sum of lower respiratory symptoms (day cough, night cough, day wheeze, night wheeze, shortness of breath: maximum score 15). They also recorded the best of three PEFR measurements in the morning and evening, and every month underwent a bronchial provocation challenge to inhaled methacholine.

Nonparametric analysis was used for the definition of symptom and PEFR episodes. The upper respiratory tract (URT) and lower respiratory tract (LRT) symptom episodes were defined as 2 or more days above the child's median score preceded by 1 day at or below the median score and followed by 2 days at or below the median score, with the maximum score for the episode being greater or equal to 2 above the median. A PEFR episode was defined as a fall in morning PEF of greater than 12 centiles below that subject's median for at least 2 consecutive days, where the PEF had been greater than the twelfth centile below that subjects median for one day before and 2 days after the episode. The PEFR data were corrected for the children's increase in height over the course of the study. Thus the number of episodes (expressed as a frequency per 12 months), the average severity of episodes (maximum score), and the episode duration (length in days) were calculated. Data was log-transformed prior to analysis.

Of the 104 children who entered the study 52 received BDP and 52 placebo, of whom 94 completed (50 BDP, 44 placebo). During the treatment period the pulmonary function was consistently higher in the BDP group compared to the placebo group, with the difference in means of FEV_1 (BDP-placebo), adjusted for pretreatment FEV_1, being 0.09 L (p = 0.001). The PD_{20} to methacholine was likewise significantly increased in the BDP group compared to the placebo group, with the ratio of means (BDP/placebo), adjusted for pre-treatment log PD_{20}, being 1.7 (95% CI 1.2, 2.4; p = 0.007).

There was no difference between the BDP- and placebo-treated groups in the frequency of LRT symptom episodes per year (6.5 vs. 6.9, p = 0.7), severity of LRT episodes as measured by maximum symptom score (4.8 vs. 5.2, p = 0.3), or duration in days of LRT episodes (9.0 vs. 8.3, p = 0.6) For PEFR episodes there was likewise no difference between the BDP- and placebo-treated groups in the frequency of episodes per year (5.1 vs. 5.0, p = 0.8), severity of episodes as measured by maximum PEFR (181.4 vs. 168.8 L/min, p = 0.2), or duration in days of episodes (13.1 vs. 13.6, p = 0.7). Post-hoc calculations gave the study an 80% power to detect a 33% difference in respiratory episodes at the two-sided 5% significance level.

Studies in Immediate Preschool Children

A major limitation of studies in preschool children is the relative lack of objective outcome measures. Unlike studies in older children or adults in whom pulmonary function testing is relatively straightforward, studies in preschool children rely on subjective measures such as parent-reported symptoms or need for hospital admission. Furthermore, the limited lung function assessments that are technically feasible in the preschool age group (such as the rapid thoracoabdominal compression technique) do not lend themselves to repeated measurements in the community. For a condition as episodic as VAW there is a lack of a repeatable objective outcome measure such as change in PEFR. A pleasing irony is that this lack of repeatable objective outcome measures has encouraged the use of measures such as frequency of wheezing exacerbations, need for oral corticosteroids, emergency room visits, and hospitalizations. This, combined with the anatomical factors that contribute to the increased incidence of wheezing at this age group, and the higher frequency of symptomatic viral infections in this age group, has resulted in a bias towards studies on the effects of treatment on virus-induced asthma exacerbations.

In the early 1990s Bisgaard and colleagues (6) first demonstrated that regular budesonide could improve symptoms in infants with severe recurrent wheezing. In a double-blind, placebo-controlled, parallel group design the effect of budesonide 800 μg/day via metered-dose inhaler with spacer and facemask was assessed in a group of 77 children aged 11–36 months with physician-confirmed wheeze on at least three occasions during the preceding 12 months. An asthma exacerbation was not predefined but was quantified by the number of days the patient required oral prednisolone. The proportion of days on prednisolone decreased significantly in those receiving regular budesonide. After 8 weeks the placebo-treated children had received prednisolone on 5.1% of days in the preceding 2 weeks, compared to 0% in the budesonide-treated group (p = 0.01).

Since then a number of other investigators have demonstrated broadly similar benefits for children with persistent symptoms with breakthrough virus exacerbations. For example, Connett et al. (18) reported the effect of regular budesonide in a randomized double-blind parallel group study of 40 infants with troublesome asthma. Subjects were aged 1–3 years of age (mean 1.8 years) with a history of at least 6 months of troublesome asthma thought to be responsive to bronchodilators, and had respiratory symptoms on at least 3 days per week during the 2-week run in. Inhaled budesonide was administered via holding spacer and mask, with the dosage of corticosteroid being adjusted by the supervising physician to between 200 and 400 μg twice a day. Forty children entered the study (BUD 20 and placebo 20) of which 13 in each group completed the 6 months of the study. There were small but statistically significant benefits for the corticosteroid-treated group for day or nighttime cough, but no benefit for wheeze or any other outcomes. There were three hospitalizations in the BUD group and eight in the placebo group.

In a subsequent study, Bisgaard (5) reported the effects of fluticasone propionate in a large multicenter study of 237 children aged 12–48 months with a history of recurrent wheeze or asthma symptoms, with symptoms on 7 of the 14 days preceding entry into the study. The study was a randomized controlled, double-blind, parallel group trial over 12 weeks. Three groups of infants received via a metered dose inhaler and spacer one of the following: fluticasone propionate 50 μg twice daily, fluticasone propionate 100 μg twice daily, or placebo. An exacerbation of asthma was defined as a worsening of the child's asthmatic symptoms that required a change in medication and/or required the parents to seek medical advice. Over the 12 weeks of the study, 37% of patients receiving placebo had one or more exacerbation, compared to 26% of patients receiving fluticasone propionate 50 μg twice daily ($p < 0.05$) and 20% of patients receiving fluticasone propionate 100 μg twice daily (compared to placebo, $p = 0.03$).

In a single-center, randomized, double-blind parallel group study of regular budesonide in 38 asthmatic children aged 2–5 years, regular budesonide 400 μg twice daily via a metal spacer had a beneficial effect on asthma exacerbation rates (57). For the purpose of this study, the diagnosis was made empirically on the basis of recurrent asthma symptoms and a clinical improvement with regular inhaled corticosteroids that relapsed during interruption of treatment. At entry patients were required to have significant symptoms on at least 7 of 14 consecutive days, and it is noteworthy that the subjects were symptomatic on 95% of days during the run in period. Thus, by definition, the subjects in this study had persistent symptoms and obtained benefit from regular inhaled corticosteroids. Children were randomized to receive either budesonide 400 μg twice daily or placebo by metered-dose inhaler and metal spacer. Over the 8 weeks of the study, 12 exacerbations occurred in children receiving budesonide compared with 29 in those receiving placebo, from which exacerbation rates of 3.7 per year vs. 9.3 per year were extrapolated ($p = 0.006$). The children in this study are likely to represent exclusively patients with persistent symptoms with acute exacerbations, as opposed to episodes of viral-associated wheezing.

Chavasse and colleagues (14) have demonstrated that regular steroids are beneficial in infants with persistent wheezing and an atopic tendency. In a randomized, double-blind, placebo-controlled, parallel group study, a group of infants aged 3–12 months of age with a documented history of persistent wheeze or cough or recurrent wheeze, and a family history (first degree relative) of an atopic condition, were randomized to receive either Fluticasone 300 μg by metered-dose inhaler and spacer or placebo for 12 weeks. Exacerbation days were defined on attainment of a symptom score, but there was no significant difference in exacerbation days between the fluticasone-treated and placebo-treated groups.

Similar results have been reported with the use of nebulized corticosteroids. Early studies assessing the use of nebulized BDP did not show benefit (76), probably because of the solubility of BDP. In contrast, there is some evidence that nebulized budesonide may be effective at this age group. de Blic and colleagues reported a randomized, double-blind, parallel group study in infants younger than 30 months of age with a diagnosis of asthma, based on at least three exacerbations of dyspnea associated with wheezing during the 12 months preceding the study (20). An asthma exacerbation was defined as the requirement for oral corticosteroids on 2 or more consecutive days. Patients were randomized to receive either budesonide 1mg twice daily via nebulizer and open facemask, or placebo. Over the 12 weeks of the study there was no significant difference in the median number of exacerbations per patient, but there were significant differences in the percentage of patients with at least one exacerbation: 40% in the budesonide-treated group vs. 83% in the placebo group ($p = 0.01$). There were similar significant benefits in reported daytime and nighttime symptoms and duration of oral corticosteroid therapy. The authors attempted to differentiate between what they classified as recurrent asthma as opposed to persistent asthma, on the basis of either daily symptoms for at least 15 days before entry into the study, or one exacerbation per month requiring oral corticosteroids during the 3 months prior to entry into the study. Cox regression analysis that suggested there was a significant influence on the type of asthma, with the subjects labeled as having persistent asthma having more likely (hazard ratio = 4.47) to have an exacerbation sooner than subjects labeled as having recurrent asthma, but even adjusting for this influence budesonide still had a significant effect compared to placebo ($p = 0.01$).

All of the above studies had a requirement for interval or chronic symptoms, suggestive of a more classic asthma phenotype with virus exacerbation, rather than pure isolated VAW. In contrast those studies that have attempted to identify and treat subjects with isolated VAW have shown little if any benefit.

Wilson et al. (91) assessed the effect of continuous budesonide 200 µg twice a day by large-volume spacer in a double-blind parallel group study in 41 children aged 0.7–6.0 years of age (mean, 1.9 years). All had troublesome wheezing episodes in association with viral infections, with no or minimal symptoms between episodes. The subjects were recruited over the winter, and duration of the study was 4 months. There was no significant effect on symptom score. There was no significant difference in the mean number of wheezing episodes (BUD 2.6 vs. placebo 2.4) or in duration of episodes (BUD 8.0 vs. placebo 8.6 days), or in hospitalizations (1 per group). De Baets et al. (19) reported a randomized double-blind crossover comparison of disodium cromoglycate (DSCG) 10 mg three times a day with BDP 100 µg three times a day via a large-volume spacer for 2 months. Fifteen infants of median age 56 months (range, 43–66 months) with a history of frequent episodes of virally induced bronchial obstruction and recurrent hospitalizations were recruited. An acute episode was defined as 5 days or more of cough or wheeze requiring an increase in rescue medication. The frequency of wheezing episodes was significantly lower while receiving BDP (7 vs. 16, p < 0.005).

Thus the large well-powered studies in preschool children with persistent symptoms are consistent with those in adults, demonstrating benefit from regular inhaled corticosteroids and an approximately 50% decrease in asthma exacerbations. However, as with the results with older children, the results of regular treatment in preschool children with isolated VAW are less convincing

Studies in Infants and Toddlers

There is little evidence that the use of regular inhaled corticosteroids in infants less than 18 months of age is beneficial. The population at this age is heterogeneous, including infants with respiratory syncytial virus (RSV) bronchiolitis, postbronchiolitis wheezing, classic virus-associated wheezing, and viral exacerbations in infants destined to develop classic asthma. Most important, the effects and after effects of RSV are most marked in this age group. This is compounded by the uncertainties over drug delivery at this age, with all drugs being administered via a mask, either from a metered-dose inhaler or nebulizer. Neither the studies reported by Van Bever (84) nor by Stick (75) in infants less than 18 months reported any benefits, while the study by Noble (59) reported minimal benefit in the small number of children who completed the trial.

Van Bever (84) assessed the effects of regular nebulized budesonide 0.5mg twice daily in 23 infants aged 3–17 months in a randomized double-blind crossover trial, with each treatment arm lasting 1 month each. There were no significant differences between budesonide and placebo treatment periods. Noble (59) reported a randomized, double-blind placebo-controlled crossover comparison of budesonide 150 µg twice daily via holding spacer and mask in 20 subjects aged 4–17 months (mean 11 months) with a history of recurrent cough and/or wheeze for greater than 2 months and for 3 or more days per week. Treatment was for 6 weeks per treatment, with the last 3 weeks of treatment being used for analysis. There were small but statistically significant improvements in daytime wheeze and cough symptom scores, and a parental preference for the corticosteroid, but no effect on exacerbations. Over 60% had a family history of atopy, and with emphasis on interval symptoms over 2 months it is unlikely that many of these children had virus-associated wheezing.

Stick et al. (75) likewise measured the effects of regular beclometasone dipropionate 200 µg twice a day via large volume spacer and mask in a double-blind parallel group study of 50 infants of median age 12 months (range, 5–18 months). In addition to symptoms and rate of wheezing episodes, they also measured pulmonary function and histamine responsiveness using the rapid thoracoabdominal compression technique. Infants were included if they had three discrete episodes of wheezing, or one episode of wheezing of greater than 4 weeks. Fifty infants were recruited, of whom 23 of the BDP group and 15 of the placebo group completed the 8 weeks of the study. There were no significant benefits for corticosteroids in symptoms, pulmonary function, or bronchial responsiveness.

Conclusions

Taken together it is clear from the studies in adults, school-aged children, and immediate preschool children that regular inhaled corticosteroids decrease the frequency of asthma exacerbations in those with persistent symptoms. Assuming that the majority of these exacerbations are virus-induced, inhaled corticosteroids would appear to ameliorate virus-induced asthma attacks. However, evidence for a beneficial effect for regular inhaled corticosteroids in subjects without persistent symptoms, and isolated virus-associated wheezing, is lacking.

H. Inhaled Corticosteroids: Intermittent

Given the beneficial effects of intermittent oral corticosteroids in virus-induced asthma exacerbations, a logical extension would be that intermittent use of inhaled corticosteroids might also be beneficial but with less systemic side effects. The data to date have been poorly supportive of such an action because the majority of studies have been relatively small and underpowered. The one adequately controlled study shows clear benefit. To date there have beer four studies (18,78,79,90), all in young children, assessing whether commencing inhaled corticosteroids at the onset of either a URTI or wheezing was beneficial. There are two studies, one in children (30) and one in adults (28), assessing the stratagem of increasing the dosage of inhaled corticosteroids in asthmatic subjects already receiving regular inhaled corticosteroids.

IV. Commencing Inhaled Corticosteroids at Onset of Symptoms

As previously noted, the pattern of VAW may have no interval symptoms at all, but a sudden increase in symptoms and decrease in PEFR at onset of respiratory viral infection. It therefore seems illogical to administer continuous prophylactic therapy to individuals with few interval symptoms. There will be a trade off between potential benefits from continuous therapy and the difficulties of administering regular therapy in preschool children, with the added concerns over possible side effects. In this situation the potential benefits of continuous therapy will decrease with decreasing frequency of wheezing episodes. Three groups of investigators have assessed commencing therapy at onset of viral URTI in children who did not necessarily have interval symptoms (18,79,90), while one group has assessed such a strategy in infants with a more classic asthmatic picture with interval symptoms and virus exacerbations (78).

Wilson and Silverman (90), in a randomized, double-blind random crossover study in children aged 1–5 years, compared BDP 750 μg three times daily or placebo via large-volume spacer for 5 days at the onset of a wheezing attack. At entry all subjects had had at least two separate wheezing episodes requiring beta$_2$ agonists within the preceding 3 months; seven were receiving concomitant regular inhaled corticosteroids, six were receiving regular sodium cromoglycate. Each subject aimed to complete four acute episodes, with either BDP or placebo for two episodes each. In all, 24 children completed 35 pairs of treatment, and there was no difference in hospitalization rate between the two treatments (four in each group), although there was a nonsignificant decrease in need for oral corticosteroids (BDP three courses, placebo six courses). In the 18 attacks that did not require either oral corticosteroids or hospitalization, there were small but significant benefits for BDP in decreasing mean daytime and nighttime symptom scores, and there was a significant parental preference for the corticosteroid (BDP 19 vs. placebo 9).

Connett and Lenney (18) in a double-blind random-order crossover study compared inhaled budesonide with placebo for 7 days for acute wheezing episodes in children aged 1–5 years of age. Treatment was budesonide 800 μg twice daily or placebo via large-volume spacer using the mouthpiece; or (if patients were too young to use the mouthpiece) budesonide 1600 μg twice daily or placebo via large-volume spacer with mask. All were reported to wheeze after URTIs, had wheezed on at least two occasions, and were receiving no concomitant prophylactic medication. Subjects commenced therapy at the onset of an URTI with either budesonide or placebo, with the opposite treatment for the subsequent URTI. Twenty-five children completed 28 pairs of treatment, and again there was a nonsignificant decrease in need for oral corticosteroids (BUD two courses, placebo eight courses) and a significant parental preference for the corticosteroid (BUD 12 vs. placebo 6). There were small but significant decreases in day- and nighttime symptom scores when receiving the corticosteroid, and a trend in favor of shorter duration of symptoms.

Svedmyr and colleagues (78) investigated the effect of commencing inhaled budesonide at the onset of an URTI in 26 children aged 3–10 years. All children had a history of asthma with regular deterioration during URTI, and 22 of them were atopic on skin prick testing. At the first sign of URTI the parents commenced budesonide 200 μg or placebo four times a day for 3 days, then three times daily for 3 days, and finally twice daily for the last 3 days. The children were randomized in a double-blind manner to alternate between budesonide and placebo for URTI episodes. Over the course of 2 years 67 protocol valid episodes were recorded. Both morning and evening PEFR were significantly higher during budesonide treatment (104% predicted) than placebo (96% predicted) ($p = 0.015$ and 0.02, respectively), although PEFR values in the placebo-treated children were no different from normal values. Nine children visited the emergency room 11 times because of asthma: 8 while receiving placebo and 3 while receiving budesonide, and 5 courses of oral corticosteroids were administered, all when receiving placebo. There were no significant benefits for budesonide treatment for symptom score variables.

The same authors have performed a similar study of parallel group design, also randomized, double-blind, and placebo-controlled (79). Subjects were aged 1–3 years and had parent-reported wheezing, noisy breathing, and cough with nearly every URTI. Between infections the children had no or minimal symptoms. Subjects commenced placebo or treatment at the first sign of a URTI: initially budesonide 400 μg four times a day by large-volume spacer and face mask for the first 3 days, and then 400 μg twice daily for the last 7 days. Parents completed a daily symptom diary scored 0–3 for both asthma and URTI. Fifty-five children entered the study, although data were available on only 52. Over the 12 months of the study a total of 265 URTI episodes were identified. Parent reported that mean asthma symptom scores were significantly lower in the budesonidetreated children than placebo over each 10 day episode (0.38 vs. 0.55, p = 0.03), but there was no effect on URTI scores. Over the course of the study there were 39 emergency room visits (budesonide 16 vs. placebo 23, p = NS) necessitating 31 courses of oral corticosteroids (budesonide 14 vs. placebo 17, p = NS) and 8 hospitalizations (budesonide 6 vs. placebo 2, p = NS).

None except the last study (79) had prestudy power calculations, and the first three appear underpowered to detect modest differences between treatments. However, there is a consistency of findings, with all four demonstrating nonsignificant decreases in need for oral corticosteroids. Three of the studies were of crossover design and one parallel group, and all had respiratory symptoms exacerbated by URTI. The population in the first report by Svedmyr (78) were asthmatic with URTI exacerbations, while the other three reports were on children with a more classic pattern of pure VAW. Nevertheless a rough post hoc analysis does not seem inappropriate. Combining all 4 studies, 19 courses of oral corticosteroids were administered during 250 wheezing episodes while receiving inhaled corticosteroids, compared to 36 courses of corticosteroids during 239 wheezing episodes while receiving placebo (chi squared = 4.2; p < 0.04). Taken together all four studies appear to decrease the need for course of oral corticosteroids. Even when all four studies are combined, the number of hospitalizations is still too small for meaningful interpretation.

V. Increasing the Dosage of Inhaled Corticosteroids

The two studies in which the dosage of inhaled corticosteroid has been increased at first glance appear to give contradictory findings, but this reflects sample size and inappropriate power to detect differences.

The first study reported by Garrett (30) determined the effect of doubling the dosage of inhaled corticosteroids at the onset of an asthma exacerbation in a group of 28 asthmatic children aged 6–14 years in a randomized, double-blind, crossover study. All were receiving regular inhaled corticosteroids at a dosage of less than 400 µg twice daily BDP equivalent at entry and were maintained on their usual dosage. Subjects were randomized to either double the dosage of inhaled corticosteroid or administer a placebo if any of the following occurred: their PEFR measurement fell below 80% of normal; they had doubled their usual daily requirement for beta$_2$ medication; or they were awoken at night by their asthma. Eighteen exacerbation pairs were suitable for analysis, but there was no suggestion of benefit in any of the outcome variables measured including morning PEFR, evening PEFR, and symptom scores. No power calculations are given for this study, and it appears underpowered to detect any real differences between treatment options.

In contrast, an adequately powered study, which increased the dosage of inhaled corticosteroid fivefold at onset of asthma exacerbation, has demonstrated significant benefit in adults (28). In a randomized controlled, double-blind, double-dummy, three parallel group study, 213 adults with moderate asthma (FEV_1 between 50% and 90% predicted) and requiring 500–1000 µg/day BDP equivalent were randomized to one of the following: regular budesonide 100 µg twice daily; regular budesonide 400 µg twice daily; or budesonide 100 µg twice daily plus (at onset of a respiratory exacerbation) extra budesonide 200 µg four times daily for 7 days (total dosage = 1000 µg/day). Patients completed 1 month of high-dosage budesonide (800 µg twice daily) before proceeding to randomization to 6 months of treatment. A respiratory exacerbation was defined as a decrease in PEFR of >30% below baseline on 2 consecutive days.

Over the 6 months of study, 32.2% of subjects receiving budesonide 100 µg twice daily had at least one exacerbation, compared to 16.4% of those receiving 400 µg budesonide twice daily (p = 0.015) and 18% of those receiving budesonide 200 µg twice daily increased to 1000 µg/day at onset of a respiratory exacerbation (p = 0.025). There were no significant differences in outcome variables between those receiving budesonide 400 µg twice daily and those who received 100 µg twice daily increasing to 1000 µg/day when symptomatic. This was unlikely to be simply due to improvements in asthma control, given that there were no major significant differences in spirometry between the three groups over the course of the study. There was a small statistically significant benefit in mean morning PEFR in those receiving the regular higher-dosage budesonide by the end of the study. If anything, however, the patients receiving budesonide 200 µg twice daily with an additional 400 µg per day had slightly lower mean morning PEFR than those receiving budesonide 100 µg twice alone.

It is clear from these results that a stratagem of increasing inhaled corticosteroid dosage fivefold at worsening of respiratory symptoms is effective at decreasing the frequency of asthma exacerbations in adult asthmatics. All subjects were required to be labeled as having asthma, to be receiving regular inhaled corticosteroids at relatively high dosages, and still require $beta_2$ agonists on a daily basis. Thus they were a group with relatively severe asthma, and yet most of the subjects in the study reported by Foresi did not have an asthma exacerbation during the 6 month treatment period. Even in those subjects receiving budesonide 100 µg twice daily, only 32% had one or more respiratory exacerbation in 6 months. The report does not permit the calculation of the number needed to treat to prevent one respiratory exacerbation, but it can be calculated that approximately seven such asthmatics need to be treated with a fivefold increase in inhaled corticosteroid to prevent one or more asthma exacerbations per 6 months. Few conclusions can be drawn from the small study in children, although the absence of even a trend in benefit for doubling the inhaled corticosteroids would suggest that an increase of greater magnitude is needed. It is difficult to determine the maintenance dosage of inhaled corticosteroid from Garrett's report, but it is likely to be greater than that in Foresi's study. Yet 75% of the children reported by Garrett had at least one exacerbation during the 6 months of the study. Both studies required a diagnosis of asthma, persistent symptoms, and a need for maintenance inhaled corticosteroids at entry, so again these findings should not be extrapolated to subjects with intermittent viral-associated wheezing without chronic symptoms. Given such significant reservations over the power of the study reported by Garrett, it can be concluded that increasing the dosage of inhaled corticosteroids at onset of respiratory symptoms will result in a modest decrease in asthma exacerbations.

VI. Addition of Long-Acting β_2-Agonists in Subjects Already Receiving Inhaled Corticosteroids

A series of pivotal studies has demonstrated the benefits of the addition of a LABA in addition to regular inhaled corticosteroids in the control of asthma symptoms. The first reports (34,93) demonstrated that the addition of long-acting beta$_2$ was superior to doubling the dosage of inhaled corticosteroid for control of symptoms. However, the landmark FACET study included predefined definitions for mild and severe exacerbations of asthma in its outcome measures (61). In a randomized, double-blind, parallel group multicenter study of moderate to severe asthma, all of which patients were receiving inhaled corticosteroids at entry, a total of 852 patients were randomized into four equal groups comparing budesonide at either low dosage (100 μg twice daily) or high dosage (400 μg twice daily) with in addition either placebo or eformoterol 12 μg twice daily. A mild asthma exacerbation was defined as more than 1 day with one of the following: morning PEFR of less than 20% below baseline; the use of more than three additional inhalations of terbutaline in 24 hours compared with baseline; or nocturnal awakening due to asthma. A severe exacerbation was defined as either requiring oral corticosteroids or a decrease in morning PEFR of >30% below the baseline on 2 consecutive days.

There was a consistent decrease in the number of mild and severe asthma exacerbations by increasing the dosage of budesonide or by adding eformoterol. The highest rate of severe exacerbations was seen in those receiving low-dosage budesonide alone (0.91 exacerbations a year) followed by the low-dosage budesonide plus eformoterol (0.67), the higher-dosage budesonide plus placebo (0.46), with the lowest rate being seen in those receiving high-dosage budesonide plus eformoterol (0.34 exacerbations per year). A similar trend was seen for mild exacerbations, again with the combination of the higher-dosage budesonide and eformoterol reducing the rate of severe exacerbations by almost two-thirds compared to the low-dosage budesonide alone. For mild exacerbations there was no significant difference in benefit between adding in eformoterol to the low-dosage budesonide, or increasing the higher-dosage budesonide. In contrast, for the severe exacerbations, increasing the dosage of budesonide was significantly more beneficial than the addition of eformoterol.

The authors of the FACET study have done a more detailed descriptive analysis of the 425 severe exacerbations documented in the study (82). It is pleasing that the description, both on symptoms and on change in PEFR seen during acute exacerbation, is very similar to those previously reported in children with documented virus infection in association with wheezing (41).

Decreases in asthma exacerbation rates have been reported for patients with milder asthma in the OPTIMA study: a double-blind, randomized parallel group multicenter study of asthmatics receiving either no inhaled corticosteroids at all, or if they were receiving inhaled corticosteroids the dosage was less than 400 μg BDP equivalent per day (60). All subjects had evidence of asthma demonstrated by one of the following during the 2 week run in period: two or more inhalations per week of β_2 inhaler; PEFR variability of >15%; or >12% increase in FEV_1 after inhalation of a β_2-agonist. A total of 698 subjects were receiving no corticosteroids, and they were randomly assigned to one of the following: budesonide l00 μg twice daily, budesonide 100 μg plus eformoterol 4.5 μg twice daily, or placebo twice daily. A total of 1272 subjects were receiving corticosteroids at study entry, and were randomized to one of the following: budesonide 100 μg twice daily budesonide 100 μg plus eformoterol 4.5 μg twice daily, budesonide 200 μg twice daily or budesonide 200 μg plus 4.5 μg eformoterol twice daily. The primary outcome variable was the time to the first asthma exacerbation, defined as one of the following: a need for oral corticosteroid treatment: a hospital admission or emergency treatment for asthma; or a decrease in morning PEFR of >25% from baseline on 2 consecutive days.

For subjects not receiving corticosteroids prior to entry to the study, receiving budesonide alone decreased the risk of first asthma exacerbation by 60% (RR = 0.40, 95% CI = 0.27–0.59) compared to patients receiving placebo. Over the year of the study the exacerbation rate decreased from 0.77 for placebo to 0.29 per year for budesonide (RR = 0.38, 95% CI = 0.25-0.57). However, there was no additional benefit from the addition of eformoterol on asthma exacerbation rate.

In the group previously receiving inhaled corticosteroids, there was a nonsignificant trend in the reduction of the rate of severe exacerbations from 0.96 per year to 0.92 per year with increasing the dosage of budesonide from 100 to 200 μg twice daily (RR = 0.82, 95% CI = 0.67-1.01). However, the addition of eformoterol to the lower dosage of budesonide decreased the rate of exacerbations to 0.56 per year, and to the higher dosage of budesonide decreased the rate to 0.36 exacerbations per year (overall RR = 0.48, 95% CI = 0.39–0.59). Of greater significance was that the addition of eformoterol to the lower dosage of budesonide was significantly more effective in decreasing the risk of a severe exacerbation than doubling the dosage of budesonide (RR = 0.71, 95% CI = 0.52–0.86). Thus, in this large study of patients with mild asthma, a low dosage of inhaled corticosteroids alone is sufficient to decrease the rate of asthma exacerbations. However, the addition of a long-acting $beta_2$ gave significantly greater benefit, and that benefit was significantly greater than doubling the dosage of inhaled corticosteroids from 100 to 200 μg budesonide twice daily.

Similar trends have been reported in a meta-analysis of nine randomized controlled studies comparing the addition of salmeterol to an inhaled corticosteroid, with increasing the dosage of inhaled corticosteroid (68). The pooled results demonstrated a decreased risk of any asthma exacerbation (mild, moderate, or severe) of 2.73% (95% CI = 0.43–5.04) and of a moderate or severe asthma exacerbation of 2.42% (95% CI = 0.24–4.60). Although the magnitude of effect appears significantly lower than that reported for eformoterol, there is consistency in decreasing the rate of exacerbations from adding a long-acting β_2-agonists compared to increasing the dosage of inhaled corticosteroid.

It is noteworthy that all studies to date demonstrating benefit for the addition of a LABA to regular inhaled corticosteroids in decreasing asthma exacerbation rates have been performed in adults. Those studies that have addressed the addition of a LABA in children have not demonstrated significant benefit (87).

VII. Leukotriene Receptor Antagonists

Leukotriene receptor antagonists (LTRA) and inhibitors were the first new therapeutic option in asthma management since the introduction of inhaled corticosteroids in the early 1970s. Leukotrienes are produced by inflammatory cells in the lungs, including eosinophils and mast cells. They result in bronchoconstriction, increased mucus secretion, and increased airway vascular permeability. Studies in adult and children have demonstrated benefits in asthma control from LTRAs. Both LTRAs and inhibitors are attractive therapy to the treatment of asthma since they appear to have both a bronchodilator and anti-inflammatory role.

Currently zileuton is the only available leukotriene inhibitor, but there are limited data available on the effect on asthma exacerbations (39,48). There are three LTRAs available: zafirlukast, pranlukast, and montelukast. In placebo-controlled studies in adults with moderate to severe asthma (mean FEV_1 between 60% and 68% predicted) both zafirlukast (56,77) and montelukast (65) showed modest benefits in baseline lung function and symptoms. Either need for medical assistance (77) or asthma exacerbations was significantly decreased. The designs of these studies were unrealistic in current practice, given that these moderately severe asthmatics were receiving no current inhaled corticosteroids to treat their asthma. Direct comparisons of, for example, montelukast with an inhaled corticosteroid (for example, inhaled beclomethasone) and placebo demonstrate that although montelukast has an affect in decreasing asthma exacerbation, it is less efficacious than an inhaled corticosteroid, even at a relatively modest dosage. Malstrom and colleagues (49) reported a randomized, double-blind, double-dummy, three-way parallel group study comparing montelukast 10 mg once daily with beclomethasone 400 µg per day via metered-dose inhaler and spacer or placebo in nearly 900 adult patients with asthma and an FEV_1 of between 50% and 85% predicted. Patients receiving placebo had an asthma exacerbation on 26.1% of days, compared to 15.2% of days in those receiving montelukast ($p < 0.05$) or 9.7% for patients receiving beclomethasone ($p < 0.05$).

Asthma exacerbations were significantly less frequent in the beclomethasone-treated group than in the montelukast-treated group ($p < 0.05$). Asthma attacks (defined as requiring oral corticosteroids or an unscheduled medical contact) were significantly less frequent in those who received either beclomethasone (10.1%) or montelukast (15.6%) than in those receiving placebo (27.3%). Although there was a trend for the beclomethasone-treated subjects to have fewer attacks than the montelukast-treated subjects, this did not reach statistical significance. Thus, it appears that in patients with chronic asthma, regular inhaled corticosteroids, albeit at a modest dosage, are superior to LTRAs in reducing asthma exacerbations.

Montelukast has demonstrated significant benefits compared to placebo in both 2–5-year-old (44) and 6–14-year old (45) children. In a multicenter, randomized, double-blind, parallel group study, 336 asthmatics aged 6–14 years received either oral montelukast 5 mg a day or matching placebo. Entry criteria were a FEV_1 of between 50% and 85% of predicted value, with >15% reversibility following administration of a β_2 inhaler, and predefined daytime symptoms and requirement for beta$_2$ inhaler. An asthma exacerbation day was defined as a decrease of >20% in baseline morning PEFR, or an increase in β_2-agonist use of 70% from baseline, or an increase of >50% in asthma symptom scores. Over the 8 weeks of the study, 95.5% of subjects receiving placebo had an asthma exacerbation, compared to 84.8% of those receiving montelukast (p = 0.002), while subjects receiving placebo had 25.6% of days with an asthma exacerbation, compared to 20.6% days of those receiving montelukast (p = 0.05). Thus there is evidence of benefit in decreasing asthma exacerbations in these subjects with strictly defined asthma, but the effect is modest.

Perhaps the greatest scope for any new therapy is in the preschool child with marked symptoms in association with viral upper respiratory infections. The use of an oral preparation such as a leukotriene receptor antagonist would be particularly attractive due to the difficulties in drug delivery by the inhaled route in this population. Knorr et al. (44) reported a large double-blind, multinational, parallel-group study comparing montelukast 4 mg a day and placebo in 689 patients aged 2–5 years. All patients had at least three episodes of physician-witnessed asthma symptoms during the preceding year. In addition, patients had to be symptomatic on at least 8 of the preceding 14 days of the baseline period, and have used a beta$_2$ agonist on at least 8 of those 14 days. Thus, this group of patients were more persistent than intermittent in their symptoms. An asthma attack was defined as either worsening asthma symptoms requiring oral corticosteroids or an unscheduled medical review. Over the 12 weeks of the study, 28% of the patient receiving placebo required oral corticosteroid rescue, compared to 19% in the montelukast-treated group (p = 0.008), but there was no difference in the number of patients experiencing one or more asthma attack (22% vs. 26%).

Thus the LTRAs appear effective in decreasing asthma exacerbations in symptomatic asthmatic subjects spanning a wide age range: from preschool children, through school-aged children, and into adulthood. Unfortunately the findings are least clear in the preschool age group, which has the greatest difficulties with all current therapies. Although the need for oral corticosteroid rescue was decreased, there was no effect on the asthma exacerbation rate. Furthermore all the studies to date across the age groups have been in subjects with predefined chronic symptoms and features suggestive of asthma, as opposed to pure virus-associated wheezing, and the findings cannot be extrapolated to this group of subjects. The one study whose inclusion criteria might possibly contain subjects with pure virus-associated wheeze is that in preschool children aged 2–5 years (44), where the beneficial effects were least clear-cut. Head-to-head comparisons in older subjects with symptomatic asthma clearly demonstrate inhaled corticosteroids to be superior to LTRAs in decreasing the frequency of asthma exacerbations (49), with a trend to decreasing more severe asthma attacks.

VIII. Anti-Immunoglobulin E Antibody (Omalizumab)

Omalizumab is a murine recombinant monoclonal humanized antibody that acts by forming complexes with the ε3 domain of the Fc fragment of human IgE. It is an effective treatment of asthma in adults (11,72) and children (54) requiring regular ICS. Two near identical studies in adults containing a total of over 1000 subjects requiring medium dosages of ICS (500–1200 μg BDP/day) have shown very similar results, demonstrating an ability to decrease need for ICS with a concomitant decrease in the number of asthma exacerbations (11,72). Omalizumab was administered every 2 or 4 weeks subcutaneously (the dosage was dependent on subject's weight and serum total IgE) for a total of 7 months in both studies. In the first 16 weeks the dosage of ICS was kept stable; in the subsequent 12 weeks the dosage of ICS was decreased as symptoms allowed. An asthma exacerbation was defined as the need for oral corticosteroids or a doubling in the dosage BDP. Omalizumab decreased the rate of asthma exacerbations by approximately 50%, both during the initial phase with stable ICS dosing (0.39 vs. 0.66, $p = 0.003$ and 0.36 vs. 0.75; $p < 0.001$ respectively), and when the dosages of ICS were being reduced (rate 0.28 vs. 0.54; $p = 0.006$ and 0.28 vs. 0.66; $p < 0.001$). In a similar study in 334 allergic asthmatic children aged 6–12 years requiring regular ICS, Milgrom and colleagues (54) reported a similar reduction in need for ICS and a decrease in the rate of asthma exacerbations from 39% over 12 weeks to 18%.

IX. Conclusions

Regular beta$_2$ agonists without concomitan ICS are ineffective in decreasing episodes of virus-induce asthma (86), and may even increase the rate of such exacerbations (83). The addition of regular LABA in addition to regular either low- or high-dosage ICS decreases the frequency of exacerbations. Viewed purely from the perspective of asthma exacerbations, there is greater benefit from increasing the dosage ICS than adding a LABA (61). Both the cromolyn nedocromil (15) and the LTRA montelukast (49) decrease the frequency of asthma exacerbations, but magnitude of effect is not as great as that for ICS, and is possibly significantly worse. The anti-immunoglobulin E antibody omalizumab reduces the rate of asthma exacerbations by 50% in asthmatic subjects requiring medium dosages of ICS, but there is no evidence at this stage for its use in the absence of ICS.

Thus corticosteroids, whether oral or inhaled, appear to be the treatment of choice for virus-induced asthma exacerbations. Short courses of oral corticosteroids administered at the onset of URTI symptoms in children with a mixture of RVIW and persistent asthma decrease the frequency of wheezing attacks, emergency room visits, and hospitalizations (10). There is overwhelming evidence of their benefit in established acute asthma exacerbations (50,66,67). Clearly their side effects preclude their long-term use in the vast majority of asthmatics.

Short courses of high-dosage inhaled corticosteroids are also beneficial in established acute asthma exacerbations (25). More important is that there is clear and consistent evidence from studies in adults (49,60), school-aged children (15), and immediate preschool age children (7,57) that regular low-dosage inhaled corticosteroids decrease the frequency of asthma exacerbations in those with persistent symptoms by approximately 50% compared to placebo. In adults there is a further approximately 50% decrease in asthma exacerbations when high-dosage of ICS (800/μg per day) and low-dosage ICS (200 μg/day) are compared (28). These effects are in addition to the well-documented improvements on symptom control, pulmonary function, and bronchial hyperresponsiveness. Assuming that the majority of these exacerbations are virus-induced, inhaled corticosteroids would appear to ameliorate virus-induced asthma attacks. Furthermore, there is evidence in children that commencing high-dosage ICS at the onset of either URTI symptoms or lower airway symptoms decreases the need for subsequent courses of oral corticosteroids, and evidence in adults that increasing the dosage of ICS in asthmatics with persistent symptoms and an acute exacerbation is beneficial (28). Thus ICS are effective both at preventing and at treating virus-induced asthma exacerbations in those with persistent symptoms.

However, evidence for a beneficial effect for regular inhaled corticosteroids in subjects without persistent symptoms, and pure VAW, is lacking. Studies that have attempted to identify this subgroup of subjects are confined to infancy (75) and childhood (19,23,91) and do not appear to have a major effect on the frequency of virus induced asthma attacks (23,75,84). Although there may be some minor benefits in pulmonary function and nonspecific bronchial hyperresponsiveness, these benefits do not affect the frequency of asthma exacerbations (23). Indeed it is arguable that the potential side effects of treatment outweigh the improvements in pulmonary function (23). There appear to be no such studies in adulthood.

It is interesting to speculate why there is a discrepancy between the response to regular inhaled corticosteroids of virus-associated exacerbations in those with persistent symptoms and those without. There are limited bronchoalveolar data in children suggesting that those with atopic asthma have increased numbers of mast cells and eosinophils compared to children with isolated viral-associated wheeze (74). There is also a suggestion that asthma in childhood may have a more significant neutrophil involvement than in adults (32,51), and that this possibly reflects a greater proportion of subjects without persistent symptoms. Eosinophilic infiltration of the bronchial mucosa appears to be a characteristic of all forms of adult asthma including atopic asthma, nonatopic asthma, and occupational asthma and now is believed to be the major contributor to airway damage. Corticosteroids decrease airway eosinophil recruitment, possibly through inhibition of lymphocyte production of IL-5, inhibit eosinophil activation so decreasing release of inflammatory mediators, and increase eosinophil apoptosis (2).

Given that oral corticosteroids have an effect on VAW, an alternative explanation is that the studies assessing regular ICS in pure VAW may not have administered sufficient ICS. However, the study in children reported by Doull (23) administered 400 μg of BDP, higher than reported to be beneficial in adults (49,60) It is possible that pure VAW requires a higher dosage of ICS to affect exacerbations than persistent asthma.

The different responses to regular inhaled corticosteroids reported may reflect differences in the underlying pathophysiology. Two possibilities warrant consideration. It is possible that the underlying inflammatory response during acute virus-associated wheezing exacerbations differs between the two phenotypes, and that the response observed reflects the differential response to corticosteroids of differing inflammatory cells. An alternative is that regular corticosteroids may simply shift the baseline by decreasing the chronic airway inflammation seen even in mild persistent asthma, so that a relatively greater viral hit is required to induce symptoms of an exacerbation. Furthermore, the reported beneficial effects of inhaled corticosteroids on asthma exacerbations in those with persistent symptoms may be due to their relatively greater effects on eosinophilic inflammation. There is clearly an urgent need for studies comparing the airway inflammatory response in subjects with persistent asthma and those with only virus-associated exacerbations.

References

1. Anonymous. Determination of dose-response relationship for nebulised ipratropium bromide in asthmatic children. J Pediatr 1984; 105:1002–1005.
2. Barnes PJ, Pedersen S, Busse WW. Efficacy and safety of inhaled corticosteroids. Am J Respir Crit Care Med 1998; 157:1S–53S.
3. Barnes PJ Anti-inflammatory therapy in asthma. Annu Rev Med 1993; 44:229–249.
4. Bertelsen A, Andersen JB, Busch P, et al. Nebulised sodium cromoglycate in the treatment of wheezy bronchitis. Allergy 1986; 41:266–270.
5. Bisgaard H, Gillies J, Groenewald M, Maddern C. The effect of inhaled Fluticasone propionate in the treatment of young asthmatic children. A dose comparison study. Am J Respir Crit Care Med 1999; 160:126–131.
6. Bisgaard H, Munck SL, Nielson JP, Peterson W, Ohlsson SV. Inhaled budesonide for treatment of reccurent wheezing in early childhood. Lancet 1990; 336:649–651.
7. Bisgaard H, Nielsen KG. Bronchoprotection with a leukotriene receptor antagonist in asthmatic pre-school children. Am J Respir Crit Care Med 2000; 162:187–190.
8. Brightling CE, Bradding P, Symon FA, Holgate ST, Wardlaw A J, Pavord ID. Mast-cell infiltration of airway smooth muscle in asthma. N Engl J Med 2002; 346:1699–1705.
9. British Thoracic Society. The British guidelines on asthma management. Thorax 1997; 52 (Suppl. 1):S1–S21.
10. Brunette MG, Lands L, Thibodeau L-P. Childhood asthma: Prevention of attacks with short term corticosteroid treatment of upper respiratory tract infection. Pediatrics 1988; 81:624–629.
11. Busse W, Corren J, Lanier Q, et al. Omalizumab, anti-IgE recombinant humanised monoclonal antibody, for the treatment of severe allergic asthma. J Allergy Clin Immunol 2001; 108:184–190.
12. Busse WW. What role for inhaled steroids in chronic asthma? Chest 1993; 104:1565–1571.
13. Cade A, Brownlee KG, Conway SP, Haigh D, Short A, Brown J, Dassu D, Mason SA, Phillips A, Eglin R, Graham M, Chetcuti A, Chatrath M, Hudson N, Thomas A, Chetcuti PAJ Randomised placebo controlled trial of nebulised corticosteroids in acute respiratory syncytial viral bronchiolitis Arch Dis Child 2000; 82:126–130.

14. Chavasse RJ, Bastion-Lee Y, Richtr H, Hilliard T, Seddon P. Persistent wheezing in infants with an atopic tendency responds to inhaled Fluticasone. Arch Dis Child 2001; 85:143–148.

15. Childhood Asthma Management Program Research Group. Long-term effects of budesonide or nedocromil in children with asthma. N Engl J Med 2000; 343:1054–1063.

16. Clough JB, Holgate ST. Episodes of respiratory morbidity occuring in children with cough and wheeze. Am J Resp Crit Care Med 1994;149:48–53.

17. Cogswell JJ, Simpkiss MJ. Nebulised sodium cromoglycate in recurrently wheezy preschool children. Arch Dis Child 1985; 60:736–738.

18. Connett G, Lenney W. Prevention of viral induced asthma attacks using inhaled budesonide. Arch Dis Child 1993; 68:85–87.

19. De Baets F, Van Daele S, Franckx H, Vinaimont F. Inhaled steroids compared with disodium cromoglycate in preschool children with episodic viral wheeze. Pediatr Pulmonol 1998; 25:361–366.

20. De Blic J, Delacourt C, Le Bourgeois M, Mahut B, Ostinelli J, Caswell C, Scheinmann P. Efficacy of nebulised budesonide in treatment of severe infantile asthma: a double-blind study. J Allergy Clin Immunol 1996; 98:14–20.

21. Djukanovic R, Roche WR, Wilson JW, Beasley CRW, Twentyman OP, Howarth PH, Holgate ST. Mucosal inflammation in asthma. Am Rev Respir Dis 1990; 142:434–457.

22. Dolan LR, Short-term, high-dose, systemic steroids in children with asthma: effect on the hypothalamic pituitary axis. J Allergy Clin Immunol 1987; 80:81–87.

23. Doull IJM Lampe F, Smith S, Schreiber J, Freezer NJ, Holgate ST. The effect of inhaled corticosteroids on episodes of viral associated wheezing in school age children. Br Med J 1997; 315:858–862.

24. Doull IJM, Freezer NJ, Holgate ST. Growth of prepubertal children with mild asthma treated with inhaled beclomethasone dipropionate. Am J Respir Crit Care Med 1995; 151:1715–1719.

25. Edmonds ML, Camargo CA Jr, Pollack CV Jr, Rowe BH Early use of inhaled corticosteroids in the emergency department treatment of acute asthma (Cochrane Review). In: The Cochrane Library. Issue 2, 2002.

26. Evans DJ, Taylor DA, Zetterstrom O, Chung F, O'Connor BJ, Barnes PJ. A comparison of low-dose inhaled budesonide plus theophylline and high-dose inhaled budesonide for moderate asthma. N Engl J Med 1997; 337:1412–1419.

27. Farr BM, Gwaltney JM, Hendley JO, Hayden FG, Naclerio RM, McBride T, Doyle WJ, Sorrentino JV, Riker DK, Proud D. A randomized controlled trial of glucocorticoid prophylaxis against experimental rhinovirus infection. J Infect Dis 1990; 162:1173–1177.

28. Foresi A, Morelli MC, Catena E. Low dose budesonide with the addition of an increased dose during exacerbations is effective in long-term asthma control. Chest 2000; 117: 440–446.

29. Fraenkel DJ, Bardin PG, Sanderson G, Lampe F, Johnston SL, Holgate ST. Lower airways inflammation during rhinovirus colds in normal and in asthmatic subjects. Am J Respir Crit Care Med 1995; 151:879–886.

30. Garrett J, Williams S, Wong C, Holdaway D. Treatment of acute asthmatic exacerbations with an increased dose of inhaled steroid. Arch Dis Child 1998; 79:12–177.

31. Geller-Berstein C, Levin S. Nebulised sodium cromoglycate and the treatment of wheezy bronchitis in infants and young children. Respiration 1982; 43:294–298

32. Gibson PG, Norzila MZ, Fakes K, Simpson J, Henry RL. Pattern of airway inflammation and its determinance in children with acute severe asthma. Pediatr Pulmonol 1999; 28: 2617–2670.

33. Godden DJ, Ross S, Abdalla M, McMurray D, Douglas A, Oldman D, Friend JA, Legge JS, Douglas JG. Outcome of wheeze in childhood. Symptoms and pulmonary function 25 years later. Am J Respir Crit Care Med 1994; 149:106–112.
34. Greening AP, Ind PW, Northfield M, Shore G. Added Salmeterol versus higher dose corticosteroid in asthma patients with symptoms on existing inhaled corticosteroid. Lancet 1994; 344:219–224.
35. Guidelines for the Diagnosis and Management of Asthma. 1997. Expert Panel Report, No. 2. National Institutes of Health. Bethesda, MD: NIH Publication No. 97–4051.
36. Haahtela, TM, Jarvinen T, Kava K, et al. Comparison of a beta 2-agonist, terbutaline, with an inhaled corticosteroid, budesonide, in newly detected asthma. N Engl J Med 1991; 325:388–392.
37. Henry RL, Hiller EJ, Molmer AD, et al. Nebulised Ipratropium bromide and sodium cromoglycate in the first two years of life. Arch Dis Child 1984; 59:54–57.
38. Henry RL, Milner AD, Stokes GM. Ineffectiveness of ipratropium bromide in acute bronchiolitis. Arch Dis Child 1983; 58:925–926.
39. Israel E, Cohn J, Dube L, Drazen JM. Effect of treatment with Ziluton. A 5-Lipoxygenase inhibitor, in patients with asthma. A randomised controlled trial. Zileuton Clinical Trial Group. JAMA 1996; 275:931–936.
40. Jeffery PK, Godfrey RW, Ädelroth E, Nelson F, Rogers A, Johansson S-A. Effects of treatment on airway inflammation and thickening of basement membrane reticular collagen in asthma. Am Rev Respir Dis 1992; 145:890–899.
41. Johnston SL, Pattemore PK, Sanderson G, Smith S, Lampe F, Josephs L, Symington P, O'Toole S, Myint SH, Tyrell DAJ, Holgate ST. Community study of role of viral infections in exacerbations of asthma in 9–11 year old children. Br Med J 1995; 310: 1225–1228.
42. Kerrebijn KF; Van Essen-Zandvliet EE, Neijens HJ. Effect of long term treatment with inhaled corticosteroids and beta agonists on the bronchial responsiveness in children with asthma. J Allergy Clin Immunol 1987; 79:653–659.
43. Klein R, Waldman D, Kershar H, Berger W, Coulson A, Katz RM, Rachelefsky GS, Siegel SC. Treatment of chronic childhood asthma with, beclomethasone dipropionate aerosol: a double blind crossover trial in non-steroid dependent patients. Pediatrics 1977; 60:7–13.
44. Knorr B, Franchi LM, Bisgaard H, Vermeulen JH, LeSouef P, Santanello N, Michelle TM, Reiss TF, Nguegen HH, Bratton DL. Montelukast, a leukotriene receptor antagonist, for the treatment of persistent asthma in children aged 2 to 5 years. Pediatrics 2001; 108.
45. Knorr B, Matz J, Bernstein JA, Ngueyen HH, Seidenberg BC, Reiss T, Becker A. Montelukast for chronic asthma in 6 to 14 year old children. A randomised, double blind trial. JAMA 1998; 279:1181–1186.
46. König P, Eigen H, Ellis MH, Ellis E, Blake K, Feller D, Shapiro G, Welch M, Scott C. The effect of nedocromil sodium on childhood asthma during the viral season. Am J Respir Crit Care Med 1995; 152:1879–1886.
47. Laitinen, LA, Laitinen A, Haahtela T. A comparative study of the effects of an inhaled corticosteroid, budesonide, and a β_2-agonist, terbutaline, on airway inflammation in newly diagnosed asthma: a randomized, double-blind, parallel-group controlled trial. J Allergy Clin Immunol 1992; 90:32–42.
48. Liu MC, Dube LM, Lancaster J. Acute and chronic effects of a 5-Lipoxygenase inhibitor in asthma: a six month randomised multi-centre trial. Zileuton Study Group. J Allergy Clin Immunol 1996; 98:859–871.

49. Malstrom K, Rodrigeuz-Gomez G, Guerra J, Villaran C, Pineiro A, Wei LX, Siedenberg BC, Reiss TF. Oral montelukast, inhaled beclomethasone, and placebo for chronic asthma. A randomised controlled trial. Ann Intern Med 1999; 130:487–495.

50. Manser R, Reid D, Abramson M. Corticosteroids for acute severe asthma in hospitalised patients (Cochrane Review). In: The Cochrane Library, Issue 2, 2002.

51. Marguet C, Jouen-boedes F, Dean TP, Warner JO. Bronchoalveolar cell profiles in children with asthma, infantile wheeze, chronic cough, or cystic fibrosis. Am J Respir Crit Care Med 1999; 159:1533–1540.

52. Martinez FD, Wright AL, Taussig LM, Holberg CJ, Halonen M, Morgan WJ. Asthma and wheezing in the first six years of life. N Engl J Med 1995; 332:133–138.

53. Milgrom H, Frick RB, Jr., Su JQ, Reimann JD, Bush RK, Watrous ML, Metzger WJ. Treatment of allergic asthma with monoclonal anti IgE antibody. N Engl J Med 1999; 341:1966–1973.

54. Milgrom H, Berger W, Nayak A, et al. Treatment of childhood asthma with anti-immunoglobulin E antibody (Omalizurnab). Pediatrics 2001; 108:e36.

55. Milner AD. The role of corticosteroids in bronchiolitis and croup. Thorax 1997 52: 595–597.

56. Nathan RA, Burnstein JA, Bielory L, et al. Zafirlukast improves asthma symptoms and quality of life in patients with moderate reversible air flow obstruction. J Allergy Clin Immunol 1998; 102:935–942.

57. Neilsen KG, Bisgaard H. The effect of inhaled budesonide on symptoms, lung function, and cold air methacholine responsiveness in 2–5 year old asthmatic children. Am J Respir Crit Care Med 2000; 162:1500–1506.

58. Nicholson KG, Kent J, Ireland DC. Respiratory viruses in the exacerbations of asthma in adults. Br Med J 1993; 307:982–986.

59. Noble V, Ruggins NR, Everard ML, Milner AD. Inhaled budesonide for chronic wheezing under 18 months of age. Arch Dis Child 1992; 67:285–288.

60. O'Byrne PM, Barnes PJ, Rodriguez-Roison R, Runnerstrom E, Sandstrom T, Svensson K, Tattersfield A. Low dose inhaled budesonide and eformoterol in mild persistent asthma. The Optima randomized trial. Am J Respir Crit Care Med 2001; 164:1392–1397.

61. Pauwells RA, Claes-Goran L, Postma DS, Tattersfield AE, O'Byrne P, Barnes PJ, Ullman A. Effects of inhaled eformoterol and budesonide on exacerbations of asthma. N Engl J Med 1997; 337; 1405–1411.

62. Pierrepoint MJ, Doull IJM. Inflammation in asthma: the basis for rational therapy. Curr Paediatr 2000; 10:145–149.

63. Plotnick LH, Ducharme FM. Combined inhaled anticholinergics and beta2-agonists for initial treatment of acute asthma in children (Cochrane Review). In: The Cochrane Library, Issue 2, 2002.

64. Racineux JL, Troussier J, Tureant A. Comparison of bronchodilator effects of salbutamol and theophylline. Bull Eur Physiopathol Respir 1981; 17:799–806.

65. Reiss TF, Chervinsky P, Dockhorn RJ, Shingo S, Seidenberg B, Edwards TB. Montelukast, a once daily leukotrine receptor antagonist, in the treatment of chronic asthma. Arch Intern Med 1998; 158:1213–1220.

66. Rowe BH, Keller JL, Oxman AD. Effectiveness of steroid therapy in acute exacerbations of asthma: a meta-analysis. Am J Emerg Med 1992; 10:301–310.

67. Rowe BH, Spooner CH, Ducharme FM, Bretzlaff JA, Bota GW. Carticosteroids for preventing relapse following acute exacerbations of asthma (Cochrane Review). In: The Cochrane Library, Issue 2, 2002.

68. Shrewsbury S, Pyke S, Britton M. Meta-analysis of increased dose of inhaled steroid or addition of Salmeterol in symptomatic children (MIASMA). Br Med J 2000; 320: 1368–1373.

69. Silverman M. Inhaled sodium cromoglycate. Thorax 2001; 56:585–586.

70. Silverman M. Out of the mouths of babes and sucklings: lessons from early childhood asthma. Thorax 1993; 48:1200–1204.

71. Simons FER. A comparison of Beclamethasone, Salmeterol and placebo in children with asthma. Canadian, beclamethasone diapropionate–salmeterol Zinafoate study group. N Engl J Med 1997; 337:1659–1665.

72. Soler M, Matz J, Townley R, Buhl R, O'Brien J, Fox H, Thirlwell J, Bupta N, Della Cioppa G. The anti-IgE antibody omalizumab reduces exacerbations and steroid requirements in allergic asthmatics. Eur Respir J 2001; 18:254–261.

73. Speight ANP, Lee DA, Hey EN. Underdiagnosis and undertreatment of asthma in childhood. Br Med J 1983; 286:1253–1256.

74. Stevenson EC, Turner G, Heaney LG, Shock BC, Taylor R, Gallagher T, Ennis M, Sheilds MD. Bronchoalveolar lavage findings suggest two different forms of childhood asthma. Clin Exp Allergy 1997; 27:1027–1035.

75. Stick SM, Burton PR, Clough JB, Cox M, LeSouef PN, Sly PD. The effects of inhaled beclomethasone dipropionate on lung function and histamine responsiveness in recurrently wheezy infants. Arch Dis Child 1995;73:327–332.

76. Storr J, Lenney CA, Lenney W. Nebulize beclomethasone dipropionate in preschool asthma. Arch Dis Child 1986, 61; 270–273.

77. Suissa S, Dennis R, Burnst P, Sheehy O, Wood-Dauphinee S. Effectiveness of the leukotrine receptor antagonist zafirlukast for mild to moderate asthma. A randomised, double blind placebo controlled trial. Ann Intern Med 1997; 126:177–183.

78. Svedmyr J, Nyberg E, Asbrink-Nilsson E, Hedlin G. Intermittent treatment with inhaled steroids for deterioration of asthma due to upper respiratory tract infections. Acta Paediatr 1995; 84:884–888.

79. Svedmyr J, Nyberg E, Thunqvist P, Asbrink-Nilsson E, Hedlin G. Prophylactic intermittent treatment with inhaled corticosteroids of asthma exacerbations due to airway infections in toddlers. Acta Paediatr 1999; 88:42–47.

80. Tarlo S, Broder I, Spence L. A prospective study of respiratorty infection in adult asthmatics and their normal spouses. Clin Allergy 1979;9:293–301.

81. Tasche MJA, Uijen JHJM, Bernsen RMD, de Jongste JC, van der Wouden JC. Inhaled disodium cromoglycate (DSCG) as maintenance therapy in children with asthma: a systematic review. Thorax 2000; 55:913–920.

82. Tattersfield AE, Postma DS, Barnes PJ, Svensson K, Bauer C, O'Byrne PM, Lofdahl C, Pauwels RA, Ullman A. Exacerbations of asthma. A descriptive study of 425 severe exacerbations. Am J Resp Crit Care Med 1999; 160:594–599

83. Taylor DR, Sears MR, Herbison GP, Flannery EM, Print CG, Lake DC, Yates DM, Lucas MK, Li Q. Regular inhaled beta agonist in asthma: effects on exacerbations and lung function. Thorax 1993; 48:134–138.

84. Van Bever HP, Schuddinck L, Wojciechowski M, Stevens WJ. Aerosolized budesonide in asthmatic infants: a double blind study. Pediatr Pulmonol 1990; 9:177–180.

85. Van Essen-Zandvliet EE, Hughes MD, Waalkens HJ, Duiverman EJ, Pocock SJ, Kerrebijn KF. Effects of 22 months of treatment with inhaled corticosteroids and/or beta 2 agonists on lung function, airway responsivness and symptoms in children with asthma. Am Rev Respir Dis 1992; 146:547–554.

86. Verberne AA, Frost C, Roorda RJ, van der Laag H, Kerrebijn KF, Dutch Paediatric

Asthma Study Group. One year treatment with salmeterol compared with beclomethasone in children with asthma. Am J Respir Crit Care Med 1997; 156:688–695.

87. Verveme AAPH, Frost C, Duiverman EJ, et al. Additional of salmeterol versus doubling the dose of beclamethasone in children with asthma. Am J Respir Crit Care Med 1998; 158:213–219.

88. Ward MJ, Fentem PH, Roderick-Smith WH, Davis D. Ipratropium bromide in acute asthma. Br Med J 1981; 282:598–600.

89. Williams H, McNicol KN. Prevalence, natural history and relationship of wheezy bronchitis and asthma in children. An epidemiological study. Br Med J 1969; iv:321–325.

90. Wilson NM, Silverman M. Treatment of episodic asthma in preschool children using intermittent high dose inhaled steroids. Arch Dis Child 1990, 65;407–410.

91. Wilson NM, Sloper K, Silverman M. Effect of continuous treatment with topical corticosteroid on episodic viral wheeze in preschool children. Arch Dis Child 1995; 72: 317–320.

92. Wolfe JD, Tashkin DP, Calvarese B, Simmons M. Bronchodilator effects of terbutaline and aminophylline alone and in combination in asthmatic patients. N Engl J Med 1978; 298:363–367.

93. Woolcock A, Lundback B, Ringdal N, Jacques LA. Comparison of addition of Salmeterol to inhaled steroids with doubling of the dose of inhaled steroids. Am J Respir Crit Care Med 1996; 153:1481–1488.

SUBJECT INDEX

A

Activation cytokines, sources and actions, 175
Activator protein-1 (AP-1)
  airway inflammation, 207–209
  respiratory syncytial virus, 215
Acute asthma, *Chlamydia/Mycoplasma*, 611–616
Acute asthma exacerbations
  adenoviruses, 123
  HCoV, 439
  human coronaviruses, 123
  human rhinoviruses, 439
  influenza A, 123
  influenza B, 123
  influenza C, 123
  lower airways, respiratory virus infection, 117–133
  parainfluenza viruses, 123–124
  respiratory syncytial virus, 122
  rhinovirus, 122–124
  viral agents, 122–124
Acute bacterial sinusitis, 541
Acute otitis media, 20
  adults, 502–504
  defined, 543–544
  virus occurrence in, 544–545
Acute respiratory infection, clinically defined syndrome spectrum, 430–431

Acute respiratory viral infections, airway hyperreactivity, 344–346
Acute sinusitis, 504
  diagnosis, 542
  inflammation and pathophysiology, 541–542
  symptoms, 542
  treatment, 542–543
Acute viral sinusitis, defined, 540–541
Acute virus-induced wheeze, young children
  family impact, 443
  public health burden, 444
Adamantanes, common cold, 687–688
Adaptive immune response, birth *vs.* adults, 107
ADCC, 24, 280
Adenovirus-based gene therapy, 290
Adenoviruses, 25–28, 144
  acute asthma exacerbations, 123
  airway cell infection, 153–154
  classification, 26
  epidemiology, 27–28
  pathogenesis and immunity, 28
  proteins, 25
  replication, 26
  structure and replication, 25–26
  underdeveloped countries, 28
Adenovirus infection
  bone marrow transplant recipients, 496
  military, 499

741